Wound, Ostomy and Continence Nurses Society™

Core Curriculum

WOUND MANAGEMENT

Wound, Ostomy and Continence Nurses Society™

Core Curriculum

WOUND MANAGEMENT

EDITED BY:

Dorothy B. Doughty, MN, RN, CWOCN, FAAN
WOC Nurse Clinician
Emory University Hospital
Atlanta, Georgia

Laurie L. McNichol, MSN, RN, GNP, CWOCN, CWON-AP
Clinical Nurse Specialist and WOC Nurse
Cone Health
Greensboro, North Carolina

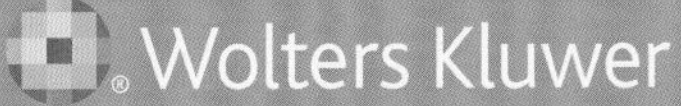

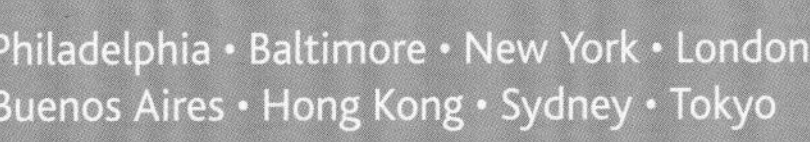

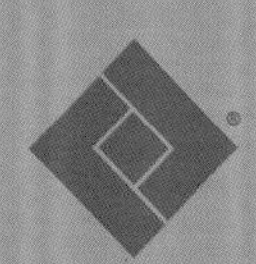

Wound
Ostomy and
Continence
Nurses
Society®

Executive Editor: Shannon W. Magee
Senior Product Development Editor: Emilie Moyer
Editorial Assistant: Kathryn Leyendecker
Senior Marketing Manager: Mark Wiragh
Senior Production Project Manager: Cynthia Rudy
Design Coordinator: Teresa Mallon
Manufacturing Coordinator: Kathleen Brown
Prepress Vendor: SPi Global

9 8 7 6 5 4 3

Printed in China

Cataloging-in-Publication Data available on request from the Publisher.
ISBN: 978-1-4511-9440-1

LWW.com

CCS0317

For my parents, Howard and Theresa Lovejoy, who taught me the importance of faithfulness, perseverance, and lifelong learning. For my husband, Ed, who has shown me there are infinite possibilities and that the journey is a thousand times better together. For those gifts, I am forever grateful.

—Laurie McNichol

To my husband, Mac, who is the "wind beneath my wings"!

—Dorothy Doughty

And special thanks and tremendous gratitude to Tom Conville, who went above and beyond to "make this happen"!

TRIBUTE

Dr. JoAnn Maklebust, the lead author of Chapter 19, passed away on November 16, 2014, shortly after completing this impressive chapter. We are deeply indebted to her for this chapter and for the many other important contributions she has made to nursing, especially to the field of pressure ulcer prevention and treatment. For those of you who did not have the pleasure of knowing Dr. Maklebust, we would like to share some words as a tribute to her memory.

Dr. Maklebust's professional nursing career spanned more than 58 years. She graduated from the University of Michigan School of Nursing in 1956 and earned the Masters of Science in Nursing at Wayne State University in Detroit, Michigan. JoAnn was an expert on pressure ulcers and was a founding member of the National Pressure Ulcer Advisory Panel (NPUAP). She and her colleague and friend, Mary Sieggreen, coauthored books on pressure ulcer prevention and treatment. JoAnn also published more than 100 articles. Over the course of her career, Dr. Maklebust received 26 professional nursing awards. At the age of 78, despite failing health, she pursued doctoral study at Maryville University, and at the age of 80, graduated with her Doctor of Nursing Practice (DNP) degree. Upon completing the DNP degree, she immediately set her mind to the task of writing the chapter presented in this book.

JoAnn was a consummate clinician, mentor, and leader. She was generous with her time and her knowledge. When it came to pressure ulcers, she favored the protective and healing balm of good nursing care over the trumped-up claims of wound care products. She believed so much in the power and influence of the bedside nurse that she would give of herself without hesitation. If a nurse needed something from her she was right there to offer it. She derived a great sense of personal satisfaction in seeing the success of others and had an uncanny ability to inspire others to better themselves as professionals, to go to school, to help others, to think critically, and to do more to improve the care of patients, especially those at risk for pressure ulcers.

The problem of pressure ulcers was most abhorrent to Dr. Maklebust. We can sense this from the title of one article she authored: "Pressure Ulcers: The Great Insult." Personal conversations with Dr. Maklebust revealed the depth of compassion she felt for patients with pressure ulcers. This compassion was grounded in a deep understanding and appreciation of the inherent dignity of all human beings. From her point of view, pressure ulcers wounded not only the bodily tissues but also wounded deeply the dignity of the person.

Most remarkable about Dr. Maklebust was her courage and perseverance. She was always willing to speak the truth about pressure ulcer prevention and to take on every challenge and stick to it until she saw a positive result. For example, when she was a member of the NPUAP, she embraced the challenge of getting CMS to change their ruling in favor of reimbursing for pressure ulcer dressings in the home care setting.

If Dr. Maklebust were here to offer you some advice about pressure ulcer prevention and treatment, we believe she would encourage you to use wound care products judiciously, use compassion generously, and use critical thinking continuously.

Morris A. Magnan and Mary Sieggreen

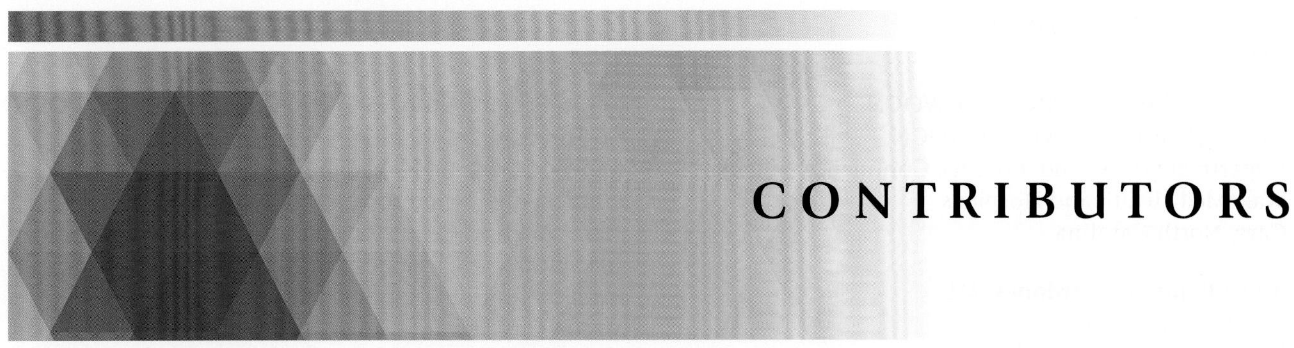

CONTRIBUTORS

Ashwin Agarwal, BS
Medical Student
Duke University School of Medicine
Durham, North Carolina

Lizabeth E. Andrew, MS
Retired
Newnan, Georgia

Elizabeth A. Ayello, PhD, RN, ACNS-BC, CWON, ETNN, MAPWCA, FAAN
Faculty
Excelsior College School of Nursing
Albany, New York
Clinical Editor
Advances in Skin and Wound Care
New York, New York

Sharon Baranoski, MSN, RN, CWCN, APN-CCNS, FAAN
President
Wound Care Dynamics, Inc.
Shorewood, Illinois

Barbara M. Bates-Jensen, PhD, RN, FAAN
Professor of Nursing and Medicine
University of California, Los Angeles
Los Angeles, California

Carole Bauer, MSN, RN, ANP-BC, OCN, CWOCN
Wound, Ostomy and Continence Nurse Practitioner
Karmanos Cancer Center
Detroit, Michigan

Janice M. Beitz, PhD, RN, CS, CNOR, CWOCN, CRNP, MAPWCA, FAAN
Director
WOC Nursing Education Program
Professor
Rutgers University School of Nursing–Camden
Camden, New Jersey

Phyllis A. Bonham, PhD, MSN, RN, CWOCN, DPNAP, FAAN
WOC Nurse Consultant
Professor Emerita
College of Nursing
Medical University of South Carolina
Charleston, South Carolina

David M. Brienza, PhD
Professor
University of Pittsburgh
School of Health and Rehabilitation Sciences
Pittsburgh, Pennsylvania

C. Tod Brindle, MSN, RN, CWOCN, Clin IV
Nurse Clinician
Wound Care Team
VCU Medical Center
Richmond, Virginia

Ruth A. Bryant, RN, MS, CWOCN
Scholar in Residence
Washington State University
Providence Health Care
Spokane, Washington

Michele (Shelly) Burdette-Taylor, PhD, RN-BC, MSN, CWCN, CFCN
CEO of TayLORD Health, LLC
Advanced Wound Care
Sharp Memorial Hospital
San Diego, California
Faculty
School of Nursing, Community Health
University of Alaska
Anchorage, Alaska

Joanna J. Burgess, BSN, RN, CWOCN
Nursing Specialty Services, CWOCN
Department of Wound, Ostomy, Continence Nursing
WakeMed Health and Hospitals
Cary, North Carolina

Adela Rambi G. Cardones, MD
Assistant Professor
Department of Dermatology
Duke University
Staff Physician
Durham VA Medical Center
Durham, North Carolina

Linda J. Cowan, PhD, ARNP, FNP-BC, CWS
Research Health Scientist
Center of Innovation for Disability and Rehabilitation Research
North Florida/South Georgia Veterans Health System
Clinical Associate Professor
Adult and Elderly Department
College of Nursing
University of Florida
Gainesville, Florida

Suzanne Creehan, MSN, RN, CWON
Program Manager
Wound Care Team
VCU Medical Center
Richmond, Virginia

David R. Crumbley, MSN, RN, CWCN
Assistant Clinical Professor
Auburn University School of Nursing
Auburn, Alabama

Barbara A. Dale, BSN, RN, CHHN, CWOCN
Director of Wound Care
Quality Home Health
Livingston, Tennessee

Becky Dorner, RD, LD, FAND
President
Becky Dorner & Associates, Inc.
Nutrition Consulting Services, Inc.
Naples, Florida

Dorothy B. Doughty, MN, RN, CWOCN, FAAN
WOC Nurse Clinician
Emory University Hospital
Atlanta, Georgia

Kevin R. Emmons, DrNP, RN, AGPCNP-BC, CWCN
Clinical Assistant Professor
Wound Faculty
Rutgers University School of Nursing–Camden
Camden, New Jersey

JoAnn Ermer-Seltun, MS, RN, ARNP, FNP-BC, CWOCN
Co-Director and Faculty
webWOC Nursing Education Program
Minneapolis, Minnesota
Mercy Medical Center Advanced Wound Center and Continence Clinic
Bladder Control Solutions, LLC
Mason City, Iowa

Jane Fellows, MSN, RN, CWOCN
Ostomy/Wound Clinical Nurse Specialist
Duke University Medical Center
Durham, North Carolina

Bonny Flemister, MSN, RN, CWOCN, ANP, GNP-BC
Independent Consultant
Kilgore, Texas

Lynn Fong, BSN, RN, CWOCN
WOC Nurse Clinician
Sharp Memorial Hospital, Wound Care
San Diego, California

Elizabeth Friedrich, MPH, RD, CSG, LDN, FAND
President
Friedrich Nutrition Consulting
Salisbury, North Carolina

Kelly A. Jaszarowski, MSN, RN, CNS, ANP, CWOCN
Clinical Instructor
R. B. Turnbull, Jr., MD WOC Nursing Education Program
Cleveland Clinic
Cleveland, Ohio
WOC/ET Consultant
Washington, Illinois

Jan Johnson, MSN, ANP-BC, CWOCN
Nurse Practitioner
Wound Management Clinic
Department of Dermatology
Duke University Medical Center
Durham, North Carolina

Lee Ann Krapfl, BSN, RN, CWOCN
Wound, Ostomy, and Continence Nurse Specialist
Mercy Medical Center
Dubuque, Iowa

Carolyn Lund, RN, MS, FAAN
Neonatal Clinical Nurse Specialist
UCSF Benioff Children's Hospital Oakland
Oakland, California

Dianne Mackey, MSN, RN, CWOCN
Staff Educator
Home Health, Hospice, and Palliative Care
San Diego, California

Morris A. Magnan, PhD, RN
Clinical Nurse Specialist
Karmanos Cancer Center
Detroit, Michigan

JoAnn Maklebust, MSN, RN, APRN, AOCN, FAAN
Nurse Practitioner, Surgical Oncology
Karmanos Cancer Institute, Patient Services
Detroit, Michigan

Laurie L. McNichol, MSN, RN, GNP, CWOCN, CWON-AP
Clinical Nurse Specialist and WOC Nurse
Cone Health
Greensboro, North Carolina

Yvette Mier, BSN, RN, CWOCN
Certified Wound, Ostomy and Continence Nurse
Outpatient Wound Treatment Center
WellStar Kennestone Regional Medical Center
Marietta, Georgia

Susan S. Morello, BSN, RN, CWOCN, CBN
Clinical Consultant
Omaha, Nebraska

Asfandyar Mufti, BMSc
Medical Student
Faculty of Medicine
University of Ottawa
Ottawa, Ontario, Canada

Rose W. Murphree, DNP, RN, CWOCN, CFCN
Director
Wound, Ostomy and Continence Nursing Education Center
Nell Hodgson Woodruff School of Nursing
Emory University
Atlanta, Georgia

Debra S. Netsch, DNP, APRN-CNP, FNP-BC, CWOCN
Nurse Practitioner and WOC Nurse
Mankato Clinic, Ltd.
Mankato, Minnesota
Co-Director and Faculty
webWOC Nurse Education Program
Minneapolis, Minnesota

Denise Nix, MS, RN, CWOCN
Consultant
Minnesota Hospital Association
Minneapolis, Minnesota

C. W. J. Oomens, PhD, Ir
Associate Professor
Biomedical Engineering Department
Eindhoven University of Technology
Eindhoven, The Netherlands

Benjamin F. Peirce, RN, CWOCN
Wound Technology Network, Inc.
Hollywood, Florida

Barbara Pieper, PhD, RN, CWOCN, ACNS-BC, FAAN
Professor
Nurse Practitioner
College of Nursing
Wayne State University
Detroit, Michigan

Mary Ellen Posthauer, RD, CD, LD, FAND
President
MEP Healthcare Dietary Services, Inc.
Evansville, Indiana

Janet M. Ramundo, MSN, RN, CWOCN
Instructor
Wound, Ostomy, and Continence Nursing Education Center
Emory University
Atlanta, Georgia

Laurie M. Rappl, PT, DPT, CWS
Clinical Manager
Aurix Systems by Nuo Therapeutics
Gaithersburg, Maryland

Michelle C. Rice, MSN, RN, CWOCN
Ostomy/Wound Clinical Nurse Specialist
Department of Advanced Clinical Practice
Duke University Hospital
Durham, North Carolina

Bonnie Sue Rolstad, MS, RN, CWOCN
President and Faculty
webWOC Nursing Education Program
Minneapolis, Minnesota

Barbara Rozenboom, BSN, RN, CWON
Wound Ostomy Nurse
Unity Point at Home
Urbandale, Iowa

Gregory Schultz, PhD
Professor
Department of Obstetrics and Gynecology
Institute for Wound Research
University of Florida
Gainesville, Florida

R. Gary Sibbald, BSc, MD, Med, FRCPC(Med), FRCPC(Derm), MACP, FAAD, MAPWCA
Professor
Public Health and Medicine
University of Toronto
Toronto, Canada

Charleen Singh, MSN/Ed, RN, FNP-BC, CWOCN
WOCN Coordinator
Stanford Children's Health
Palo Alto, California

Joyce K. Stechmiller, PhD, ACNP-BC, FAAN
Department Chair and Associate Professor
Adult and Elderly Department
University of Florida College of Nursing
Gainesville, Florida

Debra M. Thayer, MS, RN, CWOCN
Senior Technical Service Specialist
3M Critical and Chronic Care Solutions Division
3M Health Care
St. Paul, Minnesota

Freya van Driessche, BS, MS
Wound Research Fellow
Department of Dermatology and Cutaneous Surgery
Miller School of Medicine
University of Miami
Miami, Florida

Lia van Rijswijk, MSN, RN, CWCN
Clinical Editor
Ostomy Wound Management
Newtown, Pennsylvania

Myra Varnado, BS, RN, CWOCN, CFCN
Chief Nursing Officer
Wound Care Specialists
Metairie, Louisiana

Carolyn Watts, MSN, RN, CWON
Senior Associate in Surgery
Clinical Nurse Specialist
Section of Surgical Sciences
School of Medicine
Vanderbilt University Medical Center
Nashville, Tennessee

Dot Weir, RN, CWON, CWS
Wound Clinician
Osceola Regional Medical Center
Orlando, Florida

Stephanie S. Yates, MSN, RN, ANP-BC, CWOCN
Wound, Ostomy and Continence Nurse Practitioner
Clinical Nurse Specialist
Duke University
Durham, North Carolina

FOREWORD

It is an honor to be invited to write the foreword to the *Wound, Ostomy and Continence Nurses Society™ Core Curricula*. Having served 22 years as a Wound, Ostomy and Continence (WOC) Nursing Program Director, I can attest as to how valuable a resource these books will be to students, faculty, preceptors, and all clinicians caring for people with wounds, ostomies, and incontinence.

Terms currently popular in health care refer to patient-centered and patient-focused care. For those of you entering the wonderful WOC nursing specialty, know this: the patient has always been the focus of WOC nursing! In fact, our specialty grew from a need identified by patients themselves. As colorectal and urologic surgeries advanced, so did the number of people living with ostomies. In 1958, Akron, Ohio native Norma N. Gill joined her surgeon, Rupert B. Turnbull, Jr., MD, in founding what was then coined by Dr. Turnbull as enterostomal therapy (ET).

Beginning in 1948, when she was a 28-year-old mother of two young children, Norma began a long odyssey battling mucosal ulcerative colitis. She manifested all the gastrointestinal symptoms, including massive bouts of bloody diarrhea associated with this disease, along with many of the extraintestinal manifestations, such as uveitis, iritis, and extensive pyoderma gangrenosum on her face, chest, abdomen, and legs. During a brief remission in 1951, much to the amazement of Norma and her husband Ted, she became pregnant. The pregnancy was fraught with complications, the need for numerous blood transfusions, and fear for the lives of both mother and child throughout. Despite all of these life-threatening occurrences, in June 1952, Norma gave birth to a healthy baby girl. The complications continued after her baby's birth, and Norma's response to treatment was spotty at best. In October 1954, she was admitted to the Cleveland Clinic, and there her life was saved and history forever changed. Dr. Turnbull operated to remove Norma's colon and create an ileostomy. Her postoperative course after ileostomy was rocky, and she had to undergo some additional operations to remove her rectum and have plastic surgery performed on her face.

Despite all of this, Norma began to feel better—incredibly better. As she was resuming her role as a wife and mother, she felt the need, as we now say, to "pay it forward." Norma wanted to help others who were facing the same challenges she had endured and emerged stronger than she had been before her illness. Her journey began with the Akron physicians and hospital she had come to know well during her illness. Norma started from scratch and cobbled together an inventory of the limited equipment available at the time. Soon she had many referrals from the surgeons and knew she had found her calling. In 1958, during an appointment with Dr. Turnbull, she told him what she was doing in Akron to help people with new ostomies and fistulae. He was impressed and called her a couple of months later to offer her a job at the Cleveland Clinic.

August 1958 is when the seeds for the modern specialty of WOC nursing were planted. It was not long before the word was out, and surgeons began requesting that their staff come to train with Norma and Dr. Turnbull. The R.B. Turnbull, Jr. School of Enterostomal Therapy (now WOC Nursing) was established. After her long work day in Cleveland, Norma would return to Akron and see patients in hospitals there before heading home to her family and doing it all again the next day.

There was a child in an Akron hospital who always remembered her first encounter with Norma. Here was a woman who commanded respect. The surgeon, head nurse, and staff nurses, as well as the girl's mom, crowded around the bed as Norma taught the proper way to care for a new ileal conduit. That child grew up well adjusted to her new stoma, and thanks to a great family and the one and only Norma Gill, that child grew up to be me! The baby who was predicted never to be born to Norma and Ted is Sally Gill-Thompson—one of my best friends and a famous ET practitioner in her own right.

After establishment of the formal program in Cleveland, other ET schools soon opened, and graduates from the United States and abroad spread the word across the globe. Professional organizations were established, and admission criteria became more stringent as health care became more complex. ET nurses became well respected for their skills and experience caring for people with complex ostomies and fistulae. It was a natural extension of our practice to embrace wound and continence care, and with a painful good-bye to our ET designation in the 1990s, we became known as WOC nurses to better reflect our practice. As you embark on your studies of WOC nursing, take time to reflect and appreciate the wonderful legacy you are continuing with your specialty practice.

Norma will be watching.

Paula Erwin-Toth, MSN, RN, CWOCN, CNS, FAAN

PREFACE

The WOCN Society has funded development and publication of the WOC Nursing Core Curriculum to support both WOC nursing education and WOC nursing practice. The content is based on the curriculum blueprint developed by the WOC Nursing Education Program Directors and approved by the WOCN Society's Accreditation Committee and Board of Directors, and the content is organized in a manner to support learning by the novice practitioner or student in an accredited wound care program. Specifically, the wound section begins with the characteristics of normal skin, the physiology of wound healing, and principles of wound assessment and wound management, and then moves to skin and wound care for specific patient populations and for specific types of wounds. However, the text is also designed to support the knowledgeable wound care practitioner; there are chapters on thermal wounds, surgical wound management, oncologic lesions, palliative care, and fistula management, in addition to in-depth content related to pressure ulcer prevention and management and the pathology and management of venous, arterial, and neuropathic wounds.

The chapters in the wound text are written by clinicians, most of whom are wound care nurses; this section of the core curriculum is written "by wound care clinicians, for wound care clinicians." As editors, we are very grateful to our extremely knowledgeable and committed contributors, and we thank each of them for saying "yes" to the opportunity to elevate practice through their writing. Each chapter begins with curriculum objectives addressed in the specific chapter, and a topical outline to give the reader a quick overview of the content covered in that chapter. Throughout the chapter, clinical pearls are embedded to highlight key "take home" messages. Each chapter also includes multiple illustrations, tables, and boxes to facilitate understanding. Finally, there are questions and answers at the end of each chapter to support the individual's self-assessment of knowledge.

ACKNOWLEDGMENTS

The Wound, Ostomy and Continence Nurses Society™ (WOCN®) wishes to thank all of the clinical experts who munificently shared their time and expertise to create this textbook. The Society would like to especially acknowledge the consulting editors, Dorothy Doughty and Laurie McNichol, for their inspiration, knowledge, and unwavering commitment to the development of this resource and to the field of wound, ostomy and continence nursing.

The WOCN Society would like to acknowledge Hollister Incorporated for providing a commercially supported educational grant for the development of this textbook.

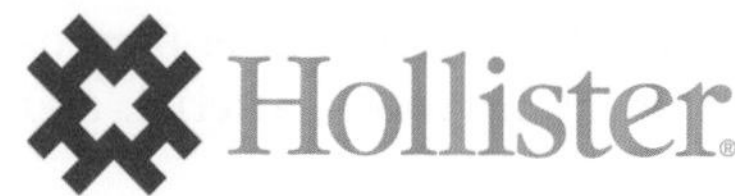

CONTENTS

PART 1

General Concepts

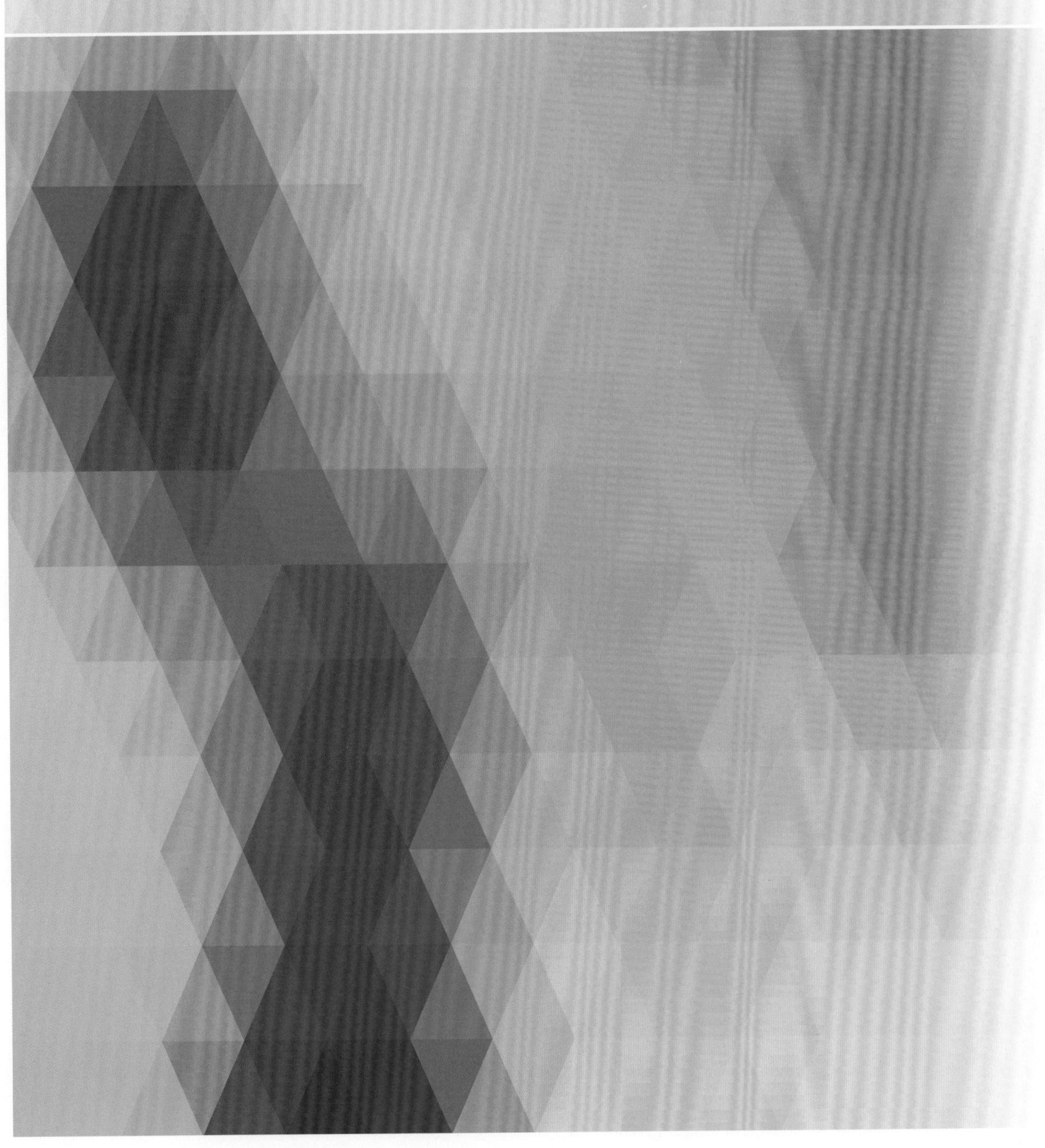

CHAPTER 1

Anatomy and Physiology of the Skin

Asfandyar Mufti, Elizabeth A. Ayello, and R. Gary Sibbald

OBJECTIVES

1. Describe the anatomy and physiology of the skin and soft tissue, changes across the lifespan, and implications for maintenance of skin health.
2. Describe common skin conditions to include pathology, presentation, and management.
3. Use accurate dermatologic terminology to describe skin lesions and wounds.

Topic Outline

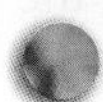 **Anatomy and Physiology of the Skin**

- Epidermis
  - Stratum Basale
  - Stratum Spinosum
  - Stratum Granulosum
  - Stratum Lucidum
  - Stratum Corneum
- Dermis
  - Papillary Dermis
  - Reticular Dermis
  - Epidermal Appendages
- Subcutaneous Tissue
- Muscle

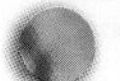 **Functions of the Skin and Soft Tissue**

- Thermoregulation and Regulation of Cutaneous Blood Flow
- Insulation
- Immunity
- Immune Surveillance
  - Langerhans' Cells
- Sensory Perception
- Barrier Function/Protection
- Synthesis of Vitamin D

Skin Changes throughout Life

- Infants and Children
- Older Adults
  - Thermoregulation
  - Cell Turnover Time

Common Skin Conditions in the Elderly

- Photoaging
- Actinic Keratosis
- Basal Cell Carcinoma
- Squamous Cell Carcinoma
- Cutaneous Horn
- Seborrheic Keratoses
- Nevi (Moles)
- Melanoma

Skin Immune System

- Allergic Contact Dermatitis
- Impact of Aging

Skin and Vitamin D Production

Permeability and Dermal Absorption

Skin Assessment

- Skin Color
- Skin Temperature
- Skin Turgor
- Moisture Status
- Skin Integrity

Principles for Using Skin Care Products

Conclusion

The skin is the largest organ in the human body and serves the critical function of maintaining a barrier between the internal and external environments. Anatomically, the skin is divided into two major components: the epidermis and dermis. The epidermis is the outermost layer of the skin, and the dermis is deep to the epidermis. The subcutaneous tissue lies beneath the dermis and is sometimes known as the hypodermis, although it is not a primary layer of the skin (Fig. 1-1).

CLINICAL PEARL

The skin is the largest organ in the body and serves the critical function of maintaining a barrier between the internal and external environments.

Anatomy and Physiology of the Skin

As noted, the skin itself is divided into two major layers, the epidermis and dermis; each layer has unique structures and functions.

Epidermis

The epidermis is a stratified squamous epithelial structure, with four to five distinct and well-defined stratified layers. The layers are, from the base to external environment, as follows: stratum basale (also known as stratum germinativum), stratum spinosum, stratum granulosum, stratum lucidum (present only in areas of thicker skin, such as palms of hand and plantar surface of feet), and stratum corneum (see Fig. 1-1). The layers of the epidermis contain migrating epithelial cells (keratinocytes) that are undergoing differentiation to prepare them to provide an effective barrier once they reach the skin surface (stratum corneum). In addition to keratinocytes, the epidermis contains other cell types that are important for both the structural integrity and function of the skin: melanocytes, Langerhans' cells, and Merkel's cells.

Stratum Basale

The deepest layer of the epidermis is known as the *stratum basale* or *stratum germinativum* and ranges from one to three cells in thickness. The *stratum basale* is the reproductive layer of the epidermis and is characterized by proliferating keratinocytes. When a basal cell divides, one cell begins upward migration and the other cell remains in the basal layer to continue the reproductive cycle. As these keratinocytes migrate towards the stratum corneum (outermost epidermal layer), they undergo a maturation process involving a number of morphological and biochemical changes; this is known as *terminal differentiation or keratinization*. Once terminal differentiation is complete, all that remains is a layer of tightly packed dead cells. The stratum basale also contains melanocytes, which are responsible for producing the pigment *melanin*. Morphologically, melanocytes have dendrites extending from their cell bodies and contain organelles known as melanosomes. As the name suggests, melanosomes contain melanin that is produced from the amino acid tyrosine. In addition to being responsible for each individual's unique skin color, melanin also has photoprotective properties; it can absorb harmful ultraviolet light and protect cells against DNA damage. Migrating keratinocytes in the *stratum spinosum* are protected from harmful UV light by the melanosomes, which move along the

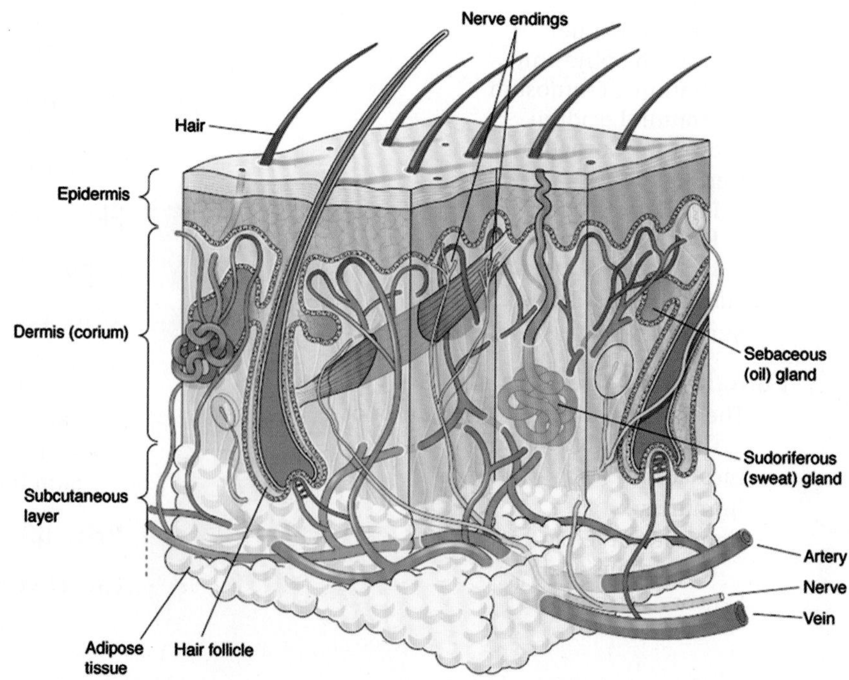

FIGURE 1-1. Cross section of skin and soft tissue. (Reprinted with permission from Cohen, B. J., & Taylor, J. (2005). *Memmler's structure and function of the human body* (8th ed.). Philadelphia, PA: Lippincott Williams & Wilkins.)

dendrites of the melanocytes to the periphery to provide enhanced pigment dispersion and photoprotection (as evidenced by hyperpigmentation, or tanning).

Stratum Spinosum

Above the *stratum basale* lies the *stratum spinosum.* In addition to keratinocytes, this cell layer contains immune cells known as *Langerhans' cells (LH cells).* These LH cells are dendritic in nature and are usually classified as phagocytic and *antigen-presenting cells* (APCs).

Stratum Granulosum

Moving further towards the surface of the epidermis, the next cell layer is the *stratum granulosum*. The stratum granulosum is composed of flattened keratinocytes that have distinct darkly staining keratohyalin granules. The cells within this epidermal layer contain organelles known as *Odland bodies*, which contribute significantly to the barrier function of the epidermis. Odland bodies contain lipids and enzymes that are discharged into the extracellular space. These lipids and enzymes form a lipophilic layer between the stratum granulosum and the stratum corneum that acts as a barrier to water loss. Defects in this lipophilic barrier are now hypothesized to be the major defect in atopic dermatitis, which is characterized by structural abnormalities or lower levels of normal lipids including ceramides.

CLINICAL PEARL

Keratinocytes in the stratum granulosum layer release lipids such as ceramides; these lipids help to maintain the normal brick and mortar configuration of the skin.

Stratum Lucidum

This layer is found between the stratum corneum and the stratum granulosum; the stratum lucidum consists of translucent cells seen only on the palms of the hands and soles of the feet. This layer is not present on thinner skin in other body regions.

Stratum Corneum

The outermost layer of the epidermis is known as the *stratum corneum*. The cells in this layer are terminally differentiated keratinocytes, also known as corneocytes; they are flat, keratinized, and dead, with no nuclei or organelles. The stratum corneum varies in thickness, depending on the region of the body. It is thickest on the soles of the feet or palms of the hands.

Retained nuclei in the stratum corneum are present only when the cells from the basal layer of the skin migrate more quickly to the skin surface. For example, in active psoriasis, transit time is cut in half (from the usual 28 days to 14 days); this results in reduced differentiation of the keratinocytes and retained nuclei, and the silver white scale characteristic of psoriatic plaque.

CLINICAL PEARL

New skin cells (keratinocytes) are produced in the basal layer and then migrate to the surface; as they migrate, they lose the nucleus and undergo terminal differentiation to enable them to provide an effective barrier once they reach the surface.

Dermis

Below the epidermis is a layer of connective tissue known as the *dermis*, which is the major anatomic component of the skin. The epidermis and the dermis connect to each other via projections that allow them to interlock with one another, which adds mechanical strength and reduces the risk of skin tears. Rete ridges from the epidermis and dermal papillae from the dermis interdigitate, much like the visual interface between ocean waves and the air. The interface between dermal papillae and epidermal rete ridges is known as the dermal–epidermal junction (see Fig. 1-1).

Papillary Dermis

The dermis is composed of two distinct layers: reticular and papillary. The papillary layer is the uppermost layer of the dermis and the layer immediately below the epidermis. This layer of the dermis is composed primarily of loose areolar connective tissue, capillary loops, and nerve terminals including Meissner's corpuscles (mechanoreceptors). One of the main functions of the papillary layer is to supply nutrients to the avascular *stratum basale* layer of the overlying epidermis. The capillary loops of the papillary dermis provide perfusion required to support epidermal cell mitosis and the differentiation of keratinocytes required for normal barrier function.

Reticular Dermis

The reticular layer is the bottom layer of the dermis. This layer contains most of the connective tissue proteins that give the skin its strength and elasticity. These proteins, such as collagen and elastin fibers, are embedded in a glycosaminoglycan (mucopolysaccharide) network. As is true of the epidermis, the dermis contains a number of different cells, especially in the reticular layer. Key cells include the fibroblasts, mast cells, and macrophages. Fibroblasts are responsible for the synthesis of connective tissue and extracellular matrix, specifically the production of collagen (dermal building blocks) and elastin (tensile strength); they also produce laminin, a key component of basement membrane, and fibronectin, which binds extracellular matrix proteins. Mast cells are granulated immune cells that are situated throughout the dermis and are responsible for the release of histamine, leukotrienes, prostaglandins, and various chemotactic agents. Excessive release of histamine and other inflammatory mediators can cause hives along with allergic rhinitis and asthma. Lastly, the dermis contains macrophages, a key component of the innate immune system. The macrophages normally function to remove extracellular debris and engulf pathogens, and they play an essential role in normal wound healing. In addition to a rich vascular network of arteries, arterioles, capillaries, venules, and veins, the dermis has an extensive lymphatic system and multiple sensory nerves.

CLINICAL PEARL

The dermis contains cells critical to immune function and to healing, such as macrophages and fibroblasts.

Epidermal Appendages

The hair follicles, sweat glands, and sebaceous glands are anatomically located deep in the dermis and are lined with the basal layer of the epidermis. The epidermal and dermal structures are capable of reproduction throughout life; however, the epidermal appendages are not capable of reproduction. If an injury extends past the hair follicles, sebaceous glands, and sweat glands, those structures cannot be reproduced.

CLINICAL PEARL

Epidermal structures and most dermal structures are capable of regeneration; the epidermal appendages, subcutaneous tissue, and muscle do *not* have the ability to regenerate, and wounds involving loss of these structures will heal by scar formation.

Subcutaneous Tissue

Underneath the dermis is a layer of subcutaneous fat, often referred to as *hypodermis*. It provides insulation and acts to separate the skin from underlying muscle, tendons, bone, and joints. The subcutaneous tissue also plays a critical role in pressure redistribution; individuals who have very minimal subcutaneous tissue are at much higher risk for pressure ulcer development if they become bedbound or chairbound. Individuals who are morbidly obese are also at higher risk for pressure ulcer development and for impaired healing; this is because the excess subcutaneous tissue increases interface pressures between the skin and the bed or chair, and subcutaneous tissue is poorly perfused and therefore slow to heal (NPUAP, EPUAP, PPPIA, 2014). Subcutaneous tissue lacks the capacity for reproduction; if a wound extends to the subcutaneous tissue layer, the defect must heal by scar formation.

Muscle

The layer of soft tissue deep to the hypodermis and immediately adjacent to the bone is the muscle layer; this layer has a higher metabolic rate than either the skin or subcutaneous tissue and is the layer most impacted by unrelieved pressure over a bony prominence. Current evidence suggests that most pressure ulcers begin at the muscle–bone interface (NPUAP, EPUAP, PPPIA, 2014).

Functions of the Skin and Soft Tissue

The most critical function of the skin is its role as a barrier between the internal and external environments; however, it has a number of additional functions, and each of these is briefly described.

Thermoregulation and Regulation of Cutaneous Blood Flow

The ability of the skin to control blood flow is vital for thermoregulation and maintenance of physiologic body temperature. Cutaneous blood flow is primarily controlled by the sympathetic nervous system with noradrenaline and adrenaline being the primary neurotransmitters (Charkoudian, 2003). In the skin, the release of noradrenaline or adrenaline leads to vasoconstriction, which decreases cutaneous blood flow. When the levels of noradrenaline and adrenaline are reduced, the result is vasodilation and an increase in cutaneous blood flow.

The skin responds rapidly to restore thermal equilibrium when there is an increase or decrease in core body temperature. For example, during exercise or episodes of severe hyperthermia, blood flow to the skin can increase to as much as 6,000 to 8,000 mL/min (Johnson & Proppe, 2011; Rowell, 2011; Taylor et al., 1984). In comparison, resting blood flow to the skin is approximately 250 mL/min (Johnson et al., 1986; Johnson & Proppe, 2011). Cutaneous vasodilation provides for increased heat dissipation, thus returning core body temperature towards normal.

The opposite is true for severe cold exposure and hypothermia. The resulting cutaneous vasoconstriction significantly decreases blood flow to the skin, thus reducing heat dissipation. If this compensatory mechanism is insufficient to restore thermal homeostasis, shivering begins. The contraction of skeletal muscles involved in shivering generates heat that helps to maintain core body temperature (Charkoudian, 2003).

Insulation

Insulation and conservation of heat is another very important function of the skin. In nonobese individuals, ≥80% of the total body adipose tissue is stored in the hypodermis. Due to the decreased perfusion and water content of adipose tissue, it does not conduct heat as efficiently and thus acts as a very efficient insulating layer.

Immunity

The skin is exposed to a wide variety of pathogens and foreign bodies, and one of its major functions is to maintain a barrier against pathogenic invasion and thus against infection. An intact stratum corneum provides a mechanical barrier to pathogenic invasion. In addition, the skin produces *antimicrobial peptides (AMPs)* that provide a second level of protection should the barrier be breached (Goodarzi et al., 2007). Over 20 different AMPs have been identified to date, and different AMPs are effective against bacteria, viruses, and fungi. Most AMPs have unique mechanisms of action; however, they can be categorized into general categories. For example, some AMPs disrupt the cell membranes of pathogens without harming human cell membranes, while others stimulate the host immune system via chemotactic and angiogenic agents (Gallo, 2008).

CLINICAL PEARL

In addition to providing a structural barrier to pathogen invasion, the skin produces a number of AMPs that provide a secondary level of protection.

Immune Surveillance

Langerhans' Cells

Langerhans' cells (LCs) are found mainly in the *stratum spinosum* layer of the epidermis. They are dendritic in morphology and act as *antigen-presenting cells*. In addition to their phagocytic properties, they present foreign antigens to lymphocytes, thus activating the cell-mediated immune system. Interaction with the T lymphocytes results in activation of the LCs themselves, which triggers the release of different chemotactic agents (Bennett et al., 2007). Although LCs are primarily found in the epidermis, once they are activated by a foreign antigen, they move to local lymph nodes via the lymphatic vessels in the dermis. In the lymph nodes, T lymphocytes specific to the foreign antigen undergo clonal proliferation that leads to an extensive cell-mediated immune response (Burns et al., 2010). The presence of LCs in the skin accounts for the high incidence of contact allergic dermatitis caused by topical medications, especially in persons with leg ulcers. Chemicals in direct contact with the skin are more likely to cause an allergic response as compared to those given via the oral or parenteral routes.

Sensory Perception

The skin possesses a number of afferent sensory receptors that respond to various environmental stimuli. These receptors are spread throughout the different layers of the skin and can detect touch, pressure, temperature, pain, and itch. Touch and pressure sensation is mediated by a class of receptors known as *mechanoreceptors*. There are four different mechanoreceptors in the skin: Merkel's receptor, Meissner's receptor, pacinian corpuscle, and Ruffini's corpuscle. Merkel's receptors are primarily located in the basal layer of the epidermis, whereas Meissner's receptors are predominantly found in the dermal papillae (Halata et al., 2003; Winkelmann, 1959).

Barrier Function/Protection

One of the main functions of the skin is to maintain a barrier between the internal and external environments, thus protecting against invasion by external pathogens and environmental irritants and against excessive water loss from the internal environment. This barrier function is dependent on both an intact stratum corneum and on normal lipid production. Lipids found in the extracellular matrix of the stratum corneum are secreted by Odland bodies located primarily in the upper stratum spinosum and stratum granulosum. The Odland bodies are secreted by the keratinocytes during the process of terminal differentiation. The lipids released by Odland bodies serve to fill the gaps between the corneocytes (terminally differentiated keratinocytes), thus contributing the "mortar" to the brick and mortar configuration of the intact stratum corneum (the corneocytes are the bricks). The skin lipids also bind water, normally maintaining skin water content at 10% or higher. Thus, an intact barrier both excludes pathogens and irritants and retains water. The barrier function of the skin is usually measured objectively by "transepidermal water loss" (TEWL); when the barrier function of the skin is compromised, TEWL rises (Fluhr et al., 2006).

CLINICAL PEARL

Normal barrier function is dependent on intact keratinocytes and on normal levels of skin lipids. Barrier function is reflected by "TEWL."

Protection against pathogenic invasion is also supported by the acidic pH of the skin, the AMPs, and the immune components of the skin. The pH of the skin is normally 4 to 6.5; this "acid mantle" inhibits pathogenic growth (Yosipovitch & Hu, 2003). In addition, the AMPs and the immune system of the skin provide additional "secondary" protection against pathogenic invasion. The corneocytes (terminally differentiated keratinocytes) embedded in the extracellular matrix also contribute to the mechanical rigidity and frictional resistance protection of the skin; these are two of the most important functions of these surface keratinocytes.

Synthesis of Vitamin D

In the presence of ultraviolet sunlight, the skin can synthesize vitamin D_3 from 7-dehydrocholesterol. While the role of vitamin D in bone health and calcium absorption is well known, it has other roles of equal importance. These include immunocompetence, protection against some cancers, and genome control of cell proliferation and differentiation during the wound healing process (Berger et al., 1988; Kaminski & Drinane, 2014; Matusomoto et al., 1991; Norman, 1998; Xiao et al., 1995). Vitamin D is believed to express genes in keratinocytes that code for antimicrobial receptors and cathelicidin, an AMP that eradicates microbes found on wound surfaces (Bikel, 2008; Kaminski & Drinane, 2014; Norman, 1996; Schauber et al., 2007; Segaert, 2008).

Skin Changes throughout Life

There are a number of skin changes that occur across the lifespan that impact on skin health and wound healing.

Infants and Children

While the structural components of the skin remain similar across the age continuum, specific characteristics and functions are not as well developed in the newborn compared to an adult. For example, the skin of a newborn is thinner and more permeable than adult skin, and there is a higher ratio of surface area to total body weight. These changes place infants at higher risk for fluid loss (Jarvis, 2012) and for increased systemic absorption of topically applied substances.

Temperature regulation is less effective among infants and children, often resulting in higher fevers than adults. In addition, the eccrine sweat glands' ability to increase heat induced sweat production is only minimally developed in children (Jarvis, 2014). The subcutaneous layer is thinner and less developed, and infants and children are less able to shiver; thus, they need to be protected from the cold (Jarvis, 2014). At puberty, the skin becomes more mature; the epidermis thickens and there is increased oil and sweat production (Jarvis, 2014). See Chapter 12 for more detailed information on the care of Skin and Wounds for the Neonatal and Pediatric Populations.

CLINICAL PEARL

Infant skin is thinner, which places them at greater risk for systemic absorption of topically applied substances.

When assessing the skin of an infant, it is important to differentiate between normal skin color variations and bruises that could suggest child abuse. For example, African American, Asian American, Indian, and Hispanic newborns may exhibit Mongolian spots, a blue-black area of discoloration most typically found on the buttocks. Similar lesions can occur around the eye (Nevus of Ito) and in the shoulder region (unilateral Nevus of Ito). Another skin color variation is café au lait, an oval patch of light brown pigmentation; while limited café au lait spots are considered normal, the presence of five or more is associated with increased incidence of neurofibromatosis. Another congenital color variation is port-wine stain (nevus flammeus), a flat dark red-blue-purple patch usually found on the face or the scalp. Infants and children with Down syndrome may have cutis marmorata, a reticulated red or blue pattern of mottling seen on the extremities that is more prominent when the child is in a cooler environment (Jarvis, 2014).

Older Adults

Aging is associated with multiple changes in the structure and function of the skin (see also Chapter 13, Skin and Wound Care for Geriatric Population). A summary is presented in Table 1-1.

Skin functions that decline with aging will be briefly discussed.

TABLE 1-1 Structural Changes in Aging Skin

Skin Layer	Structural Change
Epidermis	• ↓ Melanocytes • ↓ Langerhans' cells • Flattening of dermal–epidermal junction • ↓ Epidermal thickness
Dermis	• ↓ Fibroblasts • ↓ Mast cells • ↓ Papillary capillary network • ↓ Collagen • ↓ Elastin

Sources: Montagna, W., & Carlisle, K. (1979). Structural changes in aging human skin. Structural changes in aging human skin. *The Journal of Investigative Dermatology*, *73*, 47–53; Fenske, N. A., & Lober, C. W. (1986). Structural and functional changes of normal aging skin. *Journal of the American Academy of Dermatology*, *15*(4), 571–585; National Pressure Ulcer Advisory Panel, European Pressure Ulcer Advisory Panel, and Pan Pacific Pressure Ulcer Advisory Panel. (2014). Prevention and Treatment of Pressure Ulcers: Clinical Practice Guideline. NPUAP, Washington, DC.

Thermoregulation

As an individual ages, both endogenous and exogenous factors lead to changes in thermoregulation. Body heat is generated by endogenous factors such as metabolic rate and physical activity. As muscle mass is lost and physical activity decreases, there is a decline in metabolism and energy production. This results in a decreased ability to maintain thermal homeostasis, specifically a slower and/or incomplete adaptation to temperature change. Elderly individuals have thinner skin and most also lose body fat, resulting in less insulation against cold and less ability to radiate metabolic heat. Even in the summer months, the elderly may wear a sweater or need a blanket. The elderly are also much more prone to heat stroke as aging skin has fewer sweat glands, and thus, the temperature regulation of the skin is decreased. In addition, elderly skin is drier, so older persons need to be encouraged to drink water and avoid extremes in temperatures. In regard to the reduced metabolic rate among the elderly, it is interesting to note that a high-protein meal can increase the metabolic rate by 30% or more, whereas a high-carbohydrate meal will only increase energy production by 4% (Guyton, 1991).

Cell Turnover Time

Aging is also associated with an increase in time required for renewal of the stratum corneum, due to a reduced rate of epidermal mitosis; specifically, renewal of the stratum corneum takes an average of 30 as opposed to 20 days. Wound healing is also prolonged in the middle aged and elderly adult.

CLINICAL PEARL

Aging is associated with prolonged time required for replacement of the stratum corneum by new cells, due to slower rate of epidermal mitosis; this results in thinner skin and delayed healing.

Common Skin Conditions in the Elderly

There are a number of skin conditions, both benign and malignant, that are much more common in the elderly.

Photoaging

Photoaging is a major cause of premature aging in persons who have experienced excessive sun exposure (Bolognia, 1995). Benign changes in the skin caused by photoaging include wrinkling, telangiectasia (threadlike blood vessels), thinning of the skin (atrophy of the dermis and epidermis), and pigmentary changes (hyper- and hypopigmentation). Collectively, these changes are often referred to as poikiloderma (telangiectasia, pigment change, atrophy). This type of change is more common in persons with blonde or red hair, blue eyes, and skin that burns rather than tans. Fitzpatrick (1975, 1986, 2007) outlined four Caucasian skin types based on the skin's response to ultraviolet radiation. The four Fitzpatrick classes of skin color are as follows:

- Category 1 (always burns, never tans)
- Category 2 (usually burns, tans slightly)
- Category 3 (sometimes burns, tans uniformly)
- Category 4 (rarely burns, always tans) (Fitzpatrick, 1975, 1986, 2007)

Two other skin types, skin color category type 5 (Asian skin) and skin color category type 6 (deeply pigmented Black skin), were subsequently added to this classification (Fitzpatrick, 1986; 2007).

Changes in skin pigmentation are common among the elderly; some are due to natural aging but many are due to photoaging. The difference in natural aging and photoaging can be easily illustrated, by comparing the skin on the buttocks (which is rarely if ever exposed to the sun) to the skin on the face, in terms of wrinkling, pigmentary changes, telangiectasia, and enlarged sebaceous glands (sebaceous hyperplasia). In addition to the mottled pigmentation caused by photodamage, there is hypopigmentation related to reduced numbers and function of melanocytes, and increased risk of bruising due to capillary fragility. Purpuric lesions (bruises caused by minor trauma) are indicative of increased risk for skin tears; hypopigmentation related to diminished melanocyte function is indicative of increased risk for melanoma and its precursors.

Actinic Keratosis

Those individuals with Celtic-type skin are much more prone to precancerous and cancerous changes in the skin, including palpable scaly red papular areas known as actinic keratosis (solar keratosis) (Fig. 1-2). The presence of these premalignant lesions should alert the clinician to also inspect the skin carefully for cancerous lesions.

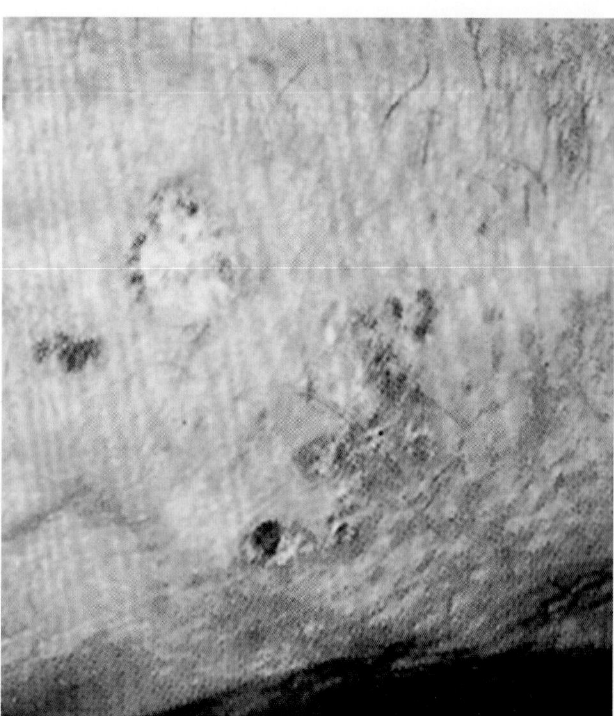

FIGURE 1-2. Actinic keratosis. (Reprinted with permission from Sauer, G. C. (1985). *Manual of skin diseases* (5th ed.). Philadelphia, PA: JB Lippincott.)

Basal Cell Carcinoma

The most common skin cancer is basal cell carcinoma (BCC), which most commonly presents as a "pearl-like" translucent papule with potential central ulceration (Fig. 1-3). There is also frequently a surface telangiectasia traversing the edge of the lesion. These lesions are common on sun-exposed areas of the face, especially the nose, forehead, and ears. Less common variants of basal cell carcinoma include superficial BCC, sclerosing BCC, morpheaform BCC, and pigmented BCC.

> **CLINICAL PEARL**
>
> The most common type of skin cancer is BCC, which presents clinically as a "pearl-like" translucent papule with central ulceration. The second most common type is squamous cell carcinoma (SCC), which presents clinically as an enlarging keratotic papule.

Squamous Cell Carcinoma

The second most common skin cancer is SCC. These lesions begin as keratotic papules that gradually enlarge in an irregular way and may become painful (Fig. 1-4). They are most common around the lips (especially the lower lip, as a result of sun damage or smoking), the ears, other areas on the face, or exposed skin on the back of the hands or arms. Both SCC and BCC may appear on the legs in the elderly and may be mistakenly diagnosed as skin ulcers (venous and mixed arterial/venous ulcers). For this

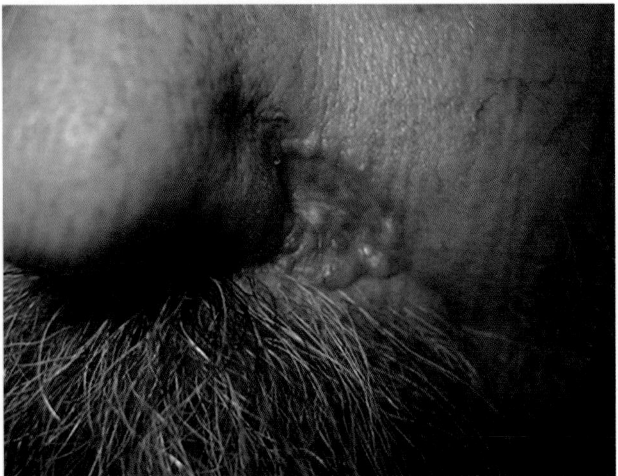

FIGURE 1-3. Basal cell carcinoma.

reason, the wound clinician must maintain a high index of suspicion and should not hesitate to biopsy a nonhealing wound. Previous studies have documented that wounds that are healable and are appropriately managed should demonstrate a 30% reduction in size by week 4 of treatment (and should heal by week 12). Wounds that fail to demonstrate appropriate progress should be biopsied at the edge to rule out skin cancer (Falanga & Sabolinski, 1999). Clinical lesions suspicious of SCCs around the lips, on the nose, or on the ears should be biopsied and treated accordingly.

SCCs on the legs may arise from old burn scars, osteomyelitis sinuses, the edge of previous skin grafts, or old radiotherapy sites. Early diagnosis is critical because failure to accurately diagnose the lesion can result in locally invasive or metastatic disease. An accurate differential diagnosis is therefore critical to avoid the tragic consequences of treating a cancerous leg lesion as a venous or mixed arterial/venous ulcer. For more information on accurate assessment of leg wounds, see Chapters 21 to 24 (Venous Ulcers, Arterial Ulcers, Neuropathic Ulcers, Differential Assessment) and Chapter 29 (Oncologic Lesions).

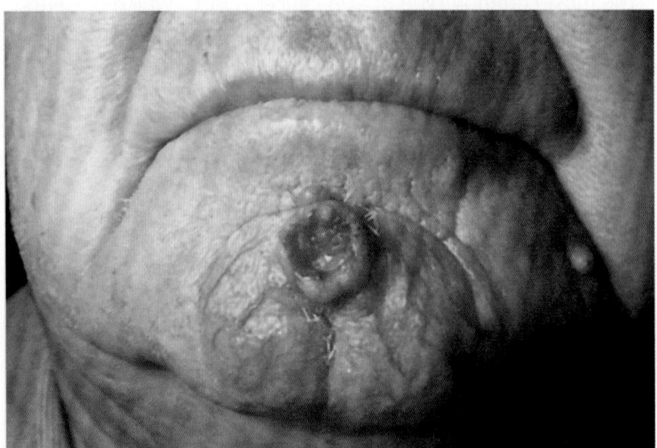

FIGURE 1-4. Squamous cell carcinoma. (Reprinted with permission from Weber, J. R. N., & Kelley J. R. N. (2003). *Health assessment in nursing* (2nd ed.). Philadelphia, PA: Lippincott Williams & Wilkins.)

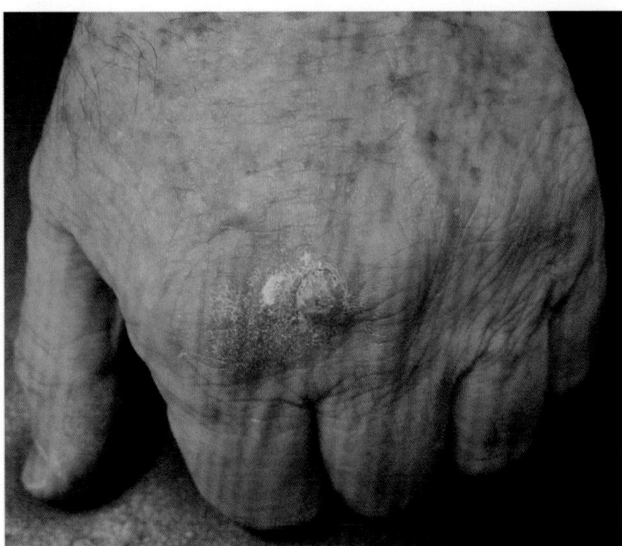

FIGURE 1-5. Cutaneous horn.

CLINICAL PEARL

Both BCC and SCC may occur on the legs in the elderly and may be mistaken for a venous ulcer or other chronic ulcer.

Cutaneous Horn

Another common lesion in the elderly is the cutaneous horn (Fig. 1-5). These are caused by an irregular and often vertical growth of keratin over a tissue base that varies in terms of pathology. The lesions may be hard and *can* become painful. Cutaneous horns may have a thick or very narrow tapered keratotic column (the "horn"). About 60% of these lesions are benign with a wart or seborrheic keratosis (SK) at the base. Another 20% are premalignant, with an actinic keratosis histologically at the base. Unfortunately, the remaining 20% are frankly malignant. The malignant lesions are most commonly caused by Bowen's disease (SCC that spreads horizontally without vertical invasion) or an early SCC (Copcu et al., 2004; Korkut et al., 1997).

Seborrheic Keratoses

SK are common but benign skin lesions in the elderly that have the appearance of a "stuck-on barnacle" (Hafner & Vogt, 2008; Noiles & Ronald, 2007) (Fig. 1-6). The lesions contain keratin with horn cysts that, if examined closely or viewed under the dermatoscope, might have the appearance of grains of sand within the surface. The lesions may be small and white (often referred to as stucco keratosis); these are more common on the head, neck, distal hands, or arms (Yeatman et al., 1997). They may also present as large, pigmented eruptive lesions that commonly occur on the trunk but can also occur on the face, backs of the

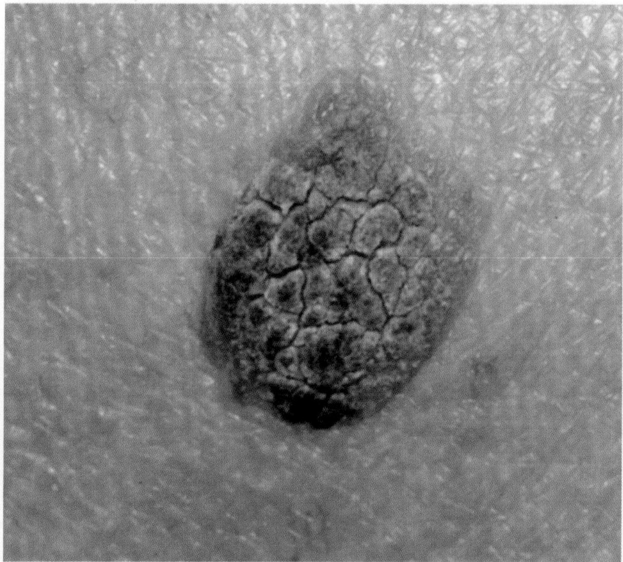

FIGURE 1-6. Seborrheic keratosis.

hands, or other areas that are socially visible, and can be potentially disfiguring.

Nevi (Moles)

Moles are very common, typically benign lesions, especially among Caucasian individuals (Fig. 1-7). Congenital nevi are moles that are present on the skin at birth. As an individual grows, the congenital nevi may become more darkly pigmented, but the growth and pigmentation is regular and even. Congenital nevi are usually divided into three categories based on their size. When these nevi are under 1.5 cm in diameter, they are referred to as "small," and the risk of malignant transformation is extremely low. When the size of these lesions is 1.5 to 19.5 cm in diameter, they are referred to as "medium," but the risk of malignant transformation remains low (Bittencourt et al., 2000; Habif, 2004). When the diameter of these lesions exceeds 20 cm, they are classified as "large" and the risk of malignant transformation is significant (Egan et al., 1998, Zaal et al., 2005). Most nevi develop in late childhood as small brown dots, gradually enlarge in the teen years and the early 20s, and often persist until age 50; at this point, they start to lose their pigment, become elevated and soft, become neuroid nevi, and disappear with time (James et al., 2006). Congenital giant hairy pigmented nevi over 20 cm should be watched more carefully for malignant transformation, as these nevi carry a 5% to 15% lifetime risk of melanoma (Esterly, 1996). Unfortunately, simply removing the surface of these lesions does not eliminate the malignant potential. Melanocytes are spindle cells that, by their shape, are well adapted for mobility and secondary spread of malignant cells. This is why melanocytic tumors (melanoma) can metastasize hematogenously (through the blood stream) to other organs (liver and brain) as well as regional lymph nodes, as detected via a sentinel lymph node biopsy.

FIGURE 1-7. Benign nevus (mole). (Reprinted with permission from Goodheart, H. P. (2003). *Goodheart's photoguide of common skin disorders* (2nd ed.). Philadelphia, PA: Lippincott Williams & Wilkins.)

In addition to normal nevi, some individuals have slightly larger and irregular dysplastic nevi. They evolve in childhood and early adult life, are characterized by a much more irregular surface, and can develop into melanoma. Dysplastic nevi when fully developed are slightly larger than normal nevi (e.g., the size of an eraser on the end of a pencil) and have irregular pigmentation (e.g., light brown and/or dark brown with often pink coloration [the pink is more common in very fair individuals]). The risk of melanoma increases in the presence of dysplastic nevi. The more nevi present, the greater the risk of malignant transformation or the de novo appearance of a melanoma. Individuals can be classified as having a few nevi, an average of 30 to 50 nevi, a moderately increased number of nevi (50 to 100), or markedly increased number of nevi with more than 100 nevi. In addition to a genetic predisposition, the cumulative sun exposure in childhood is linked to the number of nevi that form on the arms of adults (Gallagher & Mclean, 1995).

Melanoma

The presence of dysplastic nevi along with blistering sun burns, blue eyes, and fair hair all predispose individuals to melanoma. It is also believed that melanoma is more common in individuals who have intermittent but intense sun exposure (e.g., sun exposure related to tropical holidays), as opposed to the prolonged but moderate amount of sun exposure experienced by the farmer or fisherman. The most common melanoma is superficial spreading melanoma (70%), which is more common in younger individuals and usually occurs on the backs of males and lower legs of females (Fig. 1-8). The characteristics of a melanoma can be remembered best by the letters ABCDE. This includes the following:

A = asymmetry (one side does not look like the other)
B = irregular border (blurred, uneven, or "notched" edges)
C = variable and uneven color

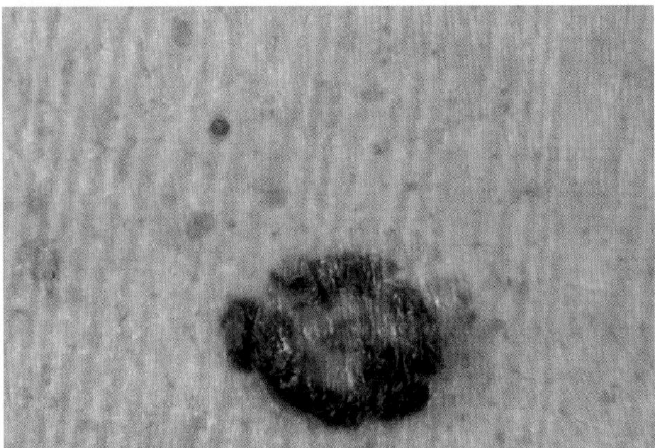

FIGURE 1-8. Superficial spreading melanoma. (Reprinted with permission from Goodheart, H. P. (2003). *Goodheart's photoguide of common skin disorders* (2nd ed.). Philadelphia, PA: Lippincott.)

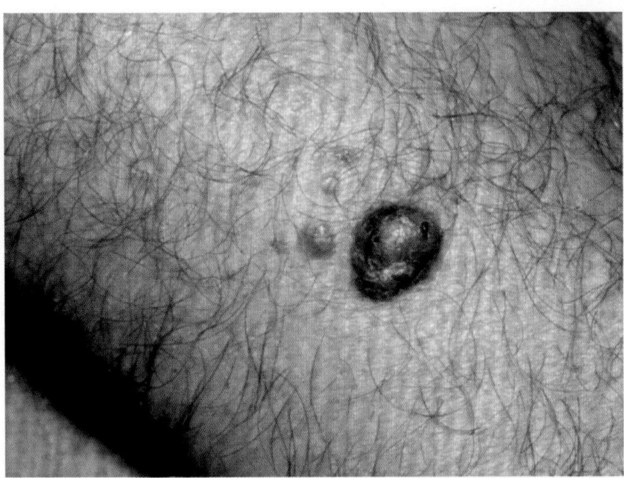

FIGURE 1-9. Nodular melanoma. (Reprinted with permission from Goodheart, H. P. (2003). *Goodheart's photoguide of common skin disorders* (2nd ed.). Philadelphia, PA: Lippincott.)

D = diameter >6 mm (the size of an eraser on the end of a pencil) that requires more attention
E = evolving lesion (is worth further evaluation) (Abbasi et al., 2004; Rigel et al., 2005)

CLINICAL PEARL

The acronym ABCDE should be used to help differentiate a melanoma from a benign nevus. A = asymmetry; B = border irregularity; C = variable uneven color; D = diameter >6 mm; E = evolving lesion.

Around 20% to 50% of superficial spreading melanomas arise in existing nevi and 50% to 80% on what appears to be clinically normal skin; however, it is important to remember that abnormal melanocytes exist throughout the body although they are concentrated in existing nevi.

The second most common melanoma is the lentigo maligna melanoma. This type of melanoma accounts for 10% to 15% of melanomas and is most common on the face but occasionally involves other exposed body areas. It is seen more commonly in the elderly, and, in this case, sun exposure is both the initiator and promoter of the malignancy. These melanomas do *not* arise within preexisting nevi but rather occur de novo. Early lesions are often undetected because they can be confused with solar lentigines (freckles from sun damage that are larger than the usual freckles seen in young individuals) or a large SK. Nodular melanoma is relatively uncommon, accounting for about 10% to 15% of melanomas; these lesions lack a vertical growth phase, are invasive almost from their onset, and are elevated above the level of the skin (Kelly et al., 2003). These lesions can be darkly pigmented and quickly growing or may present without pigment or as an ulcer (Fig. 1-9). Nodular melanomas can be confused with other ulcerative lesions, which again underscores the importance of early biopsy for any wound that has an atypical location or appearance especially if it is also not healing at the expected rate. The least common melanocytic malignancy is a subungual melanoma (acrolentiginous melanoma) (Levit et al., 2000). These are often seen under the fingernails or distal locations in individuals with darkly pigmented skin (Fitzpatrick group). Again, a high index of suspicion is critical, because these lesions tend to metastasize early.

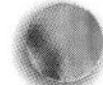

Skin Immune System

The skin is the most efficient immune organ in the body; thus, allergic reactions to drugs applied topically are much more likely and more common than allergic reactions to drugs ingested systemically. A key component of the skin's immune system is the LCs; these cells are located in the epidermis and are responsible for processing antigens (Bos & Kapsenberg, 1993). The LCs then "present" the antigen to the lymphocytes and migrate to regional lymph nodes, where they continue to process antigens and also recruit activated T cells, triggering a more generalized inflammatory response.

Allergic Contact Dermatitis

This is why poison ivy and poison oak are two of the most potent contact allergens known (Gladman, 2006; Lee and Arriola, 1999). When the skin is exposed to one of these agents, a type 4 allergic reaction occurs that is similar to the reaction that occurs with a tuberculin test. If the exposure is an initial (sensitizing) exposure, the rash is typically delayed, sometimes for up to 3 weeks (depending on the level of response by the LCs). If the person has already been sensitized, blistering can occur at the site of contact within a few hours. External allergens usually cause linear types of blistering, and poison ivy or poison oak more commonly involves the lower legs or arms where the skin is relatively thin and often unprotected in hot weather. The poison ivy Rhus antigen is a resin that becomes fixed to the skin within a few minutes. The dermatitis can spread to other parts of the body through contact with inanimate objects contaminated with the resin, such as a bicycle, clothing, or tools. The poison ivy antigen is processed by lymphocytes and

Langerhans' cell at the site of skin contact. The sensitized lymphocytes then migrate to the regional lymph nodes and recruit other lymphocytes that become sensitized; these lymphocytes have the potential to migrate to distal skin sites, thus causing the rash to become generalized. Contact with inanimate objects can cause new skin sites to react; these objects should therefore be washed thoroughly with a surface active agent to remove resin that could cause further skin sensitization (Gladman, 2006; Lee & Arriola, 1999).

Impact of Aging

Aging is associated with a loss of immune system responsiveness. The decrease in cell-mediated immunity is a probable contributing factor to the increased risk of viral infections and malignancy among older individuals. One example would be chickenpox. When this disorder is acquired at a young age, the child's immune system typically handles the virus very effectively. However, if primary infection occurs at an older age (e.g., in an individual over 20 years of age), the acute varicella illness is often much more severe. This is why varicella vaccination is recommended for individuals without evidence of previous chickenpox, especially immigrants moving to northern climates, where the indoor winter habitat facilitates the spread of varicella. Aging reduces immunity to the varicella virus and allows activation of the previously dormant virus, which results in outbreaks of varicella zoster (shingles) along a nerve pathway (dermatome). The elderly individual who develops shingles is also at greater risk for nerve damage resulting in painful postherpetic neuralgia. This excruciating neuropathic pain has a very negative effect on quality of life and requires prompt intervention (Woo et al., 2008).

CLINICAL PEARL

Aging is associated with diminished immunocompetence of the skin; this is one factor contributing to the increased risk for shingles (varicella zoster) among the elderly.

Skin and Vitamin D production

As explained earlier, the skin plays an important role in vitamin D metabolism. The precursor to vitamin D, 7-dehydrocholesterol, is abundantly present in the skin (Crissey et al., 2003). Vitamin D is produced photochemically when ultraviolet light acts on 7-dehydrocholesterol. Vitamin D is further metabolized in the liver and finally activated in the kidney (Holick et al., 1987). Vitamin D deficiency has been documented in individuals who lack UV exposure, including elderly individuals in nursing homes and individuals living in northern climates; vitamin D levels should be checked and supplementation provided for individuals who are unable to obtain sun exposure and who are vitamin D deficient. It should be noted that the amount of UV exposure required for vitamin D metabolism can be obtained with minimal outdoor exposure. There are concerns that vitamin D deficiency may become more common due to the increased use of sunscreen, especially products with sun protection factors (SPFs) over 15 that block most of the photoactivated vitamin D_3 production (Institute of Medicine [US] Committee to Review Dietary Reference Intakes for Vitamin D and Calcium [2011]). Routine use of sunscreen should be promoted in all situations where there is the risk of burning and subsequent increased risk of skin cancer development; however, limited sun exposure should be encouraged in order to assure normal vitamin D metabolism (Holick et al., 1995; Marks et al., 1995).

Permeability and Dermal Absorption

The permeability of the skin to topically applied agents varies, depending on the age of the person and the anatomic area and characteristics of the skin. As noted, the skin of infants and elders is thin and fragile with increased permeability to some but not all chemicals. Therefore, clinicians need to use caution when recommending topical medications that can be systemically absorbed.

Percutaneous absorption varies depending on the anatomic site. For example, if the absorption of topical steroids on the forearms is considered to be 1, the absorption rate on the palmar surface of the hand is 0.83, and the absorption rate on the plantar aspect of the foot is 0.14. This means that the absorption rate on the forearm is six times that on the plantar surface of the foot. A lower potency steroid could be used on the forearm to obtain the same results as a much greater potency steroid on the plantar surface of the foot. Using the same comparator, the cheeks and forehead are much more permeable than the forearms, absorbing 8 to 13 times the amount of steroid, due in part to increased vascularity and in part to the thinner skin. The number of hair follicles in the area is another factor to consider, due to increased absorption along the hair follicle. An extreme example of high absorptive capacity is the scrotum. It will absorb 42 times the amount compared to the forearm, because the skin surface is very thin with a large surface area (due to folds), there is a prominent vascular network, and there are a large number of hair follicles facilitating absorption. In addition, proximity to the inner thighs and external genitalia creates a relatively occlusive environment for the scrotum (Feldmann & Maibach, 1967).

CLINICAL PEARL

Percutaneous absorption of medications such as steroids depends on the anatomic site; the rate of absorption over the scrotum is 42 times greater than over the forearm!

Skin Assessment

While most clinicians would agree that skin assessment is part of a physical examination, there is a lack of consensus as to what should be included in a basic skin assessment.

Common practice might include the following five components: skin color, temperature, turgor, moisture status, and integrity. In addition to the general physical assessment and specific skin assessment, factors that impact on skin health should be assessed, such as comorbidities, vitamin and mineral deficiencies that are manifested in skin changes, and smoking.

Skin Color

Normal variations in skin color have already been described earlier in this chapter in relation to the continuum of aging from birth to death. Skin color assessment must be based on the individual's normal skin color, with attention to areas in which there are color changes. Ayello et al. (2014) have developed a photo guide for assessing brown (Fitzpatrick category 5 dark brown/yellow) skin for changes related to moisture-associated skin damage (MASD), specifically incontinence-associated dermatitis or IAD, which can be downloaded from www.woundpedia.com.

Changes in skin color, either darkening or lightening, can be indicative of pathology. For example, a brownish gray discoloration of the lower limb(s) may be caused by hemosiderin staining in persons with venous disease and frequently precedes the development of a venous ulcer (Fig. 1-10). Atrophie blanche (Fig. 1-11) is manifest by white star-shaped patches (scars) just above the medial malleolus in the patient with vascular disease (typically chronic venous insufficiency). In contrast, pallor with leg raising or cyanosis and dependent rubor are characteristic of arterial insufficiency.

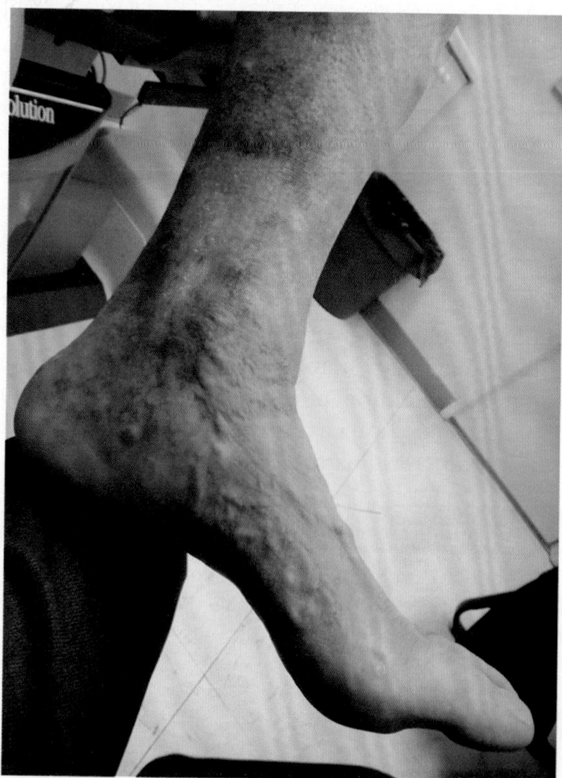

FIGURE 1-10. Hemosiderin staining. (Courtesy of Dr. Afsaneh Alavi.)

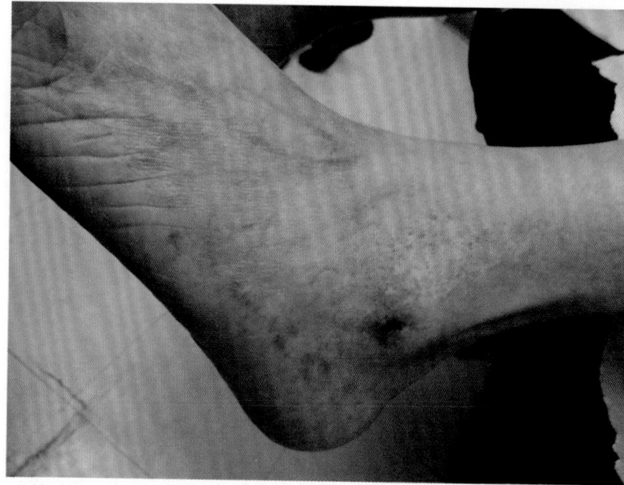

FIGURE 1-11. Atrophie blanche. (Courtesy of Dr. Afsaneh Alavi.)

Skin Temperature

Normal skin is "warm to touch"; ischemic skin is typically cool to touch, and areas of trauma, deep and surrounding infection, and deep inflammation are frequently warmer than adjacent skin (Sibbald et al., 2011). Routine assessment of plantar surface temperature using a dermal thermometer can identify persons at immediate risk for diabetic or other neurotropic foot ulcers due to repetitive trauma. Randomized controlled trials (RCTs) provide evidence that routine assessment (by the patient and by clinicians) can reduce the incidence of ulcers in persons with diabetes mellitus and neuropathy as outlined in three randomized controlled trials comparing daily monitoring of plantar foot temperatures compared to diabetic education or enhanced foot screening practices. See Chapter 23 for further discussion of plantar surface temperature monitoring in the management of the patient with neuropathy (Arad et al., 2011; Armstrong et al., 2007; Armstrong & Lavery, 1997; Houghton et al., 2013; Lavery et al., 2004; Lavery et al., 2007).

The use of an infrared thermometer can also detect skin temperature elevation due to periwound infection that can contribute to prompt detection and treatment of the infection (Sibbald et al., 2006). In fact, elevated skin temperature was the individual criterion most indicative of periwound infection involving the deep and surrounding wound tissues (Woo & Sibbald, 2009). Mufti et al. (2015) validated less expensive (<$100) infrared thermometers available on eBay as equivalent to the gold standard Dermatemp thermometer. These findings support the validity of low-cost thermometers as appropriate diagnostic tools for clinicians in everyday practice, and we believe these devices should be included in every wound care nurse's "toolkit." See Chapter 10 for further discussion of the assessment and management of superficial and deep wound infections.

Skin Turgor

Skin turgor refers to the skin's resiliency and ability to quickly return to its original state. The clinician uses two fingers to gently lift a portion of the patient's skin, ideally over the sternum. The rate at which the skin returns to its original state reflects skin turgor. Failure of the skin to rapidly resume its original state is a common sign of dehydration; however, altered skin turgor is also a common finding in the elderly.

Moisture Status

As mentioned earlier in this chapter, one of the functions of skin is maintenance of moisture balance; normally, the stratum corneum has a water content that ranges from 10% to 15 % (Dealy, 2009).When TEWL is excessive (>15%), the result is dry skin (xerosis) (Dealy, 2009). Dry skin is believed to be more vulnerable to damage and local injury from pressure and shear. Conversely, skin that is too moist is also more vulnerable to pressure injury as well as MASD (see Chapters 17 and 18 on pressure ulcers and MASD).

The simplest way to assess skin for moisture content is by visual inspection; dry skin frequently appears flaky and dull, while overhydrated skin appears moist and may be lighter in color than the surrounding skin. Touch can also be used to detect skin that is overly dry or overly moist. In the future, instruments may be available at the bedside to assess subepidermal moisture levels. There is emerging evidence that higher subepidermal moisture levels may be indicative of increased risk for pressure ulcer development, especially in individuals with darkly pigmented skin. Research is ongoing to verify the significance of these findings and to develop simple tools that would allow the clinician to measure subepidermal moisture at the bedside (Bates-Jensen et al., 2009).

Skin Integrity

A critical element of skin assessment is prompt identification of any breaks in skin integrity. If there are any lesions or ulcerations, the clinician needs to determine the type of damage/cause of the lesion, which provides guidance as to correction or treatment of the causative factors (the critical first step in management of any wound) (Schultz et al., 2003). The wound nurse should base diagnosis/classification of any lesion or wound on a comprehensive history and physical exam as well as any indicated diagnostic studies. The correct classification system should be used for the type of chronic wound identified. For example, the NPUAP pressure ulcer category/staging system (see Chapter 18) should only be applied for pressure ulcers and not for skin tears (see Chapter 17 for the ISTAP Classification system). When the diagnosis/classification is unclear, consultation with a dermatologist should be initiated.

Skin status is also affected by micronutrient deficiencies, and the signs of micronutrient deficiency are not always recognized. Kaminski and Drinane (2014) have provided a succinct summary of some of the micronutrient deficiencies that can impact on wound healing and that are manifest by skin changes; these are outlined in Table 1-2. See Chapter 6, nutritional assessment and support, for more detailed description of the role that vitamins and minerals play in skin and tissue integrity and wound healing.

The clinician should carefully describe the morphology of any skin lesion using standardized dermatologic terminology (Table 1-3).

CLINICAL PEARL

It is critical for the wound nurse to use standard dermatologic terminology when documenting skin lesions and wound status.

TABLE 1-2 Skin Changes Resulting from Micronutrient Deficiencies

Vitamin Deficiencies		
Vitamin	**Clinical Presentation**	**Characteristics**
B_2		Angular stomatitis is a moist crack in the mucosa at the angle of the upper and lower lips. It is a sign of vitamin B_2 deficiency, usually accompanied by magenta-colored glossitis.
B_3	A B	(A) Pellagra is a vitamin B_3 deficiency. Early signs are a crepe paper appearance to the skin, as illustrated here. Thin islands of epidermis are separated by rivulets. (B) Advanced pellagra is the typical alligator skin noted in sun-exposed areas of niacin-deficient individuals. In the past, farmers working with an open collar developed these legions on their superior chest/inferior neck.

(Continued)

TABLE 1-2 Skin Changes Resulting from Micronutrient Deficiencies (*Continued*)

C	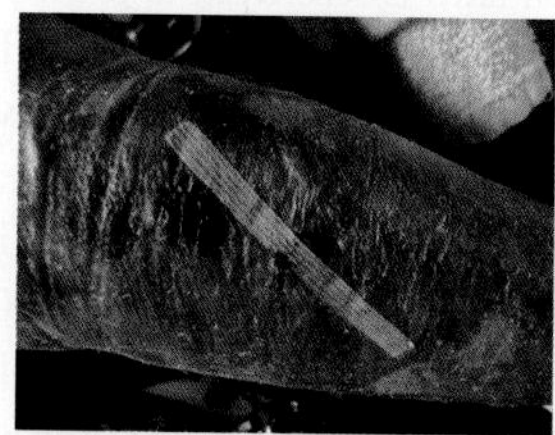	Profound chronic scurvy leaves the skin susceptible to a typical triangular skin tear. This may be a sign of scurvy and not a condition in itself; the patient should be assessed for other indicators of vitamin C deficiency and treatment should be initiated.
C	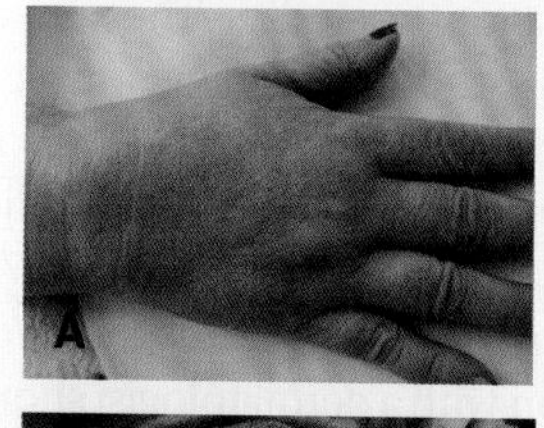 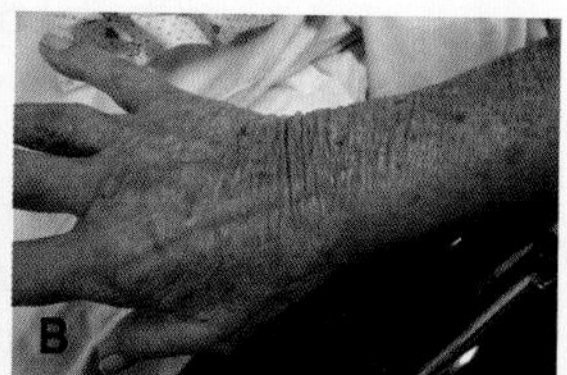 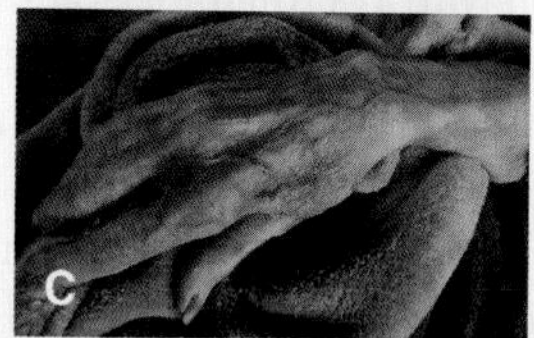 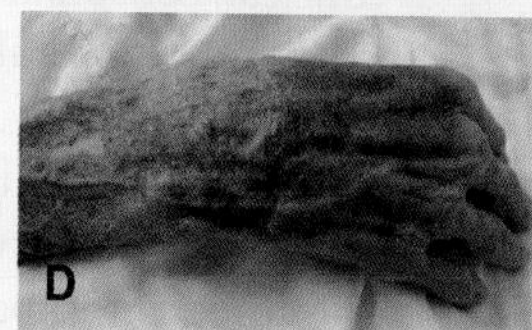	Chronic scurvy can be staged by observing the thickness of the dermis and its transparency. Early stages prevent direct observation of the tendrils of extensor tendons and the venous plexus over the tendon sheath. The skin becomes progressively transparent with stage IV, featuring a slightly opaque, transparent epidermis revealing an unobstructed view of the deeper anatomy. (A) Normal dermis; (B) +1; (C) +2; (D) +3; and (E) +4.
	Minerals and other micronutrients	
Name	**Clinical Presentation**	**Characteristics**
Zinc	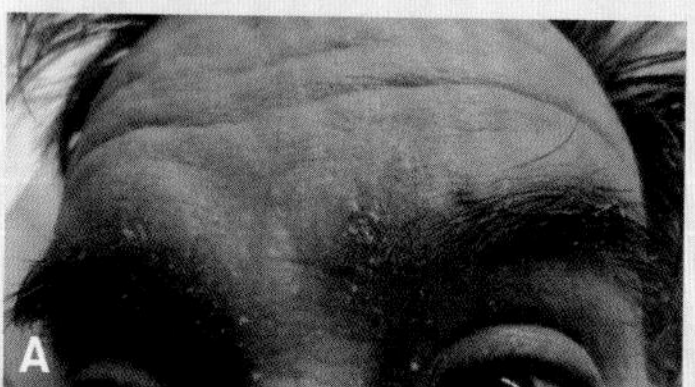 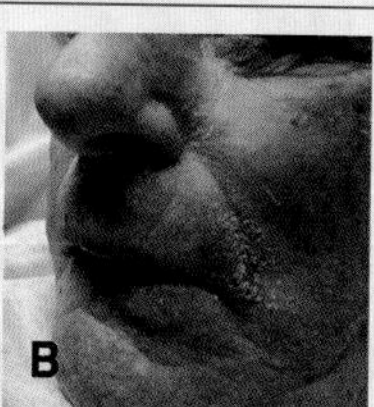	Zinc rash is a seborrheic-like reddish, flakey condition best seen along the lateral eyebrow (A) and the nasal labial folds (B).
Fatty acids	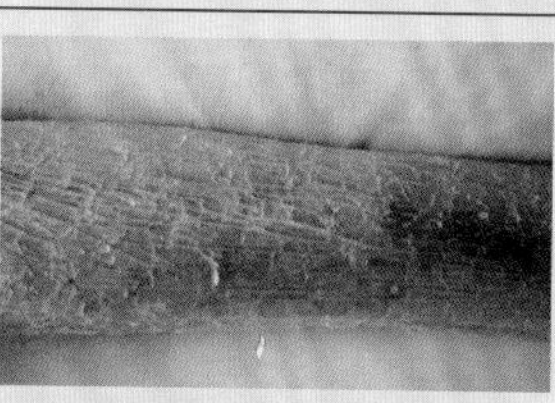	Essential fatty acid deficiency presents as a large "snowflake" exfoliated condition of the epidermis. It typically starts with the anterior area of the lower extremities. It can progress to involve the entire body. These "snowflakes" can be released by gentle rubbing and gathered off the surface of the mattress.
Glucosamine	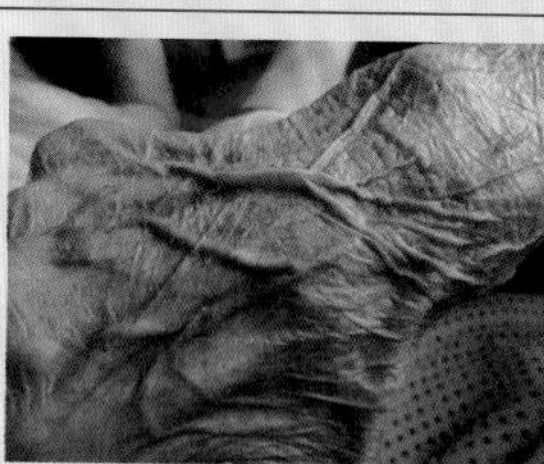	A deficiency in glucosamine and other intracellular constituents responsible for local hydration results in prolonged tenting of the skin despite normal hydration on physical examination.

Reprinted with permission from Kaminski, M. V., Jr., & Drinane, J. J. (2014). Learning the oral and cutaneous signs of micronutrient deficiencies. *Journal of Wound Ostomy & Continence Nursing, 41*(2), 127–135.

TABLE 1-3 Common Dermatologic Terminology, Lesions

Group	Lesion Type	Definition
Flat 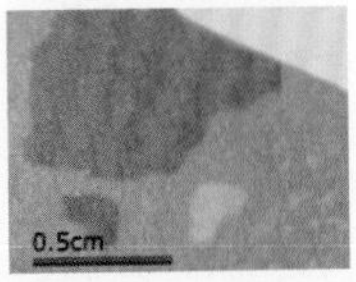	Macule 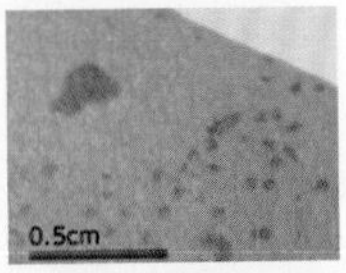	A flat, generally <0.5 cm area of skin or mucous membranes with different color from surrounding tissue. Macules may have nonpalpable, fine scale (Fig. 3-1).
	Patch* 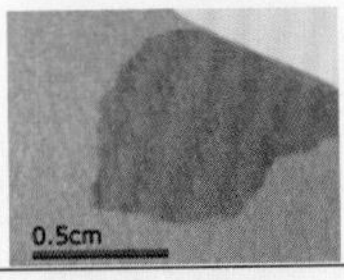	A flat, generally >0.5 cm area of skin or mucous membranes with different color from surrounding tissue. Patches may have nonpalpable, fine scale.
Raised and smooth 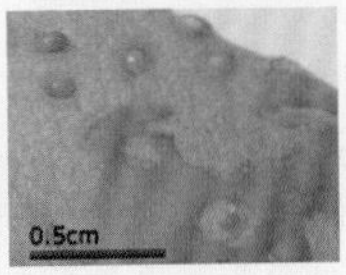	Papule 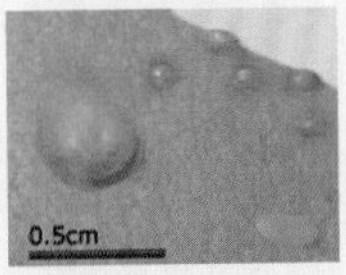	A discrete, solid, elevated body usually <0.5 cm in diameter. Papules are further classified by shape, size, color, and surface change (Fig. 3-3).
	Plaque 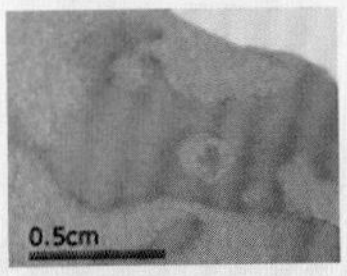	A discrete, solid, elevated body, usually broader than it is thick, measuring more than 0.5 cm in diameter. Plaques may be further classified by shape, size, color, and surface change (Fig. 3-4).
	Nodule 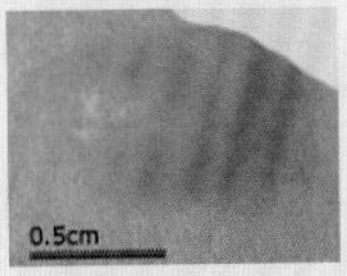	A dermal or subcutaneous firm, well-defined lesion usually >0.5 cm in diameter (Fig. 3-5).
	Cyst 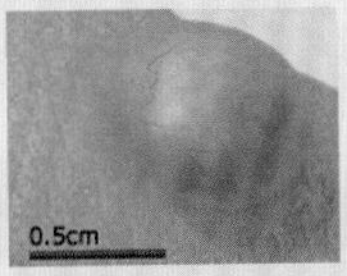	A closed cavity or sac containing fluid or semisolid material. A cyst may have an epithelial, endothelial, or membranous lining (Fig. 3-6).
Surface change 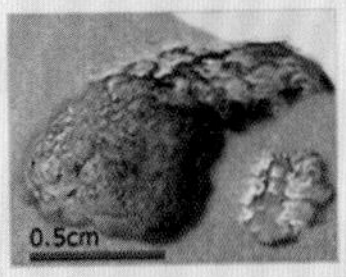	Crust 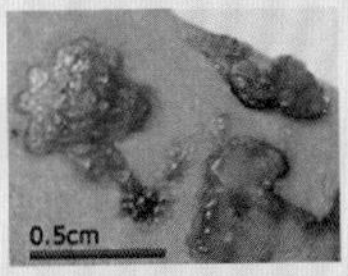	A hardened layer that results when serum, blood, or purulent exudate dries on the skin surface. Crusts may be thin or thick and can have varying color. Crusts are yellow-brown when formed from dried serum, green or yellow-green when formed from purulent exudate, or red-black when formed by blood (Fig. 3-7).
	Scale 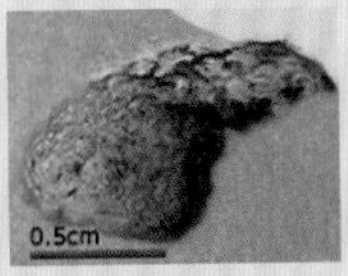	Excess stratum corneum accumulated in flakes or plates. Scale usually has a white or gray color (Fig. 3-8).

(Continued)

TABLE 1-3 Common Dermatologic Terminology, Lesions (*Continued*)

Group	Lesion Type	Definition
Fluid-filled 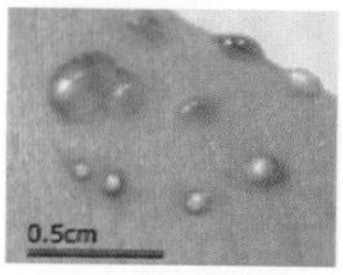	Abscess 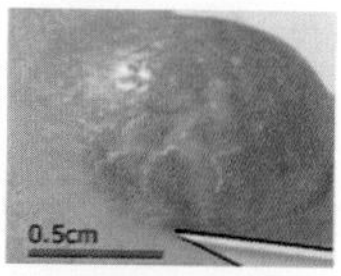	A localized accumulation of pus in the dermis or subcutaneous tissue. Frequently red, warm, and tender (Fig. 3-9).
	Bulla 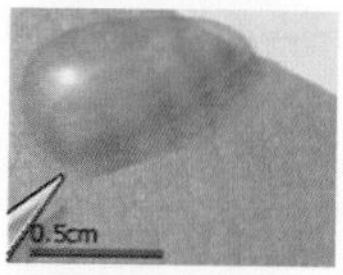	A fluid-filled blister >0.5 cm in diameter. Fluid can be clear, serous, hemorrhagic, or pus filled (Fig. 3-10).
	Pustule 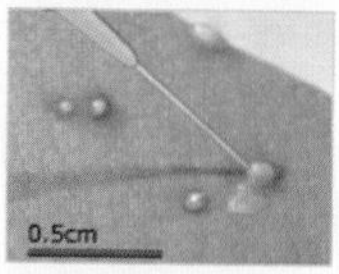	A circumscribed elevation that contains pus. Pustules are usually <0.5 cm in diameter (Fig. 3-11).
	Vesicle 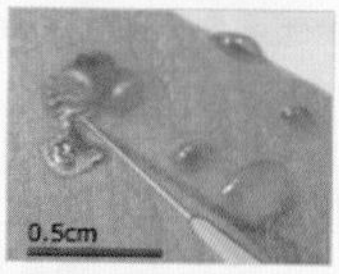	Fluid-filled cavity or elevation <0.5 cm in diameter. Fluid may be clear, serous, hemorrhagic, or pus filled (Fig. 3-12).
Red blanchable 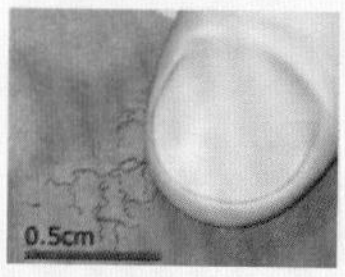	Erythema 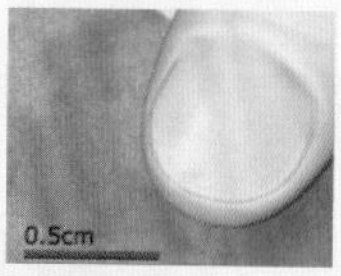	Localized, blanchable redness of the skin or mucous membranes (Fig. 3-13).
	Erythroderma 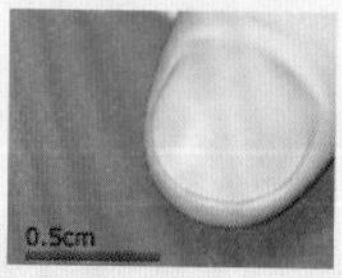	Generalized, blanchable redness of the skin that may be associated with desquamation (Fig.3-14).
	Telangiectasia 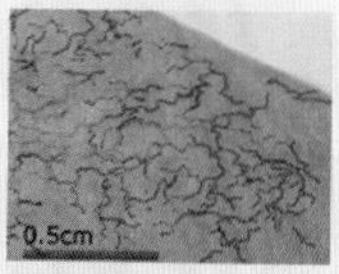	Visible, persistent dilation of small, superficial cutaneous blood vessels. Telangiectasias will blanch (Fig. 3-15).
Purpuric 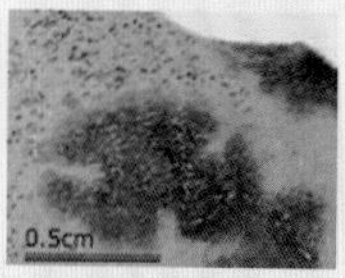	Ecchymosis 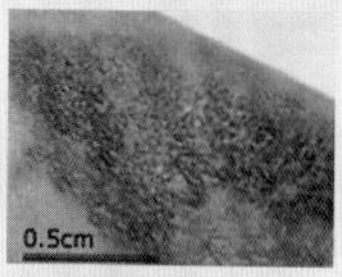	Extravasation of blood into the skin or mucous membranes. Area of flat color change may progress over time from blue-black to brown-yellow or green (Fig. 3-16).
	Petechiae 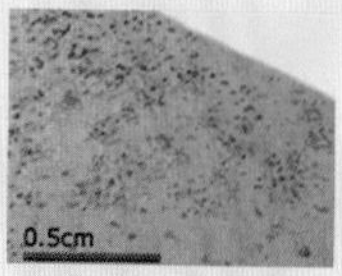	Tiny 1–2 mm, initially purpuric, nonblanchable macules resulting from tiny hemorrhages (Fig. 3-17).
	Palpable purpura 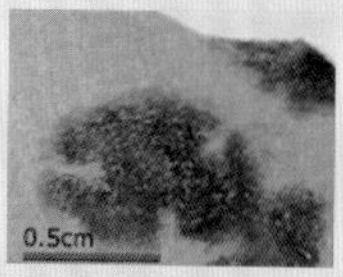	Raised and palpable, nonblanchable, red or violaceous discoloration of skin or mucous membranes due to vascular inflammation in the skin and extravasation of red blood cells (Fig. 3-18).

TABLE 1-3 Common Dermatologic Terminology, Lesions (*Continued*)

Group	Lesion Type	Definition
Sunken	Atrophy	A thinning of tissue defined by its location, such as epidermal atrophy, dermal atrophy, or subcutaneous atrophy (Fig. 3-19).
	Erosion	A localized loss of the epidermal or mucosal epithelium (Fig. 3-20).
	Ulcer	A circumscribed loss of the epidermis and at least upper dermis. Ulcers are further classified by their depth, border/shape, edge, and tissue at its base (Fig. 3-21).
Gangrene	Gangrene	Necrotic, usually black, tissue due to obstruction, diminution, or loss of blood supply. Gangrene may be wet or dry (Fig. 3-22).
Eschar	Eschar	An adherent thick, dry, black crust (Fig. 3-23).

*When used to describe an early clinical stage of cutaneous T-cell lymphoma (mycosis fungoides), the term patch may include fine textural change such as "cigarette paper" thinning, poikilodermatous atrophy, or slickness secondary to follicular loss (Fig. 3-2).
From Craft, N., Fox L. P. (2010). *VisualDx: Essential adult dermatology*. Philadelphia, PA: Lippincott Williams & Wilkins.

Principles for Using Skin Care Products

As mentioned previously, the skin has an acid mantle that needs to be maintained for proper barrier function; thus, skin care products and skin care routines should be designed to maintain this acidic pH. For example, use of alkaline soaps and cleansers should be avoided; pH-balanced no rinse cleansers are generally the preferred agent for routine bathing. Overly frequent bathing should also be avoided, especially with hot water, due to the potential for dehydration of the stratum corneum and depletion of the normal lipid levels of the skin (with resultant compromise of the barrier function of the skin). After showering or bathing, moisturizing products (emollients and humectants) should be applied to the skin while the skin is still moist rather than allowing it to dry completely. Emollients provide lipids to fill in the gaps between the skin cells and to retard water loss, thus helping to maintain the moisture content of the stratum corneum within the normal range of 10% to 15%. Emollients have a softening and moisturizing effect on the skin; this category includes products such as silicone, dimethicone, lanolin, and ceramides. Humectants "work" by actively attracting water to the skin and are designed for use with very dry rough skin (xerosis). This category includes agents with urea, lactic acid, glycerin, and alpha hydroxy acids. For patients at risk or who have MASD, moisture barrier products are an essential element of care; these products are discussed in detail in Chapter 17.

When selecting skin and wound care products, clinicians must remember that the skin plays an important role in immunity and the skin is very susceptible to allergic reactions. When selecting products for skin care, it is important to avoid using products on the skin that have ingredients that are known sensitizers (likely to cause allergic reactions). The clinician must determine the ingredients in skin and wound care products and must be alert to known sensitizers. For example, neomycin is one of the ingredients in some triple antibiotic creams; the other two are polymyxin and gramicidin (Menezes de Pádua et al., 2005). Triple antibiotic ointment has bacitracin (former allergen of the year for the American Academy of Dermatology) instead of gramicidin in the cream formulations. Neomycin has two sensitizers, with 60% of the allergic reactions due to the neomycin sugars and 40% of the allergic reactions caused by the deoxystreptamine backbone (Chung & Carson, 1975; Rietschel & Fowler, 1995; Schorr & Ridgway, 1997; Sibbald et al., 2012). This backbone is common to all aminoglycoside antibiotics from the same class: gentamicin, amikacin, and tobramycin. The development of an allergy to the deoxystreptamine backbone eliminates a large number of systemic antibiotics as well as topical agents. Common sensitizers other than neomycin include bacitracin, lanolin, and Pentalyn H (Katz & Fisher, 1987; Wakelin et al., 2001). Natural lanolin is found in some emollient creams and moisturizers and is a common sensitizer in persons with leg ulcers; chemically modified lanolin may be less likely to cause a sensitivity reaction. Pentalyn H is found in the adhesives of some hydrocolloid ostomy skin barriers, and its allergic potential cross-reacts with colophony. In addition to avoidance of sensitizing agents, it is best to avoid topical antibiotic agents with a systemic counterpart due to the development of resistant organisms that eliminate the effectiveness of the related systemic agent. If a patient is being treated with a topical antimicrobial and there is no improvement in wound status within 2 weeks, the patient and wound should be assessed for bacterial resistance.

Conclusion

An assessment of the multiple functions and appropriate care of the skin is an important competency for wound care nurses. In this chapter, we have provided an overview of skin functions as well as the normal attributes of the skin including changes from birth to old age. Elements of a skin assessment include the five components of physical assessment: skin color, temperature, turgor, moisture status, and integrity. Factors to consider in a holistic assessment of a person at risk for skin injury have been reviewed.

Skin care treatment plans need to be based on the normal characteristics of the skin including maintaining the acidic pH, managing moisture balance, protecting the skin from barrier disruption, and avoidance of skin sensitizers. The remaining chapters in this book will build on this foundation as specific skin and wound conditions will be addressed.

REFERENCES

Abbasi, N. R., Shaw, H. M., Rigel, D. S., et al. (2004). Early diagnosis of cutaneous melanoma: Revisiting the ABCD criteria. *JAMA, 292*(22), 2771–2776.

Arad, Y., Fonseca, V., Peters, A., et al. (2011). Beyond the monofilament for the insensate diabetic foot. Asystematic review of randomized trials to prevent the occurrence of plantar foot ulcers in patients with diabetes. *Diabetes Care, 34*(4), 1041–1046.

Armstrong, D. G., & Lavery, L. A. (1997). Predicting neuropathic ulceration with infrared dermal thermometry. *Journal of the American Podiatric Medical Association, 87*(7), 336–337.

Armstrong, D. G., Holtz-Neiderer, K., Wendel, C., et al. (2007). Skin temperature monitoring reduces the risk for diabetic foot ulceration in high-risk patients. *The American Journal of Medicine, 120*(12), 1042–1046.

Ayello, E. A., Sibbald, R. G., Quiambao, P. C. H, et al. (2014). Introducing a moisture-associated skin assessment photo guide for brown pigmented skin. *WCET Journal, 34*(2), 18–25.

Bates-Jensen, B. M., McCreath, H. E., Pongquan, V. (2009). Subepidermal moisture is associated with early pressure ulcer damage in nursing home residents with dark skin tones. *Journal of Wound Ostomy & Continence Nursing, 36*(3), 277–284.

Bennett, C. L., Noordegraaf, M., Martina, C. A., et al. (2007). Langerhans cells are required for efficient presentation of topically applied hapten to T cells. *The Journal of Immunology, 179*(10), 6830–6835.

Berger, U., Wilson, P., McClelland, R. A., et al. (1988). Immunocytochemical detection of 1-25-dihydroxyvitamin D receptors in normal human tissue. *The Journal of Clinical Endocrinology and Metabolism, 67*(3), 607–613.

Bikel, D. D. (2008). Chapter 3. Vitamin D: Production, metabolism, and mechanisms of action. In F. Singer (Ed.), *Diseases of bone and mineral metabolism*. Retrieved June 6, 2010, from http://www.endotext.org

Bittencourt, F. V., Marghoob, A. A., Kopf, A. W., et al. (2000). Large congenital melanocytic nevi and the risk for development of malignant melanoma and neurocutaneous melanocytosis. *Pediatrics, 106*(4), 736–741.

Bolognia, J. L. (1995). Aging skin. *The American Journal of Medicine, 98*(suppl 1A), 1A–99S.

Bos, J. D., & Kapsenberg, M. L. (1993). The skin immune system: Progress in cutaneous biology. *Immunology Today, 14*(2), 75–78.

Burns, T., Breathnach, S., Cox, N, et al. (2010) *Rook's textbook of dermatology, 4 volume set (Vol. 1)*. Hoboken, NJ: John Wiley & Sons.

Charkoudian, N. (2003). Skin blood flow in adult human thermoregulation: how it works, when it does not, and why. Mayo Clinic Proceedings 78(5), 603–612.

Chung, C. W., & Carson, T. R. (1975). Sensitization potentials and immunologic specifications of neomycins. *The Journal of Investigative Dermatology, 64*(3), 158–164.

Copcu, E, Nazan, S., & Nil, C. (2004). Cutaneous horns: Are these lesions as innocent as they seem to be? *World Journal of Surgical Oncology, 2*(1), 18.

Craft, N., Fox, L. P., & Visual, D. X. (2010). *Essential adult dermatology*. Philadelphia, PA: Wolters Kluwer Health, Lippincott Williams & Wilkins.

Crissey, S. D., Ange, K. D., Jacobsen, K. L., et al. (2003). Serum concentrations of lipids, vitamin D metabolites, retinol, retinyl esters, tocopherols and selected carotenoids in twelve captive wild felid species at four zoos. *The Journal of Nutrition, 133*(1), 160–166.

Dealy C. (2009). Skin care and pressure ulcers. *Advances in Skin and Wound Care, 22*(9), 421–428.

Egan, C. L., Oliveria, S. A., Elenitsas, R., et al. (1998). Cutaneous melanoma risk and phenotypic changes in large congenital nevi: A follow-up study of 46 patients. *Journal of the American Academy of Dermatology, 39*(6), 923–932.

Esterly, N., (ed). (1996). Management of congenital melanocytic nevi: A decade later. *Pediatric Dermatology, 13*, 312–340

Falanga, V., & Sabolinski, M. (1999). A bilayered living skin construct (APLIGRAF) accelerates complete closure of hard-to-heal venous ulcers. *Wound Repair and Regeneration, 7*(4), 201–207.

Feldmann, R. J., & Maibach, H. I. (1967). Regional variation in percutaneous penetration of 14C cortisol in man. *Journal of Investigative Dermatology, 48*(2), 181–183.

Fenske, N. A., & Lober, C. W. (1986). Structural and functional changes of normal aging skin. *Journal of the American Academy of Dermatology, 15*(4), 571–585.

Fitzpatrick, T. B. (1975). Soleil et peau (Sun and skin). *Journal de Médecine Esthétique (in French), 2*, 33–34.

Fitzpatrick, T. B. (1986). Ultraviolet-induced pigmentary changes: Benefits and hazards. *Current Problems in Dermatology, 15*, 25–38.

Fitzpatrick Skin Type Classification Scale. (November 2007). Skin INc. Retrieved July 13, 2014, from http://www.skininc.com. skinscience/physiology/10764816.html

Fluhr, J. W., Feingold, K. R., & Elias, P. M. (2006). Transepidermal water loss reflects permeability barrier status: Validation in human and rodent in vivo and ex vivo models. *Experimental Dermatology, 15*(7), 483–492.

Gallagher, R. P., & McLean, D. I. (1995). The epidemiology of acquired melanocytic nevi. A brief review. *Dermatologic Clinics, 13*(3), 595–603.

Gallo, R. L. (2008). Sounding the alarm: Multiple functions of host defense peptides. *Journal of Investigative Dermatology, 128*(1), 5–6.

Gladman, A. C. (2006). Toxicodendron dermatitis: Poison ivy, oak, and sumac. *Wilderness & Environmental Medicine, 17*(2), 120–128.

Goodarzi, H., Trowbridge, J., & Gallo, R. L. (2007). Innate immunity: A cutaneous perspective. *Clinical Reviews in Allergy & Immunology, 33*(1–2), 15–26.

Guyton, A. C. (1991). *Textbook of medical physiology* (8th ed.). Philadelphia, PA: Saunders, 1991.

Habif, T. P. (2004). Nevi and malignant melanoma. *Clinical dermatology: A color guide to diagnosis and therapy* (4th ed., pp. 776–777). Edinburgh, U.K.: Mosby.

Hafner, C., & Vogt, T. (2008). Seborrheic keratosis. *JDDG: Journal der Deutschen Dermatologischen Gesellschaft, 6*, 664–677. doi: 10.1111/j.1610-0387.2008.06788

Halata, Z., Grim, M., & Bauman, K. I. (2003). Friedrich Sigmund Merkel and his "Merkel cell", morphology, development, and physiology: Review and new results. *The Anatomical Record. Part A, Discoveries in Molecular, Cellular, and Evolutionary Biology, 271*(1), 225–239.

Holick, M. F., Smith, E., & Pincus, S. (1987). Skin as the site of vitamin D synthesis and target tissue for 1, 25-dihydroxyvitamin D3: use of calcitriol (1, 25-dihydroxyvitamin D3) for treatment of psoriasis. *Archives of Dermatology, 123*(12), 1677–1683a.

Holick, M. F., Matsuoka, L. Y., & Wortsman, J. (1995). Regular use of sunscreen on vitamin D levels. *Archives of Dermatology 131*(11), 1337–1338.

Houghton, V. J., Bower, V. M., & Chant, D. C. (2013). Is an increase in skin temperature predictive of neuropathic foot ulceration in people with diabetes? A systematic review and meta-analysis. *Journal of Foot and Ankle Research, 6*(1), 31.

Institute of Medicine (US) Committee to Review Dietary Reference Intakes for Vitamin D and Calcium. (2011). 8, implications and special concerns. In A. C. Ross, C. L. Taylor, A. L. Yaktine (Eds.), et al. *Dietary reference intakes for calcium and vitamin D*. Washington, DC: National Academies Press.

James, W. D., Berger, T. G., Elston, D. (2006). *Andrews' diseases of the skin: Clinical dermatology*. Philadelphia, PA: Saunders Elsevier.

Jarvis, C. (2012). *Physical examination & health assessment* (6th ed.). St. Louis, MO: Elsevier.

Johnson, J. M., Brengelmann, G., Hales, J, et al. (1986). *Regulation of the cutaneous circulation*. Paper presented at the Federation proceedings.

Johnson, J. M., & Proppe, D. W. (2011). Cardiovascular adjustments to heat stress. *Comprehensive Physiology*: 215–243. DOI:10.1002/cphy.cp040111

Kaminski, M. N., & Drinane, J. J. (2014). Learning the oral and cutaneous signs of micronutrient deficiencies. *Journal of Wound, Ostomy and Nursing Care, 41*(2), 127–135.

Katz, B. E., & Fisher, A. A. (1987). Bacitracin: A unique topical antibiotic sensitizer. *Journal of the American Academy of Dermatology, 17*(6), 1016–1024.

Kelly, J. W., Chamberlain, A. J., Staples, M. P., et al. (2003). Nodular melanoma. No longer as simple as ABC. *Australian Family Physician, 32*, 706–709.

Korkut, T., Tan, N. B., & Oztan, Y. (1997). Giant cutaneous horn: A patient report. *Annals of Plastic Surgery, 39*(6), 654–655.

Lavery, L. A., Higgins, K. R., Lanctot, D. R., et al. (2004). Home monitoring of foot skin temperatures to prevent ulceration. *Diabetes Care, 27*(11), 2642–2647.

Lavery, L. A., Higgins, K. R., Lanctot, D. R., et al. (2007). Preventing diabetic foot ulcer recurrence in high-risk patients: use of temperature monitoring as a self assessment tool. *Diabetes Care, 30*(1), 14–20.

Lee, N. P., & Arriola, E. R. (1999). Poison ivy, oak, and sumac dermatitis. *Western Journal of Medicine, 171*(5-6), 354.

Levit, E. K., Kagen, M. H., Scher, R. K., et al. (2000). The ABC rule for clinical detection of subungual melanoma. *Journal of the American Academy of Dermatology, 42*(2), 269–274.

Marks, R., Foley, P. A., Jolley, D., et al. (1995). The effect of regular sunscreen use on vitamin D levels in an Australian population: Results of a randomized controlled trial. *Archives of Dermatology, 131*(4), 415–421.

Matusomoto, K. Y., Azuma, Y., Kiyoki, M, et al. (1991). Involvement of endogenously produced 1,25-dihydroxyvitamin D-3 in the growth and differentiation of human keratinocytes. *Biochimica et Biophysica Acta, 1092*(3), 311–318.

Menezes de Pádua, C. A., Schnuch, A., Lessmann, H., et al. (2005). Contact allergy to neomycin sulfate: Results of a multifactorial analysis. *Pharmacoepidemiology and Drug Safety, 14*(10), 725–733.

Montagna, W., Carlisle, K. (1979). Structural changes in aging human skin. Structural changes in aging human skin. *The Journal of Investigative Dermatology, 73*, 47–53.

Mufti, A., Coutts, P., Sibbald, R. G. (2015). Infrared skin thermometry: A low cost tool for diabetic foot self monitoring and routine wound care practice. *Advances in Skin and Wound Care, 28*(1), 37–44.

Noiles, K., Ronald, V. (2007). Are all seborrheic keratoses benign? Review of the typical lesion and its variants. *Journal of Cutaneous Medicine and Surgery, 12*(5), 203–210.

National Pressure Ulcer Advisory Panel, European Pressure Ulcer Advisory Panel and Pan Pacific Pressure Injury Alliance. (2014). *Prevention and treatment of pressure ulcers: Clinical practice guideline*. In H. Emily (Ed.). Osborne Park, Western Australia: Cambridge Media.

Norman, A. W. (1998). Sunlight, season, skin pigmentation, vitamin D and 25-hydroxyvitamin D: integral components of the vitamin D endocrine system. *American Journal Clinical Nutrition, 67*(6), 1108–1110.

Norman, A. W. (1996). Vitamin D. In E. E. Ziegler & I. J. Filer, (Eds), *Present knowledge in nutrition* (pp. 120–129). Washington, DC: International Life Sciences Institute.

Rietschel, R. L., & Fowler, J. F. (1995). *Reactions to topical antimicrobials in Fisher's contact dermatitis* (4th ed., pp. 205–225). Baltimore, MD: Williams & Wilkins.

Rigel, D. S., Friedman, R. J., Kopf, A. W., et al. (2005). ABCDE—an evolving concept in the early detection of melanoma. *Archives of Dermatology, 141*(8), 1032–1034.

Rowell, L. B. (2011). *Cardiovascular adjustments to thermal stress. Comprehensive Physiology*.

Schauber, J., Dorschner, R. A., Coda, A. B., et al. (2007). Injury enhances TRL2 function and antimicrobial peptide expression through a vitamin D-dependent mechanism. *Journal Clinical Investigation, 117*, 803–811.

Schorr, W. F., & Ridgway, H. B. (1997). Tobramycin-neomycin cross sensitivity. *Contact Dermatitis, 3*(3):133–137.

Schultz, G. S., Sibbald, R. C., Falanga, V., et al. (2003). Wound bed preparation: A systematic approach to wound management. *Wound Repair and Regeneration, 11*(Suppl 1):S1–S28.

Segaert, S. (2008). Vitamin D regulation of cathelicidin in the skin: Toward a renaissance of vitamin D in dermatology? *Journal of Investigative Dermatology, 126*(4), 816–824.

Sibbald, R. G., Alavi, A., Sussman, G, et al. (2012). Chapter 17, Dermatological aspects of wound care (pp. 207–222). In D. L. Krasner, G. T. Rodeheaver, R. G. Sibbald (Eds.), et al. *Chronic Wound Care 5. A clinical source book for healthcare professional*, Volume 1 Malvern, PA: HMP Communications.

Sibbald, R. G., Goodman, L., Woo, K. Y., et al. (2011). Special considerations in wound bed preparation 2011: An update. *Advances in Skin and Wound Care, 24*(9), 415–436.

Sibbald, R. G., Woo, K., & Ayello, E. A. (2006). Increased bacterial burden and infection: The story of NERDS and STONES. *Advances in Skin & Wound Care, 19*(8), 447–461.

Taylor, W. F., Johnson, J. M., Oleary, D., et al. (1984). Effect of high local temperature on reflex cutaneous vasodilation. *Journal of Applied Physiology: Respiratory, Environmental and Exercise Physiology, 57*, 191–196.

Wakelin, S. H., Smith, H., White, I. R., et al. (2001). A retrospective analysis of contact allergy to lanolin. *British Journal of Dermatology, 145*(1), 28–31.

Winkelmann, R. (1959). *The erogenous zones: Their nerve supply and its significance*. Paper presented at the Proceedings of the staff meetings. Rochester, MN: Mayo Clinic.

Woo, K. Y., Harding, K., Price, P., et al. (2008). Minimising wound-related pain at dressing change: Evidence-informed practice. *International Wound Journal, 5*(2), 144–157.

Woo, K. Y., & Sibbald, R. G. (2009). A cross-validation study of using NERDS and TONEES to assess bacterial burden. *Ostomy Wound Management, 55*(8), 40–48.

Xiao, Q. T., Chen, T. C., Holick, M. F. (1995). 1,25-Dihydroxyvitamin D 3: A novel agent for enhancing wound. *Journal of Cellular Biochemistry, 59*(1), 53–56.

Yeatman, J. M., Kilkenny, M., & Marks, R. (1997). The prevalence of seborrhoeic keratoses in an Australian population: Does exposure to sunlight play a part in their frequency? *British Journal of Dermatology, 137*(3), 411–414.

Yosipovitch, G., & Hu, J. (2003). Clinical features-free CME-the importance of skin pH-here's what you need to educate patients about regarding skin pH, so that they can protect themselves. *Skin and Aging-Journal of Geriatric Dermatology, 11*(3), 88–94.

Zaal, L. H., Mooi, W. J., Klip, H., et al. (2005). Risk of malignant transformation of congenital melanocytic nevi: A retrospective nationwide study from The Netherlands. *Plastic and Reconstructive Surgery 116*(7), 1902–1909.

QUESTIONS

1. Which structure of the skin provides the body with photoprotective properties by absorbing harmful ultraviolet light?
A. Melanin
B. Langerhans' cells
C. Odland bodies
D. Stratum lucidum

2. What is a unique function of the layer of epidermis known as the stratum basale?
A. Providing immunity via Langerhans' cells
B. Producing new epithelial cells
C. Releasing lipids to help maintain normal brick and mortar skin configuration
D. Protecting the palms of the hands and soles of the feet

3. Which cells located in the dermis produce collagen (dermal building blocks) and elastin (tensile strength) critical to immune function and healing?
A. Leukotrienes
B. Prostaglandins
C. Macrophages
D. Fibroblasts

4. Which patient's wound would the wound care nurse expect to heal by scar formation?
A. A head wound extending beyond the hair follicles
B. A shallow wound on the hand caused by cutting a bagel in half
C. A superficial pressure ulcer
D. A first-degree burn

5. Which layer of tissue if very minimal in a patient's body places the patient at high risk for pressure ulcer development?
A. Epidermis
B. Subcutaneous tissue
C. Muscle
D. Epidermal appendages

6. Which of the following statements accurately describes how the skin functions as a barrier between the internal and external environments?
A. The skin lipids bind water, normally maintaining skin water content at 20% or higher.
B. When the barrier function of the skin is compromised, transepidermal water loss (TEWL) rises.
C. Protection against pathogenic invasion is supported by an alkaline pH of the skin.
D. Merkel's receptors embedded in the extracellular matrix contribute to the mechanical rigidity and frictional resistance protection of the skin.

7. The nurse assessing the skin of patients in a nursing home keeps in mind the structural changes that occur in aging skin. What is one of these changes?
A. Increase in melanocytes
B. Rounding of dermal–epidermal junction
C. Increase in mast cells
D. Decrease in collagen

8. The wound care nurse assesses the skin of a patient and documents "angular stomatitis accompanied by magenta-colored glossitis." What vitamin deficiency would the nurse suspect?

A. B_2
B. B_3
C. C
D. D

9. The nurse uses the acronym ABCDE to distinguish a melanoma from a benign nevus. Based on this acronym, what is a distinguishing characteristic of melanoma?

A. B = A regular border
B. C = Consistent red or black color
C. D= Diameter greater than 4 mm
D. E = Evolving lesion

10. On which body site would the transdermal application of a medication obtain the greatest percutaneous absorption?

A. Plantar surface of the foot
B. Forearm
C. Forehead
D. Hand

11. Which principle of skin care product use would the wound care nurse include in a teaching plan for a patient with a leg wound?

A. Use alkaline soaps and cleansers to neutralize acidic skin.
B. Do not use products on the skin that have known sensitizers.
C. Bathe frequently using water that is as hot as tolerated.
D. Allow skin to dry completely before applying moisturizers.

ANSWERS: 1.**A**, 2.**B**, 3.**D**, 4.**A**, 5.**B**, 6.**B**, 7.**D**, 8.**A**, 9.**D**, 10.**C**, 11.**B**

CHAPTER 2

Wound Healing

Janice M. Beitz

OBJECTIVES

1. Differentiate between acute and chronic wounds to include implications for management.
2. Describe the physiology of partial-thickness and full-thickness wound healing and identify implications for nursing management.

Topic Outline

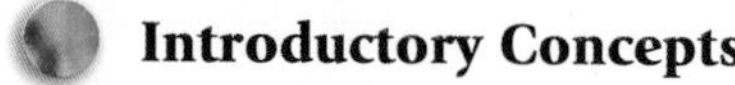

Introductory Concepts

Phases of Wound Healing
- Hemostasis
- Inflammation
- Proliferation
- Maturation

Mechanisms of Wound Healing

Types of Wound Closure

Acute versus Chronic Wounds

Aging and Wound Healing

Partial- versus Full-Thickness Wound Healing

Wound Healing: Risk Factors for Nonhealing
- Perfusion and Oxygenation
- Glycemic Control
- Comorbidities
- Nutritional Status
- Tobacco Use
- Spinal Cord Injury
- Infection

Psychological Factors and Wound Healing

Implications for Optimal Wound Care

Future Directions for Wound Healing Therapies

Conclusion

Introductory Concepts

A wound represents a disruption in the normal structure and function of the skin and underlying soft tissues and can be related to a variety of etiologies (e.g., trauma, surgery, sustained pressure, vascular disease, infection, etc.). Human beings sustain wounds across their lifespan that range from a simple knee abrasion to a major surgical incision. With most acute wounds (abrasions, lacerations, or surgical incisions), no excessive concern is necessary since humans are "programmed" to heal and acute injury triggers the repair process. However, when an acute wound fails to heal normally or a wound develops as a result of a chronic condition (e.g., a venous or arterial ulcer), the patient's quality of life can be seriously affected, and the costs of care can increase substantively. Since both acute and chronic wounds affect millions of people internationally, it is critical for contemporary clinicians to have a good understanding of wound healing mechanisms and the pathogenesis of chronic wounds. This chapter provides an overview of the processes and components of wound healing, describes the various types and phases of healing, distinguishes between the repair processes for acute and chronic wounds, and describes factors affecting wound healing.

Phases of Wound Healing

In an acute wound such as a surgical incision, wounding generates a cellular response. This response involves activation of specialized cells including platelets, macrophages, keratinocytes, fibroblasts, and endothelial cells. Simultaneously, cytokines (nonantibody proteins) and growth factors are released that coordinate and control the activities of the cells responsible for repair, thus promoting wound healing. Under normal conditions, bleeding will be quickly controlled and the wound will heal in an orderly, effective manner. The repair process for acute wounds involves four major phases: hemostasis, inflammation, proliferation or regeneration, and maturation (remodeling) (Fig. 2-1) (Bainbridge, 2013).

CLINICAL PEARL

In an acute wound such as a surgical incision, the "order of repair" is a brief inflammatory phase, epithelial resurfacing and granulation tissue formation, and remodeling.

Hemostasis

The hemostasis phase commences immediately following wounding. Small vessels in the wound constrict, and activated platelets aggregate within the damaged blood vessels, triggering the clotting cascade. The activated platelets release a myriad of growth factors and cytokines that control and expedite the wound healing process (e.g., platelet-derived growth factor); the activated platelets also help to create the fibrin structure that serves as the scaffold for cell migration during the initial repair process. Notably, larger blood vessels do not constrict, and additional measures are typically required to stop the bleeding from these vessels (e.g., manual pressure, electrocautery, suturing, etc.) (Armstrong & Meyr, 2012, 2013).

CLINICAL PEARL

With acute injury, bleeding and clotting cause release of growth factors, which initiates the repair process.

Inflammation

Once the fibrin matrix has been established and bleeding has been controlled, the cytokines and growth factors initiate the inflammatory phase. The goal of the inflammatory phase is establishment of a clean wound bed (i.e., elimination of necrotic tissue and establishment of bacterial control). During this phase, neutrophils and monocytes are chemoattracted to the wounded area. Initially, neutrophils are predominant, and their primary effect is elimination of bacteria via enzymatic activity. As the inflammatory process continues, the number and activity of neutrophils decrease and the number and activity of macrophages (derived from tissue monocytes) increase; macrophages eliminate the dead bacteria, neutrophils, and cellular debris. In addition, macrophages release other cytokines that promote transition from the inflammatory phase into the proliferative phase of repair (e.g., vascular endothelial growth factor [VEGF], which promotes development of new blood vessels, or neoangiogenesis, and platelet derived growth factor [PDGF], which promotes fibroblast activity and synthesis of collagen and other connective tissue proteins, also known as fibroplasia). Macrophages are essential during the early phases of repair, and impaired macrophage activity, as seen in uncontrolled diabetes, is associated with impaired wound healing (Miao et al., 2012). In contrast, normal macrophage activity contributes to rapid resolution of the inflammatory phase, followed by transition into the proliferative phase with formation of healthy durable scar tissue (He & Marneros, 2013).

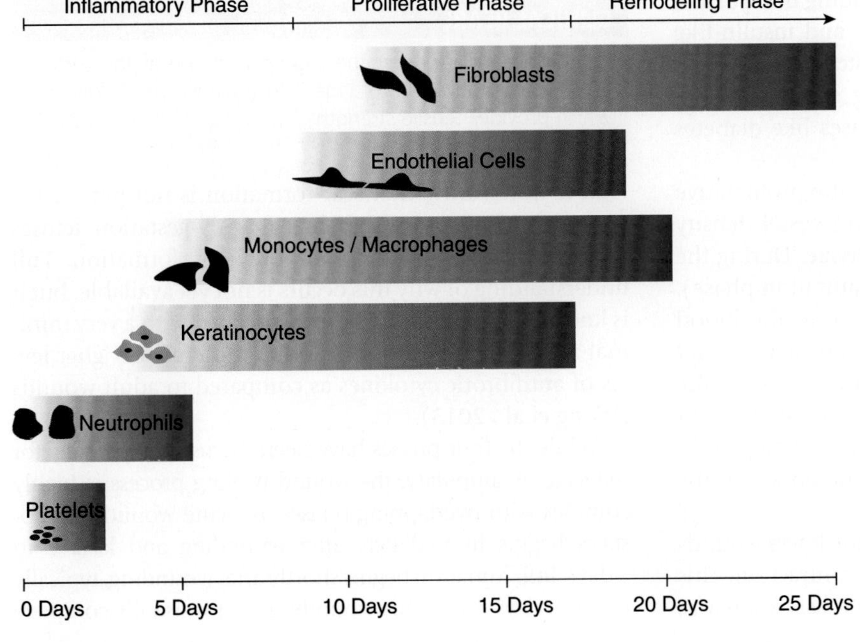

FIGURE 2-1. Phases of healing with associated cellular activity. Note that in this model, hemostasis and inflammation are considered one phase.

Proliferation

The proliferation or regeneration phase begins with fibroblast migration to the area, which occurs in response to cellular signaling; this is followed by formation of a new extracellular matrix (ECM) (granulation tissue). Fibroblasts are the cells responsible for synthesis of new connective tissue proteins; they are normally found primarily in the dermal layer of uninjured tissue, and their usual function is to repair any damage to the connective tissue, also known as the ECM. They are summoned to the specific wound site by the growth factors and cytokines released during the inflammatory phase: PDGF, interleukin-I beta (IL-1β), and tumor necrosis factor alpha (TNF-α). These chemoattractants actually direct the fibroblast to the correct area by binding to specific areas on the cell surface; this helps the fibroblasts to orient themselves within the wound (Bainbridge, 2013). Once on-site and correctly oriented within the wound bed, the fibroblasts work to synthesize connective tissue proteins such as collagen, which is the most abundant family of proteins in the body (Bootun, 2012). The newly formed granulation tissue is comprised primarily of newly formed blood vessels and provisional collagen (type III collagen), which lacks tensile strength and acts primarily as a filler and scaffold.

At the same time collagen is being synthesized, angiogenesis is occurring, which provides the new blood vessels that are essential to cellular activity and wound healing. Angiogenesis actually begins immediately after injury, because the activated platelets trigger angiogenic growth factors such as VEGF. However, there is another cell that also plays a vital role in neoangiogenesis. Endothelial progenitor cells (EPCs), normally located in the bone marrow, are recruited via the circulation to the area bordering the wound; they are then incorporated into the tissue and contribute to growth of new blood vessels (Demidova-Rice et al., 2012). EPC activity is mediated by substances that are well known to affect wound healing including nitric oxide, VEGF, matrix metalloproteases (MMPs), and insulin-like growth factor. Some authors have suggested that it is deficiencies in these intermediate signaling substances that contribute to wound chronicity in diseases like diabetes (Demidova-Rice et al., 2012).

Angiogenesis is quite vigorous during the proliferative phase of wound healing, which results in vessel density that far exceeds that needed by normal tissue. During the final phase of repair (the remodeling/maturation phase), most of the newly formed vessels disappear; the blood vessel bed is essentially "pruned back" to normal vascular density (DiPietro, 2013). (This explains the change in the color of the scar tissue, from bright red to pale pink or white.) The ability to stimulate and control angiogenesis is predicted to be an important therapeutic option in the future (Yoo & Kwon, 2013).

Another component of repair for full-thickness wounds closing by secondary intention is wound contraction. This process is dependent on specialized fibroblasts known as myofibroblasts. Myofibroblasts are specialized cells with characteristics of both fibroblasts and smooth muscle cells. Because they generate contractile force, they are able to pull the edges of the wound together to reduce the size of the defect (Bainbridge, 2013).

Maturation

The final phase of wound healing is the maturation, or remodeling phase. As the provisional collagen matrix is replaced with a stronger form of collagen (type 1), the cells responsible for collagen synthesis and angiogenesis undergo apoptosis. Wound strength increases significantly during the remodeling phase as the type 3 collagen is replaced with type 1 collagen (from minimal tensile strength at 21 days' postacute wounding to 60% or more at 2 to 3 months' postacute wounding). In a normally healing wound, 80% of original tensile strength will be achieved, and this is the maximum strength that can be obtained; 100% tensile strength is not a possibility because the normal soft tissue (dermis, subcutaneous, and/or muscle) has been replaced with scar tissue (Gantwerker & Hom, 2012). In an open full-thickness wound, the contraction that began during the proliferative phase will also continue; contraction contributes to healing by reducing the size of the defect. Normally, there is a fine balance between the proliferation of new (type 1) collagen and breakdown of the old (type 3) collagen; however, in some situations, there is insufficient breakdown of the old collagen or overproduction of the new collagen, resulting in a hypertrophic scar or a keloid. Conversely, if the proliferation of new (type 1) collagen is impaired by factors such as cancer chemotherapy, malnutrition, or steroids, the wound is at high risk for dehiscence or recurrent breakdown (because the "old" type 3 collagen lacks tensile strength) (Goldberg & Diegelmann, 2012).

CLINICAL PEARL

Remodeling occurs after the wound is closed at the surface and involves conversion of type 3 collagen to type 1 collagen, which provides tensile strength.

It is noteworthy that scar formation is not part of the wound healing process in utero. Early-gestation fetuses repair cutaneous wounds without scar formation. Full understanding of why this occurs is not yet available, but it is known that fetal wounds are associated with a very minimal inflammatory response and that there are higher levels of antifibrotic cytokines as compared to adult wounds (Wong et al., 2013).

While the four phases have been discussed separately for the sake of simplicity, the wound healing process is highly complex with overlapping phases. In acute wounds, hemostasis begins immediately after wounding and lasts 1 to 2 days; inflammation begins shortly after wounding, typically peaks at days 3 to 5 postwounding, and is usually complete by day 10; proliferation begins at day 1 postinjury and is typically complete by days 21 to 30. Remodeling actually begins during the proliferative phase and can last for up to 2 years (Gantwerker & Hom, 2012). The time frame for the phases of wound healing differs substantially for chronic wounds.

CLINICAL PEARL

Maximum tensile strength for a full-thickness wound healing by scar tissue formation is 80% of original tissue strength.

Mechanisms of Wound Healing

Three main mechanisms typify the healing process: connective tissue deposition (also known as granulation tissue formation), contraction, and epithelialization. Whether all three mechanisms are necessary depends on the type and nature of the wound. For example, an acute surgical wound that is closed by a surgeon using sutures and clips up to skin level (called primary intention) will close by migration of epithelial cells (epithelial resurfacing) across the minimal gaps in the skin surface (concurrent with the inflammatory phase) and by formation of enough granulation tissue to knit the tissue layers together. No tissue contraction is necessary or possible, because all tissue layers have been approximated. In contrast, a large open chronic wound such as a dehisced incision or full-thickness pressure ulcer requires formation of a substantial amount of granulation tissue, and contraction can play a critical and beneficial role in healing by reducing the size of the defect. This wound closing by secondary intention will also require significant epithelial resurfacing once it has filled with granulation tissue. This type of wound is likely to have a broader scar when closed (Fig. 2-2).

CLINICAL PEARL

The "order of repair" for an open wound healing by secondary intention is a (sometimes prolonged) inflammatory phase, then granulation tissue formation followed by epithelial resurfacing, and finally remodeling.

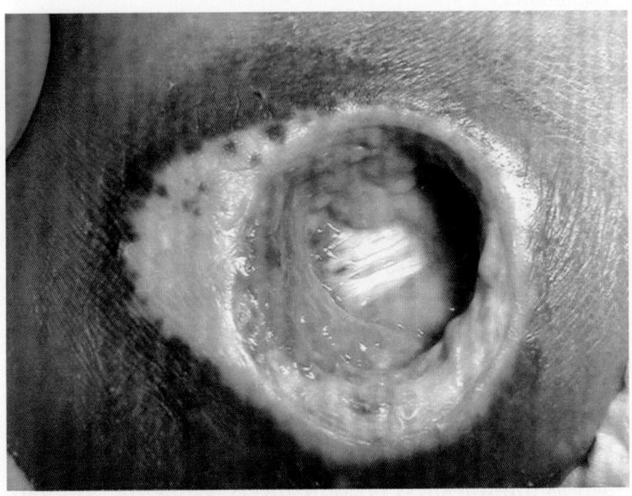

A

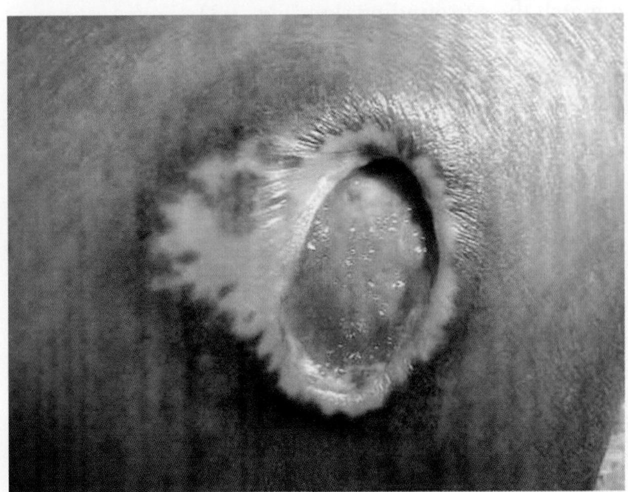

B

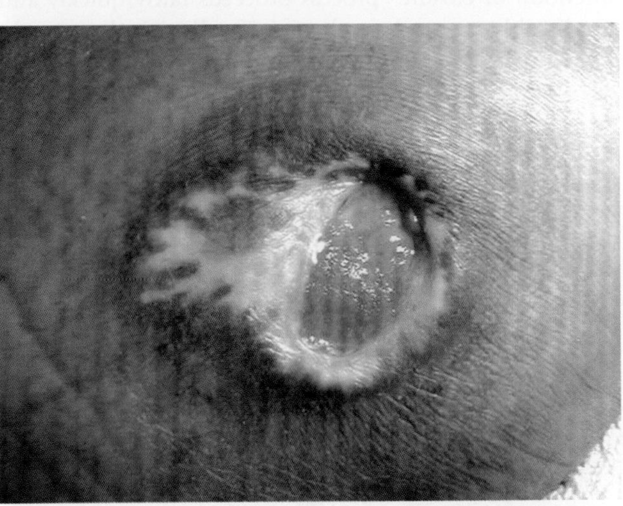

C

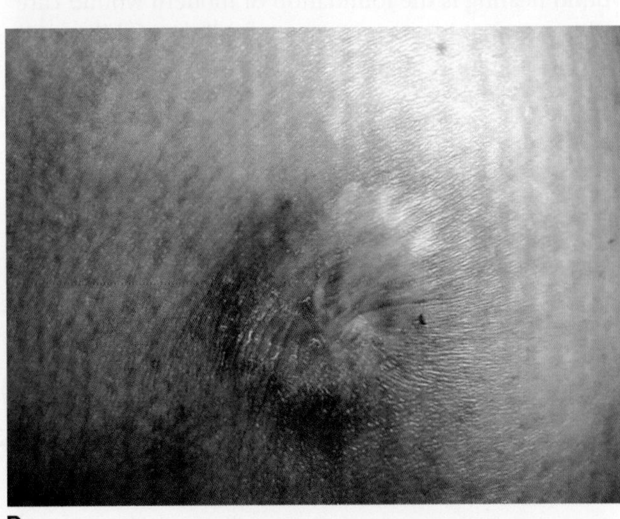

D

FIGURE 2-2. Series of photos showing progress in full-thickness wound healing: **(A)** contraction, **(B, C)** granulation tissue formation, and **(D)** epithelialization. (Photos copyright © B. M. Bates-Jensen.)

Superficial (partial-thickness) wounds such as abrasions or skin graft donor sites heal by regeneration as opposed to scar formation, because the structures in the epidermis and the superficial dermis can replace themselves. This means that partial-thickness wounds heal by reepithelialization; granulation tissue formation is not needed and does not occur, nor does contraction. If the wound extends into the dermis, the fibroblasts normally present in that skin layer will repair the dermal defect at the same time that epithelialization is occurring at the wound surface (Goldberg & Diegelmann, 2012). Partial-thickness wound healing involves two major phases; the first phase is epithelial resurfacing, which involves a marked increase in the rate of keratinocyte mitosis and changes in cell structure and function that permit lateral migration. Once the wound surface has been reepithelialized, lateral migration ceases due to a phenomenon known as contact inhibition, and vertical migration resumes, which gradually reestablishes normal epidermal thickness. It should be noted that the neoepidermis in all humans is bright pink in color, but gradually repigments to match the surrounding skin (Fig. 2-3).

CLINICAL PEARL

Superficial (partial-thickness) wounds heal by epithelial resurfacing and reestablishment of normal skin thickness; there is no scar formation.

As discussed, all wounds heal through some combination of the three critical processes: epithelialization, granulation tissue formation, and contraction. Interestingly, the factors that promote normal healing are essential for each of these processes and are the same as those identified by Winter (1962) in his seminal work on wound epithelialization in porcine models: (a) wound hydration, (b) blood supply, and (c) infection minimization. Moist wound healing is the foundation of modern wound care and is essential for maintenance of cellular viability and for cell migration. A dry wound bed compromises cell viability by eliminating the interstitial fluid environment critical to normal cellular function and also makes it much more difficult for cells to migrate across the wound surface. Normal perfusion is equally important, since all phases of wound repair are oxygen dependent and since blood flow is also the vehicle for delivery of the nutrients required for repair; thus, vascular health and neoangiogenesis are critical to wound healing. A third "essential element" of wound management is control of bacterial loads; infection is a major impediment to repair due to the negative effects of bacteria and their toxins on the repair process (Gantwerker & Hom, 2012; White et al., 2012). In summary, wound healing is facilitated by a wound bed that is free of dead tissue and debris, well vascularized, uninfected, and moist (Armstrong & Meyr, 2014).

CLINICAL PEARL

Moist wound healing is the foundation of modern wound care and is essential for maintenance of cell viability and cell migration.

Types of Wound Closure

Specific terminology is used to describe the various ways in which full-thickness wounds heal, with surgical wounds as the reference point. Primary closure or primary intention refers to wounds closed by sutures or skin staples at the time of surgery. All layers of tissue are approximated, which means that minimal amounts of granulation tissue and new epithelium are required for healing. Secondary closure or intention involves closure of an abdominal wound to fascia level and intentionally leaving upper layers open to granulate in over time. Secondary intention can also refer to nonsurgical wounds filling in over time such as full-thickness pressure ulcers. While the "primary intention or closure" process proceeds fairly quickly and predictably, secondary closure usually involves weeks of requisite granulation tissue deposition and wound

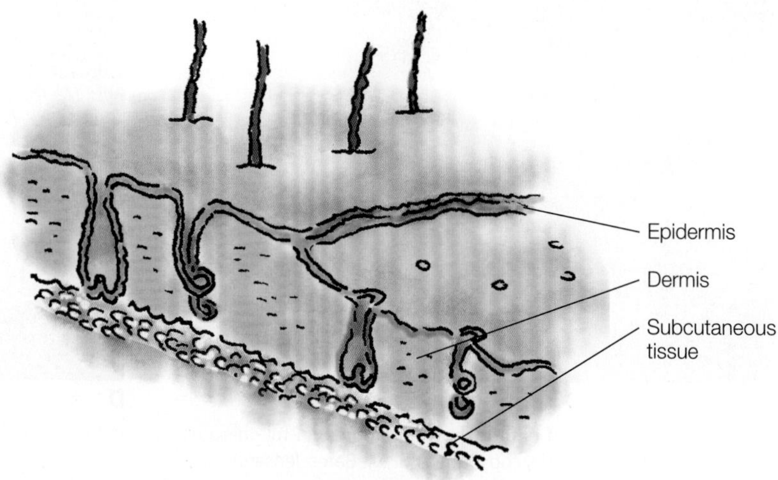

FIGURE 2-3. Partial-thickness wound.

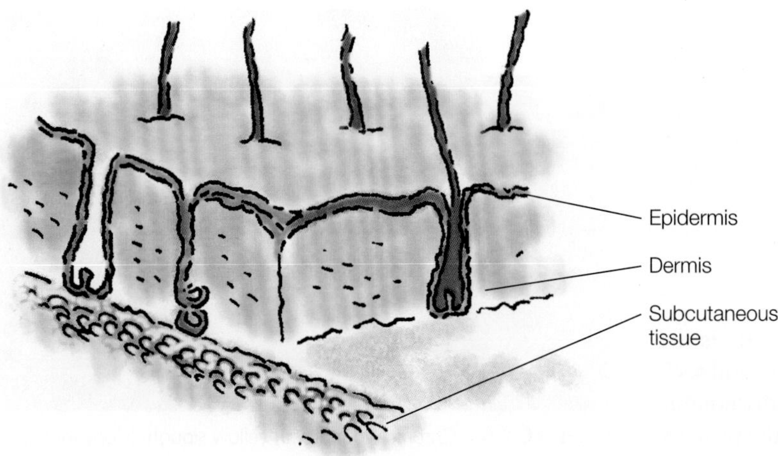

FIGURE 2-4. Full-thickness wound.

contraction, followed by eventual slow epithelialization. The scar in secondary closure is often wider than primary closure (Armstrong & Meyr, 2014; Yao et al., 2013). Wounds that are considered dirty or contaminated with foreign debris or bacteria $>10^5$/g of tissue may be left open to heal by secondary intention to reduce the risk of deep wound infection (Goldberg & Diegelmann, 2012; Shanahan, 2013) (Fig. 2-4).

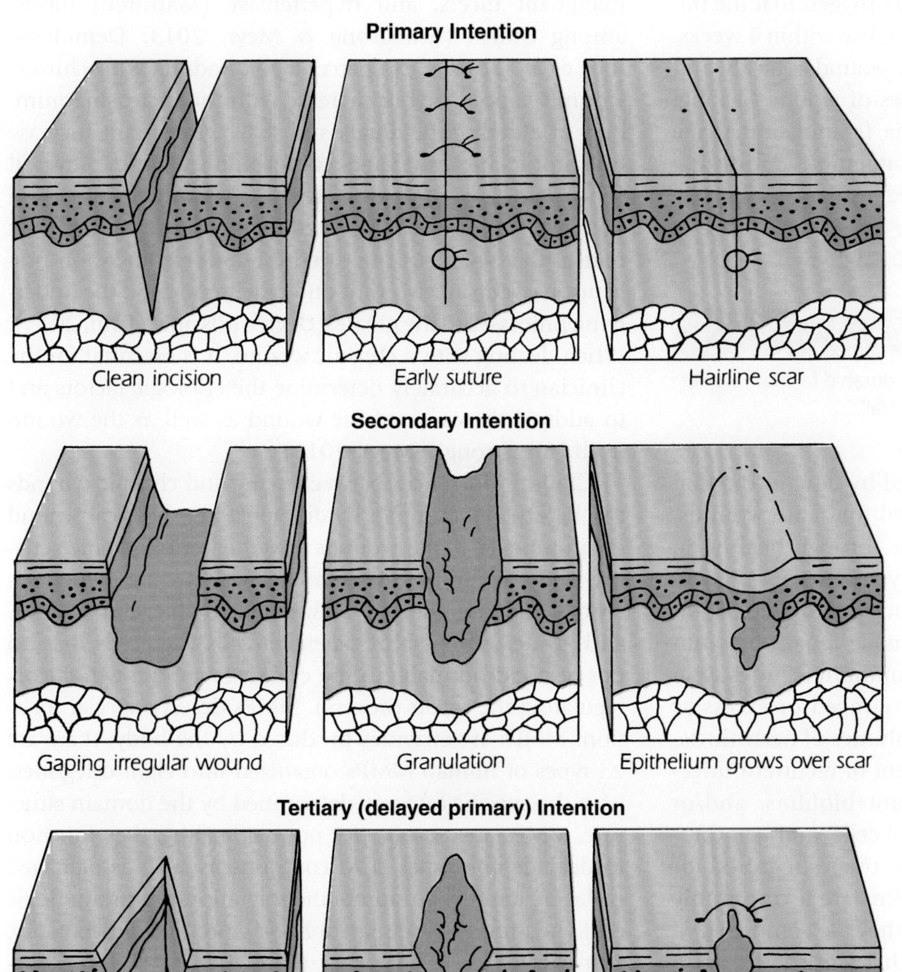

FIGURE 2-5. Types of wound healing/closure: primary, secondary, and tertiary intention. (Adapted from Smeltzer, S. C., Bare, B. G., Hinkle, J. L., et al. (2010). *Brunner & Suddarth's Textbook of Medical–Surgical Nursing* (12th ed., p. 474) Philadelphia, PA: Lippincott Williams & Wilkins.)

A third option is tertiary intention or closure. If a wound is too contaminated or infected to permit primary closure, the surgeon may keep the wound at secondary closure level until antibiotic therapy and manual cleansing reduce the bacterial burden to <10^5 organisms/g of tissue. The wound is then closed via delayed primary closure (Goldberg & Diegelmann, 2012) (Fig. 2-5).

Acute versus Chronic Wounds

Differing definitions of acute versus chronic wounds are available from various authors and professional wound societies; however, a common core of descriptors is discernable upon review. It is first important to realize that the primary difference is in the nature of the repair process as opposed to a specific time frame (Armstrong & Meyr, 2012). An acute wound is a wound that heals in an orderly, timely, and durable manner and that does not require long-term follow-up. In general, acute wounds have a clearly identifiable mechanism of injury such as trauma or surgery (Armstrong & Meyr, 2012; Paul, 2013). Some sources suggest that the trajectory for acute wound healing is complete within 4 weeks. Whatever the exact time frame, acute wounds quickly and efficiently proceed through the phases of wound healing: hemostasis, inflammation, fibroplasia (granulation tissue formation), epithelialization, and maturation (Armstrong & Meyr, 2012). Risk factors for delayed healing are typically minimal, and the wound proceeds to a predictable state of tissue repair (Demidova-Rice et al., 2012).

CLINICAL PEARL

Acute wounds heal in a predictable and durable fashion, while chronic wounds frequently plateau or "stall."

Chronic wounds are characterized by descriptors that are the "opposite" of those just used for acute wounds. A chronic wound does not progress through healing in an orderly and timely manner; they commonly plateau or "stall" at some point due to various pathologic conditions, and as a result, predictable tissue repair does not occur (Armstrong & Meyr, 2013). Common features typifying chronic wounds include a prolonged or excessive inflammatory phase (due to large volumes of necrotic tissue or high bacterial loads), persistent or recurrent infection, the formation of drug-resistant biofilms, and/or the failure of fibroblasts, endothelial cells, and keratinocytes to produce the new vessels and tissues required for durable closure of the defect. Biofilms are a commonly encountered impediment to repair; they are comprised of complex communities of bacteria that work together to generate an extracellular polymeric substance that shields them from host defenses, most antiseptics, and antibiotics. Biofilms frequently present as a recurrent film or thin layer of slough and must be promptly recognized and effectively managed if wound healing is to progress

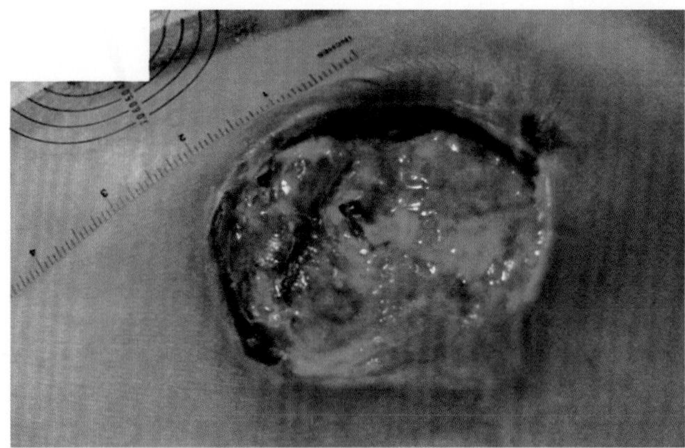

FIGURE 2-6. Chronic wound with yellow slough. (Copyright © C. Sussman.)

(Demidova-Rice et al., 2012; Griswold, 2012; Percival et al., 2012) (Fig. 2-6).

Chronic wound types include venous ulcers, ischemic ulcers, pressure ulcers, neuropathic (diabetic) ulcers, malignant ulcers, and hypertensive (Martorell) ulcers, among others (Armstrong & Meyr, 2013; Demidova-Rice et al., 2012). The percentage of adults with chronic wounds is predicted to increase with the increasing numbers of elderly individuals and the concomitant increase in chronic illness-related comorbidities. Since physical functioning, psychological health, social interaction, and financial stability are impacted by a chronic wound, it is critical that we focus our attention and resources on prevention of chronic wounds and amelioration of the underlying processes to the greatest degree possible (Paul, 2013). When dealing with a chronic wound, it is essential for the clinician to accurately determine the etiologic factors and to address the cause of the wound as well as the wound itself (Armstrong & Meyr, 2013).

Clinical differences between acute and chronic wounds can be explained in part by differences in the local wound environments. Acute wounds have higher mitogenic activity, while chronic wounds are characterized by higher levels of proinflammatory cytokines, elevated levels of MMPs, and greater numbers of senescent cells (i.e., cells that do not respond normally to the cytokines and growth factors regulating the repair process). MMPs deserve special mention. MMPs are enzymes produced by the body; there are 23 types of human MMPs organized into eight categories, with the specific category determined by the domain structure. MMPs are *necessary* for normal healing; they function to degrade abnormal ECM components such as damaged collagen, and they promote the migration of immunologic cells (neutrophils and macrophages) into the injured tissue. Normal healing is characterized by high MMP levels during the inflammatory phase and markedly reduced levels during the proliferative phase. In contrast, chronic wounds are frequently characterized by persistently high MMP levels, which contribute to breakdown of growth factors and impaired collagen synthesis (Rohl & Murray, 2013). Thus,

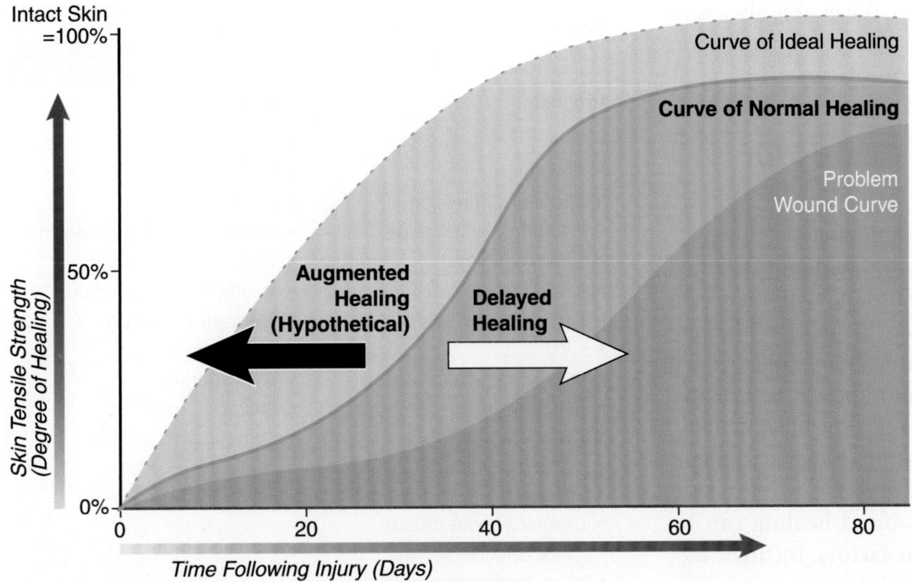

FIGURE 2-7. Healing trajectories of normal, problem, and hypothetical "ideal" wounds.

one focus of ongoing wound-related research is methods to control and modify MMP levels throughout the repair process (McCarty et al., 2012); currently available therapies for MMP modification will be discussed in Chapter 11.

Another characteristic of the chronic wound microenvironment is insufficient expression of fibronectin, chondroitin sulfate, and tenascin, all of which are critical to normal cell migration. In addition, chronic wounds are characterized by alterations in the ECM that can result in matrix instability and impaired synthesis of collagen and other connective tissue proteins. For example, hyperglycemia can increase MMP production, cause degradation of the ECM, and reduce the cell to cell interaction that is critical to normal repair (Demidova-Rice et al., 2012).

One strategy that is sometimes used to convert a "chronic" wound into an "acute" wound is surgical debridement (Goldberg & Diegelmann, 2012). Debridement induces acute tissue injury and bleeding, which results in hemostasis and activation of the many regulatory processes that normally control repair. However, it is equally important to address the systemic factors that caused the chronic wound if healing is to occur and recurrence is to be prevented (Fig. 2-7).

CLINICAL PEARL

A strategy sometimes used to convert a chronic wound into an acute wound is surgical debridement.

 Aging and Wound Healing

While age is commonly noted as a potential risk factor for poor wound healing, it is clear from the literature that *age itself* is not a risk factor for failure to heal. In general, wound healing in healthy older adults may be delayed but is not defective. For example, healing of acute surgical wounds is not problematic for most older patients. Indeed, fibroblast activity in response to cytokines is not affected by age and tensile wound strength seems to be unaffected in elders. "The accumulation of collagen in wounds does not seem to differ with age. In fact, the formation and quality of scarring may *improve* with age" (Thomas & Burkemper, 2013, p. xvi). Thus, it appears that any problems with wound healing associated with advanced age are most likely due to the multiple comorbidities that affect some older adults (Sgonc & Gruber, 2013).

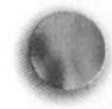 Partial- versus Full-Thickness Wound Healing

Another perspective on wound healing relates to the depth of affected tissue. The deeper the tissue layers affected, the greater number of wound healing mechanisms required. From this perspective, wounds are classified as either partial or full thickness. More specifically, wounds confined to the epidermal and dermal layers are considered to be partial thickness, while wounds that extend through the dermis are considered full thickness. As previously noted, partial-thickness wounds heal by epithelialization alone; in contrast, full-thickness wounds require granulation tissue formation to fill the soft tissue defect and may require contraction to reduce the size of the defect, followed by epithelial resurfacing.

As an example, a Stage II pressure ulcer is by definition a partial-thickness wound that heals by epithelialization, while a Stage III or IV pressure ulcer is a full-thickness lesion that requires granulation, contraction, and epithelialization. Deep tissue injury (bruising under intact skin) and unstageable pressure ulcers most often represent full-thickness damage. Because the repair process for full-thickness wounds is quite extensive and may require months or even years for completion, the goal is always to either prevent the pressure ulcer or to prevent progression of a Stage II ulcer to a Stage III/IV wound.

 Wound Healing: Risk Factors for Nonhealing

Wounds that fail to heal normally are labeled "chronic," and, as noted, these wounds are associated with marked alterations in the patient's quality of life and with increased morbidity and even mortality. There is usually not one single factor that results in impaired healing; rather, it is a constellation of factors that interact to impair chemotaxis, tissue oxygenation, myofibroblast and fibroblast activity, development of provisional and mature collagen, and epithelialization (Armstrong & Meyr, 2012).

The factors known to impede wound healing can be categorized as intrinsic and extrinsic factors. Intrinsic factors include factors such as advanced age, immune compromise (either innate or induced), psychological stress, hereditary skin disorders (e.g., epidermolysis bullosa), and disease states/comorbidities (e.g., diabetes and neuropathy, chronic obstructive pulmonary disease [COPD], cardiovascular disease, peripheral arterial disease, acute and chronic kidney disease, liver failure, alcoholism, malignant disease, and spinal cord disease). Extrinsic factors include factors such as infection (local and systemic), malnutrition, insufficient perfusion/oxygenation, smoking, chemotherapy, radiation therapy, and selected medications (e.g., steroids, anticoagulants, angiogenesis inhibitors) (Armstrong & Meyr, 2012; Gantwerker & Hom, 2012) (**Table 2-1**). Since immunosuppressive agents such as steroids and antirejection drugs are commonly administered for inflammatory bowel disease, rheumatoid arthritis, and organ transplant, these disease states have also been associated with impaired wound healing (Bootun, 2012).

TABLE 2-1 Factors Affecting Wound Healing

Intrinsic	Extrinsic
• Age	• Smoking
• Alcoholism	• Radiation
• Immunosuppression	• Chemotherapy
• Hereditary skin disease	• Infection (local or systemic)
• Chronic disease:	• Poor nutritional intake
• COPD	• Insufficient oxygenation
• CAD	• Medication therapy
• CVD	• Anticoagulants
• Liver failure	• Cyclosporine
• Renal failure	• Steroids
• Renal insufficiency	• Immobility (e.g., SCI)
• Diabetes mellitus	
• Peripheral vascular disease	
• Chronic venous disease	
• Sickle cell disease	
• Vasculitic/thrombotic disorders	
• Pain	
• Psychological stress	

Sources: Armstrong & Meyr (2012), Avila et al. (2012), Bootun (2013), Demidova-Rice et al. (2012), Gantwerker & Hom (2012), Woo (2012a, 2012b).

CLINICAL PEARL

Failure to heal is frequently due to systemic factors such as impaired perfusion, malnutrition, smoking, and poor glycemic control.

Perfusion and Oxygenation

Though the list of intrinsic factors (those relating to the patient's health) and extrinsic factors is formidable, some risk factors are particularly important. For example, adequate perfusion and oxygenation are critical for normal wound healing. Oxygen is required for inflammation, angiogenesis, collagen synthesis, and epithelialization. Thus, any alterations in oxygenation due to arterial disease, vasoconstriction, hypotension, vasopressors, advanced lung disease, severe anemia, or edematous states such as anasarca can be deleterious to wound healing. Any condition associated with impaired perfusion results in reduced delivery of critical cells and nutrients to the injured tissues and compromised removal of metabolic wastes (Armstrong & Meyr, 2012; Gantwerker & Hom, 2012), *in addition to* the adverse effects on tissue oxygenation. The critical role of oxygen in wound healing has been observed by mountain climbers who noted the inability to clear skin infections at high altitude. In addition, Eisenbud (2012) points out that the most common chronic wounds (arterial, venous, diabetic, and pressure) develop or are perpetuated due to inadequate tissue oxygen levels (Eisenbud, 2012). Not surprisingly, delivery of high concentrations of oxygen (hyperbaric oxygen therapy [HBOT]) is an effective treatment for chronic wounds caused or perpetuated by hypoxia, so long as there is sufficient plasma flow to deliver the oxygen to the wound site (Bhutani & Vishwanath, 2012). Adequate tissue oxygen levels are also needed for maintenance of normal nitric oxide (NO) levels, and abnormal NO levels are associated with excessive inflammation and impaired collagen synthesis (Park et al., 2013).

Glycemic Control

Another factor critical to wound healing is glycemic level. Hyperglycemia can impair every major aspect of the repair process, specifically inflammation, granulation tissue formation, development of tensile strength, and epithelial resurfacing. Thus, tight glucose control is an essential element of care for the wound clinician. Tight glycemic control has been associated with reduced wound complications in cardiovascular surgery patients, and tight glucose control is somewhat easier to maintain in the acute care setting; the staff can control dietary intake, medication administration, and glucose monitoring and can increase the frequency of glucose monitoring and implement insulin drips if needed. In the home care and outpatient setting, the clinician must work with the patient as well as other members of the health care team to establish appropriate goals for glycemic control and to consider short-term contracts for adherence to the patient-controlled elements of the management plan. The American Diabetes Association (2014) suggests an A1C goal of 6.5 to 7.0 (random glucose 140 to 154 mg/dL) for individuals with long life expectancy, no significant cardiovascular disease, and no significant problems with hypoglycemia and an A1C goal of <*8.0* (random glucose 183 mg/dL) for patients with limited life expectancy, history of severe hypoglycemia, and major comorbidities. In addition to the issues with hyperglycemia, diabetes is important because it is associated with vasculopathy, neuropathy, and immune dysfunction. Diminished macro- and microvascular blood supply, diminished sensory awareness of acute or repetitive injury/infection, and cellular dysfunction (especially macrophage dysfunction) in the presence of prolonged hyperglycemia increase the risk for both wound development and impaired healing.

Comorbidities

Other chronic disease states can have a profound and negative impact on wound healing. Cardiovascular disease (coronary artery disease [CAD] and associated heart failure and lower extremity arterial disease [LEAD]) can significantly reduce the amount of blood delivered to the distal extremities, resulting in chronic tissue ischemia. Conversely, venous insufficiency can impair venous return, resulting in chronic edema and changes in the soft tissues that increase vulnerability to minor trauma; the chronic edema then impairs delivery of oxygen to the traumatized tissues, which delays healing. Advanced COPD can also reduce tissue oxygen levels to a degree that impairs wound healing (Armstrong & Meyr, 2012).

Nutritional Status

Malnutrition, and most especially inadequate protein intake, is a major risk factor for impaired healing. Malnourished individuals lack the available nutrients to synthesize the connective tissue proteins (such as collagen) required for wound repair. Nutritional management must address intake of sufficient calories and protein to promote healing, but must also include attention to critical micronutrients (key vitamins and minerals.) For example, ascorbic acid (vitamin C) plays an important role in all phases of wound healing; in addition to its antioxidant properties, it is a cofactor in collagen synthesis and helps to regulate normal cellular apoptosis (Morres, 2013). Other nutrients that contribute to wound healing include trace elements such as magnesium, copper, zinc, and iron, specific amino acids such as arginine and glutamine, and possibly vitamins A and E (Rocchetti & Braga, 2012).

Tobacco Use

Tobacco use is profoundly detrimental to wound healing. Cigarette smoking promotes prolonged vasoconstriction through the effects of nicotine and other noxious substances. The impact is especially negative for patients with lower extremity wounds, since arterial insufficiency is a common causative factor for these wounds; for these patients, smoking cessation is sometimes the factor that determines whether the wound will heal or whether amputation will be required. However, smoking also has a significant detrimental effect in trunk wounds of relatively healthy patients. This is illustrated by the findings of a retrospective chart review of 597 caesarean deliveries with 30 cases of wound dehiscence; smoking was independently and significantly associated with wound complications (OR 5.32, 95% CI: 1.77 to 15.97, $p < 0.01$) (Avila et al., 2012).

Renal and hepatic failure can also increase risk for failure to heal, and advanced renal failure is also sometimes associated with the development of severe chronic wounds (e.g., calciphylaxis). The poor healing associated with advanced kidney and liver disease may be due to retention of metabolic wastes or to aberrations in mineral and electrolyte levels.

Spinal Cord Injury

Spinal cord injury is another comorbidity that increases both the risk for skin breakdown and the risk of impaired healing. The immobility and sensory loss associated with cord injury markedly increase the risk for pressure ulcer development, and for many patients, it is difficult to commit to the offloading typically required for wound healing. In addition, there are studies showing that healing below the level of injury is impaired as compared to healing above the level of injury; these differences and the implications for care are discussed further in Chapter 15.

Infection

Infection, especially if occult and/or untreated, can cause severe inhibition of wound healing; high levels of bacteria can cause additional tissue damage, and the inflammatory mediators and toxins associated with bacterial infections result in prolongation of the inflammatory phase of repair and delay in collagen synthesis and epithelial resurfacing. Thus, an effective management program for any wound requires prompt identification and effective treatment of any wound infection. It should be noted that superficial therapies such as antimicrobial dressings are insufficient therapy for invasive infection.

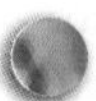 Psychological Factors and Wound Healing

The effect of psychological health on wound healing deserves special attention. Known psychological influences on wound healing include stress, coping style, positive affect, environmental enrichment, and social support. Psychological factors exert physiologic effects on conditions such as vessel size and leukocyte distribution through mediators such as oxytocin, vasopressin, epinephrine, and cortisol (Broadbent & Koschwanez, 2012). Chronic stress in particular has been shown to have immunosuppressive effects and to compromise wound healing. Recent reviews have suggested that psychological interventions such as relaxation can actually help wounds heal faster (Gouvin & Kiecolt-Glaser, 2012).

Pain is another factor with profound impact on wound healing. In response to painful stimuli, pain fibers release pain neuropeptides (e.g., substance P and neurokinin A) that activate immunoactive cells and trigger release of proinflammatory cytokines. The stress response that is associated with pain also triggers release of glucocorticoid hormones, and cortisol can reduce signaling for and production of growth factors (Woo, 2012a, 2012b).

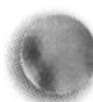 Implications for Optimal Wound Care

Clinician understanding of the intrinsic and extrinsic factors affecting wound healing is critical because it provides a basis for intervention. Whenever possible, the factors impeding prompt wound healing must be addressed and eradicated or ameliorated to the extent possible.

In general, comorbidities must be well managed. For example, good and consistent glycemic control is imperative for the patient with diabetes, any cardiovascular or pulmonary disease must be addressed, and renal and hepatic function must be optimized.

Measures to optimize perfusion are critical. For persons who are smokers, smoking cessation programs and nicotine replacement therapy may be essential interventions. Persons with arterial compromise need to understand the importance of using requisite therapies *and* not smoking. Conversely, venous insufficiency clients need to understand why compression is critical to optimal healing and need to faithfully adhere to ambulation, compression, and elevation therapies.

Nutritional repletion is also essential; the wound care nurse must obtain or complete a baseline assessment of nutritional status and must monitor nutrient intake, weight trends, and relevant laboratory findings (such as albumin and prealbumin). Baseline interventions include provision of adequate protein, calories, and micronutrients; if these interventions are insufficient, additional measures should be considered, such as protein supplements. In selected situations, anabolic steroids such as oxandrolone may be considered for promotion of weight gain and wound healing (Bauman et al., 2013). Chapter 6 addresses the nutritional aspects of wound healing and wound management in detail. Wound healing is also dependent on maintaining a moist but balanced wound environment to support the cellular activities essential to repair. A variety of wound dressings can address the objective of maintaining appropriate moisture levels in the wound bed (Newton, 2013); specific options and considerations are discussed in detail in Chapter 8. Individuals who are immunosuppressed may require additional interventions to promote healing; for example, a trial of topical vitamin A may be warranted for a patient who requires chronic corticosteroid therapy and whose wound is not progressing or progressing very slowly. Immunocompromised persons may also benefit from the use of dressings with antimicrobial and anti-inflammatory effects, since they are at high risk for both superficial and invasive wound infection; products to be considered include but are not limited to silver dressings, cadexomer iodine dressings, dressings impregnated with polyhexamethylene biguanide, dressings impregnated with methylene blue and crystal violet, and dressings with medicinal honey (Majtan, 2014; White et al., 2012). Prevention and management of wound infection is addressed in detail in Chapter 10.

Attention to psychological state is also vitally important; clinical depression and other psychological conditions have been associated with self-induced wounding (factitious wounds) (Sansone & Sansone, 2013). Clinical psychologists, psychiatrists, or psychiatric advanced practice nurses should be consulted, since effective use of pharmacologic and cognitive therapies can help interrupt the cycle of wounding and improve healing outcomes.

As noted in Chapter 4, the goal for wound care is dependent on the ability to substantially correct the etiologic factors and the systemic factors affecting healing. In situations where these factors can*not* be corrected, the goal for wound care should be modified to focus on maintenance or simply on symptom management.

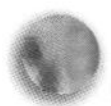 Future Directions for Wound Healing Therapies

Our understanding of the wound repair process and the factors controlling healing continue to evolve and to inform our clinical practice. A major area for future research related to wound healing is epigenetic regulation. Epigenetics is the study of the interaction between environmental factors and the genome of the individual cell; these interactions involve cell signaling, which produces persistent and heritable changes in gene expression even though the DNA is not changed. Epigenetics is relevant to wound care, because disease states can affect epigenetic processes in ways that contribute to chronic wounds (Mann & Mann, 2013). Current data suggest that stem cell therapy may be one approach to alteration of epigenetic signaling in a way that promotes improved wound healing (Chen et al., 2012; Ti et al., 2014).

Another focus of study is the role of microRNAs in the regulation of wound healing. It is known that these substances act as key regulators of gene expression and that they therefore impact on wound healing. Ongoing research may provide the basis for development of microRNA-targeted wound healing therapies (Lai & Siu, 2014; Mills & Cowin, 2013; Ning & Andl, 2013).

Conclusion

This chapter has addressed the major physiologic processes involved in wound repair (hemostasis, inflammation, granulation tissue formation and contraction, and epithelialization) and has compared and contrasted the repair process for acute and chronic wounds and for full-thickness and partial-thickness wounds. Systemic factors affecting healing have been addressed, along with implications for provider intervention.

REFERENCES

American Diabetes Association. (2014). Standards of medical care in diabetes-2014. *Diabetes Care, 37* (Suppl 1), S14–S80.

Armstrong, D. G., & Meyr, A. J. (2012). Wound healing and risk factors for non-healing. *Uptodate.* Accessed January 31, 2014 at www.uptodate.com/contents/wound-healing-and-riskfactors-for-non-healing?source

Armstrong, D. G., & Meyr, A. J. (2013). Clinical assessment of wounds. *Uptodate.* Accessed January 31, 2014 at www.uptodate.com/contents/clinical-assessment-of-wounds?source

Armstrong, D. G., & Meyr, A. J. (2014). Basic principles of wound management. *Uptodate.* Accessed January 31, 2014 at www.uptodate.com/contents/basic-principles-of-wound-management?source

Avila, C., Bhangoo, R., Figuerua, R., et al. (2012). Association of smoking with wound complications after cesarean delivery. *Journal of Maternal-Fetal and Neonatal Medicine, 25*(8), 1250–1253.

Bainbridge, P. (2013). Wound healing and the role of fibroblasts. *Journal of Wound Care, 22*(8), 407–412.

Bauman, W. A., Spungen, A. M., Collins, J. F., et al. (2013). The effect of oxandrolone on the healing of chronic pressure ulcers in persons with a spinal cord injury. *Annals of Internal Medicine, 158*(10), 718–726.

Bhutani, S., & Vishwanath, G. (2012). Hyperbaric oxygen and wound healing. *Indian Journal of Plastic Surgery, 45*(2), 316–324.

Bootun, R. (2013). Effects of immunosuppressive therapy on wound healing. *International Wound Journal, 10*, 98–104.

Broadbent, E., & Koschwanez, H. E. (2012). The psychology of wound healing. *Current Opinion in Psychiatry, 25*(2), 135–140.

Chen, C., Corselli, M., Peault, B., et al. (2012). Human blood-vessel-derived stem cells for tissue repair and regeneration. *Journal of Biomedicine and Biotechnology*, 9, article ID 597439, doi: 10.1155/2012/597439

Demidova-Rice, T. N., Hamblin, M. R., & Herman, I. M. (2012). Acute and impaired wound healing: Pathophysiology and current methods for drug delivery, Part 1: Normal and chronic wounds: Biology, causes, and approaches to care. *Advances in Skin and Wound Care, 25*(7), 304–312.

DiPietro, L. A. (2013). Angiogenesis and scar formation in healing wounds. *Current Opinion in Rheumatology, 25*, 87–91.

Eisenbud, D. E. (2012). Oxygen in wound healing. Nutrient, antibiotic, signaling molecule, and therapeutic agent. *Clinics in Plastic Surgery, 39*, 293–310.

Gantwerker, E. A., & Hom, D. B. (2012). Skin: Histology and physiology of wound healing. *Clinics in Plastic Surgery, 39*(1), 85–97.

Goldberg, S. R., & Diegelmann, R. F. (2012). Wound healing primer. *Critical Care Nursing Clinics of North America, 24*, 165–178.

Gouvin, J. P., Kiecolt-Glaser, J. K. (2012). The impact of psychological stress on wound healing: Methods and mechanisms. *Critical Care Nursing Clinics of North America, 24*, 201–213.

Griswold, J. A. (2012). Why diabetic wounds do not heal. *Texas Heart Institute Journal, 39*(6), 860–861.

He, L., & Marneros, A. G. (2013). Macrophages are essential for the early wound healing response and the formation of a fibrovascular scar. *American Journal of Pathology, 182*(6), 2407–2417.

Lai, W., & Siu, P. M. (2014). Micro RNAs as regulators of cutaneous wound healing. *Journal of Bioscience, 38*(3), 519–524.

Majtan, J. (2014). Honey: An immunomodulator in wound healing. *Wound Repair and Regeneration, 22*, 187–192.

Mann, J., & Mann, D. (2013). Epigenetic regulation of wound healing and fibrosis. *Current Opinion in Rheumatology, 25*(1), 101–107.

McCarty, S. M., Cochrane, C. A., Clegg, P. D., et al. (2012). The role of endogenous and exogenous enzymes in chronic wounds: A focus on the implications of aberrant levels of both host and bacterial proteases in wound healing. *Wound Repair and Regeneration, 20*(2), 125–136.

Miao, M., Niu, Y., Xie, T., et al. (2012). Diabetes-impaired wound healing and altered macrophage activation: A possible pathophysiologic correlation. *Wound Repair and Regeneration, 20*, 203–213.

Mills, S. J., & Cowin, A. J. (2013). Micro RNAs and their roles in wound repair and regeneration. *Wound Practice and Research, 21*(1), 26–39.

Morres, J. (2013). Vitamin C: A wound healing perspective. *Wound Care*, S6–S11.

Newton, H. (2013). An introduction to wound healing and dressings. *British Journal of Healthcare Management, 19*(6), 270–273.

Ning, M. S., & Andl, T. (2013). Control by a hair's breadth: The role of micro RNAs in the skin. *Cellular and Molecular Life Sciences, 70*, 1149–1169.

Park, J. E., Abrams, M. J., Efron, P. A., et al. (2013). Excessive nitric oxide impairs wound collagen accumulation. *Journal of Surgical Research, 183*, 487–492.

Paul, J. (2013). Characteristics of chronic wounds that itch. *Advances in Skin and Wound Care, 26*(7), 320–332.

Percival, S. L., Hill, K. E., Williams, D. W., et al. (2012). A review of the scientific evidence for biofilms in wounds. *Wound Repair and Regeneration, 20*, 647–657.

Rocchetti, S., & Braga, M. (2012). Glycemia, nutrition and wound healing. *Nutritional Therapy and Metabolism, 30*(3), 121–128.

Rohl, J., & Murray, R. Z. (2013). Matrix metalloproteases during wound healing—a double edged sword. *Wound Practice and Research, 21*(4), 174–182.

Sansone, R. A., & Sansone, L. A. (2013). Preventing wounds from healing: Clinical prevalence and relationship to borderline personality. *Innovations in Clinical Neuroscience, 10*(11–12), 23–27.

Sgonc, R., & Gruber, J. (2013). Age-related aspects of cutaneous wound healing: A mini-review. *Gerontology, 59*, 159–164.

Shanahan, D. R. (2013). Inaugural professorial lecture: The progression of trauma wound care—why delay wound closure? *Journal of Wound Care, 22*(4), 194–196.

Thomas, D. R., & Burkemper, N. M. (2013). Aging skin and wound healing. *Clinics in Geriatric Medicine, 29*(2), xi–xx.

Ti, D., Li, M., Fu, X., et al. (2014). Causes and consequences of epigenetic regulation in wound healing. *Wound Repair and Regeneration, 22*, 305–312.

White, R., Cooper, R., & Edwards-Jones, V. (2012). What is the role of biofilms in wound healing? *Wounds, 8*(2), 20–24.

Winter, G. (1962). Formation of the scab and the rate of epithelialization of superficial wounds in the skin of young domestic pig. *Nature, 193*, 293.

Wong, V. W., Gurtner, G. C., & Longaker, M. T. (2013). Wound healing: A paradigm for regeneration. *Mayo Clinic Proceedings, 88*(9), 1022–1031.

Woo, K. Y. (2012a). Chronic wound-associated pain, psychological stress, and wound healing. *Surgical Technology International, 22*(12), 57–65.

Woo, K. Y. (2012b). Exploring the effects of pain and stress on wound healing. *Advances in Skin and Wound Care, 25*(1), 38–44.

Yao, K., Bae, L., & Yew, W. (2013). Post-operative wound management. *Australian Family Physician, 42*(12), 867–870.

Yoo, S. Y., & Kwon, S. M. (2013). Angiogenesis and its therapeutic opportunities. *Mediators of Inflammation*, 11, Article ID 127170.

QUESTIONS

1. The incision of a postoperative cardiac surgery patient is in the inflammatory phase of wound healing. What is one mechanism of healing occurring in this phase?

A. Neutrophils and monocytes are chemoattracted to the wounded area.
B. Fibroblasts migrate to the area in response to cellular signaling.
C. A new extracellular matrix (granulation tissue) is formed.
D. Cells responsible for collagen synthesis and angiogenesis undergo apoptosis.

2. The WOC nurse is explaining the phases of wound healing to a patient who has a sutured laceration. Which statement accurately describes the typical time frame for proliferation to occur?

A. 1 to 2 days
B. 3 to 5 days
C. 21 to 30 days
D. 1 to 2 years

3. A patient has a full-thickness pressure ulcer on the back of his head. What order of healing would occur with this wound?

A. Epithelial resurfacing—granulation tissue formation
B. Reepithelialization—granulation tissue formation—remodeling
C. Epithelial resurfacing—scar formation—remodeling
D. Inflammatory phase—granulation tissue formation—epithelial resurfacing—remodeling

4. What process is the foundation of modern wound care and is essential for maintenance of cellular viability and cell migration?

A. Dry wound preparation
B. Moist wound healing
C. Antibacterial soaks
D. Aggressive surgical debridement

5. The WOC nurse is assessing a surgical wound that is too contaminated to permit primary closure. What is the expected recommendation for treatment of this wound?

A. Keep the wound at secondary closure level until bacterial burden is decreased to $<10^5$ organisms/g of tissue; then close via delayed primary closure.
B. Close the wound using sutures or skin staples at time of surgery; reopen the wound in 2 to 3 days and allow to heal by tertiary closure.
C. Close the wound to fascia level, and intentionally leave upper layers open to granulate in over time.
D. Allow the wound to fill in naturally over time, and close the wound with stitches after granulation tissue forms if necessary.

6. A patient who has diabetes mellitus has chronic foot ulcers. What is a characteristic of the healing phase of these types of wounds?

A. There is a shortened inflammatory phase in chronic wounds.
B. Biofilms do not commonly occur in chronic wounds.
C. Chronic wounds heal in an orderly, timely, and durable manner.
D. Chronic wounds commonly plateau at some point in the healing process.

7. The WOC nurse is explaining the difference between acute and chronic wounds to a patient diagnosed with hypertensive ulcers. What is one clinical characteristic of a chronic wound?

A. Higher mitogenic activity than acute wounds
B. Lower levels of proinflammatory cytokines than acute wounds
C. Elevated levels of matrix metalloproteases (MMPs)
D. Decreased numbers of senescent cells than acute wounds

8. What is the primary reasoning for using debridement to convert a "chronic" wound into an "acute" wound?
   A. Debridement removes eschar that inhibits healing.
   B. Debridement causes bleeding and clotting and activates repair processes.
   C. Debridement prevents slowing of wound healing due to microbial activity.
   D. Debridement increases MMP levels during the proliferative phase.

9. The WOC nurse is assessing risk factors for delayed wound healing for patients on a surgical ward. What is a known intrinsic factor?
   A. Alcoholism
   B. Radiation treatment
   C. Poor nutritional intake
   D. Medication therapy

10. Which patient would the WOC nurse consider most "at risk" for delayed wound healing?
   A. A 75-year-old female with a surgical incision
   B. A 60-year-old male with hypotension
   C. A 40-year-old female with multiple sclerosis
   D. A 5-year-old male with an unintentional wound

11. Special populations require modification of the wound treatment plan. Which statement accurately describes an intervention based on the intrinsic or extrinsic factors related to the patient?
   A. Smokers should use additional compression and elevation therapies.
   B. Anabolic steroids may be considered for patients with spinal cord injuries.
   C. Individuals who are immunosuppressed may benefit from a trial of topical vitamin B.
   D. Immunocompromised persons may benefit from the use of dressings with antimicrobial and anti-inflammatory effects.

ANSWERS: 1.**A**, 2.**C**, 3.**D**, 4.**B**, 5.**A**, 6.**D**, 7.**C**, 8.**B**, 9.**A**, 10.**B**, 11.**D**

CHAPTER 3

Assessment of the Patient with a Wound

Barbara M. Bates-Jensen

OBJECTIVES

1. Conduct a comprehensive assessment of the patient with compromised skin or soft tissue integrity to include history, physical examination, and appropriate diagnostic studies.
2. Use assessment data to determine the following:
   - Factors causing or contributing to the alteration in skin/soft tissue integrity
   - Potential for healing and any systemic conditions that would interfere with healing
   - Wound characteristics (to include phase of wound healing) and implications for wound management
3. Develop an individualized plan of care based on assessment data and current evidence-based guidelines that addresses each of the following factors:
   - Correction or amelioration of etiologic factors
   - Attention to systemic factors affecting repair process
   - Evidence-based topical therapy
   - Pain management
   - Patient and caregiver education
   - Use data from serial wound assessments to identify wound deterioration or failure to progress

Topic Outline

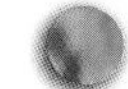 Introduction

Assessment of the patient with a wound includes assessment of the patient's overall health status and ability to heal, skin status, wound etiology and severity, and wound status, to include stage of healing. Assessment includes a focused history and physical examination, selected diagnostic studies when indicated, followed by interpretation and synthesis of the data, and communication of findings to other health care providers. Communication of wound assessment data is best accomplished using a standardized language and approach: use of standardized wound assessment tools, structured narrative wound notes, and/or photodocumentation. Multiple clinical practice guidelines for wound management include recommendations for the use of standardized wound assessment at baseline and at frequent intervals to determine wound treatment response and wound progress (Hopf et al., 2006; National Pressure Ulcer Advisory Panel/National Pressure Ulcer Advisory Panel, 2014; Robson et al., 2006; Steed et al., 2006; Whitney et al., 2006; Wound Ostomy Continence Nurses Society, 2010). An initial assessment of the wound provides the foundation for development of an appropriate management plan and also provides the baseline data that permit determination of progress in healing during subsequent evaluations. In this chapter, aspects of assessment of the patient with a wound are presented including guidelines for skin inspection, guidelines for obtaining a focused history and review of systems, factors to be included in general physical examination and assessment of wound status and wound severity, pertinent laboratory values and diagnostic tests, parameters to be included in assessment of wound-related pain, evaluation of progress in wound healing, and strategies for improving wound documentation, including photodocumentation.

Type and Frequency of Assessment

There are two general types of wound assessment, initial or baseline assessment and serial or follow-up assessments. The initial assessment provides the foundation for deciding treatment options and the plan of care and must include determination of wound etiology, assessment of systemic factors affecting the ability to heal, patient and caregiver goals, and wound status; the initial data permit comparison with follow-up data that allows caregivers to determine whether the wound is progressing or deteriorating. The baseline assessment should be performed when the wound is first observed or identified. The baseline assessment must be comprehensive, encompassing all aspects of the wound and the patient's ability to heal from a systemic perspective. Failure to address all aspects of wound development and wound status during the baseline assessment can compromise the appropriateness of the care plan and the ability to determine intermediary outcomes (progress vs. deterioration) during wound treatment. Follow-up assessments provide comparison data, which allow clinicians to determine wound response to treatment; these "serial" assessments should be performed at least weekly, with dressing changes, whenever a change occurs in the wound, or more frequently if so stipulated by health care facility policy. Follow-along assessments should be compared to either the baseline assessment data or the prior follow-along assessment.

Assessment should be performed by a licensed registered nurse, advanced practice nurse, physician's assistant, physical therapist, podiatrist, or physician with the requisite knowledge and skill in wound care. It should be noted that knowledge about wound assessment and wound healing has grown tremendously in the last 5 years, and the average nonspecialist clinician lacks current knowledge regarding clinical practice guidelines, correct wound-related terminology, and basic wound characteristics. Thus, a challenge for wound care clinicians is providing continuous, timely, multidisciplinary education on wound assessment.

Skin Inspection and Assessment

Inspection is different from assessment. Inspection involves visually observing the skin and any wound sites for specific conditions and monitoring for any changes over time. Inspection can be performed by trained licensed practical nurses, physical therapy assistants, nurse aides, family members, home caregivers, and the patient. Skin inspection should occur whenever a patient is admitted to any health care organization and on a routine basis thereafter. Inspection occurs more frequently than assessments, usually daily or every shift. Because inspection occurs on a more frequent basis, it is a critical "first-line" tool for identifying early indicators of skin or wound deterioration that require further assessment. As an example, if a nurse's aide discovers a new reddened area over the sacrum while providing incontinence care, she/he should notify the registered nurse, who should conduct an assessment of the area and the patient to determine the etiology of the lesion and any changes needed in the existing care plan. Similarly, if a family caregiver notices increased wound drainage and odor from a surgical incision, the health care provider should be notified and an assessment scheduled to evaluate for possible infection.

Skin Inspection

Skin inspection involves visually observing all body parts without the presence of clothing, undergarments, or shoes; in-depth skin assessment includes inspection of the feet; key pressure areas such as the buttocks, sacrum, shoulders, knees, ankles, heels, and occiput; the perineal and perianal skin; the skin between any body folds or crevasses; and the skin underneath all medical devices. Specific conditions to observe for include areas of skin loss, areas of redness or other skin discoloration, edema, rash, increased skin temperature or moisture, and, in the case of a wound, new or increased drainage. If a wound dressing is present and not due to be changed, the dressing should be observed for intactness and any signs of excess wound drainage, rash, or skin discoloration on the surrounding skin (Nix, 2011). If the dressing is dry and intact, dressing status should be documented, and it is not necessary to remove the dressing. The one exception to this is a protective dressing applied to the sacrococcygeal area; current guidelines stipulate that the protective dressing should be lifted daily to permit skin inspection and then replaced.

Skin inspection can be accomplished as part of routine care. For example, the buttocks, sacrum, and perineal areas are easily inspected during incontinence care, when transferring the patient from bed to chair, or when getting the patient dressed. Inspection of the elbows and arms can occur when the intravenous site is checked or when dressing the patient. In acute care settings, top to toe skin inspection is typically performed at the beginning and ending of a shift, which allows team members to share findings between the outgoing and incoming team. Those who conduct the skin inspection must report any abnormalities in skin condition; at a minimum, skin status reports should include any change in skin condition, areas of discoloration, presence of rash, and wounds (Nix, 2011). In some institutions, this process is codified as part of the shift hand-off report and as part of required communication when transferring patients between areas. The Turn on Transfer (ToT) program involves both a verbal report of skin status and a brief visual inspection of the sacrum and heels by both delivering and receiving nurses. Routine skin and wound inspection coupled with standardized communication regarding skin and wound status is an essential baseline component of an effective skin and wound care program.

Skin Assessment

Skin *assessment* involves palpation in addition to inspection, followed by interpretation of patterns and trends in the data. As with skin inspection, assessment should involve particular attention to bony prominences, lower extremities, skin folds and crevasses, and the skin under medical devices. In addition to inspecting for visible changes in color, integrity, and lesions, the clinician should gently palpate to identify areas of altered skin texture/roughness; callus formation; presence of induration; presence, severity, and type of edema; areas of skin temperature changes (using the backs of the fingers); and areas of tenderness. Skin turgor is a measure of skin hydration and is assessed by gently pinching a fold of skin (typically at the sternum or forehead) and noting how quickly it returns to baseline status. Palpation is also used to test for capillary refill (a measure of perfusion) and for blanchability of any erythematous areas; the examiner presses a finger firmly against the area of erythema for 5 seconds and then lifts the finger and observes the tissues for blanching followed by a return of color to the area. Nonblanchable erythema is indicative of some level of tissue damage and inflammation involving the skin and soft tissues; nonblanchable erythema over a bony prominence is classified as a Stage I pressure ulcer. For areas that are erythematous but blanchable, it is important to provide off-loading and to monitor the intensity of the erythema and the blanch response as an ongoing measure of treatment success. If the erythema progresses from blanchable to nonblanchable, it signifies worsening of skin and soft tissue condition.

Skin Assessment in Persons with Dark Skin Tones

Assessment of skin discoloration in persons with dark skin tones is more complicated. Dark skin tones may not exhibit a visible blanch response, and it is difficult to detect changes in skin color due to hyperemia, even for expert clinicians. Use of good lighting is essential for skin assessment of persons with dark skin tones. The clinician should observe for a deepening of normal ethnic skin color or a purple, blue, or gray discoloration to the skin. Additional indicators of ischemic (pressure) damage include pain, change in skin texture (e.g., features similar to peau d'orange skin), edema, and increased warmth. In areas of previous full-thickness wounds, the scar tissue will be lighter in color as compared to the person's normal ethnic skin color as there are no melanocytes in the scar tissue.

CLINICAL PEARL

Assessment of skin status in the person with darkly pigmented skin must include palpation as well as inspection.

Assessment (and documentation) of any skin lesions should include location, distribution, and arrangement of any rash and use of appropriate terminology to describe primary and secondary skin lesions. Primary skin lesions are classified both by type of the lesion and size of the lesion. Macules and patches are erythematous flat skin discolorations (<1.0 cm and >1.0 cm, respectively), while papules or plaques are raised erythematous skin areas (<1.0 cm and >1.0 cm, respectively). Nodules and tumors represent solid areas of excess tissue growth, vesicles and bulla are clear fluid-filled blisters (<1.0 cm and >1.0 cm, respectively), and pustules are pus-filled blisters. Key secondary skin lesions include scale, lichenification, keloids, hypertrophic scars, erosions, fissures, excoriation, denudation, crusts, and atrophy. (See Chapter 1 for further discussion of common dermatologic lesions and appropriate dermatologic terminology.)

Documentation of Skin Status

Documentation of the skin inspection must communicate any deviations from normal and may consist of a simple checklist or flow sheet, a body diagram, or narrative notes indicating "dressing intact" or "skin warm, dry, and intact; no lesions." Figures 3-1 and 3-2 provide examples of two types of skin inspection documentation forms. When findings differ from previous inspections, the changes must be communicated to other members of the health care team and documented in the patient's record.

An initial full body or head-to-toe skin assessment is particularly critical at the point of admission to a health care facility; a key responsibility of the admitting nurse is prompt identification of any existing wound or other

Skin Observation Form

Name: ______________________________ Date: ____/____/____

	BODY LOCATION See body diagrams below if unsure of location												
SKIN CONDITION check if present	SACRUM or COCCYX (Tailbone)	Right BUTTOCK	Left BUTTOCK	Right ISCHIUM (Bottom of Gluteal fold)	Left ISCHIUM (Bottom of Gluteal fold)	Right HIP	Left HIP	Right HEEL	Left HEEL	Right inner ANKLE	Left inner ANKLE	Right outer ANKLE	Right outer ANKLE
Normal Skin													
Redness													
Bruise													
Rash													
Blister													
Open wound													
Other:													

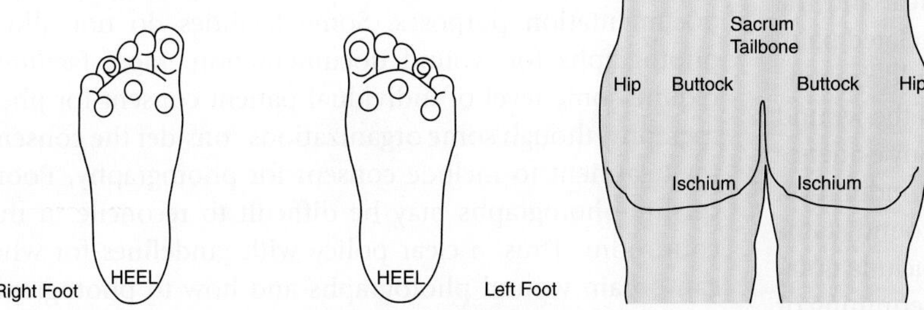

FIGURE 3-1. Sample of skin inspection documentation form.

Skin Observation Form—Instructions: Observe skin daily & record if condition is present

Name: ______________________________ Month: ______________________________ Year: ________

Body Location	Day:	1	2	3	4	5	6	7	8	9	10	11	12	13	14	15	16	17	18	19	20	21	22	23	24	25	26	27	28	29	30	31
	Skin Condition																															
Sacrum or Tailbone	Redness																															
	Bruise																															
	Wound																															
Right Buttock	Redness																															
	Bruise																															
	Wound																															
Left Buttock	Redness																															
	Bruise																															
	Wound																															
Right Ischium (At gluteal fold)	Redness																															
	Bruise																															
	Wound																															
Left Ischium (At gluteal fold)	Redness																															
	Bruise																															
	Wound																															
Right Hip	Redness																															
	Bruise																															
	Wound																															
Left Hip	Redness																															
	Bruise																															
	Wound																															
Right Heel	Redness																															
	Bruise																															
	Wound																															
Left Heel	Redness																															
	Bruise																															
	Wound																															
Other Locations:	Redness																															
	Bruise																															
	Wound																															

FIGURE 3-2. Another sample of skin inspection documentation form.

skin condition. Documentation of pressure-related lesions that are "present on admission" is essential, because the Centers for Medicare and Medicaid Services (CMS) no longer provide reimbursement and payment for full-thickness pressure ulcers that develop while the patient is in the hospital (CMS, 2008; CMS, 2009).

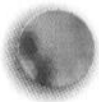

Assessment and Documentation of Wound Status

General Concepts

Assessment and documentation of wound status is an important nursing responsibility and is best accomplished with the use of a standardized wound assessment instrument (Bates-Jensen & Sussman, 2012; NPUAP/EPUAP, 2014). Use of a standardized wound assessment instrument guides the assessment process and provides continuity in communication about the wound. Initial documentation must include probable etiology, wound duration and previous treatments, and wound status, as well as documentation regarding systemic factors affecting ability to heal and the patient's concerns and goals, including wound-related pain. Documentation at each dressing change should include notations about wound location, appearance of the wound bed, volume and characteristics of exudate, and any evidence of infection, such as periwound erythema and induration (CMS, 2009). A thorough documentation of wound status should be conducted at least weekly and must include notations about wound dimensions and depth; undermining or pocketing and tunneling; description of wound base, wound edges, and surrounding tissues; volume and characteristics of exudate; and healing characteristics of the wound. Each of these parameters is discussed in greater depth later in this chapter. Maintaining wound assessment documentation in the same physical place in the electronic or paper medical record facilitates comparative evaluation and interpretation of serial assessment findings. Serial assessment data provide insight regarding wound progress or deterioration, which impact treatment plans. For example, as the amount of necrotic tissue decreases, the focus of topical therapy shifts from debridement to maintenance of a moist wound surface and exudate control.

Photography has also been used to enhance wound assessment and documentation and to provide visual assessment of wounds over time. It is important to maximize the accuracy of wound photographs in order to ensure that they are meaningful. Photography guidelines include the following:

- Place the patient in the same position for all photographs.
- Take the photograph from the same angle.
- Take a close-up photograph of the wound and then a second photograph showing the wound and the body part. Try to take the close-up photograph from a standard distance from the wound (e.g., use a string at the base of the camera to assure consistency in the distance of the close-up photograph).
- Include a ruler with centimeters and a color guide in the photograph.
- Include a label with date, anatomic location, and patient identification (ID) number (use a nonidentifiable ID that meets Health Insurance Portability and Accountability Act [HIPAA] regulations) in the photograph.
- Obtain patient authorization according to facility policy prior to photography.
- Use a digital camera with a density of at least 1.5 megapixels, but 3 megapixels or greater is better for picture clarity.
- Assure adherence to infection control policies. For example, prepare the wound for photography; then remove gloves, wash hands, retrieve the camera, and take the photograph without touching anything around the wound. Return the camera to a safe location, wash hands and don gloves, and complete wound care.
- Download the photographs to the patient's record, and delete the photograph from the camera.

There are some nuances to wound photography for documentation purposes. Some facilities do not allow photographs for wound documentation. Most facilities require some level of individual patient consent for photography, though some organizations consider the consent for treatment to include consent for photography. Poor-quality photographs may be difficult to reconcile in the courtroom. Thus, a clear policy with guidelines for who can obtain wound photographs and how to photograph wounds is important for the facility (Nix, 2011). From a risk management perspective, it is useful, at a minimum, to obtain a photograph of the wound at admission and upon discharge from the organization.

A major benefit of wound photodocumentation is its potential use in telemedicine. Photography can increase access to expert wound care for people who live in rural areas or areas with limited access to wound experts, and it has been used to supplement wound assessment data. For example, photography has been used to reliably detect callus and foot ulceration in persons with diabetes, to quantify granulation tissue in healing wounds, and to enhance wound assessment by wound experts using telehealth modalities (Hazenberg et al., 2012; Houghton et al., 2000; Iizaka et al., 2013; Russell Localio et al., 2006). Some investigators have suggested that photography does not replace in-person assessment as they have not found strong agreement between assessments conducted in person compared to assessment by photograph (Terris et al., 2011). Others have found strong agreement between in-person and photographic approaches to wound assessment (Houghton et al., 2000; Jesada et al., 2013). There are also cameras with lasers that measure the length, width, and depth of the wound and use these measurements to compute wound size. These devices provide more comprehensive photodocumentation and have been shown to improve accuracy and reliability of wound size measurements (Kecelj et al., 2008; Miller et al., 2012).

Wound Etiology

An essential element of initial assessment for the patient with a wound is determination of wound etiology; this allows implementation of a treatment plan that includes measures to correct or ameliorate the causative factors. Critical clues to etiology of trunk wounds include wound location, wound depth and contours, and patient history (e.g., exposure to prolonged pressure vs. exposure to moisture and/or friction) (Bryant, 2011). Critical clues to the etiology of lower extremity wounds include pain pattern, location, and appearance of wound bed and surrounding tissue. See Table 3-1 for etiologic clues for common types of trunk wounds and leg ulcers.

CLINICAL PEARL

Determination of wound etiology is a critical "first step" in wound assessment. If etiology is unclear, appropriate referrals and testing must be initiated.

TABLE 3-1 Clues Regarding Wound Etiology

	Pathological Factors	Typical Location	Typical Clinical Manifestations
Pressure ulcers	Any disease or condition that leads to limited mobility and/or exposure to shear force Skin and soft tissue compression by medical device	Sacrum, coccyx, buttocks, ischial tuberosities, trochanters, heels. Can occur over any bony prominence Most common locations: sacrum and heels Under medical device	• Evidence of ischemic damage: purple discoloration of skin progressing to full-thickness skin loss surrounded by blanchable or nonblanchable erythema • Round ulcer; may be irregular if large • Tunneling/undermining or pocketing may be evident • Progression to a deep crater (subcutaneous tissue to the fascia) to exposure of the muscle, bone, or supporting structures (i.e., tendon) • Surrounding skin may appear with deepening of ethnic skin tone or erythema, induration, warmth, possible mottling
Incontinence-associated dermatitis	Damage caused by maceration + friction or exposure to irritants and pathogens	Buttocks, coccyx, perineum, perianal area, and upper/inner thighs	• Diffuse, intense blanchable erythema • Superficial skin loss (patchy or extensive) • Secondary candidiasis common (maculopapular rash with central patch or plaque formation and distinct satellite lesions at periphery)
Intertriginous dermatitis (ITD)	Maceration within body folds due to trapped moisture + friction or mechanical stretch	Linear breaks at the base of the body fold or matching lesions on either side of the body fold • Natal cleft • Under breast tissue • Under pannus • Axillae	• Linear break in the skin at the base of the body fold • Superficial "kissing" ulcers on opposing sides of skin folds

Venous ulcers	Compromised venous return resulting in soft tissue changes that render them vulnerable to ulceration	Lower extremity: calf superior to the medial or lateral malleolus, typically in the "gaiter" area	• Shallow ulcers with ruddy wound base (may also present with combination of red tissue and thin layer yellow film, i.e., biofilm)
			• Moderate to large amounts of exudate
			• If no coexisting arterial disease: warm feet, good pulses, ABI > 0.8
			• Surrounding skin may exhibit any or all of the following:
			  • Hemosiderin staining
			  • Edema
			  • Dermatitis (scaling, crusting, weeping, erythema, inflammation)
			• Pain typically worsened by dependency and relieved by elevation

(*Continued*)

TABLE 3-1 Clues Regarding Wound Etiology (*Continued*)

	Pathological Factors	Typical Location	Typical Clinical Manifestations
Arterial ulcers	Lower extremity arterial disease causes severe tissue ischemia, resulting in spontaneous necrosis or nonhealing wounds (LEAD).	Tips of toes and/or forefoot Nonhealing wounds involving lower leg or foot	• Ulcers are full thickness, typically round, with punched-out appearance or a distinct border. • Ulcer base pale or necrotic • Typically minimal exudate • Pain worsened by activity and elevation and relieved by rest and dependency
Neuropathic ulcers (diabetic foot ulcers)	Damage to nerve endings results in sensory loss, foot deformities, very dry skin.	Plantar aspect of foot, metatarsal heads, areas of foot in contact with shoe	• Typically full-thickness ulcers with possible tunneling or undermining • Red wet base common but may also present with necrotic tissue • Commonly located within or under callus • May not be painful; may present with neuropathic ("pins and needles," "electric shock") pain that is frequently worse at night
Skin tears	Fragile skin with loss of normal cohesion between epidermal and dermal layers	Usually located on forearm or lower extremity (shin). May be present in other locations after falls	• Superficial injury/ulcer to the epidermis/dermis • May present with viable skin flap that covers the wound, partial skin flap, necrotic flap that has to be removed, or no flap • Bruising of surrounding skin common; bleeding also common • Fragile surrounding skin

Systemic Health Status

In addition to determination of wound etiology and wound status, the initial assessment must include assessment of the individual's overall health status, with particular attention to systemic factors and lifestyle factors affecting repair. This involves a focused history and physical examination. Data can be obtained from the patient, patient's family or significant others, caregivers, other health care providers, and the medical record.

Focused Patient History

The patient history information is collected through an interview with key stakeholders (e.g., patient, family, significant others, and caregivers). A focused history is one that targets areas that are most pertinent to patients with wounds, that is, systemic factors and lifestyle factors affecting the repair process.

The interview usually begins with discussion of the "chief complaint," that is, the problem that brought the individual to the clinic or provider, and the duration of the problem. The wound care nurse should investigate the patient's goals, understanding of the etiologic factors contributing to the wound and the interventions required to enhance healing, wound-related concerns, and wound-related symptoms. Helpful questions to ask include the following:

- How did you hope I could help you today?
- When did you first notice the wound? How often have you had wounds?
- What do you think caused your wound? Why do you think it started when it did?
- Does the wound occur in a certain place or under certain circumstances? Is it associated with any specific activity?
- How long do you think the wound will last? What do you think will be required to get the wound to heal?
- What symptoms/problems are you experiencing related to the wound?

Specific questions to be asked in regard to wound-related symptoms include the following:

- What is the location and what are the characteristics of the symptom(s)? (Where do you feel the wound? Show me where it hurts. Do you feel it anywhere else? What does it feel like?)
- How severe is the symptom? When does the symptom appear/what is the timing of the symptom? What are the antecedents and consequences of the symptom(s)? What makes it better? Worse?
- How does the wound interfere with your usual activities? How bad is it?

The next component of the interview is a review of the patient's past health history. Information about management of and response to past problems provides an indication of the patient's potential response to current treatment of the problem. Much of this information may be available in the patient's medical record. If not available, the following general information should be obtained: past general health, accidents or injuries with any associated disabilities, hospitalizations, surgeries, major acute or chronic illnesses, medications, and allergies. Current health information includes allergies (environmental, food, drug), habits, medications, and sleep and exercise patterns.

CLINICAL PEARL

In conducting the health history, it is essential to ask about allergies, as there are a number of potential allergens in wound care products and topical antibiotics.

The nurse should evaluate current and past habits, including alcohol, tobacco, substance, drug, and caffeine use. Alcohol, tobacco, and substance use, in particular, present significant problems for tissue perfusion and nutrition for wound healing. The patient should also be asked about nicotine patches or other common smoking cessation aides in use as these products may also affect tissue perfusion. A full medication profile must be obtained, including prescription, homeopathic or alternative products, and over-the-counter medications, to include names, dosages, frequency, intended effect, and compliance with the regimen.

It is important to assess the patient's usual routine and patterns of activity; one approach is to ask the patient to describe a usual day's activities. Exercise patterns influence wound healing and exercise and mobility are key factors for preventing many wounds. Usual daily (and weekend) activities provide insight into the patient's lifestyle and potential health risks. The nurse should also ask about sleep patterns and whether the patient perceives the sleep to be adequate and satisfactory. The nurse should ask the patient where he or she usually sleeps; patients with severe arterial insufficiency may sleep sitting up in recliner chairs because of the pain associated with the disease. Likewise, patients with chronic obstructive pulmonary disease (COPD) may sleep sitting up because of difficulty breathing in the supine position.

The family health history provides information about the general health of the patient's relatives and family. Family health information is helpful in the identification of genetic, familial, or environmental illnesses. Specific areas to target are diabetes mellitus, heart disease, and stroke. Each of these diseases can impair wound healing in an existing wound and is a risk factor for further wounding. If the patient has a family history of these diseases, he or she may have early signs of the disease as yet undiagnosed and is at higher risk of eventual disease development.

It is important to ask about the patient's sociologic, psychological, and nutritional status. Sociologic data fall into seven areas: relationships with family and significant others, environment, occupational history, economic status and resources, educational level, daily life, and patterns of health care.

Relationships with family and significant others include gathering information on the patient's position and role in the family, the persons living with the patient, the persons to whom the patient relates, and any recent family changes or crises. The role of the patient within the family may dictate treatment decisions. For example, the truck driver with venous ulcers may also be responsible for financial security of the family; thus, it is unrealistic to expect compliance with a care plan that includes restricted driving time. The family support system should be assessed by asking the following questions: Who will change the wound dressing and perform procedures? Who prepares meals? Who will transport the patient to the clinic?

Environment plays a significant role in the health and illness of individuals; thus, the nurse should ask about the home, community, and work environments. Home care patients present challenging environments for wound repair. For example, the homeless patient living alone with a dog on the street will require different management strategies than will the middle-aged man living with a spouse and family in a three-bedroom house in the suburbs. The community environment may provide additional resources for the patient, such as senior citizens' centers, health fairs, or the neighborhood grocery store that delivers to the home. In contrast, the community may also pose significant hazards such as danger from street crime, fall risk because of poorly kept sidewalks or no sidewalks, and inadequate access to healthy food options (prolific fast food restaurants, no healthy options, limited access to fresh fruits/vegetables at local markets).

The work environment and occupational history provides information on the ability of the patient to eliminate certain risk factors for impaired healing. For example, the clerk whose job requires prolonged standing and who has a venous ulcer will need assistance with work setting modifications. Economic status and resources impact on the ability to obtain needed treatment and supplies; it is therefore important to identify patients with inadequate resources (including inadequate health insurance) and to make appropriate referrals for financial assistance.

The educational level of the patient suggests potential health literacy level and learning style, and education is a critical component of wound care for every patient. Thus, patients should be asked about their preferred learning approaches (written materials, audiovisuals, verbal explanations, or demonstrations). Assessment of usual health care and access provides insight into usual attention to health maintenance.

The psychological history includes an assessment of the patient's cognitive abilities (including learning style, memory, comprehension), responses to illness (coping patterns, reaction to illness), response to care (compliance), and cultural implications for care. If there are any concerns as to cognition, the clinician should administer a mental status examination to quantify cognitive status. Previous coping patterns and reactions to illness can be identified with questions such as the following: Have you had difficulties with wound healing in the past? Do you have a history of chronic wounds? A history of recurrent or nonhealing wounds suggests potential problems with adherence to treatment regimens.

Assessment should also identify cultural issues that might impact care and adherence to recommended treatment regimens. The nurse should ask about wound care beliefs and preferences and usual health care resources and providers. It is also important to determine the persons to be involved in the patient's care.

Nutrition plays a major role in wound healing (see Chapter 6 for Nutrition information). Thus, it is important to ask about the patient's usual nutrient intake and any recent unplanned weight loss. Queries regarding foods and fluids ingested during the past 24 hours are an effective means of determining nutritional intake patterns. The nurse should pay particular attention to protein intake and to fruit and vegetable consumption and should also ask about over-the-counter vitamin/mineral and nutritional supplements.

Review of Systems

The systems review portion of the patient history and the physical assessment of each system provide information important for wound diagnosis and on comorbidities that may impair wound healing. Table 3-2 provides guidelines for systems review focused on factors affecting wound development and wound healing, and Chapters 6, 21, and 22 provide in-depth guidelines for assessment of nutritional status, arterial perfusion, venous return, and lymphatic function. The reader should consult physical assessment texts for more in-depth and comprehensive physical assessment parameters and guidelines.

CLINICAL PEARL

Wound healing is a systemic phenomenon; thus, the assessment includes assessment of the many systems that impact on tissue integrity and wound healing.

TABLE 3-2 Systems Review and Assessment

System	Impact on Repair	Factors to Address in History Taking	Parameters to Include in Physical Assessment (if indicated)
Respiratory	Responsible for oxygenation of blood (normal tissue oxygen levels essential for wound repair and infection control)	Cystic fibrosis COPD Lung cancer Pneumonia Post-op status Asthma (consider management/use of steroids/impact of steroids on repair) Current and past tobacco use (attempts to stop tobacco use, willingness to consider smoking cessation, etc.)	Color of mucous membranes/nail beds Lung sounds Pulse oximetry $TcPO_2$ levels if available Pulmonary function tests
Cardiac	Perfusion of tissues	CAD/history of MI Heart failure (to include medications and adherence to medication regimen) HTN (level of control; medications) Hyperlipidemia Cardiac surgery Current and past tobacco use (attempts to stop tobacco use, willingness to consider smoking cessation, etc.)	Pulses (brachial, radial) BP Heart sounds Edema (dependent vs. lower extremity—note dependent edema in patient on bedrest will be in sacral area; unilateral vs. bilateral; severity) Indicators of heart failure (bilateral edema, activity intolerance, shortness of breath, etc.) Advanced practice: auscultation for bruits
Gastrointestinal	Responsible for digestion/absorption of nutrients and fluids	Food and fluid intake (oral, enteral, TPN) Recent unplanned weight loss (% change in weight) Diarrhea (cause?) Fecal incontinence (especially if patient has trunk wound)	Weight and weight trends Indicators of vitamin and mineral deficiencies S/S dehydration (dry MM, reduced skin turgor) Perianal skin status

TABLE 3-2 Systems Review and Assessment (*Continued*)

System	Impact on Repair	Factors to Address in History Taking	Parameters to Include in Physical Assessment (if indicated)
Genitourinary	Elimination of protein waste/ excess fluid and electrolytes	ESRD and management approach (dialysis? protein restriction?) Coexisting DM and HTN? Urinary incontinence	Edema Perineal skin status if patient incontinent UA results BUN/creatinine
Peripheral vascular system	Delivers blood to tissues; returns venous blood and lymph to circulation	LEAD/PAD Vascular surgery (bypass procedures, stent placement, sclerotherapy, etc.) Amputations DVT Chronic venous insufficiency Past arterial or venous ulcers Lymphedema Claudication and level of activity associated with pain Pruritus	Peripheral pulses (femoral, popliteal, DP, PT)—presence and quality (0 = nonpalpable; 1+ = barely palpable; 2+ = normal; 3+ = full; 4+ = bounding) Ankle–brachial index Trophic changes in skin, hair, nails Symmetry of limbs/ evidence calf muscle atrophy Elevational pallor or cyanosis/dependent rubor Temperature of skin on lower extremities Capillary refill Edema (unilateral vs. bilateral, pitting vs. nonpitting), severity using established scale (1+ = 2 mm induration; 2+ = 4 mm induration; 3+ = 6 mm induration; 4+ = 8 mm induration) Varicosities Ankle flare Hemosiderosis Lipodermatosclerosis Atrophie blanche Venous dermatitis Skin changes consistent with lymphedema (cobblestone texture, papillomatous lesions)
Musculoskeletal	Responsible for normal movement and ambulation	Spinal cord injury (level of injury and functional status; assess wheelchair cushion and sleep surface cushion) CVA Parkinson's Arthritis MS	Gait and ambulatory stability ROM Deformities Ability to turn/move self in bed Ability to move extremities
Endocrine	Maintains normal glucose control	DM • Type/duration • Management (diet, insulin, oral agents) • Control (HgbA1C levels, range of values for random glucose checks) • Complications (paresthesias, neuropathy, retinopathy, nephropathy) • Knowledge level/understanding of relationship between glycemic control and wound healing	Gait Results of monofilament testing of sensory function Deformities/callus formation Footwear (appropriateness of fit, abnormal wear patterns) Skin temperature Fissures (heels, between toes)
Medications/ therapies interfering with healing		History of radiation to the involved area Current or recently completed chemotherapy Steroids (>30 mg/day for more than 30 days)	

Although this review of systems with physical assessment guidelines is not inclusive, it provides a framework of those areas of most concern to the clinician managing patients with wounds. The wound nurse must remember that wounds will not heal if there is inadequate systemic support; thus, assessment of perfusion status, nutritional status, use of tobacco products, and glycemic control are of particularly critical importance. In addition, as noted previously, the wound nurse must ask about all medications being consumed and must ask specifically about steroids and agents known to be cytotoxic (such as chemotherapeutic agents) as well as past history of radiation to the area of the wound. Finally, the wound nurse must conduct an open discussion of patient/caregiver goals in relation to the wound and their willingness to adhere to any required lifestyle modifications (such as smoking cessation, tight glycemic control, or consistent off-loading).

CLINICAL PEARL

Intermittent claudication is characterized by reproducible pain or fatigue that is precipitated by a predictable level of activity or elevation and relieved by rest and dependency.

Clinicians can complete the general history, systems review, and physical assessment in about 30 to 40 minutes for a patient with a single wound. An experienced clinician can perform a basic physical assessment in 10 to 15 minutes. Typically, not all information is gathered at the same time. Portions of the history and physical assessment may be gathered over a period of several days, during several clinic visits, or during multiple home visits.

Wound History and Wound Severity

The first step in assessing wound severity is to obtain a detailed wound history and determine how the wound occurred. The wound history should include questions about the onset, duration, and past treatment of the wound. (How long has the wound been present? Have you had previous wounds? How has the wound been treated? What was the response to treatment? What disciplines have been involved in the management of the wound?) It is very important to ask about previous therapy and response in order to avoid repetition of unsuccessful interventions. The patient should be queried regarding his or her understanding of the cause of the wound and their specific wound-related concerns (e.g., exudate, odor, and pain). Wound duration is an important assessment characteristic; current evidence indicates that the longer the diabetic foot ulcer or leg ulcer has been present, the less likely it is to heal within a 12- to 20-week time frame (Kantor & Margolis, 1998, 2000a, 2000b, 2000c; Lantis et al., 2013; Margolis et al., 2004; Margolis, Hoffstad, Allen-Taylor, Berlin, 2002; Margolis et al., 2003b; Robson et al., 2000). Specifically, wounds older than 12 months were significantly less likely to heal within a 12- to 20-week time frame. Wound duration is also an important prognostic indicator for healing of pressure ulcers. Brandeis et al. (1990) showed that pressure ulcer healing was most likely to occur during the first 3 months of therapy, with 32% of stage 3 ulcers and 23% of stage 4 ulcers healing during the 3-month time frame (Brandeis et al., 1990).

CLINICAL PEARL

Data indicate that wound duration is an indicator of potential for healing; the longer the duration of the wound, the less likely it is to heal.

Assessment of wound severity refers to the use of a classification system for diagnosing the severity of tissue trauma by determining the tissue layers involved in the wound. Classification systems such as determining partial- or full-thickness depth, staging pressure ulcers, and grading diabetic ulcers provide objective communication regarding wound severity and the tissue layers involved in the injury. Determining wound severity involves evaluating the wound for depth of tissue involvement and classifying the wound according to an established and accepted system.

Open wounds are classified by depth and level of skin and tissue injury. Partial-thickness wounds involve the epidermis and *part* of the dermis. These lesions are shallow; present as a pink or red shallow ulcer, an abrasion, or a fluid-filled blister; and heal without scar tissue. Full-thickness wounds involve the epidermis, extend all the way through the dermis, and may involve subcutaneous fat tissues, muscle, and underlying structures such as tendons, ligaments, and bones. Full-thickness wounds may be divided into shallow full-thickness wounds (those involving epidermal, dermal structures, and subcutaneous tissues) and deep full-thickness wounds (those involving muscle and underlying structures). Of note, once a wound is full thickness, it will heal with scar tissue formation. Depth of full-thickness wounds depends in part on the anatomic location of the wound; for instance, a full-thickness wound on the calyx of the ear can be very shallow and still involve the epidermis, dermis, and underlying tissues, while a full-thickness wound on the buttocks may be much deeper because the anatomy of the buttock includes adipose tissue and muscle, and the tissue layers in this area are thicker. To determine whether or not the wound is partial or full thickness, the nurse should observe the wound bed for evidence of dermal appendages such as hair follicles, which appear as small red dots within a pale wound bed; the presence of dermal appendages is consistent with a partial thickness wound. The depth of the wound should be evaluated within the context of the anatomic location, recalling that the epidermis is the thinnest on the eyelids at 0.05 mm and the thickest on the palms of the hands and soles of the feet at 1.5 mm and the dermis also varies in thickness from 0.3 mm on the eyelid to 3.0 mm on the back. Average thickness of the epidermal dermal layers combined is 2 mm (0.2 cm); thus, *in general,* a partial-thickness wound is <0.2 cm in depth and a full-thickness wound is >0.2 cm in depth. If the wound is deep full thickness, the nurse should note the additional tissues and structures involved in the wound. Wounds of specific etiology are often further categorized. Pressure ulcers are commonly classified according to grading or staging systems based on the depth of tissue destruction. The National Pressure Ulcer Advisory Panel (NPUAP)/European Pressure Ulcer Advisory Panel (EPUAP) staging classification system is most commonly used to describe depth of tissue damage (NPUAP/EPUAP, 2014). Staging systems measure only one characteristic of the wound, anatomic depth, and should not be viewed as a complete assessment independent of other wound characteristics. Staging systems are best used as a diagnostic tool for indicating wound severity. Chapter 18 presents pressure ulcer staging criteria according to the NPUAP/EPUAP. Pressure ulcer stage is determined by observing the level of visible tissue involvement where a Stage I pressure ulcer and suspected deep tissue injury (DTI) are defined as discoloration of the skin over a bony prominence, erythema, or redness and maroon or purple, respectively. In persons with dark skin tones, the nurse should observe for a deepening of normal ethnic skin color or purple, blue, or gray skin discoloration. A Stage II pressure ulcer is a partial-thickness ulcer with damage to the epidermis and part of the dermis, and Stages III and IV pressure ulcer represent full-thickness ulcers involving deeper tissues and structures such as subcutaneous fat, muscle, tendon, and bone. Diabetic foot ulcers are classified using one of two systems: the Wagner Ulcer Classification System (Wagner, 1981) or the University of Texas System (Armstrong & Harkless, 1998) (see Chapter 23). The Wagner Ulcer Classification System is based on wound depth and the extent of tissue necrosis. The Wagner system includes six grades, progressing from 0 to 5 in order of severity of breakdown. The University of Texas System addresses ulcer depth and also includes the presence of infection and ischemia (Armstrong & Harkless, 1998). Wounds of increasing grade and stage are less likely to heal without vascular repair or amputation (see Chapter 23).

Assessment of Wound Status

The physical examination of the wound is essential for determining baseline wound attributes for comparison with later, follow-along assessments to determine wound progress and response to treatment. Assessment of wound status also provides direction for treatment.

Location

The nurse should first identify the location of the wound using accurate anatomical terms. Body diagrams are a frequently used and helpful tool for documentation of wound location. Location may also be identified by choosing the anatomic site from a list of anatomic locations. It is important to be specific with anatomic terminology. For example, documenting a wound on the "ankle" is not helpful as the wound could be located on the medial or lateral ankle on either the right or left leg. Accurate documentation of wound location allows all clinicians to determine progress (or deterioration) of specific wounds over time and provides a clear (and legally defensible) record, whereas vague or inaccurate documentation of wound location in a patient with multiple wounds can result in confusion as to which wounds are improving and which are plateaued or deteriorating (Fig. 3-3). In addition, anatomic location of the wound is a key determinant of probable wound etiology:

- Wounds caused by arterial insufficiency generally occur at the tips of toes and distal foot, the areas most distal to the heart.
- Venous leg ulcers typically occur on the calf superior to the medial or lateral malleolus.
- Most pressure ulcers occur over bony prominences with the sacral area and heels being the most common locations. Other pressure areas include right and left inner buttocks, ischial tuberosities, trochanters, knees, medial and lateral malleoli, shoulders, and occiput.
- Neuropathic ulcers typically develop on the plantar surface of the foot, most commonly over the metatarsal head of the great or second toe.
- Moisture-associated skin damage: Incontinence-associated dermatitis occurs over the perineal area, buttocks, groin, and possibly in the natal cleft.
- Moisture-associated skin damage: Intertriginous dermatitis occurs within skin folds where there is trapped moisture and may present as a linear break at the base of the fold or as "kissing lesions" on the opposing sides of the fold.
- Friction damage occurs over the fleshy prominences in contact with the seating or lying surface and is typically superficial (partial thickness).
- Skin tears typically occur on the forearms or shins.

Shape

Wound shape, which also helps to determine the overall size of the wound, is determined by evaluating the perimeter of the wound. Shape of the wound is related to wound contraction: As wounds heal, they often change shape and may begin to assume a more regular, circular/oval shape. Wounds that are butterfly shaped or mirror image lesions over the sacrum have been associated with rapid evolution and mortality in one study and have been suggested as a characteristic of terminal pressure ulcers related to skin failure (Kennedy, 1989; Langemo & Brown, 2006; Levine, 2013; Sibbald et al., 2009). Shape of the wound is also associated with specific wound etiology. Wounds that are round, with a punched out appearance, are often arterial in origin. Venous leg ulcers often have an irregular or an oval shape. Intertriginous dermatitis, a type of

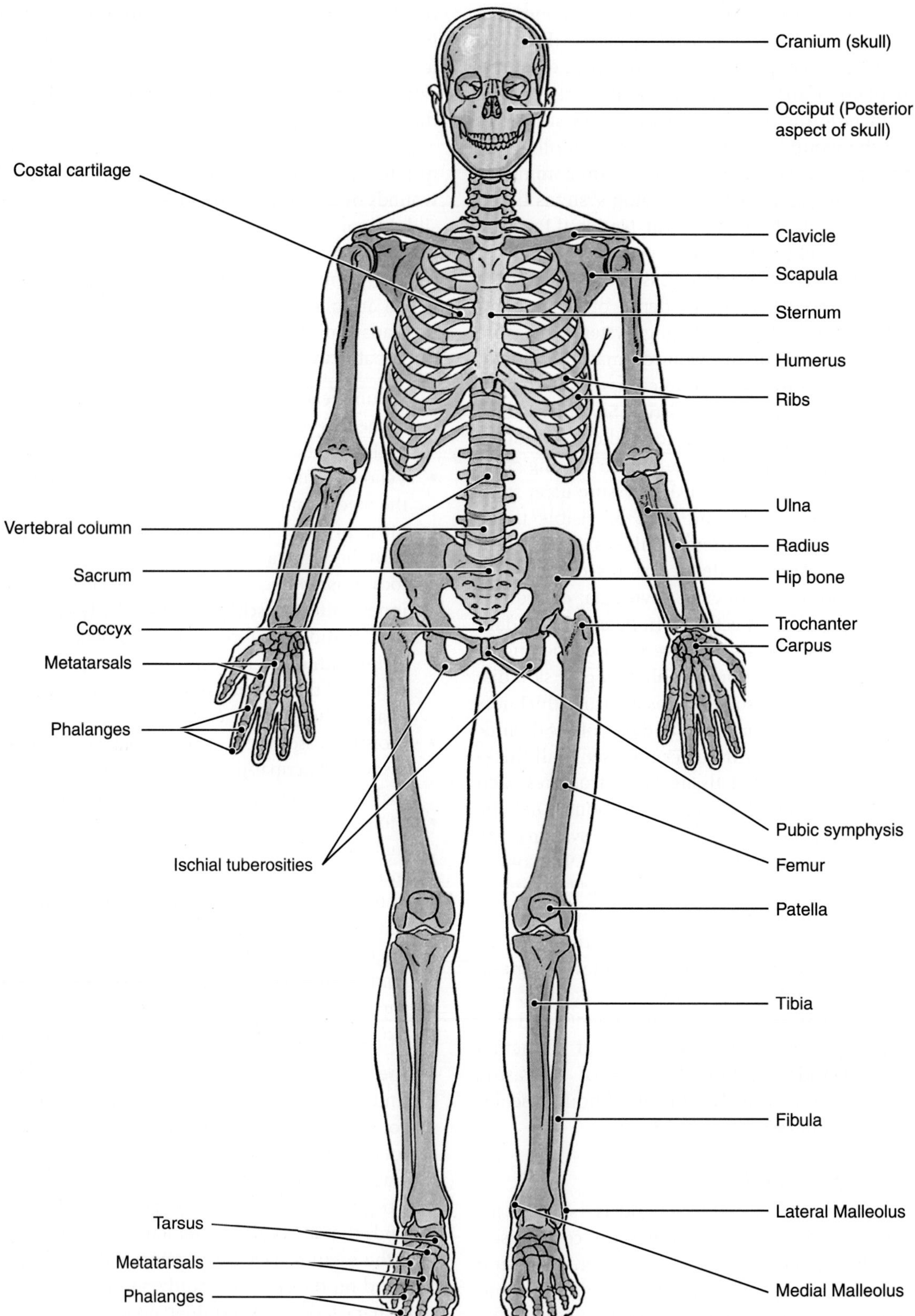

FIGURE 3-3. Chart of anatomic locations/bony prominences.

moisture-associated skin damage, often presents on the buttocks area with "kissing" lesions where two nearly identical wounds present on each buttock at the site where the buttocks touch each other, or as a linear wound in the gluteal cleft.

Size

Wound size can be determined by measuring (in cm) the length and width (perpendicular to the length) of the wound surface that is visible; the nurse can then determine surface area by multiplying the length by the width.

It can be difficult to determine where to measure size on some wounds, because the edge of the wound may be hard to visualize or the edge may be irregular. Use of the same reference points for determining size improves the reliability and meaningfulness of the measurements. In clinical practice, one of two reference points are used: the longest aspect of the wound and the widest aspect of the wound (perpendicular to the length), or the greatest length of the wound from head to toe (or using a clock face to represent the body, 12 o' clock—the head, to 6 o' clock—the feet) and the greatest width of the wound from side to side (or 3 o' clock to 9 o' clock) (Fig. 3-4). Depth is determined by placement of a cotton-tipped applicator or commercial measuring device at the deepest part of the wound. Kantor and Margolis (1998) have shown that simple wound measurements (length, width, length × width for surface area) are highly correlated with more difficult planimetric wound area calculations. The use of simple wound measurements to monitor and predict healing can be used effectively and with confidence in the clinical setting.

Predicting Wound Healing

Multiple studies have demonstrated a clear and significant relationship between rate of change in wound size at four weeks and healing at 12 and 20 weeks (Cardinal et al., 2008; Cardinal et al., 2009a; Kantor & Margolis, 2000a, 2000b, 2000c; Lantis et al., 2013; Margolis, Allen-Taylor, Hoffstad, Berlin, 2002; Margolis et al., 2003b; Robson et al., 2000; Van Rijswijk, 1993; Van Rijswijk & Multicenter Leg Ulcer Study Group, 1993; Van Rijswijk & Polansky, 1994). Van Rijswijk et al. (1993) showed that >30% reduction in surface area of venous leg ulcers at two weeks was a significant predictor of time required for healing. Kantor and Margolis (2000a, 2000b, 2000c) found that percent change in wound area in diabetic foot ulcers and venous ulcers during the first 4 weeks was the best predictor for healing by 24 weeks. Other studies have confirmed that the percent change in wound area or wound trajectory during the first 4 weeks is a predictor of healing at 12 or 24 weeks for both diabetic foot ulcers and venous leg ulcers (Lantis et al., 2013; Margolis, Allen-Taylor, Hoffstad, Berlin, 2002; Robson et al., 2000).

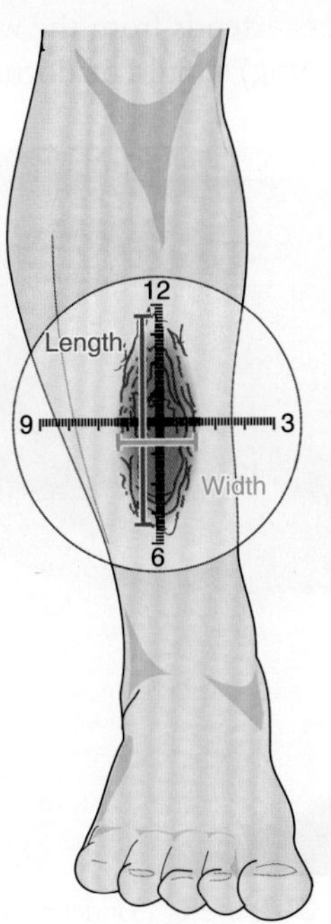

FIGURE 3-4. Wound measurement (length × width).

> **CLINICAL PEARL**
>
> Percent reduction in wound area during the first 4 weeks of appropriate management is an important predictor of healing.

Other markers of size have also demonstrated ability to predict healing at 12 or 24 weeks. In addition to percent area reduction, healing rates of 0.11cm/week or greater have been shown to be predictive of healing for both diabetic foot and venous leg ulcers. Venous ulcers with initial wound area < 10 cm^2 and < 12 months' duration have a 78% chance of healing at week 24 compared to those with initial wound area > 10 cm^2 and > 12 months' duration, which have a 78% chance of nonhealing (Margolis et al., 2004). Other investigators have used more complicated size measures and calculations. Log healing rate, log wound area ratio (Lantis et al., 2013; Margolis et al., 2004; Robson et al., 2000), linear wound margin advance, and mean adjusted wound margin advance (Cardinal et al., 2008, 2009b) are more complicated to calculate, but have also shown ability to predict healing at 12 and 20 weeks based on healing progress at 4 weeks, and this is true for a wide variety of wounds.

Early work in this area found similar results and is the basis for conducting a comprehensive evaluation of the wound's response to therapy at least every 2 weeks. Two clinical studies found that full-thickness pressure ulcers that decreased 47% and 39% in size during the first 2 weeks of treatment were much more likely to heal and were distinguishable from those that did not heal (Sheehan et al., 2003; Van Rijswijk, 1993; Van Rijswijk & Polansky, 1994). Other clinical studies of predictors of healing for leg ulcers found that a >30% reduction in ulcer area after 2 weeks of treatment was a significant predictor of healing (Arnold et al., 1994; Van Rijswijk, 1993). In addition, a retrospective study of prognostic factors for venous ulcer healing found that 40% healing by week 3 predicted more than 70% of the outcomes correctly. Kantor and Margolis report that the percentage of change in area over the first 4 weeks of treatment represents a practical and predictive measure of complete wound healing (Kantor & Margolis, 2000a, 2000b, 2000c). Sheehan et al. (2003) studied diabetic foot ulcers and found that 82% of ulcers with a documented 50% reduction in size at 4 weeks healed, whereas those with a percent change of 25% failed to heal. Of equal importance, the sensitivity of the finding of 50% reduction was 91%, and the negative predictive value was also 91%. (The high negative predictive value indicates that those who do not fall in the healer group have a high likelihood of failure to heal.) The findings related to the rate of reduction in wound size as a predictor of healing within a 12- to 20-week time frame are strong and consistent. The conclusion supported by these studies is that pressure ulcers and leg ulcers (venous and diabetic) that fail to demonstrate a significant reduction in size (30% to 50%) during the first 2 to 4 weeks of therapy are much less likely to heal than ulcers that show a 30% to 50% reduction in wound area. Evaluation of the rate of wound area reduction should be part of all routine wound practice to determine those wounds that require referral for more aggressive therapy.

Depth

As noted, the depth of the wound is measured using a cotton-tipped applicator, which is placed vertically at the deepest part of the wound; a pen is used to draw a line on the applicator at the parallel plane to the skin and then compared to a measuring device. Multiple measures of depth within the wound can increase reliability of depth evaluation.

Edges

Assessment of wound edges is one of the most important components of the wound assessment. When assessing wound edges, the nurse should use observation and palpation to determine the following:

- Are the edges clear and distinct, or indistinct and diffuse? (Edges are indistinct when there are areas where the normal tissues blend into the wound bed). Well-defined edges are clear and distinct from normal skin and can be outlined easily on a transparent piece of plastic.
- Are the edges attached or unattached to the wound bed? Edges that are even with the skin surface and the wound base are attached to the base of the wound; this means that the wound is flat at the edge, with no appreciable depth. Edges that are not attached to the base of the wound imply a wound with some depth of tissue involvement. The wound that is a crater or has a bowl/boat shape with sides and depth is a wound with edges that are not attached to the wound base.
- Are the wound edges open and proliferative, or closed and rolled under? (Fig. 3-5) The edges of chronic wounds frequently become rolled under and thickened to palpation; the development of closed and rolled wound edges is termed epibole. Wounds of long duration may continue to undergo thickening and fibrosis of the wound edges, causing the edge to feel hard, rigid, and indurated to palpation. Hyperkeratosis is the callus-like tissue that may form around the wound edges; this is especially common with neuropathic diabetic foot ulcers. The chronic wound edge achieves a unique coloring over time due to hemosiderin deposits from breakdown of cells and tissues. The pigment turns a grayish brown hue in persons with both dark and light skin tones.

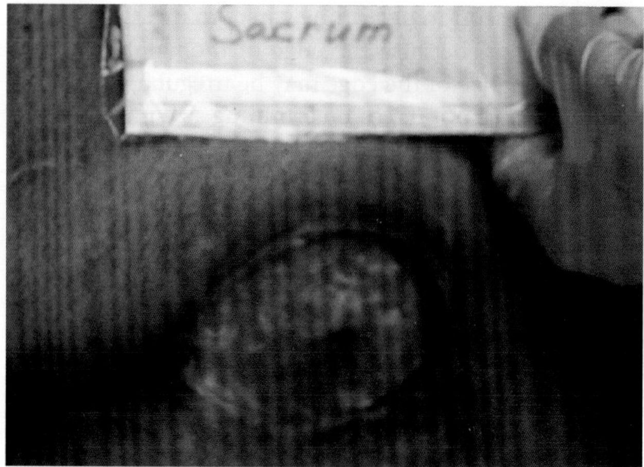

FIGURE 3-5. Wound edges (closed vs. open).

CLINICAL PEARL

Assessment of wound edges is one of the most important components of wound assessment.

Undermining/Tunneling

Undermining, or pocketing, and tunneling represent the loss of tissue underneath an intact skin surface (Figs. 3-6 and 3-7). Undermining and tunneling are measured using a cotton-tipped applicator, which is gently inserted under the edge of the wound and, without undue pressure, advanced as far as possible; the tip of the applicator is then elevated so that it can be seen or felt on the surface of the skin, the surface is marked with a pen, and the distance from the mark on the skin to the edge of the wound is measured. This process is continued all around the wound. The extent of undermining is determined by noting the per cent of the wound edge involved in the process and the distance the process extends from the wound edge; undermining (and tunneling) should be documented in terms of

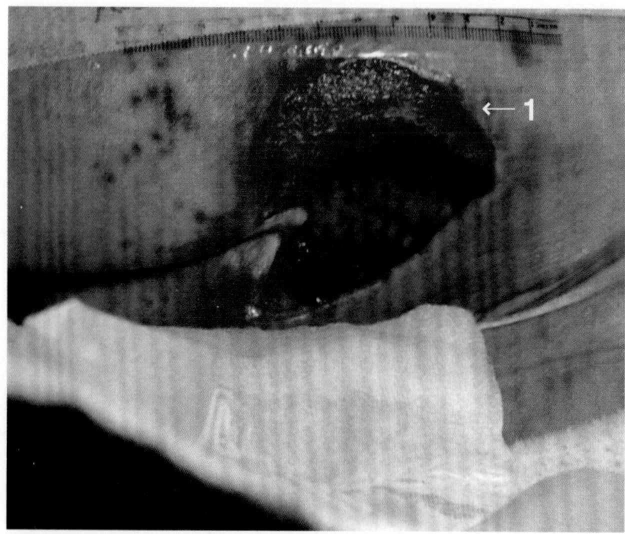

FIGURE 3-6. Undermining.

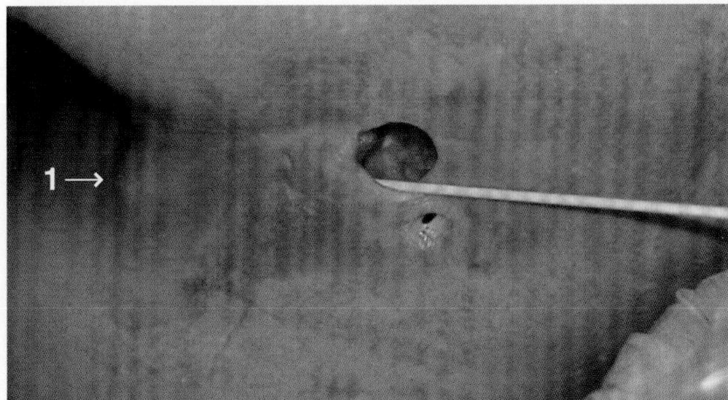

FIGURE 3-7. Tunneling.

location (using clockface) and extension from wound edge (e.g., undermining 3 to 6 o'clock extending 2 to 4 cm from wound edge). Tunneling may occur at other sites besides the wound edge, such as the base of the wound. Tunneling presents as a narrow tract whereas undermining presents as a lip or pocket. Another noninvasive method of assessment of wound pockets is the use of ultrasound to evaluate the undermined tissues. Ultrasonography provides a visual picture of the impaired tissues and can be repeated to monitor for improvement (Ueta et al., 2011). Ultrasound has also been used to evaluate skin thickness over bony prominences in persons with spinal cord injury (Yalcin et al., 2013) and to detect heel ulcers (Helvig & Nichols, 2012).

CLINICAL PEARL

Undermining or tunneling should be documented in terms of location (by clockface) and extension from wound edge.

Necrosis

Necrosis is dead, devitalized tissue. Necrotic tissue should be assessed and documented in terms of amount, color, consistency or moisture content, and adherence to the wound bed. The amount of necrotic tissue present in the wound is evaluated by one of two methods. One method involves using clinical judgment to estimate the percentage of the wound covered with necrosis. (Picture the wound as a pie and divide it into four [25%] quadrants; look at each quadrant and judge how much necrosis is present; estimate the percentage of necrosis in each quadrant, and sum the percentages.) A second method involves actual linear measurements of the necrotic tissue. (Measure the length and width of the necrosis and multiply to determine surface area of necrosis.) Others have used a variety of methods for determining the area of necrotic tissue using computerized planimetry and portable wound measurement systems and have compared results obtained with these systems to visual estimation; data indicate that visual estimation is reliable and consequently a valid technique for daily practice (Laplaud et al., 2010).

The level and type of tissue death influence the clinical appearance of the necrotic tissue. For example, necrosis of the subcutaneous fat typically results in formation of stringy,

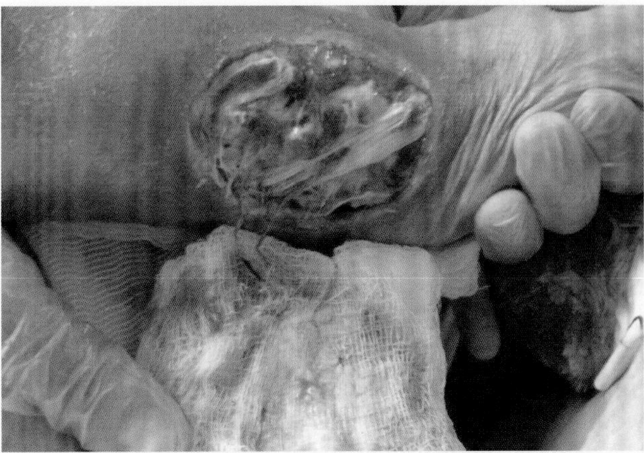

FIGURE 3-8. Slough.

yellow slough, while muscle necrosis results in dead tissue that may be thicker and more tenacious. Necrotic tissue is typically described based on the characteristics of color, consistency, and adherence. Color varies as necrosis worsens, from white/gray nonviable tissue, to yellow slough, and finally to black eschar (Figs. 3-8 and 3-9 A and B). Consistency refers to the cohesiveness of the debris (i.e., thin or thick, stringy or clumpy, moist or dry); typically more advanced

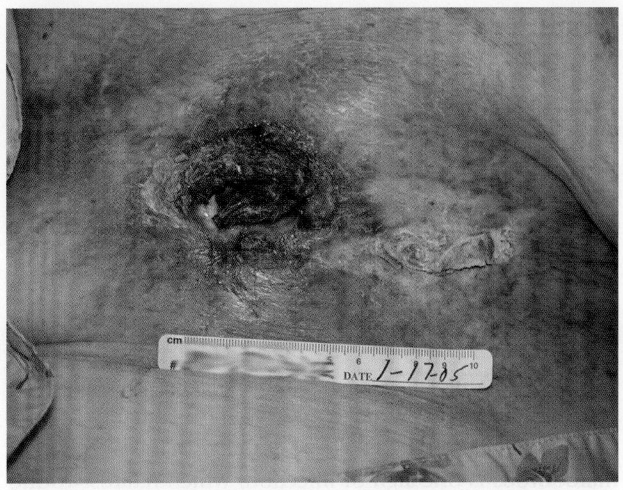

A

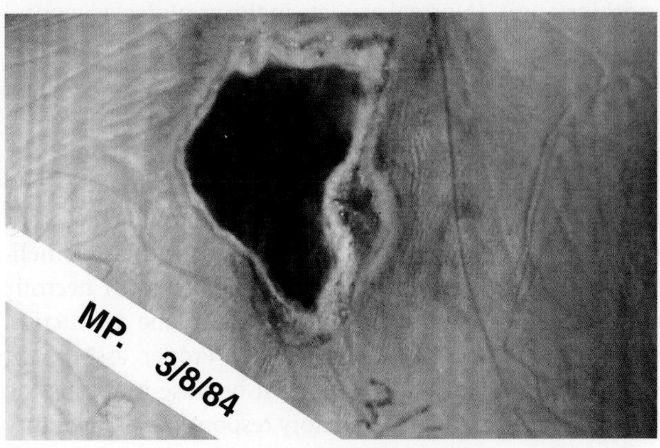

B

FIGURE 3-9. **A, B.** Eschar.

necrosis is thick and dry. *Adherence* refers to the adhesiveness of the necrotic debris to the wound bed tissues and the ease with which the two may be separated. The adherence of the necrotic tissue has major implications for best approaches to debridement, as discussed in Chapter 9. The characteristics of the necrotic tissue change with wound duration, additional trauma and tissue death, and debridement.

The terms *slough* and *eschar* refer to different levels of necrosis and are described according to color, consistency, and adherence. Slough is yellow or tan and may present as thin, mucinous, or stringy fibrin-like material scattered throughout the wound bed or clustered in the base of the wound. In contrast, eschar is associated with deeper tissue damage and is usually black, gray, or brown in color. It may be loosely or firmly adherent to the wound tissues and may be soggy, soft, hard, crusty or leathery in texture. A soft, soggy eschar is usually strongly attached to the base of the wound but may be lifting from (and loose from) the edges of the wound. A hard, crusty leathery eschar is strongly attached to the base and edges of the wound and is sometimes mistaken for a scab. Evidence of underlying tissue necrosis may appear before a wound is apparent, for example, the purple or maroon skin discoloration known as sDTI.

Exudate Type and Amount

Wound exudate (also known as wound fluid, wound drainage) is an important assessment feature, because the volume and characteristics of the exudate contribute to assessment for wound infection, appropriateness of topical therapy, and progress in wound healing. In the acute wound, exudate is tied to wound healing; the volume of exudate should be minimal progressing to none over days 1 to 4 postinjury, and the drainage should be serosanguinous in nature. In chronic wounds, the presence of moderate to large amounts of drainage that persists even after necrotic tissue has been debrided and infection has been treated suggests prolonged inflammation with failure to move to the proliferative phase of wound healing. High volume drainage that is purulent or malodorous is one sign of infection, which retards wound healing, causes odor, and should be treated aggressively in most instances. (Normal exudate in the noninfected wound is usually serous or serosanguinous in nature.) In the infected wound, the exudate may thicken, become purulent, and persist in moderate to large amounts. Examples of exudate changes associated with wound infection include the thick, malodorously sweet-smelling, green drainage associated with *Pseudomonas* infection or the ammonia-like odor characteristic of *Proteus* infection. Wounds with foul-smelling drainage are generally infected or filled with necrotic debris, and healing time is prolonged as tissue destruction progresses (Seiler & Stahelin, 1995). Proper assessment of wound exudate is also important because it affirms the body's brief, normal inflammatory response to tissue injury and is a key consideration in determination of appropriate wound therapy. However, the wound nurse should be aware that exudate is one of the most distressing symptoms for patients with wounds.

Accurate assessment of exudate volume and characteristics is frequently challenging, due to variability resulting from wound size and absorptive capacity of dressings being used. What might be considered a large amount of drainage for a smaller wound may be considered a small amount for a larger wound, making clinically meaningful assessment of exudate difficult. Evaluating exudate type is sometimes confusing, due to the fact that some dressing materials interact with or trap wound fluid to produce exudate with the color and consistency of purulent drainage. For example, both hydrocolloid and alginate dressings mimic a purulent drainage on removal of the dressing. Therefore, assessment of exudate should be undertaken after removal of the wound dressing and wound cleansing with normal saline or water. To judge the amount of exudate in the wound, the nurse should observe both the wound itself and the dressing removed from the wound. (Is the wound surface moist? Dry and desiccated? Macerated due to pooled exudate? Is the dressing completely saturated, 50% saturated, or minimally wet?) The nurse must also take into consideration the absorptive properties of the dressing and the length of time the dressing has been in contact with the wound. For example, the clinician might determine that the alginate dressing was 50% saturated following 24 hours of contact with the wound; based on these data, the clinician might estimate the volume of exudate for this wound as "moderate." Clinical judgment of the amount of wound drainage requires some experience with expected volume of wound exudate in relation to phase of wound healing and type of wound as well as knowledge of absorptive capacity and normal wear time of topical dressings.

CLINICAL PEARL

Assessment of exudate type and volume is an important aspect of wound assessment, but can be confounded by wound size and types of dressings.

Surrounding Skin Characteristics

The tissues surrounding the wound are often the first indication of impending further tissue damage; thus, the nurse should routinely assess the tissues within 4 cm of the wound edges for presence and extent of erythema, edema, induration, maceration, and denudement. Nonblanchable erythema or deep purple, blue, or black discoloration may herald impending extension of the wound due to additional pressure damage; induration (abnormal firmness or hardness of the tissues) is another potential indicator of impending breakdown. (To assess for periwound induration, the wound nurse should gently palpate and "pinch" the tissues, moving from healthy tissue and toward the wound margins.) It is usual to feel slight firmness at the wound edge itself. Normal tissues feel soft and spongy; induration feels hard and firm to the touch. The combination of erythema

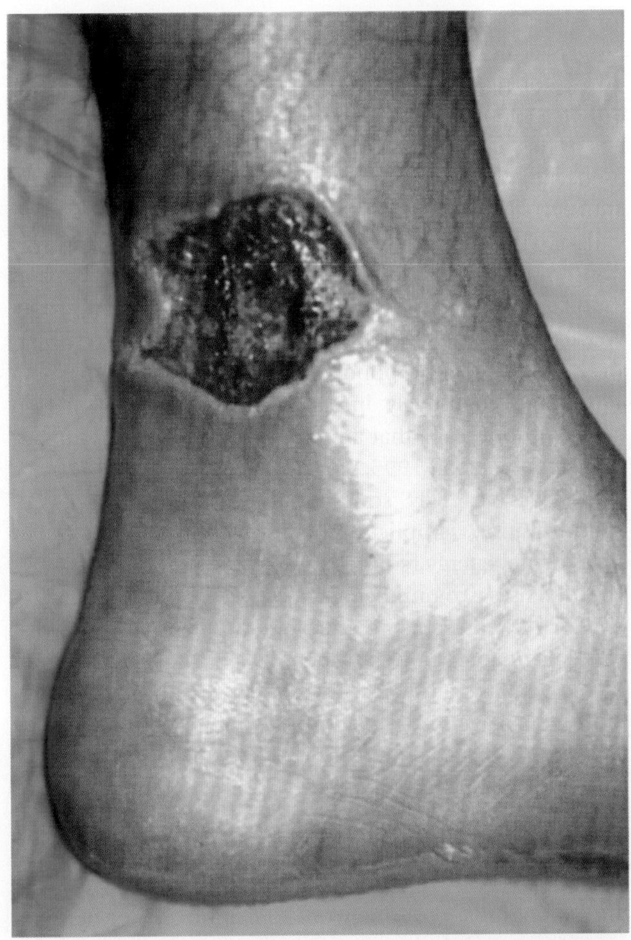

A

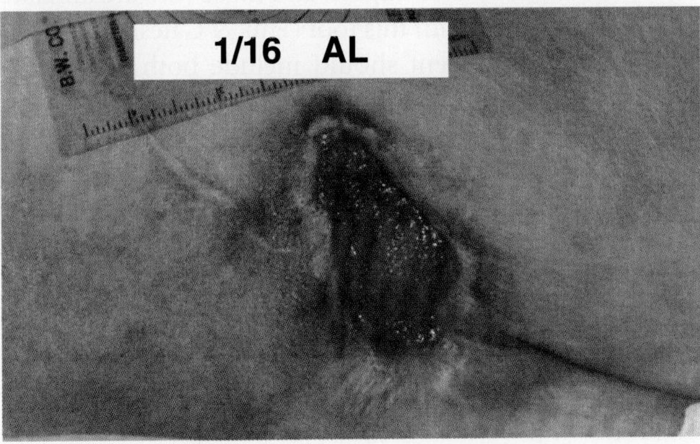

B

FIGURE 3-10. A, B. Granulation tissue.

and induration extending circumferentially around the wound is typically indicative of invasive wound infection. Periwound edema presents an impediment to repair, because it interferes with tissue oxygenation; therefore, the wound nurse should be alert to this finding and should undertake further assessment to determine the extent and severity of the edema, including palpation to determine whether the edema is pitting and to rule out crepitus. Crepitus is the accumulation of air or gas in tissues; is palpated as a grating, popping, or cracking sensation; and is usually indicative of anaerobic infection. Macerated skin is a signal that wound exudate is not being effectively controlled and mandates a change in either dressing type or dressing change frequency. A positive finding is the extension of new epithelium from the wound edge toward the wound center; the new skin is pink and dry, lacks pigmentation, and typically mirrors the outline of the original wound.

Granulation Tissue and Epithelialization

Granulation and epithelial tissues are markers of wound health. They signal the proliferative phase of wound healing and usually foretell wound closure. Granulation tissue is the growth of small blood vessels and connective tissue into the wound cavity. The granulation tissue is healthy when it is bright, beefy red, shiny, and granular with a velvety appearance (Fig. 3-10 A and B). The tissue looks "bumpy" and may bleed easily. Unhealthy granulation tissue, resulting from poor vascular supply or high bacterial loads, appears pale pink or blanched to a dull, dusky red. Usually, the first layer of granulation tissue to be laid down in the wound is pale pink, and, as the granulation tissue deepens and thickens, the color becomes bright, beefy red. The percentage of the wound that is filled with granulation tissue and the characteristics of the granulation tissue are indicators of wound health. The nurse should estimate the percentage of the wound with granulation tissue; while this is easier when the same clinician is performing serial assessments, it is important even if this is the first time the wound has been seen, because it provides data that will be used for comparison at the next assessment.

It is critically important to differentiate between wounds with a pink/red but nongranulating base and wounds that are actively granulating; a pink red smooth base is frequently seen in wounds that have "plateaued" and are not healing, whereas granulation tissue is an indicator of healing. Thus, a viable but nongranulating wound requires further evaluation to determine the reasons for failure to heal (Fig. 3-11).

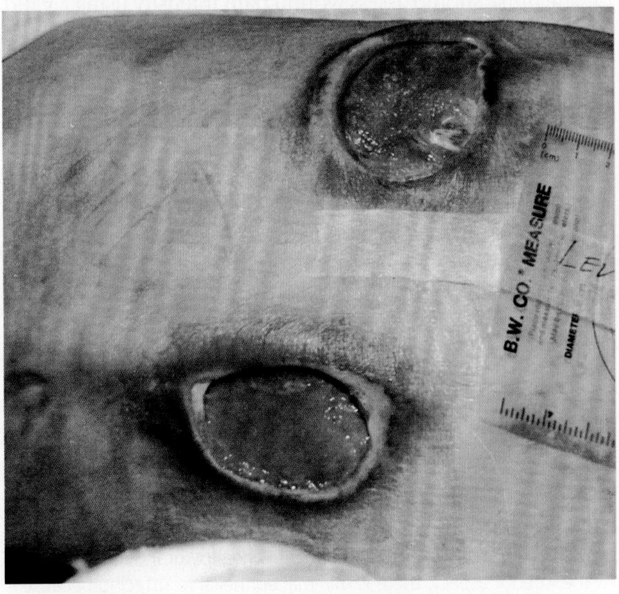

FIGURE 3-11. Viable nongranulating wound bed.

As explained in Chapter 2, partial-thickness wounds heal by epidermal resurfacing and regeneration, specifically the proliferation and migration of epithelial cells from the wound edges and the hair follicles distributed throughout the wound bed. In contrast, full-thickness wounds heal by scar formation: the tissue defect fills with granulation tissue, the edges contract, and the wound is resurfaced by epithelialization. Therefore, epithelialization may occur throughout the wound bed in partial-thickness wounds but only from the wound edges in full-thickness wounds. The new epithelium is pink and dry in people of all races (Fig. 3-12); progress in epithelialization is assessed by determining the percentage of the wound that is covered by new epithelium and the distance from the wound edge to which the new epithelium extends. A transparent measuring guide can be used to help determine the percentage of wound involvement and the distance to which the epithelial tissue extends across the wound.

CLINICAL PEARL

Granulation tissue formation and reepithelialization are indicators of wound healing.

Wound Pain Assessment

Wound assessment would not be complete without an assessment of wound pain, to include the location, distribution, type, quality and intensity, and any aggravating or relieving factors (Krasner, 2011). Location of the pain may include the wound bed itself as well as surrounding skin and tissues. Distribution of the pain may be diffuse or specific to the wound area. The patient should be asked to describe the type of pain. Descriptors such as aching, throbbing, sharp, and dull are characteristic of nociceptive pain, while neuropathic pain is usually described as burning, tingling, "pins and needles," and "electric shock" in nature.

The nurse should assess wound pain intensity using a valid pain severity assessment tool. Pain intensity is commonly measured quantitatively using a visual analog scale (VAS), FACES scale, numerical rating scale (NRS), or verbal descriptor scale (VDS) (Freeman et al., 2001). The VAS is a 0- to 100-mm numbered line with ratio scale properties. It has demonstrated high validity and reliability when used with hospitalized patients (Wewers & Lowe, 1990). However, it may be difficult for children and frail elders, with or without cognitive impairment, to follow the instructions for use of the VAS. The FACES scale consists of six cartoon faces ordered from smiling to crying (Bieri et al., 1990; Wong & Baker, 1988). The FACES scale has been used extensively with pediatric populations. A version for use with adults and cognitively impaired elders uses oval-shaped faces, without tears, that are more adult-like in appearance (Simon & Malabar, 1995; Stuppy, 1998; Taylor et al., 2003). Advantages of FACES scales are the ease and quickness of administration, simplicity, the correlation with VAS, and little mental energy required by the patient (Stuppy, 1998). The NRS uses two number anchors, most typically 0 and 10, in which 0 represents no pain and 10 represents the worst pain imaginable (Paice & Cohen, 1997). The NRS is administered verbally, allowing for use over the phone and with those who have visual or physical impairments such that use of other tools is difficult or not possible. The VDS uses adjectives that reflect extremes of pain and are ranked in order of severity (Manz et al., 2000). Each adjective is given a number that reflects the patient's pain intensity. In general, a VDS is easy to administer and understand. However, the patient must pick one word to describe his or her pain even if no word choice accurately describes it. Furthermore, individuals with limited English and those who are illiterate may have difficulty with this tool (Fink & Gates, 2014).

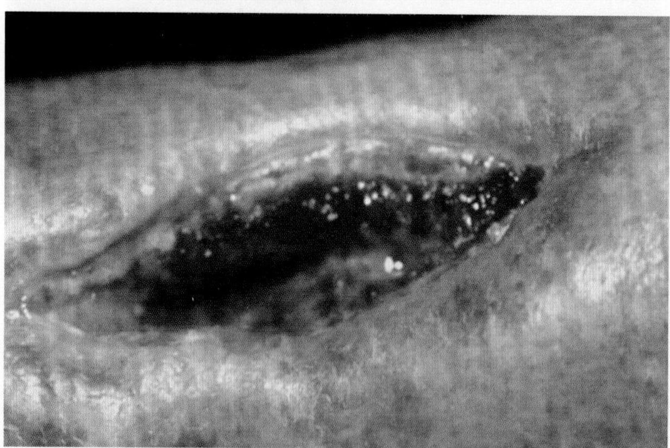

FIGURE 3-12. Epithelial resurfacing. Note epithelial resurfacing at superior aspect of wound, where there is healthy granulation tissue. At the inferior aspect, there is minimal epithelial resurfacing because of poor quality granulation. At the left side of the wound, there is *no* epithelial resurfacing because there is no granulation tissue.

The pain assessment should include both procedural and nonprocedural wound pain. Procedural wound pain is pain experienced during procedures such as dressing changes, repositioning, and debridement (Krasner, 1995; Merskey & Bogduk, 1994). Nonprocedural pain is the pain associated with living with an open wound (Krasner, 1995; Merskey & Bogduk, 1994); it may be "around-the-clock" pain that interferes significantly with activities of daily living and quality of life. The patient should also be asked about pain management strategies and should be queried regarding exacerbating and relieving factors. (What reduces or relieves wound pain? What makes the wound pain worse? How do you manage the pain?) A pain diary can pinpoint the time(s) of day and the activity(ies) associated with pain relief and aggravation, which assists the wound nurse to develop an effective plan for pain management. All pain management strategies, both behavioral and pharmaceutical, should be evaluated in terms of effectiveness. (Is the strategy/medication effective? For how long?) In general, procedural pain can be managed with premedication and with changes in wound care procedures and products. In contrast, around-the-clock pain typically requires around-the-clock analgesia, topical or systemic or both. A pain diary can be useful in monitoring and assessing treatment responses.

CLINICAL PEARL

Assessment of wound-related pain must include type of pain, severity, and exacerbating and relieving factors.

It should be noted that pain patterns and factors exacerbating or reducing the pain are an important aspect of differential assessment. Pain relief for painful venous ulcers typically occurs when the legs are elevated and edema is lessened. In contrast, pain relief for arterial ulcers occurs when the legs are placed in a dependent position as this supports arterial blood flow. Patients with diabetic foot ulcers may complain of tingling or burning sensations, which signal neuropathic pain as compared to nociceptive pain.

Pain related to chronic wounds affects the patient's quality of life, and pain is reported by patients with all types of chronic wounds (Roth et al., 2004; Woo, 2012). If pain is a significant factor for the patient and the goals of care are to improve quality of life, it may also be prudent to conduct a quality of life assessment. There are now several tools available for assessment of quality of life that are specific for patients with wounds (Engelhardt et al., 2014; Gorecki et al., 2011, 2013, 2014).

Wound Inspection

Wound inspection involves observing the wound for signs of complications such as infection, deterioration, or increase in severity and can be conducted by caregivers, family members, the patient, and health care workers. Inspection for infection includes looking for increased wound drainage or purulent drainage, need for more frequent dressing changes due to increased volume of exudate, periwound erythema and induration, foul odor from the wound, and elevated patient temperature. Any increase in bleeding, wound pain, wound size, visible depth, or necrotic tissue should be reported, as should evidence of foreign objects visible in the wound. The inspection findings should be reported to the licensed health care provider for evaluation and determination regarding whether additional assessment is indicated.

Chronic wounds may exhibit signs of wound infection differently than acute wounds often due to immunosuppression of the patient. The classic signs of infection in acute wounds (redness, swelling or edema, pain, increase in temperature, and purulent exudate) are not generally present in chronic wound infection. Signs of chronic wound infection include delayed healing or deterioration of the wound (despite appropriate treatment), pale or dark red and friable granulation tissue, pocketing or tunneling at the base of the wound, and foul odor (Gardner et al., 2001). Chronic wounds are all contaminated with microorganisms, and chronic wounds have been shown to heal in the presence of high levels of microorganisms in contrast to acute wounds; however, excessively high levels of bacteria (critical colonization) impair healing and must be treated, typically with antimicrobial dressings (see Chapter 10). A robust assessment of wound characteristics is important in monitoring for infection.

Follow-Along Serial Assessments

Performing a complete baseline assessment of multiple wound characteristics allows the development of an appropriate care plan. However, baseline assessment and implementation of an appropriate management plan must be followed with ongoing serial assessments to determine responsiveness to therapy. Evaluation of the wound at scheduled intervals allows the provider to determine progress in healing versus a plateau or deterioration in wound status and to revise the treatment plan as appropriate; it often provides an indication of the patient's overall health as well. In many cases, the improvement or deterioration in wound status reflects a change in the patient's overall health status. Progressive monitoring of changes in wound characteristics is also important to determine whether the treatment is effective in meeting the goals for the patient—controlling odor, managing exudate, preventing infection, preparing a clean wound bed, reducing surface area, or minimizing pain. Serial assessment data involving multiple wound characteristics reflect the wound's progression through the wound healing phases. Wounds in the inflammatory phase have differing characteristics than those in the proliferative or remodeling phase of healing, and progress is measured differently for a wound in the inflammatory phase and a wound in the proliferative phase. Monitoring for specific wound characteristic changes as a measure of progression through the wound healing phases is important in providing treatment to support wound closure.

One way to monitor and interpret changes in wound characteristics over time is use of a standardized wound assessment tool. Use of a systematic approach with a comprehensive assessment tool is helpful for tracking and communicating findings and for organizing the assessment process. There are few tools available that encompass multiple wound characteristics to evaluate overall wound status and healing. Two available tools are the Pressure Ulcer Scale for Healing (PUSH) and the Bates-Jensen Wound Assessment Tool (BWAT).

The Pressure Ulcer Scale for Healing (PUSH) is a tool originally developed to measure pressure ulcer healing by the NPUAP (Bartolucci & Thomas, 1997; Stotts et al., 2001; Thomas et al., 1997). It was first developed as a tool for measurement of pressure ulcer healing and has since been evaluated for use in assessment of venous and diabetic ulcer healing (Edwards et al., 2005; Gardner et al., 2011; Hon et al., 2010; Ratliff, 2005). The PUSH tool incorporates surface area measurements, exudate amount, and surface appearance. These wound characteristics were chosen based on principal component analysis to define the best model of healing (Bartolucci & Thomas, 1997; Thomas et al., 1997). The clinician measures the size of the wound, calculates the surface area (length times width), and chooses the appropriate size category on the tool (0 to 10). Exudate is evaluated as none (0), light (1), moderate (2), or heavy (3). Tissue type choices include

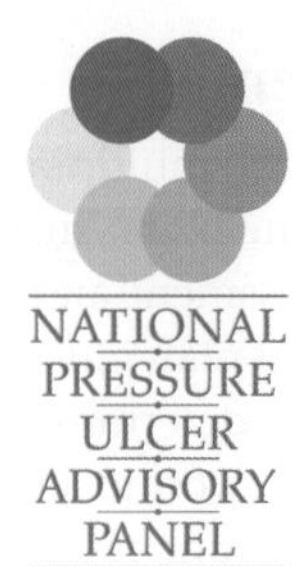

Pressure Ulcer Scale for Healing (PUSH)

PUSH Tool 3.0

Patient Name_______________________________ Patient ID# ______________

Ulcer Location _______________________________ Date ______________

Directions:

Observe and measure the pressure ulcer. Categorize the ulcer with respect to surface area, exudate, and type of wound tissue. Record a sub-score for each of these ulcer characteristics. Add the sub-scores to obtain the total score. A comparison of total scores measured over time provides an indication of the improvement or deterioration in pressure ulcer healing.

LENGTH × WIDTH (in cm²)	0 0	1 < 0.3	2 0.3 – 0.6	3 0.7 – 1.0	4 1.1 – 2.0	5 2.1 – 3.0	**Sub-score**
		6 3.1 – 4.0	7 4.1 – 8.0	8 8.1 – 12.0	9 12.1 – 24.0	10 > 24.0	
EXUDATE AMOUNT	0 None	1 Light	2 Moderate	3 Heavy			**Sub-score**
TISSUE TYPE	0 Closed	1 Epithelial Tissue	2 Granulation Tissue	3 Slough	4 Necrotic Tissue		**Sub-score**
							TOTAL SCORE

Length × Width: Measure the greatest length (head to toe) and the greatest width (side to side) using a centimeter ruler. Multiply these two measurements (length x width) to obtain an estimate of surface area in square centimeters (cm²). Caveat: Do not guess! Always use a centimeter ruler and always use the same method each time the ulcer is measured.

Exudate Amount: Estimate the amount of exudate (drainage) present after removal of the dressing and before applying any topical agent to the ulcer. Estimate the exudate (drainage) as none, light, moderate, or heavy.

Tissue Type: This refers to the types of tissue that are present in the wound (ulcer) bed. Score as a "4" if there is any necrotic tissue present. Score as a "3" if there is any amount of slough present and necrotic tissue is absent. Score as a "2" if the wound is clean and contains granulation tissue. A superficial wound that is reepithelializing is scored as a "1". When the wound is closed, score as a "0".

- 4 – **Necrotic Tissue (Eschar):** black, brown, or tan tissue that adheres firmly to the wound bed or ulcer edges and may be either firmer or softer than surrounding skin.
- 3 – **Slough:** yellow or white tissue that adheres to the ulcer bed in strings or thick clumps, or is mucinous.
- 2 – **Granulation Tissue:** pink or beefy red tissue with a shiny, moist, granular appearance.
- 1 – **Epithelial Tissue:** for superficial ulcers, new pink or shiny tissue (skin) that grows in from the edges or as islands on the ulcer surface.
- 0 – **Closed/Resurfaced:** the wound is completely covered with epithelium (new skin).

www.npuap.org
11F

PUSH Tool Version 3.0: 9/15/98

FIGURE 3-13. PUSH tool. (Used with permission of the National Pressure Ulcer Advisory Panel, 2014.)

closed (0), epithelial tissue (1), granulation tissue (2), slough (3), and necrotic tissue (4). The three subscores are then summed for a total score. Total PUSH scores can be monitored over time for healing or wound degeneration. Aspects of the PUSH tool are included in the Minimum Data Set Assessment, the mandated multidomain assessment instrument used for persons admitted to any CMS-certified long-term care facility. The PUSH tool offers a quick assessment to predict healing outcomes (Fig. 3-13). The PUSH tool is best used as a method for predicting wound healing. Assessment of additional wound characteristics may still be needed, to develop a comprehensive treatment plan for wounds.

The BWAT includes additional wound characteristics that may be helpful in designing a plan of care for the wound. The BWAT (Fig. 3-14) was originally developed as the Pressure Sore Status Tool in 1990 by Bates-Jensen (Bates-Jensen & McNees, 1995, 1996; Bates-Jensen et al., 1992), using a Delphi iterative process with a multidisciplinary panel of experts in wound healing, and subsequently revised in 2001 and 2006. The tool requires evaluation of 13 wound characteristics with a numerical rating scale and rates them from best (1) to worst possible (5). The BWAT includes location and shape (nonscored items), size, depth, edges, undermining or pockets, necrotic tissue type, necrotic tissue amount, exudate type, exudate amount, surrounding skin color, peripheral tissue edema, peripheral tissue induration, granulation tissue, and epithelialization. The 13 wound characteristics appear with descriptors rated on a scale of 1 (best for that characteristic) to 5 (worst attribute of the characteristic). It is recommended that wounds be scored initially for a baseline assessment and at regular intervals to evaluate therapy and healing progress. Once a wound has been assessed for each item on the BWAT, the 13 item scores can be summed for a total score. The total score can then be monitored to determine progress in healing or degeneration of the wound. Total scores range from 9 (skin intact but always at risk for further damage) to 65 (profound tissue degeneration). The BWAT is widely used in a variety of health care settings with all chronic wounds (Bolton et al., 2004; De Laat et al., 2005).

An additional benefit associated with the assignment of numeric values to items on the BWAT is that it assists in setting interim wound healing goals. Clinical experience shows that not all wounds heal and certainly not always in the same setting. The BWAT allows for goal setting as appropriate to the health care setting and the individual patient and wound. For example, the patient with a large, necrotic, full-thickness wound in acute care will probably not be in the facility long enough for the wound to heal completely. However, the BWAT enables clinicians to set intermediate or secondary goals, such as "Necrotic tissue in the wound will decrease in amount and type." The BWAT allows for monitoring of improvement or deterioration in individual characteristics as well as the total score. This in turn enables assessment of the patient's response to specific treatments. For example, the characteristics of necrotic tissue type and amount may be tracked with exudate type and amount to evaluate the response to debridement or infection management. The ability to track wound symptoms such as exudate allows evaluation of interventions designed to alleviate distressing wound symptoms and as such is useful.

There is also a pictorial guide for training health professionals in use of the BWAT (Harris et al., 2010). The BWAT Pictorial Guide includes 102 photographs of a variety of wound types, not just pressure ulcers, illustrating each descriptor for each of the BWAT items. Validation of the photographic content was accomplished in a three-stage consensus process working with nurses specializing in wound care.

In addition to being used to identify specific wound treatments, the BWAT has been used to describe characteristics of recurrent pressure ulcers in persons with spinal cord injury as these ulcers have not been well described. Because the BWAT evaluates multiple wound characteristics, it is particularly well suited for describing specific wound characteristics in special populations or wounds. For example, recurrent pressure ulcers in persons with spinal cord injury tend to occur at the same anatomic location as the original ulcer and present as full-thickness ulcers with a mean BWAT score of 33.63, with minimal exudate, and with nearly half presenting with undermining (48%) and necrotic slough (50%) (Bates-Jensen et al., 2009). The BWAT has also been used as an outcome measure examining the use of negative pressure wound therapy for pressure ulcers in a long-term acute care setting (de Leon et al., 2009), and a change in total BWAT score at one week predicts 50% wound healing as evidenced by change in surface area (Bates-Jensen, 1999). The BWAT is incorporated into several health care organizational electronic medical records (EMR) and lends itself well to EMR in terms of data entry and data access for reports.

To assist clinicians in assessing wound bed preparation prior to application of advanced technology therapy, Falanga and colleagues developed the Wound Bed Score (WBS) to specifically address wound bed preparation (Falanga, 2008; Falanga et al., 2006). The WBS consists of a score for wound bed appearance (based on granulation tissue, fibrinous tissue, and presence of eschar) and a wound exudate score (based on exudate control, exudate amount, and dressing requirements). Additional items relating to the surrounding skin (healing edges, edema, periwound dermatitis, and callus) are also included. Each item receives a score from 0 (worst score) to 2 (best score) with all items summed for a total score. The WBS has been used in venous ulcers and correlated with healing (Falanga et al., 2006). The instrument can be used at the bedside to determine the likelihood that wound closure will occur. The higher the score, the more favorable

BATES-JENSEN WOUND ASSESSMENT TOOL

Instructions for use

General Guidelines:

Fill out the attached rating sheet to assess a wound's status after reading the definitions and methods of assessment described below. Evaluate once a week and whenever a change occurs in the wound. Rate according to each item by picking the response that best describes the wound and entering that score in the item score column for the appropriate date. When you have rated the wound on all items, determine the total score by adding together the 13-item scores. The HIGHER the total score, the more severe the wound status. Plot total score on the Wound Status Continuum to determine progress. If the wound has healed/resolved, score items 1,2,3 and 4 as =0.

Specific Instructions:

1. **Size**: Use ruler to measure the longest and widest aspect of the wound surface in centimeters; multiply length × width. Score as = 0 if wound healed/resolved.

2. **Depth**: Pick the depth, thickness, most appropriate to the wound using these additional descriptions, score as =0 if wound healed/resolved:

   1 = tissues damaged but no break in skin surface.
   2 = superficial, abrasion, blister or shallow crater. Even with, &/or elevated above skin surface (e.g., hyperplasia).
   3 = deep crater with or without undermining of adjacent tissue.
   4 = visualization of tissue layers not possible due to necrosis.
   5 = supporting structures include tendon, joint capsule.

3. **Edges**: Score as = 0 if wound healed/resolved. Use this guide:

   Indistinct, diffuse = unable to clearly distinguish wound outline.
   Attached = even or flush with wound base, no sides or walls present; flat.
   Not attached = sides or walls are present; floor or base of wound is deeper than edge.
   Rolled under, thickened = soft to firm and flexible to touch.
   Hyperkeratosis = callous-like tissue formation around wound & at edges.
   Fibrotic, scarred = hard, rigid to touch.

4. **Undermining**: Score as = 0 if wound healed/resolved. Assess by inserting a cotton tipped applicator under the wound edge; advance it as far as it will go without using undue force; raise the tip of the applicator so it may be seen or felt on the surface of the skin; mark the surface with a pen; measure the distance from the mark on the skin to the edge of the wound. Continue process around the wound. Then use a transparent metric measuring guide with concentric circles divided into 4 (25%) pie-shaped quadrants to help determine percent of wound involved.

5. **Necrotic Tissue Type**: Pick the type of necrotic tissue that is predominant in the wound according to color, consistency and adherence using this guide:

   White/gray non-viable tissue = may appear prior to wound opening; skin surface is white or gray.
   Non-adherent, yellow slough = thin, mucinous substance; scattered throughout wound bed; easily separated from wound tissue.
   Loosely adherent, yellow slough = thick, stringy, clumps of debris; attached to wound tissue.
   Adherent, soft, black eschar = soggy tissue; strongly attached to tissue in center or base of wound.
   Firmly adherent, hard/black eschar = firm, crusty tissue; strongly attached to wound base and edges (like a hard scab).

FIGURE 3-14. Bates-Jensen Wound Assessment Tool (BWAT). (Copyright © 2001 Barbara Bates-Jensen.)

6. **Necrotic Tissue Amount**: Use a transparent metric measuring guide with concentric circles divided into 4 (25%) pie-shaped quadrants to help determine percent of wound involved.

7. **Exudate Type**: Some dressings interact with wound drainage to produce a gel or trap liquid. Before assessing exudate type, gently cleanse wound with normal saline or water. Pick the exudate type that is predominant in the wound according to color and consistency, using this guide:

Bloody	=	thin, bright red
Serosanguineous	=	thin, watery pale red to pink
Serous	=	thin, watery, clear
Purulent	=	thin or thick, opaque tan to yellow or green may have offensive odor

8. **Exudate Amount**: Use a transparent metric measuring guide with concentric circles divided into 4 (25%) pie-shaped quadrants to determine percent of dressing involved with exudate. Use this guide:

None	=	wound tissues dry.
Scant	=	wound tissues moist; no measurable exudate.
Small	=	wound tissues wet; moisture evenly distributed in wound; drainage involves ≤ 25% dressing.
Moderate	=	wound tissues saturated; drainage may or may not be evenly distributed in wound; drainage involves > 25% to ≤ 75% dressing.
Large	=	wound tissues bathed in fluid; drainage freely expressed; may or may not be evenly distributed in wound; drainage involves > 75% dressing.

9. **Skin Color Surrounding Wound**: Assess tissues within 4cm of wound edge. Dark-skinned persons show the colors "bright red" and "dark red" as a deepening of normal ethnic skin color or a purple hue. As healing occurs in dark-skinned persons, the new skin is pink and may never darken.

10. **Peripheral Tissue Edema & Induration**: Assess tissues within 4cm of wound edge. Non-pitting edema appears as skin that is shiny and taut. Identify pitting edema by firmly pressing a finger down into the tissues and waiting for 5 seconds, on release of pressure, tissues fail to resume previous position and an indentation appears. Induration is abnormal firmness of tissues with margins. Assess by gently pinching the tissues. Induration results in an inability to pinch the tissues. Use a transparent metric measuring guide to determine how far edema or induration extends beyond wound.

11. **Granulation Tissue**: Granulation tissue is the growth of small blood vessels and connective tissue to fill in full thickness wounds. Tissue is healthy when bright, beefy red, shiny and granular with a velvety appearance. Poor vascular supply appears as pale pink or blanched to dull, dusky red color.

12. **Epithelialization**: Epithelialization is the process of epidermal resurfacing and appears as pink or red skin. In partial thickness wounds it can occur throughout the wound bed as well as from the wound edges. In full thickness wounds it occurs from the edges only. Use a transparent metric measuring guide with concentric circles divided into 4 (25%) pie-shaped quadrants to help determine percent of wound involved and to measure the distance the epithelial tissue extends into the wound.

FIGURE 3-14. *(Continued)*

BATES-JENSEN WOUND ASSESSMENT TOOL NAME

Complete the rating sheet to assess wound status. Evaluate each item by picking the response that best describes the wound and entering the score in the item score column for the appropriate date. If the wound has healed/resolved, score items 1,2,3, & 4 as =0.

Location: Anatomic site. Circle, identify right **(R)** or left **(L)** and use **"X"** to mark site on body diagrams:

____ Sacrum & coccyx ____ Lateral ankle
____ Trochanter ____ Medial ankle
____ Ischial tuberosity ____ Heel
____ Buttock ____ Other site: ____________

Shape: Overall wound pattern; assess by observing perimeter and depth.
Circle and date appropriate description:

____ Irregular ____ Linear or elongated
____ Round/oval ____ Bowl/boat
____ Square/rectangle ____ Butterfly Other Shape

Item	Assessment	Date Score	Date Score	Date Score
1. Size*	*0 = Healed, resolved wound 1 = Length x width <4 sq cm 2 = Length x width 4--<16 sq cm 3 = Length x width 16.1--<36 sq cm 4 = Length x width 36.1--<80 sq cm 5 = Length x width >80 sq cm			
2. Depth*	*0 = Healed, resolved wound 1 = Non-blanchable erythema on intact skin 2 = Partial thickness skin loss involving epidermis &/or dermis 3 = Full thickness skin loss involving damage or necrosis of subcutaneous tissue; may extend down to but not through underlying fascia; &/or mixed partial & full thickness &/or tissue layers obscured by granulation tissue 4 = Obscured by necrosis 5 = Full thickness skin loss with extensive destruction, tissue necrosis or damage to muscle, bone or supporting structures			
3. Edges*	*0 = Healed, resolved wound 1 = Indistinct, diffuse, none clearly visible 2 = Distinct, outline clearly visible, attached, even with wound base 3 = Well-defined, not attached to wound base 4 = Well-defined, not attached to base, rolled under, thickened 5 = Well-defined, fibrotic, scarred or hyperkeratotic			
4. Under-mining*	*0 = Healed, resolved wound 1 = None present 2 =Undermining < 2 cm in any area 3 = Undermining 2-4 cm involving < 50% wound margins 4 = Undermining 2-4 cm involving > 50% wound margins 5 = Undermining > 4 cm or Tunneling in any area			
5. Necrotic Tissue Type	1 = None visible 2 = White/grey non-viable tissue &/or non-adherent yellow slough 3 = Loosely adherent yellow slough 4 = Adherent, soft, black eschar 5 = Firmly adherent, hard, black eschar			
6. Necrotic Tissue Amount	1 = None visible 2 = < 25% of wound bed covered 3 = 25% to 50% of wound covered 4 = > 50% and < 75% of wound covered 5 = 75% to 100% of wound covered			

FIGURE 3-14. *(Continued)*

Item	Assessment	Date Score	Date Score	Date Score
7. Exudate Type	1 = None 2 = Bloody 3 = Serosanguineous: thin, watery, pale red/pink 4 = Serous: thin, watery, clear 5 = Purulent: thin or thick, opaque, tan/yellow, with or without odor			
8. Exudate Amount	1 = None, dry wound 2 = Scant, wound moist but no observable exudate 3 = Small 4 = Moderate 5 = Large			
9. Skin Color Surrounding Wound	1 = Pink or normal for ethnic group 2 = Bright red &/or blanches to touch 3 = White or grey pallor orhypopigmented 4 = Dark red or purple &/or non-blanchable 5 = Black or hyperpigmented			
10. Peripheral Tissue Edema	1 = No swelling or edema 2 = Non-pitting edema extends <4 cm around wound 3 = Non-pitting edema extends >4 cm around wound 4 = Pitting edema extends < 4 cm around wound 5 = Crepitus and/or pitting edema extends >4 cm around wound			
11. Peripheral Tissue Induration	1 = None present 2 = Induration, < 2 cm around wound 3 = Induration 2-4 cm extending < 50% around wound 4 = Induration 2-4 cm extending > 50% around wound 5 = Induration > 4 cm in any area around wound			
12. Granulation Tissue	1 = Skin intact or partial thickness wound 2 = Bright, beefy red; 75% to 100% of wound filled &/or tissue overgrowth 3 = Bright, beefy red; < 75% & > 25% of wound filled 4 = Pink, &/or dull, dusky red &/or fills ≤ 25% of wound 5 = No granulation tissue present			
13. Epithelialization	1 = 100% wound covered, surface intact 2 = 75% to <100% wound covered &/or epithelial tissue extends >0.5 cm into wound bed 3 = 50% to <75% wound covered &/or epithelial tissue extends to <0.5 cm into wound bed 4 = 25% to < 50% wound covered 5 = < 25% wound covered			
	TOTAL SCORE			
	SIGNATURE			

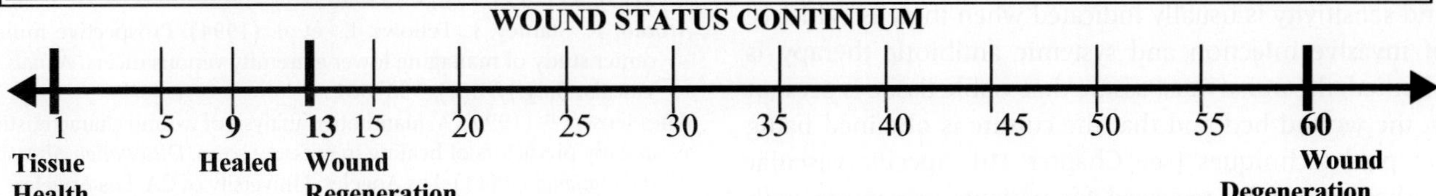

Plot the total score on the Wound Status Continuum by putting an "X" on the line and the date beneath the line. Plot multiple scores with their dates to see-at-a-glance regeneration or degeneration of the wound.

FIGURE 3-14. *(Continued)*

the wound outcome and total scores are divided into 4 quartiles: scores up to 9, scores of 10 and 11, scores of 12 and 13, and scores of 14 to 16. For each quartile increase, there is a 22% increased chance of healing (Falanga et al., 2006).

Wound healing assessment tools provide a framework for assessment and documentation of wound healing, with an attempt at quantification of multiple wound characteristics. Thus, their use should promote more meaningful communication among health care professionals involved in wound care. An objective method of assessing wound healing and monitoring changes over time also allows for evaluation of the care plan and may be used to guide and direct therapy. For example, if a specific treatment modality is in use and the patient's wound status, as determined with the wound healing tool, has not changed in two weeks, reevaluation of the plan of care is warranted.

Laboratory and Diagnostic Tests

Specific laboratory and diagnostic tests to be included in a comprehensive assessment include data on nutrition, glucose management, and tissue oxygenation and perfusion. Nutritional parameters typically include evaluation of serum albumin. Serum albumin is a measure of protein available for healing; a normal level is >3.5 mg/dL. Additional measures of nutrition include prealbumin levels and total lymphocyte count. Clinicians should evaluate laboratory values such as arterial blood gases and transcutaneous oximetry to assess tissue perfusion and oxygenation abilities. Review of laboratory values is also prudent in determining the level of diabetic control. Normal glucose levels are 80 to 120 mg/dL. Concentrations of 180 to 250 mg/dL or higher indicate that glucose levels are out of control. The goal is to maintain fasting blood glucose concentrations lower than 140mg/dL and a glycosylated hemoglobin concentration (HgbA1C) lower than 7%. The HgbA1C helps to determine the level of glucose control the patient has had over the last 2 to 3 months. The wound nurse should also evaluate hemoglobin and hematocrit for possible anemia; significant anemia compromises oxygen delivery to the tissues and mandates treatment in situations where the goal is wound healing. Wound culture and sensitivity is usually indicated when there is evidence of invasive infection and systemic antibiotic therapy is planned; the nurse must assure that viable tissue is present in the wound bed and that the culture is obtained using accepted techniques (see Chapter 10). Specific vascular studies should be reviewed for patients presenting with lower leg ulcers and diabetic foot ulcers. Laser Doppler flow studies provide data on both arterial and venous systems and in particular microflow disorders (Belcaro et al., 2007). For ulcers of arterial origin, arterial duplex scans, segmental pressures including toe pressures, pulse volume recordings, magnetic resonance angiography, and rapid sequence CT scans are noninvasive macrocirculation studies that may be ordered. An interventional angiogram and MRA (magnetic resonance angiography) are more specific diagnostic tests for arterial ulcers.

While many diagnostic tests are available for evaluating patients with venous ulcers, the duplex scan is essential and is the primary assessment tool (Ennis, 2012). Duplex scanning is a routine test used to rule out acute deep vein thrombosis in the hospital setting. Duplex scanning is noninvasive and portable, and accuracy is generally reported as over 90% for detecting femoral–popliteal thrombosis (Miller et al., 1996). There are four important components of all duplex scans, and these include visualization of the vein, compressibility of the vein wall, spontaneous venous flow, and the ability to augment flow with a compression force distal to the probe. Venous outflow can also be measured with impedance and/or strain gauge plethysmography (Hirai et al., 1985; Ting et al., 1999).

Assessment of the patient with a wound is complicated by multiple factors that influence the etiology of the wound and wound healing. Attention to all assessment parameters is crucial in developing a plan of care that results in optimal outcomes.

Conclusion

Accurate and comprehensive assessment of the individual with a wound is foundational to effective management. The initial assessment must include determination of wound etiology, assessment of the individual's ability to heal (systems review), determination of wound-related concerns and priorities from the perspective of the patient and caregiver, and in-depth assessment of wound status. Follow-up assessments focus on progress in wound healing. Structured wound assessment tools have been proven to be of significant benefit in objectively documenting progress (or deterioration) in healing.

REFERENCES

Armstrong, D. G., & Harkless, L. B. (1998, May). Validation of a diabetic wound classification system. The contribution of depth, infection, and ischemia to risk of amputation. *Diabetes Care, 21*(5), 855–859, PMID: 9589255.

Arnold, T., Stanley, J., Fellows, E., et al. (1994). Prospective multicenter study of managing lower extremity venous ulcers. *Annals of Vascular Surgery, 8*(4), 356–362.

Bates-Jensen, B. (1999). A quantitative analysis of wound characteristics as early predictors of healing in pressure sores. *Dissertation Abstracts International, 59*(11), Los Angeles: University of CA, Los Angeles.

Bates-Jensen, B., Guihan, M., Garber, S. L., et al. Characteristics of recurrent pressure ulcers in veterans with spinal cord injury. (2009). *The Journal of Spinal Cord Medicine, 32*(1), 34–42.

Bates-Jensen, B. M., & McNees, P. (1996). The wound intelligence system: Early issues and findings from multi-site tests. *Ostomy/Wound Management, 42*(Suppl 7A), 1–7.

Bates-Jensen, B., & McNees, P. (1995). Toward an intelligent wound assessment system. *Ostomy/Wound Management, 41*(Suppl 7A), 80–88.

Bates-Jensen, B. M., & Sussman, C. (2012). Tools to measure wound healing. In C. Sussman. & B. M. Bates-Jensen (Eds.), *Wound care: A collaborative practice manual for health care practitioners* (4th ed.). Baltimore, MD: Lippincott Williams & Wilkins.

Bates-Jensen, B. M., Vredevoe, D., & Brecht, M. L. (1992). Validity and reliability of the pressure sore status tool. *Decubitus, 5*(6), 20–28.

Bartolucci, A. A., & Thomas D. R. (1997). Using principal component analysis to describe wound status. *Advances in Wound Care, 10*(5), 93–95.

Belcaro, G., Cesarone, M. R., Errichi, B. M., et al. (2007). Improvement of microcirculation and healing of venous hypertension and ulcers with Crystacide: evaluation with a microcirculatory model, including free radicals, laser doppler flux, and PO2/PCO2 measurements. *Angiology, 58*(3), 323–328.

Bieri, D., Reeve, R., Champion, G., et al. (1990). The Faces Pain Scale for the self assessment of the severity of pain experienced by children: Development, initial validation, and preliminary investigation for ratio scale properties. *Pain, 41*, 139–150.

Bolton, L., McNees, P., Van Rijswijk, L., et al. (2004). Wound-healing outcomes using standardized assessment and care in clinical practice. *Journal of Wound, Ostomy, and Continence Nursing, 31*(2), 65–71.

Brandeis, G., Morris, J., Nash, D., et al. (1990). The epidemiology and natural history of pressure ulcers in elderly nursing home residents. *Journal of the American Medical Association, 264*(22), 2905–2909.

Bryant, R. A. (2011). Types of skin damage and differential diagnosis. In R. A. Bryant & D. P. Nix (Eds.), *Acute & chronic wounds* (pp. 83–84). St. Louis, MO: Elsevier Mosby.

Cardinal, M., Eisenbud, D. E., & Armstrong, D. G. (2009a). Wound shape geometry measurements correlate to eventual wound healing. *Wound Repair and Regeneration, 17*(2), 173–178.

Cardinal, M., Eisenbud, D. E., Phillips, T., et al. (2008). Early healing rates and wound area measurements are reliable predictors of later complete wound closure. *Wound Repair and Regeneration, 16*, 19–22.

Cardinal, M., Phillips, T., Eisenbud, D. E., et al. (2009b). Nonlinear modeling of venous leg ulcer healing rates, *BMC Dermatology, 9*, 2.

Centers for Medicare & Medicaid Services (CMS) (2009). Proposed Fiscal Year 2009 Payment, Policy Changes for Inpatient Stays in General Acute Care Hospitals. Available at http://www.cms.hhs.gov/apps/media/press/factsheet.asp. Accessed August 4, 2014.

Centers for Medicare & Medicaid Services. (2008.) Medicare Program; Proposed Changes to the Hospital Inpatient Prospective Payment Systems and Fiscal Year 2009 Rates; Proposed Changes to Disclosure of Physician Ownership in Hospitals and Physician Self-Referral Rules; Proposed Collection of Information Regarding Financial Relationships Between Hospitals and Physicians: Proposed Rule. *Federal Register, 73*(84), 23550. Available at http://edocket.access.gpo.gov/2008/pdf/08-1135.pdf. Accessed August 4, 2010.

De Laat, E. H., Scholte, O. P., Reimer, W. H., et al. (2005). Pressure ulcers: Diagnostics and interventions aimed at wound-related complaints: A review of the literature. *Journal of Clinical Nursing, 14*(4), 464–472.

de Leon, J. M., Barnes, S., Nagel, M., et al. (2009 Mar). Cost-effectiveness of negative pressure wound therapy for postsurgical patients in long-term acute care. *Advances in Skin and Wound Care, 22*(3), 122–127.

Edwards, H., Courtney, M., Finlayson, K., et al. (2005). Improved healing rates for chronic venous leg ulcers: pilot study results from a randomized controlled trial of a community nursing intervention. *International Journal of Nursing Practice, 11*(4), 169–176.

Engelhardt, M., Spech, E., Diener, H., et al. (2014 Sep). Validation of the disease-specific quality of life Wuerzburg Wound Score in patients with chronic leg ulcer. *Journal of Vascular Diseases, 43*(5), 372–379.

Ennis, W. J., Borhani, M., & Meneses, P. (2012). Management and diagnosis of vascular ulcers. In C. Sussman, & B. M. Bates-Jensen (Eds.), *Wound care: A collaborative practice manual for health care practitioners* (4th ed.), Baltimore, MD: Lippincott Williams & Wilkins.

Falanga, V., Saap, L. J., & Ozonoff, A. (2006). Wound bed score and its correlation with healing of chronic wounds. *Dermatology Therapy, 19*, 383–390.

Falanga, V. (2008). Measurements in wound healing. *The International Journal of Lower Extremity Wounds, 7*(1), 9–11.

Fink, R., & Gates, R. (2014). Pain assessment. In B. R. Ferrell & N. Coyle (Eds.), *Textbook of palliative nursing* (2nd ed.), New York: Oxford University Press.

Freeman, K., Smyth, C., Dallam, L., et al. (2001.) Pain measurement scales: A comparison of the visual analogue and faces rating scales in measuring pressure ulcer pain. *Journal of Wound, Ostomy, and Continence Nursing, 28*(6), 290–296.

Gardner, S. E., Hillis, S. L., & Frantz, R. A. (2011). A prospective study of the PUSH tool in diabetic foot ulcers. *Journal of Wound, Ostomy, and Continence Nursing, 38*(4), 385–393.

Gardner, S. E., & Frantz, R. A., & Doebbeling, B. N. (2001). The validity of the clinical signs and symptoms used to identify localized chronic wound infection. *Wound Repair and Regeneration, 9*(3), 178–186.

Gorecki, C., Closs, S. J., Nixon, J., et al. (2011). Patient-reported pressure ulcer pain: A mixed-methods systematic review. *Journal of Pain and Symptom Management, 42*(3), 443–459.

Gorecki, C., Brown, J. M., Cano, S., et al. (2013, Jun). Development and validation of a new patient-reported outcome measure for patients with pressure ulcers: the PU-QOL instrument. *Health and Quality of Life Outcomes, 11*, 95.

Gorecki, C., Nixon, J., Lamping, D. L., et al. (2014, Jan). Patient-reported outcome measures for chronic wounds with particular reference to pressure ulcer research: A systematic review. *International Journal of Nursing Studies, 51*(1), 157–165.

Harris, C., Bates-Jensen, B., Parslow, N., et al. (2010, May-Jun). Bates-Jensen wound assessment tool: Pictorial guide validation project. *Journal of Wound, Ostomy, and Continence Nursing, 37*(3), 253–259.

Hazenberg, C. E. V. B., Van Baal, J. G., Manning, E., et al. (2012). The validity and reliability of diagnosing foot ulcers and pre-ulcerative lesions in diabetes using advanced digital photography. *Diabetes Technology and Therapeutics, 12*, 1011–1017.

Helvig, E. I., Nichols, L. W. (2012, Sep-Oct). Use of high-frequency ultrasound to detect heel pressure injury in elders. *Journal of Wound, Ostomy, and Continence Nursing, 39*(5), 500–508.

Hirai, M., Yoshinaga M., & Nakayama, R. (1985). Assessment of venous insufficiency using photoplethysmography: A comparison to strain gauge plethysmography. *Angiology, 36*(11), 795–801.

Hon, J., Lagden, K., McLaren, A. M., et al. (2010). A prospective, multicenter study to validate use of the Pressure Ulcer Scale for Healing (PUSH(c)) in patients with diabetic, venous, and pressure ulcers. *Ostomy/Wound Management, 56*(2), 26–36.

Hopf, H. W., Ueno, C., Aslam, R., et al. (2006). Guidelines for the treatment of arterial insufficiency ulcers. *Wound Repair and Regeneration, 14*(6), 93–710.

Houghton, P. E., Kincaid, C. B., Campbell, K., et al. (2000). Photographic assessment of the appearance of chronic pressure and leg ulcers. *Ostomy/Wound Management, 46*(4), 20–30.

Iizaka, S., Kaitani, T., Sugama, J., et al. (2013). Predictive validity of granulation tissue color measured by digital image analysis for deep pressure ulcer healing: A multicenter prospective cohort study. *Wound Repair and Regeneration, 21*, 25–34.

Jesada, E. C., Warren, J. O., Goodman, D., et al. (2013). Staging and defining characteristics of pressure ulcers using photographs by staff nurses in acute care settings. *Journal of Wound, Ostomy, and Continence Nursing, 40*(2), 150–156.

Kantor, J., & Margolis, D. J. (1998). Efficacy and prognostic value of simple wound measurements. *Archives of Dermatology, 134*(12), 1571–1574.

Kantor, J., & Margolis, D. J. (2000a). Expected healing rates for chronic wounds. *Wounds: A Compendium of Clinical Research and Practice, 12*(6), 155–158.

Kantor, J., & Margolis, D. J. (2000b). A multicentre study of percentage change in venous leg ulcer are as a prognostic index of healing at 24 week. *British Journal of Dermatology, 142*, 960–964.

Kantor, J., & Margolis, D. J. (2000c). Expected healing rates for chronic wounds. *Wounds, 12*, 155–158

Kantor, J., & Margolis, D. J. (2000d). The accuracy of using a wound care specialty clinic database to study diabetic neuropathic foot ulcer. *Wound Repair and Regeneration, 8*, 169–173.

Kecelj, N., Perme, M. P., Jezersek, M., et al. (2008). Initial healing rates as predictive factors of venous ulcer healing: The use of a laser-based three-dimensional ulcer measurement. *Wound Repair and Regeneration, 16*, 507–512.

Kennedy, K. L. (1989). The prevalence of pressure ulcers in an intermediate care facility. *Decubitus, 2*(2), 44–45.

Krasner, D. (2011). Wound pain: Impact and assessment. In R. A. Bryant & D. P. Nix (Eds.), *Acute and chronic wounds* (pp. 368–379), St. Louis, MO: Elsevier Mosby.

Krasner, D. (1995). The chronic wound pain experience: A conceptual model. *Ostomy/Wound Management. 41*(3), 20.

Langemo, D. K., & Brown, G. (2006). Skin fails too: Acute, chronic, and end-stage skin failure. *Advances in Skin and Wound Care, 19*(4), 206–11.

Lantis, J. C., Marston, W. A., Farber, A., et al. (2013). The influence of patient and wound variables on healing of venous leg ulcers in a randomized controlled trial of growth-arrested allogeneic keratinocytes and fibroblasts. *Journal of Vascular Surgery, 58*(2), 433–439.

Laplaud, A., Blaizot, X., Gaillard, C., et al. (2010). Wound debridement: Comparative reliability of three methods for measuring fibrin percentage in chronic wounds. *Wound Repair and Regeneration. 18*, 13–20.

Levine, J. (2013). CMS recognizes the Kennedy Terminal Ulcer in long-term care hospitals. http://www.jeffreymlevinemd.com/unavoidable-kennedy-ulcer-in-long-term-care-hospitals/. Last accessed August 20, 2014.

Manz, B. D., Moser, R., Nusser-Gerlach, M. A., et al. (2000). Pain assessment in the cognitively impaired and unimpaired elderly. *Pain Management Nursing, 1*(4), 106–115.

Margolis, D. J., Allen-Taylor, L., Hoffstad, O., et al. (2004). The accuracy of venous leg ulcer prognostic models in a wound care system. *Wound Repair and Regeneration, 12*, 163–168.

Margolis, D. J., Gelfand, J. M., Hoffstad, O., et al. (2003a). Surrogate end points for the treatment of diabetic neuropathic foot ulcers. *Diabetes Care, 26*, 1696–1700.

Margolis, D. J., Taylor, L. A., Hoffstad, O., et al. (2003b). Diabetic neuropathic foot ulcers: Predicting who will not heal. *The American Journal of Medicine, 115*, 627–631.

Margolis, D. J., Taylor, L. A., Hoffstad, O., et al. (2002). Diabetic neuropathic foot ulcer: The association of wound size, wound duration, and wound grade. *Diabetes Care, 25*, 1835–1839.

Merskey, H., & Bogduk, N. (1994). Classification of chronic pain: Description of chronic pain syndromes and definitions of pain terms. *IASP task force on taxonomy* (2nd ed.), Seattle, WA: IASP Press.

Miller, N., et al. (1996). A prospective study comparing duplex scan and venography for diagnosis of lower-extremity deep vein thrombosis. *Cardiovascular Surgery, 4*(4), 505–508.

Miller, C., Karimi, L., Donohue, L., et al. (2012). Interrater and intrarater reliability of silhouette wound imaging device, *Advances in Skin and Wound Care, 25*(11), 513–518.

National Pressure Ulcer Advisory Panel, European Pressure Ulcer Advisory Panel & Pan Pacific Pressure Injury Alliance. (2014). Prevention and treatment of pressure ulcers. In Emily Haesler (Ed.), *Clinical Practice Guideline*. Perth, Australia: Cambridge Media.

Nix, D. P. (2011). Skin and wound inspection and assessment. In R. A. Bryant & D. P. Nix (Eds.), *Acute and chronic wounds* (pp. 108–121). St. Louis, MO: Elsevier Mosby.

Paice, J. A., Cohen, F. L. (1997). Validity of a verbally administered numeric rating scale to measure cancer pain intensity. *Cancer Nursing, 20*, 88–93.

Ratliff, C. R. (2005). Use of the PUSH tool to measure venous ulcer healing. *Ostomy/Wound Management, 51*(5), 58–63.

Robson, M. C., Cooper, D. M., Aslam, R., et al. (2006). Guidelines for the treatment of venous ulcers. *Wound Repair and Regeneration, 14*(6), 649–662.

Robson, M. C., Hill, D. P., Woodske, M. E., et al. (2000, Jul). Wound healing trajectories as predictors of effectiveness of therapeutic agents. *Archives of Surgery, 135*(7), 773–777.

Roth, R. S., Lowery, J. C., Hamill, J. B. (2004). Assessing persistent pain and its relation to affective distress, depressive symptoms, and pain catastrophizing in patients with chronic wounds; a pilot study. *American Journal of Physical Medicine and Rehabilitation, 83*(11), 827–834.

Russell Localio, A., Margolis, D. J., Kagan, S. H., et al. (2006). Use of photographs for the identification of pressure ulcer in elderly hospitalized patients: Validity and reliability. *Wound Repair and Regeneration, 14*, 506–513.

Seiler, W. D., & Stahelin, H. B. (1995). Identification of factors that impair wound healing: A possible approach to wound healing research. *Wounds, 6*, 101–106.

Sheehan, P. J. P., Caselli, A., Gurini, J. M., et al. (2003). Percent change in wound area of diabetic foot ulcers over a 4-week period is a robust predictor of complete healing in a 12-week prospective trial. *Diabetes Care, 26*, 1879–1882.

Sibbald, R. G., Krasner, D. L., Lutz, J. B., et al. (2009, October). The SCALE expert panel: Skin changes at life's end. *Final Consensus Document, 1*.

Simon, W., & Malabar, R. (1995). Assessing pain in elderly patients who can't respond verbally. *Journal of Advanced Nursing, 22*(4), 663–669.

Steed, D. L., Attinger, C., Colaizzi, T., et al. (2006). Guidelines for the treatment of diabetic ulcers. *Wound Repair and Regeneration, 14*(6), 680–692.

Stotts, N. A., Thomas, D. R., Frantz, R., et al. (2001). An instrument to measure healing in pressure ulcers: Development and validation of the Pressure Ulcer Scale for Healing (PUSH). *The Journals of Gerontology Series A: Medical Sciences, 56*(12), M795–M799.

Stuppy, D. J. (1998). The Faces Pain Scale: Reliability and validity with mature adults. *Applied Nursing Research, 11*, 84–89.

Taylor, L. J., Herr, K., & Paice, J. A. (2003). Pain intensity assessment: A comparison of selected pain intensity scales for use in cognitively intact and cognitively impaired African American older adults. *Pain Management Nursing, 4*, 87–95.

Terris, D. D., Woo, C., Jarczok, M. N., et al. (2011). Comparison of in-person and digital photograph assessment of stage III and IV pressure ulcers among veterans with spinal cord injuries. *Journal of Rehabilitation Research and Development, 48*, 215–224.

Thomas, D. R., Rodeheaver, G. T., Bartolucci, A. A., et al. (1997). Pressure Ulcer Scale for Healing: Derivation and validation of the PUSH tool. *Advances in Wound Care, 10*(5), 96–101.

Ting, A. C., et al. (1999). Air plethysmography in chronic venous insufficiency: Clinical diagnosis and quantitative assessment. *Angiology, 50*(10), 831–836.

Ueta, M., Sugama, J., Konya, C., et al. (2011). Use of ultrasound in assessment of necrotic tissue in pressure ulcers with adjacent undermining. *Journal of Wound Care, 20*(11), 503–504, 506, 508, passim

Van Rijswijk, L., & Multi-center leg ulcer study group. (1993). Full-thickness leg ulcers: Patient demographics and predictors of healing. *The Journal of Family Practice, 36*(6), 625–632.

Van Rijswijk, L., & Polansky, M. (1994). Predictors of time to healing deep pressure ulcers. *Ostomy Wound Management, 40*(8), 40–48.

Van Rijswijk, L. (1993). Full-thickness pressure ulcers: Patient and wound healing characteristics. *Decubitus, 6*(1), 16–21.

Wagner, F. E. W. (1981). The dysvascular foot: A system for diagnosis and treatment. *Foot and Ankle,* (2), 64–122.

Wewers, M. E., & Lowe, N. K. (1990). A critical review of visual analogue scales in the measurement of clinical phenomena. *Research in Nursing and Health, 13,* 227–236.

Whitney, J., Phillips, L., Aslam, R., et al. (2006). Guidelines for the treatment of pressure ulcers. *Wound Repair and Regeneration, 14*(6), 663–679.

Wong, D., & Baker, C. (1988). Pain in children: Comparison of assessment scales. *Pediatric Nursing, 14,* 9–17.

Woo, K. Y. (2012). Exploring the effects of pain and stress on wound healing. *Advances in Skin and Wound Care, 25*(1), 38–44.

Wound Ostomy Continence Nurses Society (WOCN). (2010). Guideline for management of pressure ulcers. WOCN clinical practice guideline series #2, Glenview, IL.

Yalcin, E., Akyuz, M., Onder, B., et al. (2013, May). Skin thickness on bony prominences measured by ultrasonography in patients with spinal cord injury. *The Journal of Spinal Cord Medicine, 36*(3), 225–230.

QUESTIONS

1. A wound care nurse is performing a follow-up assessment of a patient's wound. What data would the nurse gather that is usually not included in the initial assessment?

A. Wound etiology
B. Systemic factors affecting the ability to heal
C. Patient and caregiver goals
D. Wound response to treatment plan

2. A wound care nurse gently pinches a fold of skin over the patient's sternum and notes how quickly it returns to normal. The nurse is assessing for:

A. Skin turgor
B. Edema
C. Capillary refill
D. Erythema

3. The nurse uses palpation to test a patient's skin for blanchability of an erythematous area. Which statement correctly identifies a key finding of this assessment?

A. Blanchable erythema is indicative of some level of tissue damage and inflammation involving the skin and soft tissues.
B. Blanchable erythema over a bony prominence is classified as a stage 1 pressure ulcer.
C. Erythema progressing from blanchable to nonblanchable signifies worsening skin condition.
D. An area of erythema that is nonblanchable needs off-loading to monitor the intensity of the erythema.

4. Following a baseline skin assessment, a wound care nurse notes the following data: raised erythematous skin area on right forearm; lesions are 1.5 cm. What type of skin lesion would the nurse document?

A. Macule
B. Patches
C. Plaques
D. Papules

5. The wound care nurse is documenting a pressure ulcer located on a patient's heel by using photography. Which of the following is a recommended guideline when using this technique?

A. Take the photograph from different angles.
B. Take a close-up photograph of the wound and a second showing the wound and body part.
C. Place the patient in different positions for the photographs.
D. Use a digital camera with a density of at least 6 megapixels.

6. A wound care nurse is assessing a patient who is receiving silver sulfadiazine as a topical therapy for a wound. For which adverse effect should the nurse monitor this patient?

A. Allergic reaction
B. Edema
C. Erythema
D. Fissures

7. A wound care nurse measures a patient's ankle-brachial index (ABI), and records a value of 0.78. What condition does this reading indicate?

A. Dehydration
B. Fluid and electrolyte imbalances
C. Edema
D. Arterial insufficiency

8. The wound care nurse assesses a patient's wound as a shallow full-thickness wound. This classification indicates what type of tissue involvement?

A. Epidermis and part of the dermis
B. Epidermal, dermal structures, and subcutaneous tissues
C. Muscle and underlying structures
D. Epidermal tissue only

9. Which statement accurately describes a wound edge condition and its etiology?

A. Edges are distinct when there are areas where the normal tissues blend into the wound bed.
B. The edges of chronic wounds frequently are open and proliferative with thickening and fibrosis present.
C. Edges that are even with the skin surface and the wound base are attached to the base of the wound.
D. The wound that is a crater (bowl/boat shape with sides and depth) is a wound with edges that are attached to the wound base.

10. The wound care nurse is assessing tunneling in a patient's wound. Which step in the procedure is performed correctly?

A. The nurse inserts a cotton-tipped applicator under the edge of the wound and advances as far as possible.
B. The nurse uses a pen to make a mark on the applicator at the surface line of the wound.
C. The nurse determines undermining by noting the percent of the wound depth involved in the process and the distance the process extends from the wound base.
D. When documenting, the nurse distinguishes undermining as presenting with a narrow tract and tunneling presenting as a lip or pocket.

11. Which statement accurately describes the characteristics and implications of necrotic tissue in a wound bed?

A. Necrosis of muscle tissue typically results in the formation of stringy, yellow slough.
B. Consistency refers to the cohesiveness of the debris; typically more advanced necrosis is thin and wet.
C. A hard, crusty leathery eschar is not attached to the base and edges of the wound and is sometimes mistaken as a scab.
D. Color varies as necrosis worsens, from white/gray nonviable tissue, to yellow slough, and finally to black eschar.

12. The wound care nurse assessing a patient's wound notes a combination of erythema and induration extending circumferentially around the wound. These data are indicative of:

A. Invasive wound infection
B. Crepitus
C. Formation of granulation tissue
D. Wound dehiscence

ANSWERS: 1.**D**, 2.**A**, 3.**C**, 4.**C**, 5.**B**, 6.**A**, 7.**D**, 8.**B**, 9.**C**, 10.**A**, 11.**D**, 12.**A**

CHAPTER 4

General Principles of Wound Management

Goal Setting and Systemic Support

Lee Ann Krapfl and Benjamin F. Peirce

OBJECTIVES

1. Use assessment data to determine the following:
   - Factors causing or contributing to the alteration in skin/soft tissue integrity
   - Potential for healing and any systemic conditions that would interfere with healing
   - Wound characteristics (to include phase of wound healing) and implications for wound management
2. Establish appropriate wound care goals based on wound healability and patient priorities.
3. Develop an individualized plan of care based on assessment data and current evidence-based guidelines that addresses each of the following factors:
   - Correction or amelioration of etiologic factors
   - Attention to systemic factors affecting the repair process
   - Evidence-based topical therapy
   - Pain management
   - Patient and caregiver education
4. Discuss challenges to seamless care and strategies to address those challenges.

Topic Outline

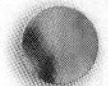 Goal Setting

Goal setting is a foundational "first step" in development of an effective plan of care. Goals should be established following comprehensive assessment and prior to care plan development. As pointed out in current literature, patient and caregiver involvement in goal setting and care planning is essential, and patient involvement is actually mandated in various setting-dependent regulations. However, the reality is that patient involvement is often cursory; the result is that the provider goals are not aligned with the patient's goals, and outcomes are compromised. Goals and care plan specifics must be mutual if the desired outcomes are to be achieved, because many components of the care plan are patient dependent and require the patient to modify lifestyle behaviors in order to manage the underlying disease process as well as the wound itself.

Impact of Chronic Disease

Chronic wounds are often manifestations of chronic disease; thus, goal setting and care planning must include measures to manage the disease in addition to wound care procedures. Many wound care providers focus almost exclusively on treatment of the wound; however, as is discussed further in this chapter, the first priority in wound management is correction of etiologic and contributing factors, and most of the work in managing these condition(s) rests with the patient. This means that wound care clinicians must broaden their focus both in goal setting and care planning and must include strategies to correct causative conditions and to optimize the patient's ability to heal; this requires attention to factors such as glycemic control, smoking cessation, nutritional intake, and possible off-loading or elevation of the affected area. For many of the most common and costly conditions associated with chronic wounds, patients need to modify and monitor behavior in three areas: medication management, diet, and lifestyle. Medications are a key component of managing the most common conditions including diabetes, cardiovascular conditions, and chronic obstructive pulmonary disease (COPD); yet patients are frequently inconsistent in terms of taking the right medications at the right time. Dietary modifications, exercise regimens, and smoking cessation are other elements of management that are frequently "prescribed" as essential components of a wound management plan. In everyday practice, it is common for clinicians to "tell" patients what to do and to expect them to follow the instructions provided. While it is true that patient behaviors in each of these areas have significant impact on effective disease management, changing these behaviors in real life can be very challenging for patients and families; thus, it is critical for the clinician to talk "with" the patient, to be able to explain the impact of certain conditions and behaviors on the potential for wound healing, and to truly "hear" the patient's goals and priorities as they relate to overall wound management. For example, the patient with a neuropathic ulcer must be willing to consistently "off-load" the ulcer via a contact cast or removable cast walker if the wound is to heal; however, if the patient is the sole support for his or her family, the patient's ability to manage his or her job may be as important or more important to him or her than getting the wound to heal. The clinician working with this patient must be able to establish an open dialog, and must be able to assist the patient to prioritize goals and to determine what he or she can do and is willing to do to promote wound healing. Ideally, the clinician and patient will work together to establish realistic goals and a realistic care plan to which the patient can commit.

CLINICAL PEARL

Chronic wounds are manifestations of chronic disease; effective management requires disease management as well as wound care.

One challenge in promoting effective self-management of many chronic diseases is the insidious and slow nature of disease progression, and the cumulative and delayed effects of nonadherence to the plan of care. In general, nonadherence does not produce an immediate negative consequence. If the patient became violently ill following a deviation from the plan of care, then that alone could prove to be a powerful motivator. However, in most cases the negative effects of nonadherence manifest many weeks, months, or years later, and this can be a major barrier in getting patients to identify and change behavior. Fortunately, in the area of wound care, the effects of adherence or nonadherence do manifest relatively quickly in terms of wound progress or deterioration. This means that short-term contracts can be beneficial to both the clinician and patient. For example, the clinician might conduct a thorough baseline assessment followed by a clear and open discussion with the patient regarding the elements of care required for wound healing. The clinician might ask the patient if he or she would be willing and able to commit to 3 to 4 weeks of smoking cessation or tight glucose control or consistent off-loading, during which time the clinical team would also commit their resources to promotion of wound healing. Typically, within that time frame there is clearly visible progress, and in many cases this serves to reinforce the recommended change in behavior.

Another common challenge in team-based goal setting is the difficulty some patients have in articulating clear and reasonable goals; this is particularly common among patients with unstable chronic conditions who have experienced significant recent changes in health status and lifestyle. These individuals may have a hard time being realistic in what they can hope to achieve because they basically "want their life back." Clinicians skilled at working with patients with chronic diseases note that one effective tactic is to have the patient reflect back to where he or she was last month or last quarter, and to use this as a basis for short-term goal setting. Establishment of attainable short-term goals increases the likelihood that the patient will experience initial success, which increases his or her self-confidence and provides the needed motivation to sustain changed behaviors.

Working with patients to articulate realistic goals is both a science and an art. It requires knowledge of the various disease processes/comorbidities, effective communication skills, and the ability to educate and motivate in language the patient can understand.

Types of Goals

There are three broad types of goals related to wound management: wound healing, wound maintenance, and patient comfort. When establishing a plan of care, it is essential to first determine whether or not wound healing is a realistic goal.

Healing

Wound clinicians are frequently confronted with wounds labeled as nonhealing, based on the fact that they have been open for a matter of weeks or months and have not closed using traditional strategies. The reasons for the failure to heal are of course varied, but most often include failure to correctly identify and correct etiologic factors and/or inadequate attention to the systemic factors affecting the repair process. In most cases, once all of the etiologic factors have been accurately identified and addressed, systemic support is provided, and topical care is delivered that is evidence based and individualized, the wound will go on to closure.

Maintenance

Unfortunately, situations do exist where the wound will never close, in spite of consistent appropriate management by the clinical team; this is usually due to inability to correct etiologic factors or noncorrectable systemic barriers (e.g., an individual with severe arterial disease who is not a candidate for revascularization, or a patient with advanced dementia who is no longer taking adequate nutrition and hydration and for whom enteral or parenteral nutrition is deemed to be unsafe or against the patient's wishes) (Teno et al., 2012). However, just because the wound is determined to have a very low probability of closure does not suggest that the individual is terminal or end of life. Patients can and do manage open wounds for years. For example, a wound with underlying osteomyelitis or a wound occurring in a previously radiated field will not close without surgical intervention. If the patient is a poor surgical risk, or refuses surgical intervention, he or she needs to know that wound closure is not a realistic goal. In situations where wound healing is very unlikely but the patient is not end of life, the goal becomes maintenance. The clinician should work with the patient and caregiver to develop a plan of care that prevents infection and minimizes deterioration, and the plan should be designed knowing that this will be a lifelong issue for the patient (Maida, 2013). It should be noted that goals can change if there are changes in the conditions preventing repair; for example, changes in a patient's psychosocial situation may positively affect his/her ability and willingness to adhere to key elements of the management program, and this would then result in a change in goals (from maintenance to healing).

Comfort

Finally, there are circumstances in which palliative care is the focus, such as when the chronic disease state is end stage and is no longer deemed responsive to medical treatment, or when the patient is terminally ill. In these situations, the focus of care should be based on the patient's and family's wishes for end-of-life care. In most cases, the primary goal of management becomes comfort; even if the patient retains some ability to heal, he or she may not live long enough to obtain wound closure. In addition, the individual may not wish to spend his or her final weeks or months of life focusing time, energy, and resources on his or her wound; an inappropriate focus on wound healing can result in expectations and care directives that adversely affect the patient's quality of life (Tippett, 2014). (For example, frequent repositioning of an end-of-life patient may cause additional pain and distress for both the patient and family and may be contrary to the patient's and family's goals for end-of-life care.) Because many clinicians automatically establish a "healing" goal and fail to involve the patient and family in the goal-setting process, WOC nurses are frequently asked to make recommendations on topical treatment when it seems that the individual has little healing potential due to poorly controlled or advanced stages of chronic illness. It is not unusual for these patients and families to be totally unaware of the low healing potential because no one in the health care system has ever previously brought up the issue. Thus it is critical for the wound care nurse to consider whether or not the etiologic factors and systemic factors affecting healing can be corrected, whether the patient and family are able and willing to adhere to the elements of care for which they are responsible, and whether or not the patient is end of life.

CLINICAL PEARL

There are three types of wound management goals: wound healing, wound maintenance, and comfort.

It is helpful to promptly identify situations in which healing is not likely to occur or is not the focus of care. The knowledgeable wound care clinician can usually identify situations in which the goal should be maintenance or comfort based on the data obtained during the initial assessment; critical assessment parameters and decision-making factors include whether or not the causative factors and systemic factors affecting repair can be corrected, whether or not the patient and family are able and willing to adhere to the elements of care for which they are responsible, and whether or not the patient is end of life (Lavery et al., 2008; Apelqvist, 2012). It is critical to discuss assessment findings and care goals openly with the patient, family, and caregivers, since the goal should guide decision making at each patient contact to ensure that wound care decisions are realistic and appropriate for the patient situation. When the wound care goal is comfort or maintenance, the interventions should be focused on symptom alleviation (pain management, exudate containment, odor control, and bleeding prevention), prevention of infection, and establishment of simple, atraumatic care procedures. Expensive and complex treatment modalities are typically impractical and unnecessary. On the other hand, selected advanced wound care dressings might prove to be therapeutic in meeting comfort and maintenance goals by minimizing dressing changes, reducing pain, managing exudate, minimizing odor, reducing infection, and minimizing bleeding and trauma. Bulky gauze dressings may limit the patient's ability to be as mobile and active as possible, while advanced wound care dressings may prove to be lower profile and less cumbersome, permitting activities that may enhance their quality of life. When goals are determined to be maintenance or comfort, evaluation of the plan of care should be based on whether the symptoms are being successfully managed, rather than whether or not healing is occurring. While wound improvement or even healing does occasionally occur even among end-of-life patients, it should not be the focus or the expectation of care in these situations. Indeed, it is important to educate both the patient and staff regarding the fact that deterioration of the wound is not usually caused by any failure on the part of the staff and/or family, but rather by overall systems failure and skin organ failure. Making this clear to the patient and family can help prepare them and assure that they do not feel that their loved one received poor-quality care.

CLINICAL PEARL

Even when wound healing is unlikely, it is possible to establish measurable goals and a plan of care that enhances quality of life.

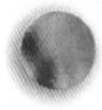

General Principles in Treatment Planning

Wound care is often focused primarily on topical treatment; however, this is only one element of comprehensive wound management. The majority of chronic wounds begin as minor traumatic injuries that would heal in a few days in a healthy individual but progress to serious nonhealing wounds in patients with underlying chronic disease (Demidova-Rice et al., 2012). Healing of these chronic wounds requires a comprehensive approach to management that includes correction of etiologic factors and attention to systemic factors that affect healing as well as topical therapy. Chronic wounds are complicated and challenging and are best managed with a holistic approach involving a variety of disciplines. The familiar saying goes that we need to treat the whole patient and not just the hole in the patient; a nonhealing wound is frequently indicative of underlying multiorgan disease that is poorly controlled. The wound and its progression toward healing is the window through which we can view the broader health of the patient.

A comprehensive plan of care should address three areas: (1) correction of etiologic factors; (2) provision of systemic support for healing, and (3) topical treatment that creates and maintains an optimal healing environment. This plan is like a three-legged stool. Without all three legs, the plan will fail. Healing will be jeopardized, the risk for complications is increased, and recurrence is likely.

CLINICAL PEARL

A comprehensive plan of care is like a three-legged stool: correction of etiologic factors, systemic support, and evidence-based topical therapy.

Correction of Etiologic Factors

Correctly identifying the etiology of the wound is key to developing a comprehensive management plan. Failure to adequately address the causative factor(s) will result in failure to heal, even if systemic support is provided and topical therapy is appropriate. Thus, initial assessment and intervention must include identification of the etiologic factor(s) and initiation of measures to address those factors; for example, the most critical intervention in the management plan for a pressure ulcer is to eliminate or minimize the pressure that caused the wound. Typically, a thorough assessment of the wound and surrounding tissue provides definitive clues as to etiology, because most wounds present in a predictable location and with classic characteristics. It is equally important to obtain a detailed patient history when possible, because the patient history serves to confirm or correct initial impressions. In situations where the etiology is *not* clear, selected diagnostic tests or consults are necessary. Table 4-1 provides a summary of the interventions required for the most commonly encountered wounds; the pathology, presentation, and management of each of these is covered in greater depth in upcoming chapters.

Systemic Support for Healing

Wound healing is a systemic process that requires increased calorie, protein, and vitamin/mineral intake, sufficient

TABLE 4-1 Correction of Etiologic Factors

Etiologic Factor	Critical Interventions
Pressure/shear	• Pressure redistribution surfaces • Routine repositioning to off-load the ulcer
Friction	• Gentle skin care and repositioning • Low friction surface
Moisture-associated skin damage	• Bladder/ bowel retraining/toileting programs • Urine and stool containment • Skin care to include cleansing, moisturizing, and protection • Management of diaphoresis
Venous insufficiency (lower extremity venous disease)	• Leg elevation • Compression wraps/stockings
Arterial insufficiency (lower extremity arterial disease)	• Vascular consult (revascularization) • Counseling re: smoking cessation (if applicable)
Neuropathy	• Off-loading • Tight glycemic control
Autoimmune disease	• Anti-inflammatory agents (topical vs. systemic)
Infectious agents (bacterial, fungal, viral)	• Antimicrobial therapy (topical vs. systemic)

blood flow and oxygenation to support the repair process, and relatively normal glycemic levels. Since many chronic wounds are associated with disease states impacting perfusion and oxygenation, nutritional status, and blood glucose levels, the body's ability to heal the wound may be significantly impaired; multiple poorly controlled comorbidities are also associated with compromised healing. Thus, assessment and correction of systemic conditions that adversely affect repair is the second priority in wound management. Box 4-1 lists factors to consider in providing systemic support for healing.

Tissue Perfusion and Oxygenation

Well-oxygenated blood and the ability to perfuse the tissues with that oxygen-rich blood are critical to wound healing. Hypoxic cells cannot support tissue repair or mount a defense against bacterial invasion; thus, any condition that affects blood volume, oxygenation, or tissue perfusion compromises wound healing and places the patient at increased risk of infection. This includes such conditions as severe anemia, hypovolemia and hypotension, sepsis, lower extremity arterial disease (LEAD), edema, lower extremity venous disease (LEVD), severe COPD, and radiation damage (Kapetanaki et al., 2013; Wright et al., 2014). Obesity should also be considered as a high-risk condition since adipose tissue is poorly perfused (Pierpont et al., 2014). In addition, many obese patients suffer from sleep apnea, which can further impact tissue oxygenation. Measures to improve perfusion and oxygenation must be individualized for the patient and the wound. For example, the patient with LEAD should be referred for vascular testing and possible revascularization procedures. General measures to improve tissue oxygenation include use of nasal oxygen for patients who are hypoxic, maintenance of adequate hydration to reduce blood viscosity, and management of edema through elevation and compression. Sleep apnea monitoring would be helpful in patients afflicted with this disorder.

Smoking Cessation

Tobacco can be smoked, chewed, or sniffed, and the method of intake is significant, because some of the health risks associated with smoking are related to the nicotine and others are related to the smoke. Nicotine causes vasoconstriction, increases blood coagulability, and binds to vitamin C; each of these effects has a negative impact on wound healing, and these negative effects occur with smokeless tobacco as well as use of cigarettes. Tobacco smoke creates carbon monoxide and tar, which binds to hemoglobin and impairs oxygenation; thus, smoking is much more deleterious than is use of smokeless tobacco, because the hypoxia caused by the smoke adds to the vasoconstrictive and coagulability effects of the nicotine to create significant impairment to wound healing. Inhaling secondhand smoke can have a similar effect on wound repair, and individuals who live in homes where there are smokers frequently experience delayed healing.

BOX 4-1. Factors to Consider in Providing Systemic Support

A. Tissue perfusion and oxygenation
B. Smoking cessation
C. Nutritional support
D. Glycemic control
E. Corticosteroids
F. Age and comorbidities

The risks to general health posed by tobacco smoking are well documented. As health care providers, our goal should always be to move the patient toward total smoking cessation. However, it is essential for the health care provider to recognize and appreciate the addictive nature of tobacco products and to be empathetic and supportive of the patient who is contemplating modifications in his/her tobacco use. The clinician should counsel the patient regarding strategies that have been shown to be effective, such as behavior modification, acupuncture, medications, and nicotine replacement. There are various nicotine replacement products such as nicotine spray, gum, inhalers, lozenges, and patches that may be recommended as a pathway to cessation.

Electronic cigarettes, commonly referred to as e-cigarettes, are a new approach to nicotine replacement; however, the benefits of these products as compared to conventional cigarettes are controversial. While the toxic chemicals in tobacco smoke have been eliminated, there are other known toxins in the cartridges (Weinberg & Segelnick, 2011). Current evidence suggests that e-cigarettes may help to suppress the urge to smoke and may be a useful tool in smoking cessation programs; however, the overall effect of e-cigarettes and nicotine vaporization on wound healing has yet to be determined. Thus the clinician must remain alert to updated research findings and must use these to guide practice.

Another agent that patients smoke is marijuana, and its use may increase since at least 23 states have now legalized some form of medical marijuana (Legal Medical Marijuana States and DC, 2014). The active components of cannabis can be effective in treating pain, nausea and vomiting, and loss of appetite associated with various clinical conditions, and inhalation of the drug through smoking provides a rapid onset of the therapeutic effects. However, marijuana smoke also contains carbon monoxide and tars, which adversely affect oxygenation, and marijuana smoke contains 50% to 70% more carcinogenic hydrocarbons than does tobacco smoke. In addition, marijuana smoke is commonly inhaled deeper and held longer than tobacco smoke, so there is increased exposure to these toxins (Marijuana: Drugs and Supplements, 2014). Therefore, smoking marijuana should be discouraged in patients with open wounds. It is interesting to note that the tetrahydrocannabinol (THC) in marijuana acts as a smooth muscle relaxant, which contributes to vasodilation, reduced blood pressure, and increased blood flow to the tissues (Cardiovascular Effects of Cannabis, 2014), and THC can be ingested orally or vaporized and applied directly to the skin (thus eliminating the adverse effects of marijuana smoke). However, there is only anecdotal evidence to support the potential positive effects of oral or percutaneous THC on wound healing; further research is essential before any recommendations can be made (Jones, 2002).

Nutritional Support

The body requires essential nutrients in order to synthesize new tissue and fight infection; thus, assessment of the patient's nutritional status and provision of the macronutrients and micronutrients required for repair is a critical aspect of wound management. Chapter 6 details the specific nutrients needed to support wound healing, and provides step-by-step guidelines for nutritional assessment and intervention. In general, any patient with a wound requires adequate calories, additional protein, and sufficient intake of critical vitamins and minerals (e.g., vitamin C, zinc, and iron) (Kaminski & Drinane, 2014). Adding a multivitamin with mineral supplement is sometimes recommended as an easy way to ensure adequate intake of these micronutrients.

The wound clinician should also consider that many patients with chronic illnesses have preexisting unmet nutritional needs for a variety of reasons. It should never be assumed that nutritional needs are being met, even when the patient is obese, as the patient's diet may consist primarily of high-calorie foods of poor nutritional value. There is increasing recognition that food deserts exist, particularly in large, urban centers; these are communities where easy access to food is limited to processed foods high in sodium, calories, and fat. Thus, many individuals ingest adequate or excessive calories and may "appear" to be well nourished or overnourished, when in fact their intake of protein and essential micronutrients is totally inadequate.

With any type of injury or infection, there is an increase in the metabolic rate, and thus there is an increased need for calories. Typically, patients who are trying to heal open wounds should not be on a weight-loss diet, as reduced caloric intake may also limit intake of essential nutrients required for wound healing. A good rule of thumb is to recommend caloric restriction only in situations where the expertise of a qualified nutritional expert is available.

All patients with chronic wounds should have their nutritional status evaluated. Whenever the wound nurse suspects a nutritional deficiency, the appropriate action is to refer the patient for nutritional assessment, if that service is available. Unfortunately, in some settings, such as home health care, the nurse may be the person tasked with this assessment. Chapter 6 details the components of a nutritional assessment and provides simple guidelines the nurse can use to develop a "prescription" for nutritional intervention. Simple strategies for obtaining accurate data regarding current intake include the "24-hour recall" method (asking the patient to relay everything he/she ate or drank in the past 24 hours) and asking the patient to keep a diet journal for 3 days. In addition to assisting the nurse to identify nutritional deficiencies, such a journal can provide insight regarding simple ways to increase protein intake by modifying the foods the patient is already eating. For example, use of powdered milk is an inexpensive, easy way to add protein to many foods, including creamed soups, cereals, puddings, and shakes.

Glycemic Control

Wound healing is frequently impaired in patients with diabetes for a number of reasons. For example, diabetes may result in vascular compromise that increases the risk for LEAD and impaired healing of lower extremity wounds; this is more common among individuals with long-standing and poorly controlled diabetes and will be discussed further in Chapter 22. However, the most common negative effect of diabetes is hyperglycemia, which negatively impacts bacterial control and all phases of wound healing. Therefore, management of wounds in patients with diabetes must include measures aimed at consistent control of blood glucose levels. Goals for glycemic control are affected by the patient's life expectancy, advanced complications or extensive comorbidities, and history of severe hypoglycemia. For younger patients with long life expectancy, limited complications and comorbid conditions, and no history of severe hypoglycemia, the American Diabetes Association recommends the following: A1C 6.5% to 7.0% (mean plasma glucose 140 to 154 mg/dL). For individuals with limited life expectancy, advanced comorbidities or complications, or history of severe hypoglycemia, a less stringent goal is recommended: A1C <8.0% with a mean plasma glucose of 183 (American Diabetes Association, 2014).

Measures for maintaining adherence to established goals include (1) self-monitoring and tracking of blood glucose levels, (2) adherence to the prescribed diabetic diet and exercise regime, and (3) medication management. Diabetes is a progressive disease. Effective self-management can slow the progression but will not completely halt it (Standards of Medical Care in Diabetes, 2014). Management is complex and requires a collaborative multidisciplinary approach, particularly if there is a patient history of poor or inconsistent adherence. Individuals must assume an active role in their plan of care to be successful. Providing self-management education and support are vital components of diabetes care, and the WOC nurse is in a key position to reinforce that education. The presence of a potentially life- or limb-threatening wound might be a powerful motivator for the patient. The WOC nurse might be the right person, in the right place, at the right time to provide the necessary feedback, positive reinforcement, and support that the patient needs. Depending on the care setting, it may be helpful to consult other resources such as a dietician and/or diabetic educator to assist with comprehensive assessment, teaching, and support. Patients must not only demonstrate the ability to correctly self-monitor their blood glucose but must also be able to use the results to adjust their medication, diet, and exercise therapy. Collaboration with the patient's primary physician is necessary to determine the desired A1C goals and to help the patient develop an algorithm for self-adjustment of insulin based on the results of blood glucose monitoring.

Certainly, different practice settings present unique opportunities and challenges. For example, in the acute care setting, diet and activity can be more closely controlled, blood glucose levels can be closely monitored, and medications are adjusted by staff. The challenge is that it is not always easy to determine the patient's level of understanding and motivation for self-management post-discharge. On the other hand, the home care or outpatient setting provides a much better opportunity to assess the patient's ability to self-manage his or her diabetes. If the outcome is less than optimal, the wound care nurse can share observations of both positive and negative behaviors and can relate those behaviors to wound care outcomes; this may impact the patient's willingness to establish short-term goals and contracts for diabetes self-management and wound care.

Corticosteroids

Any medication that suppresses the body's immune response can impair wound healing. The therapeutic effects of these drugs block the normal inflammatory response, which is the first phase of wound healing. In addition to delaying healing, corticosteroids can increase the risk of infection. The negative effects appear to be both time and dose dependent; doses of more than 30 mg/day for more than 30 days are particularly damaging to repair.

There is some evidence to support the use of vitamin A (retinoids) to counteract the negative effects of steroids on wound healing. The mechanism of action is not fully understood, since vitamin A has no beneficial effects in patients who are not taking steroids. Current thinking is that the beneficial effect is related to enhanced leukocyte migration associated with the use of vitamin A. The recommended dose is 25,000 international units orally per day for up to 10 days. An alternative method of administration is topical application of up to 100,000 IU (Wicke et al., 2000). Topical preparations are thought to pose less of a risk of impacting the desired systemic effect of the steroid. Caution should be taken with patients with liver disease due to potential toxicity.

Topical antimicrobial ointments and dressings may be useful adjuncts because of the higher risk of infection posed by these drugs.

Patients on long-term steroids often have very thin and fragile epidermis, or steroid-dependent skin changes. Minimizing the use of tapes and adhesive products in wound management is appropriate to reduce the risk of periwound trauma. The use of adhesive remover products, tape anchors, stretchable netting material, and silicone-based adhesives are all useful tools in protection of fragile skin.

Age and Comorbidities

Advanced age and the presence of comorbidities, such as renal or hepatic disease, often adversely affect wound healing. Although healthy elderly people retain the ability to heal their wounds, age-related changes and delays do occur in all phases of wound healing. In addition, advanced age is associated with a marked increase in the prevalence of comorbidities and use of medications that affect healing (Sgonc & Gruber, 2013). Any acute exacerbation in a systemic condition, such as acute or chronic kidney disease or a newly occurring viral or bacterial infection, can cause a wound to stall or deteriorate, as the calories, protein, and energy needed to support wound healing are deployed to fight other systemic battles. While comorbid conditions cannot be totally eliminated or reversed, it is frequently possible to minimize their effects through appropriate multidisciplinary management. It is also important to recognize and communicate with the patient that wound healing will be delayed. In summary, to maximize wound healing in a patient of advanced age or with multiple comorbidities, it is important to optimize the person's overall health state by reducing stress, managing pain, assuring adequate sleep, and maximizing activity levels. In addition to systemic factors, the local wound environment must be optimized.

Evidence-Based Topical Treatment

The third component of a comprehensive plan of care is evidence-based topical treatment. Chapters 7, 8, and 9 provide in-depth discussion and guidelines for wound cleansing, wound bed preparation, and dressing selection based on wound characteristics. It is worth noting that the optimal dressing at the time of initial assessment may not be the best choice later; topical therapy must change as the wound condition changes. For example, an open wound previously managed with gauze dressings may present initially with small amounts of exudate and would best be managed with a minimally absorptive dressing. However, it is common for the amount of exudate to increase within a week or two following implementation of moist wound healing, and at that point the wound will require a more absorptive dressing. Generally the goal is to manage exudate while maintaining a moist wound bed, and to achieve an optimal balance between too desiccated and too wet. In developing a plan for topical therapy, the clinician must also consider the frequency of dressing change. Wound healing is disrupted whenever the dressing is removed, so reduced frequency of dressing changes is usually both beneficial to healing and easier for the patient and caregivers. Because the condition of the wound can change quickly, topical therapy should be reevaluated with each dressing change. This may seem obvious to the knowledgeable wound care nurse, but reluctance to alter the treatment in spite of failure to progress is a common problem among practitioners. Serial assessments are essential and should prompt adjustments in the topical therapy in response to changes in wound depth, exudate, and bioburden.

The importance of comprehensive serial assessments has implications other than modifications in dressing selection. Serial assessments are the basis for prompt recognition of a plateau in wound healing or deterioration in wound status. There is substantial evidence to indicate that absence of progress for two consecutive weeks (despite appropriate management) is indicative of a problem and mandates reassessment of the entire management plan. Reassessment must include attention to etiologic factors and systemic support as well as topical therapy; too often providers rush to change the dressing, when that might not be the reason for the plateau or deterioration. Comprehensive reassessment must include confirmation of the etiology and a reevaluation of measures in place to address etiology, and must include consideration of the possibility that there are additional etiologic factors that have not been recognized and corrected. Reassessment must also address the measures in place to optimize systemic conditions affecting repair; for example, nutritional status, glycemic control, tobacco use, and current medications must be reevaluated, as well as management of any comorbid conditions. Finally, wound status should be critically reassessed in light of current topical therapy, with particular attention to exudate control, maintenance of a moist wound bed, protection of the healing wound from trauma and bacterial invasion, and control of bacterial burden. For example, in assessing the patient with a nonhealing sacral pressure ulcer, it is important to determine whether or not the wound is being consistently off-loaded, whether the patient has stopped smoking, and whether or not the patient's nutritional intake provides adequate support for healing. Changing the topical dressing will not provide healing if the patient is not adherent to the other critical elements of care. Engaging the patient in a meaningful discussion of the factors delaying healing, the patient's role in managing those factors, the barriers to their adherence, and strategies for overcoming those barriers can help the patient achieve his or her overall goals and promote wound healing.

Strategies to Promote Seamless Transitions in Care

Most chronic wounds do not heal in a matter of days but over weeks or even months. This means that the patient may transition from acute care to home health or outpatient care, and care for the same wound may be delivered by many different practitioners in varied practice settings. A substantial and growing body of research suggests that patients transitioning across sites of care are often unprepared to manage their condition, receive conflicting instructions on condition management, have problems reaching a clinician who has access to their plan of care, and have little input into their own plan of care (Coleman et al., 2006; Naylor et al., 2004). This has a number of implications for wound care clinicians. Clearly, the goal is to make the transition from one care setting and provider to another care setting and provider as seamless as possible, and that requires attention to the way in which wound care is ordered and communicated, and to the principles underlying collaborative practice.

CLINICAL PEARL

Assuring seamless transition between one care setting and another is a critical element of patient-centered care.

Products and Protocols

When ordering wound care products for a patient moving from one setting to another, it is important to recognize that wound care protocols vary between practice settings and this can have an impact on the patient's understanding of and adherence to the wound management plan. Sometimes this variability exists because of patient acuity. For example, in the acute care setting, wounds are usually being debrided or treated for infection, and in these situations it is critical for the staff to provide frequent wound assessment and at least daily dressing changes. Thus, in the acute care setting, advanced dressings designed to stay in place for several days may not be the best choice and may not be used. In contrast, wound care in the home setting is generally less acute, and reduced frequency of dressing changes is both therapeutically appropriate and more cost-effective. In addition, the goal in home care is for the patient or family to become independent in wound care, so simplicity and ease of application is another factor to be considered for the wound care nurse in this setting. Use of products and protocols that are easy for the patient or caregiver to obtain and to follow is particularly important for the patient with a potentially long-standing wound in which maintenance is the goal. For example, an order for an alginate filler dressing and an adhesive foam cover dressing that is changed only twice a week is much more "user friendly" than an order for damp gauze filler and dry gauze/tape cover dressing changed twice daily. In addition to differences in wound care protocols, there are differences in product availability among care settings. Many acute care facilities, clinics, and home health agencies have adopted product formularies and decision tools that guide product selection as a means to help improve consistency while controlling costs. As patients transition across these sites of care, products available in one setting may not necessarily be available in the next one.

These differences in protocols and formularies can present a major problem when the patient is transitioned from one care setting to another, particularly if the provider coordinating the transition fails to take these differences into consideration and writes orders for a home care patient based on the care provided in the acute care setting.

CLINICAL PEARL

Challenges to seamless care include differences in wound care protocols and priorities, differences in product formularies, and lack of communication between care settings and providers.

Wound care nurses can help improve continuity of care for patients transitioning to another care setting by considering product availability in the next setting when coordinating discharge plans and obtaining discharge wound care orders. If the patients will be purchasing their own supplies, it is also important to consider the patient's financial resources (including third-party payer coverage), and any preferred provider for durable medical equipment (DME) and wound care supplies, including dressings. Specific strategies the wound care nurse can employ to promote seamless transitions include the following. (1) Meet with wound clinicians in other care settings to ascertain product availability, and work together to develop product "cross-walks" that simplify selection decisions as patients transition from one care setting to the next. (2) If there is a certain dressing type or category that is frequently ordered for community dwelling patients, meet with local DME providers to ensure the product is available. (3) Foster a principle-based approach to topical therapy, and utilize appropriate alternatives or substitutions for preferred products that are not available, at least for the short term. (4) Work with ordering providers to assure that wound care orders are appropriate for the setting to which the patient is being transferred, that orders are clear and protocols are as simple as possible, and that any product orders are written in generic terms (e.g., alginate dressing, foam dressing, etc.). The wound care nurse is often viewed as a community resource, and these community connections and relationships help everyone deliver the best and most seamless care.

Clear Communication

There are a number of other strategies the wound care nurse can employ to promote patient-centered care and seamless transition of care. For example, as the patient transitions between patient care settings, there is the potential for errors due to gaps in communication. The effective wound care nurse provides clear instructions to the staff of the "receiving" agency, maintains communication with the patient and family/caregivers, and provides contact information to the staff of the receiving agency, so that they can obtain any needed clarification of discharge orders.

Wound care nurses are often involved in planning and providing care for patients whose dressing change procedures are initially very complex; in these situations, it is important to remember to simplify the procedures as soon as appropriate. For care provided by patients and/or family members, it is even more important to keep procedures and protocols simple. The more complicated the procedure, the less likely it will be followed consistently, and using multiple products when a single product will work not only complicates the procedure but also adds to the cost of care.

The wound nurse must remember that all members of the health care team, including the family/caregivers, have an important role in promotion of wound healing. Often, the people closest to the patient can play a very important role in influencing, motivating, and reinforcing behavior change. In the inpatient setting, the bedside caregivers, such as nursing assistants, are of particular importance to patient outcomes; they are usually the people responsible for turning and repositioning, incontinence care, bathing, and feeding, and their care frequently "makes the difference" in terms of outcomes. Thus, they should be included in educational programs and in recognition and reward programs.

As noted, many agencies develop "formularies" for wound care products; this can help to standardize care, simplify decision making, and reduce supply costs. The wound care nurses can play a key leadership role in development of an appropriate formulary for their facility or agency. In most wound care clinicians' ideal world, the dressing options would be endless; however, the current reality is that agencies are no longer able to maintain large inventories of diverse products to meet every possible need. Instead, agencies are utilizing group purchasing organizations in order to take advantage of "bulk rates," and product formularies are being developed with the goal of providing optimal care at the best price. Wound care nurses are well equipped to assist with formulary decisions; they utilize a principle-based approach to product selection and can therefore assist the agency to select products that are both therapeutically appropriate and cost-effective. The wound nurse can then develop wound care protocols based on formulary products and can educate the staff as to "which protocol/product" to use in which situation.

Conclusion

Effective patient-centered wound care involves mutual establishment of appropriate goals (healing vs maintenance or comfort); when the goal is healing, the wound care nurse must coordinate development of a comprehensive plan of care that includes identification and correction of etiologic factors, attention to the systemic factors and conditions affecting repair, and evidence-based topical therapy. On an agency-wide basis, the wound care nurse uses his/her extensive knowledge of the principles and evidence underlying wound care along with his/her knowledge of the various dressings and therapies currently available to develop formularies and protocols that provide for care that is both therapeutically appropriate and cost-effective. Finally, the wound care nurse is prepared to promote seamless transitions in care by establishing collegial relationships with care providers in other agencies and by working with the ordering provider to assure that discharge/transition orders for wound care are clear and appropriate for the setting to which the patient is being transitioned, as simple as possible, and written in generic terms.

REFERENCES

American Diabetes Association. (2014). Standards of medical care in diabetes. *Diabetes Care, 37*(Suppl 1), S14–S80.

Apelqvist J. (2012, June). Diagnostics and treatment of the diabetic foot. *Endocrine, 41*(3), 384–397.

Cardiovascular Effects of Cannabis. (2014). *Independent drug monitoring unit.* Retrieved from http://www.idmu.co.uk/canncardio.htm

Coleman, E. A., Parry, C., Chalmers, S., et al. (2006). The care transitions intervention: Results of a randomized controlled trial. *Archives of Internal Medicine, 166*, 1822–1828.

Demidova-Rice T. N., Hamblin M. R., & Herman I. M. (2012, July). Acute and impaired wound healing: Pathophysiology and current methods for drug delivery. Part 1: Normal and chronic wounds: Biology, causes and approaches to care. *Advances in Skin & Wound Care, 25*(7), 304–314.

Jones R. T. (2002, November). Cardiovascular system effects of marijuana. *Journal of Clinical Pharmacology, 42*(S1), S58–S63.

Kaminski M. V., & Drinane J. J. (2014). Learning the oral and cutaneous signs of micronutrient deficiencies. *Journal of Wound Ostomy & Continence Nurses Society, 41*(2), 127–135.

Kapetanaki M. G., Mora A. L., & Rojas M. (2013, January). Influence of age on wound healing and fibrosis. *Journal of Pathology, 229*(2), 310–322. Retrieved from http://onlinelibrary.wiley.com/doi/10.1002/path.4122/full

Lavery L. A., Seaman J. W., Barnes S. A., et al. (2008, January). Prediction of healing for postoperative diabetic foot wounds based on early wound area progression. *Diabetes Care, 31*(1), 26–29.

Legal Medical Marijuana States and DC. (2014). LegalMarijuanaStates. Procon.org. Retrieved from http://medicalmarijuana.procon.org/view.resource.php?resourceID=000881

Maida V. (2013, March). Wound management in patients with advanced illness. *Current Opinion in Supportive and Palliative Care, 7*(1), 73–79.

Marijuana (*Cannabis sativa*): Drugs and supplements. (2014). *The Mayo Clinic 2014*. Retrieved from http://www.mayoclinic.org/drugs-supplements/marijuana/background/hrb-20059701

Naylor M. D., Brooten D. A., Campbell R. L., et al. (2004). Transitional care of older adults hospitalized with heart failure: A randomized controlled trial. *Journal of the American Geriatrics Society, 52*, 675–684.

Pierpont Y. N., Dinh T. P., Salas R. E., et al. (2014, February). Obesity and surgical wound healing: A current review. *International Scholarly Research Notices: Obesity, 2014*(638936), 1–13. Retrieved from http://www.hindawi.com/journals/isrn/2014/638936/abs

Sgonc R., & Gruber J. (2013). Age-related aspects of cutaneous wound healing: A mini review. *Gerontology, 59*(2), 159–164. Retrieved from http://www.karger.com/Article/Fulltext/342344

Standards of Medical Care in Diabetes. (2014, January). *Diabetes Care, 37*(Suppl 1), 1–67. Retrieved from http://care.diabetesjournals.org/content/37/Supplement_1/S14.full.pdf+html

Teno J. M., Gozalo P., Mitchell S. L., et al. (2012, May 12). Feeding tubes and the prevention or healing of pressure ulcers. *Archives of Internal Medicine, 172*(9), 697–701.

Tippett A. (2014). *Palliative wound care.* Presentation at the Northern Illinois WOCN Nurse Conference. Retrieved from http://www.niawocn.org/downloadables/2014%20wocnmeeting/PALLIATIVE%20WOUND%20CARE%20%20wocn%202014.pdf

Weinberg M. A., & Segelnick, S. L. (2011). A profile of electronic cigarettes. *U.S. Pharmacist, 36*(7), 37–41. Retrieved from http://www.uspharmacist.com/content/d/feature/c/29050

Wicke C., Halliday B., Allen D., et al. (2000). Effects of steroids and retinoids on wound healing. *Archives of Surgery, 135*(11), 1265–1270. Retrieved from http://archsurg.jamanetwork.com/article.aspx?articleid=390751

Wright J. A., Richards T., & Srai S. K. S. (2014, July). The role of iron in skin and cutaneous wound healing. *Frontiers in Pharmacology, 5*(156). doi:10.3389/fphar.2014.00156. Retrieved from http://www.ncbi.nlm.nih.gov/pmc/articles/PMC4091310/

QUESTIONS

1. What should be the focus of wound management for a patient with chronic wounds who has terminal cancer?
- A. Wound healing
- B. Wound maintenance
- C. Comfort
- D. Correction of etiological factors

2. What critical intervention should the wound nurse recommend to manage chronic wounds of a diabetic patient diagnosed with neuropathy?
- A. Compression wraps/stockings
- B. Tight glycemic control
- C. Anti-inflammatory agents
- D. Antimicrobial therapy

3. What would a wound nurse recommend as an intervention to manage a chronic wound for a patient with severe chronic obstructive pulmonary disease (COPD)?
- A. Use of nasal oxygen
- B. Reduction of fluid intake
- C. Weight loss counseling
- D. Use of corticosteroids

4. A wound nurse is devising a care plan for a patient with a dehisced incision. Which strategy is recommended to promote wound healing?
- A. Use of marijuana
- B. Replacing tobacco cigarettes with e-cigarettes
- C. Use of anticoagulants to improve perfusion
- D. Increasing calories in the diet

5. Which macronutrient would the wound nurse increase in the diet of a patient to promote wound healing?
A. Protein
B. Essential minerals such as zinc
C. Fat
D. Vitamins

6. Based on the American Diabetes Association goal for glycemic control, what glucose level would the wound nurse recommend for a young patient with a long life expectancy who has limited complications and no history of severe hypoglycemia?
A. AIC 5.5% to 6.0%
B. AIC 6.0% to 6.5%
C. AIC 6.5% to 7.0%
D. AIC 7.0% to 7.5%

7. The wound nurse is devising a care plan for a patient with chronic wounds who has been on long-term corticosteroid use for rheumatoid arthritis. What is a recommended strategy to promote wound healing?
A. Increase the dosage of the corticosteroid.
B. Apply 25,000 international units of vitamin A to the wound daily for 10 days.
C. Avoid the use of topical antimicrobial ointments and dressings.
D. Avoid the use of adhesive remover products and silicone-based adhesives.

8. When devising a treatment plan for patients with chronic wounds, the wound nurse should keep in mind that:
A. Chronic wounds are manifestations of acute conditions
B. Dressings heal wounds
C. Overall health of the patient must be addressed to promote healing
D. Topical therapy should be used as a last resort

9. What is the chief priority of the wound nurse to promote seamless transition of care for a patient moving from an acute care facility to a home care setting?
A. Clear communication regarding care plan and goals
B. Ordering wound care products
C. Assessing the condition of the wound
D. Providing counseling to the patient

10. Which of the following is an effective strategy for promoting a seamless transition between care settings for patients with chronic wounds?
A. Use of different wound care protocols and priorities for each facility in the system
B. Selection of products based on cost considerations alone
C. Wound care orders that specify trade names/ brand of dressing
D. Generic wound care orders and frequent communication with other providers

ANSWERS: 1.C, 2.**B**, 3.**A**, 4.**D**, 5.**A**, 6.**C**, 7.**B**, 8.**C**, 9.**A**, 10.**D**

CHAPTER 5

Patient and Caregiver Education

Significance and Guidelines

Lia van Rijswijk

OBJECTIVES

1. Develop an individualized plan of care based on assessment data and current evidence-based guidelines that addresses each of the following factors:
   - Correction or amelioration of etiologic factors
   - Attention to systemic factors affecting repair process
   - Evidence-based topical therapy
   - Pain management
   - Patient and caregiver education
2. Discuss common challenges in patient and caregiver education.
3. Use the nursing process to develop an appropriate teaching plan for an individual patient and/or caregiver.
4. Identify resources for patient and caregiver education.

Topic Outline

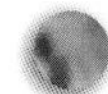 Introduction and Requirements

Throughout this core curriculum, there have been frequent references to the importance of patient and family education, and the role of the wound care nurse in providing that education; this chapter will provide a framework the wound care nurse can use to assure appropriate and effective instruction regarding wound prevention and wound management.

Education has been a core function of nursing for as long as nursing has been recognized as a unique discipline. The National League of Nursing (previously known as the National League of Nursing Education) observed as early as 1918 that nurses are agents for the promotion of health and the prevention of illness in all settings in which they practice (National League of Nursing Education, 1937). The brochure developed by the American Hospital Association to explain "The Patient Care Partnership: Understanding Expectations, Rights and Responsibilities" (American Hospital Association, 2001) includes several specific patient rights that relate to information and education. All State Nurse Practice Acts include teaching within the scope of nursing practice responsibilities and the American Nurses Association's Scope and Standards of Practice (American Nurses Association [ANA], 2010) provides detailed measurement criteria for health education. Specifically, registered nurses are expected to provide health education using methods that are appropriate to the situation and to the patient's developmental level, learning needs, learning readiness, ability to learn, language preference, and culture while seeking opportunities for feedback and evaluation of effectiveness (ANA, 2010). According to the ANA, the role of the Advanced Practice Registered Nurse includes designing health information and education materials by synthesizing all relevant theories and information and helping patients to access quality health information (ANA, 2010). Thus, in addition to being an effective teacher, the Certified Wound Care Nurse (CWCN) will usually be expected to develop appropriate teaching

TABLE 5-1 Education Assessment and Implementation Recommendations in Select Chronic Wound Guidelines*

Title (Author)	Recommendation (Level of Evidence or Strength of Recommendation**)
Guideline for prevention and management of pressure ulcers. (WOCN)	• Educate patient/caregiver about the causes and risk factors for pressure ulcer development and ways to minimize risk. **(C)**
Pressure ulcer prevention. In: Evidence-based geriatric nursing protocols for best practice. (Ayello)	• Teach patient, caregivers, and staff the prevention protocol **(N/A)**
Prevention and treatment of pressure ulcers: clinical practice guideline. (NPUAP/EPUAP)	• Assess the individual's/family member's knowledge and belief about developing and healing pressure ulcers **(C)** • Teach the individual and his/her family about the normal healing process and keep them informed about progress (or lack of progress) toward healing, including signs and symptoms that should be brought to the professional's attention. **(C)** • Education about the role of repositioning in pressure ulcer prevention should be offered to all persons involved in the care of individuals at risk of pressure ulcer development, including the individual and significant others (where possible). **(C)**
Association for the Advancement of Wound Care guideline of pressure ulcer guidelines. (AAWC)	• Conduct Psychosocial and Quality of Life Assessment (including cognition, and barriers to self-care/learning) **(A)** • Develop and implement organized, structured, and comprehensive training programs for health care personnel, patients, families, and all caregivers for prevention and treatment of pressure ulcers **(B)**
(1) Risk assessment & prevention of pressure ulcers. (2) Risk assessment & prevention of pressure ulcers 2011 supplement. (RNOA)	• An educational program for prevention of pressure ulcers should incorporate the principles of adult learning and the level of information provided, and the mode of delivery must be flexible to accommodate the needs of the adult learner. Program evaluation is a critical component of the program planning process. **(IIb)**
SOLUTIONS wound care algorithm. (ConvaTec)	• Provide patient and/or caregiver teaching and support (venous ulcer) **(A)** • Provide patient and/or caregiver teaching and support (arterial/venous ulcers, diabetic foot ulcers) **(C)**
Association for the Advancement of Wound Care venous ulcer guideline. (AAWC)	• Provide patient education including cause of skin breakdown, smoking cessation, how and why to use compression and leg elevation **(A)**
Guideline for management of wounds in patients with lower-extremity venous disease. (WOCN)	• Educate patients that compression stockings or other compression wraps/bandages must be worn every day for the prevention of venous edema and venous leg ulcer recurrence. **(A)**
Assessment and management of foot ulcers for people with diabetes. (RNAO)	• Provide health education to optimize diabetes management, foot care, and ulcer care. **(Ia)**
Guideline for management of wounds in patients with lower-extremity neuropathic disease. (WOCN)	• Educate patients and caregivers, focusing on daily self-care measures, early recognition and reporting of potential foot problems **(N/A)**

*All available at Agency for Healthcare Research and Quality Guideline clearinghouse: www.guideline.gov

**See Individual guideline for specific level of evidence/recommendation scheme. Level of evidence/strength of recommendation ranges from high/strong (A or Ia) to low (C or IV)

EPUAP, European Pressure Ulcer Advisory Panel; NPUAP, National Pressure Ulcer Advisory Panel; WOCN, Wound Ostomy Continence Nurses Association; RNAO, Registered Nurses' Association of Ontario.

plans and educational materials for in- and outpatients with wounds and can also be expected to be involved in education of staff members.

Original research examining the effects of patient education on wound prevention and treatment outcomes is limited (Dorresteijn et al., 2012); despite this, all guidelines for chronic wound prevention and management currently available through the Department of Health and Human Services' (DHHS) Agency for Healthcare Research and Quality (AHRQ) guideline clearinghouse Web site contain patient and caregiver education recommendations, albeit with varying levels of evidence and strength of recommendations (Table 5-1). In other words, patient and caregiver education is an integral component of nursing, the CWCN role, and evidence-based care.

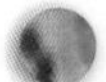

Goals of Care and Education

The ultimate goal of patient and caregiver education is to assist patients to implement behaviors that help them meet their goals for care. "The success of the nurse's efforts at teaching depends not on how much information has been imparted but rather on how much the person has learned" (Bastable, 2006). Thus education involves both teaching and learning with the goal of helping people to achieve optimal independence in their self-care and health. The goals of education change when the goals of care change and can range from recognizing the signs and symptoms of an infection and being able to change a dressing to preventing the development or recurrence of a wound.

CLINICAL PEARL

The goal of patient and caregiver education is to affect behavior.

Assessment

Every nursing process, including teaching and development of instructional content and materials, begins with a complete and thorough assessment of the learner. Using the ANA measurement criteria described, the wound care nurse needs to begin by understanding *what* the patient or caregiver needs to learn to help meet the goals of care. For assessment (and evaluation) purposes, the Health Belief Model (HBM) (Rosenstock et al., 1988) can provide a useful framework. Originally developed to predict and explain health behavior, this model is also useful in explaining the role of culture, values, and beliefs in predicting outcomes and adherence to the plan of care (Edelman et al., 2014). The model postulates that the likelihood of a person implementing recommended behaviors is affected by a number of factors; these factors are categorized as individual perception variables, modifying variables, and variables determining likelihood of action (Table 5-2). Although the predictive value of each factor varies, the effect of *perceived benefits* and *perceived barriers* on likelihood of action has consistently been observed in a wide variety of studies (Carpenter, 2010). For example, when researchers investigated factors influencing patient concordance with compression stocking use to prevent venous leg ulcer recurrence, they found only two factors that differed significantly between persons who did and did not wear compression stockings daily: the belief that wearing stockings was worthwhile and the belief that stockings were uncomfortable to wear (Jull et al., 2004).

CLINICAL PEARL

The factors most likely to affect adherence to care recommendations are the individual's perceptions of the *benefits* and *barriers* associated with the recommendation.

The take-home message from these studies is the importance of assessing each individual from the perspective of his/her beliefs and priorities related to the care recommendations. Open-ended questions are more effective than "yes/no" questions when trying to identify gaps in knowledge, understand a patient's culture (Rankin & Stallings, 1996), and explore the factors in all three dimensions of the HBM that may be barriers or facilitators to self-care and optimal health. Good examples of open-ended questions that address the individual's *beliefs about and understanding* of the disease process, potential *modifying factors,* and perceived ability to *implement care recommendations* include the following:

- What do you think caused your wound? Why do you think it started when it did?
- How severe is it? How does the wound affect you?
- What are you most worried about?
- If you didn't have this wound, what would you be doing right now? What would you like to do when the wound is healed? Do you think it will take a long or short time for the wound to heal?
- Do you know anyone who had a similar problem and what happened to him/her?
- What are your goals for care of this wound?
- What kind of treatment do you think is needed to get the wound to heal?
- How do you feel about the care recommendations that have been made (e.g., smoking cessation, tight glucose control, offloading)?

Demographic and psychosocial variables are important to assess since they are known to affect outcomes of care. For example, researchers found that leg elevation, use of compression hosiery, social support, and self-efficacy all significantly affected the risk of venous ulcer recurrence

TABLE 5-2 Using the Health Belief Model

Individual Perceptions	Modifying Factors	Likelihood of Action Variables
• Beliefs about susceptibility to... (e.g., venous ulcer recurrence) **plus** • Beliefs about seriousness of... (e.g., what happens if I get another wound?) **equals** • Perceived threat of... (e.g., what are the risks when I develop another venous ulcer?)	• Demographic variables (e.g., age, race, ethnicity) • Sociopsychological variables (e.g., personality, socioeconomic status, peer and reference group pressure) • Structural variables (e.g., knowledge about disease/condition)	• Perceived Benefits of Action (e.g., no wound pain and clinic visits) **minus** • Perceived Barriers to Action (e.g., compression stockings too warm, expensive, difficult to apply) **equals** • **Likelihood of taking action** (e.g., wearing compression stockings daily)

Adapted from Rosenstock, I. M., Strecher, K. J., & Becker, M. H. (1988). The social learning theory and Health Belief Model. *Health Education Quarterly, 15,* 175–183, with permission.

(Finlayson et al., 2011). In a study examining risk factors for pressure ulcer development in Spinal Cord Injury (SCI) patients, level of injury and shorter time since injury increased the risk of having a pressure ulcer at the time of the study; however, so did being black, being male, not having a high school diploma, and having a household income <$ 25,000 per year (Saunders et al., 2010). These observations are not surprising since demographic and psychosociologic variables have a profound impact on health literacy.

Health literacy is usually defined as the degree to which individuals have the capacity to obtain, process, and understand basic health information and services; efforts to improve health literacy have been an area of increased focus in recent years, and are included in the 2010 Affordable Care Act (Koh et al., 2012). Studies suggest that many patients who have or are at risk for a chronic wound have the same demographic characteristics as persons found to have the highest rates of limited literacy and health illiteracy. Specifically, studies show that one in four adults (25%) has a low level of health literacy, and this number increases to 37.9% for persons >50 years of age (Paasche-Orlow et al., 2005). The percentage of adults with limited health literacy continues to increase with increasing age. These data have profound implications for the wound care nurse. Conservatively, the wound care nurse should expect that at least 40% of her/his wound care patients will have limited ability to obtain, process, and understand information and instructions regarding their care. Low health literacy is associated with a number of adverse health outcomes; these include reduced ability to take medication correctly, reduced ability to interpret labels and health messaging, poorer health outcomes and health status among the elderly, less effective use of health care services, and higher all-cause mortality rates (Berkman et al., 2011).

CLINICAL PEARL

Health literacy is defined as an individual's ability to understand and process health-related information ... 40% of individuals >50 years of age have limited health literacy.

Several methods and tools are available to assist the clinician in screening for health literacy (**Table 5-3**). Depending on the care setting and the assessment goals, the wound nurse may choose either a detailed and extensive assessment tool or a few simple screening questions. For example, in one study involving a random sample of VA patients (average age 61 years) it was found that a single question ("How confident are you filling out medical forms by yourself?") effectively identified individuals with inadequate, though not marginal, health literacy skills (Chew et al., 2008). In addition to determining the individual's health literacy, current level of knowledge regarding the disease process, wound, and treatment plan, goals for care, and willingness to modify lifestyle behaviors, the nurse must consider whether the patient or caregiver is physically and emotionally capable of providing and learning the care. For example, is the patient or caregiver physically capable of applying compression hosiery or changing position to relieve pressure? Is the person with a new SCI emotionally ready to discuss the injury and its impact, let alone pressure ulcer prevention strategies?

Teaching Goals and Objectives

Prior to initiating a teaching session or developing an educational program or materials, it is important to consider (1) the teaching goal and objectives based on the goals of care, (2) assessment findings, and (3) in most situations, the principles of adult (andragogy) or older adult (geragogy) learning. Adults are generally self-directed, have a lifetime of experience they want to use and share, need to know why they should learn something and how it benefits them, may have difficulty with someone telling them what to do (self-concept), are life-, task- and problem-centered, and respond more to internal priorities than to external motivators (Knowles et al., 1998). When teaching older adults, the wound nurse may need to make adaptations to accommodate normal physical and cognitive changes associated with aging: for example, written instructions should be at least 14-point font and good lighting should be provided, hearing aids should be in and on, and information should be provided in shorter teaching sessions with more repetition. At the same time, the wound nurse

TABLE 5-3 Health Literacy Assessment and Screening Tools

Title/Name	Availability
Rapid Estimate of Adult Literacy in Medicine, shorter version (REALM-R)	Tool and directions available at AHRQ Web site: http://www.ahrq.gov/professionals/quality-patient-safety/pharmhealthlit/realm-r.html
Single Item Literacy Screener (to identify adults in need of help with printed materials)	Tool and directions available at: http://www.champ-program.org/static/SILS_Tool.pdf
The Newest Vital Sign (health literacy tool)	Available in English and Spanish at: http://www.pfizer.com/health/literacy/public_policy_researchers/nvs_toolkit/
Short Test of Functional Health Literacy in Adults (STOFHLA)	Available (PdF) at: http://www.reginfo.gov/public/do/DownloadDocument?documentID...1 and at: http://www.peppercornbooks.com/

should be aware that the vast majority of older adults retain the ability to learn and should avoid assumptions of cognitive decline (ageism) (Bastable, 2006).

Most chronic wound conditions develop as a result of several complex interactions; thus, providing effective education in regard to wound management or wound prevention is not easy. For example, to help an individual patient prevent the development of a pressure ulcer following discharge (goal of care and education), the patient needs to meet a variety of objectives in the cognitive (knowledge), affective (emotions, feelings), and behavioral or psychomotor domain. Specifically, the patient and/or caregiver needs at least a basic understanding of the role of immobility, shear damage, moisture, and malnutrition on skin and tissue health, and needs to verbalize and demonstrate the critical measures for prevention: correct positioning, moisture management, and nutritional intake.

A systematic literature review of cancer patient education strategies has shown that, regardless of strategy used, structured, culturally appropriate, and patient-specific teachings are more effective than unstructured ad hoc teaching methods (Friedman et al., 2011). *Teaching plans are invaluable to organize the objectives, content, teaching/learning activities, and evaluation methods,* in part because it requires the wound care nurse to examine the teaching/learning process related to specific areas (Beitz, 2007).

CLINICAL PEARL

Teaching plans are invaluable.

Instructional objectives must be clearly defined and should clearly delineate what it is that the patient/caregiver needs to be able to *do, explain, discuss, etc.* Verbs used in instructional objectives should be measurable, can be classified based on the behavioral objective domain classifications (cognitive, affective and psychomotor), and can be found in textbooks (Bastable, 2006). The wound care nurse can also use Bloom's Taxonomy verbs, which are available online from a variety of sources.

The third element in developing a teaching plan is to divide the overall content and skills to be learned into individual "lessons" that are manageable. A sample teaching plan for pressure ulcer prevention is as follows:

- Day 1—The patient can explain the relationship between pressure and skin breakdown (cognition/comprehension)
- Day 2—The patient independently shifts weight using appropriate techniques while sitting and lying down (behavioral/psychomotor)
- Day 3—The patient asks questions and discusses the importance of preventing pressure ulcers (affective/responding).

An optimal teaching plan also includes evaluation methods, for example, the learner answers questions correctly and demonstrates appropriate off-loading techniques.

The most effective individual teaching plans are based on assessment findings. It is of course important to address identified structural variables (knowledge gaps), but, as mentioned, the effect of perceived benefits and perceived barriers (see **Table 5-2**) on likelihood of action is profound (Carpenter, 2010) and must be considered in the teaching objectives and content. For example, if the patient has indicated that his life is very hectic and he sometimes forgets to take his medication, the nurse should assume that remembering to shift weight may be an important barrier to achieving the overall goal of care and strategies that may work for him need to be explored. Similarly, if the patient has stated that her goal is to get the plantar surface wound to heal, but she has also explained that she has to work, cannot take time off, and has a high deductible health insurance plan and financial concerns, an effective management plan must include exploring off-loading devices and strategies that will reduce these barriers to implementing the recommended plan of care.

Teaching Strategies and Implementation

Teaching strategies and implementation methods are detailed in the teaching plan. Multiple teaching strategies (e.g., computer technology, audio- and videotapes, written materials, demonstrations) are generally more effective than is verbal teaching alone (Friedman et al., 2011). In one study involving the ability of patients at risk for foot ulcers to recall information, videos were found to be more effective than written material only (Gravely et al., 2011). Although every person learns differently, most learn best when exposed to information in more than one mode; for example, a combination of visual, auditory, reading/writing, and kinesthetic (experience and practice) information (Fleming & Mills, 1992). An advantage to one-on-one patient/caregiver teaching strategies is the ability to readily adapt the information to meet individual needs and goals. Immediate responses can be solicited, learning evaluated, and modifications made. It is, however, important to make sure that the patient does not feel that he/she is "put on the spot" or that his/her knowledge is tested. During demonstrations/return demonstrations of psychomotor skills, it is especially important for the learner to know that he or she is not expected to perform the task flawlessly—only practice will build competence (Bastable, 2006).

Because one-on-one education is very time intensive, other educational materials (videos, printed materials) are widely used in health care to complement face-to-face teaching. It is critical for the wound nurse to carefully assess all written and audiovisual materials to assure appropriate reading level and comprehension. As previously noted, population assessments have shown that a large percentage of people have health literacy limitations and they are unable to understand many of the educational materials used today.

CLINICAL PEARL

Do not reinvent the wheel—use what is known and available.

Written materials can be readily assessed for appropriateness of reading level using one of several reading level analysis tools: for example, the Flesch Reading Ease Formula and Flesch-Kincaid Grade level are included in word processing software tools. Most health education materials are written at a 10th grade reading level; however, 21% of adults in the United States read below a 5th grade level and 19% of high school graduates cannot read (U.S. Department of Education, 2007). There is obviously a profound "disconnect" between many educational products available today and what we know about health literacy. In a recent analysis of written materials used to teach patients about skin care and pressure ulcer prevention, researchers found that most materials were written at an 8th or 10th grade reading level and none of the materials were appropriate teaching tools for low-literacy patients (Wilson, 2003).

Although reading levels are important, it is only one consideration in developing appropriate health education materials. All educational materials (e.g., videos, printed materials) should be prepared using health literacy universal precautions (Brach et al., 2012). *A health literate health care organization simplifies all communication to the greatest extent possible* and verifies comprehension with everyone; they do not make assumptions about who understands or needs extra assistance. Fortunately, there are many resources to help the wound care nurse prepare education materials that meet the needs of patients using scientific principles of health communication that go beyond determining reading levels (**Table 5-4**).

CLINICAL PEARL

All educational materials should be prepared using health literacy universal precautions (keep it simple!)

Evaluation

Evaluating the success of educational efforts is determined by the extent to which learning occurred; evaluation of patient/caregiver learning is based on the objectives outlined in the teaching plan and whether or not the goals of care are met. Can the patient safely and correctly shift weight or apply compression stockings (objectives), *and/or* did he or she implement this practice into his or her daily life (goals of care/action) (see **Table 5-2**)? In evaluating individual patient/caregiver learning, it is necessary to ask open-ended questions and to observe return demonstrations.

In evaluating an overall educational program, the wound nurse must determine whether the educational tools that were developed meet the desired objectives. Fortunately, many of the resources available for development of health communication tools also contain strategies for testing and evaluation (see **Table 5-4**) and AHRQ has developed a Patient Education Materials Assessment Tool (PEMAT) and User's Guide (Shoemaker et al., 2013). In general, an educational evaluation can range from a simple formative evaluation of the process used to a more complex impact evaluation (Abruzzese, 1978; Bastable, 2006). A guiding question for a total program evaluation may be "How well did patient education activities implemented throughout the year meet the goals established for a clinic's patient education program?" (Bastable, 2006). While difficult to use for a specific health care area (e.g., the wound clinic), from a health care systems perspective the Centers for Medicare and

TABLE 5-4 Resources to Improve Educational Outcomes and Develop Health Literate Education Communications

Publisher and Title	Purpose	Availability
Centers for Disease Control and Prevention (CDC) Clear Communication Index	Tool for developing and assessing CDC Public Communication Products	http://www.cdc.gov/ccindex/pdf/clear-communication-user-guide.pdf
CDC Clear Communication Index Score Sheet	Helps evaluate appropriateness of communication products	http://www.cdc.gov/healthliteracy/pdf/fillable-form-may-2013.pdf
DHHS office of Disease Prevention and Health Promotion Literacy Online Guide	Overview of how to deliver online health information	http://www.health.gov/healthliteracyonline/
National Patient Safety Foundation Ask Me 3	Patient education program designed to promote communication between health care providers and patients.	http://www.npsf.org/for-health-careprofessionals/programs/ask-me-3/
AHRQ Health Literacy Universal Precautions Toolkit	Toolkit to help improve spoken and written communication, patient self-management, and supportive systems.	http://www.ahrq.gov/qual/literacy/
CDC—Simply Put	Guide for creating easy-to-understand teaching materials	http://www.cdc.gov/healthliteracy/pdf/simply_put.pdf

Medicaid Services (CMS) Hospital Consumer Assessment of Healthcare Providers and Systems (HCAHPS) survey outcomes also contain information that may be useful in evaluating teaching strategies. For example, patients are asked to rate how often nurses and doctors listened carefully, explained things in a way they could understand, and are asked how well they understood their care when leaving the hospital. (CMS, 2014). *The sheer number of communication questions in the HCAHPS survey serves as yet another reminder that patient/caregiver education affects patient outcomes!*

The entire process of patient/caregiver education, from assessment to evaluation, is cyclical, and evaluation findings should be put to good use and lead to education improvements wherever they are needed. In this case, we can practice what we preach when teaching psychomotor skills to patients: "Practice makes perfect."

CLINICAL PEARL

Learning and teaching improve with practice.

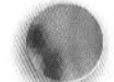

Conclusion

Patient and caregiver education is an integral component of evidence-based practice and the wound care nurse role. The goal of education is to influence patient/caregiver behavior, and we have learned over the past few decades that adjustments in behavior require more than delivery of information. There are a number of studies that demonstrate a complex and significant relationship between individual perceptions, psychosocial variables, and perceived benefits and barriers of specific actions and interventions; all of these factors must be considered when developing an effective education plan. We have also learned a lot about health literate communications strategies, and providers are encouraged to follow health literacy universal precautions when developing educational materials and approaches.

Fortunately, patient and caregiver education involves the same basic steps as the nursing process (with which wound care nurses are very familiar), and research examining health behavior can be used to assure that we are asking the right questions and developing appropriate objectives to meet the goal of care. In addition, there are multiple tools available to guide the nurse in designing effective educational programs, including those developed by the Agency for Health Research and Quality (AHRQ) and the Centers for Disease Control and Prevention (CDC).

REFERENCES

Abruzzese, R. S. (1978). *Nursing staff development: Strategies for success.* St. Louis, MO: Mosby-Year Book.

American Hospital Association. (2001). *The patient care partnership: Understanding expectations, rights, and responsibilities.* Atlanta, GA: Author.

American Nurses Association. (2010). *Nursing: Scope and standards of practice* (2nd ed.). Silver Springs, MD: Author.

Bastable, S. B. (2006). *Essentials of patient education.* Sudbury, MA: Jones & Bartlett.

Beitz, J. (2007). Health promotion and health education. In M. J. Morison, C. J. Moffatt, & P. J. Franks (Eds.), *Leg ulcers: A problem-based learning approach.* Edinburg, UK: Mosby Elsevier.

Berkman N. D., Sheridan S. L., Donahue, K. E., et al. (2011). Low health literacy and health outcomes: An updated systematic review. *Annals of Internal Medicine, 155*(2), 97–107.

Brach, C., Keller, D., Hernandez, L. M., et al. (2012). *Ten attributes of health literate health care organizations.* Washington, DC: Institute of Medicine. Available at: http://iom.edu/~/media/Files/Perspectives-Files/2012/Discussion-Papers/BPH_Ten_HLit_Attributes.pdf

Carpenter, C. J. (2010). A meta-analysis of the effectiveness of Health Belief Model variables in predicting behavior. *Health Communication,* DOI: 10.1080/10410236.2010.521906

Centers for Medicare and Medicaid Services. (2014). Hospital consumer assessment of health care providers and systems. *Survey Instruments.* Baltimore, MD. Available at: http://www.hcahpsonline.org/surveyinstrument.aspx. Accessed September 1, 2014.

Chew, L. D., Griffin, J. M., Partin, M. R., et al. (2008). Validation of screening questions for limited health literacy in a large VA outpatient population. *Journal of General Internal Medicine, 23*(5), 561–566. DOI: 10.1007/s11606-008-0520-5

Dorresteijn, J. A., Kriegsman, D. M. W., Assendelft, W. J. J., et al. (2012). Patient education for preventing diabetic foot ulceration. *The Cochrane Library.* DOI: 10.1002/14651858.CD001488.pub4

Edelman, C. L., Kuzma, E. C., & Mandle, C. L. (2014). *Health promotion throughout the life span* (8th ed.). St. Louis, MO: Elsevier Mosby.

Finlayson, K., Edwards, H., & Courtney, M. (2011). Relationships between preventive activities, psychosocial factors and recurrence of venous leg ulcers: a prospective study. *Journal of Advanced Nursing, 67*(10), 2180–2190. DOI 10.1007/s13187-010-0183-x

Fleming, N. D., & Mills, C. (1992). Helping students understand how they learn. *The Teaching Professor, 7*(4), Madison, WI: Magma Publications.

Friedman, A. J., Cosby, R., Boyko, S., et al. (2011). Effective teaching strategies and methods of delivery for patient education: A systematic review and practice guideline recommendations. *Journal of Cancer Education, 26,* 12–21.

Gravely, S. S., Hensley, B. K., & Hagood-Thompson, C. (2011). Comparison of three types of diabetic foot ulcer education plans to determine patient recall of education. *Journal of Vascular Nursing, 29*(3), 113–119.

Jull, A. B., Mitchell, N., Arroll, J., et al. (2004). Factors influencing concordance with compression stockings after venous leg ulcer healing. *Journal of Wound Care, 13*(3), 90–92.

Knowles, M. S., Holton, E. F., & Swanson, R. A. (1998). *The Adult learner.* Houston, TX: Gulf Publishing.

Koh, H. K., Berwic, D. M., Clancy, C. M., et al. (2012). New Federal policy initiatives to boost health literacy can help the nation move beyond the cycle of costly "crisis care." *Health Affairs, 31*(2), 434–443. DOI: 10.1377/hlthaff.2011.1169

National League of Nursing Education. (1937). *A curriculum guide for schools of nursing.* New York, NY: Author.

Paasche-Orlow, M. K., Parker, R. M., Gazmararian, J. A., et al. (2005). The prevalence of limited health literacy. *Journal of General Internal Medicine,20*(2),175–184.DOI:10.1111/j.1525-1497.2005.40245.x

Rankin, S. H., & Stallings, K. D. (1996). *Patient education: Issues, principles, practices* (3rd ed.). Philadelphia, PA: Lippincott-Raven.

Rosenstock, I. M., Strecher, K. J., & Becker, M. H. (1988). The social learning theory and Health Belief Model. *Health Education Quarterly, 15,* 175–183.

Saunders, L. L., Krause, J. S., Peters, B. A., et al. (2010). The relationship of pressure ulcers, race, and socioeconomic conditions after spinal cord injury. *Journal of Spinal Cord Medicine, 33*(4), 387–395.

Shoemaker, S. J., Wolf, M. S., & Brach, C. (2013). *The Patient Education Materials Assessment Tool (PEMAT) and user's guide*. Rockville, MD: Agency for Health Care Quality and Research. Available at: http://www.ahrq.gov/pemat. Accessed September 1, 2014.

United States Department of Education, National Center for Education Statistics. (2007). *The condition of education 2007.* (NCES 2007-064), Indicator 18. Available at: http://nces.ed.gov/pubs2007/2007064.pdf

Wilson, F. L. (2003). Assessing the readability of skin care and pressure ulcer patient education materials. *Journal of Wound Ostomy & Continence Nursing, 30*(4), 224–230.

QUESTIONS

1. What is the ultimate goal of patient and caregiver education?

A. Imparting as much information as possible to the patient
B. Helping patients achieve optimal independence in self-care and health
C. Helping patients recognize signs and symptoms of infection
D. Teaching patients how to manage the health care system

2. The wound care nurse consults the Health Belief Model when planning teaching to prevent pressure ulcer development for a patient on bed rest. Which factor represents a modifying variable of behavior based on this health belief framework?

A. Belief about susceptibility to pressure ulcer development
B. Perceived threat of developing a pressure ulcer
C. Perceived benefit of techniques used to prevent pressure ulcers
D. Psychosociologic variables of the patient affecting the treatment plan

3. The wound care nurse is interviewing a diabetic patient who has a surgical wound that is showing signs of dehiscence. Which interview question best addresses the individual's understanding of the disease process?

A. "What are your goals for care of this wound?"
B. "How does this wound affect you?"
C. "What role do you think having diabetes played in this wound condition?"
D. "Do you feel you are able to follow the treatment plan we discussed?"

4. Which of the following is an example of a psychosociologic variable that may impact health literacy?

A. Economic status
B. Individual perceptions of health
C. Beliefs about the seriousness of the problem
D. Perceived benefits of action

5. Which of the following is an accurate statistic that should be considered when creating a teaching plan for a patient with a wound?

A. Fifty percent of adults over 50 years of age have a low level of health literacy.
B. One in four adults has a low level of health literacy.
C. At least 20% of wound care patients have a low level of health literacy.
D. Sixty percent of patients treated for wounds have incomes <$25,000.

6. Which information about adult learners should the wound care nurse consider when devising a teaching plan for wound care?

A. Adults are easily motivated to learn a new skill.
B. Adults may have difficulty with someone telling them what to do.
C. Adults are not problem centered; rather, they focus on the big picture.
D. Adults respond more to external motivators than to internal priorities.

7. A wound care nurse is teaching a 70-year-old patient how to care for a new stoma. Which teaching approach modification would be appropriate for this patient?

A. Information should be provided in longer teaching sessions.
B. Written instructions should be 10-point font or higher.
C. Teaching sessions should be short with more repetition.
D. Assume that the vast majority of older adults experience cognitive decline.

8. Which teaching strategy is designed to meet a teaching objective based on the psychomotor domain?

A. The nurse requests a return demonstration of a dressing change.
B. The nurse provides written brochures explaining stoma care.
C. The nurse assesses if the patient values his or her health enough to stop smoking.
D. The nurse describes the process of wound healing to a patient.

9. Which teaching strategy should be followed when performing discharge planning for hospitalized patients?
   A. Instructional objectives should be broadly defined and applicable to all patients.
   B. The teaching plan should be limited to one or two lessons that are manageable.
   C. Verbal teaching is generally more effective than using multiple teaching strategies.
   D. Individual teaching plans should be based on assessment findings and should identify and consider structural variables.

10. Evaluation of the teaching plan is based on:
   A. Learned psychomotor skills
   B. Assessment as to whether objectives outlined in the teaching plan have been met
   C. Treatment progress
   D. Patient satisfaction

ANSWERS: 1.**B**, 2.**C**, 3.**C**, 4.**A**, 5.**B**, 6.**B**, 7.**C**, 8.**A**, 9.**D**, 10.**B**

CHAPTER 6

Nutritional Assessment and Support in Relation to Wound Healing

Becky Dorner, Mary Ellen Posthauer, and Elizabeth Friedrich

OBJECTIVES

1. Develop an individualized plan of care based on assessment data and current evidence-based guidelines that addresses each of the following factors:
   - Correction or amelioration of etiologic factors
   - Attention to systemic factors affecting the repair process
   - Evidence-based topical therapy
   - Pain management
   - Patient and caregiver education
2. Discuss the key factors to be included in a nutritional assessment, and the potential value of a structured screening tool.
3. Describe current guidelines for nutritional support of the patient with or at risk for skin breakdown, including guidelines for caloric intake, protein intake, fluid intake, and micronutrient intake.

Topic Outline

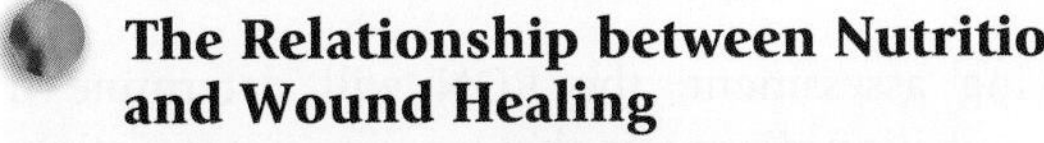

The Relationship between Nutrition and Wound Healing

Nutrition is believed to play an important role in both prevention and treatment of wounds. While there is limited research related to the role of nutrition in wound healing (Choo et al., 2013), there is clinical consensus that nutritional support is an important aspect of a comprehensive care plan for pressure ulcer prevention and for wound management (Dorner et al., 2009). The majority of studies regarding nutrition and wound care are related to pressure ulcers; thus, nutrition management for the prevention and treatment of pressure ulcers is the major focus of this chapter (Posthauer & Schols, 2014). Adequate calories, protein, fluids, vitamins, and minerals are needed by the body to maintain tissue integrity and prevent tissue breakdown; inadequate intake of essential nutrients over time can result in nutritional deficiencies that affect skin integrity. Of particular importance is inadequate intake of protein and calories, which can result in protein energy malnutrition (PEM). PEM alters body composition and the normal pathways by which the body uses protein and fat for fuel (Litchford, 2010); as a result, the body breaks down muscle tissue for energy, and there is a loss of lean body mass (Demling, 2009). In addition, inadequate daily intake of energy can result in inadequate intake of vitamins and minerals.

Malnutrition is associated with many adverse outcomes, including increased risk of pressure ulcers and impaired wound healing (National Pressure Ulcer Advisory Panel, 2014). Providing adequate amounts of calories, protein, vitamins, and minerals in the diet is one key to preventing and treating both malnutrition and pressure ulcers.

CLINICAL PEARL

Preventing and/or treating malnutrition is widely recognized as a key to prevention of pressure ulcers and promotion of wound healing.

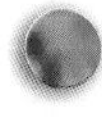

Identifying Individuals with Compromised Nutritional Status

Nutrition Screening

Nutrition screening is the process of identifying characteristics that are known to be associated with nutrition problems (Posthauer & Thomas, 2012). The nutrition-screening process is used to identify individuals at nutritional risk, which should prompt referrals to the appropriate health care professionals for more in-depth assessment. Most nutrition-screening tools are composed of a few simple questions that can be asked by a nurse or any qualified health care professional when the patient is admitted to a health care facility or home health care agency. Screening tools should be quick and easy to use, and valid and reliable for the population served.

Several validated nutrition-screening tools are available, including the Mini-Nutritional Assessment (MNA), the Malnutrition Universal Screening Tool (MUST), the Malnutrition-Screening Tool (MST), and the Subjective Global Assessment (SGA). The MNA has been validated in elderly populations residing in long-term care or community settings and is easy to use when assessing older individuals with pressure ulcers and comorbidities (Hengstermann et al., 2007; Kaiser, 2009) (Fig. 6-1).

Once an individual has been identified as at risk for nutritional compromise, it is imperative to assure prompt referral to a registered dietitian nutritionist (RDN), who will complete the nutritional assessment and determine the nutritional plan of care. Additional indicators for RDN referral include presence of a pressure ulcer or chronic wound that is deteriorating or not healing and comorbidities such as diabetes, chronic kidney disease, heart failure, and chronic obstructive pulmonary disease (COPD). Individuals assessed as being at risk for pressure ulcer development per the Braden Scale or Norton Scale should also be referred to the RDN for a comprehensive nutrition assessment. Finally, individuals with unique dietary circumstances (such as those following vegan diets) or those with limited economic resources or chewing or swallowing problems are candidates for nutrition assessment.

Nutrition Assessment and Follow-Up

Nutrition assessment is a systematic method for obtaining, verifying, and interpreting the data needed to identity nutrition-related problems, their causes, and their significance (Academy of Nutrition and Dietetics, 2013). Using nutrition assessment data, the RDN is able to determine whether a nutrition diagnosis (problem) exists. The nutrition assessment is grouped into five domains (Academy of Nutrition and Dietetics, 2013):

- Food-/nutrition-related history (nutrient intake, food behaviors, etc.)
- Anthropometric measurements (height, weight, body composition, body mass index, weight history)
- Biochemical data, medical tests, and procedures (CBC, CMP, lipid profile, HgbA1C, etc.)
- Nutrition-focused physical findings (overall appearance and any signs and symptoms of nutritional deficiencies or excesses)
- General client history (medical history, weight history, social and socioeconomic history)

Following assessment, the RDN will determine if there is a nutrition diagnosis that requires intervention. Unintended weight loss, PEM, and poor food or fluid intake are all indicators of nutritional deficiencies that increase the risk for pressure ulcer development and/or impaired healing. Most individuals with pressure ulcers will require nutritional intervention. Other health professionals, including speech language pathologists and occupational therapists, may recommend interventions that can increase food and nutrient intake, such as a change in positioning for ease of swallowing or the addition of a self-help feeding device. Frequent monitoring

Mini Nutritional Assessment
MNA®

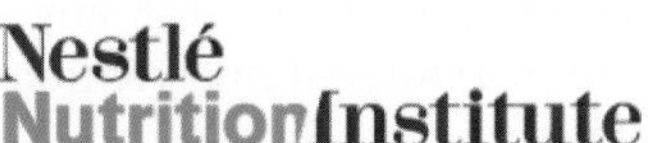

Last name: First name:

Sex: Age: Weight, kg: Height, cm: Date:

Complete the screen by filling in the boxes with the appropriate numbers. Total the numbers for the final screening score.

Screening

A Has food intake declined over the past 3 months due to loss of appetite, digestive problems, chewing or swallowing difficulties?
0 = severe decrease in food intake
1 = moderate decrease in food intake
2 = no decrease in food intake ☐

B Weight loss during the last 3 months
0 = weight loss greater than 3 kg (6.6 lbs)
1 = does not know
2 = weight loss between 1 and 3 kg (2.2 and 6.6 lbs)
3 = no weight loss ☐

C Mobility
0 = bed or chair bound
1 = able to get out of bed / chair but does not go out
2 = goes out ☐

D Has suffered psychological stress or acute disease in the past 3 months?
0 = Yes 2 = no ☐

E Neuropsychological problems
0 = severe dementia or depression
1 = mild dementia
2 = no psychological problems ☐

F1 Body Mass Index (BMI) (weight in kg) / (height in m^2)
0 = BMI less than 19
1 = BMI 19 to less than 21
2 = BMI 21 to less than 23
3 = BMI 23 or greater ☐

IF BMI IS NOT AVAILABLE, REPLACE QUESTION F1 WITH QUESTION F2.
DO NOT ANSWER QUESTION F2 IF QUESTION F1 IS ALREADY COMPLETED.

F2 Calf circumference (CC) in cm
0 = CC less than 31
3 = CC 31 or greater ☐

Screening score (max. 14 points)

12 - 14 points: Normal nutritional status
8 - 11 points: At risk of malnutrition
0 - 7 points: Malnourished ☐☐

References
1. Vellas B, Villars H, Abellan G, et al. Overview of the MNA® - Its History and Challenges. *J Nutr Health Aging* 2006;**10**:456-465.
2. Rubenstein LZ, Harker JO, Salva A, Guigoz Y, Vellas B. Screening for Undernutrition in Geriatric Practice: Developing the Short-Form Mini Nutritional Assessment (MNA®-SF). *J Geront* 2001;**56A**: M366–377.
3. Guigoz Y. The Mini-Nutritional Assessment (MNA®) Review of the Literature - What does it tell us? *J Nutr Health Aging* 2006; **10**:466–487.
4. Kaiser MJ, Bauer JM, Ramsch C, et al. Validation of the Mini Nutritional Assessment Short-Form (MNA®-SF): A practical tool for identification of nutritional status. *J Nutr Health Aging* 2009; **13**:782–788.

For more information: www.mna-elderly.com

FIGURE 6-1. Mini-Nutritional Assessment (MNA). MRA is Société des Produits Nestlé S.A., Vevey, Switzerland, Trademark Owners. Copyright © Nestlé. www.mna-elderly.com.

and evaluation is necessary for any patient at nutritional risk, to determine if interventions are having their intended effect.

CLINICAL PEARL

The RDN should be routinely consulted for assistance with management of individuals at risk for or demonstrating evidence of undernutrition.

Food-/Nutrition-Related History and Client History

Information about an individual's food-related history, medical history, and socioeconomic status can provide important clues to overall nutritional status and potential for improvement in nutritional status. For example:

- An individual's ability to perform activities of daily living (ADLs) and instrumental activities of daily living (IADLs) may affect his or her ability to access nutritious food. For community-dwelling individuals who have no mealtime assistance, this can have a significant impact on food consumption.
- Individuals with chewing and/or swallowing problems are at risk for inadequate intake of food and fluids.
- Individuals who have food allergies or intolerances may be unable to consume some nutritious foods. For example, those with lactose intolerance may not be able to consume milk or cheese, which are excellent sources of protein.
- Cognitive impairment can affect the individual's ability to obtain and prepare food and his/her ability to focus on eating.
- Medications (including prescription, over-the-counter, and herbal supplements) can impair appetite, cause dry mouth and/or GI distress, or produce other side effects that adversely affect nutrient intake.
- Socioeconomic status can affect access to food. Referral to appropriate sources for economic assistance or supplemental food may be necessary.
- Comorbidities like diabetes and chronic kidney disease can necessitate dietary restrictions that affect an individual's food choices.

It is important to remember, particularly when dealing with food habits and access to food, to treat the whole person, not just the pressure ulcer or wound; this requires sensitivity to individual and cultural preferences as well as to economic issues and food availability.

Anthropometric Data

Height and weight, including weight history over time, are critical elements of the nutritional assessment for every individual with pressure ulcers or at risk for developing pressure ulcers. This information is used to estimate daily calorie, protein, and fluid needs and to assess nutritional status over time. One key indicator of undernutrition is unintended weight loss (defined as 5% of body weight in 30 days or 10% of body weight in 180 days) (Sullivan et al., 2004; Thomas, 2008); slow weight loss over time (sometimes called insidious weight loss) can also indicate a nutritional deficiency. Height and weight are also used to determine body mass index (BMI); individuals with a low BMI (< 22) may be at higher risk for pressure ulcers (Horn et al., 2004). See **Tables 6-1, 6-2,** and **6-3** for classification of weight status based on BMI.

TABLE 6-1 Calculation of BMI

BMI is calculated the same way for both adults and children. The calculation is based on the following formulas:

Measurement Units	Formula and Calculation
Kilograms and meters (or centimeters)	Formula: weight (kg)/[height (m)]^2 With the metric system, the formula for BMI is weight in kilograms divided by height in meters squared. Since height is commonly measured in centimeters, divide height in centimeters by 100 to obtain height in meters. Example: weight = 68 kg, height = 165 cm (1.65 m) Calculation: 68 ÷ (1.65)^2 = 24.98
Pounds and inches	Formula: weight (lb) / [height (in.)]^2 × 703 Calculate BMI by dividing weight in pounds (lbs) by height in inches (in.) squared and multiplying by a conversion factor of 703. Example: weight = 150 pounds, height = 5′5″ (65″) Calculation: [150 ÷ (65)^2] × 703 = 24.96

Interpretation of BMI for adults

For adults 20 years old and older, BMI is interpreted using standard weight status categories that are the same for all ages and for both men and women. For children and teens, on the other hand, the interpretation of BMI is both age and sex specific.

Source: Centers for Disease Control and Prevention (2014).

CLINICAL PEARL

Unintended weight loss is a common indicator of malnutrition; thus, ongoing monitoring of patient weight and prompt response to unintended weight loss is a critical element of a nutritional management program.

TABLE 6-2 BMI Classification for Adults

BMI	Weight Status
Below 18.5	Underweight
18.5–24.9	Normal
25.0–29.9	Overweight
30.0 and above	Obese

Source: Centers for Disease Control and Prevention (2014).

TABLE 6-3 BMI Classification Based on Height

Height	Weight Range	BMI	Weight Status
5′9″	124 pounds or less	Below 18.5	Underweight
	125–168 pounds	18.5–24.9	Normal
	169–202 pounds	25.0–29.9	Overweight
	203 pounds or more	30 or higher	Obese

Source: Centers for Disease Control and Prevention (2014).

Biochemical Data

Serum albumin and prealbumin have historically been used to determine visceral protein status; however, it is critical to realize that there is no laboratory test that can provide a "stand-alone" assessment of an individual's nutritional status (Dorner et al., 2009). It is now recognized that many acute and chronic diseases can contribute to inflammation and that inflammation results in reduced levels of hepatic proteins like albumin and prealbumin. Inflammation exerts a significant effect on serum levels of hepatic proteins by altering metabolism of those proteins and by causing capillaries to become "leaky," thus permitting proteins to pass through the capillary walls and into surrounding tissues (Furhman et al., 2004). Serum levels of albumin, prealbumin, and transferrin are therefore reduced in conditions causing inflammation, such as infection, injury, or trauma; as the individual recovers from the inflammatory condition, levels of hepatic proteins rise back toward normal (Litchford et al., 2014). Thus in many cases, hepatic protein levels are indicative of inflammation related to acute or chronic disease, as opposed to poor nutritional status (White et al., 2012). Albumin and prealbumin may correlate with overall prognosis, but frequently do not correlate well with nutritional status; thus, their usefulness in nutritional assessment is limited (Covinsky et al., 2002; Johnson & Merlini, 2007; White et al., 2012). While albumin and prealbumin levels are still commonly used to diagnose malnutrition, these laboratory tests should not be used as a "stand-alone" basis for nutrition interventions (Collins & Friedrich, 2013).

Identification and classification of anemia is an important element of assessment, because adequate levels of iron are required for collagen formation, oxygen transport, and new cell generation, and low iron stores can adversely affect wound healing. A nutritional anemia profile can help identify and classify anemia (Academy of Nutrition and Dietetics, 2013); **Table 6-4** outlines the types of anemia based on lab results.

CLINICAL PEARL

Identification of malnutrition should not be based solely on lab values such as albumin and prealbumin, but on a comprehensive evaluation that includes weight history, protein and calorie intake, and overall health status.

Another element of assessment is hydration status; an electrolyte and renal profile can be used to help identify overhydration or dehydration (Academy of Nutrition and Dietetics, 2013). Lab values that are used to evaluate hydration status include serum BUN, sodium, and serum osmolality (Academy of Nutrition and Dietetics, 2013).

Nutrition-Focused Physical Assessment

Compromised nutritional status can manifest as a specific constellation of physical symptoms; thus, an emerging area of nutrition assessment is nutrition-focused physical assessment (NFPA) (Litchford, 2012). NFPA involves hands-on assessment of the individual specific to nutrition-related components of health (Litchford, 2012) and can help the nutrition and dietetics practitioner to identify the individual with compromised nutritional status. The International Dietetics and Nutrition Terminology Reference Manual defines nutrition-focused physical findings as "physical appearance, muscle and fat wasting, swallow function, appetite, and affect" (Academy of Nutrition and Dietetics, 2013). **Table 6-5** outlines some common physical signs and symptoms of undernutrition.

Identifying Protein Energy Malnutrition

The definition of protein–energy malnutrition has evolved in recent years. It is now recognized as a complex syndrome that manifests in different ways. As a result of this new understanding, the definition of the condition and the diagnostic criteria have been subject to intense scientific scrutiny. In 2012, the Academy of Nutrition and Dietetics (Academy) and the American Society for Parenteral and Enteral Nutrition (ASPEN) published a joint consensus statement on the identification and documentation of adult malnutrition (White et al., 2012). The statement proposed a three-pronged definition of malnutrition based on etiology (White et al., 2012), as follows:

1. **Malnutrition in the context of social or environmental circumstances (starvation-related malnutrition):** This may be pure starvation due to financial or social reasons, or starvation caused by anorexia nervosa.
2. **Malnutrition in the context of acute illness or injury:** This includes malnutrition associated with organ failure, pancreatic cancer, rheumatoid arthritis, or sarcopenic obesity.
3. **Malnutrition in the context of chronic illness**: This includes malnutrition associated with major infections, burns, trauma, or closed head injury.

The Academy/ASPEN consensus statement, in addition to providing a definition of malnutrition, suggests the following criteria for diagnosis:

- Insufficient energy intake
- Weight loss
- Loss of muscle mass
- Loss of subcutaneous fat
- Localized or generalized fluid accumulation that may sometimes mask weight loss
- Diminished functional status as measured by handgrip strength

TABLE 6-4 Classification and Management of Anemia

Laboratory Tests and Nutrition Interventions Related to Anemia

Lab Test	Normal Values	Iron Deficiency (Microcytic)	Folate Deficiency (Macrocytic)	B_{12} Deficiency (Macrocytic)	Anemia of Chronic Disease
Hemoglobin (Hgb)	Female: 12–16 g/dL Male: 14–18 g/dL	↓	↓	↓	↓
Hematocrit (Hct)	Female: 37%–47% Male: 42%–52%	↓	↓	↓	↓
Mean corpuscular volume (MCV)	80–95 μg	↓	↑	Normal or increased	Normal
Mean corpuscular hemoglobin (MCH)	27–31 pg	↓	↑	↑	Normal
Serum iron (Fe)	Female: 60–160 μg/dL Male: 80–180 μg/dL	↓	↑	↑	↓
Total iron-binding capacity (TIBC)	250–460 μg/dL	↑	N/A	N/A	↓
Ferritin	Male: 12–300 ng/mL Female: 10–150 ng/mL	<12 ng/mL	>300 ng/mL	>300 ng/mL	Normal or increased
Serum B_{12}	160–950 pg/mL	Normal	↓	↓	Normal
Folate	5–25 μg/dL	Normal	↓	↑	Normal or decreased
Nutrition interventions		Increase iron-rich foods, particularly heme sources. Include a vitamin C source with meals to increase iron absorption. Limit coffee, tea, nuts, which may inhibit iron absorption. A multivitamin with iron is recommended for individuals with mild to moderate deficiency. For individuals with severe deficiency, an iron supplement is needed.	Increase folate-rich foods (fresh fruits/vegetables). Folate supplementation may be required for individuals with impaired absorption. Folate may mask a vitamin B_{12} deficiency, so serum B_{12} levels should always be checked prior to administering folate supplements.	Increase amounts of B_{12}-containing foods in the diet based on individual patient references. Supplementation with intramuscular injections or oral B_{12} is almost always recommended, due to the risk of irreversible neuropathy associated with B_{12} deficiency.	There is no nutritional therapy that will treat this type of anemia. The only treatment for this type of anemia is to correct the underlying condition or disease causing the anemia. Taking additional iron or vitamins does not help as the body is unable to absorb the additional nutrients.

Reprinted from Dorner, B. (2012). *The complete guide to nutrition care for pressure ulcer prevention and treatment*. Naples, FL: Becky Dorner & Associates, Inc., with permission.

TABLE 6-5 Signs and Symptoms of Undernutrition

Physical Signs of Malnutrition

Signs	Possible Causes
HAIR	
Dull, dry, lack of natural shine, easily plucked	Protein–energy deficiency Essential fatty acid (EFA) deficiency
Thin, sparse: alopecia	Zinc, biotin, protein deficiency
Color changes, depigmentation, lack luster	Other nutrient deficiencies: manganese, copper
Easily plucked with no pain	Protein deficiency
Corkscrew hair; unemerged, coiled hairs	Vitamin C deficiency
EYES	
Small, yellowish nodules around eyes	Hyperlipidemia
White rings around both eyes	
Angular inflammation of eyelids, "grittiness" under eye lids ulcerations of cornea	Riboflavin deficiency
Pale eye and mucous membranes	Vitamin B_{12}, folacin, and/or iron deficiency
Night blindness, chronic dry eye, dull or soft cornea	Vitamin A, zinc deficiency
Redness and fissures of eyelid corners; red and inflamed conjunctiva, swollen and sticky eyelids	Riboflavin/pyridoxine deficiency
Ring of fine blood vessels around cornea	General poor nutrition
Bitot's spots (white spots in eyes)	Vitamin A deficiency
LIPS	
Redness and swelling of mouth	Niacin, riboflavin, iron, and/or pyridoxine deficiency
Angular fissures, scars at corner of mouth	Niacin, riboflavin, iron, and/or pyridoxine deficiency
Soreness, burning lips, pallor	Pyridoxine deficiency
GUMS	
Spongy, swollen, bleed easily, redness	Vitamin C deficiency
Gingivitis	Vitamin C, niacin deficiency
MOUTH	
Cheilosis, angular scars	Riboflavin, iron, niacin, pyridoxine deficiency
Soreness, burning	Riboflavin deficiency
TONGUE	
Sores, swollen, scarlet, raw, "beef tongue"	Folacin, niacin deficiency
Soreness, burning tongue, purplish color	Riboflavin deficiency
Smooth with papillae (small projections)	Riboflavin, vitamin B_{12}, pyridoxine, niacin, folate, protein, iron deficiency
Glossitis	Iron, zinc, riboflavin, pyridoxine deficiency

TABLE 6-5 Signs and Symptoms of Undernutrition (*Continued*)

TASTE	
Sense of taste diminished	Zinc deficiency
TEETH	
Gray-brown spots, mottling	Increased fluoride intake
Missing or erupting abnormally	Generally poor nutrition
FACE	
Skin color loss, dark cheeks and eyes, enlarged parotid glands, scaling of skin around nostrils	Protein–energy deficiency, specifically niacin, riboflavin, and pyridoxine deficiencies
Pallor	Iron, folacin, vitamin B_{12}, and vitamin C deficiencies
Hyperpigmentation	Niacin deficiency
NECK	
Thyroid enlargement	Iodine deficiency
Symptoms of hypothyroidism	Iodine deficiency
NAILS	
Brittle, banding	Protein deficiency
Spoon shaped	Iron deficiency, protein deficiency
Central line ridges	Folate, iron deficiencies, malnutrition
SKIN	
Slow wound healing	Zinc, vitamin C, protein deficiency; malnutrition
Psoriasis	Biotin deficiency
Eczema, lesions	Riboflavin, zinc deficiency
Scaling of the scalp, dandruff, oiliness of the scalp, lips, and nose	Biotin deficiency, pyridoxine, zinc, riboflavin, essential fatty acids deficiency; vitamin A excess or deficiency
Petechiae (purple or red pinpoint hemorrhages in the skin)	Vitamin C
Dryness, mosaic, sandpaper feel, flakiness	Increased or decreased vitamin A
Follicular hyperkeratosis (gooseflesh)	Vitamin A deficiency
Dark, dry, scaly skin	Niacin deficiency
Lack of fat under skin, cellophane appearance	Protein–energy deficiency, vitamin C deficiency
Bilateral edema	Protein–energy, vitamin C deficiency
Yellow colored	Beta carotene excess, B_{12} deficiency
Cutaneous flushing	Side effect of niacin treatment
Body edema; round swollen face	Protein, thiamin deficiency
Pallor, fatigue, depression, apathy	Iron, folate deficiency
GASTROINTESTINAL	
Anorexia, flatulence, diarrhea	Vitamin B_{12}, folate deficiency

(*Continued*)

TABLE 6-5 Signs and Symptoms of Undernutrition (*Continued*)

Signs	Possible Causes
MUSCULAR SYSTEM	
Weakness	Phosphorus or potassium deficiency, vitamin C, vitamin D deficiency
Wasted appearance	Protein–energy deficiency
Calf tenderness, absent knee jerks, foot and wrist drops	Thiamin deficiency
Peripheral neuropathy, tingling, "pins and needles"	Folacin, pyridoxine, pantothenic acid, phosphate, thiamine, B_{12} deficiencies
Muscle twitching, convulsions, tetany	Magnesium or pyridoxine excess or deficiency, calcium, vitamin D deficiencies
Muscle cramps	Chloride decreased, sodium deficiency; calcium, vitamin D, magnesium, potassium deficiencies
Muscle pain	Biotin, vitamin D deficiency
SKELETAL SYSTEM	
Demineralization of bone	Calcium, phosphorus, vitamin D deficiencies
Epiphyseal enlargement of leg and knee, bowed legs	Vitamin D deficiency
Bone tenderness	Vitamin D deficiency
NERVOUS SYSTEM	
Listlessness	Protein–energy deficiency
Loss of position and vibratory sense, decrease and loss of ankle and knee reflexes, depression, inability to concentrate, defective memory, delirium	Thiamin, vitamin B_{12} deficiencies
Seizures, memory impairment, and behavioral disturbances	Magnesium, zinc deficiencies
Peripheral neuropathy, dementia	Pyridoxine deficiency
Dementia	Niacin, vitamin B_{12} deficiencies

Reprinted from Dietetics in Health Care Communities, *Pocket Resource for Nutrition Assessment 2013*, with permission.

BOX 6-1. Proposed Clinical Characteristics Used to Identify and Categorize Malnutrition*

1. **Energy intake**: Malnutrition is the result of inadequate food and nutrient intake or assimilation; thus, recent intake compared to estimated requirements is a primary criterion for defining malnutrition. The clinician may obtain or review the food and nutrition history and estimate optimum energy needs; energy needs should be compared to estimates of energy consumed and inadequate intake should be reported as a percentage of estimated energy requirements over time.
2. **Interpretation of weight loss:** The clinician may evaluate weight in light of other clinical findings including the presence of underhydration or overhydration. The clinician may assess weight change over time reported as a percentage of weight loss from baseline.
3. **Body fat:** Loss of subcutaneous fat (e.g., orbital, triceps, fat overlying the ribs)
4. **Muscle mass:** Muscle loss (e.g., wasting of the temples [temporalis muscle], clavicles [pectoralis and deltoids], shoulders [deltoids], interosseous muscles, scapula [latissimus dorsi, trapezious, deltoids], thigh [quadriceps], and calf [gastrocnemius])
5. **Fluid accumulation:** The clinician may evaluate generalized or localized fluid accumulation evident on exam (extremities, vulvar/scrotal edema, or ascites). Weight loss is often masked by generalized fluid retention (edema), and weight gain may be observed.
6. **Reduced grip strength:** Use standards supplied by the manufacturer of the measurement device (dynamometer).

*A minimum of two characteristics are required for a diagnosis of malnutrition. Based on criteria proposed by the Academy/A.S.P.E.N, malnutrition can be identified into one of three categories (malnutrition in the context of acute illness or injury, malnutrition in the context of chronic illness, and malnutrition in the context of environmental circumstances) and can be classified as severe or nonsevere within each category. Refer to source below for more information.
Source: Collins, N., & Friedrich, E. (February 2013). Changing the malnutrition paradigm. *Ostomy Wound Management*, *2–4*. Reprinted with permission from HMP Communications.

If an individual has two or more of these criteria, he/she meets the proposed guidelines for malnutrition. Using specific parameters related to each of these six criteria, the proposal provides guidelines for classifying the malnutrition as nonsevere or severe.

The basic characteristics used to make a malnutrition diagnosis are detailed in Box 6-1. These characteristics and criteria rely on the age-old methods of medical history, physical examination/clinical signs, anthropometric data, assessment of food and nutrient intake, and functional assessment (Collins & Friedrich, 2013). Laboratory markers of inflammation (C-reactive protein [CRP], white blood cell count, and blood glucose levels) may also be used to help determine if the condition is starvation related, chronic disease related, or acute disease or injury related. It should be noted that the Academy and A.S.P.E.N criteria are a dynamic work in progress and may change over time. ICD-9 codes for malnutrition remain unchanged, although discussion is underway regarding changes to the current language to establish consistency with etiology-based diagnostic terminology (White et al., 2012).

A comprehensive assessment to identify PEM requires more time than a simple blood draw but provides helpful data as to the type (etiology) of malnutrition, which provides guidance as to best approach to intervention (Collins & Friedrich, 2013). It is important to share the data with other members of the interdisciplinary team, as well as the planned interventions. The plan should include strategies to monitor the individual's nutritional status as they move from one care setting to another.

TABLE 6-6 Food Sources for Nutrients Critical to Healing

Nutrient	Function	Source
Calories	Supply adequate energy, prevent weight loss, preserve lean body mass	Carbohydrate, protein, and fat, with carbohydrate and fat the preferred sources
Carbohydrates	Deliver energy, spare protein	Grains, fruits, and vegetables, with complex carbohydrates the preferred source
Proteins	Contain nitrogen, which is essential for wound healing. A component of the immune system that supplies the binding material of skin, cartilage, and muscle	Meats, fish, poultry, eggs, legumes, and dairy products; choose lean meat and reduced-fat or low-fat dairy products.
Fat	Most concentrated energy source carrying the fat soluble vitamins Provides insulation under the skin and padding for bony prominences	Meats, eggs, dairy products, and vegetable oils
Fluids	Solvent for minerals and vitamins, amino acids, and glucose Help maintain body temperature and transport materials to cells and waste products from cells	Water, juices, and other beverages; fruits and vegetables contain approximately 95% water.
Vitamin C	Water-soluble, noncaloric organic nutrient essential for collagen formation and iron absorption	Citrus fruits and juices, tomatoes, potatoes, tomatoes, broccoli
Minerals: zinc and copper	Nonorganic, noncaloric nutrients Zinc is a cofactor for collagen formation, metabolizes protein, and assists in immune function. Copper assists in the formation of red blood cells and is responsible for collagen cross-linking and erythropoiesis.	Zinc: meats, liver, eggs, and seafood Copper: nuts, dried fruit, organ meats, dried beans, whole-grain cereal

Reprinted from Dietetics in Health Care Communities, *Pocket Resource for Nutrition Assessment, 2013*, with permission.

Nutrients That Play a Role in Wound Healing

For overall good health, it is important to consume all essential nutrients in the quantities recommended by the Dietary Reference Intakes. A diet that contains good sources of protein, low-fat dairy foods, fruits, vegetables, and grains (especially whole grains) can provide the essential nutrients in adequate amounts to maintain good health (U.S. Department of Agriculture, 2010). Nutrients are generally broken down into macronutrients (those needed in large amounts) and micronutrients (those needed in small amounts). Protein, carbohydrate, fat, and fluid are known as the macronutrients. Vitamins and minerals are considered micronutrients. Each nutrient plays a different role in the body, with some having more of an influence on wound healing than others. **Table 6-6** outlines the main nutrients that play a role in wound healing and their specific functions. **Table 6-7** outlines key nutrients for those on a vegan diet.

Nutritional Needs of Individuals with Pressure Ulcers

Each individual has unique nutritional needs that are based on their body size (weight), activity level, and comorbidities; the comprehensive nutrition assessment assists the RDN to identify areas of concern and to develop an individualized plan of care. The *Clinical Practice Guideline for Prevention and Treatment of Pressure Ulcers,* which was developed by multiple coordinating professional groups, provides information on specific nutritional needs for prevention and treatment of pressure ulcers in adults (National Pressure Ulcer Advisory Panel et al., 2014). These guidelines were developed following a systematic, comprehensive review of peer-based research on pressure ulcer prevention and treatment published after the year 2009. All studies meeting the inclusion criteria were reviewed for quality, summarized in evidence tables, and classified according to their level of evidence using an established classification system (Sacket, 1996). Recommendations for practice are rated according to the strength of cumulative evidence supporting the recommendation (Box 6-2).

As a general rule, food sources of nutrients are preferred over supplements, with supplements ordered if an individual cannot or will not consume adequate nutrients through food alone. Major food sources for each of the macronutrients and micronutrients are listed in **Table 6-6**. The *Clinical Practice Guideline for Prevention and Treatment of Pressure Ulcers* (NPUAP, 2014) provides the following recommendations for intake of calories, protein and amino acids, fluid, and vitamins and minerals.

CLINICAL PEARL

Patients with open wounds and patients at risk for pressure ulcers need the following: 30 to 35 cal/kg body weight/day; 1.25 to 1.5 g protein/kg body weight/day; and sufficient fluid intake (usually about 30 mL/kg body weight/day).

TABLE 6-7 Vegan Food Sources for Nutrients Critical to Healing

Nutrient	Dietary Sources	Key Points
Protein	Soy products (soy beans, edamame, tofu, tempeh, textured vegetable protein, soy protein, meat analogs) Dried beans and peas Lentils Nuts Nut butters	In the past, it was recommended that a vegan diet combines a variety of vegan foods to ensure intake of all essential amino acids at each meal. However, evidence now shows that as long as a variety of vegan sources of protein are consumed over the course of a day, all needs for essential amino acids can be met (Craig & Mangels, 2009).
Zinc	Fortified cereals Whole grains Beans Nuts	The bioavailability of zinc from vegetarian diets is lower than that from nonvegetarian diets, mainly due to the high phytic acid content of vegetarian diets, which affects zinc absorption (Craig & Mangels, 2009).
Vitamin C	Red and green pepper Citrus fruits and juices Kiwi Broccoli Strawberries Cantaloupe Cauliflower Cabbage	Intake is generally adequate for a vegan diet that includes the recommended 2 cups of fruit and 2½ cups of vegetables per day.
Vitamin B_{12}	Fortified foods and supplements	Not generally associated with wound healing, but is important because those who don't consume animal foods must consume fortified foods or supplements to meet requirements

Sources: Craig and Mangels (2009), Collins and Harris (2012), National Institutes of Health (2013a, 2013b) Unites States Department of Agriculture (2010).

BOX 6-2. Nutrition for Pressure Ulcer Prevention and Healing

Nutrition Screening

1. Screen nutritional status for each individual at risk of or with a pressure ulcer:
   - At admission to a health care setting
   - With each significant change of clinical condition
   - When progress toward pressure ulcer closure is not observed (Strength of Evidence = C)
2. Use a valid and reliable nutrition-screening tool to determine nutritional risk (Strength of Evidence = C).
3. Refer individuals found to be at risk of malnutrition and individuals with an existing pressure ulcer to a registered dietitian or an interprofessional nutrition team for a comprehensive nutrition assessment (Strength of Evidence = C).

Nutrition Assessment

1. Assess the weight status of each individual to determine weight history and identify significant weight loss (≥5% in 30 days or ≥10% in 180 days) (Strength of Evidence = C).
2. Assess the individual's ability to eat independently (Strength of Evidence = C).
3. Assess the adequacy of total nutrient intake (food, fluid, oral supplements, and enteral/parenteral feeds) (Strength of Evidence = C).

Care Planning

1. Develop an individualized nutrition care plan for individuals with or at risk of a pressure ulcer (Strength of Evidence = C).
2. Follow relevant and evidence-based guidelines on nutrition and hydration for individuals who exhibit nutritional risk and who are at risk of pressure ulcers or have an existing pressure ulcer (Strength of Evidence = C).

Energy Intake

1. Provide individualized energy intake based on underlying medical condition and level of activity (Strength of Evidence = B).
2. Provide 30 to 35 kcal/kg body weight for adults at risk of a pressure ulcer who are assessed as being at risk of malnutrition (Strength of Evidence = C).
3. Provide 30 to 35 kcal/kg body weight for adults with a pressure ulcer who are assessed as being at risk of malnutrition (Strength of Evidence = B).
4. Adjust energy intake based on weight change or level of obesity. Adults who are underweight or who have had significant unintended weight loss may need additional energy intake (Strength of Evidence = C).
5. Revise and modify/liberalize dietary restrictions when limitations result in decreased food and fluid intake. These adjustments should be made in consultation with a medical professional and managed by a registered dietitian whenever possible (Strength of Evidence = C).
6. Offer fortified foods and/or high-calorie, high-protein oral nutritional supplements between meals if nutritional requirements cannot be achieved by dietary intake (Strength of Evidence = B).
7. Consider enteral or parenteral nutritional support when oral intake is inadequate. This must be consistent with the individual's goals (Strength of Evidence = C).

BOX 6-2. Nutrition for Pressure Ulcer Prevention and Healing (*Continued*)

Protein Intake

1. Provide adequate protein for positive nitrogen balance for adults assessed to be at risk of a pressure ulcer (Strength of Evidence = C).
2. Offer 1.25 to 1.5 g protein/kg body weight daily for adults at risk of a pressure ulcer who are assessed to be at risk of malnutrition when compatible with goals of care, and reassess as condition changes (Strength of Evidence = C).
3. Provide adequate protein for positive nitrogen balance for adults with a pressure ulcer (Strength of Evidence = B).
4. Offer 1.25 to 1.5 g protein/kg body weight daily for adults with an existing pressure ulcer who are assessed to be at risk of malnutrition when compatible with goals of care, and reassess as condition changes (Strength of Evidence = B).
5. Offer high-calorie, high-protein nutritional supplements in addition to the usual diet to adults with nutritional risk and pressure ulcer risk, if nutritional requirements cannot be achieved by dietary intake (Strength of Evidence = A).
6. Assess renal function to ensure that high levels of protein are appropriate for the individual (Strength of Evidence = C).
7. Supplement with high protein, arginine, and micronutrients for adults with a pressure ulcer Category/Stage III or IV or multiple pressure ulcers when nutritional requirements cannot be met with traditional high-calorie and protein supplements (Strength of Evidence = B).

Hydration

1. Provide and encourage adequate daily fluid intake for hydration for an individual assessed to be at risk of or with a pressure ulcer. This must be consistent with the individual's comorbid conditions and goals (Strength of Evidence = C).
2. Monitor individuals for signs and symptoms of dehydration including change in weight, skin turgor, urine output, elevated serum sodium, and/or calculated serum osmolality (Strength of Evidence = C).
3. Provide additional fluid for individuals with dehydration, elevated temperature, vomiting, profuse sweating, diarrhea, or heavily exuding wounds (Strength of Evidence = C).

Vitamins and Minerals

1. Provide/encourage individuals assessed to be at risk of pressure ulcers to consume a balanced diet that includes good sources of vitamins and minerals (Strength of Evidence = C).
2. Provide/encourage an individual assessed to be at risk of a pressure ulcer to take vitamin and mineral supplements when dietary intake is poor or deficiencies are confirmed or suspected (Strength of Evidence = C).
3. Provide/encourage an individual with a pressure ulcer to consume a balanced diet that includes good sources of vitamins and minerals (Strength of Evidence = B).
4. Provide/encourage an individual with a pressure ulcer to take vitamin and mineral supplements when dietary intake is poor or deficiencies are confirmed or suspected (Strength of Evidence = B).

Adapted from National Pressure Ulcer Advisory Panel, European Pressure Ulcer Advisory Panel and Pan Pacific Pressure Injury Alliance. (2014). *Prevention and treatment of pressure ulcers: Clinical practice guideline*. In E. Haesler (Ed.), Osborne Park, Western Australia: Cambridge Media, with permission.

Energy (kilocalories)

Energy, measured in the form of kilocalories, is provided in the diet by the macronutrients, protein, carbohydrates, and fats. Providing adequate energy promotes anabolism (tissue building), nitrogen and collagen synthesis, and wound healing (Dorner et al., 2009) and acts to "spare protein" by providing alternative sources of energy. Any condition that increases the metabolic rate (e.g., infection, trauma, stress, pressure ulcers, etc.) creates a hypermetabolic state that increases energy (caloric) needs. The *Clinical Practice Guidelines on Prevention and Treatment of Pressure Ulcers* (NPUAP, 2014) recommends the following:

- Provide individualized energy intake based on underlying medical condition and level of activity (Strength of Evidence = B).
- Provide 30 to 35 kcal/kg of body weight for adults at risk of a pressure ulcer who are assessed as being at risk of malnutrition (Strength of Evidence = C).
- Provide 30 to 35 kcal/kg of body weight for adults with a pressure ulcer who are assessed as being at risk of malnutrition (Strength of Evidence = B).

Using the guidelines as a resource, the RDN will calculate the appropriate caloric intake based on the individual's nutrition assessment. An adult with unintended weight loss and low BMI may require additional calories above the 30 to 35 kcal/kg of body weight; in contrast, a severely obese individual may require a caloric range below the recommended level.

Food first before supplements is the general rule; when supplements are required, they should be offered between meals to avoid further reduction in food intake and to maximize meal consumption. The guidelines recommend and research supports measures to liberalize dietary choices, especially when meals are refused due to the type of food served (Dorner et al., 2010). For example, if a person with heart failure and pressure ulcers is refusing to eat the 2-g-sodium therapeutic diet as ordered, then moving to a less restrictive diet is appropriate.

Protein

Sufficient protein should be provided to maintain positive nitrogen balance for any individual who has a pressure ulcer or is assessed as at risk for a pressure ulcer. Clinical judgment should be used when determining the appropriate level of protein for each person, based on overall nutritional status, comorbidities, and tolerance to the interventions. Renal function is of particular concern, as high levels of protein intake may be contraindicated in patients with chronic kidney disease (Harvey, 2013). The *Clinical Practice Guidelines for Prevention and Treatment of Pressure Ulcers* (NPUAP, 2014) provides the following recommendations:

- Provide adequate protein for positive nitrogen balance for adults assessed to be at risk of a pressure ulcer (Strength of Evidence = C).

- Offer 1.25 to 1.5 g protein/kg of body weight daily for adults at risk of a pressure ulcer who are assessed to be at risk of malnutrition when compatible with goals of care, and reassess as condition changes (Strength of Evidence = C).
- Provide adequate protein for positive nitrogen balance for adults with a pressure ulcer (Strength of Evidence = B).
- Offer 1.25 to 1.5 g protein/kg of body weight for adults with an existing pressure ulcer who are assessed to be at risk of malnutrition when compatible with goals of care, and reassess as condition changes (Strength of Evidence = B).

Amino Acids

Amino acids are the building blocks of protein. In practice, specialized protein supplements with selected amino acids are often recommended to promote wound healing when standard care has proven unsuccessful. Some amino acids must be provided via dietary intake (essential or indispensable amino acids), while others can be synthesized by the body (nonessential or dispensable amino acids). Three amino acids (arginine, glutamine, and cysteine) are commonly linked to wound healing because they are conditionally indispensable—in other words, they become essential in situations causing physiologic stress, such as trauma, chronic disease, or poor dietary intake. **Table 6-8** outlines the various categories of amino acids.

In recent years, most experts have stopped short of recommending specific amino acids, such as arginine, to promote wound healing (Castellanos et al., 2006; Litchford, 2010). However, according to the 2014 National Pressure Ulcer Advisory Panel, growing evidence supports nutritional supplementation with additional protein, arginine, and micronutrients to promote pressure ulcer healing. One recent study in four nursing homes concluded that the rate of pressure ulcer healing was accelerated when a supplement enriched with protein, arginine, zinc, and vitamin C was consumed daily for at least 8 weeks (Cereda et al., 2009). Another randomized controlled trial involved well-nourished older adults with Stage III and Stage IV pressure ulcers in four European countries, using the same formula as the one used in Cereda's study. The investigators documented improved healing and concluded that a high-protein supplement with arginine and micronutrients might be associated with improved healing rates in older adults who were not malnourished (van Anholt et al., 2010). However, the studies supporting use of amino acid supplements are limited, and additional studies are needed before definitive recommendations can be made. At this time, the clinician must use his or her clinical judgment in regard to the use of supplemental amino acids.

Fluids

Adequate fluids should be provided to prevent dehydration. Individuals with draining wounds, emesis, diarrhea, or increased insensible losses due to fever, excessive perspiration, or air-fluidized beds may need additional fluids daily. Recommended fluid intake for healthy adults is 2.4 L/day for women and 3.7 L/day for men (IOM, 2004). Hydration needs are met by consuming liquids as well as the moisture (fluid) content of foods.

Fluid needs can be estimated using a number of methods including 1.0 mL/kcal consumed (TRANS Taasman DWCG, 2011) or body weight in kg × 30 mL/kg (except in those with renal or cardiac distress). Inadequate fluid intake is a common problem, especially among the elderly; simple strategies that have been proven effective are listed in Box 6-3.

TABLE 6-8 Categories of Amino Acids

Indispensible (Essential) Amino Acids (Needed in the Diet, Cannot Be Manufactured in the Body)	Dispensable (Nonessential) Amino Acids (Not Needed in the Diet, Can Be Manufactured in the Body)	Conditionally Indispensible Amino Acids
Histidine	Alanine	Arginine
*Isoleucine	Asparagine	Cysteine (cystine)
*Leucine	Aspartic acid	Glutamine
Lysine	Glutamic acid	Glycine
Methionine	Serine	Proline
Phenylalanine		Tyrosine
Threonine		
Tryptophan		
*Valine		

Key: *Branched chain amino acids; synthesis is limited in chronic disease.
Note: A conditionally indispensible amino acid is one that becomes essential in certain conditions, such as chronic disease, trauma, or poor dietary intake.
Reprinted from Dorner, B. (2012). *The complete guide to nutrition care for pressure ulcer prevention and treatment.* Naples, FL: Becky Dorner & Associates, Inc., with permission.)

BOX 6-3. Strategies to Enhance Fluid Intake

- Identify and offer the individual's favorite beverages.
- Offer a beverage following wound care treatment.
- Offer extra fluids with each medication pass.
- Keep water at the bedside and within reach.
- Offer a variety of beverages with meals.
- Offer beverages before or after physical therapy sessions.
- Monitor all individuals for signs and symptoms of dehydration.

Vitamins and Minerals

Adequate vitamins and minerals are needed for overall good health and to promote skin integrity and wound healing. However, no research has demonstrated a positive effect on wound healing of supplements of any specific micronutrients (including vitamin C, zinc, and copper). Vitamin C is a cofactor, along with iron, that contributes to the oxidation of lysine and proline, which is required for the production of collagen. A deficiency of vitamin C could delay wound healing, but mega doses of ascorbic acid have not resulted in accelerated healing (ter Reit et al., 1995). Zinc is a cofactor for collagen formation and is also necessary for protein metabolism; however, mega doses of elemental zinc above the UL of 40 mg/day is not recommended unless a deficiency is confirmed (IOM, 2006). Zinc nutritional status is difficult to measure since it is widely distributed throughout the body. Plasma and serum zinc levels are the most widely used methods of zinc assessment, but they do not necessarily reflect cellular zinc status. Therefore, a serum zinc level is not recommended to determine status. Health professionals must use clinical judgment and fully assess a person's zinc intake, potential losses, conditions that may negatively affect zinc status, and clinical indicators of significant zinc deficiency (e.g., hair loss, diarrhea, eye and skin lesions). Copper is essential for cross-linking of collagen, but high serum zinc levels interfere with copper metabolism. If an individual with wounds is consistently consuming an oral diet that is low in vitamins and minerals, a daily multivitamin with minerals could be beneficial. Also, it should be noted that most oral nutritional supplements provide additional calories, protein, vitamin C, and zinc. See **Table 6-6** for additional sources of nutrients. The 2014 *Prevention and Treatment of Pressure Ulcers: Clinical Practice Guidelines* recommends the following:

- Provide/encourage individuals assessed to be at risk of pressure ulcers to consume a balanced diet that includes good sources of vitamins and minerals (Strength of Evidence = C).
- Provide/encourage an individual assessed to be at risk of a pressure ulcer to take vitamin and mineral supplements when dietary intake is poor or deficiencies are confirmed or suspected (Strength of Evidence = C).
- Provide/encourage an individual with a pressure ulcer to consume a balanced diet that includes good sources of vitamins and minerals (Strength of Evidence = B).
- Provide/encourage an individual with a pressure ulcer to take vitamin and mineral supplements when dietary intake is poor or deficiencies are confirmed or suspected (Strength of Evidence = B).

CLINICAL PEARL

A multivitamin–mineral supplement should be recommended when inadequate intake is known or suspected.

Care Planning: Developing Nutrition Interventions to Prevent and/or Treat Pressure Ulcers

An individualized/interdisciplinary plan for nutrition should be developed in conjunction with the individual and/or caregivers and should include a discussion of the risks and benefits of recommended interventions. Interventions to help improve nutritional status might include but are not limited to the following:

- Individualized diets: Those individuals who are on therapeutic diets might benefit from a more liberal, less restrictive diet, especially if intake is poor (Dorner et al., 2010).
- Texture modifications: If chewing or swallowing problems are preventing food intake, food textures or fluid consistencies might need to be modified to maximize meal intake.
- Assistance with food preparation and/or eating, as needed.
- Improved access to food (including transportation) if financial limitations affect nutritional status.
- Targeted nutrition interventions, including fortified foods, oral nutritional supplements, or tube feeding.
- Offering six small meals daily to ensure increased caloric intake.
- Rotating the type of high-calorie/high-protein snacks offered between meals to avoid flavor fatigue.

Oral Nutritional Supplements

When an individual cannot meet their nutritional needs through consumption of meals and snacks, then other strategies are necessary. Options include adding fortified foods to meals or snacks or offering high-calorie, high-protein supplements (such as those made with milk and ice cream) in between meals.

Fortified or enhanced foods can be made in the kitchen by adding ingredients to regular foods that boost the calories and/or protein provided by the foods a person already eats. Examples include oatmeal made with whole milk or half and half, powdered milk and brown sugar, or cream soup made with whole milk or half and half.

Oral nutritional supplements (ONS) are commercial products that supply nutrients such as protein, carbohydrates, fat, vitamins, minerals, and/or amino acids.

A 2005 study showed that offering high-protein, high-calorie supplements to individuals at risk for pressure ulcers for 4 to 72 weeks was associated with a significant reduction in pressure ulcer development compared to routine care (Stratton et al., 2005). Additional research supports the value of providing ONS as a therapeutic intervention to promote healing when oral intake is inadequate (Brewer et al., 2010; Cereda et al., 2011).

Appetite Enhancers

Appetite stimulants and anabolic steroids may contribute to improved food intake and/or to treatment of unintended weight loss. There are a number of different medications available that can enhance appetite; however, more research is needed to determine their effectiveness in promoting pressure ulcer healing. In the long-term care setting, there is insufficient evidence to support the use of most appetite enhancers (Rudolph, 2009). Some evidence suggests that megestrol acetate may be of benefit in this setting; however, there are risks associated with its use, and there are no studies addressing benefits and risks if used for long periods of time (Rudolph, 2009; AMDA clinical practice guidelines, 2010). At this point in time, use of appetite enhancers should be considered on an individual basis.

Oxandrin is an anabolic steroid sometimes used to promote anabolism and weight gain in patients with significant unintended weight loss. In one study, oxandrin demonstrated an improvement in wound healing in individuals with weight loss and chronic wounds (Demling & DeSanti, 1998).

Tube Feeding and Wound Healing

When oral intake is inadequate, enteral or parenteral feeding may be recommended if it is consistent with an individual's wishes; enteral feeding is preferred over parenteral nutrition as long as the gut is functioning. One of the potential benefits of enteral nutrition is reduced risk of pressure ulcer development and/or improved wound healing; the studies included in a 2005 systematic review by Stratton and colleagues indicated that enteral feedings can reduce the risk of pressure ulcer development by 25% and may improve wound healing (Brown, 2013; Stratton et al., 2005). However, studies that have reviewed enteral nutrition for improved outcomes related to pressure ulcers have been disappointing (Dorner et al., 2009). For example, Teno and colleagues (2012) report that enteral feedings are not associated with prevention or improved healing of pressure ulcers in individuals with advanced dementia and may be associated with increased risk for other issues. Specific adverse effects associated with enteral feedings include GI complications (diarrhea, nausea, and vomiting), aspiration pneumonia, metabolic complications, and mechanical complications with tube placement (Russell, 2013; Chernoff & Seres, 2014). Given the mixed data regarding benefits, each individual should be evaluated for the risks versus benefits of tube placement. In general, if an individual is catabolic and the source of the catabolism is untreatable, such as chronic or critical illness, enteral feeding is less likely to positively affect outcome (Chernoff & Seres, 2014). The position of the Academy of Nutrition and Dietetics is that individuals have the right to request or refuse nutrition and hydration as medical treatment (Maillet et al., 2013).

CLINICAL PEARL

The decision to initiate enteral feedings must be individualized and made with caution; there are a number of potential complications associated with enteral feedings, and there is no compelling evidence of benefit in wound healing.

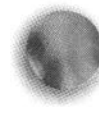

Issues That Affect Nutrition Assessment and Interventions for Pressure Ulcers and Wounds

Overweight and Obesity

Overweight and obesity are defined based on BMI. Tables 6-1, 6-2, and 6-3 outline BMI definitions. The subject of nutritional management of obese individuals with pressure ulcers raises more questions than it provides answers. There are no studies that specifically address the obese individual with pressure ulcers, so research is needed to better define appropriate caloric intake for these individuals (Dorner et al., 2009).

Historically, many RDNs have used an adjustment of actual body weight when calculating caloric needs for obese individuals. According to the Academy of Nutrition and Dietetics Evidence Analysis Library, caloric needs for healthy obese individuals are most accurately estimated by the Mifflin St. Jeor formula using *actual* body weight (Academy of Nutrition and Dietetics Evidence Analysis Library, 2006). However, it is unclear if this formula provides appropriate recommendations for the obese individual who presents with wounds or pressure ulcers. For that reason, practitioners may choose to use the 2014 *Prevention and Treatment of Pressure Ulcers: Clinical Practice Guidelines'* recommendation of 30 to 35 kcal/kg body weight, recognizing that the resulting estimates may be unrealistically high. Clinical judgment should be used to adjust caloric intake goals based on the individualized nutrition assessment.

CLINICAL PEARL

When caring for patients who are overweight or obese, wound-healing goals take priority over weight loss goals.

Standard estimates of protein and fluid needs for underweight or normal weight individuals with pressure ulcers may not apply to those who are overweight or obese. Unfortunately, there is little evidence-based guidance available for practitioners on how to estimate these needs. If applying the *Prevention and Treatment of Pressure Ulcers: Clinical Practice Guidelines* for protein and fluids, estimates may again be unrealistically high, so clinical judgment is required to make adjustments based on the individualized nutrition assessment.

Because estimating the nutritional needs of overweight and obese individuals is problematic, ongoing monitoring of calorie, protein, and fluid intake; weight; and progress in wound healing is particularly important and may be the best way to determine whether nutritional needs are being met.

Although weight loss is usually recommended for obese individuals, weight loss efforts may need to be postponed temporarily, or at least modified, to assure provision of sufficient nutrients for wound healing (Dorner et al., 2009). An obese individual with wounds should consume a diet adequate in protein and calories to meet wound-healing needs instead of a low-calorie diet designed for weight reduction (Posthauer & Thomas, 2012). Because the wound-healing process depends on an adequate flow of nutrients, reducing caloric and/or protein intake could compromise wound healing by resulting in a breakdown of lean body mass (Demling, 2009).

Vegan Diets

Vegetarian-based diets are growing in popularity as Americans focus on healthy eating; approximately 3.2% of US adults, or 7.3 million people, follow a vegetarian diet. Approximately 0.5%, or 1 million, of those are vegans, who consume no animal products at all (The Vegetarian Times, 2008). Appropriately planned vegetarian or vegan diets are healthful and nutritionally adequate (Craig & Mangels, 2009) for most people, including older adults. Vegetarian diets tend to be lower in saturated fat and cholesterol and have higher levels of dietary fiber, magnesium, potassium, vitamins C and E, folate, and several phytochemicals (Craig & Mangels, 2009) than diets that contain meat. Vegans and some other vegetarians tend to have lower intake of selected nutrients, including zinc, which is thought to have a role in wound healing. Other nutrients that may not be provided in sufficient amounts in a vegan diet include vitamin B_{12} and iron. Dry beans, nuts, peas, lentils, and tofu are all protein sources that should be encouraged for vegans. Meat analogs made of soy, microproteins, or seitan are also good sources of protein. The diet of a vegan with wounds or pressure ulcers should be evaluated for adequacy of intake related to key nutrients, with supplements ordered if a deficiency is confirmed or suspected. Table 6-7 outlines key nutrients that are important for vegans with wounds.

Oral Nutritional Supplements for Vegans

If meal intake is poor, oral nutritional supplements (ONS) may be necessary to help meet calorie, protein, and nutrient needs. Supplements for vegans should contain no dairy, meat, or egg products. Milk protein is commonly used as the base for commercial nutritional supplements available through medical supply companies and pharmacies (Nutrition Product Guides, Abbott Nutrition, 2014; Products and Applications, Nestle Nutrition, 2014); thus, it may be necessary to find alternate sources for vegan supplements.

Diabetes Mellitus

Individuals with diabetes are at increased risk for nonhealing wounds and wound infections. Poorly managed blood glucose levels can affect the ability of a wound to heal (Litchford, 2010), so glycemic control is a key issue for individuals with both wounds and diabetes.

Effective blood glucose control requires an interdisciplinary approach that addresses diet, physical activity, and medication management. According to *Nutrition Therapy Recommendations for the Management of Adults with Diabetes* (2014), there is no conclusive evidence regarding the ideal amount of carbohydrate intake for people with diabetes (Evert et al., 2014). The term "ADA diet" (e.g., "1,200-calorie ADA diet") is no longer used because the American Diabetes Association does not endorse any single diet plan (Posthauer & Thomas, 2012). It is the position of the American Diabetes Association (ADA) that no "one-size-fits-all" eating pattern is appropriate for individuals with diabetes. Total energy intake (and therefore portion size) is one important consideration. Priority should be given to coordinating food intake and administration of oral hypoglycemics or insulin for individuals on medication (Evert et al., 2014).

Older adults who are functional, are cognitively intact, and have significant life expectancy should receive diabetes care similar to younger individuals (Standards of Medical Care in Diabetes, 2014); in these individuals, the glycemic goal is usually <130 mg/dL. Glycemic control may be less important in those with life-limiting illness or substantial cognitive or functional impairment (Standards of Medical Care in Diabetes, 2014). However, those with poorly controlled diabetes may be subject to complications such as dehydration, impaired wound healing, or wound infection, so glycemic goals should be established with the goal of preventing these consequences (Standards of Medical Care in Diabetes, 2014).

Chronic Kidney Disease

Individuals with chronic kidney disease (CKD) often have comorbidities that affect their nutrition care. For example, an individual with CKD, diabetes, and wounds or pressure ulcers has complicated and conflicting nutritional needs; the diet for stage 3 or 4 CKD that is limited in calories, protein, potassium, phosphorus, sodium, and fluid may not meet the protein or nutrient needs required for wound healing. Clinical consultation with an RDN is essential when treating individuals with CKD and wounds; the RDN is prepared to provide in-depth assessment of the risks versus the benefits of therapeutic diets, especially for older adults (Dorner et al., 2010).

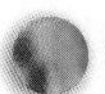 Conclusion

Nutrition plays a key role in the prevention and treatment of wounds. The majority of evidence-based research related to nutrition has been done in people with pressure ulcers. Early identification of individuals at risk for malnutrition and/or pressure ulcers as well as identification of malnutrition and/or pressure ulcers is critical and should prompt a referral to the RDN. Comprehensive assessment by an RDN can identify medical, nutritional, and situational problems that can contribute to poor nutritional status and increase the risk for further complications. Nutrition interventions to prevent or treat pressure ulcers should be individualized based on medical and nutrition diagnoses and situational factors and formulated to improve the individual's quality of life. Regular monitoring and evaluation by the interdisciplinary team is needed to assess the effects of interventions. Each member of the health care team has a specific role in the care and treatment of individuals with wounds, and interdisciplinary collaboration, communication, and continuity are essential elements of effective care for the individual with wounds.

REFERENCES

Academy of Nutrition and Dietetics Evidence Analysis Library. (2006). *Adult weight management guideline*. Retrieved July 11, 2014 from http://andevidencelibrary.com/topic.cfm?cat=2798

Academy of Nutrition and Dietetics. (2013). *Pocket guide for international dietetics and nutrition terminology (IDNT) reference manual* (4th ed.). Chicago, IL: Academy of Nutrition and Dietetics.

American Medical Directors Association. (2010). *Altered nutritional status in long-term care setting clinical practice guideline*. Columbia, MD: American Medical Directors Association.

Brown, B. (2013). Patient selection and indications for enteral feedings. In P. Charney, A. Malone (Eds.), *Pocket guide to enteral nutrition* (2nd ed., pp. 14–51). Chicago, IL: Academy of Nutrition and Dietetics.

Brewer, S., Desneves, K., Pearce, L., et al. (2010). Effect of an arginine-containing nutritional supplement on pressure ulcer healing in community spinal patients. *Journal of Wound Care, 19*(7), 311–316.

Castellanos, V., Litchford, M., Campbell, W. (2006). Modular protein supplements and their application to long-term care. *Nutrition in Clinical Practice, 21*, 485–504.

Centers for Disease Control and Prevention Web site. Reviewed September 13, 2001. *About BMI for adults*. Retrieved July 14, 2014 from http://www.cdc.gov/healthyweight/assessing/bmi/adult_bmi/index.html#Interpreted

Cereda, E., Gini, A., Pedrolli, C., et al. (2009). Disease-specific, versus standard, nutritional support for the treatment of pressure ulcers in institutionalized older adults: A randomized controlled trial. *Journal of the American Geriatrics Society, 57*(8), 1395–1402.

Cereda, E., Klersy, C., Rondanelli, M., et al. (2011). Energy balance in patients with pressure ulcers: A systematic review and meta-analysis of observational studies. *Journal of the American Dietetic Association, 111*, 1868–1876.

Chernoff R., & Seres D. (2014). Nutritional support for the older adult. In Chernoff R. *Geriatric nutrition* (4th ed., pp. 465–485). Burlington, MA: Jones and Bartlett Learning.

Choo, S., Hyter, M., & Watson, R. (2013). The effectiveness of nutritional interventions and the treatment of pressure ulcers-a systematic literature review. *International Journal of Nursing Practice, 19*(suppl 1), 19–27.

Collins, N., & Friedrich, E. (2013). Changing the malnutrition paradigm. *Ostomy Wound Management*, 58, 2–4.

Collins, N., & Harris, C. (2012). Nutrition411-are vegetarian diets adequate for wound healing? *Ostomy Wound Management, 14–18.*

Covinsky, K. E., Covinsky, M. H., & Palmer, R. M. (2002). Serum albumin concentration and clinical assessments of nutrition status in hospitalized older people; different sides of different coins? *Journal of the American Geriatric Society, 50*, 631–637.

Craig, W. J., & Mangels, A. R. (2009). Position of the American Dietetic Association: Vegetarian diets. *Journal of the American Dietetic Association, 109*, 1266–1282.

Demling, R. H. (2009). Nutrition, anabolism, and the wound healing process: An overview. *Eplasty, 9*, e9. Retrieved July 11, 2014 from http://www.ncbi.nlm.nih.gov/pmc/articles/PMC2642618/

Demling, R., & DeSanti, L. (1998). Closure of the nonhealing wound corresponds with correction of weight loss using the anabolic agent oxandrolone. *Ostomy Wound Management, 44*, 58–62.

Dorner, B. (2012). *The complete guide to nutrition care for pressure ulcers: Prevention and treatment.* Naples, FL: Becky Dorner & Associates, Inc.

Dorner, B., Friedrich, E., & Posthauer M. E. (2010). Position of the American Dietetic Association: Liberalization of the diet prescription improves quality of life for older adults in long-term care. *Journal of the American Dietetic Association, 110*, 1549–1553.

Dorner, B., Posthauer, M. E., & Thomas, D. (2009). *The role of nutrition in pressure ulcer prevention and treatment: National Pressure Ulcer Advisory Panel White Paper.* Retrieved July 11, 2014 from http://www.npuap.org/wp-content/uploads/2012/03/Nutrition-White-Paper-Website-Version.pdf

Evert, A. B., Boucher, J. L., Cypress, M., et al. (2014). Nutrition therapy recommendations for the management of adults with diabetes. *Diabetes Care, 37*(s1), S120–S143.

Furhman, M. P., Charney, P., & Mueller, C. (2004). *Journal of the American Dietetic Association, 104*, 1258–1264.

Harvey, K. S. (2013). Nutrition management in chronic kidney disease stages 1 through 4. In L. Byham-Gray, J. Stover, K. Wiesen, (Eds.), *A clinical guide to nutrition care in chronic kidney disease* (2nd ed., pp. 25–37). Chicago, IL: Academy of Nutrition and Dietetics.

Hengstermann, S., Fischer A., Steinhagen-Thiessen, E., et al. (2007). Nutrition status and pressure ulcer: What we need for nutrition screening. *Journal of Parenteral Enteral Nutrition, 31*(4), 288.

Horn, S. D., Bender, S. A., Ferguson, M. L., et al. (2004). The National Pressure Ulcer Long-Term Care Study: Pressure ulcer development in long-term care residents. *Journal of the American Geriatrics Society, 52*(3), 359–367.

Institute of Medicine. (2004) [cited 2013 September]. *Dietary Reference Intakes for Water, Potassium, Sodium, Chloride, and Sulfate National Academy of Sciences*, Available from http://www.iom.edu/Reports/2004/Dietary-Reference-Intakes-Water-Potassium-Sodium-Chloride-and-Sulfate.aspx

Institute of Medicine. (2006). *Dietary reference intakes: The essential guide to nutrient requirements*. Washington, DC: National Academy of Sciences.

Johnson, A. M., & Merlini, G. Clinical indications for plasma protein assays: Transthyretin (prealbumin) in inflammation and malnutrition. *Clinical Chemistry and Laboratory Medicine*, 2007, *45*(3), 419–426.

Kaiser, M. J., Bauer, J. M., Ramsch, C., et al. (2009). Validation of the mini nutritional assessment short-form (MNA-SF): A practical tool for identification of nutritional status. *Journal of Nutritional Health and Aging, 13*, 782–788.

Litchford, M. D., Dorner, B., & Posthauer, M. E. (2014). Malnutrition as a precursor of pressure ulcers. *Advances in Wound care, 3*(1), 54–63.

Litchford, M. D. (2012). *Nutrition focused physical assessment: Making clinical connections*. Greensboro, NC: Case Software.

Litchford, M. D. (2010). *The advanced practitioner's guide to nutrition and wounds*. Greensboro, NC: Case Software.

Maillet, J. O., Schwartz, D. B., Posthauer, M. E. (2013). Position of the Academy of Nutrition and Dietetics: Ethical and legal issues in feeding and hydration. *Journal of the Academy of Nutrition and Dietetics, 113*(6), 828–833.

National Institutes of Health Office of Dietary Supplements. (2013a). *Zinc fact sheet for health professionals*. Retrieved July 11, 2014 from http://ods.od.nih.gov/factsheets/Zinc-HealthProfessional/#h3

National Institutes of Health Office of Dietary Supplements. (2013b). *Vitamin C fact sheet for health professionals*. Retrieved July 11, 2014 from National Institutes of Health Office of Dietary Supplements. http://ods.od.nih.gov/factsheets/VitaminC-HealthProfessional/

National Pressure Ulcer Advisory Panel, European Pressure Ulcer Advisory Panel, and Pan Pacific Pressure Injury Alliance. (2014). In E. Haesler (Ed.), *Prevention and treatment of pressure ulcers: Clinical practice guideline*. Osborne Park, Western Australia: Cambridge Media.

Nutrition Product Guides. (2014). Retrieved June 9, 2014 from Abbott Nutrition Website, http://abbottnutrition.com/product/product-handbook-landing

Posthauer, M. E., Schols, J. M. G. A. (2014). Nutritional strategies for pressure ulcer management. In D. L. Krasner (Ed.), *Chronic wound care: The essentials* (pp. 131–144). Malvern, PA: HMP Communication, LLC.

Posthauer, M. E., & Thomas, D. R. (2012). Nutrition and wound care. In S. Baronski & E. A. Ayello (Eds.), *Wound care essentials* (3rd ed., pp. 240–264). Ambler, PA: Lippincott Williams & Wilkins.

Products and Applications. (2014). Retrieved June 9, 2014 from Nestle Nutrition Web site, http://www.nestle-nutrition.com/Products/Default.aspx

Rudolph, D. (2009). Appetite stimulants in long term care: A literature review. *The Internet Journal of Advanced Nursing Practice, 11*(1). Retrieved July 11, 2014 from http://ispub.com/IJANP/11/1/9279

Standards of Medical Care in Diabetes–2014. (2014). *Diabetes Care, 37*(S1), S14–S80.

Stratton, R. J., Ek, A. C., Engfer, M., et al. (2005). Enteral nutritional support in prevention and treatment of pressure ulcers: A systematic review and meta-analysis. *Ageing Research Reviews, 4*(3), 422–450.

Sullivan, D. H., Johnson, L. E., Bopp, M. M., et al. (2004). Prognostic significance of monthly weight fluctuations among older nursing home residents. *The Journals of Gerontology Series A, Biological Sciences and Medical Sciences, 59*(6), M633–M639.

Teno J. M., Gozalo P., Mitchell S. L., et al. (2012). Feeding tubes and the prevention or healing of pressure ulcers. *Archives of Internal Medicine, 172*(9), 697–701.

ter Riet, G., Kessels, A. G., & Knipschild, P. G. (1995). Randomized clinical trial of ascorbic acid in the treatment of pressure ulcers. *Journal of Clinical Epidemiology, 48*(12), 1453–1460.

Thomas, D. R. (2008). Unintended weight loss in older adults. *Ageing Health, 4*(2), 191–200.

Trans Tasman Dietetic Wound Care Group. Evidence date January 2010. *Evidence based practice guidelines for the nutritional management of adults with pressure injuries*. www.ttdwcg.org. 2011.

The Vegetarian Times. (2008). *Vegetarianism in America*. Retrieved July 11, 2014 from http://www.vegetariantimes.com/article/vegetarianism-in-america/

Russell M. (2013). Complications of enteral feedings. In P Charney., A Malone. *Pocket guide to enteral nutrition* (2nd ed., pp. 170–197). Chicago, IL: Academy of Nutrition and Dietetics.

Sacket, D. I. (1996). Evidence based medicine. What it is and what it isn't. *British Medical Journal, 312*, 71–72.

United States Department of Agriculture and United States Department of Health and Human Services. (2010). *Dietary guidelines for Americans 2010. (HHS Publication No HHS-ODPHP-2010-01-GDA-A)*. Retrieved July 11, 2014 from http://www.health.gov/dietaryguidelines/

van Anholt, R., Sobotka, L., Meijer, E., et al. (2010). Specific nutritional support accelerates pressure ulcer healing and reduces wound care intensity in non-malnourished patients. *Nutrition, 26*(9), 867–872.

White, J. V., Guenter, P. Jensen, G., et al. (2012). Consensus statement of the Academy of Nutrition and Dietetics/American Society for Parenteral and Enteral Nutrition: Characteristics recommended for the identification and documentation of adult malnutrition (undernutrition). *Journal of the Academy of Nutrition and Dietetics, 112*, 730–738.

QUESTIONS

1. A nutritional assessment is performed on a patient to determine if he is undernourished. What is a key indicator of undernutrition?

A. Loss of 5% of body weight in 30 days
B. Loss of 10% of body weight in 30 days
C. Loss of 25% of body weight in 180 days
D. Loss of 30% of body weight in 90 days

2. Which patient would the RDN consider at high risk for the development of pressure ulcers?

A. A patient with BMI greater than 25
B. A patient who has increased levels of hepatic proteins
C. A patient who has a BMI less than 18
D. A patient who runs marathons

3. Which patient criteria support a diagnosis of malnutrition?

A. Insufficient energy intake and increased subcutaneous fat
B. Loss of muscle mass and loss of subcutaneous fat
C. Fluid accumulation and weight gain
D. Diminished functional status and increased muscle mass

4. What is the primary reason for taking the time to perform a comprehensive assessment to identify PEM as opposed to ordering a simple blood draw to formulate a diagnosis?
   A. Blood tests do not provide a definitive diagnosis.
   B. Blood tests for malnutrition are expensive and unreliable.
   C. There are no blood tests available.
   D. There is a high incidence of false-positive results with blood tests.

5. The RDN is preparing a dietary plan for a patient diagnosed with malnutrition. Which micronutrient might the nurse include?
   A. Protein
   B. Carbohydrates
   C. Water
   D. Vitamin B

6. The RDN is explaining the role of energy in the diet to a patient diagnosed with starvation-related malnutrition. Which statement accurately describes the effect of energy on the body?
   A. "Energy is provided in the diet by micronutrients."
   B. "Providing adequate energy prevents anabolism."
   C. "Energy acts to spare protein by providing alternative sources of energy."
   D. "Conditions increasing the metabolic rate decrease energy needs."

7. The RDN is determining energy needs for a patient assessed with risk of malnutrition, who has a pressure ulcer and weights 70 kg. According to the *Clinical Practice Guidelines on Prevention and Treatment of Pressure Ulcers,* how many kcalories would the nurse recommend?
   A. 1,500
   B. 2,100
   C. 2,500
   D. 3,200

8. How many grams of protein are recommended for an adult patient at risk for a pressure ulcer and malnutrition, who weights 50 kg?
   A. 62.5
   B. 90.0
   C. 87.5
   D. 112.5

9. The RDN is determining fluid needs for a healthy adult who weighs 60 kg. What amount is recommended by the 2014 *Prevention and Treatment of Pressure Ulcers: Clinical Practice Guidelines*?
   A. 1,000 mL
   B. 1,500 mL
   C. 1,800 mL
   D. 2,000 mL

10. Which of the following statements is most accurate regarding the nutritional management of special populations?
   A. An obese individual with wounds should consume a low-calorie diet designed for weight reduction.
   B. Nutritional supplements for vegans should contain dairy, meat, or egg products.
   C. The American Diabetes Association endorses the "ADA diet" plan for individuals with diabetes.
   D. The diet for stage 3 or 4 CKD may not meet the protein or nutrient needs required for wound healing.

ANSWERS: 1.**A**, 2.**C**, 3.**B**, 4.**A**, 5.**D**, 6.**C**, 7.**B**, 8.**A**, 9.**C**, 10.**D**

CHAPTER 7

General Principles of Topical Therapy

JoAnn Ermer-Seltun and Bonnie Sue Rolstad

OBJECTIVES

1. Describe the principles underlying "moist wound healing" and "wound bed preparation."
2. Explain the impact of wound care goals on wound care management and topical therapy.
3. Develop an individualized plan of care based on assessment data and current evidence-based guidelines that addresses each of the following factors:
   - Correction or amelioration of etiologic factors
   - Attention to systemic factors affecting repair process
   - Evidence-based topical therapy
   - Pain management
   - Patient and caregiver education
4. Recommend or provide topical therapy based on best available evidence, to include:
   - Debridement of necrotic tissue when indicated
   - Identification and management of wound-related infections
   - Management of epibole and hypertrophic granulation tissue
   - Selection of dressings to manage exudate and maintain moist wound surface
5. Describe indications and procedure for chemical cauterization of closed wound edges and/or hypertrophic granulation tissue.

Topic Outline

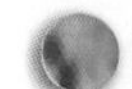 Introduction

People with chronic wounds are considered to be the latest global health care challenge, and chronic wounds now occur in epidemic proportions (Treadwell & Keast, 2010). In addition to the impact on morbidity and potential mortality, chronic wound care is estimated to cost over 50 billion dollars per year in the United States alone (Fife et al., 2012). Factors contributing to the persistence and cost of chronic wounds include a delay in proper identification and correction of etiologic factors and impediments to healing, wound care inconsistencies among practitioners and clinics, and a lack of evidence-based wound management (O'Donnell & Balk, 2011). In light of this predicament, there is a crucial need for an evidence-based, prioritized, and standardized approach to chronic wound management that can be implemented by wound care providers in a variety of settings (Gale et al., 2014). Chronic wound management must have a holistic, patient-centered focus where the etiology of the wound is identified and treated if possible, comorbidities and cofactors are reviewed and corrected when feasible, and local wound care is implemented that provides a microenvironment for healing (in curable wounds), or stabilization, if palliation is the wound care goal. This chapter focuses on wound bed preparation as it relates to providing an optimal local microenvironment; however, the wound care nurse must remember that effective therapy requires attention to all three principles: correction of causative factors, optimization of systemic factors affecting healing, and evidence-based topical therapy (Sibbald et al., 2011). A holistic approach to chronic wound management requires an interdisciplinary team and an individualized plan of care that addresses patient-/family-centered concerns and preferences.

CLINICAL PEARL

Effective wound management must include correction of etiologic factors, systemic support for healing, and evidence-based topical therapy that provides a local environment that supports repair.

 Priorities in Wound Management

An effective wound management plan must be consistent with the goals of care, individualized for the patient, and based on current evidence and scientific principles.

Establishment Appropriate Wound Care Goals

The first priority in developing an effective and individualized plan of care is to determine the cause of the wound and to classify the wound as "healable," "maintenance," or "nonhealable" (Sibbald et al., 2011). This categorization will determine the overall goals of wound care goal, which will in turn direct treatment priorities and modalities that are individualized and realistic.

Healing Goal

Individuals with "healable" wounds have the resources (physical, psychosocial and health system support) to successfully heal the wound in a reasonable time frame (and within their lifespan). In order to be classified as "healable," wounds must meet the following criteria: (1) causative factors have been identified and can be corrected and (2) there is sufficient systemic support (perfusion, nutritional support, glycemic control, etc.) to promote healing. Treatment goals for healable wounds should focus upon proper wound bed preparation as described later in the chapter using the TIME acronym as a framework.

Maintenance Goal

"Maintenance" wounds are wounds that might be healable, but the potential for healing is negated either by the individual's choice (noncompliance in edema management, poor glycemic control, lack of self-care efforts) or by insufficient health care resources to correct the causative factors and provide sufficient systemic support and topical therapy to optimize healing. For these wounds, care is focused on wound stabilization and prevention of complications.

Comfort Goal

The "nonhealable" wound cannot proceed through the wound healing phases due to limited tissue perfusion, inability to effectively correct etiologic factors, or end-of-life status. For these patients, comfort and symptom management are the primary focus of care.

Therefore, classification of the "healability" of a wound will determine whether the global goal is wound closure, wound stabilization (along with effective pain and symptom control), or comfort (management of wound-related symptoms as opposed to wound healing). For patients at end of life and patients in palliative care, comfort is the primary goal. Palliative care is a complex care model that is patient and family centered (Emmons & Lachman, 2010; Letizia et al., 2010). The ultimate goal in palliative wound care is to improve the quality of life for those with life-threatening or debilitating disorders through symptom control and improvement of psychosocial well-being, via a multidisciplinary team approach (Emmons & Lachman, 2010). Patients receiving palliative wound care commonly have "nonhealable" or "maintenance" wounds; however, some have wounds that are "healable" from the perspective of ability to correct etiologic factors and systemic status supporting wound healing (Sibbald et al., 2011). The determination of wound care goals in this situation is impacted significantly by patient goals; some patients choose palliation because the care required to heal the wound costs them too much effort in respect to altering their lifestyle or in regards to the financial or psychosocial costs of care. Chapter 33 further describes the concept of palliative care and the primary goals in palliative chronic wound management.

CLINICAL PEARL

Classification of a wound in terms of "healability" determines whether the goal is wound closure, stabilization, or comfort.

Establishment of Individualized Wound Care Plan

Once the "healability" of the wound is determined, the next priority is to assure that the plan of care is patient centered and individualized. The plan must address the patient's unique risk factors, comorbidities, and quality of life issues; must include consideration of their circle of care or support system and their ability to access care; and must address personal concerns such as pain control, activities of daily living, psychosocial well-being, and financial constraints (Sibbald et al., 2011). Likewise, specific dressing selection is based upon the characteristics of the wound (type of tissue, depth of tissue destruction, amount of drainage, presence of odor or pain, evidence of critical colonization or infection) but must be consistent with the principles of wound bed preparation (Fig. 7-1). The plan of care should be written and a permanent part of the health care record, reevaluated at least every 30 days, and updated/modified whenever there is no measurable progress for 2 to 3 weeks and whenever there is a significant change in the patient's health care status (Sibbald et al., 2011). The wound care nurse must be cognizant of common barriers to effective wound care and must do everything possible to eliminate these barriers: inappropriate or non–patient-centered goals, depression, pain, anxiety, complicated treatment modalities, impaired cognition or dexterity, financial barriers and lack of resources, lack of confidence, or skepticism and lack of knowledge due to inadequate or ineffective patient education (Nix & Peirce, 2012).

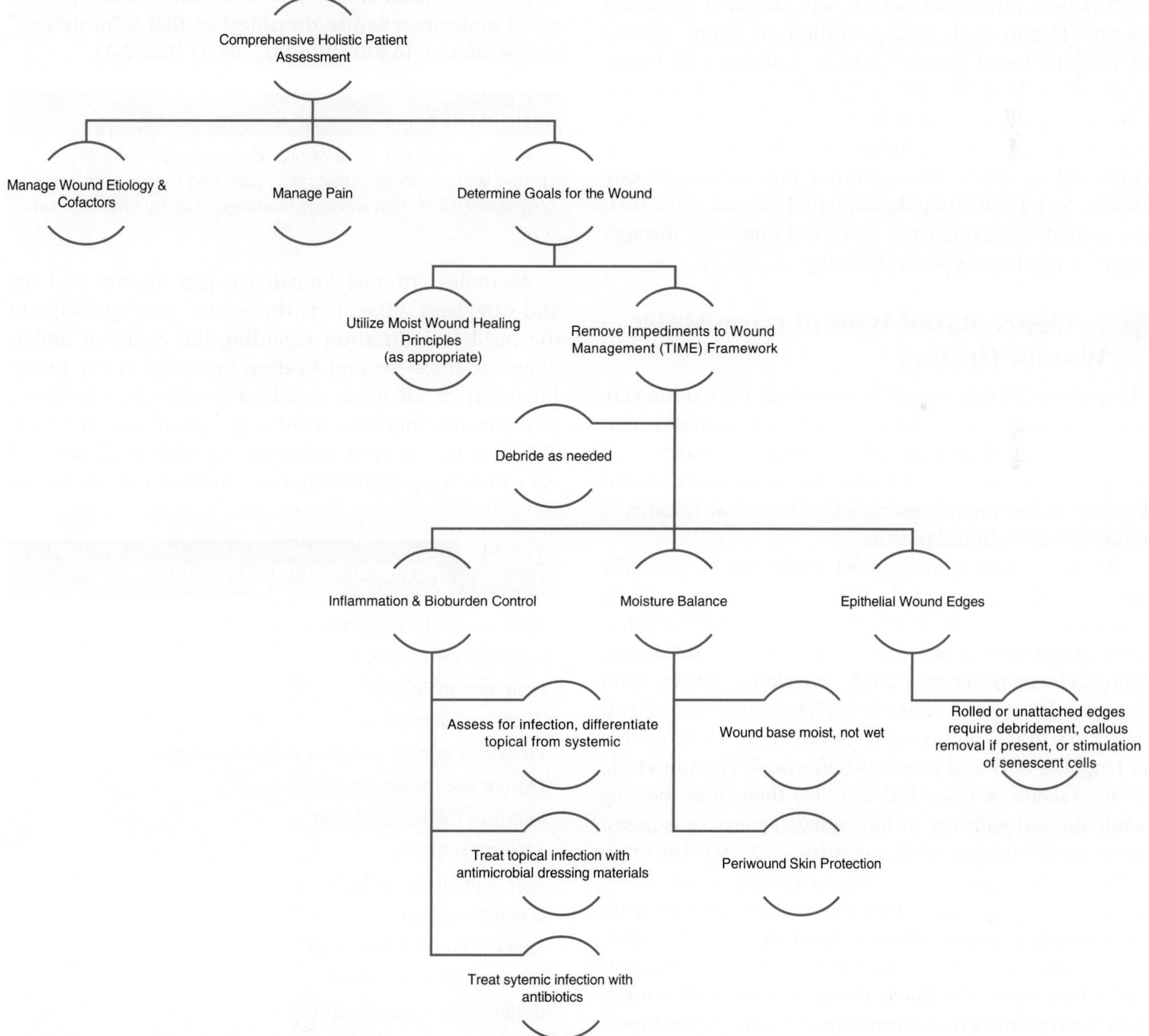

FIGURE 7-1. Decision tree for wound management. (From Woo, K. Y., Krasner, D. L., & Sibbald, R. G. (2014). Pain in people with chronic wounds: Clinical Strategies for decreasing pain and improving quality of life. In D. L. Krasner (Ed.), *Chronic wound care: The essentials. A clinical source book for healthcare professionals* (pp. 111–122). Malvern, PA: HMP Communications. Reprinted with permission of HMP Communications, LLC.)

Evidence-Based Wound Care

A model for evidence based medicine was proposed by Sackett et al. (2000) that involves clinical decision making based on the following essential elements: best available clinical evidence (clinical practice guidelines); clinical expertise (wound certification); and patient preferences. These three elements must drive the wound plan of care.

The importance of care that is evidence based and patient centered is underscored by the federal health care payment reform initiatives included in the 2010 Affordable Care Act (US). Health care systems are challenged to establish Accountable Care Organizations (ACOs) that are reimbursed based on quality-of-care metrics and population-level outcomes (Flattau et al., 2013). ACOs that provide the best quality of care with the least amount of resources, as evidenced by positive clinical outcomes and high patient satisfaction scores, will receive a monetary reward (Flattau et al., 2013). In the near future, the use of evidence-based clinical practice guidelines (Whitney et al., 2006; WOCN, 2010, 2011, 2012, 2014) and best practice to guide care for various types of chronic wounds may be mandated and linked to reimbursement (Gale et al., 2014). Now is the opportune time for wound care experts to improve population-based wound outcomes, the patient care experience, and fiscal outcomes through improved delivery systems (Flattau et al., 2013).

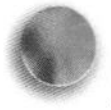

Evidence-Based Wound Care: Moist Wound Healing

The purpose of this section is to provide the wound care specialist with high-level evidence that includes randomised controlled trials (RCTs), bench research, and sentinel references related to the science of moist wound healing and to provide examples of how that research is translated into clinical practice.

Wounds healing in a moist environment generally heal faster (Brolmann et al., 2013; Jones & Fennie, 2007; Vloemans et al., 2014; Wiechula, 2003), with fewer infections (Brolmann et al., 2013; Hutchinson & McGuckin, 1990; Vloemans et al., 2014; Wiechula, 2003), with less pain (Brolmann et al., 2013; Vloemans et al., 2014; Wiechula, 2003) and scarring, (Hein et al., 1998; Michie & Hugill, 1994) and more cost-effectively (Bolton et al., 1996; Xakellis & Chrischilles, 1992) than those healing while dressed with dry or impregnated gauze or exposed to the air (Ovington, 2002; van Rijswijk, 2004). The original research supporting this statement was published over a half century ago and continues to be confirmed with increasingly rigorous research (Brolmann et al., 2013; Vloemans et al., 2014). Since the original research was published, clinical trials involving thousands of wounds have been published confirming the benefits of moisture in the physiologic wound environment. Yet today, this knowledge has not fully transferred into clinical practice. Even experts in the field incorrectly combine moisture-retentive and non–moisture-retentive dressings into the "occlusive" dressing groups of controlled studies, mistaking modern dressings for "occlusive" or moisture-retentive dressings (Ubbink et al., 2008). In fact, one of the most prevalent dressings in use today is plain gauze, a porous material that dehydrates the wound within 4 hours of application (even when moistened with saline) (Colwell et al., 1993). Barriers to clinical practice change are multifaceted and likely include tradition, the concern about infection that is contraindicated by evidence, availability and low purchase price of gauze, an incomplete understanding of moist wound healing practices, the unit cost of modern dressings as opposed to gauze, and the complexity of numerous moist wound healing product choices available. This lag in knowledge transfer means that today's patient and caregiver may yet believe that the best way to manage the acute or chronic wound is to expose the wound to air (i.e., to avoid moisture-retentive dressings) so that a "protective" scab is allowed to form (Bolton, 2004) (Box 7-1).

CLINICAL PEARL

Wounds managed in a moist environment generally heal faster, with fewer infections, less pain and scarring, and more cost-effectively than wounds managed in a dry environment.

Awareness of this knowledge gap among patients and caregivers alike alerts the wound care specialist to the need for education regarding the evidence underlying the moist wound healing therapies in use today. Inclusion of all team members is critical as evidence provides the foundation for appropriate interventions. The benefits of early intervention with evidence and education for patients/families usually results in greater

BOX 7-1. Advantages of Moist Wound Healing

- Prevents wound desiccation
- Enhances cell migration
- Promotes angiogenesis
- Augments autolysis
- Provides a protective barrier to external threats
- Lessens risk for wound infection
- Improves thermoregulation
- Fosters pH balance
- May alter biological factors
- Diminishes fibrosis
- Reduces dressing frequency
- Enhances patient comfort
- Better cosmetic appearance
- Saves nursing time
- Cuts cost

patient adherence. The patient and family who initially wanted to leave the wound exposed to air to form a protective scab will be favorably inclined to provide moist wound care because they understand the benefits. When the collaborative team and staff understand the evidence, system change is facilitated; specifically, processes, procedures, and care pathways are changed, resulting in reduced wound care product costs and improved patient outcomes.

CLINICAL PEARL

The concepts of moist wound healing have not been fully translated into clinical practice; therefore, the wound nurse must be prepared to educate other staff members as well as patients/families as to the benefits of moist wound healing.

Moist Wound Healing: The Evidence

Knowledge of the repair process for both partial-thickness and full-thickness wounds leads to an understanding of the importance of hydration for all living tissue. Biology teaches that cells living within a fluid environment are actively involved in the destruction of any debris; they are also observed to migrate freely, to reproduce, and to contribute actively to tissue repair and proliferation. All of these functions are critical to the repair process. When a wound occurs, the protective barrier of the skin is compromised. Since one of the primary functions of the skin is protection, skin injury and skin loss result in exposure of the underlying tissue to the external environment where dehydration occurs. Without intervention to restore and maintain the protective barrier, the dehydration results in cell death and tissue desiccation. It has been stated that "Perhaps the single most pertinent parameter of the local wound environment relative to tissue viability and proliferation is that of tissue hydration" (Ovington & Eisenbud, 2004). Therefore, monitoring and maintenance of moisture in the wound is a primary goal for the wound care specialist.

CLINICAL PEARL

"Perhaps the single most pertinent parameter of the local wound environment relative to tissue viability and proliferation is that of tissue hydration" (Ovington & Eisenbud, 2004).

Moist wound healing was practiced for centuries, as reflected by ancient literature. The Sumerians before 2000 BC and, later, the Egyptians documented the use of moist wound healing with "occlusive poultices" made of honey, resin, and/or grease-coated lint (Manjo, 1975). In 1846 a surgeon, Robert Liston, documented the use of lint dressings soaked in water and covered with oiled silk (Bishop, 1959). However, moist wound healing was replaced by "dry wound care" and a focus on antiseptics in the 1860s, due to concerns that a moist environment increased the risk for wound infection; while this was later proven to be untrue, that perception has persisted and, as noted, still influences wound care beliefs and procedures. In the mid-1950s, the practice of moist wound healing reemerged, and Gilje (1948) published a paper indicating that venous ulcerations healed faster under "tape" than under gauze. Odland (1958) reported his observation that blisters healed faster when unbroken.

The seminal publication on the benefits of moist wound healing in soft tissue injuries is credited to George Winter in 1962. Winter demonstrated that porcine partial-thickness wounds covered with a polyethylene film epithelialized twice as fast as those exposed to the air. He also reported an increased rate of regeneration in the underlying connective tissue, indicating that a moist wound environment positively affected the deeper structures as well. A year later, Hinman and Maibach (1963) reported on a study of partial-thickness wounds created on human volunteers; they found faster epithelialization among the wounds that were occluded. Some 30 years after Winter's publication, De Coninck et al. (1996) repeated Winter's work with full-thickness wounds utilizing a semipermeable polyurethane film dressing. They also reported a shorter time to healing among wounds managed with the moisture-retentive dressing.

In addition to reduced time to closure, Winter (1962), and later Rogers (2000), demonstrated that moist wound healing prevented trauma to wounds. They demonstrated that allowing gauze to dry onto the surface of the wound causes trauma to the healing tissue with removal; specifically, they found that the new blood vessels and newly formed tissue became attached to the dry gauze and were forcibly removed during dressing changes, thereby reinjuring the wound and delaying closure. In addition to these negative effects on the healing wound, Ovington (2002) later reported that gauze (wet or dry) is not an effective barrier to bacteria. She demonstrated that 64 layers of gauze were required in order to reach a "barrier" level. Hutchinson and McGuckin (1990) confirmed the clinical relevance of this finding; in a meta-analysis of 35 controlled studies involving acute and chronic wounds, they reported a significant reduction in the incidence of infections with moisture-retentive dressings, that is, 3.2% infections in 1,013 wounds dressed with moisture-retentive dressings compared to 7.6% infections in 1,421 wounds covered with non–moisture-retentive dressings. This is most likely due in part to the effects of the cell death and tissue desiccation caused by wound dehydration; the dead tissue provides nutrients for the bacteria that are able to access the wound through the portals in the dressing. In addition, the wound is continually reinjured during the process of dressing removal. Thus the use of gauze is associated with tissue desiccation, bacterial invasion, and repetitive injury. Finally, the overall cost of gauze is usually greater than the cost of moisture-retentive dressings, because the cost of therapy is much greater than the cost of the dressing itself (Bolton et al., 1996; Xakellis & Chrischilles, 1992). Gauze is less expensive per unit dressing than moisture-retentive dressings, but significantly more expensive per venous or pressure ulcer patient healed or per total cost of management for a period of time, such as 12 weeks (Kerstein et al., 2001). The increased dressing change frequency and longer healing times associated with gauze increase the labor and cost required for gauze-based wound care (Ovington, 2002; Kerstein et al., 2001). The wound care specialist today should realize that gauze remains a mainstay in wound care because of availability and familiarity as opposed to care outcomes or cost of care (Bolton, 2004; Ovington, 2002).

CLINICAL PEARL

The wound care clinician should realize that gauze remains a mainstay of wound care because of availability and familiarity as opposed to care outcomes or cost-effectiveness.

Physiologically, Winter's (1962) results indicated that epithelial cellular migration (i.e., wound resurfacing) and extracellular matrix (ECM) formation (i.e., wound filling) occur optimally in a moist environment with living cells. Those wounds dressed with gauze or exposed to the air require twice the time to heal because of tissue desiccation, surface cell death, and development of a scab. The presence of a scab inhibits epithelial cell migration and requires that the cells delve downward (i.e., under the scab) in order to contact living fibrous tissue and continue their journey to complete wound resurfacing. Healing in this manner increases the depth or length of the original injury and the time required to heal the wound (Fig. 7-2A and B). An everyday example of this process may be seen when a person has a biking injury resulting in a wound on the knee. The injury bleeds and is cleansed. When gauze is applied to the wound and taped, the wound continues to dry out under the porous material until a scab forms. Once the "protective" scab is in place and drainage stops, the dressing may be discontinued. During removal, the patient may see bleeding as the gauze is forcibly removed from an embedded clot. One day during a shower, the scab falls off and there is a completely healed wound below! In order to close this wound, epithelial cells delved downward under the scab to contact moist tissue so that they could migrate, proliferate and eventually resurface the wound. In contrast, if a moisture-retentive dressing had been applied, the epidermal cells would have been able to proliferate and to migrate over the moist surface of the wound until the multiple migrating epidermal cells contacted other migrating epidermal cells. At that point, contact inhibition would occur, causing cessation of lateral migration and resumption of vertical migration, which gradually reestablishes epidermal thickness.

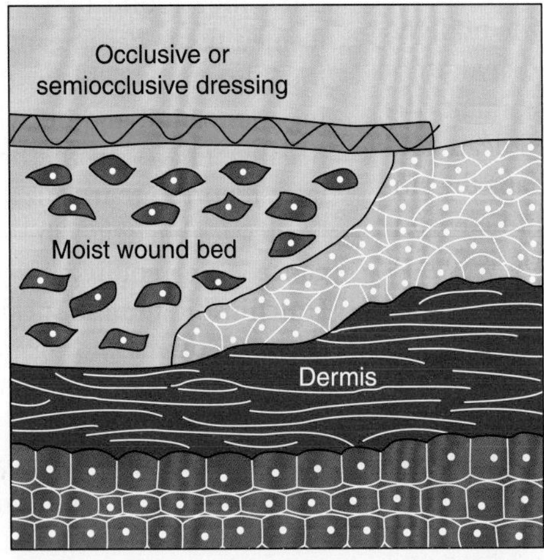

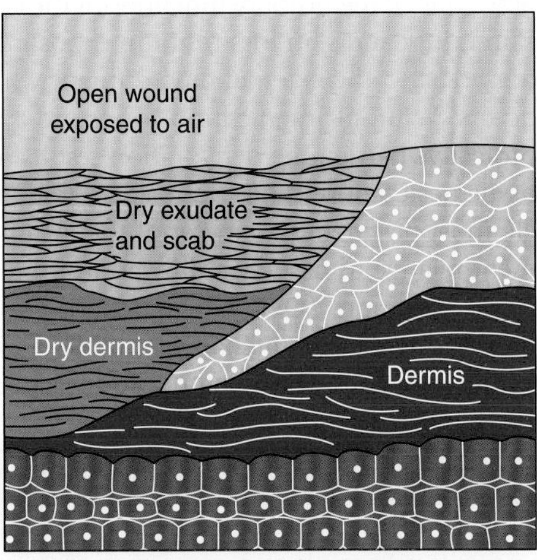

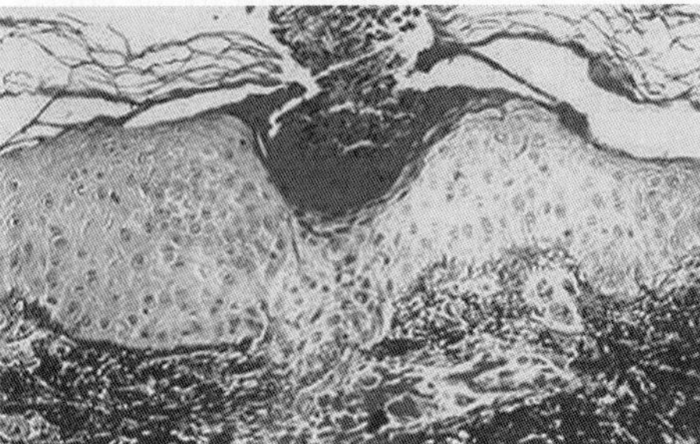

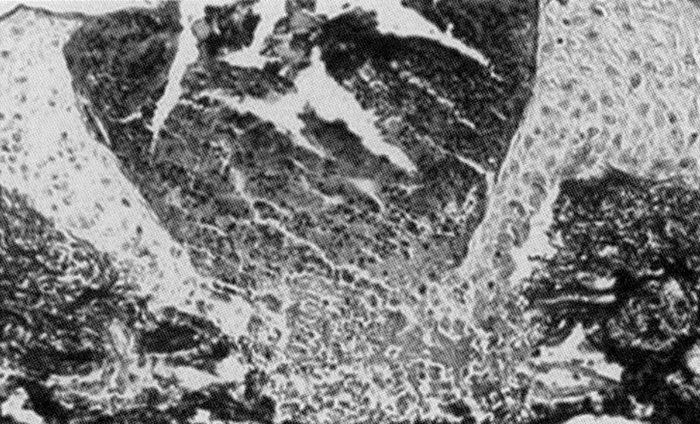

FIGURE 7-2. A. Wound healing in moist versus dry environment. **B.** Histology of a human incision covered with a moisture-retentive dressing and another of identical depth protected, but air exposed. (From Bryant, R., & Nix, D. (2012). *Acute and chronic wounds, current management concepts* (4th ed). New York: Mosby, reprinted with permission of Elsevier.)

CLINICAL PEARL

Presence of a scab or dry wound surface requires the cells involved in repair to tunnel down to a moist tissue layer in order to continue the repair process.

Maintenance of a moist wound surface also promotes full-thickness wound repair. Dyson et al. (1992) reported that the inflammatory and proliferative phases of wound healing were shortened by use of moist wound healing as opposed to dry conditions. They also showed that revascularization occurred at a faster rate and in a more orderly manner in wounds managed in a moist environment. Increased production of collagen in the wound was also reported in a moist environment. Field and Kerstei (1994) and Singh et al. (2004) later confirmed that moist wound management facilitates healing, supports the breakdown of avascular tissue and fibrin (autolytic debridement), reduces pain, and does not increase the risk of infection. Subsequent research supports the concept that wounds managed in a moist environment heal faster with less pain, fewer infections, and less scarring (Alvarez et al., 1983; Bolton & van Rijswijk, 1991; Brolmann et al., 2013; Cherry & Ryan, 1985; Hutchinson & McGuckin, 1990; Hefton & Staiano-Coico, 1989; Hein et al., 1998; Hopf et al., 2006; Kerstein et al., 2001; Pirone et al., 1990; Varghese et al., 1986). There is also reduced risk of infection when moisture-retentive dressings are utilized to maintain a physiologic, protected wound environment where exogenous microorganisms are prohibited from entering the wound (Bolton, 2004; Hutchinson, 1994; Hutchinson & McGuckin, 1990). For a complete discussion of wound healing cellular activities, please see Chapter 2.

Moisture Balance

A moist wound healing environment is defined as one that maintains moisture balance at the interface between the wound and the dressing by use of therapies that maintain, absorb, or donate moisture. Wounds may be dry, moist, or heavily exudative. Topical therapies are available to address each situation, with the goal of maintaining a moist surface, while avoiding the accumulation and pooling of exudate. Conceptually, a dry wound usually requires moisture donation (i.e., a hydrogel). A wound with a limited volume of exudate requires a dressing that can absorb the excess exudate without dehydrating the wound surface; good dressings in these situations include hydrocolloids and foams. Wounds with high-volume exudate require dressings that are highly absorptive in order to manage the exudate and prevent maceration of the wound surface (Brolmann et al., 2013; Junker et al., 2013). For further information on specific wound dressings, please refer to Chapter 8.

CLINICAL PEARL

Moisture balance is critical to wound healing, and requires a balancing act between absorption of exudate (which impairs healing) and prevention of desiccation (which also impairs healing).

Moisture-Retentive Dressings

The dressings and advanced therapies used to maintain moisture balance at the wound surface are most accurately termed "moisture retentive," meaning they are designed to maintain continuous moisture at the wound–dressing interface and to prevent desiccation of the wound surface. Other less precise terms related to wound care dressings include the word occlusive (i.e., semiocclusive and occlusive dressings). Occlusive dressings permit no gaseous exchange between the wound and the environment, which means moisture vapor cannot escape from the wound bed; semiocclusive dressings permit limited moisture vapor transfer. Very few dressings are totally occlusive; the major subset in the occlusive or mostly occlusive category is hydrocolloid dressings. The term occlusive should be limited to dressings that *are* occlusive, because such dressings are generally considered to be contraindicated for use in infected wounds due to lack of data as to safety in these conditions; in contrast, moisture-retentive dressings are very appropriately used for infected as well as noninfected wounds. Moisture-retentive dressings are not occlusive to all moisture; they allow evaporation of some moisture from the skin and wound. Dressings with limited moisture vapor transmission (i.e., ≤30 g moisture vapor transmission/square meter of dressing/hour) have been reported to optimize healing of a wide variety of acute and chronic animal and human wounds (Bolton, 2007; Bolton & van Rijswijk, 1990). In addition to maintaining an optimally moist wound surface, some moisture-retentive dressings are impermeable to viruses and bacteria, thus providing high-level protection against infection (Bowler et al., 1993).

CLINICAL PEARL

Occlusive and moisture retentive are not synonymous terms; most moisture-retentive dressings permit evaporation of moisture from the skin and wound and are therefore *not* occlusive.

Moisture-retentive dressings are designed with a backing that is permeable to vapors but impermeable to fluids; this allows for evaporative loss of the moisture that is continually diffusing and evaporating through the skin, while keeping the wound bed moist and protected from external sources of moisture The rate at which the outer layer of a dressing allows moisture to evaporate through its membrane is known as the moisture vapor transmission rate (MVTR). As noted above, the ideal MVTR of the outer dressing material for most wounds is less than about 30 g/m^2/h. This is more than the MVTR of intact skin at most body sites, but less than the rates of moisture vapor transmission permitted by most fibrous, foam, or gauze dressings (Bolton, 2007). Dressings with lower MVTR help to maintain a moist wound surface (Bolton, 2007; Bolton & van Rijswijk, 1990), but can increase the risk of maceration in a highly exudative wound; in contrast, dressings with higher MVTR are beneficial in management of highly exudative wounds but could permit dehydration of the wound surface when there is minimal exudate. Thus the MVTR of a dressing is a key consideration for the wound nurse who is selecting a dressing for a specific wound. MVTR is a dressing characteristic very commonly seen on packages or inserts, particularly for transparent film dressings. These dressings have relatively low MVTRs and are frequently used to protect unbroken skin where fluid accumulation is unlikely. As the patient perspires, the moisture typically evaporates through the dressing film. If the patient has a wound with significant exudate, an absorptive dressing must be used over the wound to manage the drainage, and the transparent film can be used as the cover dressing; the film provides protection against fluid invasion and provides appropriate moisture vapor management for the periwound skin. When the patient has a wound, dressings that transmit less moisture vapor than the average wound loses retain wound moisture, fostering optimal wound healing (Bolton, 2007; Bolton & van Rijswijk, 1990; Junker et al., 2013). Moisture-retentive dressings can reduce open wound pain and infection rates compared to gauze (Brolmann et al., 2013).

Exudate Management

Appropriate moisture balance at the wound surface includes management of wound exudate as well as prevention of dehydration. Wound exudate is composed primarily of water, but electrolytes, nutrients, protein digesting enzymes (matrix metalloproteinases [MMPs]), growth factors, neutrophils, macrophages, platelets and microorganisms are also present (Romanelli et al., 2010). All open wounds contain microorganisms, as does wound exudate, but the presence of microorganisms does not necessarily signal infection; infection occurs when the bacterial loads overwhelm host defenses and is manifest by additional findings such as wound deterioration and periwound erythema and induration.

The fluid produced by an acute wound is typically "prorepair," containing large amounts of growth factors and other substances supporting ECM production. In contrast, the fluid produced by a chronic wound is typically "proinflammatory" and contains large concentrations of cytokines and proteases that tend to maintain the wound in an inflammatory state. This imbalanced and proinflammatory exudate contributes to the chronicity of nonhealing wounds and requires effective management with absorptive dressings and other topical therapies. Issues related to chronic wound exudate are discussed further in the section on impediments to wound healing.

CLINICAL PEARL

Acute wound fluid is typically "prorepair," while chronic wound fluid is usually "proinflammatory" due to high concentrations of inflammatory cytokines and proteases.

In summary, there is strong evidence that moist wound healing results in increased healing rates, decreased healing time, improved scar appearance, reduced pain, reduced infection, and reduced cost of care (Jones & San Miguel, 2006; Nemeth et al., 1991; Ovington, 2007; Romanelli et al., 2010; Tur & Bolton, 2014). In addition, new therapies are emerging that involve the use of moist wound healing products to deliver antimicrobials, analgesics and a host of bioactive molecules (i.e., growth factors and micrografts) (Junker et al., 2013). It is important for the wound nurse to remember that moist wound healing refers to the wound base only; the periwound skin should remain dry and protected from excessive moisture or dryness.

Clinical Application

1. Current evidence strongly supports **maintenance of a moist wound base when the goal is healing**. Wound healing is enhanced in a moist environment, and moisture-retentive dressings are designed with this goal in mind. They protect the wound from external contaminants while maintaining balanced moisture at the wound base via absorption, moisture donation, and/or moisture retention.

   Caution: Moist wound healing may be contraindicated in the patient with stable, dry eschar and a poorly vascularized noninfected wound of the lower extremity (see Chapter 22).
2. Care should also be designed to **protect the periwound skin from maceration and mechanical injury**. In a wound with well-controlled moisture balance and less frequent dressing changes, periwound skin may not require additional skin protection. However, in most situations routine protection of the periwound skin, with either a liquid film barrier or a moisture barrier ointment, is indicated. Wounds on the trunk are typically managed with adhesive dressings; in this situation, a liquid film barrier is the best option for periwound skin protection. In contrast, moisture barrier ointments are a good choice for protection of the skin surrounding extremity wounds being managed with wrap dressings.
3. A third critical element of effective wound management is **ongoing monitoring of exudate levels, with adjustments in topical therapy as needed**. Wound

exudate levels are affected by many factors, and the volume of exudate changes throughout the healing process and in response to changes in bacterial loads. Exudate levels are generally the highest during the early inflammatory phase of healing and typically increase when there is wound infection (either local or invasive) (Golinko et al., 2009). A critical aspect of therapeutic topical wound care is effective management of exudate while maintaining a moist wound surface; this requires careful "matching" of the dressing (and its absorptive qualities) with the wound (and volume of exudate). One type of dressing is not likely to fit all the phases of healing. The wound nurse should expect changes in wound status and wound requirements and should provide routine follow-up in order to adjust protocols based on moisture balance, patient concerns, or other considerations.

4. Another key point is the need to **anticipate the need for patient/family and health care provider/team education**. The evidence related to moist wound healing has not been fully translated into clinical practice; thus the plan of care must include teaching related to the science of moist wound healing.
5. Finally, **clinical decision making that is research based and patient centered** (i.e., reflects the goals and priorities of the patient and family) **is recognized as evidence based** (Institute of Medicine, 2008).

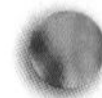

Wound Bed Preparation: TIME Framework

Acute wounds heal at a predictable rate as they go through the healing cascade from injury to hemostasis, inflammation, proliferation (repair), and the maturation (remodeling) phases. In contrast, chronic wounds fail to proceed or "get stuck" in the repair process and fail durable closure. People who suffer from chronic wounds are considered to be the latest epidemic health care problem globally (Treadwell & Keast, 2010), and chronic wound care is estimated to cost over 50 billion dollars per year in the United States alone (Fife et al., 2012).

The goal then is to move the chronic wound to an acute state in order to promote healing. In 2003, a group of health care providers (physicians and nurses) and scientists developed a straightforward framework to identify and then remove or correct the intrinsic and extrinsic impediments to repair most commonly affecting chronic wounds (Schultz et al., 2003). The acronym TIME (Table 7-1) reflects this simple and structured framework for addressing barriers to chronic wound healing and for identifying key clinical assessments and treatment options for optimal wound bed preparation (Schultz & Dowsett, 2012). This internationally recognized concept (EWMA, 2004) provides a comprehensive approach to wound bed preparation and provides guidance to clinicians for promoting healing in a TIMEly fashion.

TABLE 7-1 TIME Framework for Chronic Wound Management

Clinical Observations	Proposed Pathophysiology	WBP Clinical Actions	Effect of WBP Actions	Clinical Outcome
Tissue nonviable or deficient	Defective matrix and cell debris	Debridement (episodic or continuous): Autolytic, sharp surgical, enzymatic, mechanical or biological Biological agents	Restoration of wound base and functional extracellular matrix proteins	Viable wound base
Infection or inflammation	High bacterial counts or prolonged inflammation ↑Inflammatory cytokines ↑Protease activity ↓Growth factor activity	Remove infected foci Topical/systemic: Antimicrobials Anti-inflammatories Protease inhibition	Low bacterial counts or controlled inflammation: ↓Inflammatory cytokines ↓Protease activity ↑Growth factor activity	Bacterial balance and reduced inflammation
Moisture imbalance	Desiccation slows epithelial cell migration	Apply moisture-balancing dressings	Restored epithelial cell migration, desiccation avoided	Moisture balance
	Excessive fluid causes maceration of wound margin	Compression, negative pressure or other methods of removing fluid	Edema, excessive fluid controlled, maceration avoided	
Edge of wound—nonadvancing or undermining	Nonmigration of keratinocytes Nonresponsive wound cells and abnormalities in extracellular matrix or abnormal protease activity	Reassess cause or consider corrective therapies: Debridement Skin grafts Biological agents Adjunctive therapies	Migration of keratinocytes and responsive wound cells. Restoration of appropriate protease profile	Advancing edge of wound

The TIME concept is dynamic, not linear; as the wound "gets stuck" or progresses through the phases of wound healing, different aspects of the framework will necessitate attention. For example, a necrotic wound that has been debrided and is now free of devitalized tissue but begins to drain excessively as a result of inflammation caused by biofilm formation requires attention to both the underlying critical colonization and the resulting problem with moisture balance. The TIME framework also enables clinicians to evaluate the therapeutic value of a specific intervention; for example, sharp debridement may result in establishment of a viable wound bed and also in reduced bioburden as evidenced by diminished volumes of exudate. (EWMA, 2004).

CLINICAL PEARL

The TIME framework provides guidance to the clinician in eliminating common barriers to wound healing and thus assuring a local environment that promotes repair. T = Tissue Management; I = Control of Inflammation/Infection; M = Moisture Balance; and E = Edge Advancement.

T = Tissue Management

The concept of tissue management is removal of nonviable and unhealthy tissue from the wound bed, in order to promote transition from the inflammatory phase into the proliferative phase. Types of tissue to be addressed in wound management include nonviable tissue, biofilm, hypergranulation tissue, and hypertrophic scar.

Nonviable Tissue

It is well accepted by wound care specialists that the removal of nonviable tissue such as slough, eschar, fibrin, or callus benefits wound healing. Yet the importance of thorough debridement in promotion of wound healing was not fully appreciated until landmark randomized clinical trials demonstrated higher rates of wound closure in patients with diabetic foot ulcers (Cardinal et al., 2009; Steed et al., 1996) and venous ulcers (Cardinal et al., 2009) who underwent repeated debridement to establish a clean wound bed. Frank necrotic and nonfunctional tissue is an excellent culture medium for bacterial growth and places the patient at risk for infection and even sepsis. In addition, the presence of necrotic tissue prolongs the inflammatory phase by recruiting macrophages and neutrophils, which produce inflammatory proteases and cytokines that degrade the ECM and retard wound healing (Gale et al., 2014).

Biofilm

Also, strong recent evidence suggests that the majority of chronic wounds (approximately 60%) contain bacteria embedded in an extracellular polysaccharide matrix known as a biofilm (Attinger & Wolcott, 2012; Bjarnsholt et al., 2008; Han et al., 2011; James et al., 2008; Kirketerp-Moller et al., 2008), which are not detected with normal wound culture methods (Keast et al., 2014). Biofilms are believed to be detrimental to wound healing and to degrade the ECM; sharp debridement removes the biofilm and thereby helps to control the associated inflammation and tissue damage (Keast et al., 2014; Wolcott et al., 2010). The International Wound Infection Institute (Keast et al., 2014) provides several "tips" for prevention and control of biofilms: (1) Irrigate the wound with body temperature solution at 4 to 15 psi (cold cools the wound and reduces mitotic activity), to remove surface contaminants, bacteria, exudate, and residual dressing. (2) Debride the wound of nonviable, poor-quality tissue frequently. (3) Apply an antimicrobial dressing between debridements; biofilms can reform quickly but are more vulnerable to antimicrobial agents in the 24 to 48 hours following mechanical removal. Silver and cadexomer iodine have shown bactericidal effectiveness with weakened biofilms (Aklyama et al., 2004; Rhoads et al., 2008; Wolcott et al., 2010). (4) Prevent excessive wound moisture through the use of absorptive products and manage underlying conditions that cause edema (venous insufficiency), inflammation/infection, poor compliance, and comorbidities, that is, chronic heart, renal, and/or liver failure.

CLINICAL PEARL

The first goal of topical therapy for most wounds is elimination of nonviable, inflammatory, and unhealthy tissue from the wound bed via debridement, cleansing, and appropriate use of antimicrobial agents.

Debridement moves the chronic wound to a more acute wound state by activating the healing cascade as discussed in Chapter 2; in addition, debridement reduces bioburden, the levels of inflammatory proteases and cytokines, and the numbers of senescent cells (Kirshen et al., 2006; Strohal et al., 2013). The end result is reduced risk of infection, elimination of factors that prolong the inflammatory phase, and the ability to visualize the wound base and wall. As noted before, research demonstrates that chronic wounds benefit from surgical or serial debridement to eliminate all necrotic tissue. Methods of debridement most often seen in current practice include mechanical, autolytic, chemical, biologic (maggots), sharp, hydrosurgical, and surgical. Chapter 9 provides an in-depth discussion of the principles and guidelines for debridement.

Hypergranulation

Hypergranulation is one type of inferior tissue that impedes wound healing by preventing reepithelialization. Although this is a problem commonly encountered in clinical practice, little is known about the etiology, pathology, and treatment of hypergranulation tissue; as a result, current management approaches are empiric and range from simple polyurethane foam dressings to chemical cauterization or surgical debridement. Ermer-Seltun and Netsch (2013) conducted a literature search to quantify and analyze the evidence regarding the etiology and management of hypergranulation tissue, and found 70 articles and six book chapters where this issue was discussed. Terms used to describe hypergranulation included proud flesh, exuberant granulation, hypertrophic granulation, hyperplasia of granulation, granulation hypertrophy, and overgranulation. There was limited discussion and no standardized language for description of the clinical characteristics, which are commonly reported by clinicians to include pale, boggy, edematous, friable, pedunculated, or nodular granulation tissue. All authors who addressed etiology stated that the cause of hypergranulation was unknown. Vuolu (2009) grouped the hypothesized etiologic factors into three categories: inflammatory factors (increased bioburden, foreign body such as suture, unstabilized tubes, or allergic reaction to topical treatment); occlusion and overhydration of the wound bed leading to tissue edema, excessive growth factors, and possibly a cytotoxic effect of occlusive dressings; and/or an imbalance in the molecular environment controlling repair (e.g., excessive MMPs [matrix metalloproteinases], reduced collagenase activity, or the failure of apoptosis (programmed cell death). Recommended treatment ranged from nothing to aggressive surgical excision. The most commonly reported intervention was chemical cauterization with silver nitrate, which was a point of controversy among the authors due to its caustic nature, the potential for pain if used on tissue with intact sensory fibers, absence of standardized guidelines for application, and lack of evidence regarding effectiveness. In animal studies, use of antineoplastic agents and an opioid antagonist were shown to be effective in prevention of hypergranulation tissue formation (Hardillo et al., 2001; Zagon et al., 2008); however, no human studies have been done, and these treatments are not recommended. The "wait and see approach" is also not recommended; this approach was shown to be *in*effective in management of peritubular hypergranulation and in hypergranulation related to corneal abrasions and scalp wounds. Current "best evidence" in regard to management is based on small sample sizes or case reports and includes the following: short-term use of topical steroids; application of light pressure to the hypergranulation tissue; change to a more absorptive and less occlusive dressing (with or without antimicrobial agents), such as silver alginate/hydrofiber and plain or antimicrobial foam; and collagen dressings with MMP-inhibiting properties. Interestingly, one case study reported the use of imiquimod as potentially promising for resistant hypergranulation tissue (Lain & Carrington, 2005). Use of pulse dye lasers has also shown promise; in a small case series ($n = 9$) involving scalp wounds, there was total resolution of hypergranulation with progression to reepithelialization in all subjects (Wang & Goldberg, 2007). In summary, research is needed to clearly identify the etiologic factors, clinical characteristics, and best management of hypergranulation tissue; until such research is completed and published, clinicians must use available evidence and their clinical judgment to manage this common problem (Fig. 7-3).

CLINICAL PEARL

There is a paucity of research regarding the causes and management of hypergranulation tissue; empiric approaches to management include chemical cauterization, use of absorptive and antimicrobial dressings to reduce wound bed maceration and bacterial loads, use of steroids, and debridement.

Hypertrophic Scar Tissue

Hypertrophic and keloid scar tissue represent a fourth type of inferior tissue. The last phase of wound healing, maturation or remodeling, involves degradation of the immature ECM (type 3 collagen) produced during the proliferative phase, and replacement with type 1 collagen, which provides tensile strength to the wound (see Chapter 2). A potential complication during this phase of repair is the development of hypertrophic or keloid scar tissue, which is thought to be caused by excessive synthesis of type 1 collagen and insufficient degradation of the existing ECM (type 3 collagen). One contributing factor to this imbalance in synthesis and degradation is thought to be an exaggerated and prolonged inflammatory response (Rahban & Garner, 2003; Wilgus, 2007), which results in excessive production of profibrotic cytokines such as TGFB1 and TGFB2. Hypertrophic and keloid scars appear raised, are red to pink in color, and are frequently pruritic. Hypertrophic scars are confined to the incisional site, whereas keloid scars typically extend well beyond the original borders of the wound and can be conceptualized as a progressively enlarging "collagen tumor" (Atiyeh, 2005; Slemp & Kirschner, 2006). Cosmetic and functional defects are common with keloids (Doughty & Sparks-DeFriese, 2012); they therefore require aggressive intervention and should prompt referral to plastic surgery for excision and management. Topical treatment may be at least partially effective in management of hypertrophic scarring and may be used in conjunction with other therapies after excision of keloid scars to limit recurrence; commonly used therapies include compression and silicone gel sheeting, which must be applied consistently for several months (Doughty & Sparks-DeFriese, 2012).

I = Inflammation and Infection Control

As explained in Chapter 2, the inflammatory phase of repair can be prolonged by a number of local and systemic factors: presence of nonviable tissue, high bacterial loads, impaired leukocyte function (as seen in diabetes), and other conditions resulting in reduced ability to control bacterial

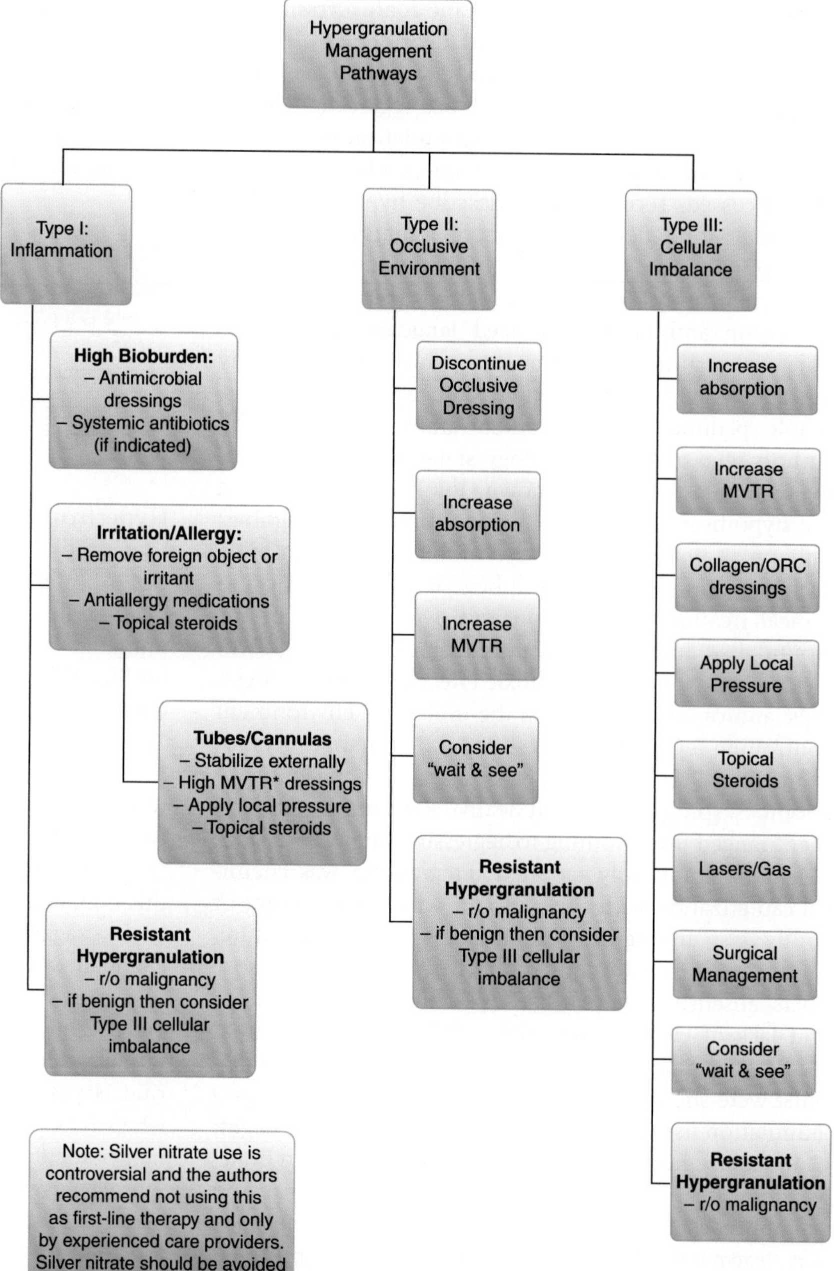

FIGURE 7-3. Possible management options for hypergranulation tissue. (Adapted with permission from Vuolo, J. (2010). Hypergranulation: Exploring possible management options. *British Journal of Nursing*, *19*(6), S4, S6–S8. British Journal of Nursing © 2010 MA Healthcare Limited. All rights reserved.)

loads (e.g., ischemia, hypoxia, anti-inflammatory medications such as steroids, and immunosuppression) (Zhao et al., 2013). Moreover, current research has identified high protease levels as the mediator for prolonged inflammation. Proteases, also known as MMPs, are enzymes that act on proteins to physically degrade them (Gibson et al., 2009); as noted throughout this text, they play an important role in normal wound healing by eliminating damaged ECM and bacteria, by promoting cell migration, and by assisting with the degradation of type 3 collagen required for normal remodeling of the ECM. MMPs are produced by host wound cells (keratinocytes, fibroblasts, and endothelial cells), and activated inflammatory cells (macrophages and neutrophils) secrete large numbers of MMPs and reactive oxygen species (ROS) into the wound bed, in order to control bacterial loads and inhibit biofilm formation (Gibson et al., 2009; Keast et al., 2014; Phillips et al., 2010). As long as there are high bacterial loads and/or biofilm present in the wound bed, the high levels of MMPs and inflammatory process will persist (Gibson et al., 2009; Keast et al., 2014). In addition, the MMPs and ROS are damaging to normal tissue, and they degrade growth factors, thus further interfering with repair (Gibson et al., 2009; Phillips et al., 2010). Interestingly, the best available biochemical marker for predicting poor wound healing is high protease levels (Cowan et al., 2014; International Consensus, 2011). There is now a point of care test designed to measure MMP levels in wound fluid; it is currently available in Europe and will soon be available in the United States (Schultz & Dowsett, 2012). This is important, because a diagnostic test will enable the clinician to promptly detect high protease levels and to intervene accordingly. Specifically, when high levels of MMPs are suspected or determined by testing, the clinician should implement collagen dressings that are designed to sequester MMPs. The collagen fibers act as "sacrificial protein substrates" since the MMPs' main function is to degrade proteins. This "sacrificial" collagen dressing thereby reduces the levels of the MMPs in the wound, thus protecting the growth factors and ECM and interrupting the cycle of inflammation (Cullen et al., 2002; Lobmann et al., 2006; Smeets et al., 2008).

CLINICAL PEARL

Management of inflammation requires management of bacterial loads, correction of wound etiologic factors, and use of dressings that reduce MMP (protease) levels.

Interestingly, regardless of the specific factors resulting in prolonged inflammation, nonhealing wounds exhibit similar biochemical traits: high levels of inflammatory cytokines and MMPs, reduced growth factor activity, and diminished quantities and response of proliferative cells (Harris et al., 1995). These traits create a hostile wound microenvironment, resulting in inflammation that can persist for months or even years if not addressed properly. In order to break the cycle, the clinician must correct wound etiology, eliminate factors contributing to persistent inflammation (nonviable tissue and high bacterial loads), and reduce MMP levels through use of MMP inhibiting dressings (as described above).

The importance of correcting wound etiology cannot be overemphasized (Harris et al., 1995); for example, studies indicate that nonhealing venous ulcers are characterized by excessive inflammation and high bacterial loads, and that the heavy bioburden disappears *without* antimicrobial interventions when the edema is eliminated with therapeutic compression and principles of moist wound healing are implemented (Harris et al., 1995; Hutchinson, 1994). In contrast, failure to correct etiologic factors results in persistent tissue damage; bacteria thrive in this environment, which results in persistent inflammation.

Wound infection (either localized or invasive) is a major cause of persistent inflammation, and infectious wound complications are addressed in detail in Chapter 10. All chronic wounds are colonized with bacterial and/or fungal organisms, and colonization does not typically result in prolonged inflammation or impaired healing. It is only when the numbers and virulence of the colonizing organisms rise to a level that interferes with repair (critical colonization) that intervention is required. Indicators of critical colonization are reflected by the mnemonic NERDS (*n*onhealing wound, increased *e*xudate, dusky *r*ed or bright red and friable tissue, *d*ebris or necrotic tissue, and odor (*s*mell) (Sibbald et al., 2006; Woo & Sibbald, 2009). The clinician should be alert to indicators of critical colonization and should intervene appropriately (e.g., with antimicrobial dressings). The clinician must closely monitor the wound to assure desired response to therapy, and must modify or discontinue the therapy when it is ineffective or no longer indicated (Sibbald et al., 2011).

CLINICAL PEARL

All wounds are colonized, but this does not interfere with healing; intervention is required only for evidence of critical colonization or invasive infection. NERDS and STONEES can be used to assess for local and invasive infection requiring treatment.

The wound clinician must also assess for indicators of invasive infection, which require prompt initiation of systemic antimicrobial therapy. The mnemonic STONEES represents the signs and symptoms of deep tissue infection: increasing *s*ize of wound, elevated *t*emperature (local or systemic), development of *o*pening that probes to underlying tissue and possibly bone, *n*ew area of breakdown, *e*rythema and *e*dema, increased levels of *e*xudate, and development of odor (*s*mell). Indicators of invasive infection require notification of the prescribing provider so that appropriate systemic antimicrobial therapy can be initiated. Ideally, a wound culture is obtained from an area of clean viable tissue prior to initiation of therapy to assure that the antimicrobial agent prescribed is effective against the infecting organism. Wound cultures must be obtained according to evidence-based protocols; see Chapter 10 for proper wound culturing techniques.

Thus, a critical aspect of effective wound management is prompt identification and treatment of wound-related infection and inflammation. Infectious complications range from surface infection (critical colonization and biofilm formation) to invasive infection (cellulitis) to osteomyelitis and even sepsis. The pathology, presentation, and management of wound-related infections is discussed in depth in Chapter 10.

M = Moisture Balance

A wound surface that is too wet or too dry is a major impediment to repair; thus a critical element of effective wound management is maintenance of a wound surface that is moist but not wet. Establishing and maintaining this "balance" can be one of the most challenging aspects of the TIME wound bed preparation model. The amount of wound exudate can change dramatically in just a few days and can negatively impact the repair process and the periwound skin by retaining bacteria and proteases at the wound surface, and by macerating the wound bed and periwound skin (Falanga, 2004). In addition, as noted earlier, excessive moisture at the wound surface may contribute to hypergranulation. Accurate assessment and description of exudate levels is therefore mandatory to appropriate dressing selection, and any sudden increase in exudate should prompt wound reassessment to identify potential causative factors (such as infection).

CLINICAL PEARL

Establishing and maintaining moisture balance is one of the most challenging aspects of chronic wound management.

Chronic wound fluid has different properties than acute wound fluid. Acute wound fluid tends to promote healing; it contains high levels of proliferative cytokines and growth factors, which promote fibroblast, endothelial cell, and keratinocyte activity. In contrast, chronic wound fluid contains high levels of inflammatory cytokines and proteolytic MMPs, which promote persistent inflammation and ECM degradation (Falanga, 2004; Gibson et al., 2009). Thus, the wound nurse is challenged to select a dressing combination that effectively absorbs the wound fluid and prevents "pooling" of exudate, while still maintaining a moist surface that promotes cell migration and wound healing (Rolstad et al., 2012). Maintaining the optimal balance between exudate management and moisture retention requires ongoing assessment and prompt response to indicators of inadequate exudate control (e.g., pooled exudate or saturated dressings) or an overly dry wound surface (e.g., adherence of dressing to the wound surface or dry wound bed).

Chapter 8 provides an in-depth discussion of types of moisture-retentive dressings and the process of dressing selection.

E = Epithelial (Edge) Advancement

As explained in Chapter 2, healing of an open wound requires filling with granulation tissue followed by resurfacing with new epithelium. A closed or compromised wound edge prevents resurfacing and is a significant impediment to repair; in contrast, an advancing wound edge of new epithelium depicts the "perfect" picture of a healing wound (Schultz & Dowsett, 2012). In order for epithelialization to occur in full-thickness wounds, there must be an open epithelial edge that permits the keratinocytes (epidermal cells) to migrate from the wound edge onto the granulating wound base. Epithelial resurfacing is a complex process that involves transformation of the cells into a migratory phenotype, breakdown of attachments to the surrounding cells and structures, and alterations in the cytoskeleton that promote migration. The ideal wound edge is attached to and flush with the wound bed, moist, and open (Fig. 7-4A). If the wound edges heal prematurely (as evidenced by a dry closed edge), epithelial migration cannot occur. It is therefore imperative for the wound specialist to assess the wound margin or edge for color, thickness and degree of attachment. The optimal epithelial rim is thin and pale pink to translucent. Wound edge abnormalities include closed edges that appear "rolled" (epibole) and may be thickened, wound edges that are unattached (as seen in undermining), and wound edges that are nonadvancing (as seen in hyperkeratotic or calloused edges). Epibole is the term commonly used to designate wound edges that have "rolled" down and under until the advancing epithelial wound edge meets the inside edge thereby halting migration (contact inhibition) (Fig. 7-4B–D). Factors thought to contribute to closed wound edges include premature keratinization, calloused edges, too little moisture in the wound bed, and an unhealthy wound bed that does not support epithelial resurfacing (e.g., absence of granulation tissue or hypergranulation tissue). Wound margins that are "unattached" are those with a space or undermining between the intact skin and the underlying wound bed; resurfacing in these wounds is delayed until the wound bed fills with granulation tissue, since keratinocytes must be able to attach to a healthy wound bed in order to migrate. The literature suggests that additional factors contributing to edge failure are those responsible for delayed healing in general: prolonged hypoxia, infection, desiccation, repetitive trauma, poor blood glucose control, and molecular imbalances such as high MMP levels (Doughty & Sparks-DeFriese, 2012; Falanga, 2004; Lansdown, 2002).

Treatment involves reestablishment of an open and proliferative wound edge. Traditionally, this has been done by chemical cauterization or surgical excision. Additional reported strategies include use of polymeric membrane dressings and foam dressings impregnated with methylene blue and crystal violet (Benskin, 2008; Hawkins-Bradley & Walden, 2002; Seeman, 2008). Wounds with significant undermining require comprehensive evidence-based management to establish and maintain a moist wound surface that supports granulation tissue until the wound edge approximates the wound bed.

CLINICAL PEARL

Treatment of closed wound edges involves reestablishment of an open and proliferative edge; anecdotal reports support use of chemical cauterization, surgical excision, and polymeric membrane or antimicrobial foam dressings.

Wounds with closed wound edges that do not respond to conservative therapies require surgical removal of the nonadvancing edge ("saucerization"); this involves removal of any callus, senescent cells, and dried exudate and establishes an open edge that promotes epithelial cell advancement (Falanga, 2004). If this does not result in

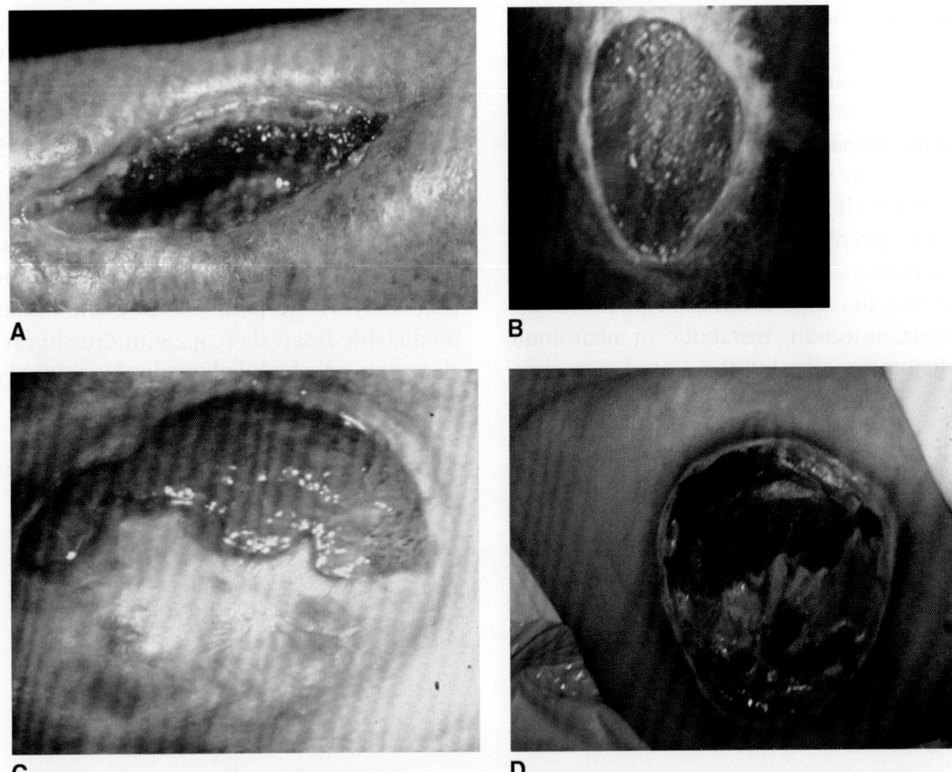

FIGURE 7-4. **A. Advancing Epithelium**: Note greater epithelial advancement from superior edge as compared to inferior edge; this is because the wound bed at the superior aspect is much healthier and more able to support cellular migration and attachment. **B. Epibole**: Wound has granulated to surface but is not epithelializing due to closed wound edges. **C. Closed vs. open wound edges**: note all epithelial resurfacing has occurred from "bottom up" because there is open wound edge at the inferior aspect of the wound while the edges at the superior aspect of the wound are closed. **D. Closed Wound Edges**: All wound edges closed and will have to be opened once the wound has granulated to surface. (From Woo, K. Y., Krasner, D. L., & Sibbald, R. G. (2014). Pain in people with chronic wounds: Clinical Strategies for decreasing pain and improving quality of life. In D. L. Krasner (Ed.), *Chronic wound care: The essentials. A clinical source book for healthcare professionals*. Malvern, PA: HMP Communications. Reprinted with permission of HMP Communications, LLC.)

epithelial resurfacing, the clinician must conduct a comprehensive reassessment of potential causative factors and should consider use of growth factors, skin substitutes, and other active therapies to stimulate epithelialization (Falanga, 2004; Schultz, 2012; Schultz and Dowsett, 2012).

Management of Wound-Related Pain

Pain is a very personal and subjective phenomenon, an unkind sensory and emotional experience that affects one's physical, psychological, and spiritual well-being and social functioning. Pain is what the person says it is and strikes whenever the person says it does (McCaffery & Pasero, 1999). The phenomenon of pain is often influenced by one's ethnicity, culture, level of support systems, past medical history, and previous pain experiences. Unmanaged or poorly managed pain can dramatically and negatively affect one's quality of life (Dallam et al., 1995; Krasner, 1997; Szor & Bourguignon, 1999; Woo, 2008; Woo et al., 2008a, 2008b). Moreover, research has linked pain to poor wound healing due to initiation of the stress response, which activates sympathetic activity and vasoconstriction; this contributes to tissue ischemia (Woo, 2008) and altered immune function/increased risk of infection (Kiecolt-Glaser et al., 1995) due to the production of cortisol and catecholamines. Any patient with a wound is at risk for acute or chronic pain of varying severity (Shukla et al., 2005). Unfortunately, pain is too often not addressed or undertreated (Hollinworth, 1995). A wise wound care clinician should always assume anyone with a wound has some level of discomfort. Gathering an accurate and thorough assessment is the first step in developing successful management strategies to reduce or eliminate pain. Chapter 3 provides a thorough discussion on systematic pain assessment; the discussion in this chapter will focus on pain prevention and management in acute and chronic wounds.

Nociceptive versus Neuropathic Pain

Wound associated pain can be nociceptive or neuropathic as well as persistent or episodic. Nociceptive pain is caused by a disruption or inflammation in tissue that stimulates somatic (skin, fascia, muscles, ligaments, joints or bones) or visceral (viscera or peritoneum) pain receptors. Nociceptive pain is considered to be a normal physiological response to a known painful stimulus. It is often described as dull, sharp, gnawing, aching, or throbbing. It can be acute, as seen in surgical or traumatic wounds, or chronic, as exhibited in long-standing venous disease or pressure ulcers. Of note, over time, persistent inflammation associated with chronic wounds may result in heightened sensitivity involving the wound itself (primary hyperalgesia) and/or the periwound tissue (secondary hyperalgesia) (WUWHS, 2004). In contrast, neuropathic pain is an abnormal physiological response that develops when pain pathways are damaged by trauma, infection, metabolic or neurologic disorders, or malignancies affecting the central or peripheral nervous system. Neuropathic pain is often described as burning, shooting, electric shock like, pins and needles, prickling, or tingling and is frequently the cause of chronic pain. Even nonnoxious stimuli such as a light touch can elicit an exaggerated painful response called allodynia.

Krasner (1995) developed a conceptual framework to describe the patient's chronic wound experience, in which she classified wound related pain as episodic (cyclic or noncyclic) or persistent (as seen in chronic wound pain) (Fig. 7-5). Acute pain that is cyclic occurs at regular or predictable intervals (e.g., with dressing removal, wound cleansing, or scheduled turning/positional changes) while

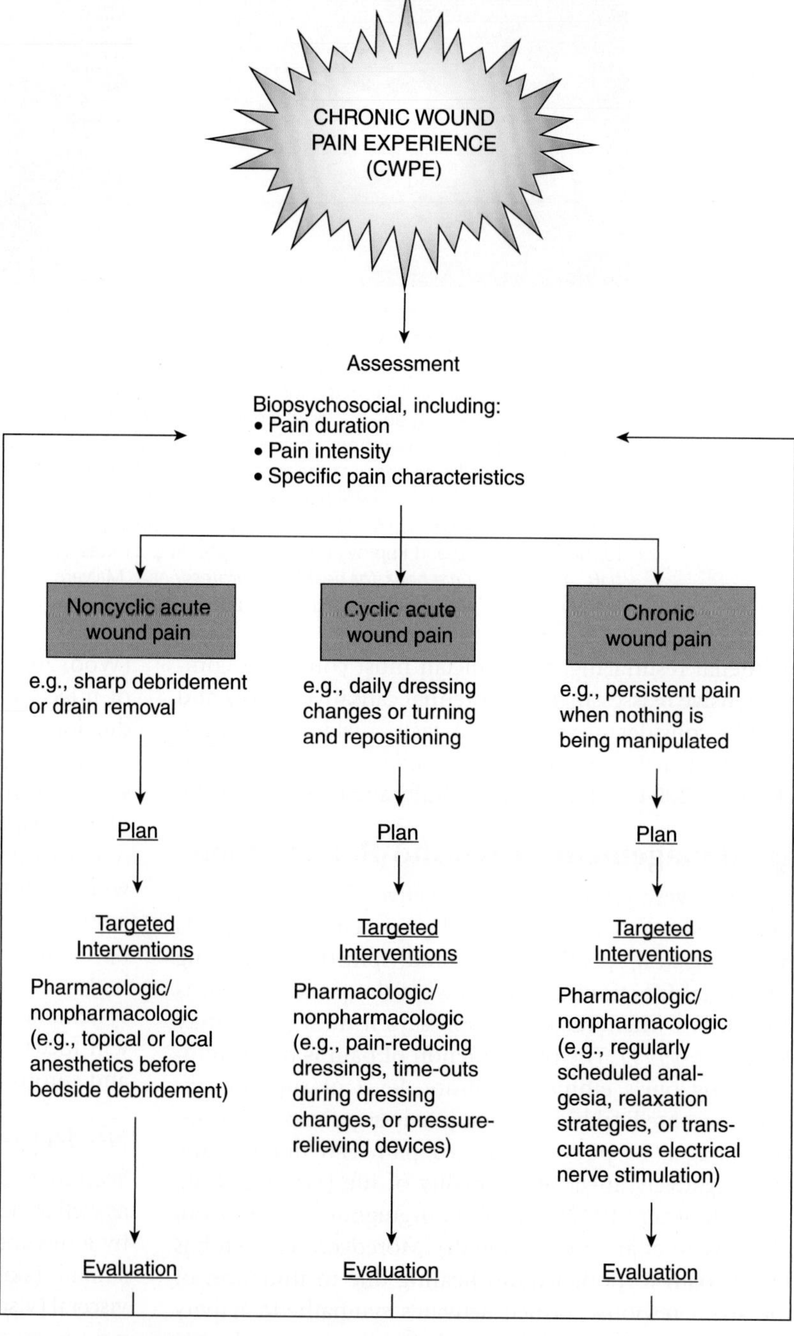

FIGURE 7-5. Chronic wound pain model. (From Woo, K. Y., Krasner, D. L., & Sibbald, R. G. (2014). Pain in people with chronic wounds: Clinical strategies for decreasing pain and improving quality of life. In D. L. Krasner (Ed.), *Chronic wound care: The essentials. A clinical source book for healthcare professionals*. Malvern, PA: HMP Communications. Reprinted with permission of HMP Communications, LLC.)

acute noncyclic pain is less predictable and associated with procedures and factors such as excisional debridement, biopsy, drain removal, coughing, dressing slippage, and/or friction. Persistent or chronic wound pain is usually related to the underlying cause of the wound (i.e., pressure, arterial insufficiency, venous congestion, neuropathy, vasculitis), aggravating factors (i.e., maceration, inflammation, edema, infection), or other pathologies (i.e., malignancy, dermatological conditions, rheumatoid arthritis). Often persistent or chronic wound pain is described as background pain. Background pain is noted at rest and is usually persistent, with potential periodic exacerbations due to care procedures or other factors. Woo and Sibbald (2008) provide an additional model of the complexity of chronic wound pain that includes causative factors, wound-related factors, and patient-centered concerns and guides the clinician in development of an individualized, strategic plan for managing chronic wound pain (Fig. 7-6).

CLINICAL PEARL

Wound-related pain is a major concern for most patients and may be either nociceptive or neuropathic and either persistent or episodic in nature.

Management Options

Wound-associated pain management must be individualized (patient-centered) and multifaceted and must address both background pain and cyclic and noncyclic triggers. The goal is to prevent pain or its exacerbation when possible, relieve or limit pain and discomfort, enhance function, and ultimately restore quality of life. A stepwise approach is necessary along with proper utilization of pharmacotherapy as mainstay therapy. Pain management begins with a comprehensive assessment that includes pain duration, intensity, and specific pain characteristics (see Chapter 3; Figs. 7-6 and 7-7).

Analgesic Medications

Pharmacological agents are selected based upon the type of pain and severity and in collaboration with the patient's primary care provider. The World Health Organization (2014) provides an analgesic three-step ladder (www.who.int/cancer/palliative/painladder/en) that was designed for management of cancer pain but is also suitable for nociceptive cyclic and chronic wound (background) pain (WUWHS, 2007; Woo et al., 2014) (see Fig. 7-7). The ladder guides the prescriber to begin with pharmacological interventions at the least benign level based upon the intensity of pain. If pain control is inadequate, then the ladder guides the clinician to add medication with greater potency alone or in

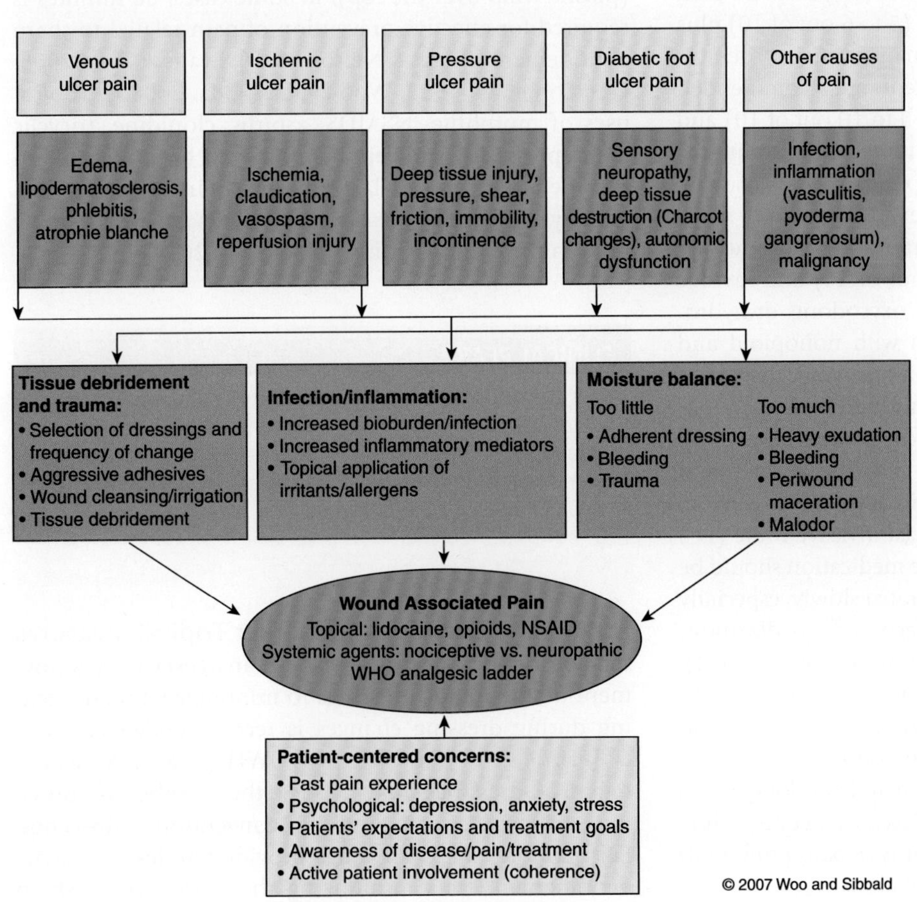

FIGURE 7-6. Wound-associated pain model. (Copyright K. Y. Woo and R. Gary Sibbald, 2007.)

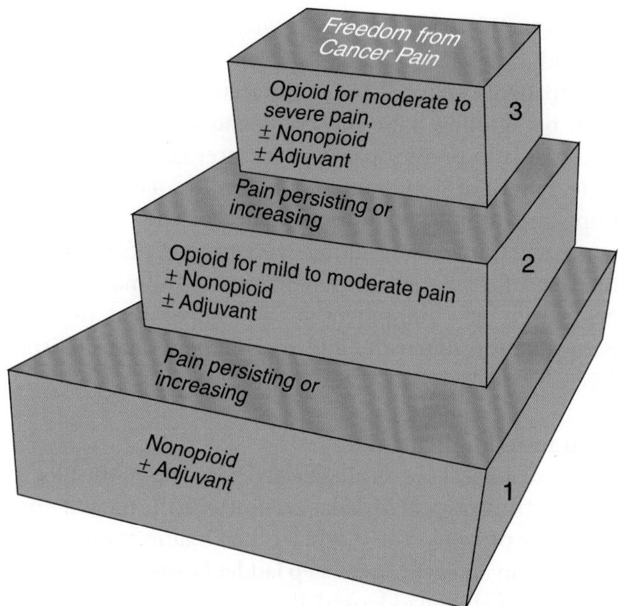

FIGURE 7-7. WHO analgesic ladder. (From World Health Organization. (1996). *Cancer pain relief: With a guide to opioid availability* (2nd ed., p. 15). Geneva, Switzerland: Author, with permission. Copyright © World Health Organization. All rights reserved.)

combination with other drugs until adequate pain control is reported. Step 1 on the ladder involves nonopioid analgesics such as acetaminophen, acetylsalicylic acid, or nonsteroidal anti-inflammatory drugs (NSAIDS) for mild pain (1 to 4 out of 10) to moderate pain (5 to 6 out of 10) plus or minus adjuvant therapy to help manage anxiety, depression, or neuropathic pain. Step 2 agents are recommended for pain that is moderate to severe (5 to 10 out of 10) and for less severe pain that is refractory to step 1 interventions; agents at this level include weak opioids such as codeine for those who have limited opioid exposure, with or without a nonopioid and adjuvant therapy. Step 3 agents are required for severe pain (8 to 10 out of 10) and involve stronger opioids such as morphine, oxycodone, or hydromorphone in possible conjunction with nonopioid and adjuvant therapy. Selection of pharmacologic agents is impacted by the patient's age, comorbidities (e.g., renal/liver status), and possible drug-to-drug interactions with concurrent medications including over-the-counter and herbal remedies, in addition to pain severity. In general, prescribers need to start with the least invasive route (i.e., oral, patches, creams). Moreover, the medication should be prescribed at the lowest dose and titrated slowly, especially in the elderly, to avoid adverse effects such as dizziness, drowsiness, delirium, nausea, or vomiting (AGS, 2012). Side effects are common with analgesics; thus, it is critical to provide ongoing monitoring and education of patients and caregivers regarding their occurrence (**Table 7-2**). Patients with chronic wound-related pain benefit from long-acting formulations with breakthrough doses as needed while those with more acute or procedural-type pain profit with regular dosing of short-acting formulations.

Adjuvant Medications

Adjuvant therapies are often utilized in combination with analgesics for neuropathic pain or for management of other symptoms such as anxiety or depression (see **Table 7-2**). Tricyclic antidepressants such as amitriptyline, nortriptyline, or doxepin are often recommended for milder neuropathic pain (burning/stinging pain) while antiepileptics such as gabapentin, pregabalin, and carbamazepine are used for more severe nerve damage (shooting/stabbing pain). Topical lidocaine patches 5% have also proven to be beneficial for neuropathic pain (Woo et al., 2014).

Topical anesthetics and dressings with nonadherent/atraumatic interfaces are crucial in managing procedural (cyclic and noncyclic nociceptive) pain. Topical analgesia is widely utilized prior to debridement but there is a paucity of evidence for its safe use. These agents come in multiple forms: jelly, cream, ointment, liquid, and patches. Lidocaine (2% to 4% jelly) is the most commonly used agent though it is considered "off label" for use on open wounds in the United States. It should be used with caution, particularly in large wounds, because systemic absorption could cause neurologic or cardiovascular adverse side effects. The agent with the strongest evidence is EMLA cream (Eutectic Mixture of Local Anesthetics consisting of lidocaine/prilocaine, AstraZeneca, Wilmington, Delaware). The EMLA cream must be in contact with the wound for a minimum of 20 minutes under occlusion (plastic wrap over the top); in some cases, 60 minutes is required for effective prevention of pain related to sharp debridement (Briggs & Nelson, 2010; Evans & Gray, 2005; Hansson et al., 1993; Woo et al., 2008a, 2008b). Topical uses of morphine, NSAIDS, aspirin, clonidine, tricyclic antidepressants, and capsaicin have all been reported in the literature, but all lack pharmacokinetic, safety and efficacy evidence; at present these agents are not routinely used in the clinical setting (Woo et al., 2014).

CLINICAL PEARL

Effective management of wound-related pain involves appropriate use of analgesic and adjuvant medications, use of nonadherent dressings and atraumatic wound care, and adjunctive nonpharmacologic therapies, including the option to call "time out" during wound care.

Atraumatic Dressings and Other Topical Measures

In addition to topical and systemic analgesia, the employment of atraumatic dressings to minimize pain and itching during dressing changes is recommended (NPUAP & EPUAP, 2014; Paul, 2013; WUWHS, 2007). Moisture-retentive dressings may reduce the number of dressing changes as compared to conventional dressings. Furthermore, these dressings provide painless, autolytic debridement, thus minimizing the frequency of sharp

TABLE 7-2 Analgesics: Mode of Action, Dosage, and Side Effects

Medication	Mode of Action	Dosage	Side Effects
Nonopioid			
Acetaminophen	Affects nitric oxide cycle, antipyretic property	325–650 mg q4h up to a maximum of 4 g/d in healthy people	Do not exceed 4 g/d to avoid liver toxicity
Acetylsalicylic acid (ASA)	Inhibits the enzyme cyclooxygenase (COX)	325–650 mg q4–6h up to 4 g/d	Gastritis, gastrointestinal bleeding; acute renal failure; may interact with anticoagulants
NSAIDs and COX-2 selective NSAIDs	Inhibit COX	Common NSAIDs: *Ibuprofen 200–400 mg q4–bh* *Ketoprofen 25–50 mg q6–8h* *Naproxen 250 mg q6h* Common COX-2 NSAIDs: *Celecoxib 200–400 mg od* *Rofecoxib 25–50 mg od* *Meloxicam 7.5–15 mg od*	Similar as ASA, fewer side effects with COX-2 NSAIDs
Coanalgesic (Adjuvant)			
Tricyclic antidepressant (TCA)	Inhibit serotonin and NE reuptake; block sodium channels	Common TCAs: *Amitriptyline, doxepin, nortriptyline 10–25 mg q hs titrate up to 150–200 mg/d*	Dry mouth; drowsiness; orthostatic hypotension
Anticonvulsants	Most agents block sodium channels; unknown for gabapentin	Common anticonvulsants: *Carbamazepine 100 mg od to maximum dose 1,200 mg/d, gabapentin 100 mg TID titrate up to 3,000 mg/d*	Drowsiness; dizziness; fatigue
Opioids (CR/SR)			
Morphine	Gold standard mu agonist	For patients who are opioid naive, start on morphine 2.5–10 mg po q4h with 10% of total daily dose (TDD) q1h as needed	
Codeine	Weak mu agonist; 0.125 as potent as morphine; convert to active analgesic by enzyme CYP2D6	Codeine 100 mg = morphine 10 mg ~10:1)	
Oxycodone (may be combined with ASA or acetaminophen)	Mu and kappa agonist; 2× as potent as morphine	Oxycodone 5 mg or Percocet 1 tab (5/325) = morphine 10 mg (1:2)	Constipation; delirium; sedation; nausea; vomiting; urinary retention
Hydromorphone	5–7.5× as potent as morphine	Hydromorphone 2 mg = morphine 10 mg (1:5)	
Methadone	Mu and delta agonist; blocks NMDA; 10x more potent than morphine	Variable	

Legend: h, hour; d, day; q, every; od, daily; hs, evening; TID, three times a day; NSAID, nonsteroidal anti-inflammatory drug; NE, norepinephrine; po, by mouth.

debridement. Low-adhesive or nonadhesive dressings (e.g., silicone or gel adhesive dressings) do not adhere to moist wound beds and therefore significantly reduce pain related to dressing removal (Woo et al., 2008a; WUWHS, 2007). For wounds with moderate to large amounts of exudate, hydrofibers and alginates minimize trauma and dressing frequency as compared to gauze type dressings (dry, wet to dry, or wet to damp), which adhere to the wound base, disrupt granulation tissue, and require frequent dressing changes, all of which promote pain. In contrast, wounds that are dry/desiccated benefit from hydrogels or other moisture-retentive dressing to minimize dressing adherence. The application of antimicrobial dressings may also help to reduce pain, due to reduction in bacterial loads and inflammation (WUWHS, 2007).

Protection of the periwound skin should be a routine consideration in topical therapy; liquid film barriers and moisture barrier ointments can be used to protect the skin from maceration and tape stripping. In addition, it is important to assure that selected dressings provide effective exudate management and that drainage is not allowed to pool on the skin (Woo et al., 2014; WUWHS, 2007). Gentle cleansing with use of noncytotoxic agents such as saline or water is recommended as opposed to abrasive techniques or harsh cleansers (Woo et al., 2014; WUWHS, 2007).

Adjunctive Therapies

Other patient-oriented nonpharmacologic approaches such as diversional activities (relaxation, touch, slow rhythmic breathing, imagery, aromatherapy, music, hypnosis, stress reduction and relaxation activities) can be used to reduce wound-related pain; in addition, the individual should be given the option to call a "time out" during wound related procedures (WUWHS, 2007). Patient education regarding wound care, dressings, and pain management is also essential for reduction of anxiety (which increases pain), adherence to "wound-friendly" care (moist as opposed to dry wound care), and appropriate use of analgesics. Specifically, patients must be assured that the prescribed analgesics will not lead to addiction, and should be educated regarding prevention and management of side effects related to analgesics, as well as the negative effects of pain on wound healing. Building rapport through active listening and mutual respect as well as an invitation to participate in their wound care decisions (timing of dressing changes, removing the dressing themselves, choice of diversional activities, etc.) are effective patient empowerment methods.

In summary, pain is a complex, subjective, biopsychosocial experience that greatly impacts the quality of life in patients with wounds. It is vital for wound care clinicians to collaborate with the primary care provider or pain specialist to properly assess and manage cyclic, noncyclic, and persistent pain in order to promote wound healing and improved quality of life.

Clinical Application

The World Union of Wound Healing Society (2004) has developed and updated (2007) a consensus document that outlines evidence-informed practice recommendations on the assessment and management of wound-related pain at dressing procedures. Key points are as follows (WUWHS, 2007):

- Identify and treat the cause of the chronic wound and address concerns expressed by the patient, including a pain assessment at each visit.
- Evaluate and document pain intensity and characteristics on a regular basis (before, during, and after dressing-related procedures).
- Cleanse the wound gently; avoid the use of abrasive wipes and cold solutions.
- Select an appropriate method of wound debridement, and include the potential for causing wound-related pain.
- Choose dressings that minimize trauma and pain during application and removal.
- Treat infections that may cause wound-related pain and inhibit healing.
- Treat local factors that may induce wound-related pain (e.g., inflammation, trauma, pressure, maceration).
- Select an appropriate dressing to minimize wound-related pain based on wear time, moisture balance, healing potential, and periwound maceration.
- Evaluate each patient's need for pharmacological (topical/systemic agents) and nonpharmacological strategies to minimize wound-related pain.
- Involve and empower patients to optimize pain management.
- Health care providers should ensure wound-related pain control for every patient.

Conclusion

In summary, effective wound management begins with identification of wound-related goals; when the goal is comfort or maintenance, the focus in topical therapy is symptom management and complication prevention. When the goal is healing, management must involve correction of etiologic and contributing factors, systemic support for healing, and evidence-based topical therapy. Evidence-based topical therapy should adhere to the concepts outlined in the TIME framework for wound management: removal of nonviable and unhealthy tissue; control of bacterial loads to prevent infection and persistent inflammation; management of moisture to assure a wound surface that is moist but not wet; and measures to maintain an open and advancing wound edge. For all patients with wounds, effective pain management is a critical aspect of management and involves appropriate use of both pharmacologic and nonpharmacologic interventions.

Acknowledgments

The chapter authors would like to acknowledge Laura Bolton, PhD, for helping us translate the compelling clinical evidence summarized in this chapter into practical information that can help inform wound care decisions and improve outcomes for the patients we all serve.

REFERENCES

Alvarez, O. M., Mertz, P. M., & Eaglstein, W. H. (1983). The effect of occlusive dressings on collagen synthesis and re-epithelialization in superficial wounds. *Journal of Surgical Research, 35*, 142–148.

Atiyeh, B. S., Costaglila, M., & Haye, K. S. (2005). Keloid or hypertrophic scar: The controversy. *Annals of Plastic Surgery, 54*(6), 676–680.

American Geriatrics Society (AGS) Panel. (2012). AGS Panel on the Pharmacological management of persistent pain in older persons. *Journal of the American Geriatrics Society, 57*, 1331–1346.

Attinger, C., & Wolcott, R. (2012). Clinically addressing biofilm in chronic wounds. *Advances in Wound Care (New Rochelle), 1*(13), 127–132.

Aklyama, H., Oono, T., Saito, M., et al. (2004). Assessment of cadexomer iodine against *Staphylococcus aureus* biofilm in vivo and in vitro using confocal laser scanning microscopy. *Journal of Dermatology, 31*(7), 529–534.

Benskin, L. (2008). Solving the closed wound edge problem in venous ulcers using polymeric membrane dressings. Scientific and Clinical Abstracts from the 40th Annual Wound, Ostomy and Continence Nurses Annual Conference: Orlando, Florida: June 21–25, 2008: Practice Innovation Abstracts: Wound-Product Selection and Innovations. *Journal of Wound, Ostomy, and Continence Nursing, 35*(3), S30–S31.

Bishop, W. J. (1959). *A history of surgical dressings*. Chesterfield, UK: Robinsons & Sons.

Bjarnsholt, T., Kirketerp-Moller, K., Jensen, P. O., et al. (2008). Why chronic wounds will not heal: A novel hypothesis. *Wound Repair and Regeneration, 16*(1), 2–10.

Bolton, L. (2004). Moist wound healing from past to present. In D. T. Rovee & H. I. Maibach (Eds.), *The epidermis in wound healing. Dermatology: Clinical and Basic Sciences Series* (pp. 89–100). Boca Raton, FL: CRC Press.

Bolton, L. L. (2007). Evidence-based report card: Operational definition of moist wound healing. *Journal of Wound, Ostomy, and Continence Nursing, 34*(1), 23–29.

Bolton, L., McNees, P., van Rijswijk, L., et al.; Wound Outcomes Study Group. (2004). Wound-healing outcomes using standardized assessment and care in clinical practice. *Journal of Wound, Ostomy, and Continence Nursing, 31*(2), 65–71.

Bolton, L., & van Rijswijk, L. (1991). Wound dressings: Meeting clinical and biological needs. *Dermatology Nursing, 3*, 146–161.

Bolton, L. L., & van Rijswijk, L. (1990). Wound dressings: Meeting clinical and biological needs. *Dermatology Nursing, 2*(3), 146–161.

Bolton, L., van Rijswijk, L., & Shaffer, F. (1996). Quality wound care equals cost effective wound care: A clinical model. *Nursing Management, 27*(7), 30, 320–337.

Bowler, P. G., Delargy, H., Prince, D., et al. (1993). The viral barrier properties of some occlusive dressings and their role in infection control. *Wounds, 5*(1), 1-8.

Briggs, M., & Nelson, E. A. (2010). Topical agents or dressings for pain in venous leg ulcers. *Cochrane Database of Systematic Reviews* (4), DC001177.

Brolmann, F. E., Eskes, A. M., Goslings, J. C., et al. (2013). TREMBRANDT study group. Randomized clinical trial of donor-site wound dressings after split-skin grafting. *British Journal of Surgery, 100*(5), 619–627.

Cardinal, M., Eisenbud, D. E., Armstrong, D. G., et al. (2009). Serial surgical debridement: A retrospective study on clinical outcomes in chronic lower extremity wounds. *Wound Repair Regeneration, 17*(3), 306–311.

Cherry, G., & Ryan, T. J. (1985). Enhanced wound angiogenesis with a new hydrocolloid dressing. In T. J. Ryan (Ed.), *An environment for healing. The role of occlusion*. Royal Society of Medicine International Congress and Symposium Series No. 88. (pp. 61–68). London, UK: Royal Society of Medicine.

Colwell, J., Foreman, M. D., & Trotter, J. P. (1993). A comparison of the efficacy and cost-effectiveness of two methods of managing pressure ulcers. *Decubitus, 6*(4), 28–36.

Cowan, L., Stechmiller, J., Phillips, P., et al. (2014). Science of wound healing: Translation of bench science into advances for chronic wound care. In D. Krasner (Ed.), *Chronic wound care: The essentials*. Malvern, PA: HMP Communications.

Cullen, B., Watt, P., Lundqvist, C., et al. (2002). The role of oxidized regenerated cellulose/collagen in chronic wound repair and its potential mechanism of action. *International Journal of Biochemistry and Cell Biology, 34*(12), 1544–1556.

Dallam, L., Smyth, C., Jackson, B., et al. (1995). Pressure ulcer pain: Assessment and quantification. *Journal of Wound Ostomy Continence Nursing, 22*(5), 211–218.

De Coninck, A., Draye, J. P., Van Strubarq, A., et al. (1996). Healing of full-thickness wounds in pigs: Effects of occlusive and non-occlusive dressings associated with gel vehicle. *Journal of Dermatological Science, 13*(3), 202–211.

Doughty, D. B., & Sparks-DeFriese, B. (2012). Wound healing physiology. In R. A. Bryant & D. P. Nix (Eds.), *Acute and chronic wounds: Current management concepts* (4th ed., pp. 71–81). St. Louis, MO: Mosby.

Dyson, M., Young, S. R., Hart, J., et al. (1992). Comparison of the effects of moist and dry conditions on the process of angiogenesis during dermal repair. *Journal of Investigative Dermatology, 99*, 729.

Emmons, K. R., & Lachman, V. D. (2010). Palliative wound care: A concept analysis. *Journal of Wound Ostomy Continence Nursing, 37*(6), 639–646.

Ermer-Seltun, J., & Netsch, D. (2013). Hypergranulation tissue management: Is it evidence based? Poster presentation presented at the Symposium of Advance Wound Care, Denver, Co.

European Wound Management Association (EWMA). (2004). *Position Document: Wound Bed Preparation in Practice*. London, UK: Medical Education Partnership Ltd.

Evans, E., & Gray, M. (2005). Do topical analgesics reduce pain associated with wound dressing changes or debridement of chronic wounds? *Journal of Wound, Ostomy, and Continence Nursing, 32*(5), 287–290.

Falanga, V. (2004). The chronic wound: Impaired healing and solutions in the context of wound bed preparation. *Blood Cells Molecules & Diseases, 32*(1), 88–94.

Field, F. K., & Kerstei, M. D. (1994). Overview of wound healing in a moist environment. *American Journal of Surgery, 167*, 2S.

Fife, C. E., Wall, V., Carter, M., et al. (2012). Examining the relationship between physician and facility level-of-service coding in outpatient wound centers: Results of a multicenter study. *Ostomy Wound Management, 58*(3), 20–22, 24, 26–28.

Flattau, A., Thompson, M., & Meara, A. (2013). Developing and integrating a practice model for health finance reform into wound healing programs: An examination of the triple aim approach. *Ostomy Wound Management, 59*(10), 42–51.

Gale, S. S., Lurie, F., Treadwell, T., et al. (2014). DOMINATE wounds. *Journal of Wound, 26*(1), 1–12.

Gibson, D., Cullen, B., Legerstee, R., et al. (2009). MMPs made easy. *Wounds International, 1*(1). Retrieved from http://www.woundsinternational.com

Gilje, O. (1948). On taping (adhesive tape treatment) of leg ulcers. *Acta Dermato-Venereologica, 28*(5), 454–467.

Golinko, M. S., Clark, S., Rennert, R., et al. (2009). Wound emergencies: The importance of assessment, documentation, and early treatment using a wound electronic medical record. *Ostomy/Wound Manage, 55*(5), 54–61.

Han, A., Zenilman, J. M., Melendez, J. H., et al. (2011). The importance of a multifaceted approach to characterizing the microbial flora of chronic wounds. *Wound Repair and Regeneration, 19*(5), 532–541.

Hansson, C., et al. (1993). Repeated treatment with lidocaine/prilocaine cream (EMLA) as a topical anesthetic for the cleansing of venous leg ulcers. A controlled study. *Acta Dermato-Venereologica, 73*(3), 231–233.

Hardillo, J., Van Clooster, C., & Delaere, P. (2001). An investigation of airway wound healing using a novel in vivo model. *Laryngoscope, 111*(7), 1174–1182.

Harris, I., Yee, K., Walters, C., et al. (1995). Cytokine and protease levels in healing and non-healing chronic venous leg ulcers. *Experimental Dermatology, 4*(6), 342–349.

Hawkins-Bradley, B., & Walden, M. (2002). Treatment of a nonhealing wound with hypergranulation tissue and rolled edges. *Journal of Wound, Ostomy, and Continence Nursing, 29*(6), 320–324.

Hefton, J., & Staiano-Coico, L. (1989). Comparison of an occlusive and a semi-occlusive dressing and the effect of the wound exudate upon keratinocyte proliferation. *Journal of Trauma, 29*, 924–930.

Hein, N. T., Prawer, S. E., & Katz, H. I. (1998). Facilitated wound healing using transparent film dressing following Mohs micrographic surgery. *Archives of Dermatology, 124*, 903–906.

Hinman, C. D., & Maibach, H. (1963). Effect of air exposure and occlusion on experimental human skin wounds. *Nature, 200*, 377–379.

Hollinworth, H. (1995). Nurses' assessment and management of pain at wound dressing changes. *Journal of Wound Care, 4*(2), 77–83.

Hopf, H. W., et al. (2006). Guidelines for the treatment of arterial insufficiency ulcers. *Wound Repair and Regeneration, 14*(6), 693–710.

Hutchinson, J. J. (1994). A prospective clinical trial of wound dressings to investigate the rate of infection under occlusion. In *Proceedings, advances in wound management* (pp. 93–96). London, UK: Macmillan.

Hutchinson, J. J., & McGuckin, M. (1990). Occlusive dressings: A microbiologic and clinical review. *American Journal of Infectious Control, 18*(4), 257–268.

Institute of Medicine. (2008). Developing trusted clinical practice guidelines. In Selected findings from knowing what works in health care: A roadmap for the nation (pp. 1–6). Washington, DC: Academic Press.

International Consensus. (2011). *The role of proteases in wound diagnostics. An expert working group review*. London, UK: Wounds International.

James, G. A, Swogger, E., Wolcott, R., et al. (2008). Biofilms in chronic wounds. *Wound Repair and Regeneration, 16*(1), 37–44.

Jones, K. R., & Fennie, K. (2007). Factors influencing pressure ulcer healing in adults over 50: An exploratory study. *Journal of the American Medical Directors Association, 8*(6), 378–387.

Jones, A. M., & San Miguel, L. (2006). Are modern wound dressings a clinical and cost-effective alternative to the use of gauze? *Journal of Wound Care, 15*, 65–69.

Junker, J. P. E., Kamel, R. A., Caterson, E. J., et al. (2013). Clinical impact upon wound healing and inflammation in moist, wet, and dry environments. *Advances in Wound Care, 2*(7), 348–356.

Keast, D., Swanson, T., & Carville, K. (2014). Ten top tips: Understanding and managing wound biofilm. *Wounds International, 5*(2), 20–24.

Kerstein, M. D., Gemmen, E., van Rijswijk, L., et al. (2001). Cost and cost effectiveness of venous and pressure ulcer protocols of care. *Disease Management and Health Outcomes, 9*(11), 651–663.

Kiecolt-Glaser, J. K., Marucha, P. T., Malarkey, W. B., et al. (1995). Slowing of wound healing by psychological stress. *Lancet, 346* (8984), 1194–1196.

Kirketerp-Moller, K., et al. (2008). Distribution, organization, and ecology of bacteria in chronic wounds. *Journal of Clinical of Microbiology, 46*(8), 2712–2722.

Kirshen, C., Woo, K., Ayello E. A., et al. (2006). Debridement: A vital component of wound bed preparation. *Advances in Skin and Wound Care, 19*(9), 506–517.

Krasner, D. (1995). The chronic wound pain experience: A conceptual model. *Ostomy Wound Management, 41*(3), 20–25.

Krasner, D. (1997). *Carrying on despite the pain: Living with painful venous ulcers. A Heideggerian hermeneutic analysis [dissertation]*. Ann Arbor, MI: UMI.

Lain, E. L., & Carrington, P. R. (2005). Imiquimod treatment of exuberant granulation tissue in a nonhealing diabetic ulcer. *Archives of Dermatology, 141*(11), 1368–1370.

Lansdown A. B. G. (2002). Calcium: A potential central regulator in wound healing in the skin. *Wound Repair and Regeneration, 10*, 271.

Letizia, M., Uebelhor, J., & Paddack, E. (2010). Providing palliative care to seriously ill patients with nonhealing wounds. *Journal of Wound Ostomy Continence Nursing, 37*(3), 277–282.

Lobmann, R., Zemlin, C., Motzkau, M., et al. (2006). Expression of matrix metalloproteinases and growth factors in diabetic foot wounds treated with protease absorbent dressing. *Journal of Diabetes and its Complications, 20*(5), 329–335.

Manjo, G. (1975). *The healing hand: Man and wound in the ancient world*. Cambridge, MA: Harvard University Press.

McCaffery, M., & Pasero, C. (1999). How can we improve the way we perform our pain assessments to meet the needs of patients from diverse cultures? *American Journal of Nursing, 99*(8), 18.

Michie, D. D., & Hugill, J. V. (1994). Influence of occlusive and impregnated gauze dressings on incisional healing: A prospective, randomized, controlled study. *Annals of Plastic Surgery, 32*, 57–64.

Nemeth, A. J., Eaglstein, W. H., Taylor, J. R., et al. (1991). Faster healing and less pain in skin biopsy sites treated with an occlusive dressing. *Archives of Dermatology, 127*, 1679–1683.

Nix, D. P., & Peirce, B. (2012). Noncompliance, nonadherence or barriers to a sustainable plan? In R.A. Bryant & D.P. Nix (Eds.), *Acute and chronic wounds: Current management concepts* (4th ed., pp. 408–414). St. Louis, MO: Mosby.

NPUAP and EPUAP. (2014). *Prevention and treatment of pressure ulcers: Clinical Practice Guidelines*. Washington, DC: NPAUP.

Odland, G. (1958). The fine structure of the interrelationship of cells in human epidermis. *Journal of Biophysical and Biochemical Cytology, 4*, 529–535.

Ovington, L. (2007). Advances in wound dressings. *Clinics in Dermatology, 25*, 33–38.

O'Donnell, T. F., Jr., & Balk, E. M. (2011). The need for an Intersociety Consensus Guideline for venous ulcer. *Journal of Vascular Surgery, 54*(6 Suppl), 83S–90S.

Ovington, L. (2002). Hanging wet to-dry dressings out to dry. *Journal of Prevention and Healing, 15*(2), 79–84.

Ovington, L., & Eisenbud, D. (2004). Dressings and cleansing agents. In M. Morison, L. Ovington& K. Wilkie (Eds.), *Chronic wound care: A problem-based learning approach*. London, UK: Elsevier.

Paul, J. (2013). A cross-sectional study of chronic wound related pain and itching. *Ostomy Wound Manage, 59*(7), 28–34.

Phillips, P. L., Wolcott, R. D., Fletcher, J., et al. (2010). Biofilms made easy. *Wounds International, 1*(3). Retrieved from http://www.woundsinternational.com

Pirone, L., Monte, K., Shannon, R., et al. (1990). Wound healing under occlusion and non-occlusion in partial-thickness and full-thickness wounds in swine, *Wounds, 2*, 74–81.

Rahban, S. R., & Garner, W. L. (2003). Fibroproliferative scars. *Clinics in Plastic Surgery, 30*(1), 77–89.

Rhoads, D. D., Wolcott, R. D., & Percival, S. L. (2008). Biofilms in wounds: Management strategies. *Journal of Wound Care, 17*(11), 502–508.

Rogers, M. (2000). Treatment of 'angiomas': a modern commentary. *Australasian Journal of Dermatology, 41*(Suppl), S89–S91.

Rolstad, B., Bryant, R., & Nix, D. (2012). Topical management. In R. A. Bryant & D. P. Nix (Eds.), *Acute and chronic wounds: Current management concepts* (4th ed., pp. 289–305). St. Louis, MO: Mosby.

Romanelli, M., Vowden, K., & Weir, D. (2010). Exudate management made easy. *Wounds International, 1*(2), 1–6.

Sackett, D. L., Strauss, S. E., Richardson, W. S., et al. (2000). Evidence-based medicine: How to practice and teach. *Evidence based medicine* (2nd ed.). Edinburgh, NY: Churchill Livingstone.

Schultz, G. (2012). Molecular and cellular regulators. In R. A. Bryant & D. P. Nix (Eds.), *Acute and chronic wounds: Current management concepts* (4th ed., pp. 324–336). St. Louis, MO: Mosby.

Schultz, G., & Dowsett, C. (2012). Wound bed preparation revisited. *Wounds International, 3*(1), 25–29. Retrieved from http://www.woundsinternational.com/practice-development/wound-bed-preparation-revisited/page-2&print

Schultz, G. S., Sibblad, R. G., Falanga, V., et al. (2003). Wound bed preparation: A systematic approach to wound management. *Wound Repair and Regeneration, 11*(Suppl 1), S1–S28.

Semann, P. (2008). Stalled surgical wound closed quickly when switched to polymetric membrane dressing. *Journal of Wound, Ostomy, and Continence Nursing, 35*(3), S22–S23.

Shukla, D., Tripathi, A. K., Agrawal, S., et al. (2005). Pain in acute and chronic wounds: a descriptive study. *Ostomy Wound Manage, 51*(11), 47–51.

Sibbald, R. G., Goodman, L., Woo, K. Y., et al. (2011). Special considerations in wound bed preparation 2011: An update. *Advances in Skin and Wound Care, 24*(9), 415–418.

Sibbald, R. G., Woo, K. Y., & Ayello, E. (2006). Increased bacterial burden and infection: the story of NERDS and STONEES. *Advances in Skin and Wound Care, 19*(8), 447–463.

Singh, A., Halder, S., Menon, G. R., et al. (2004). Meta-analysis of randomized controlled trials on hydrocolloid occlusive dressing versus conventional gauze dressing in the healing of chronic wounds. *Asian Journal of Surgery, 27*, 326.

Slemp, A., & Kirschner, R. (2006). Keloids and scars: A review of keloids and scars, their pathogenesis, risk factors, and management. *Current Opinion in Pediatrics, 18*(4), 396–402.

Smeets, R., Ulrich, D., Unglaub, F., et al. (2008). Effect of oxidized regenerated cellulose/collagen matrix on proteases in wound exudate of patients with chronic venous ulceration. *International Wound Journal, 5*(2), 195–203.

Steed, D. L., Donohoe, D., & Webster, M. W., et al.; Diabetic Ulcer Study Group. (1996). Effect of extensive debridement and treatment on the healing of diabetic foot ulcers. *Journal of American College of Surgeons, 183*(1), 61–64.

Strohal, R., Apelqvist, J., Dissemond, J., et al. (2013). EWMA document: Debridement. *Journal of Wound Care, 22*(Suppl 1), S1–S52.

Szor, J., & Bourguignon, C. (1999). Description of pressure ulcer pain at rest and during dressing change. *Journal of Wound Ostomy Continence Nursing, 26*(3), 115–120.

Treadwell, T., & Keast, D. H. (2010). Site assessments: Early steps on the journey toward outcomes. *Wounds, 22*, 71–77.

Tur, E., & Bolton, L. (2014). Skin healing, integrating scientific advances into cosmetic practice. In A. O. Barel, M. Paye & H. I. Maibach (Eds.), *H: Handbook of cosmetic science and technology* (4th ed., p. 148). Boca Raton, FL: CRC Press.

Ubbink, D. T., Vermeulen, H., Goossens, A., et al. (2008). Occlusive vs gauze dressings for local wound care in surgical patients: A randomized clinical trial. *Archives of Surgery, 143*(10), 950–955.

Van Rijswijk, L. (2004). Bridging the gap between research and practice. *American Journal of Nursing, 104*(2), 28–30.

Varghese, M., Balin, A. K., Carter, D. M., et al. (1986). Local environment of chronic wounds under synthetic dressings, *Archives of Dermatology, 122*, 52–57.

Vloemans, A. F., Hermans, M. H., van der Wal, M. B., et al. (2014). Optimal treatment of partial thickness burns in children: A systematic review. *Burns, 40*(2), 177–190.

Vuolu, J. (2010). Hypergranulation: Exploring possible management options. *British Journal of Nursing, 19*(6), S4, S6–S8.

Wang, S. Q., & Goldberg, L. H. (2007). Pulsed dye laser for the treatment of hypergranulation tissue with chronic ulcer in postsurgical defects. *Journal of Drugs in Dermatology, 6*(12), 1191–1194.

Whitney, J., Phillips, L., Aslam, R., et al. (2006). Guidelines for the treatment of pressure ulcers. *Wound Repair and Regeneration, 14*(6), 663–679.

Wiechula, R. (2003). The use of moist wound-healing dressings in the management of split-thickness skin graft donor sites: A systematic review. *International Journal of Nursing Practice, 9*, S9–S17.

Wilgus, T. A. (2007). Regenerative healing in fetal skin: A review of the literature. *Ostomy Wound Management, 53*(6), 16–33.

Winter, G. D. (1962). Formation of the scab and the rate of epithelialization of superficial wounds in the skin of the young domestic pig. *Nature, 193*, 293–294.

Wolcott, R. D., Rumbaugh, K. P., James, G. M., et al. (2010). Biofilm maturity studies indicate sharp debridement opens a time-dependent therapeutic window. *Journal of Wound Care, 19*(8), 320–328.

Woo, K. Y. (2008). Meeting the challenges of wound-associated pain: Anticipatory pain, anxiety, stress, and wound healing. *Ostomy Wound Management, 54*(9), 10–12.

Woo, K. Y., Harding, K., Price, P., et al. (2008a). Minimizing wound-related pain at dressing change: Evidence-informed practice. *International Wound Journal, 5*(2), 144–157.

Woo, K. Y., Krasner, D. L., & Sibbald, R. G. (2014). Pain in people with chronic wounds: Clinical strategies for decreasing pain and improving quality of life. In D. L. Krasner (Ed.), *Chronic wound care: The essentials. A clinical source book for healthcare professionals* (pp. 111–122). Malvern, PA: HMP Communications.

Woo, K. Y., & Sibbald, R. G. (2008). Chronic wound pain: A conceptual model. *Advances in Skin and Wound Care, 21*(4), 175–190.

Woo, K. Y., & Sibbald, R. G. (2009). A cross-sectional validation study of using NERDS and STONEES to assess bacterial burden. *Ostomy Wound Management, 55*(8), 40–48.

Woo, K. Y., Sibbald, R. G., Fogh, K., et al. (2008b). Assessment and management of persistent (chronic) and total wound pain. *International Wound Journal, 5*(2), 205–215.

World Health Organization. (2014). WHO's pain ladder. Available at: http://www.who.int/cancer/palliative/painladder/en/. Accessed October 25, 2014.

World Union of Wound Healing Societies (WUWHS). (2004). *Principles of best practice: Minimizing pain at wound dressing-related procedures. A consensus document.* London, UK: MEP, Ltd.

World Union of Wound Healing Societies (WUWHS). (2007). *Principles of best practice: Minimizing pain at wound dressing-related procedures. A consensus document.* Toronto, ON: WoundPedia, Inc.

WOCN. (2010). *Guidelines for the prevention and management of pressure ulcers, WOCN clinical practice guideline series #2.* Mount Laurel, NJ.

WOCN. (2011). *Guideline for management of wounds in patients with lower extremity venous disease (LEVD), WOCN clinical practice guideline series #4.* Mount Laurel, NJ.

WOCN. (2012). *Guidelines for management of wounds in patients with lower extremity neuropathic disease (LEND), WOCN clinical practice guideline series #3.* Mount Laurel, NJ.

WOCN. (2014). *Guideline for management of patients with lower extremity arterial disease (LEAD), WOCN clinical practice guideline series #1.* Mount Laurel, NJ.

Xakellis, G., & Chrischilles, E. A. (1992). Hydrocolloid versus saline-gauze dressings in treating pressure ulcers: A cost effective analysis. *Archives of Physical and Medicine Rehabilitation, 73*, 463-469.

Zagon, I. S., Klocek, M. S., Griffith, J. W., et al. (2008). Prevention of exuberant granulation tissue and neovascularization in rat cornea by naltrexone. *Archives of Ophthalmology, 126*(4), 501–506.

Zhao, G., Usui, M. L., Lippman, S. I., et al. (2013). Biofilms and inflammation in chronic wounds. *Advances in Wound Care (New Rochelle), 2*(7), 389–399.

QUESTIONS

1. A wound care nurse is caring for a patient with a wound classified as "healable." What is the focus of treatment for this type of wound?
- A. Proper wound bed preparation
- B. Consistent use of debridement
- C. Wound stabilization
- D. Prevention of complications

2. The wound care nurse is using the hypergranulation management pathways to treat a wound with a Type II: occlusive environment. What is a step in the pathway management?
- A. Continue occlusive dressing.
- B. Decrease absorption.
- C. Increase moisture vapor transmission rate (MVTR).
- D. Apply topical steroids.

3. Which of the following is a general principle of moist wound healing?
- A. It stops cell migration.
- B. It augments autolysis.
- C. It increases fibrosis.
- D. It can increase the risk of infection.

4. What is a primary intervention for the wound care specialist when treating patients' wounds?
- A. Packing the wound with plain gauze to absorb excess exudate
- B. Maintaining moisture balance in the wound
- C. Exposing the wound to air to allow a protective scab to form
- D. Avoiding the use of moisture-retentive dressings

5. What is one effect of managing a wound in a moist environment?
- A. Revascularization occurs at a slower rate.
- B. Wounds heal in disorganized manner.
- C. The breakdown of avascular tissue and fibrin is slowed.
- D. Collagen production is increased.

6. For which patient would moist wound healing most likely be contraindicated?
- A. A patient with diabetes mellitus who has a noninfected leg ulcer with stable dry eschar
- B. A patient who has an infected gunshot wound in the chest with fluid-filled brown eschar
- C. A patient who has a surgical incision that is showing signs and symptoms of maceration
- D. A patient with a spinal cord injury who has a pressure ulcer on the sacrum that has wet, boggy eschar

7. The wound care nurse is following the TIME concept to promote wound healing in a timely fashion. Which statement accurately describes an aspect of healing measures based on the tissue management step of this framework?
- A. The removal of nonviable tissue prolongs wound healing time.
- B. Biofilms are beneficial to wound healing as they degrade the ECM.
- C. Hypergranulation tissue slows wound healing by preventing epithelialization.
- D. Hypertrophic scar tissue will resolve on its own when the incision heals.

8. The nurse is examining a patient's venous ulcer that is characterized by critical colonization. What does this finding signify?
- A. The wound surface is too wet or too dry.
- B. It is a characteristic of all chronic wounds and does not require intervention.
- C. Organisms are interfering with repair, and intervention is required.
- D. A closed wound edge is impeding wound repair.

9. What is a first-line treatment of a wound with a compromised wound edge?
- A. Chemical cauterization
- B. Saucerization
- C. Use of growth factors
- D. Use of skin substitutes

10. Which of the following accurately describes the occurrence of nociceptive pain?
- A. It is an abnormal physiological response that develops when pain pathways affecting the central or peripheral nervous system are damaged.
- B. It is caused by a disruption or inflammation in tissue that stimulates somatic or visceral pain receptors.
- C. It is frequently described as burning, shooting, electric shock like, pins and needles, prickling, or tingling.
- D. It is considered to be an abnormal physiological response to a known painful stimulus.

11. The nurse assessing the pain of a patient with chronic leg ulcers documents a moderately severe pain level of seven on a scale of one to ten. What analgesic would be an appropriate "first-line intervention" to treat this level of pain?
- A. Acetaminophen
- B. Oxycodone
- C. Morphine
- D. Codeine

ANSWERS: 1.**A**, 2.**C**, 3.**B**, 4.**B**, 5.**D**, 6.**A**, 7.**C**, 8.**C**, 9.**A**, 10.**B**, 11.**D**

CHAPTER 8

Wound Cleansing and Dressing Selection

Kelly A. Jaszarowski and Rose W. Murphree

OBJECTIVES

1. Develop an individualized plan of care based on assessment data and current evidence-based guidelines that addresses each of the following factors:
   - Correction or amelioration of etiologic factors
   - Attention to systemic factors affecting repair process
   - Evidence-based topical therapy
   - Pain management
   - Patient and caregiver education
2. Recommend or provide topical therapy, based on best available evidence, to include the following:
   - Debridement of necrotic tissue when indicated
   - Identification and management of wound-related infections
   - Management of epibole and hypertrophic granulation tissue
   - Selection of dressings to manage exudate and maintain moist wound surface
3. Demonstrate correct procedure for each of the following:
   - Conservative sharp wound debridement (CSWD)
   - Chemical cauterization
   - Wound cleansing/dressing application
   - Noninvasive wound culture
   - Application adjunctive therapies such as negative pressure wound therapy (NPWT)

Topic Outline

 Introduction

Wound healing requires comprehensive and holistic management that includes identification and correction of the etiologic factors (to interrupt the cycle of injury), assessment and correction of systemic factors affecting repair (perfusion, nutritional status, glycemic control, intake of antiproliferative medications, comorbidities), and evidence-based topical therapy. The goal of topical therapy is to create a local environment that supports healing, through appropriate cleansing and dressing selection. This chapter provides clear guidelines for wound cleansing and dressing selection based on the phase of healing and the specific characteristics of the wound.

> **CLINICAL PEARL**
>
> The goal of topical therapy is to create a local environment that supports healing, through appropriate cleansing and dressing selection.

Wound Cleansing

Wound bed preparation begins with cleansing and requires attention to both the cleansing agent and the technique. The approach to cleansing and the appropriate agent are determined by the stage of healing as determined by the wound assessment. Wounds in the inflammatory phase of repair are characterized by the presence of devitalized tissue (eschar and/or slough) and/or by high bacterial loads and large amounts of exudate, which can frequently be malodorous. The goal in cleansing wounds is to remove as much of the devitalized tissue, bacterial burden, and exudate as possible without damaging the viable tissue within the wound bed.

Clean Wounds

Wounds in the proliferative phase of repair are characterized by healthy tissue within the wound bed (granulation tissue and/or new epithelium), relatively low levels of bacteria, and lower volumes of exudate. The goal in cleansing of these wounds is to flush away exudate without damaging the proliferative cells and newly formed tissues. A bulb syringe can effectively deliver a gentler flush pressure (0.5 psi) for the proliferative phase wound (Atiyeh et al., 2009; Edlich et al., 2010).

> **CLINICAL PEARL**
>
> The goal in cleansing for a clean granulating wound is to flush away exudate without damaging proliferative cells and newly formed tissues; appropriate solutions include saline, commercial wound cleansers, and potable tap water.

Necrotic or Infected Wounds

Cleansing of infected or dirty wounds requires irrigation and may involve use of a cytotoxic cleansing agent. These wounds require irrigation rather than gentle flushing because irrigation is much more effective in reducing bacterial loads and in loosening and removing avascular tissue and debris. Irrigation should be done with low pressure (4 to 15 psi) for three reasons: (1) to prevent splash back and contamination of other areas/surfaces/persons, (2) to prevent invasion of the bacteria into healthy tissue or bloodstream, and (3) to prevent damage to any healthy tissue present in the wound bed. The desired irrigation force may be obtained with a 35-mL syringe and 19-gauge catheter (7 psi) (Atiyeh et al., 2009; Edlich et al., 2010) or a commercial cleanser packaged in a pressurized container that delivers the desired irrigation force. Another option for irrigating a wound is the high-pressure pulsatile lavage cleansing system. Pulsatile lavage irrigation involves delivery of an irrigating solution under pressure, from an electrically powered device, with or without suction. A critical consideration in use of pulsatile lavage is the level of irrigation force; studies examining this approach report increased risk of bacterial invasion into the soft tissues if irrigating force is excessive (>15 psi). Consequently, companies are currently working to perfect the delivery system to assure safe levels of irrigation force (Hughes et al., 2012). Another consideration is the potential for aerosolization of bacteria; the clinician must follow all manufacturers' guidelines for safe use. Whenever irrigation with any degree of pressure is used to cleanse a wound, it is essential for the wound nurse to wear appropriate personal protective equipment, including a mask and face shield.

> **CLINICAL PEARL**
>
> Cleansing of dirty or infected wounds requires 4 to 15 psi irrigating force and may involve cytotoxic solutions (antiseptics).

Agents used for cleansing dirty wounds may be either noncytotoxic (saline, potable/tap water, or commercial cleansing solutions) or cytotoxic (antiseptics such as sodium hypochlorite or acetic acid solution). Antiseptic solutions are generally preferred if the goal is to kill bacteria (e.g., a heavily necrotic and infected wound). However, the clinician must be aware that use of these agents can potentially damage viable wound tissue. In determining the best cleansing agent for a specific wound, the clinician should consider the goals of care and the status of the wound bed. When the goal is swift cleansing of the wound and >50% of the wound bed is covered with devitalized tissue or there is a large amount of malodorous exudate indicating active wound infection, an antiseptic solution is probably the best choice. Use of an antiseptic for cleansing should be a short-term intervention. Once the bacterial loads have been controlled and the volume of necrotic tissue has been reduced to <40% of the wound bed, the antiseptic should be discontinued.

Antiseptic Solutions

The discussion of antiseptic agents that follows is not considered all-encompassing (Edlich et al., 2010); for example, chlorhexidine is not discussed because it is primarily utilized for surgical skin cleansing and not wound cleansing. Studies throughout the literature clearly document the negative effects of hydrogen peroxide, particularly the cytotoxicity to wound-healing cells (Thomas et al., 2009). Data regarding use of povidone–iodine are mixed, with results depending on form and concentration (e.g., scrub vs. solution or gel and full strength vs. dilute).

Sodium Hypochlorite Solution (e.g., Dakin's, Clorpactin)

The active ingredient in these products is dilute bleach; sodium bicarbonate may be added as a buffering agent. It is available in retail stores and from vendors as a solution and as a hydrogel or impregnated gauze; solutions may also be formulated by the pharmacy to adhere to specific dilution requirements and can be mixed at home in states where this is permissible. This solution has demonstrated bactericidal effectiveness against most of the bacteria in chronic wounds and also significantly reduces wound odor. Anecdotal reports indicate that it may also facilitate debridement. As noted, there is a simple recipe that can be used at home to mix the solution; the amount of bleach to be used varies based on the desired concentration. For example, the formula for half strength Dakin's solution (0.25%) is three tablespoons + half teaspoon of regular-strength household bleach (48 mL) and half teaspoon baking soda added to 32 ounces of sterile water (or water that has been boiled); the formula for quarter strength (0.125%) Dakin's is one tablespoon + two teaspoons bleach (24 mL) + half teaspoon baking soda added to 32 ounces of water. The nurse should be aware that studies indicate reduced toxicity with quarter strength concentration; bactericidal effects are retained (Fonder et al., 2008; Heggers et al., 1991). It must be stored in the refrigerator and replaced every 48 hours. Unopened jars can be stored for up to 1 month after preparation. It should be stored away from sunlight, kept out of the reach of children, and clearly marked as poisonous to prevent accidental oral ingestion. As noted, in addition to reducing bacterial loads, sodium hypochlorite solutions are sometimes used to promote debridement. When used in this way, the hypochlorite solution is used to thoroughly moisten gauze, which is then placed into the wound bed and changed every 12 hours. Some studies suggest that it may also be effective in reducing biofilm formation (Agostinho et al., 2011; Bradley & Cunningham, 2013).

Clinical Considerations

Studies have shown sodium hypochlorite to be an effective bactericidal agent even at low concentrations; some investigators recommend 0.025% or 0.0125% as the optimal concentration for killing bacteria (*MRSA, MSSA, Escherichia coli*) while preserving fibroblasts (Agostinho et al., 2011; Bradley & Cunningham, 2013). As noted, it should be discontinued once the wound bed is clean, and a noncytotoxic solution should be utilized instead. It is inexpensive and easily made at home (as previously mentioned), which is advantageous for patients with financial concerns.

CLINICAL PEARL

If sodium hypochlorite is used for cleansing or debridement of a dirty wound, it should be discontinued when a clean wound bed is established.

The nurse must monitor the patient for any signs of an adverse or allergic reaction, which is unlikely but possible. In addition, some patients report an aversion to the smell and some patients complain of stinging or burning upon application (primarily with the stronger concentrations). Protection of the periwound skin is essential when using sodium hypochlorite as a dressing. This can be done with a liquid film barrier (for trunk wounds) or a moisture barrier ointment (for extremity wounds). The wound nurse must determine the goals of care and cleansing and must decide whether sodium hypochlorite is appropriate and, if so, whether it should be used just for cleansing or for wound packing. The nurse must also continually monitor the results and must discontinue use or change the dilution as the wound bed becomes cleaner. Finally, the wound nurse must provide clear instructions to any caregivers using this solution and must assure proper storage and replacement.

Acetic Acid

Acetic acid is sometimes used because of its bactericidal effectiveness against *Pseudomonas aeruginosa*, a common wound pathogen that may produce a classic "green" hue to the wound bed and wound exudate and a very distinct odor. The most commonly used concentration is ¼ strength, which can be formulated by mixing one cup of vinegar and three cups of distilled water. Typically, the wound is irrigated with the acetic acid using a syringe and catheter.

Clinical Considerations

Acetic acid can be easily mixed in the home setting, which makes it an inexpensive product. It can be used as a cleansing/irrigating agent alone or as a wound packing agent.

Cytotoxicity to fibroblasts is a concern when applying this product, so attention to concentration is essential. Periwound skin can be damaged if the acetic acid remains in contact for a prolonged period of time. Thus, the periwound skin should be protected with a liquid barrier film or a moisture barrier ointment if the wound is filled with acetic acid–moistened gauze. Application may cause a stinging/burning sensation or even pain. If this occurs, the acetic acid may require further dilution.

The wound nurse needs to base use of acetic acid for cleansing or packing on careful assessment of the wound, because acetic acid is not effective against other pathogens. In addition, the nurse needs to monitor for evidence of effectiveness and needs to change the wound care plan if there is poor response. The nurse also needs to monitor for any adverse or allergic reaction, though this is uncommon, and may need to discontinue use if the patient reports aversion to the smell. Clear labeling of the product is a must to prevent accidental consumption. Finally, the wound nurse should collaborate with the staff to provide ongoing monitoring of wound status and must assure that use of acetic acid is discontinued once the wound bed is clean.

Noncytotoxic Solutions

Cleansing of noninfected wounds in the proliferative phase of repair involves gentle flushing with noncytotoxic solutions, saline, tap water, or commercial wound cleansers. Normal saline (0.9%) is widely available, especially in health care facilities. It can also be prepared at home by adding two teaspoons of salt to 1,000 mL of distilled water. Commercially prepared saline is available in most retail and pharmacy stores, either in spray cans or in bottles. If the prepackaged spray can is used, the nurse must turn the nozzle to the mist feature in order to avoid aggressive cleansing with potential damage to the wound surface. Commercial wound cleansers may also be used, again with use of the mist feature as opposed to the spray feature when cleansing wounds that are viable and noninfected. When considering use of a commercial wound cleanser, the nurse should ask for data that confirms the agent is noncytotoxic. In some situations, tap water is an acceptable cleanser. A Cochrane review found very little data on the use of tap water for wound cleansing, but the data available indicated that tap water is a safe agent so long as it is potable. In clinical practice, tap water is frequently used for patients in the home with large abdominal wounds. The use of a gentle shower mist may be the most effective approach to cleansing of these wounds (Fernandez & Griffiths, 2012).

Clinical Considerations

Saline is inexpensive, widely available, and easy to use. Studies have shown effective shelf life without contamination when stored in the refrigerator in the home for up to 1 month (Fellows and Crestodina, 2006). In the hospital, open bottles of saline should be discarded after 24 hours. Saline-moistened gauze is a commonly used dressing but requires frequent monitoring and changes to prevent desiccation of the wound bed. Saline does not provide any antimicrobial effects; the nurse must constantly monitor the wound for evidence of infectious complications. The nurse must assure appropriate use of saline or commercial cleansing agents, must address appropriate disposal of open bottles of saline, and must modify the care protocol if signs of infection develop.

Dressing Selection

Once the wound has been appropriately cleansed, an appropriate dressing should be applied. Selection of the best dressing(s) for a specific wound represents another challenge for the wound nurse, as there is an abundance of dressings available on the market today. However, a clear understanding of the principles of topical therapy (as discussed in Chapter 7), coupled with knowledge of dressing functions and characteristics, will guide the nurse in effectively matching the dressing to the wound. The remainder of this chapter addresses the products currently available and provides guidance in selection of appropriate products based on wound characteristics.

Wound dressings can be divided into two general categories: those that provide passive support for wound healing and those that actively impact on the processes involved in repair. The majority of the products on the market are passive, meaning that they promote wound healing by providing exudate control, maintaining a moist wound surface, protecting the wound against trauma and pathogenic invasion, and, when indicated, reducing bacterial loads. This chapter focuses on these types of dressings. Active therapy dressings and products will be discussed in the chapter on refractory wounds (Chapter 11).

Passive dressings can be classified in several different ways. One approach is based on the form of the dressing in relationship to the contours of the wound. From this perspective, dressings can be classified as wicking agents, filler dressings, or cover dressings. Another approach to classification is based on the dressing's role in maintaining moisture balance within the wound bed. From this perspective, dressings are hydraters, absorbers, or moisture retainers. All dressings can be classified as either plain or antimicrobial, and many dressings are available in both forms. Finally, dressings can be classified based on the primary materials from which they are constructed, for example, gauze, hydrogels, alginates, foams, etc. In this chapter, we discuss dressings primarily from the perspective of their form (wick, filler, cover) and function (absorb, hydrate, retain moisture); specific dressing materials are discussed within the functional categories.

Wick versus Filler versus Cover Dressing

Wicking agents are rope dressings that are placed into tunneled areas and undermined areas to evacuate fluid. They are available in plain and antimicrobial form and in a variety of materials (alginate rope, hydrofiber rope, foam strips, textile strips, nonwoven gauze strips—impregnated with hypertonic solution or dry). There are two major clinical considerations in selecting an appropriate wicking agent: width of the tunnel and volume of exudate. When placing a wick into a narrow tunnel, the nurse should elect a wick that will not leave any dressing material behind. In other words, nonwoven gauze strips would be appropriate, but woven gauze would *not* be appropriate. Alginate ropes would also be less appropriate in this situation, since alginate fibers could be left behind. When selecting a wick for a tunnel in a highly exudative and/or infected wound, the wound nurse should consider selection of an antimicrobial wicking product or a nonwoven gauze strip impregnated with saline, which provides "active" wicking through osmotic effects.

Filler dressings are dressings that are designed to go into the wound and to accommodate to the contours of the wound, whereas cover dressings are solid "sheet-type" dressings that are designed to cover the wound. Wounds with any depth require both a filler dressing and a cover dressing, whereas surface wounds require only a cover dressing. Filler dressings and cover dressings are available in both absorptive and hydrating forms, and in plain and antimicrobial forms.

Thus, the first decision the wound nurse must make is based on the contours of the wound: is a wick required? is a filler required? or is a cover dressing all that is needed? The wound with tunnels and depth will require a wick, a filler, and a cover (Fig. 8-1); the wound with depth but no tunnels will require a filler and cover (Fig. 8-2); and the wound with no tunnels and no depth will require only a cover dressing (Fig. 8-3).

CLINICAL PEARL

Dressings can be classified as wicks, fillers, or covers; wicks are used for tunnels, fillers are required for wounds with depth or undermining, and covers are required for all wounds.

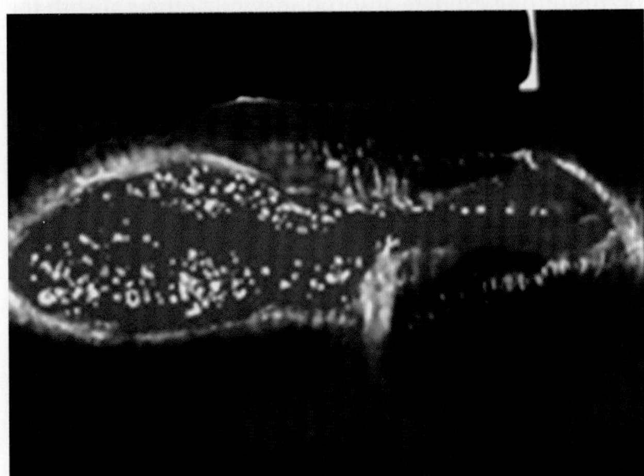

FIGURE 8-1. Wound with depth and tunnel (at 3 o'clock): needs wick, cover, filler.

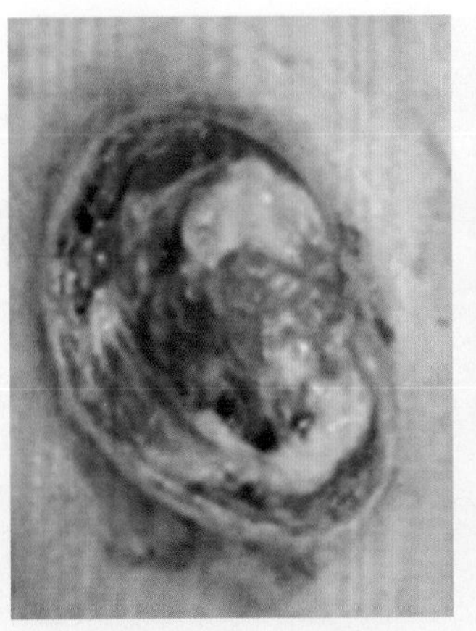

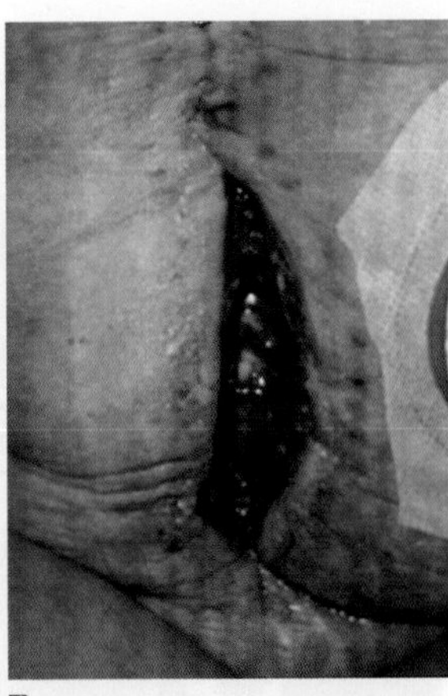

FIGURE 8-2. **A, B.** Wounds with depth: need filler and cover.

Absorber versus Hydrater versus Moisture-Retaining Dressing

As explained in detail in Chapter 7, maintenance of moisture balance at the wound surface is a key element of evidence-based topical therapy. The goal is to absorb any excess exudate and to maintain a continually moist wound surface. Very wet wounds require highly absorptive dressings, moderately wet wounds require dressings with moderate absorptive capacity, minimally wet wounds require dressings that maintain moisture but provide only limited absorption, and dry wounds require hydrating dressings. Fortunately, the wide array of dressings currently available allows the wound nurse to effectively match absorptive/hydrating capacity of the dressing to the volume of exudate produced by the wound. In selecting an appropriately absorptive dressing, the nurse must also consider frequency of dressing change. Very wet or very dry wounds may require more frequent dressing changes to maintain optimal moisture balance at the wound surface. Dressings classified as absorptive include alginates, hydrofibers, copolymer dressings, foam dressings, fabric/textile dressings, and dry gauze. Dressings classified as moisture retaining include contact layer/nonadherent dressings, hydrocolloid dressings, and transparent adhesive dressings. And, dressings classified as hydraters include hydrogel dressings and wet gauze dressings. These specific categories are discussed in more detail later in this chapter.

Thus, the second decision to be made by the wound care nurse is the degree of absorptive capacity required by the specific wound.

CLINICAL PEARL

Dressings can also be classified as hydraters or absorbers; hydraters (e.g., gels and damp gauze) are used for dry wounds, and absorbers (alginates, hydrofibers, foams) are used for wet wounds.

Antimicrobial versus Plain Dressings

Antimicrobial dressings may be needed for wounds at high risk of infection and wounds with evidence of critical colonization. Antimicrobial dressings include

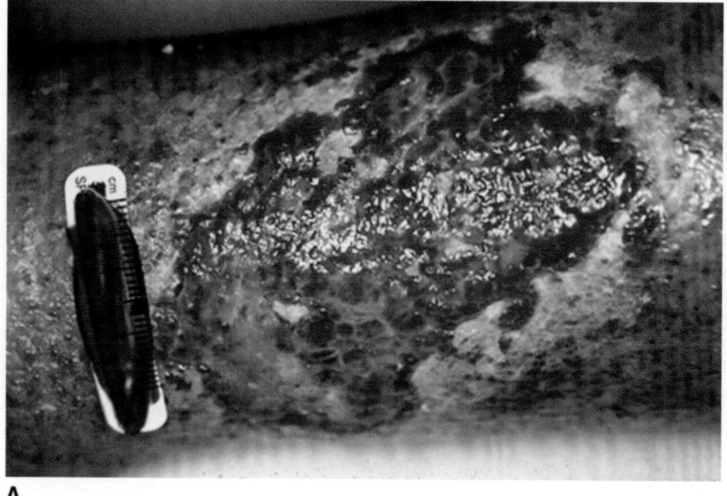

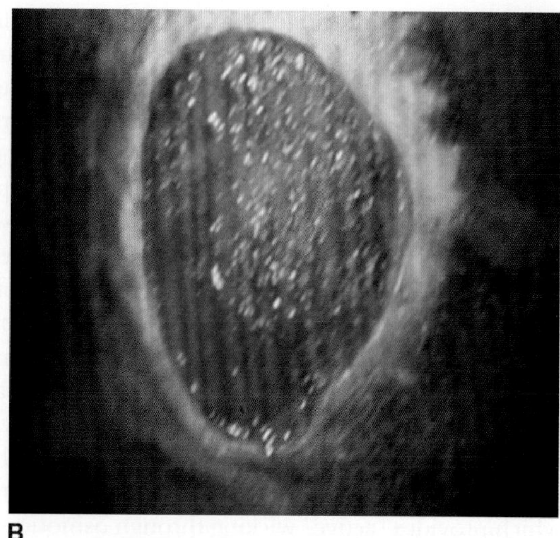

A B

FIGURE 8-3. **A, B.** Superficial/shallow wounds: need cover dressing only.

those that incorporate silver, cadexomer iodine, polyhexamethylene biguanide (PHMB), and polyvinyl alcohol (PVA) with crystal violet and methylene blue, those with medicinal honey, and those that attract and remove bacteria. All antimicrobial dressings affect a broad spectrum of organisms including essentially all known wound pathogens. Antimicrobial agents are available in various forms including creams, ointments, powder, sprays, and all forms of dressings. Each antimicrobial dressing varies in physical properties including amount and release properties of the antimicrobial, duration of antimicrobial effectiveness, absorptive capacity, management of odor, and management of pain (Vowden et al., 2011). It is these properties, along with wound status and treatment goals, that should be considered when choosing a specific dressing.

As with any therapy, length of use is determined by the wound and its progression or lack thereof. A lack of progress or a deterioration in wound status suggests the need for reassessment and change in treatment. In contrast, significant improvement in wound status usually indicates control of bacterial loads, which may signify the ability to transition away from an antimicrobial dressing. Antimicrobial dressings are available without a prescription and are effective against essentially all wound pathogens. Therefore, a wound culture is not required and antimicrobial dressings can be used in lieu of antibiotics to treat local wound infection. The risk of resistance to antimicrobial dressings is low. (A more detailed examination of these dressings can be found in Chapter 10).

CLINICAL PEARL

Antimicrobial dressings are broad spectrum; therefore, no culture is needed when using these dressings to control bacterial loads *at the wound surface*.

Specific Dressing Materials

Generic dressing classifications will be utilized for this section, and dressing categories will be listed in alphabetical order. Specific trade names will not be utilized due to the constant change in available products and WOCN's commitment to avoidance of perceived endorsement of specific products. The reader is directed to product catalogs, wound sourcebooks, and the Internet for information on specific dressings.

Calcium Alginates/Alginates

Description and Characteristics

Alginate dressings are commonly referred to as calcium alginate or seaweed dressings; they are nonwoven dressings composed of polysaccharide fibers or xerogel, which is derived from seaweed. These dressings are available in a variety of forms, including sheets and ropes. Some alginates are impregnated with antimicrobial agents such as silver. Alginate dressings absorb moderate amounts of exudate. Some form a gel as the result of an ion exchange that occurs during exudate absorption, while others absorb the exudate into the dressing so that the dressing becomes soft and moist. All alginates provide for atraumatic removal from a moist wound surface. The frequency of dressing change is dependent upon the amount of exudate and the secondary dressing utilized but typically ranges from daily to every 3 days. These dressings are indicated for wounds with moderate-to-large volumes of exudate. If the wound is highly exudative, the absorptive capacity of the alginate should be supplemented by an absorptive cover dressing. The wound nurse should follow the manufacturer's recommendations for use of the specific dressing.

The formation of a gel or a soft moist dressing permits easy and atraumatic dressing removal with wound irrigation. Because the gel or soft dressing does not adhere to the wound, there is less trauma to the wound bed and limited or no pain with dressing changes. In addition, there is less tendency on the part of staff nurses to over pack the wound. This advantage, coupled with less frequent dressing changes, may result in cost savings in terms of supplies and labor.

Clinical Considerations

Clinicians must be taught to irrigate the wound thoroughly following removal of an alginate dressing to assure removal of all dressing residue. Staff must also be taught to avoid use of alginate ropes in narrow tunnels since fragments of the dressing could be left behind. Staff should be taught not to "layer" alginate dressings as this is unnecessarily expensive. If the wound is deep and highly exudative, the staff should be taught to apply the alginate as a base (primary) dressing and to use fluffed gauze as a secondary filler for additional absorption. The wound nurse must assure that all caregivers understand that alginates are intended for exudative wounds and are inappropriate for use in relatively dry wounds. Alginates are generally considered an inappropriate choice as the primary dressing for wounds with exposed tendons, joint capsules, or bone due to the risk of tissue desiccation.

CLINICAL PEARL

Alginates (and hydrofibers) are inappropriate for dry wounds.

Contact Layers

Description and Characteristics

Contact layer dressings are well named; they are dressings that are placed onto the wound surface in direct contact with the wound bed. Contact layer dressings help to maintain a moist and protected wound surface because they are nonabsorptive. However, they are porous, which permits exudate to pass through the contact layer to a secondary dressing that provides absorption. The contact layer dressing is usually a single layer of nonadherent dressing material with perforations of varying size. Commonly used contact layer dressings include nonadherent gauze-based dressings, such as those impregnated with petrolatum derivatives or bismuth salt–based ointments, and silicone-based contact layers, including thin silicone adhesive foam (Worley, 2005). Contact layer dressings are most appropriate for surface wounds, especially extremity wounds. They are applied directly to the wound and covered with a secondary dressing. These dressings are occasionally used for wounds with depth, following the same guidelines (contact layer application followed by a secondary filler dressing and secured with a cover dressing). Contact layer dressings are most appropriate for clean wounds free of necrotic tissue as they do not create enough of a fluid environment to provide effective autolysis. They are inappropriate for third-degree burns, wounds with viscous exudate, and wounds with tunneling or undermining. Contact layer dressings may remain in the wound for as long as 1 week, depending on wound characteristics and manufacturer's recommendations. Topical medications may also be used with these dressings.

CLINICAL PEARL

Contact layers protect the wound from trauma and permit drainage to pass through the dressing for absorption by a secondary dressing.

Contact layer dressings are readily available in almost all settings, easy to apply, and effectively protect the fragile wound bed while permitting removal of exudate. Additionally, contact layer dressings are generally easy to remove, providing atraumatic and painless dressing changes. Those that are silicone based are consistently easy to remove, and those that are impregnated with petrolatum derivatives or other ointments are easy to remove so long as they are not allowed to dry out. Some contact layer dressings can be left in place when the cover or secondary dressing is changed, thus preventing disruption of the moist wound environment. This is true of silicone-based contact layers.

Clinical Considerations

Contact layer dressings cannot be effectively used in wounds with tunnels due to the inability to visualize the tunnel's end. The wound care nurse must also consider the viscosity of the drainage when considering a contact layer; some contact layer dressings have wider diameter perforations than others and would be more appropriate for thicker drainage. As noted, very viscous drainage is a contraindication to the use of these dressings. Finally, contact layer dressings do not provide a bacterial barrier. Often gauze is used as the secondary dressing, which is also permeable to bacterial invasion. Thus, contact layer dressings are sometimes suboptimal when the wound is high risk for bacterial contamination.

The wound nurse must determine whether a contact layer and secondary dressing are the best choice for a particular wound and must also consider the specific characteristics of the various contact layer dressings (e.g., potential for drying and size of perforations). It is also important to teach clinicians to carefully assess the wound at each dressing change to assure that (1) the contact layer is providing effective transfer of exudate and there is no "pooling" of the wound drainage and (2) the contact layer is maintaining a moist wound surface and is not becoming adherent to the underlying wound bed.

Composite Dressings

Description and Characteristics

Dressings that contain an absorptive layer, a cover layer, and an adhesive border are referred to as composite dressings. The cover layer may be either porous or waterproof, and the absorptive layer may extend from one end of the dressing to the other or may be an island. Composite dressings are available in a variety of sizes and combinations, with varying degrees of absorptive capacity. They are also available "plain" and with an impregnated antimicrobial agent. They are frequently used as secondary dressings but are also appropriate as primary dressings for surface wounds. The frequency of dressing change is dependent upon the specific components of the dressing, its absorptive capacity, and whether it is being used as a primary or secondary dressing. Simple composite dressings include a nonadherent gauze island dressing with a tape cover; these dressings are usually used as cover dressings. Other commercially available composite dressings combine absorptive dressings such as a hydrofiber, foam, or alginate with a cover layer that has waterproofing and moisture vapor permeability characteristics, such as a transparent adhesive or thin hydrocolloid with adhesive border. These dressings are intended for use as primary dressings.

Composite dressings are convenient and easy to apply. They are also readily available and relatively inexpensive. Dressings in which the absorptive pad extends the entire length of the dressing may be cut to fit the wound, with adhesive added to the cut end.

Clinical Considerations

Because these dressings are easy to use, they are sometimes layered on top of other advanced wound dressings, adding unnecessary cost. For example, use of an antimicrobial composite dressing as a secondary dressing is a waste of resources since the antimicrobial layer will not be in contact with the wound bed. They are also sometimes left in place for extended periods of time. Finally, other clinicians and caregivers may fail to differentiate between composite dressings with a waterproof outer layer (which would be needed for wounds exposed to urine and stool) and those that are porous, leading to inappropriate product selection.

The wound nurse must provide appropriate guidance to other clinicians and caregivers in use of composite dressings, including guidelines for product selection (composites to be used for secondary dressings vs. those to be used as primary dressings, and situations in which a waterproof outer layer is needed). The wound nurse must assure that the caregiver and/or patient understands the dressing application and costs, in addition to the expected dressing actions.

Copolymer Dressings

Description and Characteristics

Specialty absorption dressings utilizing copolymers are among the newest generation of wound care dressings (Jhong et al., 2014). The polymers bind with exudate to form a gel resulting in a super absorbent dressing. These dressings are available in multiple forms, including amorphous gel, foams, and absorptive pad dressings with a nonadherent contact layer. The pad and foam dressings prevent maceration of the wound bed and periwound skin, due to the high absorptive capacity and ability to lock the exudate within the polymer.

Clinical Considerations

Copolymer dressings may be left in place for up to 7 days, depending on the amount of drainage. Amorphous copolymer dressings require a cover dressing, while the newer pad form of these dressings may be available with an adhesive border.

Copolymer dressings may also help to control wound odor, though further study is needed (Hashely, 2011).

Foam Dressings

Description and Characteristics

Foam dressings are available in a variety of shapes and sizes, and with and without antimicrobial agents. They are also available in nonadhesive, standard and gentle adhesive, and adhesive border forms. Foam dressings are most commonly made of polyurethane and contain small, open cells for absorbing wound exudate; the absorptive capacity varies depending on the specific components of the dressing. Foam dressings can be used effectively as both primary and secondary (cover) dressings. They are appropriate for wounds with low-to-moderate volume exudate and for heavily exudative wounds. Because foam dressings maintain a moist wound surface while absorbing excess exudate, they also promote autolytic debridement of moist avascular tissue or slough (Avent, 2010). It should be noted that foams are absorptive dressings and are therefore inappropriate for use on dry wounds or wounds with minimal exudate. Foam dressings would not be effective in promoting autolysis of dry eschar because they do not donate moisture and cannot *create* a fluid environment. Frequency of dressing change is dependent upon the volume of exudate and absorptive capacity of the dressing.

Foams are extremely versatile dressings due to the variety of shapes and sizes, antimicrobial as well as plain versions, and availability of multiple adhesive options (no adhesive, border adhesive, standard adhesive, and gentle adhesive). They are appropriate for almost all exudative wounds, either as the primary dressing or as a secondary cover dressing.

CLINICAL PEARL

Foams are very versatile dressings that can be used for almost all "wet" wounds; they can be used as primary or secondary dressings and are available in multiple forms (plain and antimicrobial, and adhesive and nonadhesive).

Clinical Considerations

The wound nurse must teach other clinicians and caregivers how to use foam dressings appropriately as there are two major considerations. The first involves absorptive capacity. Manufacturers often classify a foam by the amount of exudate it is able to absorb, such as lite or extra. The clinician must consider the volume of wound exudate when selecting a foam dressing with the appropriate absorptive capacity. The second involves adhesive characteristics; the clinician must elect a nonadhesive,

adhesive, or adhesive border product based on wound location and characteristics of periwound skin and, when an adhesive product is needed, must consider whether a gentle adhesive is required. For example, the best choice for a highly exudative lower extremity ulcer with macerated periwound skin being managed with compression therapy would be a nonadhesive foam. The dressing would be secured by the compression wrap so no adhesive feature is needed and adhesion would in general be contraindicated for macerated periwound skin. In addition, a nonadhesive foam permits more moisture vapor transmission and would contribute to better exudate control. In contrast, a trunk wound would best be managed by an adhesive foam or foam with adhesive border. If the patient has very fragile skin, a gentle adhesive product should be used (e.g., a silicone- or gel-based adhesive foam).

The nurse must teach clinicians how to select and use foams appropriately. Teaching consideration must also include changing foam dressings before they become soaked with exudate as this can contribute to periwound maceration and an increased risk of bacterial invasion. Clinicians must be taught to avoid use of foam dressings on minimally draining wounds, since this could result in drying of the wound surface. These dressings are contraindicated for third-degree burns.

Gauze Dressings

Description and Characteristics

Gauze is a very commonly used dressing, despite its limitations. Gauze can be used for wound cleansing and as a wick, filler, or cover dressing. It can be moistened with saline or with an antiseptic agent, so it can be used appropriately for both clean and dirty wounds. Gauze comes in various forms, including flat dressings, some of which are precut to fit around tubes, rolled gauze, and narrow strip gauze. Gauze also comes in antimicrobial forms as well as plain. The primary characteristic to consider when selecting gauze for wound care is whether it is woven or nonwoven. Nonwoven gauze is a much better choice for dressings that will come into contact with the wound bed, because woven gauze has loose fibers that can become embedded in the wound bed and can act as foreign bodies. All gauze can be cut to fit the wound itself or opened and "fluffed" to loosely fill a wound with depth. Gauze should usually be moistened prior to placement in contact with the wound bed. Gauze has limited absorptive capacity and dries fairly rapidly; thus, it requires more frequent dressing changes. In addition, there is a tendency to over pack gauze into wounds with depth, creating the potential for trauma to the wound bed. Gauze is generally considered a less than optimal choice for a primary dressing. It is more appropriately used for a secondary (cover) dressing. If used as a primary dressing in contact with the wound bed, it is essential to adhere to the following guidelines: use a nonwoven gauze, moisten the gauze, and fluff the gauze loosely into the wound bed.

CLINICAL PEARL

Gauze may be used as a primary or secondary dressing; when used as a primary dressing, it is best to use nonwoven gauze that is moistened and to avoid overpacking.

Gauze is the wound care product most familiar to the majority of health care providers, and they are therefore comfortable with its use. However, most caregivers do not recognize the potential disadvantages of gauze and frequently use it inappropriately. Gauze is generally perceived to be less expensive than more advanced dressings. When the total cost of care is calculated, however, the increased frequency of dressing change and the cost of the labor involved in the multiple dressing changes usually means that gauze is actually *more* expensive. Gauze dressings are available in multiple shapes, sizes, and forms; in both plain and antimicrobial forms; and impregnated with saline.

Clinical Considerations

It can be difficult to teach caregivers and/or staff the difference between woven and nonwoven gauze and the appropriate uses of each. It can also be difficult to teach staff the importance of avoiding overpacking of wounds, as many have been taught incorrectly to pack wounds tightly. It is therefore critical to explain that overpacking interferes with perfusion and compromises fibroblast activity and granulation tissue development. Finally, even with optimal use, gauze is more likely to become adherent to the wound surface and to cause trauma with dressing removal.

The wound nurse must assure that gauze is used appropriately, which includes use of nonwoven rather than woven gauze in contact with the wound surface; that the gauze is loosely fluffed and not overpacked; and that the gauze in contact with the wound surface is appropriately moistened. Further, the wound nurse needs to assure that gauze strips used to wick a tunnel are used appropriately. Specifically, enough of the gauze strip is left protruding into the wound to assure easy and complete removal. Finally, the wound nurse needs to understand the comparative benefits of gauze dressings and advanced wound dressings and needs to assure that the dressing selected is the dressing most appropriate for the wound at the particular phase of healing.

Hydrocolloid Dressings

Description and Characteristics

Hydrocolloid dressings are occlusive, wafer-type dressings made of gelatin materials, such as sodium carboxymethylcellulose. The gelatin material is combined with elastomers and adhesives and applied to a carrier to create a self-adhesive. Some hydrocolloids also have a thin border of adhesive around the edge of the dressing. The constituents of the dressing interact with wound exudate to form a gel, which contributes to atraumatic removal. Because the dressing is totally occlusive, water vapor cannot escape and the dressing must absorb the moisture secreted by the skin in addition to all wound exudate. This has major implications since the absorptive capacity of the wafer dressing is limited. Specifically, these dressings are appropriate only for wounds with low-volume exudate. When the exudate overloads the absorptive capacity of the dressing, the gel spreads beyond the borders of the dressing and leakage occurs. The combination of wound exudate and trapped perspiration may create an odor when the dressing "leaks" or is removed. Because these dressings are totally occlusive, they are generally considered contraindicated for use with infected wounds, especially if there is potential anaerobic involvement. Their limited ability to manage exudate is another characteristic making them a poor choice for infected wounds, which are typically exudative. These dressings are usually a good choice for shallow wounds with minimal exudate. Hydrocolloids may also be applied to intact skin or newly resurfaced breakdown for protection, may be used under tape on fragile skin, and are frequently used to protect the periwound skin. Wear time varies from 3 to 7 days, depending on the volume of exudate. The wound nurse should also refer to the manufacturer's recommendations for the specific dressing.

CLINICAL PEARL

Hydrocolloid dressings are inappropriate for infected wounds and for exudative wounds.

Hydrocolloids are simple to apply for most clinicians and/or caregivers (peel and place). In addition, these dressings are created in varying sizes and shapes, and many are designed for specific body locations, that is, triangular shape for coccygeal area. Hydrocolloids are also available in paste or powder form. These forms may be utilized to fill in wound dead space and require a secondary dressing. Hydrocolloids may also be utilized as a secondary dressing for wounds with depth and minimal exudate. The occlusive nature of this dressing maintains a moist wound environment, which promotes autolysis of avascular tissue. The occlusive nature also insulates the wound from temperature changes and prevents contamination from excrement or bacteria. These dressings have also been utilized to cover open shingle lesions to prevent viral transmission.

Clinical Considerations

To the untrained eye, leaking gel may appear to be purulent drainage, and the odor is often mistaken as a sign of infection by those unfamiliar with the properties of this dressing. As noted, the occlusive property means this dressing is generally contraindicated when infection is known or suspected or with deep necrotic wounds. Some hydrocolloids are made with pectin and would be contraindicated for a person with known pectin allergies. Some anatomical locations can present challenges in achieving and maintaining an adhesive seal without meltdown or lifting of the edges (e.g., sacrococcygeal area). Additionally, the adhesive strength of the dressing can pose a challenge when used on fragile skin; the aggressiveness of the adhesive can result in skin stripping upon removal if the dressing has to be removed in <3 days.

The clinician must thoroughly educate caregivers in appropriate use of these dressings, as well as contraindications to use (significant exudate, suspected infection, very fragile skin in a situation where frequent dressing changes are likely). The nurse should teach caregivers to remove the dressing and thoroughly flush the wound prior to assessing for signs of infection, in order to avoid misinterpretation of the normal hydrocolloid odor as a sign of infection. Ideally, hydrocolloid dressings should be changed once or twice weekly. If wear times are <3 days, an alternative dressing should be considered.

Hydrogels

Description and Characteristics

Solid gel dressings and amorphous hydrogels are designed to hydrate the wound through the donation of water. Amorphous hydrogels are a combination of water and polymers that may be applied directly to the wound bed or to another dressing, such as gauze, creating an impregnated dressing. Amorphous hydrogels are currently available as viscous liquids and as impregnated dressings (gauze sponges, ropes, strips, etc.); these dressings are used primarily in wounds with depth or tunnels but minimal exudate (e.g., a dehisced abdominal incision). The wound nurse may elect to apply the viscous hydrogel liquid directly to the wound bed and then to cover the hydrogel with a loose layer of moistened fluffed gauze or may elect to use gel-impregnated gauze loosely fluffed into the wound bed. When using a gel dressing to hydrate a dry wound, the wound nurse must also be careful to use a moisture-retentive cover dressing, such as a transparent adhesive dressing or a hydrocolloid dressing.

Solid (wafer type) gel dressings are also now available. They may be either water based or glycerin based and are available with and without adhesive borders. The sheets can absorb varying amounts of drainage depending upon their composition, and they promote autolysis due to the fluid environment they create. These sheets offer a cooling effect, which may be beneficial for pain management. Hydrogel dressings are ideal for any wound with minimal or no exudate and are an excellent choice for management of minor burns and radiodermatitis. The frequency of dressing changes is dependent upon the specific dressing, volume of exudate, and characteristics of the secondary dressing but in general ranges from one to two times daily to every 3 days.

Hydrogels tend to be relatively inexpensive, and the application is easy for most clinicians and caregivers to understand. The solid hydrogel sheets with adhesive may allow visualization of the wound bed, which reduces the risk of premature removal during wound healing. In addition, hydrogel dressings can be safely utilized during radiation therapy, and no allergies have been associated with this dressing.

Clinical Considerations

The wound nurse must teach caregivers to use hydrogels for dry wounds and to avoid their use with wet wounds. When gel-impregnated gauze is being used, the clinician needs to remind caregivers to avoid overpacking and to use nonwoven as opposed to woven gauze when available. (See section on "Gauze Dressings" for more details.) Water-based solid gels can macerate the periwound skin; thus, the nurse must teach caregivers to protect the surrounding skin with a liquid barrier film or to cut the solid gel to fit the wound.

The wound nurse must assure use of an adequate amount of viscous gel placed into a dry wound bed as well as an appropriate secondary filler (if needed) and cover dressing. If inadequate gel is used and/or if the secondary filler and cover are absorptive rather than hydrating/moisture retentive, the dressing may dry to the wound causing trauma and pain with removal. The wound nurse should teach the caregiver to apply at least 1/8″ of hydrogel to the entire wound bed, to use a moist secondary filler when needed, and to use a moisture-retentive cover dressing. The nurse must also teach caregivers to assess the hydration and adherence of the dressing prior to removal and to rehydrate the dressing if needed.

Hydrofiber Dressings

Description and Characteristics

Hydrofiber dressings are similar to alginate dressings, and, as a result, some clinicians may incorrectly refer to these dressings as alginates. Hydrofiber dressings are composed of sodium carboxymethylcellulose and are therefore highly absorptive; the carboxymethylcellulose interacts with wound exudate to form a gel. Hydrofiber dressings are available in both plain and antimicrobial forms and in both sheet and ribbon form; they are nonadherent, which means a secondary or cover dressing is always required. Frequency of dressing change is dependent upon the volume of exudate and the cover dressing but typically ranges from daily to every 3 days.

Clinical Considerations

Because of their ability to absorb large amounts of exudate, Hydrofiber dressings are indicated for use in a variety of wounds with moderate-to-heavy exudate. Hydrofiber dressings are contraindicated in dry wounds or wounds with dry eschar and third-degree burns.

Textile Dressings

Description and Characteristics

These dressings are designed to manage moisture within the wound bed, specifically by wicking fluid away from the wound or by retaining fluid at the wound surface. They can also be used between body folds to manage moisture and prevent friction. These dressings may contain silver to reduce bacterial counts.

Clinical Considerations

With selected products, the clinician must take care to position the dressing appropriately; for example, some dressings are designed so that one surface is hydrophobic and one is hydrophilic. When using this type of dressing, the hydrophobic side is placed against the surface of a dry wound, while the hydrophilic side should be placed against the surface of a moist wound.

Transparent Film/Transparent Adhesive Dressings

Description and Characteristics

Transparent film dressings (also known as transparent adhesive dressings) are thin sheets of plastic with a layer of adhesive on one side or surface. The technology involved in production of the plastic/film renders these dressings semiocclusive or semipermeable. That is, they allow for moisture vapor transfer and atmospheric gas exchange while remaining impermeable to liquids, solids, and bacteria. They retain moisture at the wound surface because they have no absorptive capacity (a feature sometimes known as the "greenhouse effect"); this characteristic promotes autolytic debridement. Transparent film dressings are widely utilized as both primary and secondary dressings. They may be used to protect intravenous (IV) sites and newly healed wounds, as primary dressings for surface wounds that are dry or have very minimal exudate and as cover dressings for wounds with depth, especially when the wound is dry and a moisture-retentive cover dressing is needed. They are also a good cover dressing choice for wounds that are at risk for contamination from urine and stool, because they very effectively "waterproof" the dressing. Wear time is variable and depends upon wound depth, exudate, and location and whether the dressing is being used for protection, as a primary dressing, or as a cover dressing. When used as a primary dressing for a minimally exudative surface wound, a wear time of 3 to 7 days is considered adequate.

Transparent adhesive dressings are commonly utilized as the cover dressing for IV fluid cannula sites, so most clinicians are familiar with the application. Due to the moisture vapor and atmospheric gas exchange nature of these dressings, transparent film dressings may be used with necrotic and infected wounds with little risk of promoting an anaerobic environment. These dressings are available in a variety of sizes and shapes that conform to various anatomical locations. This conformability also allows the dressing to stay in place with body movement. The waterproofing feature makes these dressings an excellent choice for cover dressing.

Clinical Considerations

There is limited moisture vapor transfer from the wound bed to the external environment and these dressings have minimal to no absorptive capacity. Thus, these dressings are inappropriate as primary dressings for exudative wounds. When used to promote autolysis of desiccated tissue, the resulting liquefaction of the nonviable tissue yields an increased volume of wound exudate, which can cause maceration of the periwound skin. The liquefied nonviable tissue has been incorrectly assessed as purulent drainage. Wound care nurses, therefore, should provide education to caregivers and other health care providers regarding this phenomenon. When utilized as a secondary dressing or extra "tape" over exudative wounds, the moisture retention feature can occasionally require more frequent dressing changes. Due to the fairly aggressive adhesive feature of these dressings, removal may be a challenge. Transparent film dressings should not be "pulled back" across themselves as this action may result in skin stripping (Sussman, 2010). Instead, the dressing should be gently stretched at skin level allowing for adhesive release and then lifted.

CLINICAL PEARL

Transparent adhesive dressings have no absorptive capacity; they should be used only on dry wounds or as secondary (cover) dressings when a bacterial barrier is needed.

The wound nurse must provide proactive education of caregivers using these dressings to assure appropriate use. When these dressings are used for autolytic debridement of necrotic tissue, the nurse should avoid routine dressing changes since the goal is to create a fluid environment that supports autolysis. Instead, the clinician should monitor for lifting of the eschar and for fluid accumulation and should remove the dressing only when there is sufficient lifting of the eschar to permit sharp wound debridement or when fluid accumulation mandates dressing removal. It is critical to teach clinicians and other caregivers proper removal technique. In addition to the technique described above, it is sometimes necessary to use appropriate adhesive remover products to prevent trauma and pain with dressing removal.

BOX 8-1. Guidelines for Wound Classification

- Wounds with depth, tunnels, or undermining and moderate–large amounts of exudate: *deep/wet*
- Wounds with depth, tunnels, or undermining and minimal or no exudate: *deep/dry*
- Wounds that are shallow/superficial with no tunnels or undermining and moderate-to-large amounts of exudate: *shallow/wet*
- Wounds that are shallow/superficial with no tunnels or undermining and minimal or no exudate: *shallow/dry*

 Guidelines for Dressing Selection

Decision-making guidelines and a simple decision table can be used to facilitate product selection within a particular agency (Box 8-1 and **Table 8-1**). One effective approach to teaching staff how to use available dressings correctly is to list all of the available dressings at your agency and then

TABLE 8-1 Select Dressing Option from the Appropriate Grid

Deep Wet Wounds	Deep Dry Wounds
*Need: Absorptive filler + cover dressing to effectively manage drainage** **Filler Dressing** Options: • Calcium alginate (flat or rope) • Hydrofiber (flat or rope) • Copolymer • Gauze and specialty gauze (nonwoven, moistened, loosely fluffed) *If narrow tunnel, use "wick" **Cover Dressing** Options: • Gauze/tape (if wound exposed to contaminants, use transparent adhesive instead of tape) • Waterproof adhesive foam dressing (good choice when bacterial barrier needed)	*Need: Hydrating filler + cover dressing to provide effective moisture to the wound** **Filler Dressing** Options: • Liquid gel to wound bed + lightly fluffed damp saline gauze • Gel-soaked gauze fluffed into wound bed *If narrow tunnel, use "wick" **Cover Dressing** Options: • Gauze + transparent adhesive dressing • Waterproof adhesive foam dressing (both of these options prevent wound contamination and help keep wound bed moist)
Shallow Wet Wounds	**Shallow Dry Wounds**
Options *(may require both a primary and secondary dressing to be effective)*: • Foam dressing with adhesive border • Flat alginate + adhesive foam or alginate + wrap gauze • Hydrofiber + adhesive foam or hydrofiber + wrap gauze • Nonadherent contact layer (e.g., oil emulsion dressing, silicone weave dressing) + gauze cover • Textile dressing + wrap gauze	Options: • Solid hydrogels • Hydrocolloids • Transparent adhesive dressings • Nonadherent contact layer + gauze cover • Ointment (zinc oxide or balsam of peru/castor oil/trypsin)

place them within the appropriate category on the decision table. This will also enable you to identify any areas of duplication and/or gaps in your formulary. Streamlining your wound care formulary and simplifying the decision-making process will promote staff nurses' feelings of competence in wound care decision making and help to ensure appropriate dressing selection for individual patients.

Conclusion

The rapid advances in the science and technology underlying wound care and the myriad of advanced dressings now available enable the knowledgeable wound care nurse to provide evidence-based topical therapy to each patient with a wound. Essential parameters to be considered in dressing selection include the following: goals of treatment, depth of the wound, presence of tunnels or undermined areas, volume of exudate, need for an antimicrobial dressing, and need for a waterproof outer layer. Wounds with tunnels and depth require a wick, a filler, and a cover; wounds with depth but no tunnels require a filler and a cover; and wounds with no depth and no tunnels require only a cover. Wet wounds require absorptive dressings, while dry wounds require hydration. Wounds with signs of local infection or at high risk for infection are usually best managed with an antimicrobial primary dressing, and wounds exposed to urine or stool require a waterproof cover dressing.

REFERENCES

Agostinho, A. M., Hartman, A., Lipp, C., et al. (2011). An in vitro model for the growth and analysis of chronic wound MRSA biofilms. *Journal of Applied Microbiology, 111*(5), 1275–1282. doi: 10.1111/j.1365-2672.2011.05138.x

Atiyeh, B. S., Dibo, S. A., & Hayek, S. N. (2009). Wound cleansing, topical antiseptics and wound healing. *International Wound Journal, 6*, 420–430.

Avent, Y. (2010). Wound wise: Keep wounds moist with foam dressings. *Nursing Made Incredibly Easy!, 8*(1), 17–19.

Bradley, B. H., & Cunningham, M. (2013). Biofilms in chronic wounds and the potential role of negative pressure wound therapy: An integrative review. *Journal of Wound, Ostomy, & Continence Nursing 40*(2), pp. 143–149. doi: 10.1097/WON.0b013e31827e8481

Edlich, R. F., Rodeheaver, G. T., Thacker, J. G., et al. (2010). Revolutionary advances in the management of traumatic wounds in the emergency department during the past 40 years: Part I. *Journal of Emergency Medicine, 38*(1), 40–50. doi: 10.1016/j.jemermed.2008.09.029

Fellows, J., & Crestodina, L. (2006). Home prepared saline: A safe, cost-effective alternative for wound cleansing in home care. *Journal of Wound, Ostomy, and Continence Nursing, 33*(6), 606–609. doi: 10193-03_WJ3306-Fellows.qxd

Fernandez, R., & Griffiths, R. (2012). Water for wound cleansing: Review/Update of Cochrane database systematic review 2008. *Cochrane Database Systematic Reviews*, (2). doi: 10.1002/14651858.CD003861.pub3

Fonder, M. A., Lazarus, G. S., Cowan, D. A., et al. (2008). Treating the chronic wound: A practical approach to the care of nonhealing wounds and wound care dressings. *Journal of the American Academy of Dermatology, 58*(2), 185–206. doi: 10.1016/j.jaad.2007.08.048

Hashely, S. (2011, April). The use of superabsorbent containing fluid lock dressing to control odor in patients with malodorous ulcers in hospice population. The Symposium on Advanced Wound Care. Dallas, TX. Poster presentation.

Heggers, J. P., Sazy, J. A., Stenberg, B. D., et al. (1991). Bactericidal and wound-healing properties of sodium-hypochlorite solutions: The 1991 Lindberg Award. *Journal of Burn Care & Rehabilitation, 12I*(5), 420–424.

Hughes, M. S., Moghadamian, E. S., Yin, L-I, et al. (2012). Comparison of bulb syringe, pressurized pulsatile, and hydrosurgery debridement methods for removing bacteria from fracture implants. *Orthopedics, 35*(7), e1046–e1050. doi: 10.3928/01477447-20120621-19

Jhong, J. F., Venault, A, Liu, L. Z., et al. (2014, June 25). Introducing mixed-charge copolymers as wound dressing biomaterials. *ACS Appl Mater Interfaces, 6*(12):9858–9870. doi: 10.1021/am502382n

Sussman, G. (2010, September 1). Technology update: understanding film dressings. *Wounds International, 1*(4), 23–25.

Thomas, G. W., Rael, L. T., Bar-Or, R., et al. (2009). Mechanisms of delayed wound healing by commonly used antiseptics. *Journal of Trauma Injury, Infection, and Critical Care, 66*(1), 82–91. doi: 10.1097.TA.0b013e31818b146d

Vowden, P., Vowden, K., & Carville, K. (2011). Antimicrobial dressings made easy, *Wounds International*, (2):1.

Worley, C. (2005). So, what do I put on this wound? Making sense of the wound dressing puzzle: part 1. *Dermatology Nursing, 17*(2), 143–144.

QUESTIONS

1. A wound care nurse is initiating topical therapy for a patient with a wound infection. What is the ultimate goal of this treatment?
   A. Creating a local healing environment through wound cleansing and dressing
   B. Identifying and correcting systemic factors affecting wound repair
   C. Interrupting the cycle of injury by correcting etiologic factors
   D. Choosing the appropriate medication for the type of wound assessed

2. The wound nurse is assessing a patient's wound and documents: "wound is in the inflammatory stage with visible eschar and slough and large amounts of exudate." What is the goal in cleansing this wound?
   A. Flush away exudate without damaging the proliferative cells and newly formed tissues.
   B. Gradually scrape away dead tissue and slough without damaging healthy tissue.
   C. Remove as much devitalized tissue, bacteria, and exudate as possible without damaging viable tissue.
   D. Use a cytotoxic cleansing agent to irrigate the wound without disturbing granulation tissue.

3. The wound care nurse is monitoring the cleansing process of a necrotic wound. What technique is recommended?
   A. Use cytotoxic solution to gently flush the wound.
   B. Irrigate the wound with normal saline at < 5 psi force.
   C. Vigorously flush the wound with potable tap water.
   D. Irrigate the wound with 4 to 15 psi force; possibly with cytotoxic solution.

4. The wound care nurse is choosing a solution to irrigate a wound heavily infected with bacteria. What would be the best choice?
   A. Saline
   B. Sodium hypochlorite
   C. Potable/tap water
   D. Commercial cleansing solution

5. A patient has a gunshot wound infected with *Pseudomonas aeruginosa*. What would be the best cleansing solution for this patient?
   A. Acetic acid
   B. Sodium hypochlorite
   C. Bleach
   D. Normal saline

6. For what adverse wound condition would the nurse monitor when using saline-moistened gauze as a wound dressing?
   A. Dehiscence of the wound
   B. Tissue hypoxia
   C. Desiccation of the wound bed
   D. Hernia

7. The wound care nurse is choosing a dressing for a dehisced incision that measures 6 cm × 3 cm × 2 cm with areas of tunneling. What dressing would be an appropriate choice?
   A. "Wicking" agent, filler dressing, and cover dressing
   B. Filler dressing + cover dressing
   C. Cover dressing only
   D. Dressings are contraindicated for this type of wound.

8. A wound care nurse recommends a hydrater dressing for a wound. What would be the BEST choice?
   A. Adhesive foam dressing
   B. Calcium alginate dressing
   C. Hydrofiber dressing
   D. Hydrogel dressing

9. A patient wound requires an antimicrobial dressing. What intervention would the wound care nurse take when using this type of dressing?
   A. Obtain a culture before choosing the type of antimicrobial dressing to use on the wound.
   B. Use an antimicrobial dressing in lieu of antibiotics to treat a local wound infection.
   C. If significant improvement in wound status occurs after applying an antimicrobial dressing, use a higher dose to control bacterial load.
   D. If deterioration in wound status occurs, obtain a second culture to identify the offending organism.

10. Which type of dressing protects a wound from trauma and permits drainage to pass through to a secondary dressing?
   A. Contact layer dressing
   B. Alginate dressing
   C. Hydrofiber dressing
   D. Composite dressing

11. Which of the following is an advantage of using a foam dressing on a wound?
   A. It promotes autolysis of dry eschar.
   B. It is highly effective on minimally draining wounds.
   C. It can be used as either a primary or secondary dressing.
   D. It is one of the few dressings recommended for third-degree burns.

12. The wound nurse is choosing a dressing for a wound that is a deep, dry wound. What would be an appropriate choice?
   A. Liquid gel to wound bed plus lightly fluffed damp saline gauze
   B. Solid hydrogel dressing
   C. Transparent adhesive dressing
   D. Hydrofiber plus adhesive foam

ANSWERS: 1.**A**, 2.**C**, 3.**D**, 4.**B**, 5.**A**, 6.**C**, 7.**A**, 8.**D**, 9.**B**, 10.**A**, 11.**C**, 12.**A**

CHAPTER 9

Principles and Guidelines for Wound Debridement

Janet M. Ramundo

OBJECTIVES

1. Develop an individualized plan of care based on assessment data and current evidence-based guidelines that addresses each of the following factors:
   - Correction or amelioration of etiologic factors
   - Attention to systemic factors affecting the repair process
   - Evidence-based topical therapy
   - Pain management
   - Patient and caregiver education
2. Recommend or provide topical therapy based on best available evidence, to include
   - Debridement of necrotic tissue when indicated
   - Identification and management of wound-related infections
   - Management of epibole and hypertrophic granulation tissue
   - Selection of dressings to manage exudate and maintain moist wound surface
3. Demonstrate correct procedure for each of the following:
   - Conservative sharp wound debridement (CSWD)
   - Chemical cauterization
   - Wound cleansing/dressing application
   - Noninvasive wound culture
   - Application adjunctive therapies such as negative pressure wound therapy (NPWT)
4. Identify indications and contraindications to debridement.
5. Identify advantages, disadvantages, and guidelines for each of the following: CSWD, autolytic debridement, enzymatic debridement, chemical debridement, maggot debridement therapy, mechanical (wet to dry) debridement, ultrasonic debridement, and surgical debridement.

Topic Outline

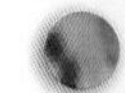 Introduction

As explained in previous chapters, elimination of necrotic tissue is a critical element of "wound bed preparation" when the goal is healing; this chapter addresses indications, contraindications, options, and guidelines for debridement. Debridement is the removal of necrotic tissue from a wound. Necrotic tissue is an impediment to healing, particularly in the chronic wound; removal of this tissue is essential to wound healing (Ramundo, 2012).

> **CLINICAL PEARL**
>
> Necrotic tissue interferes with healing and supports bacterial growth.

Necrotic tissue presents in two forms: eschar (the hard leathery form) and slough (the soft yellow form) (Figs. 9-1 and 9-2). The components of necrotic tissue include avascular tissue, fibrinous exudate, and bacteria; these substances support bacterial growth and interfere with repair. Debridement (removal of eschar and slough) is an essential component of wound bed preparation. A wound containing necrotic material remains in the inflammatory phase of wound healing and is at increased risk of infection. Debridement allows visualization of the wound base, reduces the chance for infection, reduces odor, and allows the wound healing process to continue.

Many factors must be considered when determining the best approach to debridement, including the type of necrotic material in the wound base. Wounds containing slough will respond to autolysis, enzymatic debriding agents, maggot therapy, chemical debridement, and conservative sharp wound debridement. Eschar can be removed by autolysis, enzyme application (following crosshatching of the eschar), and instrumental debridement, either conservative sharp wound debridement or surgical debridement. Infected wounds require special consideration; that is, the goal is rapid debridement that does not cause further harm to the surrounding tissue. Surgical debridement is often indicated (along with antibiotic therapy); if surgical intervention is contraindicated, "slower" approaches to debridement can be utilized (e.g., enzymatic, maggot, and conservative sharp wound debridement) so long as infection is controlled with concomitant antibiotic therapy. These methods are discussed in further detail later in this chapter.

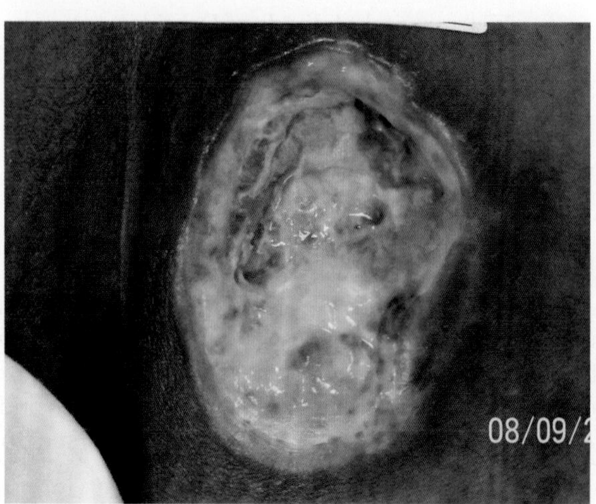

FIGURE 9-1. Slough.

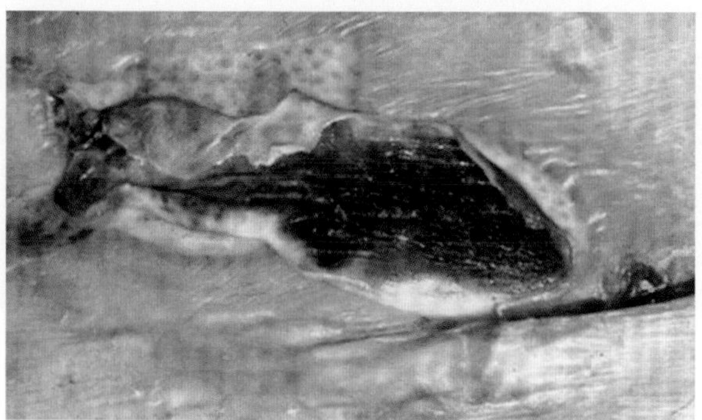

FIGURE 9-2. Eschar and slough.

Decision Making Regarding Debridement

Contraindications to Debridement

The wound nurse must be aware that there are situations in which debridement is actually contraindicated. The most important contraindication is the poorly perfused wound, such as an uninfected foot ulcer in a patient with advanced LEAD. In this situation, removal of the eschar would convert the wound from closed to open and would significantly increase the risk of infection. In addition, removal of the eschar would provide no benefit, because a poorly perfused wound does not progress to healing. Thus, current guidelines state that this wound should be left closed and monitored for any signs of infection. (Development of infection usually mandates removal of the necrotic tissue, since necrotic tissue supports bacterial growth.) Another situation in which debridement is usually contraindicated is a heel wound with dry eschar in a nonambulatory patient; the eschar is left intact as long as there are no signs of infection. Occasionally, intact eschar is left on a trunk wound as well when there are no signs of infection and other care priorities take precedence. If the eschar begins to separate or the wound shows signs of infection, then proceeding with debridement is recommended.

> **CLINICAL PEARL**
>
> Debridement is contraindicated in a closed uninfected wound that is poorly perfused and may be contraindicated in other situations in which the goal of care is maintenance or comfort as opposed to healing.

Selecting the Best Approach to Debridement

Other factors will guide the clinician in selecting the most appropriate method for removal of necrotic tissue. Foremost should be a consideration of the individual goals of care for the patient. In end-of-life care, the decision may be to forego removal of necrotic tissue and a focus on healing and to focus instead on comfort measures. Another example might be a patient with an intact eschar on the

BOX 9-1. Questions to Ask When Considering Debridement

- What are the goals of care for this patient? *Comfort versus healing*
- What is the care setting of the patient? *May impact product selection, reimbursement, safety*
- Where is the wound? *Heel ulcer must be assessed for perfusion*
- What type of necrotic tissue? *Eschar versus slough; impact on type of debridement*
- Is the wound infected? *May require concomitant antibiotic treatment*
- Who will be providing the care/performing debridement? *Skill level and license*

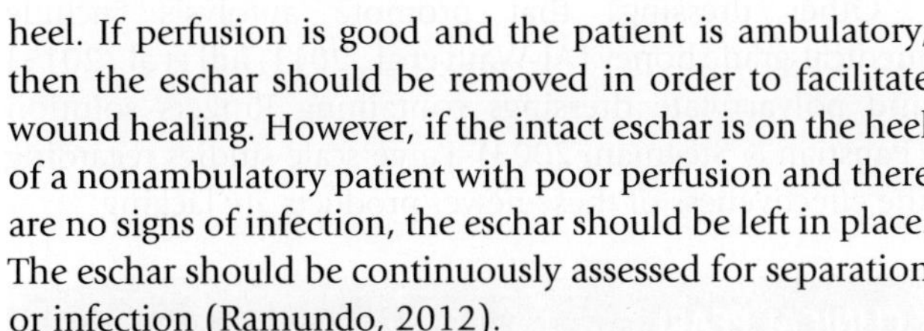

heel. If perfusion is good and the patient is ambulatory, then the eschar should be removed in order to facilitate wound healing. However, if the intact eschar is on the heel of a nonambulatory patient with poor perfusion and there are no signs of infection, the eschar should be left in place. The eschar should be continuously assessed for separation or infection (Ramundo, 2012).

Clinician level and skill will also factor into the debridement method selection process. Conservative sharp wound debridement and surgical debridement require specialized training, whereas the application of enzymes to the wound or application of dressings to enhance autolytic debridement may be safely taught to nurses, nursing assistants, and caregivers. The care setting is another important consideration. A nurse considering debridement options in home care might elect a more conservative approach to debridement than the nurse practicing in acute care, due to the difference in access to resources. Autolytic debridement and enzymatic debridement are typical choices in the home setting, whereas surgical debridement or serial conservative sharp wound debridement is frequently used in the acute care setting.

Decision making about the method of debridement is often a challenge for clinicians as there is limited guidance regarding the best methods and many factors to consider. The few studies that have been done have different end points (healing vs. amount of debridement), are limited in scope, or are in vitro (lab) studies; thus, they fail to provide any definitive evidence as to the best approach for an individual patient.

See Box 9-1 for critical questions to be addressed when considering debridement.

Progression and Maintenance of Debridement

The wound must be closely monitored during the debridement process. The wound nurse should monitor for the removal of necrotic tissue, and this should be documented at each assessment. Necrotic tissue in the wound bed is typically expressed as a percentage of the total wound bed.

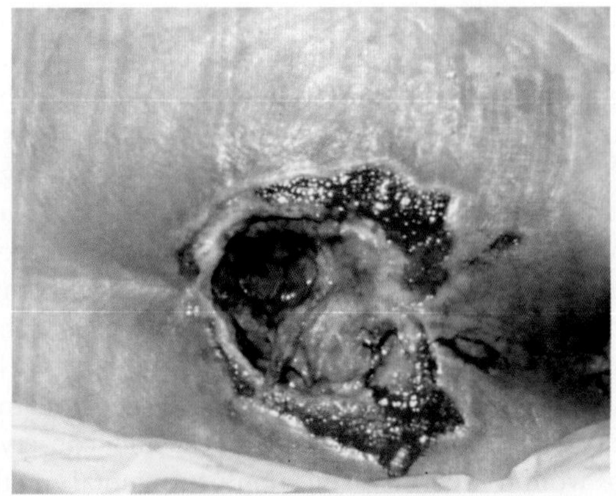

FIGURE 9-3. Soft eschar.

It should be noted that the wound dimensions typically increase as the necrotic tissue is removed from the wound. Early in the debridement process, the wound is commonly exudative; the volume of exudate typically decreases as the necrotic tissue is removed. As debridement progresses, there should be increasing exposure of healthy viable tissue in the wound base. Regardless of the type of debridement utilized, a gradual transition in the type of necrotic tissue present in the wound is typically observed. Eschar gradually softens, and densely adherent slough loosens and becomes more moist in appearance (Fig. 9-3). Postdebridement, there should also be a reduction in signs of infection (e.g., periwound erythema and induration) in an infected wound, especially when the patient is also being treated with systemic antibiotics. Typically, wound debridement is discontinued when all necrotic tissue is removed from the wound base; the wound nurse will then select appropriate topical therapy based on the characteristics of the clean wound bed.

Some clinical experts propose continuing debridement even when the wound bed is visibly free of necrotic tissue, particularly in recalcitrant wounds (those that fail to respond to moist wound healing) (Falanga et al., 2008). This theory of maintenance debridement is based on findings from clinical trials involving diabetic foot ulcers, in which healing rates were improved when sharp debridement was performed more frequently (Steed et al., 1996). Similar results were observed in a study involving 27 nursing home residents with full-thickness pressure ulcers, in which collagenase provided superior results to hydrogel even though the wounds were free of visible necrotic tissue (Milne et al., 2012). This concept requires further study to determine the effectiveness and safety of maintenance debridement and to develop guidelines for the wound nurse, who must decide whether to recommend advanced wound therapy versus maintenance debridement.

Types of Debridement

Debridement is often categorized as selective or nonselective or instrumental versus noninstrumental. Selective debridement methods remove only necrotic material from the wound bed and leave healthy tissue intact. Examples of selective debridement include autolysis, enzymatic, maggot therapy, and conservative sharp wound debridement. Nonselective debridement methods, such as surgical debridement, remove both viable and nonviable tissue from the wound bed. If the wound is debrided to the point of bleeding, it is theorized that the subsequent release of platelet-derived growth factors may stimulate wound repair. Other examples of nonselective debridement include wet-to-dry mechanical debridement, high-pressure irrigation, and ultrasound debridement. Instrumental debridement includes surgical and conservative sharp wound debridement; noninstrumental methods include autolysis, enzymatic, chemical, maggot therapy, hydrotherapy, and ultrasonic debridement. Each method of debridement has a unique mechanism of action and indications and considerations for selection and use.

CLINICAL PEARL

Surgical debridement to the point of bleeding may stimulate healing via the release of platelet-derived growth factors.

Noninstrumental Methods of Debridement

As noted, noninstrumental methods of debridement are widely used owing to their safety and availability. The various types of noninstrumental debridement are discussed individually.

Autolysis

Autolysis involves the removal of necrotic tissue by the body's own white blood cells and natural enzymes, which migrate to the wound site during the normal inflammatory process. The body's proteolytic, fibrinolytic, and collagenolytic enzymes are released to digest the devitalized tissue present in the wound while leaving the healthy tissue intact (Rodeheaver et al., 1994). Autolysis occurs naturally when the wound is kept in a moist, vascular environment with adequate leukocyte function. Because autolysis relies on white blood cells in the wound, there must be perfusion to the area and an adequate white blood cell count.

Autolysis is generally considered a safe though slow method of debridement. It is most effective on slough, and, because it is slow, it is generally considered more appropriate for noninfected wounds.

Examples of dressings that support autolysis include transparent film dressings, polyacrylate dressings, medicinal honey dressings, hydrogels (amorphous and sheet dressings), and any topical agent that adds and/or maintains a moist wound bed. Studies comparing autolysis to other methods of debridement are difficult to interpret as they use different end points as outcomes measures; many studies focus on healing rather than the effectiveness of debridement (Jull et al., 2013). Konig et al. (2005) report that autolysis compares favorably to other methods of debridement in terms of effectiveness; however, autolytic debridement is slower than some alternative methods, such as mechanical and sharp. A multicenter randomized trial conducted by Burgos et al. (2000) showed no significant difference in healing of stage III pressure ulcers managed with a hydrocolloid for autolysis and those managed with a commercially prepared topical enzyme. In contrast, another randomized study comparing the same products (hydrocolloid and enzyme) in management of stage IV pressure ulcers on the heel following surgical debridement found that the enzyme provided faster results (Müller et al., 2001). Milne et al. (2010) also compared autolytic debridement (using hydrogel) to enzymatic debridement in 27 patients with pressure ulcers and also reported faster results with the enzyme.

Other dressings that promote autolysis include medical-grade honey (Al-Waili et al., 2011; Jull et al., 2013) and polyacrylate dressings containing Ringers solution (Paustian & Stegman, 2003). Large-scale studies regarding the effectiveness of these newer products are lacking.

CLINICAL PEARL

Autolytic debridement involves breakdown of necrotic tissue via the body's own WBCs and enzymes; it requires a moist wound surface and normal WBC counts.

Guidelines for Autolytic Debridement

Typically, the wound is cleansed with normal saline or wound cleanser; the moisture retentive dressing is then applied and monitored for excessive drainage. There is typically a significant amount of drainage during the early phases of autolysis, due to liquefaction of the slough and other debris; thus, the periwound area usually needs to be protected from maceration by the application of a liquid skin barrier. Frequency of dressing changes will be determined by the amount of drainage, in accordance with the manufacturer's guidelines for the particular dressing selected. For example, although medical-grade honey dressings may generally be left in place for up to 7 days, the drainage and potential for maceration may necessitate more frequent changes. Education is essential so that the patient, family, and other caregivers will know to expect the increased drainage and to alleviate concerns that the drainage is indicative of infection. The wound should be assessed at each dressing change for reduction in the amount of necrotic tissue, volume of exudate, and any signs of infection. The time frame for results with autolysis varies depending on the size of the wound and the amount and type of necrotic tissue. Generally, the softening and separating of necrotic tissue is observed within days.

Enzymatic Debridement

Topical application of enzymes is another selective method of debridement. The only currently available enzyme debriding agent in the United States is collagenase, which is derived from clostridium bacteria. Collagenase digests the denatured collagen in necrotic tissue by dissolving the collagen "anchors" that secure the necrotic tissue to the underlying wound bed (Howes et al., 1959).

Enzymatic debridement is a safe choice with infected wounds, especially when the patient is also receiving antibiotic therapy. Collagenase can also be effectively used with selected topical antibiotics and antibacterial dressings; studies have demonstrated compatibility between collagenase and topical antibiotics, such as polymyxin B/bacitracin and mupirocin, and with selected antibacterial dressings (e.g., PVA dressings containing crystal violet and methylene blue and sodium hypochlorite solutions). However, the wound nurse must be aware that collagenase is *not* compatible with iodine products and with many silver-based products (Jovanovic et al., 2012; Konig et al., 2005; Ramundo & Gray, 2009). The length of time required to achieve debridement may range from several days to weeks. Early studies have shown collagenase to be an effective debriding agent for peripheral arterial ulcers and pressure ulcers (Boxer et al., 1969), and as noted above, recent studies indicate that collagenase may provide faster debridement when compared to autolysis (Milne et al., 2010).

Collagenase is applied to the necrotic tissue in the wound bed every 24 hours. With that in mind, the cover dressing should be one that it is practical to change every 24 hours. Care must be taken to avoid dressings with silver as this will inactivate the enzyme. Certain cleansers will also deactivate the enzymatic activity; products should be selected carefully, and the manufacturer's guidelines should be followed (Jovanovic et al., 2012).

The current manufacturer recommends a nickel thick application of the enzyme, covered with a moist normal saline dressing or a moisture-retentive dressing. The product is most effective at a wound bed pH of 6.0 to 8.0 but has been demonstrated to be effective in a pH range up to 9.5 (Shi et al., 2011). There is currently no practical way to measure pH in the wound bed; however, pH issues must be considered if the product does not appear to be effective.

CLINICAL PEARL

Enzymatic debridement requires nickel thick application of the enzyme, a moist wound environment, and avoidance of antiseptics that inactivate the enzyme, such as iodine and many silver dressings.

The enzyme should be continued as long as there is necrotic tissue visible in the wound bed; the product is generally discontinued once the wound bed is clean. Collagenase works most effectively on slough; when used on eschar, the nurse must first crosshatch the eschar to permit the collagenase to penetrate to the collagen anchoring

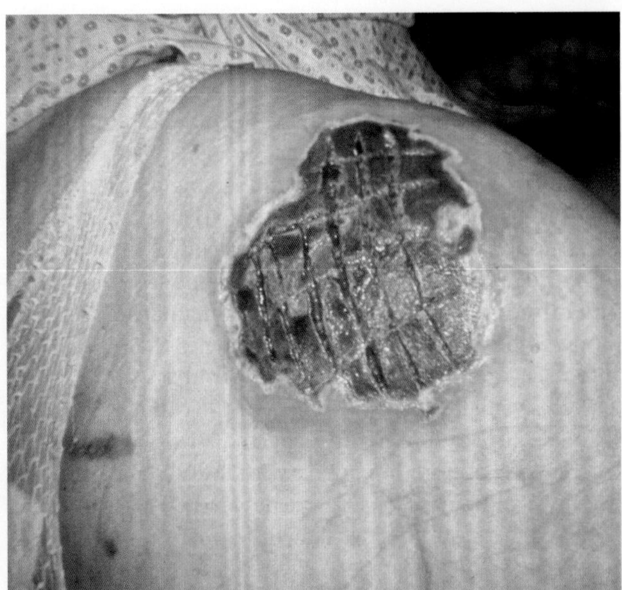

FIGURE 9-4. Eschar that has been crosshatched prior to application of enzyme.

strands (Fig. 9-4). Another option is to apply the enzyme to the periphery of the eschar (if it has begun to lift from the wound bed); this will promote further lifting of the eschar, which then allows for conservative sharp wound debridement. If prescribed for a home care patient, the patient or family member is taught the application of the product and cover dressing. Enzymes are often used in conjunction with serial conservative wound debridement. Enzymes are a prescription item, so the cost is another consideration; however, there are studies that show enzymatic debridement to be a cost-effective treatment (Waycaster & Milne, 2013; Woo et al., 2013).

Maggot Therapy

Maggot therapy is a method of debridement that involves the application of sterile larvae of the *Lucilia sericata* (green bottle fly) to a wound with necrotic tissue. The larvae secrete enzymes that digest the necrotic tissue without harming the viable tissue in the wound bed. It is often used with infected necrotic wounds, particularly if surgical debridement is not an option. Maggot therapy is often referred to as MDT (maggot debridement therapy), LDT (larval debridement therapy), or biosurgical debridement. Maggot therapy has been described in historical literature, particularly in battlefield use; its use in debridement was documented during the Civil War and in WWI. With the advent of antibiotics in the 1940s the use of MDT declined. There is renewed interest now, due to the rise in antibiotic-resistant bacteria (Courtenay, 2000).

CLINICAL PEARL

There are anecdotal reports of successful use of maggots for debridement and for biofilm removal; more data are needed.

There are many anecdotal reports of success with the use of MDT; however, large-scale studies are lacking. Some recent studies have noted successful removal of biofilm with MDT, which may hold some promise (Cowan, 2012). A large-scale study of venous ulcers (VenUS II) concluded that there was no difference in healing rates between MDT and hydrogel despite more rapid debridement in the MDT group (Dumville, 2009). Another study compared MDT to hydrogel (autolysis) in lower extremity wounds (VLU and mixed) and found improved healing rates with MDT, along with less frequent dressing changes that may factor into decision making. However, larger ulcers did not heal as well as smaller ones regardless of the choice of therapy (Mudge, 2013). In summary, maggot therapy appears to be a promising option for patients with infected wounds who are not candidates for surgery; however, it has not been shown to be more effective than other methods of debridement (Gray, 2008; Zarachi & Gergor, 2012).

Guidelines for MDT

Medical grade, sterilized maggots are applied directly to the wound and covered with a containment dressing; the recommended "dose" is approximately 5 to 8 larvae per cm^2. There are commercially available containment dressings from the distributor of the larvae, or dressings may be designed for this purpose. Typically, the periwound skin is protected with a hydrocolloid-type dressing, and a small aperture mesh dressing is applied over the wound (and the larvae) and secured to the hydrocolloid border. It is critical to assure that the cover dressing permits oxygen delivery to the wound bed, to prevent death of the larvae. Drainage will be moderate to large in volume as the necrotic tissue is liquefied.

A major concern about use of MDT is the possible aversion to this therapy by the patient and caregivers. In addition, pain and bleeding have been reported with the use of MDT (Mudge, 2013; Steenvorde & van Doorn, 2008; Steenvorde et al., 2005), so careful assessment is essential for the duration of therapy, particularly in patients on anticoagulation therapy.

Chemical Debridement

Sodium hypochlorite (Dakin's solution) has been theorized to promote debridement. Sodium hypochlorite has mostly been studied for cleansing properties rather than debridement but may be a viable option for use in an infected necrotic wound. It is thought that Dakin's solution will loosen the anchoring strands holding eschar on the wound and allow for easier removal. In addition, it is effective against most bacteria, yeast, and viruses; reduces odor; and is relatively inexpensive to use. The most common concentration is 0.25%, but this strength should not be used in a clean wound as it will destroy fibroblasts. Heggers et al. (1991) noted that at 0.0125%, the solution provides effective antimicrobial action without destroying fibroblasts. Other studies have challenged the debridement qualities of sodium hypochlorite (Thomas, 1991), and some authors state that the concentration and frequency needed to facilitate removal of necrotic tissue is impractical and possibly harmful to the wound. In clinical practice, Dakin's is typically used in heavily necrotic wounds particularly when infection and odor are a concern. Dakin's should be applied to gauze until it is moderately wet, packed lightly into the wound with a cover dressing, and changed every 12 hours. The solution should be contained in a colored bottle away from light as it breaks down easily. Commercial solutions are available now with stabilizers, which eliminate concerns about stability. Dakin's solution dressings should be considered short term while the wound is treated for infection and debrided; once concerns about infection are eliminated, another method of debridement should be considered.

CLINICAL PEARL

Chemical debridement using sodium hypochlorite and similar agents is typically reserved for wounds that are necrotic, infected, and malodorous; use remains controversial.

Hydrotherapy

Hydrotherapy involves the use of water or other fluid to cleanse and possibly loosen necrotic tissue in an attempt to remove it from the wound bed. There are few studies that look at irrigation or hydrotherapy as a method of debridement; most focus on the cleansing properties of the fluid. Historically, whirlpool has been used as a mechanical method of debridement. However, most recent guidelines do not mention whirlpool as a recommended option for debridement (NPUAP-EPUAP, 2009; Robson et al., 2006; Steed et al., 2006; WOCN, 2010, 2011, 2012, 2014). Concerns about cross-contamination as well as the development of alternate methods have largely eliminated whirlpool as a method of cleaning or debriding a wound.

Wound irrigation and pulsatile lavage involve debridement of necrotic tissue with fluid and between 4 to 15 pounds per square inch (psi) of pressure, which is adequate to remove debris from the wound bed without damaging healthy tissue or inoculating the underlying tissue with bacteria (Hopf et al., 2006; Robson et al., 2006; Steed et al., 2006; WOCN, 2010). The wound nurse should be aware that delivery of fluid under pressure can cause aerosolization and dissemination of wound bacteria over a wide area, exposing the patient and care provider to potential contamination. Consequently, the care provider should wear personal protective equipment (mask, gloves, gown, goggles) while performing irrigation (NPUAP-EPUAP, 2009). Wound irrigation may be accomplished using a 19-gauge angiocatheter and a 35-mL syringe, or with prepackaged canisters of pressurized saline or products that attach to saline bags for continuous low-pressure irrigation (WOCN, 2010).

A *pulsatile lavage* machine combines intermittent high-pressure lavage with suction to loosen necrotic tissue and facilitate its removal (Morgan & Hoelscher, 2000). Pulsatile lavage is effective for removing larger amounts of debris and should be discontinued once the wound is clean. Pulsatile lavage should be used with caution to prevent damage to blood vessels, graft sites, and exposed muscle, tendon, and bone. Patients on anticoagulant therapy should be observed carefully for any bleeding, and treatment should be discontinued immediately if bleeding occurs. Disadvantages of debridement with pulsatile lavage include cost and time. The hose and tip are designed for one-time use, and large necrotic wounds may require twice-daily treatments. Pulsatile lavage treatment should be delivered in an enclosed area separate from any other patients to prevent contamination with mist (Maragakis et al., 2004). Once the wound bed is clean, pulsed lavage is usually discontinued, and the wound is assessed for topical therapy that will support the goals of healing. Pulsed lavage is often combined with other methods of debridement such as conservative sharp wound debridement, enzyme application, or selection of a dressing that supports autolytic debridement. It is typically utilized three to seven times per week and is often performed by physical therapists who are certified in wound care.

Wet-to-Dry Gauze

Wet-to-dry debridement is a mechanical, nonselective method of debridement. This method can be painful and may damage newly formed viable tissue; it is therefore generally considered suboptimal therapy (Hopf et al., 2006; Ovington, 2001; Robson et al., 2006; Steed et al., 2006). If wet-to-dry debridement must be used, it is most appropriate with heavily necrotic and infected wounds *without* visible granulation tissue. Correct technique consists of lightly packing moistened open weave, cotton gauze in the wound bed, and allowing it to dry on the wound, to trap debris and necrotic tissue. Once dry, usually 4 to 6 hours after application, the dressing is pulled off the wound along with the trapped debris and necrotic tissue. The gauze should not be moistened prior to removal. The wound is then cleansed, and the process is repeated. Wet-to-dry gauze debridement requires dressing changes several times per day until all necrotic tissue is removed. The perception that wet–dry debridement is cost-effective may not be accurate once caregiver time is factored into the equation. Woo et al. (2013) compared the cost of various methods of debridement and noted mechanical wet-to-dry debridement as one of the most costly methods.

CLINICAL PEARL

Mechanical debridement using wet-to-dry gauze is nonselective and painful; it is generally considered contraindicated.

Moist to damp is often the method employed when gauze dressings are used and may promote autolysis; however, this approach is also not cost-effective when the time to add fluid to the dressing is factored in. In addition, there are no studies to support moist to damp gauze dressings as a method of autolytic debridement.

Ultrasound

Ultrasound uses acoustic energy to remove necrotic tissue from the wound bed and promote healing. Contact ultrasound used for debridement may be either high or low frequency and uses saline coupled with the acoustic wave to produce mechanical and thermal effects (Fig. 9-5). For example, low-frequency ultrasound with high intensity produces cavitation, which may cause breakdown of fibrin (Madhok et al., 2013; Stanisic et al., 2005). This debridement effect is *not* seen when there is no contact with the wound, as in low-frequency, low-intensity, noncontact ultrasound. A review of the literature on the use of ultrasound revealed insufficient evidence to determine its effectiveness in debridement (Cullum et al., 2010; Ramundo & Gray, 2008), although a positive impact on healing has been noted (Kavros et al., 2008).

Instrumental Methods of Debridement

Instrumental methods of debridement have the advantage of providing faster elimination of necrotic tissue. Instrumental methods include surgical approaches and conservative sharp debridement at the bedside; surgical debridement is typically a one-step approach to debridement, while conservative sharp debridement is usually used in conjunction with noninstrumental approaches.

Surgical Debridement

Surgical debridement is the nonselective removal of large amounts of necrotic tissue with a scalpel, laser, or water (hydrosurgery). It typically is performed in the operating room or special procedures area, and the patient is frequently anesthetized. It is the debridement method recommended for wounds with advancing cellulitis, wound-related sepsis, large amounts of necrotic tissue, and/or infected bone or hardware that must be removed (NPUAP-EPUAP, 2009). It is the most rapid way to remove large amounts of necrotic tissue.

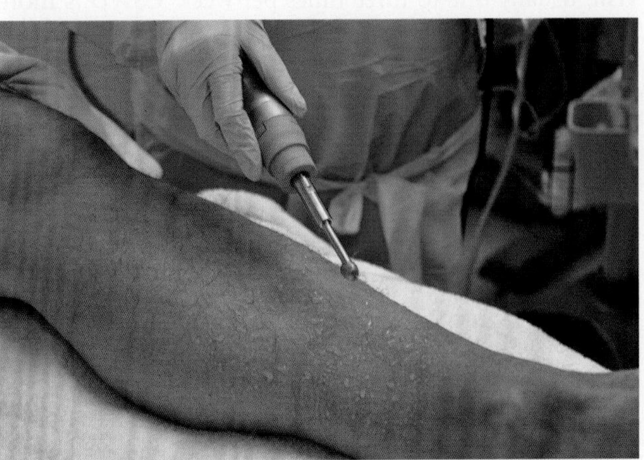

FIGURE 9-5. Contact ultrasound debridement.

Risk must be considered as the patient will likely need to have anesthesia, and there is the potential for bleeding and infection. Surgical debridement requires a high skill level and should be performed by a surgeon or advanced practice nurse with training in surgical debridement.

In additional to traditional debridement with a scalpel, new surgical methods of debridement are available. *Laser debridement,* a form of surgical debridement, uses focused beams of light to slice through tissue. Advantages of laser debridement are that the wound bed is sterilized and instantly cauterized (Flemming et al., 1986). Animal studies using a laser to debride partial-thickness burns have demonstrated results similar to those of sharp debridement but with hemostasis and no disturbance of periwound skin (Graham et al., 2002; Lam et al., 2002). Disadvantages of laser debridement include risk of injury to adjacent healthy tissue; however, newer pulsed lasers have reduced that risk (Glatter et al., 1998; Smith et al., 1997).

The *hydrosurgical water knife* is a method of surgical debridement that dispenses normal saline at high power, which provides debridement and cleansing of the wound base. This water jet device is regulated so that the clinician is able to precisely control the depth of debridement; debris from the wound is removed at the same time. The main advantage to hydrosurgery over traditional surgery is the shorter time required with similar outcomes; the shorter time contributes to the cost-effectiveness of the method (Caputo et al., 2008; Gravante et al., 2007).

Conservative Sharp Wound Debridement

Conservative sharp wound debridement (CSWD) is a method for the removal of loosely adherent necrotic tissue using sterile instruments such as scalpel, forceps, and scissors (See Box 9-2).

By definition, CSWD is confined to nonviable tissue so no blood loss is anticipated. It is typically used with other methods of debridement and done serially. For example, a wound care specialist might remove necrotic slough from a wound bed, then apply an enzyme to the wound bed along with a dressing that will support autolytic debridement. CSWD would be performed at each professional visit, usually one to three times per week. CSWD is more rapid than noninstrumental methods but slower than surgical removal. Since only necrotic tissue is removed, it is considered selective.

CLINICAL PEARL

CSWD may be used in conjunction with noninstrumental forms of debridement to facilitate wound "cleanup"; the clinician must assure that she or he is covered to do CSWD by the state nurse practice act and must rule out any conditions that would be contraindications.

BOX 9-2. CSWD Procedure

Conservative Sharp Wound Debridement Procedure

1. Review medical record to assure MD order and to rule out clotting abnormalities.
2. Perform clinical assessment to rule out contraindications such as ischemia or active cellulitis.
3. Obtain informed consent and complete time out process (if required).
4. Wash hands; apply clean gloves.
5. Set up clean field with sterile scalpel and sterile forceps/ pickups or hemostats.
6. Position the patient for comfort; drape appropriately.
7. Prep wound with povidone–iodine solution or alternative antiseptic; allow to dry.
8. Remove gloves. Sanitize the hands, and apply clean gloves.
9. Grasp loose necrotic tissue, and hold tautly so that line of dissection is clearly visualized. Use scalpel or scissors to establish plane of dissection and to cut away loose necrotic tissue.
10. Flush wound with saline following procedure, and apply appropriate dressing.

Throughout Procedure

1. Avoid all vascular structures and any structures/tissues not clearly identified.
2. Monitor patient tolerance, and discontinue procedure if evidence of pain or discomfort.
3. Control minor bleeding with direct pressure and/or silver nitrate.

Documentation

1. Wound status at the beginning and end of the procedure.
2. Procedure performed.
3. Patient tolerance and any adverse effects (bleeding or pain).

From Wound, Ostomy and Continence Nurses (WOCN Society). (2005). *Conservative sharp wound debridement: Best practice for clinicians.* Mt. Laurel, NJ: Author

Conservative sharp debridement has several advantages. It removes the necrotic tissue more quickly than the previously discussed methods, and it can be accomplished in a serial manner. This method of debridement can be combined with other debridement techniques (autolysis or enzymatic) to shorten this phase of wound care. Theoretically, a more rapid approach to debridement decreases the body's expenditure of energy during a time of high resource use.

Because of the low risk involved, conservative sharp debridement in many states is a delegated medical function that can be performed in a variety of settings by a clinician who is competent and credentialed in the technique. Therefore, conservative sharp debridement is a viable option for patients residing in nonacute care settings without the need for transfer to a hospital. A variety of requirements may need to be satisfied, depending on the nurse practice act specific to the state and the employer's requirements.

A disadvantage of conservative sharp debridement is that, depending on the size of the ulcer and the amount of necrotic tissue involved, it could conceivably take weeks to remove all of the nonviable tissue. The procedure may be uncomfortable for the patient, so the need for analgesia should be considered. Blood loss is not expected during conservative sharp debridement but remains a possibility. As a result, the patient should be assessed for factors that place him or her at risk for clotting problems if a small vessel is accidentally severed. Factors to consider include medications (e.g., anticoagulants, high-dose nonsteroidal anti-inflammatory drugs) and pathologic conditions (e.g., thrombocytopenia, impaired hepatic function, vitamin K deficiency, malnutrition). When any of these factors are present, the wound specialist should confer with the provider before proceeding with conservative sharp debridement. Another consideration prior to conservative sharp wound debridement is the presence of active wound infection; in this case, inadvertent vascular access could cause a bacteremia. Most clinicians either delay CSWD until the periwound cellulitis is under control or are very conservative when debriding these wounds to eliminate the risk of vascular access.

Professional Practice Considerations

Although debridement methods such as autolysis, wound irrigation, wet-to-dry dressings, and enzymes ideally are initiated under the direction of the provider or wound care specialist, they are procedures that can be performed by nurses, physical therapists, the patient, and caregivers. However, the more aggressive methods of debridement, specifically sharp debridement, require a greater level of skill and competence. Conservative sharp debridement should be performed only by a wound specialist or provider with demonstrated and documented competence. Although there is currently no certification for debridement, most institutions will require evidence of didactic and clinical education. In addition, many will require demonstration of competency at designated intervals. Most state boards of nursing do not address this function specifically. The wound nurse should ensure that there is a policy in place that states who is able to perform CSWD and a written procedure that is approved by the institution.

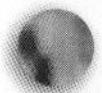

Conclusion

Debridement is a critical component of topical therapy for necrotic wounds. The wound nurse should be knowledgeable about the various methods available for debridement and should consider options based on goals of care, wound assessment, and skill level of involved clinicians. Debridement methods are often combined and modified as the wound conditions change. Continual, accurate wound assessments during the debridement phase are essential to ensure an outcome consistent with the stated wound goals.

REFERENCES

Al-Waili, N., et al. (2011). Honey for wound healing, ulcers and burns; data supporting its use in clinical practice. *The Scientific World Journal, 11*, 766–787.

Boxer, A. M., et al. (1969). Debridement of dermal ulcers and decubiti with collagenase. *Geriatrics, 24*(7), 75–86.

Burgos, A., et al. (2000). Cost, efficacy, efficiency and tolerability of collagenase ointment versus hydrocolloid occlusive dressing in the treatment of pressure ulcers: a comparative, randomised, multicenter study. *Clinical Drug Investigation, 19*(5), Available at http://link.springer.com/article/10.2165/00044011-200019050-00006. Accessed May 10, 2014.

Caputo, W. J., et al. (2008). A prospective randomised controlled clinical trial comparing hydrosurgery debridement with conventional surgical debridement in lower extremity ulcers. *International Wound Journal, 5*(2), 288–294.

Courtenay, M., Church, J., Ryan, T. (2000). Larva therapy in wound management. *Journal of Royal Society of Medicine, 93*, 72–74.

Cullum, N., Al-Kurdi, D., Bell-Syer, S. E. M. (2010). Therapeutic ultrasound for venous leg ulcers. *Cochrane Database of Systematic Reviews, 6*, CD001180. DOI: 10.1002/14651858.CD001180.pub3

Cowan, T. (2012). Visible biofilms: a controversial issue! *Journal of Wound Care, 21*(3), 106.

Dumville, J., Worthy, G., Soares, M., et al. (2009). VenUS II: a randomized controlled trial of larval therapy in the management of leg ulcers. *Health Technology Assessment, 13*(55), 1–182.

Falanga, V., et al. (2008). Maintenance debridement in the treatment of difficult to heal wounds, recommendations of an expert panel. *Ostomy Wound Management*, June(Suppl), 2–13.

Flemming, A., et al. (1986). Skin edge necrosis in irradiated tissue after carbon dioxide laser excision of tumor. *Lasers in Medical Sciences, 1*, 263–265.

Glatter, D., et al. (1998). Carbon dioxide laser ablation with immediate auto-grafting in a full-thickness porcine burn model. *Annals of Surgery, 228*(2), 257.

Graham, J. S., et al. (2002). Efficacy of laser debridement with autologous split-thickness skin grafting in promoting improved healing of deep cutaneous sulfur mustard burns. *Burns, 28*, 719.

Gravante, G., et al. (2007). Versajet hydrosurgery versus classic escharectomy for burn débridment: A prospective randomized trial. *Journal of Burn Care & Research, 28*(5), 720–724.

Gray, M. (2008). Is larval (maggot) debridement effective for removal of necrotic tissue from chronic wounds? *Journal of Wound Ostomy & Continence Nursing, 35*(4), 378.

Heggers, J., Sazy, J., Stenberg, B., et al. (1991). Bactericidal and wound-healing properties of sodium sypochlorite solutions: The 1991 Lindberg award. *Journal of Burn Care & Rehabilitation, 12*, 420–424.

Hopf, H. W., et al. (2006). Guidelines for the treatment of arterial insufficiency ulcers. *Wound Repair and Regeneration, 14*(6), 693–710.

Howes, E. L., et al. (1959). The use of clostridium histolyticum enzymes in the treatment of experimental third degree burns. *Surgery Gynecology & Obstetrics, 109*, 177.

Jovanovic, A., et al. (2012). The influence of metal salts, surfactants, and wound care products on enzymatic activity of collagenase, the wound debriding enzyme. *Wounds, 24*(9), 242–253.

Jull, A. B., et al. (2013). Honey as a topical treatment for wounds. *Cochrane Database of Systematic Reviews, 2*, CD005083.

Kavros, S. J., et al. (2008). Expedited wound healing with noncontact low frequency ultrasound in chronic wounds: A retrospective analysis. *Advances in Skin & Wound Care, 21*, 416–423.

Konig, M., et al. (2005). Enzymatic versus autolytic debridement of chronic leg ulcers: a prospective randomized trial. *Journal of Wound Care, 14*(7), 320–323.

Lam, D., Rice, P., Brown, R. (2002). The treatment of Lewisite burns with laser debridement--"lasablation". *Burns, 28*(1), 19–25.

Madhok, B. M., et al. (2013). New techniques for wound debridement. *International Wound Journal, 10*, 247–251.

Maragakis, L. L., et al. (2004). An outbreak of multidrug-resistant Acinetobacter baumannii associated with pulsatile lavage wound treatment. *Journal of American Medical Association, 292*(24), 3006–3011.

Milne, C. T., et al. (2010). A comparison of collagenase to hydrogel dressings in wound debridement. *Wounds, 22*, 270–274

Milne, C. T., et al. (2012). A comparison of collagenase to hydrogel dressings in maintenance debridement and wound closure. *Wounds, 24*(11), 317–322.

Morgan, D., & Hoelscher, J. (2000). Pulsed lavage: promoting comfort and healing in home care, *Ostomy Wound Management, 46*(4), 44–49.

Mudge, E., Price, P., Walkley, N., et al. (2014). A randomized controlled trial of larval therapy for the debridement of leg ulcers: results of a multicenter, randomized, controlled, open, observer-blind, parallel group study. *Wound Repair & Regeneration, 22*(1), 43–51.

Müller, E., et al. (2001). Economic evaluation of collagenase-containing ointment and hydrocolloid dressing in the treatment of pressure ulcers. *Pharmacoeconomics, 19*(12), 1209–1216.

National Pressure Ulcer Advisory Panal (NPUAP) and European Pressure Ulcer Advisory Panal (EPUAP). (2009). *Prevention and treatment of pressure ulcers*. Washington, DC: National Pressure Ulcer Advisory Panel.

Ovington, L. (2001). Hanging wet-to-dry dressings out to dry. *Home Healthcare Nurse, 19*(8), 477–483.

Paustian, C., & Stegman, M. R. (2003). Preparing the wound for healing: The effect of activated polyacrylate dressing on debridement. *Ostomy Wound Management, 49*(9), 34–42.

Ramundo, J. (2012). Wound debridement. In R. A. Bryant & D. P. Nix (Eds.). *Acute and chronic wounds: Current management* (4th ed.). St. Louis, MO: Mosby.

Ramundo, J., & Gray, M. (2008). Is ultrasonic mist therapy effective for debriding chronic wounds? *Journal of Wound Ostomy & Continence Nursing, 35*(6), 579.

Ramundo, J., & Gray, M. (2009). Collagenase for enzymatic debridement: A systematic review. *Journal of Wound Ostomy & Continence Nursing, 36*(6S), S4–S11.

Robson, M. C., et al. (2006). Guidelines for the treatment of venous ulcers. *Wound Repair and Regeneration, 14*(6), 649–662.

Rodeheaver, G. T., et al. (1994). Wound healing and wound management: Focus on debridement. *Advances in Wound Care, 7*(1), 22.

Shi, L., et al. (2010). The effect of various wound dressings on the activity of debriding enzymes. *Advances in Skin & Wound Care, 23*(10), 456–462.

Smith, K., et al. (1997). Depth of morphologic skin damage and viability after one, two, and three passes of a high-energy, short pulse CO_2 laser (Tru-Pulse) in pig skin. *Journal of the American Academy of Dermatology, 37*(2), 204.

Stanisic, M. C., et al. (2005). Wound debridement with 25 kHz ultrasound. *Advances in Skin & Wound Care, 18*(9), 484.

Steed, D. L., et al. (1996). Effect of extensive debridement and treatment on the healing of diabetic foot ulcer. *Journal of the American College of Surgeons, 183*, 61.

Steed, D. L., et al. (2006). Guidelines for the treatment of diabetic ulcers. *Wound Repair and Regeneration, 14*(6), 680–692.

Steenvorde, P., & van Doorn, L. P. (2008). Maggot debridement therapy: Serious bleeding can occur. Report of a case. *Journal of Wound Ostomy & Continence Nursing, 35*(4), 412.

Steenvorde, P., et al. (2005). Determining pain levels in patients treated with maggot debridement therapy. *Journal of Wound Care, 14*(10), 485.

Thomas, S. (1991). Evidence fails to justify use of hypochlorite. *Journal of Tissue Viability, 1*(1), 9–10.

Waycaster, C., Milne, C. T. (2013). Clinical and economic benefit of enzymatic debridement of pressure ulcers compared to autolytic debridement with a hydrogel dressing. *Journal of Medical Economics, 16*(7), 976–986.

Woo, K., et al. (2013). The cost of wound debridement: A Canadian perspective. *International Wound Journal.* DOI: 10.1111/iwj.12122. [Epub ahead of print]

Wound, Ostomy, and Continence Nurses (WOCN Society). (2011). *Guideline for management of wounds in patients with lower-extremity venous disease.* Mount Laurel, NJ: Author.

Wound, Ostomy and Continence Nursing (WOCN Society). (2010). *Guideline for prevention and management of pressure ulcers. Mt.* Laurel, NJ: Author.

Wound, Ostomy and Continence Nurses (WOCN Society). (2005). *Conservative sharp wound debridement: Best practice for clinicians.* Mt. Laurel, NJ: Author.

Wound, Ostomy and Continence Nurses (WOCN Society). (2014). *Guideline for management of patients with lower extremity arterial disease, WOCN Society clinical practice guideline series #1*, Mount Laurel, NJ: Author.

Wound, Ostomy and Continence Nurses (WOCN Society). (2012). *Guideline for management of patients with lower extremity neuropathic disease, WOCN Society clinical practice guideline series #1*, Mount Laurel , NJ: Author.

Zarachi, K., & Gergor, J. (2012). The efficacy of maggot debridement therapy-a review of comparative clinical trials. *International Wound Journal, 9*(5), 469–477.

QUESTIONS

1. The wound nurse is explaining to a patient why debridement was ordered to clean his pressure ulcer. Which statement by the nurse accurately explains an aspect of this process?
   A. "Debridement obscures visualization of the wound base."
   B. "Debridement increases the chance for infection."
   C. "Debridement replaces necrotic tissue with eschar."
   D. "Debridement allows the wound healing process to continue."

2. The wound nurse is recommending use of an enzymatic ointment for debridement. Which of the following is the best approach?
   A. Apply thick layer and cover with dry gauze
   B. Crosshatch eschar before application
   C. Cover with silver dressing to prevent infection
   D. Protect any viable tissue with petrolatum

3. A patient with an infected wound is scheduled for conservative sharp wound debridement. Which statement accurately describes a step in this process?
   A. Wash hands and apply sterile gloves.
   B. Prep wound with a normal saline wash.
   C. Peel off loose necrotic tissue using a scalpel.
   D. Avoid all vascular structures throughout the procedure.

4. For which patient would the wound nurse recommend a wound remain closed and monitored for signs of infection rather than ordering debridement?
   A. A patient with advanced LEAD and closed heel ulcer
   B. A patient with advanced Parkinson's disease
   C. A patient with a heel wound with dry eschar, who is ambulatory
   D. A patient with a wound that develops infection

5. Which assessment question would the nurse ask to determine product selection, reimbursement, and safety of the debridement process?
   A. What are the goals of care for this patient?
   B. What is the care setting of the patient?
   C. Where is the wound?
   D. What type of necrotic tissue is involved?

6. The wound nurse is assessing the results of debridement for a patient with a sacral pressure ulcer. Which statement accurately describes a characteristic of this progressive process?
   A. Necrotic tissue is typically expressed as centimeters in length.
   B. Wound dimensions typically decrease as the necrotic tissue is removed.
   C. Volume of exudate typically decreases as the necrotic tissue is removed.
   D. After debridement, eschar gradually hardens.

7. The wound nurse chooses nonselective debridement for a patient with a chronic wound. What process would the nurse recommend?
   A. Autolysis
   B. Enzymatic
   C. Maggot therapy
   D. Wet-to-dry mechanical

8. Which type of debridement is appropriate only for noninfected wounds?
   A. Autolysis
   B. Enzymes
   C. Chemical debridement
   D. Hydrotherapy

9. The wound nurse is choosing a debridement method for a home care patient who is also on anticoagulant therapy due to atrial fibrillation. Which method would be most appropriate for this patient?
   A. Hydrotherapy
   B. Conservative sharp wound debridement
   C. Enzymes
   D. Maggot therapy

10. A wound nurse recommends chemical debridement for a patient with a stage IV pressure ulcer. What is a disadvantage of this procedure?
    A. There is a risk for bacteremia with an infected wound.
    B. It is considered short term until concerns for infection are eliminated.
    C. There is a greater length of time needed to remove nonviable tissue.
    D. Possible loss of blood may occur.

ANSWERS: 1.**D**, 2.**B**, 3.**D**, 4.**A**, 5.**B**, 6.**C**, 7.**D**, 8.**A**, 9.**C**, 10.**B**

CHAPTER 10

Assessment and Management of Wound-Related Infections

Dot Weir and Gregory Schultz

OBJECTIVES

1. Explain why an open wound places the individual at risk for infection.
2. Differentiate among contamination, colonization, and critical colonization, to include implications for wound healing and wound management.
3. Identify indications, options, and guidelines for wound culture.
4. Describe guidelines for diagnosis and management of invasive infection.
5. Describe guidelines for diagnosis and management of osteomyelitis.
6. Discuss current guidelines for appropriate use of topical antimicrobial agents and dressings.

Topic Outline

Introduction

As discussed in Chapter 1, a key function of the skin is to maintain a boundary between the individual and the outside environment, providing an effective barrier to bacterial invasion into the deeper tissues. Specific ways in which the skin protects against bacterial invasion include the following: (1) the dry keratinized cells on the surface create a physical barrier to penetration by microorganisms; (2) the constant shedding of the keratinocytes causes shedding of any attached organisms (Cowan & Talaro, 2006); (3) the normally acidic pH (4 to 6.5) produced by the production of sebum by the sebaceous glands creates a hostile environment to microbial growth (Baranoski et al., 2011; Sussman & Bates-Jensen,

2012); (4) the breakdown of skin lipids produces toxic by-products that inhibit the growth of potential pathogens; (5) sweat inhibits microorganism growth through its low pH and high sodium concentrations; and (6) resident bacteria (e.g., *Staphylococcus epidermidis* and skin diphtheroids) inhibit colonization by more pathogenic organisms (such as *Staphylococcus aureus)* (Sussman & Bates-Jensen, 2012).

Any wound involves a break in the skin that permits access of both normal flora and pathogenic organisms, and the warmth, moisture, reduced oxygen, and nutrient-rich environment of the subepidermal tissues promotes bacterial survival and multiplication. Thus, infection is a constant risk and common complication for all types of wounds, and prevention, prompt detection, and effective management of wound-related infection is a key responsibility for the wound care nurse. That is the focus of this chapter.

CLINICAL PEARL

Any wound permits access of pathogenic organisms, and the warmth, moisture, reduced oxygen, and nutrient-rich environment of the subepidermal tissues promotes bacterial survival and multiplication—thus, infection is a constant risk and common complication for all types of wounds.

Bacteria and Wound Healing

Bioburden is the degree of microbial contamination or microbial load, that is, the number of microorganisms contaminating an object (Medical Dictionary, 2014). The most accurate definition of bioburden involves quantification relative to the object, for example, colony-forming units (CFUs) per gm of tissue or per cm^2. In clinical practice, the term bioburden is used to reflect the presence of bacteria on the wound surface and to indicate the bacterial status of a wound.

Wound healing is generally not impaired simply due to the presence of bacteria on the wound surface; the impact of the microorganisms is determined by their number, their virulence, the bacterial "mix" (numbers and types of bacteria), and the host's resistance (Bowler, 2003; Cowan & Talaro, 2006).

CLINICAL PEARL

Wound healing is not usually impaired simply by the presence of bacteria; it is the number, virulence, "mix," and host response that determine impact.

Bacterial Characteristics

The identification and description of bacteria involves microbiological procedures that use a specific language, which the clinician must be able to understand. On a microscopic level, there are numerous ways in which bacterial species are identified. On a practical level, there are commonalities in the language used in everyday practice that are important to understand. Bacteria are identified and described based on their shape, the results of their Gram stain, their need or lack of need for oxygen, and their mode of growth.

Shape

While there is great variation in the shape, size, and arrangement of bacteria, they are most basically described by one of the three most common shapes: round or ball shaped, described as a coccus (or cocci); cylindrical in shape, described as a rod or bacillus; and a spiral-shaped cylinder, known as a spirillum or spirochete, depending on the thickness and regularity of the spirals or coils. The description is broadened when there is a combination of two shapes, such as a rod that is short and plump (coccobacillus), when the bacteria are found in chains or clusters, are paired together, or are curved or twisted (biology/clc/ud/edu, 2014) (Fig. 10-1).

Gram Positive versus Gram Negative

Gram staining has been used for over a century as a method for identifying and classifying bacteria as either gram positive or gram negative. Gram staining provides rapid information for the practitioner that facilitates empirical management while awaiting the outcome of a culture.

Gram staining is named for Hans Christian Gram, the Danish scientist who developed the technique in 1884; while not infallible, it is still widely used in hospital and community laboratories today and is based on a differentiation between two major cell wall types.

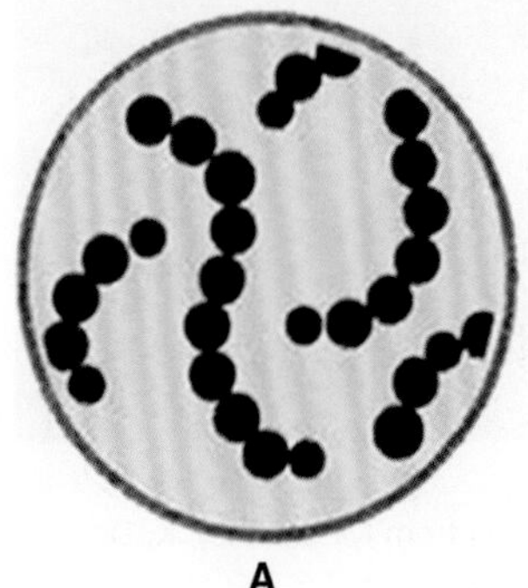

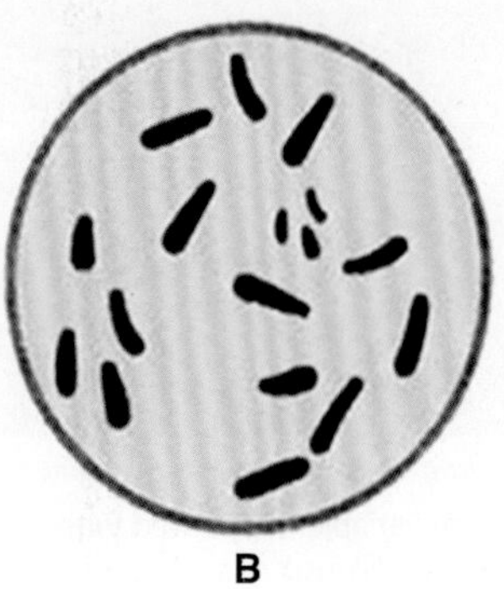

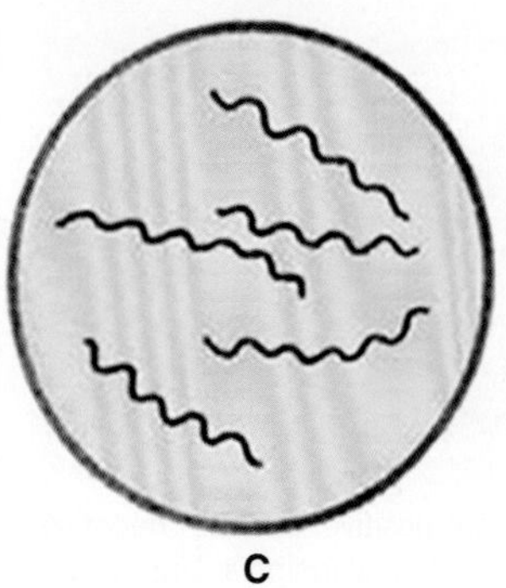

FIGURE 10-1. Shapes of bacteria. **A.** Coccus. **B.** Bacillus or rod shaped. **C.** Spirillum or spirochete.

A very basic description of the methodology is that a small sample of the bacterial culture is taken and smeared onto a slide that, when dry, is heated for a few seconds. Once cool, the smear is then flooded with the stain crystal or gentian violet, washed off, further stained with an iodine solution (Gram's iodine), and then again washed with a decolorizing agent such as alcohol or acetone. The slide is then again stained with a red dye (safranin or fuchsin) and rinsed a final time. After a final drying, the slide is examined under a microscope to identify whether the bacterial cell wall has retained the purple dye (gram positive), lost the purple color (gram negative), or retained a mix of the purple and red dyes (gram variable). Common gram-positive bacteria include various species of the genera *Streptococcus, Staphylococcus, Enterococcus, Corynebacterium,* and *Listeria*. Common gram-negative bacteria include various species of the genera *Pseudomonas, Proteus, Escherichia coli, Klebsiella, Enterobacter, Serratia, Salmonella, Shigella,* and others (Cowan & Talaro, 2006; Wikipedia, 2014; The Gram Stain, 2014) (Fig. 10-2).

CLINICAL PEARL

Bacteria are commonly identified and described based on their shape, response to Gram staining, need for oxygen, and mode of growth; Gram staining can be used to provide rapid general information to the practitioner that guides initial antibiotic therapy while awaiting definitive culture results.

Aerobic versus Anaerobic

Bacteria are further differentiated by those that survive and grow in an oxygenated environment (aerobes), those that do not require oxygen to grow and may even die in the presence of oxygen (anaerobes), and those that can use oxygen but also have anaerobic methods of energy production (facultative anaerobes) (Fig. 10-3).

Planktonic versus Biofilm

In general, clinicians discussing bacterial growth in wounds, culture results, antibiotic therapy, and bactericidal efficacy of topical dressings and agents are referring to free-floating or planktonic bacteria. Planktonic bacteria are free-living bacteria, that is, the bacteria that grow out in the laboratory flask or dish. They have been recognized for centuries, are relatively hydrophilic, and are characterized by cell walls that can be eradicated by the host's immune system and/or targeted antimicrobials. Most of the current knowledge about antibiotics is based on studies and experiments involving planktonic bacteria. The opposite mode of growth is the adherent, or sessile mode of growth, known as biofilm (Fig. 10-4).

Description of Biofilms

Biofilms are complex microbial communities; they are usually polymicrobial, containing multiple species of bacteria and fungi (biology/clc/uc/edu, 2014; Costerton et al., 1999; Dowd et al., 2008a; Trengove et al., 1996). In marked contrast to single, planktonic bacteria, which are not attached (or are only weakly attached) to the wound surface, the microorganisms in a biofilm community synthesize and secrete a matrix that firmly attaches the biofilm to either a living or nonliving surface (Stoodley et al., 2002). The matrix secreted by the organisms in the biofilm consists mainly of polysaccharide chains but also typically contains substantial amounts of bacterial DNA entwined within the polysaccharide chains. Biofilms are dynamic heterogenous communities that are continuously changing in response to factors in the immediate environment (Hall-Stoodley & Stoodley, 2009).

CLINICAL PEARL

Planktonic bacteria are free-floating organisms that are relatively easy to eradicate by WBC activity or antibiotic therapy; in contrast, biofilm bacteria are complex communities of organisms that are "protected" against WBCs and antimicrobial agents by a polymeric matrix secreted by the organisms.

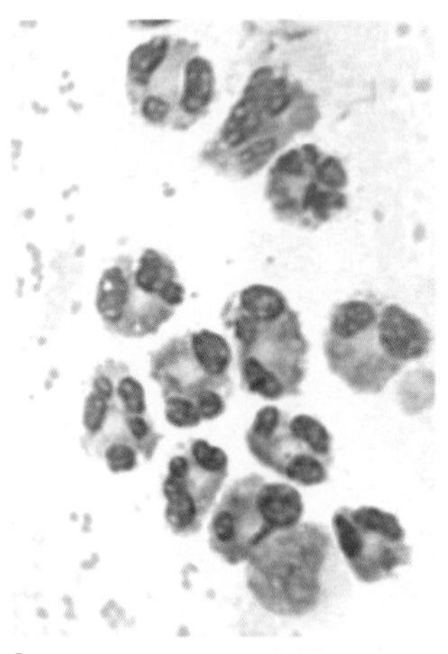
A

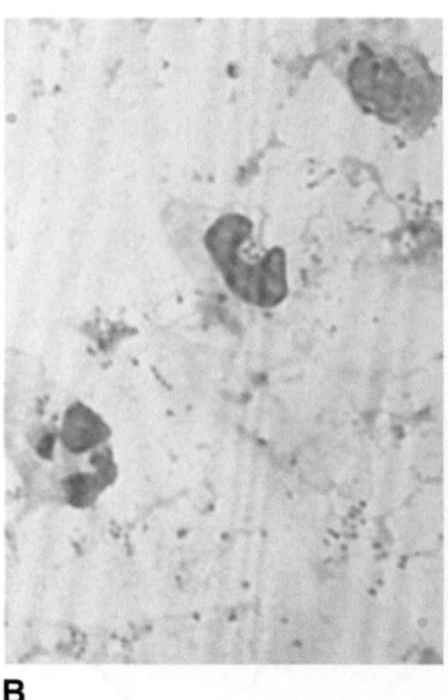
B

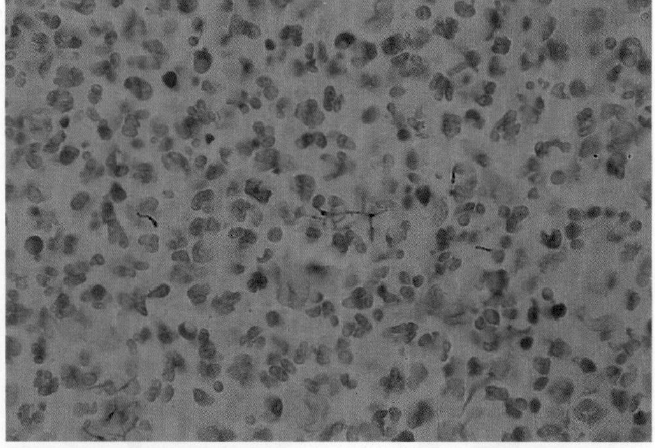
C

FIGURE 10-2. Gram staining. **A.** Gram positive. **B.** Gram negative. **C.** Gram variable. (Reprinted with permision from McClatchey, K. D. (2002). *Clinical laboratory medicine* (2nd ed). Philadelphia: Lippincott Williams & Wilkins.)

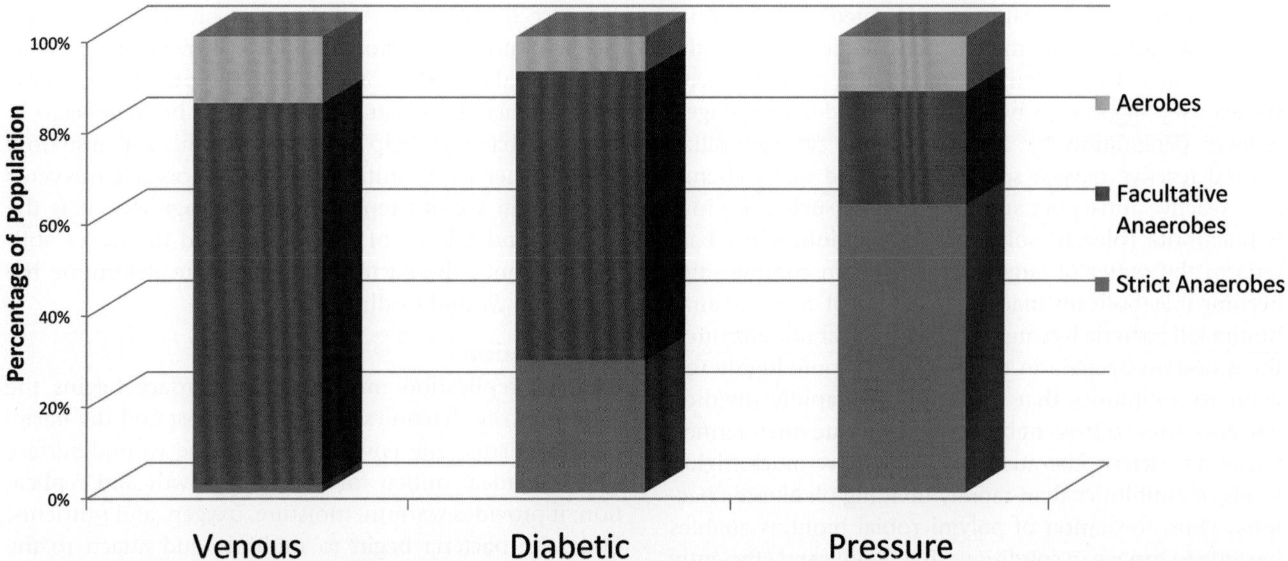

FIGURE 10-3. Aerobic versus anaerobic. Distribution of bacterial populations in chronic wounds in relation to aerotolerance. Diabetic, venous, or pressure ulcer types were analyzed separately using pyrosequencing and the resulting populations grouped into three categories based upon their suggested aerotolerance. This figure graphically illustrates the relative distribution of these functional categories among the wound types. (Used with permission from Dowd, S. E., Sun, Y., Secor, P. R., et al. (2008). Survey of bacterial diversity in chronic wounds using Pyrosequencing, DGGE, and full ribosome shotgun sequencing. *BioMed Central Microbiology*, *8*, 43. © 2008 Dowd et al; licensee BioMed Central Ltd.)

Formation of Biofilms

Biofilms begin with reversible attachment of free-floating, planktonic bacteria to a surface. As the bacteria multiply, they become more firmly attached (sessile). These multiplying planktonic bacteria produce specific molecules known as "quorum molecules"; when the concentration of "quorum molecules" reaches a sufficient threshold, it triggers a change in gene expression patterns. This change in gene expression patterns causes the bacteria to begin synthesizing and secreting components of the protective exopolymeric matrix (Costerton et al., 2003; Donlan & Costerton, 2002; Flemming et al., 2007; Sauer et al., 2002; Xavier & Foster, 2007). It is this protective matrix (or "slime") that distinguishes planktonic bacteria from biofilm bacteria.

Purpose of Biofilms

Living in polymicrobial communities that are typical of biofilms provides bacteria with many protective advantages and allows them to share their individual strengths in ways that benefit the group and increase resistance to environmental stresses (Hibbing et al., 2010; Xavier & Foster, 2007). For example, formation of the protective polymeric matrix encases the biofilm bacteria and provides an

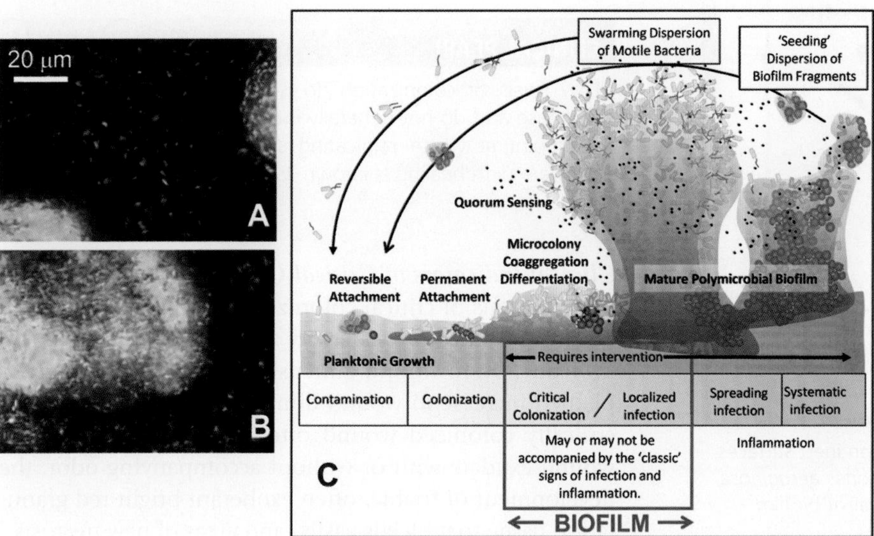

FIGURE 10-4. Biofilm. Confocal laser scanning microscopy (top view) of **(A)** planktonic *Pseudomonas aeruginosa*, **(B)** biofilm community. **(C)** Schematic representation of polymicrobial bacterial biofilm formation (side view). (Courtesy Priscilla Phillips, PhD, Assistant Professor, Kirksville College of Osteopathic Medicine. Illustration after drawing by Peg Dirckx, Center for Biofilm Engineering, Montana State University.)

evolutionary defense against natural predators: bacterial viruses, amoebae, and microbicides. Unfortunately, the tightly attached exopolymeric matrix also protects bacteria against phagocytosis by neutrophils and macrophages, reduces penetration by antibodies, and can neutralize natural reactive oxygen species (ROS) and many chemically reactive antiseptics and disinfectants, such as sodium hypochlorite (bleach) solutions. In addition, many bacteria in the center of large, mature biofilm communities become metabolically inactive, or quiescent. Since all antibiotics kill bacteria by interfering with metabolic enzymes, the quiescent bacteria in the biofilms become highly tolerant to antibiotics that efficiently kill rapidly dividing bacteria. These quiescent biofilm bacteria are often termed "persister bacteria" because they can survive much higher levels of antibiotics than rapidly dividing planktonic bacteria. Thus, formation of polymicrobial biofilms enables bacteria to survive in conditions that rapidly and efficiently kill planktonic bacteria (Fig. 10-5).

CLINICAL PEARL

Many bacteria in the center of biofilms become quiescent (metabolically inactive); these organisms are known as "persister bacteria" because they can survive much higher levels of antibiotics than can rapidly dividing planktonic bacteria.

Bacterial Loads in Chronic Wounds

There is wide agreement in the literature that all open wounds are contaminated, regardless of the age of the wound (Fig. 10-6). Contamination is defined as the presence of nonreplicating bacteria on the wound surface with no clinical host response (Browne et al., 2001; Landis et al., 2007; Stotts, 2004). The presence of some level of bacteria is actually thought to be beneficial, in that the bacteria help to stimulate the inflammatory response needed to initiate the normal cascade of events resulting in wound repair. As time progresses, it is the number and activity of the bacteria and the host's ability to balance the bacteria that seems to determine the impact on wound healing.

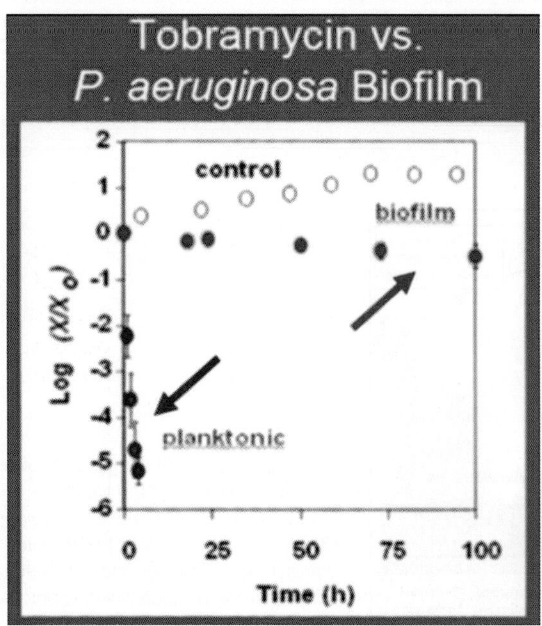

FIGURE 10-5. Antibiotics versus biofilm on inert surfaces. Tobramycin rapidly kills planktonic *Pseudomonas aeruginosa* (blue) very effectively but is not effective against biofilm *Pseudomonas* (red).

Colonization

Bacterial replication on the wound surface begins the change in the dynamics between the host and the bacterial organisms. The environment on the wound surface offers an ideal milieu for bacterial growth and replication; it provides warmth, moisture, oxygen, and nutrients. Once the bacteria begin to multiply and attach to the wound surface, the wound is considered to be colonized. However, low levels of colonization do not incite a significant host response and do not generally interfere with wound healing.

Critical Colonization

The point at which the bacteria multiplying on the surface begin to interfere with wound healing has been termed critical colonization, a term that was coined by Davis in 1996 (Davis, 1996; White & Cutting, 2006b). This concept represents a significant advance in our understanding of the relationship between bacteria and wound healing. For decades, wounds were considered to be either infected or not infected; infected wounds were typically defined as those with bacterial loads $>10^5$ (>100,000 CFU/g of tissue), and the classic host response (e.g., erythema, induration, edema, increased exudate, warmth, and pain) (Robson et al., 2006; Steed et al., 2006; Whitney et al., 2006). The awareness that pathogens can interfere with wound healing without evoking a host response is fundamental to understanding the concept of critical colonization.

CLINICAL PEARL

Low levels of colonization do not incite a significant host response and do not generally interfere with wound healing; the point at which replicating surface organisms begin to interfere with healing is known as critical colonization.

Clinical Indicators of Critical Colonization

Clinical signs of critical colonization include a plateau in the wound's healing trajectory, evidenced by minimal or no reduction in wound dimensions or by a sudden unexplained increase in wound dimensions. Additionally, the critically colonized wound often will exhibit increasing wound exudate with or without accompanying odor; the development of friable, often exuberant bright red granulation tissue that bleeds easily; and areas of new necrosis.

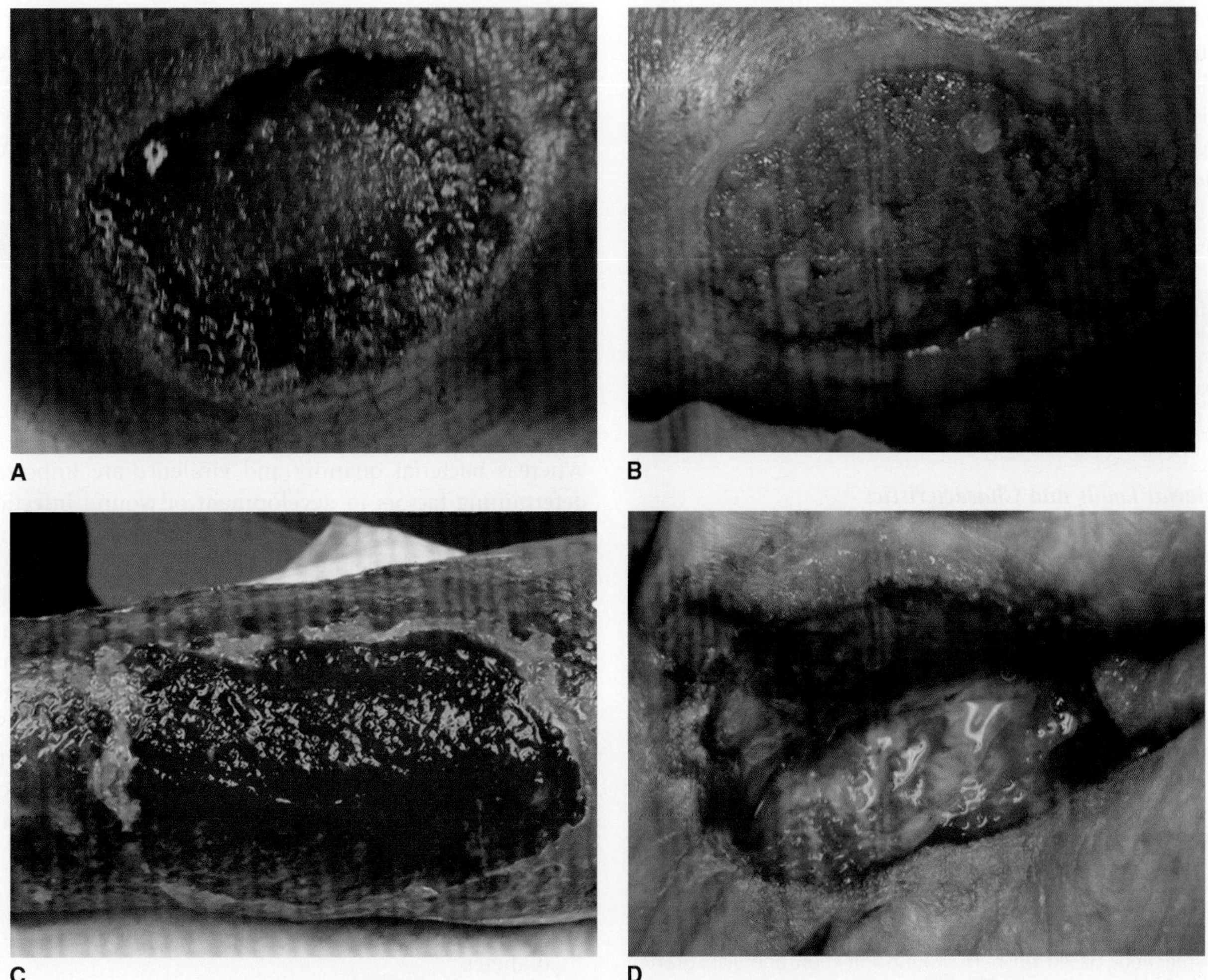

FIGURE 10-6. Bacterial loads in wounds. **A. Contamination:** The presence of bacteria on wound surfaces with no replication or multiplication of the bacteria and no clinical host response. **B. Colonization:** The act or process of establishing a colony or colonies; the spreading of species into a new habitat (www.thefreedictionary.com/colonization). Bacteria replicating; no host response. **C. Critical Colonization:** The point at which the bacteria multiplying on the surface begin to interfere with wound healing, resulting in a host response. **D. Infection:** Invasion by and multiplication of pathogenic microorganisms in a bodily part or tissue, which may produce subsequent tissue injury and progress to overt disease through a variety of cellular or toxic mechanisms (http://medical-dictionary.thefreedictionary.com/infection).

Pathology Critical Colonization

Suggested causative factors for the negative effects of critical colonization include the effects of proteases produced by the bacteria, the competition between wound healing cells and bacteria for oxygen and nutrients, the effects of exotoxins released by bacterial and fungal organisms, and the release of endotoxins caused by breakdown of the cell walls of Gram-negative organisms. In addition, rising bacterial loads stimulate white blood cell activity, and the proteases produced by the neutrophils and macrophages (especially the matrix metalloproteases, MMPs) can degrade proteins that are essential for healing. Rising bacterial loads also increase production of proinflammatory mediators including tumor necrosis factor alpha (TNFα) and interleukins such as IL-1b. Finally, bacteria can stimulate angiogenesis and contribute to the production of a deficient or corrupt matrix.

Diagnosis of Critical Colonization

In clinical practice, critical colonization is "assumed" based on the clinical findings outlined above and "confirmed" by a positive response to intervention, that is, clinical improvement and resumption of wound healing following use of an antimicrobial dressing or modality (Schultz et al., 2003; White & Cutting, 2006b).

CLINICAL PEARL

Indicators of critical colonization include a sudden unexplained plateau in wound healing, a deterioration in the quantity or quality of granulation tissue, and increased exudate; the diagnosis of critical colonization is "assumed" based on clinical findings and "confirmed" by a positive response to intervention (e.g., resumption of healing following initiation of topical antimicrobial therapy).

Invasive Wound Infection

Wound infection is described as the invasion by and multiplication of pathogenic microorganisms in a bodily part or tissue, which may produce subsequent tissue injury and progress to overt disease through a variety of cellular or toxic mechanisms (Medical Dictionary, 2014). Depending on the location of the wound and the condition of the host, the presenting signs may be subtle or profound.

CLINICAL PEARL

Depending on the location of the wound and condition of the host, the indicators of invasive wound infection may be subtle or profound.

Bacterial Loads and Characteristics

A quantitative threshold of >10^5 CFU/g of tissue biopsied has been used to define burn wound infection (Bamberg et al., 2002; Robson, 1997) and to predict skin graft failure (Robson & Krizek, 1973); however, chronic wounds have been reported to progress to closure despite levels of microorganisms as great as 10^8 CFU/g of tissue (Bamberg et al., 2002). Wound infection has also been defined in terms of bacterial load and virulence relative to the patient's level of resistance.

CLINICAL PEARL

A quantitative threshold of >10^5 CFU of bacteria per gram of tissue has been used as the "cutoff" for laboratory diagnosis of infection, based on burn wound infection and skin graft failure; however, chronic wounds have been reported to progress to closure despite levels as high as 10^8.

The majority of chronic wounds are polymicrobial. Certain pathogens (e.g., *S. aureus*, *Pseudomonas aeruginosa*, and beta-hemolytic *Streptococci*) have been cited as the most common cause of wound infection and delayed healing (Martin & Drosou, 2005). In a study of chronic leg ulcers, the investigators found no specific microorganisms most likely to result in impaired healing; however, a significantly lower probability of healing was observed if four or more bacterial groups were present in any ulcer (Trengove et al., 1996). These data provide further support for the impact of microbial interactions on overall pathogenicity; it is not just the presence of bacteria but the type and virulence of the organism(s), the interaction with other microbial agents, and the interaction with the host that determine the influence on healing of chronic wounds.

While, in general, the mere presence of bacteria is not believed to increase the risk of infection, beta-hemolytic streptococcus is an important exception to the rule; the presence of one virulent beta-hemolytic streptococcus should be considered significant and appropriate treatment initiated. In addition, some bacterial combinations may develop synergy with each other; this can result in a previously nonvirulent organism becoming virulent and causing damage to the host. Finally, antimicrobial therapy may eliminate selected organisms, allowing overgrowth of other organisms that may impair healing and result in infection.

CLINICAL PEARL

In general, the mere presence of bacteria is not believed to increase the risk of infection; beta-hemolytic streptococcus is the notable exception to this rule.

Host Resistance

Whereas bacterial quantity and virulence are important determining factors in development of wound infection, host resistance is also of notable and critical significance. Host resistance is defined as the ability of the host to mount an immune response that resists bacterial invasion and damage. This resistance can be impacted by a number of systemic and local factors, and the ability to mitigate these factors has a direct influence on the impact of the bacteria on the wound and surrounding tissues. See **Table 10-1** for lists of local and systemic factors with the potential to impact host resistance. Clinical interventions to eliminate factors adversely affecting host resistance include the following:

- Wound debridement
- Interventions to control comorbid conditions such as diabetes
- Measures to enhance tissue perfusion and oxygenation (e.g., revascularization)
- Nutritional support
- Counseling related to lifestyle changes (e.g., weight loss, smoking cessation)
- Compression therapy to eliminate interstitial edema
- Advanced wound management therapies to promote wound healing (e.g., topical biologic therapies; negative pressure wound therapy[NPWT]; hyperbaric oxygen therapy)

TABLE 10-1 Local and Systemic Factors Affecting Host Resistance to Bacteria

Local	Systemic
Size, location, and age of the wound	Poorly controlled diabetes
Necrotic tissue or foreign bodies	Inadequate vascular perfusion
Presence of scar	Edema
Previous radiation	Immunosuppressive drugs
Inadequate or improper topical treatments	Malnutrition Alcohol and/or tobacco abuse Neutrophil disorders

CLINICAL PEARL

Host resistance to infection is affected by overall systemic status and by local factors such as tissue necrosis and edema; thus, comprehensive care is required for prevention and management of infection.

Assessment and Diagnosis of Wound Infection

Determining the presence of a wound infection begins with the clinical examination. Microbiological tests can then be used to determine the specific offending organism(s) and to assure that the empirically prescribed antimicrobial agents appropriately target those organisms. However, studies indicate that reliance on clinical evaluation alone may lead to a false sense of security as to the infectious status of a wound. Serena et al. (2006) conducted a retrospective analysis of data from a phase IIB prospective, randomized, placebo-controlled clinical trial to determine the accuracy of clinical examination (as compared to biopsy) for diagnosis of infection in venous leg ulcers. Of 614 screening biopsies obtained by impeccably strict standards, 122 were found to have a colony count $>10^6$. Of the 352 patients eventually enrolled in the trial, 26% were found to have infected ulcers despite a lack of clinical signs; the investigators concluded that the incidence of infection is grossly underestimated by clinical examination.

CLINICAL PEARL

Studies suggest that clinical examination grossly underestimates the incidence of wound infection.

In guidelines published by the Wound Healing Society in 2006 (Robson et al., 2006; Steed et al., 2006; Whitney et al., 2006), the following recommendation is made: if infection is suspected in a debrided ulcer, or if epithelialization from the margin of a venous, diabetic, or pressure ulcer (or contraction of a pressure ulcer) is not progressing within 2 weeks despite appropriate compression, pressure relief, and off-loading, the type and level of infection should be determined by a tissue biopsy or a validated quantitative swab technique.

CLINICAL PEARL

If infection is suspected in a debrided ulcer, or if a chronic wound fails to progress within 2 weeks despite appropriate comprehensive management, a tissue biopsy or swab culture should be obtained to assess for infection.

Clinical Indicators of Infection

Historically, the signs and symptoms of invasive wound infection have been described as

- Rubor (redness, erythema)
- Calor (warmth)
- Dolor (pain)
- Tumor (edema/swelling)
- Presence of purulence

These classic heralding symptoms may be diminished or altered in chronic wounds or, conversely, may be mistaken for noninfectious inflammatory changes triggered by increased levels of inflammatory cytokines in the chronic wound environment. Additional clinical signs of infection in chronic wounds have been validated by Gardner et al. (2001) and include

- Serous drainage with concurrent inflammation
- Delayed healing
- Discolored and/or friable granulation tissue
- Pocketing at the base of the wound
- Foul odor
- Wound breakdown (Figs. 10-7 to 10-9)

CLINICAL PEARL

Chronic wounds may not exhibit the "classic" signs of infection (erythema, warmth, pain, swelling, and purulent drainage); the clinician should be alert to additional validated indicators, which include serous drainage with concurrent signs of inflammation, delayed healing, discolored and/or friable granulation tissue, pocketing at the base of the wound, foul odor, and wound breakdown.

The degree to which any of these 11 indicators signifies or predicts actual wound infection seems to be determined in large part by the host response; however, any patient presenting with increased wound pain, friable granulation tissue, foul odor, and wound breakdown warrants a thorough evaluation and attention to management, as these signs and symptoms showed the greatest positive predictive value for infection verified by wound culture. Invasive wound infection requires systemic antibiotic therapy and, in some situations, adjunctive topical antimicrobial therapy.

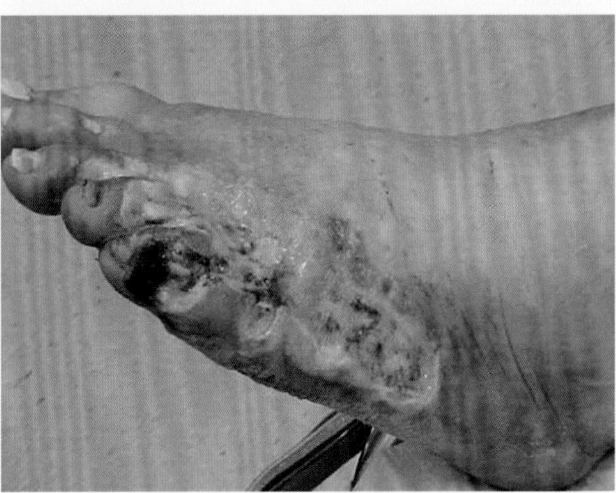

FIGURE 10-7. Infected foot.

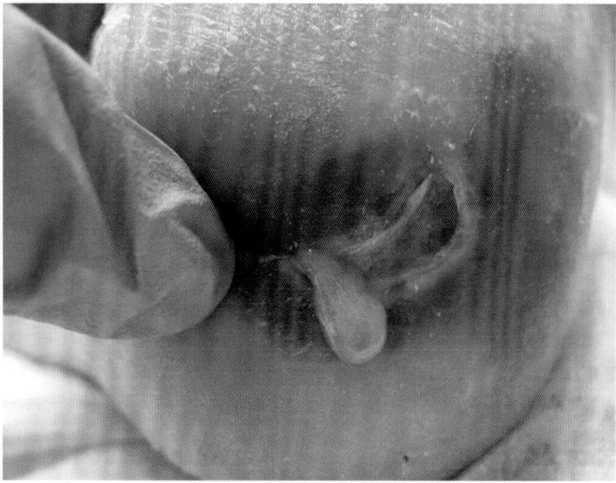

FIGURE 10-8. Purulent exudate.

Wound Cultures

Wound cultures are used to confirm or modify the plan for treatment when antibiotic therapy is indicated, and the data provided by the culture should be compared to the clinical picture. The patient presenting with clinical signs and symptoms of infection requires prompt response based on the information available at the time. Typically, treatment is initiated with antibiotics to which pathogens most commonly involved in a particular type of wound are usually sensitive; if previous cultures from the specific wound are available, the data regarding bacterial type and sensitivity can be used to guide initial treatment. The antibiotic can then be changed if indicated when culture results are obtained. Collaboration with an infectious disease specialist is recommended for wounds that culture positive for multiple types of bacteria to assure that treatment decisions are based upon current trends of known bacterial synergies and/or resistance in a particular hospital or community.

CLINICAL PEARL

Wound cultures are used to confirm or modify the plan for treatment when antibiotic therapy is indicated.

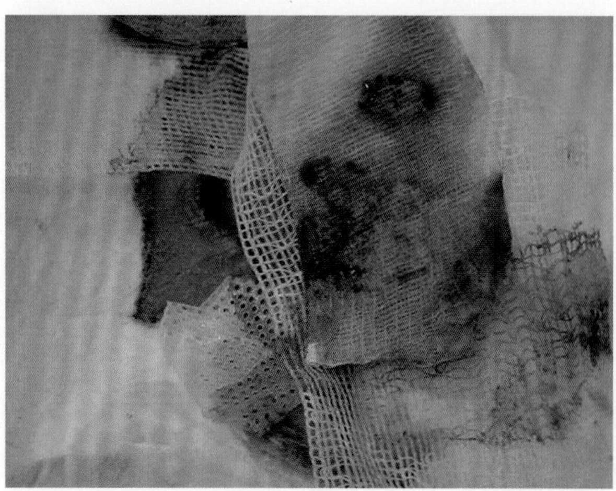

FIGURE 10-9. Exudate color change.

The appropriate method for obtaining a culture from a wound has been widely discussed and even debated over the years. The 72 hours required to obtain final results on standard laboratory cultures regardless of the method demands that the information provided be accurate so that antibiotic therapy is based on valid data. The increasing growth of resistant strains of common pathogens further confirms the critical need for antibiotic therapy based on accurate culture and sensitivity data.

Data comparing the accuracy and usability of culture results obtained by various techniques have been widely published (Drosou et al., 2003; Fernandez et al., 2008; NPUAP & PPPIA, 2014; Wikipedia, 2014). The quantitative information generated by a tissue biopsy remains the "gold standard"; and while it is the methodology most commonly used in research and clinical trials, it is likely the least often used in clinical practice.

General Guidelines

Regardless of the procedure used, there are two guidelines that are essential to accurate and valuable information. The first is adherence to the optimal time frame for transport of the specimen to the lab. Use of culture specimen containers and tubes that stabilize and fix the bacteria reduces the risk of bacterial replication or death and allows for a reasonable time frame for transport; this is particularly important for cultures obtained in the home or in an institution without a lab on the premises, such as an outpatient wound care center or skilled nursing facility. Aerobic specimens maintained in appropriate transport media will survive, and the media will not promote continued growth. Specimens obtained specifically for anaerobic culture should be placed into prereduced, anaerobically sterilized transport media (Landis et al., 2007). Secondly, and of equal or greater importance, the specimen must be carefully and accurately obtained.

CLINICAL PEARL

Regardless of the specific procedure used to obtain a wound culture, it is critical to adhere to guidelines regarding transport to the lab and to obtain the specimen from viable tissue using meticulous technique.

Specimens are obtained by three methods: tissue removal, aspiration, and swab.

Tissue Removal Technique

Tissue removal methods include standard punch biopsy and use of instruments such as a scalpel or curette to obtain tissue (Figs. 10-10 and 10-11). When obtaining tissue specimens for quantitative culture, it is important to determine the individual laboratory requirements for the size of the specimen. A 3-mm sample is required by most labs.

Another consideration when obtaining a tissue specimen for bacterial culture is the potential impact of topical and injectable anesthetic agents, which are commonly used

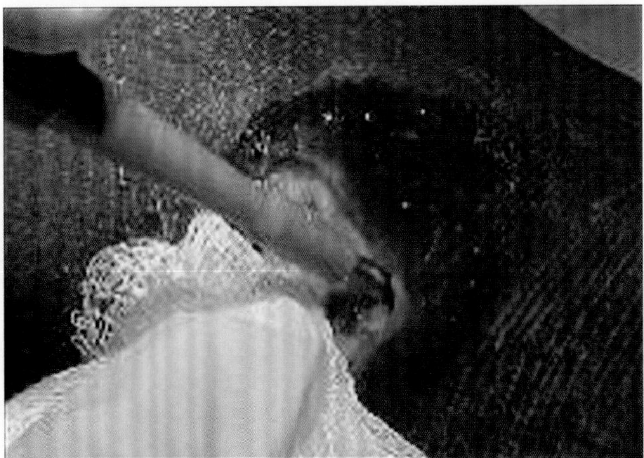

FIGURE 10-10. Punch biopsy tissue sample.

prior to tissue removal. Some of these agents have antimicrobial properties that influence bacterial survival (Berg et al., 2006; Johnson et al., 2008); however, preservative-free lidocaine 1% solution as an injectable infiltrate was found to be safe for a wound biopsy performed within 2 hours.

The major advantage of tissue cultures is the ability to identify organisms that have invaded the tissues beyond the wound surface, which optimizes antibiotic therapy. The disadvantage is that the technique is skill intensive and must be performed by a physician, podiatrist, or physician extender due to licensure restrictions. The fact that many bacterial cultures are obtained by nurses at the bedside, either in the home or institutional setting, means that tissue cultures are frequently impractical in the clinical arena. To obtain a tissue culture from a patient in these settings, the patient would have to be transported to a site where a tissue culture could be done; this would add to the cost of care and would also cause a delay in obtaining the specimen and the results. Finally, tissue culture is an invasive procedure, which means it is also more painful and commonly requires a local anesthetic in the sensate individual.

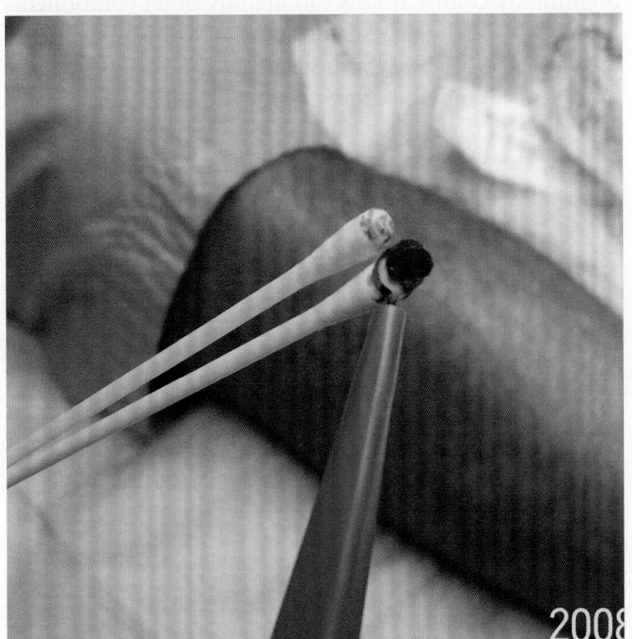

FIGURE 10-11. Curetted tissue sample.

CLINICAL PEARL

The major advantage of tissue cultures is the ability to identify organisms that have invaded the tissues beyond the wound surface, which optimizes antibiotic therapy.

Aspiration Technique

The goal of aspiration culture is to obtain fluid from the tissue below the wound bed, thereby avoiding surface contaminants. In clinical practice, this method is more commonly used to obtain a specimen from an abscess or loculated fluid collection. The skin over or adjacent to the area to be aspirated is prepared with povidone–iodine and allowed to dry for 60 seconds. The skin should then be wiped with alcohol and allowed to dry, which reduces the possibility that the specimen will be altered by the iodine on the skin surface. A 10-mL syringe with a 22-g needle should be prefilled with 0.5 mL of air and inserted through the skin toward the area to be aspirated. Suction is achieved by briskly withdrawing the plunger the length of the syringe, to the 10-mL mark. The needle is then moved backward and forward through the tissue in the area. The plunger is then released back to the 0.5-mL mark, the needle is withdrawn, and the syringe is capped and sent to the laboratory (Lee et al., 1985). (If recapping of the syringe is against agency policy, the aspirated fluid can be gently injected into a sterile container and transported.) The challenge in obtaining a culture utilizing aspiration is that, like a biopsy, it is an invasive procedure and technique is critically important, and it is not likely to be performed by the bedside care provider. Overall, it is a technique rarely mentioned for use in general practice (Fig. 10-12).

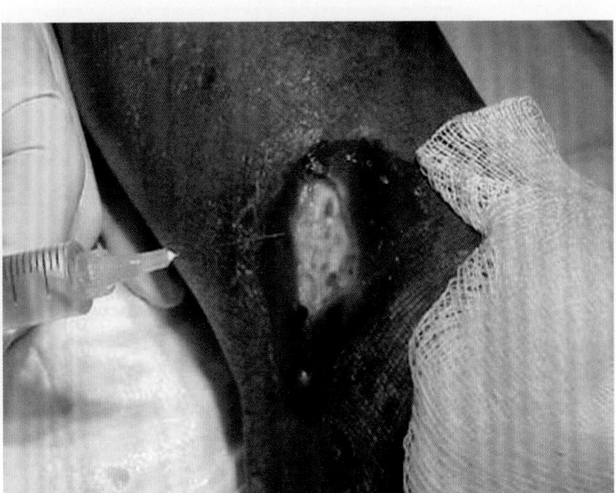

FIGURE 10-12. Aspiration.

Swab Technique

Swab cultures have historically been considered the least appropriate method for obtaining a culture due to the potential for contamination by surface debris and skin contaminants; however, as previously mentioned, swab cultures continue to be the primary method used. Because of this fact, it is imperative for clinicians to utilize optimal technique when obtaining the specimen. Modern moisture retentive wound dressings are designed to maintain an ideal environment for healing and by design are left in place for several days. Unless the dressing is designed to provide sustained antimicrobial activity, the accumulated exudate found upon removal of these dressings usually contains bacteria from the surface of the wound and the surrounding skin. Swab cultures of this accumulated exudate are likely to generate high numbers of microbes that may not reflect actual bacterial status of the wound, and can lead to initiation of systemic antibiotic therapy targeting organisms that are not negatively affecting the wound. Thus, current guidelines recommend wound cleansing prior to obtaining a swab culture: specifically, the wound surface should be cleansed with a nonpreserved, nonantimicrobial cleanser such as normal saline to remove surface debris, residual dressing material, and any coagulum easily removed from the surface. Additionally, wound debridement should be carried out if appropriate to remove necrotic and devitalized tissue, since avascular tissue also harbors high numbers of microorganisms that may not be affecting the repair process.

The two swab techniques most often described in the literature are the Z-Stroke and Levine's technique. The Z-Stroke, as the name indicates, involves starting at the top of the wound, pressing the swab into the wound surface, and moving the swab from skin edge to skin edge in a "Z" pattern down to the bottom of the wound. The inherent challenge of this technique is the probability of contamination of the swab(s) with resident bacteria from the skin as well as from any devitalized tissue remaining on the wound surface; as mentioned, this can lead to overtreatment with antibiotics that may not be warranted, subject the patient to the potential side effects of antibiotic use, and eradicate less complex bacteria while allowing more complex and pathogenic organisms to thrive.

Levine et al. (1976) described a method for obtaining a viable sample of aerobic bacteria on the surface of wounds. This method involves thoroughly cleansing the wound surface and identifying a 1-cm area of the wound that is free from necrotic tissue. The swab is rotated while applying pressure sufficient to express fluid from the wound tissue. This technique is thought to provide more accurate results than the Z-Stroke, and most certainly provides more accurate results than swabbing residual exudate at the time of dressing removal. Thus, it is the technique currently recommended for obtaining a swab culture (Fig. 10-13).

CLINICAL PEARL

Swab cultures should be obtained using Levine technique, which includes thorough irrigation of the wound bed with a noncytotoxic solution, and firmly swabbing an area of viable tissue.

Assessment of Culture Results

Final results of a wound culture generally take up to 72 hours to be reported. If Gram staining was ordered or is routinely provided as the laboratory's "standard of care," these preliminary results are available within hours and provide information that can be used to guide initial therapy. Specifically, determining whether the organism(s) is/are gram negative or gram positive provides general direction in terms of appropriate antibiotic agents. In addition, preliminary culture results can identify other components found within the specimen, such as white blood cells; the presence of WBCs indicates that the patient may be mounting an inflammatory response to the bacteria.

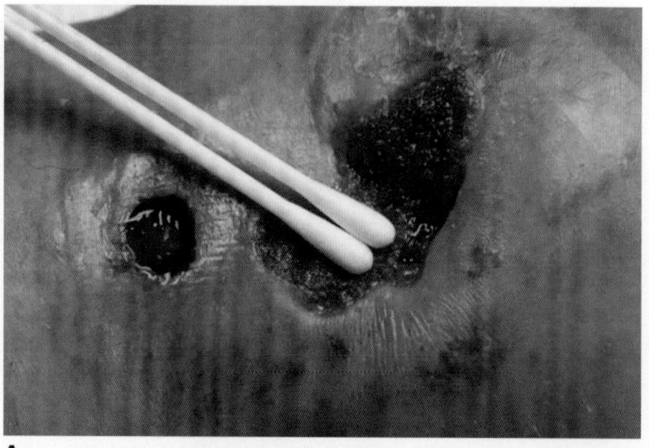

A

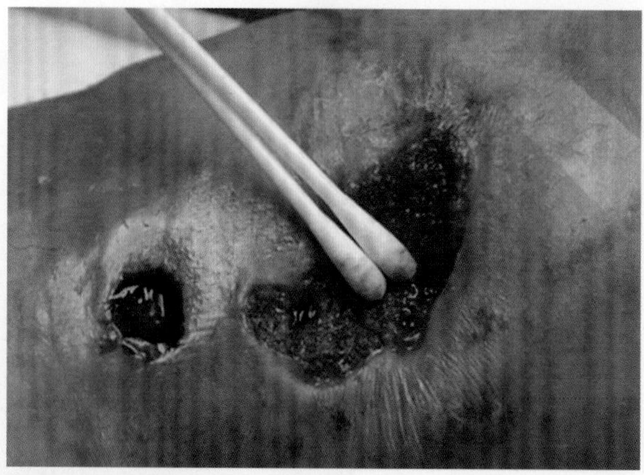

B

FIGURE 10-13. **A, B.** Levine technique. Thoroughly cleanse the wound surface, and identify a 1-cm area of the wound that is free from necrotic tissue. Rotate the swab while applying pressure sufficient to express fluid from the wound tissue.

Qualitative versus Quantitative Reports

Culture results may be classified as qualitative, semiquantitative, or quantitative, depending on the methodology used to obtain and process the specimen.

A qualitative culture is obtained by plating the specimen on solid media and identifying the organisms grown. Semiquantitative cultures are plated on solid media and then serially streaked into four quadrants. Results are reported as 1+ to 4+, identifying the number of quadrants where there was bacterial growth. Quantitative cultures are generally performed on tissue specimens, though swab specimens can also be utilized. Tissue specimens are homogenized and plated, whereas the swab specimens are serially diluted and plated. This technique allows for quantification of the number of CFU of the bacteria identified and is reported as CFU per gram of tissue for wound biopsies and CFU per cm^2 for swab cultures. As previously mentioned, soft tissue wound infections have been defined as cultures yielding $>10^5$ CFU/g or cm^2 of tissue; however, in chronic wounds, this number needs to be considered within the context of the clinical indicators previously described.

Bacterial Sensitivity Data

In addition to identification of the specific bacteria, culture results provide information regarding sensitivity of the bacterial strain to antibiotics common to the setting, laboratory, or hospital. The final culture report will identify the organism(s) grown, the sensitivity (S) or resistance (R) to the antibiotics tested, and the Minimum Inhibitory Concentration (MIC) relative to those antibiotics. The MIC identifies the lowest concentration of the antibiotic tested which resulted in inhibition or reduction of the inoculums; as a general rule, the lower the MIC the more effective the antibiotic. This information, however, must be considered in relation to the species of the bacteria, other species identified, and possible synergies that may exist. Therefore, consultation with an infectious disease specialist may be warranted in the presence of multiple organisms, significant resistance, and in the patient experiencing persistent or recurring infections.

CLINICAL PEARL

The Minimum Inhibitory Concentration (MIC) identifies the lowest concentration of antibiotics tested that produce inhibition or reduction of bacterial growth; the lower the MIC the more effective the antibiotic.

Limitations and Considerations

There are several key points the clinician should understand about standard clinical microbiology laboratory culture methods:

- Only planktonic bacteria are typically detected by standard culture techniques. Detecting bacteria in biofilm communities requires additional processing of wound samples; specifically, biofilm communities that are tightly attached to tissue samples must be dislodged and dispersed into single cells using ultrasonic energy and extensive vortexing prior to plating on agar culture dishes.
- Only a small fraction (perhaps approximately 20%) of all the bacterial species that are present in a chronic wound bed are typically detected by standard aerobic agar plating techniques. For example, identification of all bacterial species present in a series of pressure ulcers using DNA-sequencing techniques found that approximately 60% were strict anaerobic bacteria, which are very difficult to grow under standard culturing conditions (Dowd et al., 2008b, 2011).
- The polymerase chain reaction (PCR) is a molecular technique utilized to target and "amplify" bacterial DNA; this technique generates thousands to millions of copies of a particular DNA sequence, which allows them to be detected. The method relies on thermal cycling, cycles of repeated heating and cooling for melting, and then enzymatic replication of the DNA. Thus, bacteria are identified by "amplifying" a tiny sample of their DNA, without actually having to grow bacterial cultures in the microbiology laboratory. This technology is sensitive, specific, and can be completed in hours.

CLINICAL PEARL

Only planktonic bacteria are recovered/identified by wound culture; we currently lack the technology to identify biofilm bacteria; in addition, only a small percentage of the bacterial species present in a chronic wound are detected by standard culture techniques.

Therefore, standard clinical microbiology laboratory results obtained by traditional aerobic plating of wound samples provide only partial information about the actual spectrum of bacteria in the wound bed. Nevertheless, the results of standard clinical microbiology laboratory assays are usually helpful to clinicians in developing a reasonable therapy plan; wound cultures should therefore be done whenever clinical signs and symptoms indicate invasive infection requiring systemic therapy, or when a wound has failed to respond adequately to current antimicrobial therapy (either systemic or topical). However, as identification of bacteria species by DNA-sequencing techniques becomes more widely available, it is very likely that new patterns of bacterial species will be identified that correlate with, and more importantly predict, poor wound healing (Dowd et al., 2011).

CLINICAL PEARL

Despite limitations in current culture techniques, the results are usually helpful in developing a reasonable therapy plan. Therefore, cultures should be done whenever clinical signs and symptoms indicate invasive infection, or whenever a wound fails to respond to current therapy.

Osteomyelitis

Infection of the bone, or osteomyelitis, should be considered separately, as cultures taken of soft tissue may not accurately reflect bacterial penetration into bone. The absolute diagnosis of osteomyelitis is a difficult one, often resulting in expensive imaging or invasive bone biopsies. Grayson et al. (1995) reported an 89% positive predictive value (PPV) and a 56% negative predictive value (NPV) in pedal ulcers of 75 patients with 76 ulcers known to be infected, in which bone could be probed utilizing a stainless steel probe (Fig. 10-14). The authors concluded that, in patients with diabetes, the ability to probe to bone (PTB) is strongly correlated with osteomyelitis and that specialized radiologic and nuclear tests to diagnose osteomyelitis were unnecessary. Called the "poor man's bone scan," this seemingly conventional wisdom drove and continues to drive practice today.

Lavery et al. (2007) sought to assess the accuracy of the PTB test in diagnosing foot osteomyelitis. During this large 2-year study, the investigators enrolled 1,666 consecutive diabetic individuals who underwent an initial standardized detailed foot assessment followed by examinations at regular intervals. The patients were also instructed to come to the foot clinic if they developed a lower-extremity complication. Over a mean of 27.2 months, 247 patients developed a foot wound and 151 developed 199 foot infections. Osteomyelitis was found in 30 patients (in 12% with a foot wound and in 20% with a foot infection). The PTB test was found to be highly sensitive (0.87%) and specific (0.91%). While the PPV was only 0.57%, the NPV was 0.98%. The authors concluded that the PTB test, when used in a population of diabetic patients with foot wounds, had a relatively low PPV but that a negative PTB test could usually be used to exclude the diagnosis. Current guidelines recommend PTB testing, correlated with other diagnostic imaging, specifically magnetic resonance imaging (MRI), as being the most sensitive and specific noninvasive test(s) for osteomyelitis (Figs. 10-15 and 10-16).

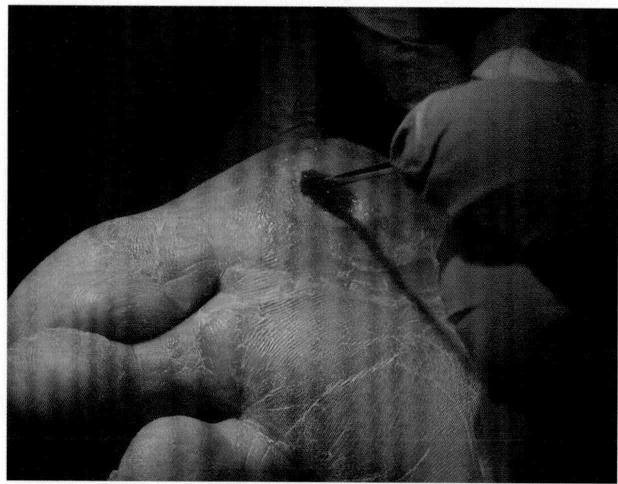

FIGURE 10-14. Probe to bone.

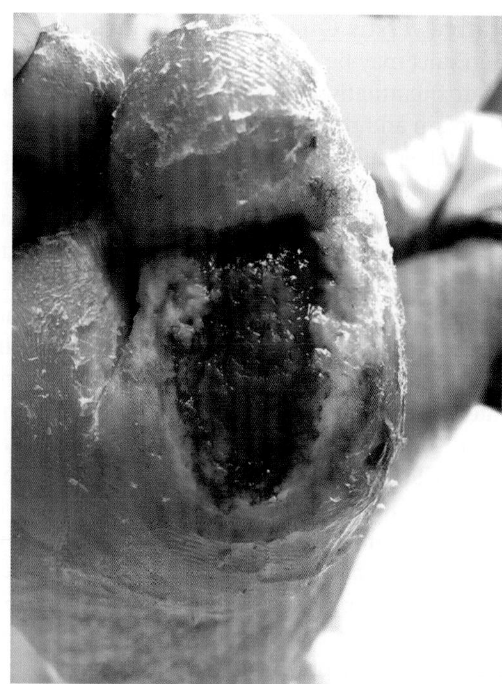

FIGURE 10-15. Plantar First Met head DFU that probed deeply.

CLINICAL PEARL

The "probe to bone" test has high negative predictive value for osteomyelitis in foot wounds; thus, this simple test can usually be used to "rule out" osteomyelitis. MRI is usually required to confirm the diagnosis of osteomyelitis in individuals with foot ulcers.

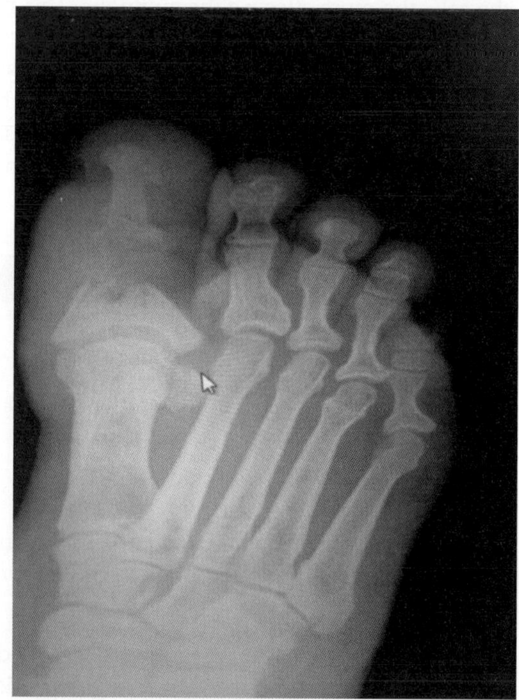

FIGURE 10-16. Correlating plain film x-ray showing bone destruction.

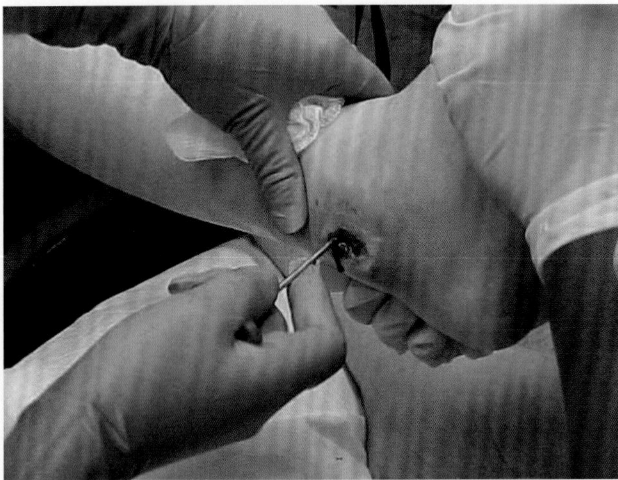

FIGURE 10-17. Bone biopsy.

The diagnosis of osteomyelitis in the bone beneath pressure ulcers is particularly problematic. In patients with deep nonhealing pressure ulcers, clinical evaluation does not accurately detect or predict the existence of underlying osteomyelitis; neither clinical evaluation nor radiologic examinations correlate well with the histopathologic diagnosis of bone infection. In addition, bone scans in the situation of deep nonhealing pressure ulcers often yield confusing results. While a bone scan is highly sensitive (almost 100%), it is poorly specific (<33%), meaning that overdiagnosis is a common problem; this is due to the tendency of the nuclear molecules to concentrate in areas of bone that are affected by pressure-induced changes and in foci of heterotopic bone ossification. Therefore, a bone scan should be used primarily for its NPV, that is, to "rule out" osteomyelitis. An accurate positive diagnosis of osteomyelitis underlying a pressure ulcer usually requires examination of bone tissue; this is best obtained intraoperatively, because osteomyelitis is likely to be a focal process, and percutaneous biopsy may fail to sample the infected bone (Steinberg & Warren, 2007) (Fig. 10-17).

CLINICAL PEARL

An accurate diagnosis of osteomyelitis in the bone underlying a pressure ulcer usually requires examination of bone tissue, which is best obtained intraoperatively (because osteomyelitis is a focal process and percutaneous bone biopsy may fail to sample the infected bone).

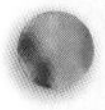

Controlling and Managing Bioburden

Bioburden management begins with careful attention to detail in the care of the patient with a chronic wound. Specifically, correction of the factors that can impair resistance to infection are essential and frequently overlooked components of the plan to control infection. Detailed evaluation and management of nutritional status, glycemic control, blood flow, edema, and exposure to trauma and pressure must be incorporated into the overall management plan and serial assessments of the patient.

The concept of wound bed preparation (Oh et al., 2011) implies comprehensive care that prepares a wound to heal and involves the foundational elements of wound care at every wound encounter as follows: cleansing, debridement of necrotic or nonviable tissue with attention to wound edges, and management and prevention of infection. Wound cleansing and debridement are covered in depth in Chapters 8 and 9 but cannot be overlooked as essential elements in management of wound bioburden. Necrotic tissue provides a breeding ground for bacterial growth and must be removed or debrided by means appropriate to the locale of care. Those wounds in which debridement is not indicated (e.g., an eschar on an ischemic heel) should be monitored frequently for signs of infection (e.g., separation and/or drainage at wound edges, erythema, induration, or fluctuance).

CLINICAL PEARL

Wound cleansing and debridement of necrotic tissue are key elements of a comprehensive plan to prevent or manage wound infection.

Wound Cleansing

All wounds should be cleansed at each dressing change, before and after debridement, and in the event of contamination using a neutral, nonirritating, nontoxic solution, and routine cleansing should be accomplished with every effort to minimize chemical and/or mechanical trauma (Schultz et al., 2003; Steed et al., 2006; Whitney et al., 2006). An exception to the requirement for routine cleansing may be the recent application of a skin graft or cellular tissue product that should be left undisturbed; in this case, the surrounding skin should be cleansed.

The choice of solution or agent used as well as the method of delivery is driven by the condition of the wound and local factors in the wound. There have been numerous citings in the literature spanning many years related to the toxicity of various solutions used for cleansing and disinfection in burn and wound care. Although definitive research is lacking, practice evidence suggests use of a nontoxic cleaning solution in combination with a delivery device that will create sufficient mechanical force to remove the surface debris without injury to healthy tissue (NPUAP & PPPIA, 2014).

Decision making relative to wound cleansing must be made based on the condition of the wound surface. The use of antiseptics has met with great scrutiny and has been the target of debate in recent years due to the perceived risks of cytotoxicity and the potential for tissue and cellular trauma associated with their use. The data against the use of antiseptics such as hydrogen peroxide, acetic acid, Dakin's solution, and povidone–iodine are based primarily on in vitro models demonstrating the toxicity of these agents to the viability of cells important to wound healing, such as fibroblasts, keratinocytes, and leukocytes. As a practical matter, the choice of solution used for wound cleansing should be made based on the presence of necrotic tissue and exudate on the wound surface, the condition and hygiene of the patient, the location of the wound, and the potential for environmental or other contamination such as incontinence.

In making the decision as to appropriate wound cleanser, the clinician should consider whether cleansing or disinfection is the desired outcome. Realistically, this decision will depend on the agent used and how it is used by the wound clinician. While packing a wound with material soaked in a particular agent may be inappropriate, use of that same solution as a cleanser or irrigation solution may be beneficial for some wounds. Thus, the wound clinician must always weigh the risks and benefits of a particular agent to a particular wound. Newer antiseptic agents such as superoxide water solutions, dilute sodium hypochlorite, and hypochlorous acid can be advantageous in management of wounds with high bacterial loads because they are able to reduce microbes on the surface of the wound without causing injury to the host wound cells.

CLINICAL PEARL

In determining the most appropriate wound cleanser, the clinician must decide whether the goal is wound cleansing or wound disinfection.

Commercially available wound cleansers contain surface active agents (surfactants) that break the bonds attaching contaminants and debris to the wound surface, allowing them to be rinsed away mechanically when the solution is sprayed or poured over the wound. The clinician should consider use of cleansing solutions with surfactants and/or antimicrobials for wounds with debris, confirmed infection, suspected infection, or suspected high levels of bacterial colonization (NPUAP & PPPIA, 2014). Any potential toxicity of these cleansers should be weighed against the need for more aggressive removal of surface debris and contaminants based on the assessment of the wound. Normal saline is an effective agent for wound cleansing when delivered with enough pressure to ensure adequate removal of surface debris. Pressures below 4 pounds per square inch (psi) are not sufficient to remove debris, and pressures exceeding 15 psi increase the risk that bacteria will be driven into the tissues (Drosou et al., 2003).

Cleansing solutions should be used at body temperature as it can take 40 minutes for a wound to return to normal temperature following cold cleansing (cleansing with room temperature solutions) and around 3 hours for leukocyte activity to recover after irrigation with a cold (room temperature) solution. The physiologic effects of hypothermia (e.g., vasoconstriction, depressed neutrophil activity, reduced ability of the cells to use oxygen free radicals to kill bacteria, and lower levels of collagen deposition) can result in impaired resistance to infection and delayed wound healing (Watret & McLean, 2014).

CLINICAL PEARL

Cleansing solutions should be warmed to body temperature to prevent interruption of leukocyte activity and impaired resistance to infection.

The use of potable water (tap water) for cleansing chronic wounds has been questioned many times. A Cochrane Review published in 2008 concluded that, based on the randomized trials available at that time, tap water is unlikely to be harmful if used for wound cleansing. The decision to use tap water to cleanse wounds should take into account the quality of water, nature of wounds, and the patient's general condition, including the presence of comorbid conditions (Fernandez et al., 2008). Recent guidelines suggest that most pressure ulcers can be cleansed with potable water (i.e., water suitable for drinking) or normal saline (NPUAP & PPPIA, 2014). If the wound is going to be cleansed as part of the patient's personal shower, the decision should also take into account the location of the wound, water conditions in a geographic area, the patient's physical condition and immune system, and the overall hygienic advantage. Patients should be advised not to immerse an open wound into a tub.

Skin cleansers, that is, those designed for use in care of the incontinent patient, should not be used as a wound cleanser. The surface-active agents in these preparations are of a concentration sufficient to emulsify and lift adherent fecal matter from the skin and therefore are damaging to the cells of an open wound.

Topical Antibiotics

Antibiotics have decreased in popularity as first-line treatments for wound management secondary to the rise of bacterial resistance. While the specific mechanism of action varies from one antibiotic to another, they generally have one, defined microbial target, which limits their effectiveness against multiple pathogens (International Consensus Group, 2012). It is agreed that antibiotics should be avoided unless there is evidence of true clinical infection; in addition, some topical antibiotics should be avoided due to the risks of hypersensitivity reactions, super infections, and increased bacterial resistance (Lipsky & Hoey, 2009). This is not to say that antibiotics should be abandoned all together; rather, they should be reserved for situations where advancing clinical infection is present, highly virulent organisms exist in the wound bed, or the host's immune response is severely compromised, such as in diabetic foot ulcer infections. In these cases, optimal therapy typically involves culture-based systemic antibiotic therapy as well as topical antimicrobial therapy. When a topical antibiotic is being considered for use in management of an infected wound, the wound team must select the specific agent based on the infecting organism and the topical agent's spectrum of bactericidal activity; if the infecting organism is unknown, it is best to obtain a culture.

CLINICAL PEARL

Antibiotics should be reserved for situations in which advancing clinical infection is present, highly virulent organisms are present in the wound bed, or there is severe immunosuppression; in these cases, optimal therapy involves culture-based systemic antibiotic therapy as well as topical antimicrobial therapy.

Perhaps the most appropriate use of topical antibiotics is for infection prophylaxis in superficial skin wounds with high risk of infection, such as those that are likely to be contaminated (accidental wounds, lacerations, abrasions, and burns). Because all traumatic wounds should be considered contaminated, use of topical antibiotics is logical for these wounds to prevent wound infection.

Antimicrobial Wound Dressings

Management and treatment of the infected and critically colonized wound is a dilemma encountered by wound clinicians with increasing frequency and is of particular concern with the rising numbers of infections caused by drug-resistant organisms. As previously discussed, careful and frequent assessment is essential to assure prompt recognition of changes in the wound that indicate either superficial or invasive infection. When the clinician realizes that sudden changes in the previously healing wound may indicate an initial host response to rising bacterial loads, she/he can initiate topical measures to reduce the bacterial load, preventing continued replication and potential invasion into the deeper tissues.

In recent years, there has been an appreciable increase in dressings that address local wound bioburden, while simultaneously managing the other needs of the wound, such as exudate and moisture balance, protection of the periwound skin, wicking of tunnels and filling of wound space, coverage, protection, and insulation. Each antimicrobial dressing option provides unique but familiar mechanisms of action that address wound care needs. The attributes of the ideal antimicrobial dressing (Maillard & Denyer, 2006) have been described as one that

- Provides sustained antimicrobial activity
- Provides a moist wound healing environment
- Allows consistent delivery of the antimicrobial over the entire surface of the wound
- Allows monitoring of the wound with minimum interference
- Manages exudate, if problematic
- Is comfortable
- Is conformable
- Provides an effective microbial barrier
- Absorbs and retains bacteria
- Avoids wound trauma on removal

The primary differentiating factor for the various dressings is the particular antimicrobial agent incorporated into the dressing. Antimicrobial agents are bound into or coated onto the dressing materials; they act as a barrier to outside contaminants in addition to interacting with wound exudate to further enhance the barrier effects and to reduce bacterial loads on the surface of the wound. Commonly used agents include silver, cadexomer iodine, honey, polyhexamethylene biguanide (PHMB), the pigments crystal violet and methylene blue, and dialkylcarbamoylchloride (DACC).

CLINICAL PEARL

In recent years, there has been an appreciable increase in the availability of dressings that address wound bioburden while simultaneously managing the other needs of the wound (e.g., exudate and moisture balance, wicking of tunnels, protection, and insulation).

Cadexomer Iodine

Many iodine preparations exist (Fig. 10-18), but not all are appropriate for wound care secondary to the cytotoxicity that may occur relative to overall concentration, release, and solubility of the iodine. Iodine has a broad spectrum of activity and works in many ways, for example, by disrupting

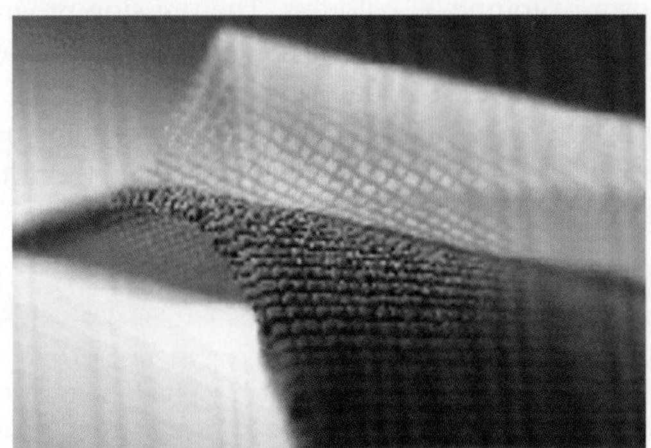

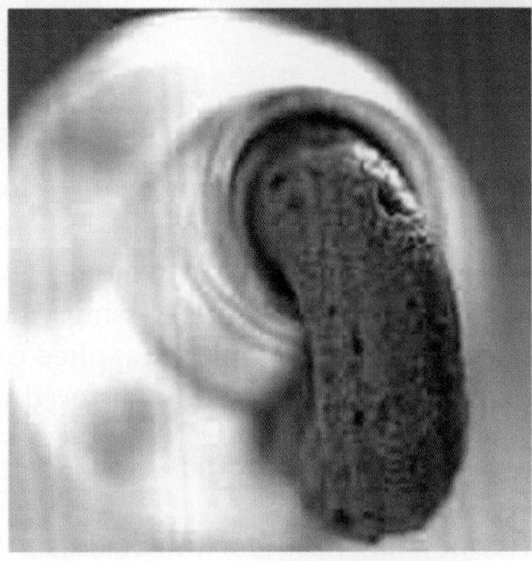

FIGURE 10-18. Cadexomer iodine.

cell walls and nuclei and by facilitating oxidative killing of microorganisms and neutrophils (Cooper et al., 1991). In vitro and in vivo studies have demonstrated iodine toxicity at the cellular level (Lineaweaver et al., 1985a, 1985b), and iodine has therefore traditionally been perceived as an inhibitor of wound healing. However, more recent studies suggest that different iodine compounds have different levels of toxicity and that the difference in toxicity associated with povidone–iodine compounds and cadexomer iodine may lie in the components of iodine delivery (Mertz et al., 1999). Specifically, a clinically beneficial iodine compound would control the speed and amount of iodine released into the wound bed, thus maintaining bactericidal effects while avoiding cytotoxicity, and would be incorporated into a dressing that permitted decreased frequency of dressing changes for the patient.

The term cadexomer iodine actually describes a delivery system rather than an antimicrobial agent. In this novel delivery system, the iodine is contained within a cadexomer starch bead. As wound exudate is absorbed, it enters the cadexomer bead, causing the openings to swell and allowing a slow, sustained release of the iodine molecules; this maintains a steady-state 0.9% concentration at the wound bed, which is nontoxic to healing wounds (Leaper & Durani, 2008). Iodine(I_2) is a potent microbicide, and the uncharged iodine molecule can penetrate the negatively charged exopolymeric matrix of most biofilms, which probably explains (at least partly) the ability of cadexomer iodine dressings to kill biofilm bacteria in laboratory experiments (Phillips et al., 2013). The microbicidal form of the iodine is brown, and iodide (I^-), which is the inactive form of iodine, is colorless. The dressing progresses from brown to colorless, which signals depletion of the iodine and acts as a signal to change the dressing. The dressing lasts for an average of 72 hours, depending on the amount of exudate, the size of the wound, and the amount of the dressing/gel used.

CLINICAL PEARL

Cadexomer iodine describes a delivery system that provides sustained release of iodine to maintain a steady-state level of iodine that is toxic to bacteria but nontoxic to the "good cells" in the wound bed.

Contraindications to use of cadexomer iodine are known allergy to iodine, dyes, or shellfish. Additionally, the structure of the cadexomer starch requires an adequate amount of exudate or moisture to allow for breakdown and release of the iodine. Thus, dry wounds without exudate may not properly activate the dressing. Additionally, iodine reduces the activity of topically applied collagenase ointment so these products should not be used simultaneously (Jovanovic et al., 2012).

Honey

The use of honey has been documented as a treatment for open wounds for centuries, having been mentioned in the Bible, the Koran, and the Torah (Fig. 10-19). It was documented for use in plasters by the Egyptians in 2000 BC, and in medical writings from 1392, and has experienced a renaissance in recent years as a topic of clinical and scientific research in wound healing. The form of medical grade honey used today differs greatly from that of the natural or culinary versions. Medical grade honey has 2 (two) general sources: *Leptospermum scoparium* (manuka), which is derived from tea plants, and *Leptospermum polygalifolium*, jelly bush honey. These forms have specific qualities related to processing that affect the end product's bacterial count, pH, enzyme activity, and overall benefit in wound care. Culinary honey uses heat to prepare the product for consumption, which invariably reduces the enzyme responsible for hydrogen peroxide production, whereas medical grade honey's gamma radiation sterilization process allows it to retain biologic activity (Pieper, 2009).

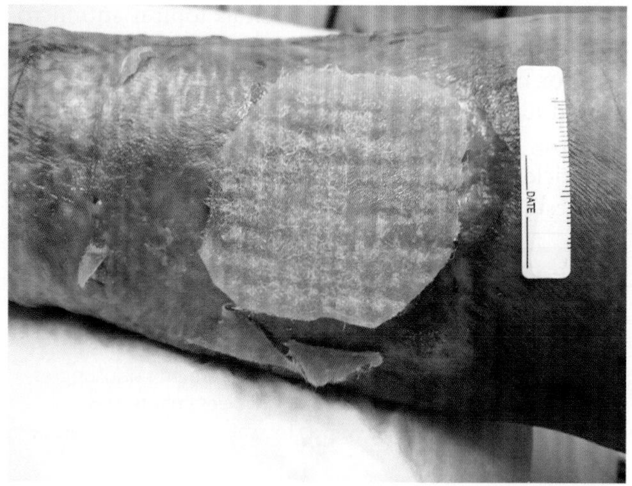

FIGURE 10-19. Honey.

Honey has demonstrated antimicrobial effects on a broad spectrum of viruses, fungi, protozoa, and over 50 species of bacteria, including clinically relevant organisms such as *Pseudomonas aeruginosa*, *S. aureus*, methicillin-resistant *Staphalococcus aureus (MRSA)*, and vancomycin-resistant *Enterococcus* (VRE) (Gethin & Cowman, 2008; Lipsky & Hoey, 2009). The antimicrobial activity of honey has been attributed to its high sugar content and low water activity, which creates an osmotic effect that dehydrates the bacteria; this effect, along with the acidic pH of 3.2 to 4.5, inhibits bacterial growth. The reduction in wound pH leads to increased oxygen release, reduced toxicity of bacterial end products, enhanced removal of abnormal wound collagen, decreased protease activity, promotion of angiogenesis, increased macrophage and fibroblast activity, and regulation of enzyme activity. The fluid shift produced by the osmotic effect also helps to create a moist wound healing environment, which reduces pain on dressing removal due to decreased potential for desiccation and adherence to the wound surface. Maintenance of a moist wound surface also promotes autolytic debridement; one study found that honey was more effective at desloughing wounds with >50% necrotic tissue than standard hydrogel, leading to statistically significant reduction in healing rates and time to epithelialization (Gethin & Cowman, 2008).

CLINICAL PEARL

Medical grade honey has unique properties that provide demonstrated antimicrobial effects, most likely as a result of osmotic activity that dehydrates the organism, and high acidity, which is generally toxic to bacteria.

Honey dressings are available in an alginate, hydrocolloid, and paste form. Dressings can be left in place for up to 7 days, but the actual wear time is determined by the volume of exudate, patient response, and soiling of secondary dressings. Reports of stinging or burning pain have been reported after initial application of the dressing to the wound bed, most likely because of the osmotic effects and the acidic pH of the dressing. Often, these symptoms are transient; however, in some cases, they persist and warrant a change in therapy. Contraindications to the use of honey include allergy to honey, and a common fear is that a sensitivity to bee venom would be a contraindication. While most clinicians will not use honey dressings for the patient with a known bee allergy, no reports of anaphylaxis have been described to date with medical grade honey wound care products (Ahmed et al., 2003; Dunford et al., 2000; Eddy & Gideonsen, 2005; Grothier & Cooper, 2011; Namias, 2003; Simon, 2006).

Polyhexamethylene Biguanide

PHMB is a biocide that has been used for many years with no known resistance (Fig. 10-20). It is used in a variety of products, including wound care dressings, contact lens cleaning solutions, perioperative cleansing products, and swimming pool cleaners (Moore & Gray, 2007; Mullder et al., 2007). The gauze sponges have also been used extensively as part of the dressing interface layer with numerous negative-pressure wound therapy devices. PHMB is a synthetic compound similar in structure to naturally occurring molecules that are produced by inflammatory cells to protect against infection. By attaching itself to the bacterial cell membrane, PHMB causes structural changes that kill the bacteria. In addition, the structural changes alter function of the efflux pumps that bacteria commonly use to pump antibiotics out of the cell; the cells are no longer able to eliminate the biocide via the efflux pumps and are thus unable to protect themselves against its bactericidal effects (Mertz et al., 1999; Moore & Gray, 2007). The incorporation of PHMB into dressings, including gauze sponges, nonadherent dressings, foams, and biosynthesized cellulose wound dressings, has been shown to provide an effective barrier to outside contamination in addition to bactericidal activity against bacteria absorbed into the dressing material. One study found that PHMB-impregnated foam showed a significant log reduction of *Pseudomonas aeruginosa* within the wound compared to standard gauze and did not allow *Pseudomonas* to colonize the PHMB-impregnated foam nor change the normal wound milieu. These results support one of the most common uses of PHMB by the wound care practitioner, which is to prevent infection in high-risk individuals (Cassinga et al., 2010). PHMB must come into direct contact with the bacterial organism. Therefore, once it is bound to a dressing material such as gauze, foam, or alginate, it can only affect bacteria that have been absorbed into the dressing (Butcher, 2012). In the case of newer wound irrigations and solutions, time of exposure is the key determinant, with at least 10 to 15 minutes of exposure required to induce optimal antimicrobial effects (Barrett et al., 2010). Therefore, clinicians utilizing PHMB in solution form should consider allowing the solution to dwell in the wound bed during the cleansing process or provide the agent as a continuous irrigation such as through the use of NPWT devices that instill or allow dwell time (Butcher, 2012).

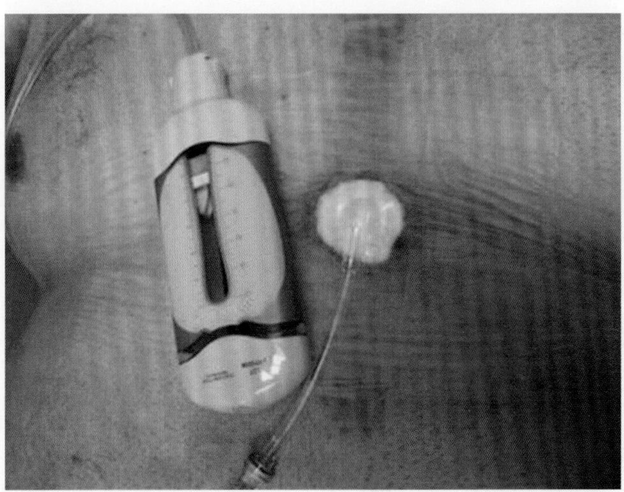

FIGURE 10-20. PHMB gauze under nonpowered NPWT device.

CLINICAL PEARL

PHMB is a biocide that has been used for many years with no known resistance; these products are generally considered more appropriate for prophylaxis or management of critical colonization than for primary treatment of an infected wound.

Contraindications to the use of PHMB include known adverse reactions to PHMB or chlorhexidine. Care should be taken to avoid saturation of PHMB impregnated gauzes with solutions other than normal saline, sterile water, or potable water, as certain antiseptic solutions such as sodium hypochlorite may result in a chemical reaction that inactivates these agents and produces a nontoxic yellow stain. Additionally, PHMB has been shown in vitro to significantly reduce the activity of exogenously applied collagenase (Jovanovic et al., 2012). Finally, because of the method of action of PHMB, it is generally considered more appropriate for prophylaxis, or for the critically colonized wound, than for primary treatment of active wound infection (Barrett et al., 2010). The frequency of dressing change is dependent upon the dressing into which the PHMB is impregnated; manufacturers' recommendations should be followed.

Methylene Blue and Gentian Violet

The pigments methylene blue crystal and gentian violet (Fig. 10-21) have been used in medicine for over 50 years as laboratory stains (Wikipedia, 2014) and as antiseptics with bacteriostatic properties against multiple clinically relevant bacteria, including resistant strains such as methicillin-resistant *S. aureus* (MRSA). One polyurethane foam dressing includes silver as an additional agent. The methylene blue and gentian violet dye molecules are bound to a polyvinyl alcohol (PVA) foam with a three-dimensional interconnected open-cell structure; when hydrated, the foam becomes a soft, conformable wound filler and contact dressing. Recently, methylene blue and gentian violet have also become available bound to polyurethane foams (open cell foams that do not require hydration). In vitro, PVA foam absorbs up to 12 times its weight in exudate (Hollister Wound Care, 2013). Coupled with its absorptive capacity, the methylene blue/gentian violet–bound foam traps and inhibits exudate-associated bacterial growth. In clinical use, the foam also has been noted to reduce hypergranulation tissue and to promote flattening of slightly rolled wound edges, particularly in venous leg ulcers; this in turn promotes epidermal edge cellular migration (Weir & Blakely, 2011). A particular advantage of gentian violet and methylene blue absorbent antibacterial dressings is compatibility with exogenously applied collagenase (Jovanovic et al., 2012). The nonrelease formulation of the dressing also prevents any harm to wound base–associated growth factors that are endogenously produced or to exogenously delivered biological agents (Jelf et al., 2008). Color change may occur in the dressing, from deep blue to a lighter blue or white caused by bacterial inhibition and depletion of the methylene blue and gentian violet components, which provides an important visual indicator to guide dressing change. The PVA dressing is changed every other day or more or less frequently, depending upon the level of exudate, and the polyurethane foam may be left in place up to 7 days.

CLINICAL PEARL

A particular advantage of methylene blue/gentian violet impregnated products is the compatibility with enzymatic agents containing collagenase.

Silver

Silver has been used for centuries (Fig. 10-22), originally in vessels used to preserve water and has had medicinal uses documented from AD 750. A renewed interest in the use of ionic silver in topical antimicrobial dressings has resulted in multiple studies to assess its ability to reduce bacterial growth and the risk of wound infection, to manage active infection, and to reduce the risk of hospital-acquired wound infections. This renewed interest is largely attributed to silver's bactericidal efficacy at low concentrations and its relatively limited toxicity to human cells. Silver has proven antimicrobial activity, which includes antibiotic-resistant bacteria such as MRSA and vancomycin-resistant enterococci (VRE). Renewed interest in clinical use has also been supported by advances in impregnation techniques and polymer technologies, resulting in numerous delivery systems in the form of dressing materials (White & Cutting, 2006). Silver is now available in amorphous hydrogels, sheet hydrogels, alginates, hydrofibers, foams, silicones, contact layers, wound powders, ointments, negative pressure foams, and irrigation solutions (silver nitrate

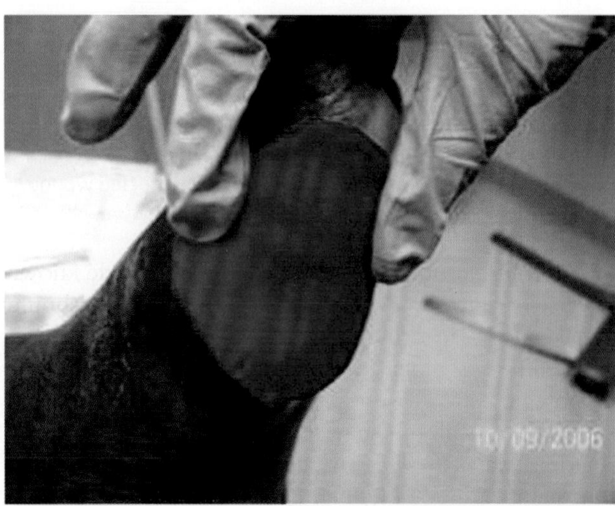

FIGURE 10-21. Methylene blue and gentian violet foam.

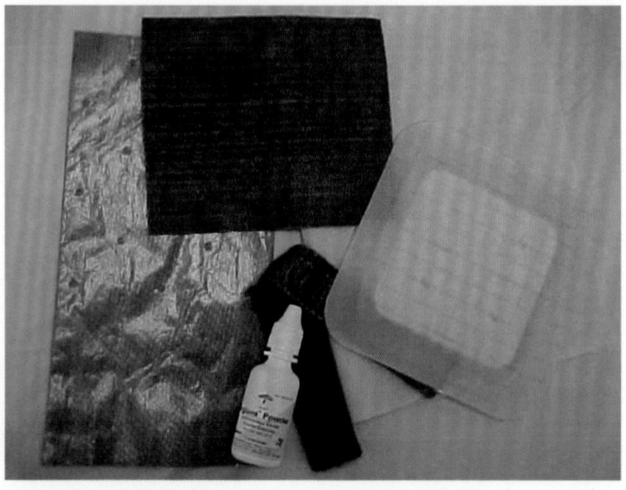

FIGURE 10-22. Examples of Silvers.

solutions); the choice of dressing for a particular wound is determined by the characteristics of the particular carrier dressing, the way silver is delivered to the wound bed, and the needs of the wound. Silver dressings "work" via one of two delivery systems: the silver may be donated to the wound bed and may therefore kill organisms on the wound surface; or the silver may be retained in the dressing and work by destroying bacteria contained in the exudate and absorbed into the carrier dressing. In order for silver to realize its total bactericidal potential, there must be controlled and sustained release of silver over time that is sufficient to cause bacterial death but within a range that prevents tissue toxicity (Cutting et al., 2009). The ability of the dressing to conform, remain in place, and provide consistent coverage of the wound bed also contributes to antimicrobial effectiveness. Again, the quantity, chemical form, delivery, release, and ability to conform influence the clinical outcomes associated with silver dressings (Expert working group consensus, 2012; Hamm, 2010; Jones et al., 2005).

CLINICAL PEARL

Silver dressings "work" through one of two mechanisms: (1) donation of silver to wound surface, with direct bactericidal activity at the wound surface, or (2) destruction of bacteria within the carrier dressing itself.

There is an abundance of information published regarding the use of silver compared to other antimicrobial agents and dressings. This is in large part related to the number of years that silver has been used in wound management; for example, silver sulfadiazine is a broad-spectrum antimicrobial that has been available for over 40 years, with extensive use in management of burn wounds. Silver sulfadiazine cream has a relatively short period of action, its penetration of burn eschar is poor, and it forms a pseudoeschar with repeated applications; as a result, frequent and often painful dressing changes are required to remove any residual cream prior to reapplication. Studies suggest that alternative methods of silver delivery may provide equally effective bacterial control with a more patient-friendly delivery system. For example, a study involving partial thickness burns showed no statistically significant difference in the rate of infection or time required for reepithelialization between burns managed with silver sulfadiazine and those managed with a silver hydrogel; however, the author reported less pain and increased patient satisfaction in the hydrogel group (Glat et al., 2009).

Silver is biologically active when it is in soluble form, that is, as Ag+ or Ag^0 clusters. Ag+ is the ionic form found in silver nitrate, silver sulfadiazine, and other ionic silver compounds. Ag^0 is the uncharged form of metallic silver present in nanocrystalline silver products. Free silver cations have a potent antimicrobial effect that destroys microorganisms immediately by blocking cellular respiration and disrupting bacterial cell membranes. Specifically, silver cations bind to tissue proteins, causing structural changes in the bacterial cell membranes that cause cell death. Silver cations also bind and denature bacterial DNA and RNA, thus inhibiting cell replication (Fong & Wood, 2006). Further, silver may increase the sensitivity of a biofilm to antibiotics and may also reduce its adhesion to the wound bed (Kostenko et al., 2010).

Concerns related to the use of silver dressings relate to the potential for development of bacterial resistance, potential for cellular toxicity, and assuring appropriate use of the right amount of silver at the right time. Percival et al. (2008) investigated the prevalence of silver resistance in bacteria from diabetic foot ulcers and found low incidence of silver-resistant genes in these bacteria; in addition, the silver-resistant genes appeared to be confined to an enteric bacterium, *Enterobacter cloacae*, which is not known to be a primary wound pathogen. There was no evidence of silver-resistant genes in common wound pathogens such as *S. aureus* and *P. aeruginosa*. These investigators also found that the wound bacteria containing silver-resistant genes were killed when challenged with silver-containing wound dressings. The toxicity of silver to normal cells and tissues has also been assessed. Silver dressings with demonstrated toxicity at 1 day in "in vitro" studies demonstrated no cytotoxicity at 1 week in "in vivo" studies; these results suggest that in vitro cytotoxicity is greater than in vivo because the silver in "in vitro" studies is not diluted by wound fluid, perfusion effects, and/or effects of the tissue reservoir or metabolism (White & Cutting, 2006a).

Considerations and contraindications related to the use of silver fall into two primary areas. Of lesser concern is the use of silver in conjunction with exogenously applied collagenase. The use of dressings with heavy metal ions is discouraged due to their impact on activity of the enzyme. The impact of silver dressings is quite variable, with in vitro reduction in activity ranging from as low as 3.8% to as high as 67% depending on the delivery system (Jovanovic et al., 2012). Thus, clinicians are encouraged to avoid silver in combination with collagenase when possible; if combined usage is being considered, the clinician should check with the drug manufacturer for specific interaction precautions.

Of greater importance from a safety perspective is the use of silver in the pediatric population, as an infant or child is at greater risk for systemic absorption of topical products and resulting toxicity (Barrett & Rutter, 1994). While there have been reports in the literature of safe use of silver in this population, those studies utilized traditional end points in wound healing trials (e.g., time to healing, pain, and length of stay), rather than risk of harm (Jester et al., 2008). The in vitro toxicity data needs to be carefully considered when considering use of silver-based products for the pediatric population (Poon & Burd, 2004; Treadwell et al., 2008). For example, silver toxicity was a reported concern in the assessment of pediatric burn patients managed with nanocrystalline silver dressings;

specifically, serum silver levels were elevated, and the elevation was closely proportional to the surface area of the wounds treated (Treadwell et al., 2008; Treadwell, 2011). An animal model has also raised questions over deposition of silver in the major organs; in some cases, serum levels of silver were noted to be 800 times greater than normal (Treadwell, 2011). When considering the use of a silver dressing for a pediatric patient, the age of the patient, size of the wound, level of silver, and delivery system should be taken into consideration. Clinicians should avoid silver dressings in neonates and should limit the use of such products in the pediatric population to no more than 2 weeks (Expert working group consensus, 2012). A thorough knowledge of the characteristics of the products to be used in this population is essential.

DACC

Dialkylcarbamoyl chloride (Weir & Brindel, 2015) (Fig. 10-23). Cell surface hydrophobicity of bacteria is a very important physicochemical feature and has a significant impact on the organism's ability to adhere to the surface of host cells or medical implants. Adhesion of bacteria to the cell surface is the first, significant step of infection. The rapid phase of adhesion depends on a variety of nonspecific, relatively weak physicochemical forces; hydrophobic interaction is assumed to be the most important of these factors (Kustos et al., 2003). When two hydrophobic particles come in contact with each other within an aqueous environment, the forces of the surrounding water molecules actually cause the particles to bind and hold together. The principles of hydrophobic interaction can be seen in daily life, such as how drops of oil may aggregate into one larger grouping when dropped into water.

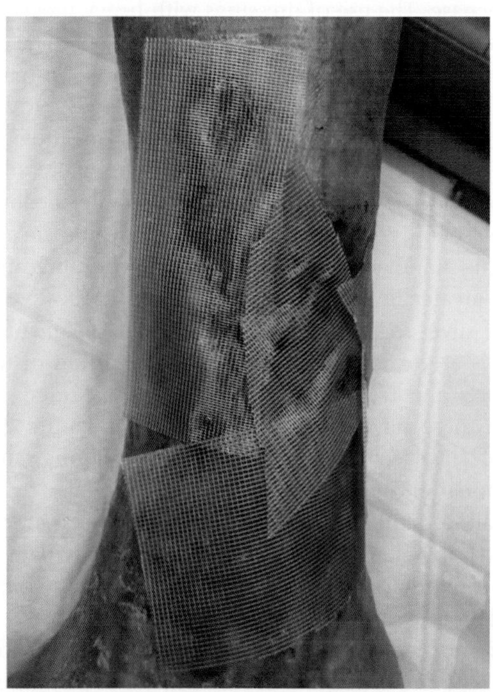

FIGURE 10-23. DACC.

Antimicrobial dressings use multiple modes of action to induce bactericidal effects and prevent bacterial replication as follows: binding to DNA, disruption of efflux pumps, disruption of bacterial cell membranes, denaturing proteins, and displacement of metallic cations in the bacterial cell wall (Hamm, 2010). Regardless of the specific mechanism of action, the end result is bacterial killing, which causes release of endotoxins, exotoxins, and cellular debris into the wound bed. This increases the inflammatory response, and the risk of inappropriate increase in MMPs activation by neutrophils (Butcher, 2011). DACC-based dressings represent a deviation from our standard approach to management of bacteria on the surface of a chronic wound. DACC "works" by physically binding the bacteria versus bacterial killing. The contact layer of the dressing is coated with a hydrophobic fatty acid derivative, which irreversibly binds with bacteria; while the bacteria are not killed, they are unable to dissociate from the surface of the dressing, which means they are rendered inactive and are then physically removed when the dressing is changed. One study used real-time PCR evaluation to measure the bacterial bioburden in wounds prior to and following use of DACC-coated dressings. The investigators found that the bacterial load at the beginning of wound treatment was 4.41 × 107 mg/tissue and at the end of therapy was 1.73 × 105 mg/tissue; this represented a 254-fold reduction in the bacterial load ($p = 0.0243$) (Gentili et al., 2012).

CLINICAL PEARL

DACC-based dressings represent a deviation from our standard approach to management of bacteria; they "work" by physically binding and removing the bacteria as opposed to killing the bacteria.

If DACC dressings are to be used effectively for wound care, appropriate levels of moisture are important, because adequate moisture at the surface of the wound is essential for optimal attachment of the bacteria to the dressing. In addition, common antiseptics and analgesics may interfere with hydrophobic attachment, including eutectic mixture of local anesthetic (EMLA) and the use of any products or topical treatments that are petrolatum-based. Therefore, if a DACC dressing is being considered for a wound that is dry and nonexudative, a hydrogel or moisture retentive cover dressing should be used to provide the moisture needed for effective use of DACC (Hamptson, 2007).

Another practical consideration in the use of hydrophobic binding dressings is frequency of dressing changes. As the dressings remove bacteria with each change, wounds with clinical signs of critical colonization or infection may require dressing changes every 12 to 24 hours to achieve the needed reduction in wound bioburden; an appropriately absorptive secondary dressing should be used to manage exudate (von Hallern & Lang, 2005). In cases of prophylaxis when there are no clinical signs of infection, dressing change frequency may be as infrequent as every 4 days (Probst & Steinenberg, 2014). Because there are no chemical agents in this dressing, safe use in children has been described. Meberg and Schoyen (1990) performed a prospective randomized study on umbilical cord disinfection, comparing use of DACC ($n = 1{,}213$) to daily cleansing with 0.5% chlorhexidine in 70% ethanol ($n = 1{,}228$), and found no difference in the rate of infections between the two groups. No adverse reactions were reported in the DACC group. The versatility of DACC dressings has led to evaluation of their potential benefit as wound fillers with NPWT. A pig model was utilized to study the efficacy of the pathogen-binding mesh (DACC) versus standard foam and gauze as related to granulation tissue formation, wound contraction, microvascular blood flow, and wound contraction (Malmsjo & Ingemansson, 2011). The authors found that pressure transduction was similar among all products, wound contraction occurred more rapidly with foam products, and the pathogen-binding mesh was associated with more rapid granulation tissue formation than gauze and demonstrated fluid-retaining qualities similar to foam. The potential benefits provided by DACC products include the fact that these dressings do not deliver any specific chemical or antimicrobial substance to the wound bed; as a result, hydrophobic bacterial-binding dressings may be used longer than the 2-week challenge period sometimes suggested for other antimicrobials (Bruce, 2012).

Conclusion

Decision making related to the management of bioburden in the chronic wound demands a thorough assessment that includes systemic risk factors as well as wound status and local risk factors and meticulous monitoring of the wound's progress in healing once a treatment decision is made. While avoidance of unnecessary systemic antibiotics is ideal, judicial use is often warranted. Although clinicians frequently rely heavily on the appearance of the wound to drive decisions regarding culture and treatment, the simple fact that a wound is not progressing may raise enough suspicion that careful assessment for excessive bioburden is prudent. Consultation with colleagues in infectious diseases should be considered when the impact of the bacterial bioburden is beyond the scope of the treating practitioner.

REFERENCES

Ahmed, A. K., Hoekstra, M. J., Hage, J. J., et al. 2003. Honey-medicated dressing: Transformation of an ancient remedy into modern therapy. *Annals of Plastic Surgery, 50*(2), 143–147.

Expert working group consensus. (2012). *International Consensus. Appropriate use of silver dressings in wounds.* London, UK: Wounds International.

Bamberg, R., Sullivan, P. K., & Conner-Kerr T. Diagnosis of wound infections: Current culturing practices of US wound care professionals. *Wounds* 2002, *14*, 314–327.

Baranoski, S., Ayello, E., Tomic-Canic, M., et al. (2011). Skin, an essential organ. In S Baranoski. & E Ayello. (Eds), *Wound care essentials: Practice principles*. Ambler, PA: Lippincott Williams & Wilkins.

Barrett, D. A., & Rutter, N. (1994). Transdermal delivery and the premature neonate. *Critical Reviews in Therapeutic Drug Carrier Systems, 11*(1), 1–30.

Barrett, S., Battacharyya, M., Butcher, M., et al. (2010). *PHMB and its potential contribution to wound management, 6*(2), 40–46. Wounds UK.

Berg, J. O., Mossner, B. K., Skov, M. N., et al. (2006). Antibacterial properties of EMLA and lidocaine in wound tissue biopsies for culturing. *Wound Repair and Regeneration, 14*(5), 581–585.

Bowler, P. G. (2003). The 10(5) bacterial growth guideline: Reassessing its clinical relevance in wound healing. *Ostomy/Wound Management, 49*(1), 44–53.

Browne, A., Dow, G., & Sibbald, R. G. (2001). Infected wounds: Definitions and controversies. In V Falanga (Ed), *Cutaneous wound healing* (pp. 203–219). London, UK: Martin Dunitz.

Butcher, M. (2011). Catch or kill. How DACC technology redefines antimicrobial management. *British Journal of Community Nursing,* (Suppl), 4–22.

Butcher, M. (2012). PHMB: An effective antimicrobial in wound bioburden management. *British Journal of Nursing, 21*, s16–s21.

Bruce, Z. (2012). *Using Cutimed Sorbact Hydroactive on chronic infected wounds, 8*(1), 119–129. Wounds UK.

Cassinga, A., Serralta, V., Davis, S., et al. (2010). The effect of an antimicrobial gauze dressing impregnated with 0.2-percent polyhexamethylene biguanide as a barrier to prevent *Pseudomonas aeruginosa* wound invasion. *Wounds, 14*, 169–176.

Cooper M. L., Laxer J. A., & Hansbrough J. F. (1991). The cytotoxic effects of commonly used topical antimicrobial agents on human fibroblasts and keratinocytes. *Journal of Trauma, 31*(6), 775–782.

Costerton, J. W., Stewart, P. S., & Greenberg, E. P. (1999). Bacterial biofilms: A common cause of persistent infections. *Science, 284*(5418), 1318–1322.

Costerton, W., Veeh, R., Shirtliff, M., et al. (2003). The application of biofilm science to the study and control of chronic bacterial infections. *Journal of Clinical Investigation, 112*(10), 1466–1477.

Cowan, D. K., & Talaro, K. P. (2006). *Infectious diseases affecting the skin and eyes. Microbiology: A Systems Approach*. New York: McGraw-Hill, 540–576.

Cutting, K., White, R., & Hoekstra, H. (2009). Topical silver-impregnated dressings and the importance of the dressing technology. *International Wound Journal, 6*(5), 396–402.

Davis E. (1996). Don't deny the chance to heal. 2nd Joint Meeting of Wound Healing Society and European Tissue Repair Society.

Donlan, R. M., Costerton, J. W. (2002). Biofilms: Survival mechanisms of clinically relevant microorganisms. *Clinical Microbiology Reviews, 15*(2), 167–193.

Dowd, S. E., Sun, Y., Secor, P. R., et al. (2008a). Survey of bacterial diversity in chronic wounds using Pyrosequencing, DGGE, and full ribosome shotgun sequencing. *BMC Microbiology, 8*(1), 43.

Dowd, S. E., Wolcott, R. D., Kennedy, J., et al. (2011). Molecular diagnostics and personalised medicine in wound care: Assessment of outcomes. *Journal of Wound Care, 20*(5), 234–239.

Dowd, S. E., Wolcott, R. D., Sun, Y., et al. (2008b). Polymicrobial nature of chronic diabetic foot ulcer biofilm infections determined using bacterial tag encoded FLX amplicon pyrosequencing (bTEFAP). *PLoS One, 3*(10), e3326.

Drosou, A., Falabella, A., Kirsner, R. S. (2003). Antiseptics on wounds: An area of controversy. *Wounds, 15*, 149–166.

Dunford, C., Cooper, R., Molan, P., et al. (2000). The use of honey in wound management. *Nursing Standard, 15*(11), 63–68.

Eddy, J. J., & Gideonsen, M. D. (2005). Topical honey for diabetic foot ulcers. *Journal of Family Practice, 54*(6), 533–535.

Fernandez, R., Griffiths, R., & Ussia, C. (2008). Water for wound cleansing. *Cochrane Database of Systematic Reviews*. CD003861.

Flemming, H. C., Neu, T. R., & Wozniak, D. J. (2007). The EPS matrix: "The house of biofilm cells". *Journal of Bacteriology, 189*(22), 7945–7947.

Fong, J., & Wood, F. (2006). Nanocrystalline silver dressings in wound management: A review. *International Journal of Nanomedicine, 1*(4), 441–449.

Gardner, S. E., Frantz, R. A., & Doebbeling, B. N. (2001). The validity of the clinical signs and symptoms used to identify localized chronic wound infection. *Wound Repair and Regeneration, 9*(3), 178–186.

Gentili, V., Gianesini, S., Balboni, P. G., et al. (2012). Panbacterial real-time PCR to evaluate bacterial burden in chronic wounds treated with Cutimed Sorbact. *European Journal of Clinical Microbiology and Infectious Diseases, 31*(7), 1523–1529.

Gethin, G., & Cowman, S. (2008). Bacteriological changes in sloughy venous leg ulcers treated with manuka honey or hydrogel: An RCT. *Journal of Wound Care, 17*(6), 241–247.

Glat, P. M., Kubat, W. D., Hsu, J. F., et al. (2009). Randomized clinical study of SilvaSorb gel in comparison to Silvadene silver sulfadiazine cream in the management of partial-thickness burns. *Journal of Burn Care and Research, 30*(2), 262–267.

Grayson, M. L., Gibbons, G. W., Balogh, K., et al. (1995). Probing to bone in infected pedal ulcers. A clinical sign of underlying osteomyelitis in diabetic patients. *JAMA, 273*(9), 721–723.

Grothier, L., & Cooper, R. (2011). Medihoney dressings made easy. *Wounds UK, 6*(2), 1–6.

Hall-Stoodley, L., & Stoodley, P. (2009). Evolving concepts in biofilm infections. *Cellular Microbiology, 11*(7), 1034–1043.

Hamm, R. (2010). Antibacterial dressings. In C Sen (Ed.), *Advances in wound care* (pp. 148–154). New Rochelle, NY: Mary Ann Liebert, Inc.

Hamptson, S. (2007). An evaluation of the efficacy of Cutimed Sorbact in different types of non-healing wounds. *Wounds UK, 3*, 1–6.

Hibbing, M. E., Fuqua, C., Parsek, M. R., et al. (2010). Bacterial competition: Surviving and thriving in the microbial jungle. *Nature Reviews Microbiology, 8*(1), 15–25.

Hollister Wound Care. (2013). Hydrofera Blue Antimicrobial Dressings Monograph.

http://biology.clc.uc.edu/courses/bio106/bacteria.htm. Accessed October 28, 2014.

http://medical-dictionary.thefreedictionary.com/bioburden. Accessed October 28, 2014.

International Consensus Group. (2012). *Appropriate use of silver dressings in wounds. An expert working group consensus*. London, UK: Wounds International. Retrieved from http://www.woundsinternational.com.

Jelf, C., Jelf, C., Aust, D., et al. (2008). *Comparison of the effects of antimicrobial wound dressings on cell viability, proliferation, and growth factor activity*. Toronto, CA: World Union of Wound Healing Societies Congress.

Jester, I., Bohn, I., Hannamann, T., et al. (2008). Comparison of two silver dressings for wound management in pediatric burns. *Wounds, 20*, 303–308.

Johnson, S. M., Saint John, B. E., & Dine, A. P. (2008). Local anesthetics as antimicrobial agents: A review. *Surgical Infections, 9*(2), 205–213.

Jones, S., Bowler, P. G., & Walker, M. (2005). Antimicrobial activity of silver-containing dressings is influenced by dressing conformability with a wound surface. *Wounds, 17*, 263–270.

Jovanovic, A., Ermis, R., Mewaldt, R., et al. (2012). The influence of metal salts, surfactants, and wound care products on enzymatic activity of collagenase, the wound debriding enzyme. *Wounds, 24*, 242–253.

Kostenko, V., Lyczak, J., Turner, K., et al. (2010). Impact of silver-containing wound dressings on bacterial biofilm viability and susceptibility to antibiotics during prolonged treatment. *Antimicrobial Agents and Chemotherapy, 54*(12), 5120–5131.

Kustos, T., Kustos, I., Kilar, F., et al. (2003). Effect of antibiotics on cell surface hydrophobicity of bacteria causing orthopedic wound infections. *Chemotherapy, 49*(5), 237–242.

Landis, S., Ryan, S., & Woo, K. (2007). Infections in chronic wounds. In D Krasner., G. T. Rodeheaver, & R. G. Sibbald (Eds.), *Chronic wound care: A clinical source book for healthcare professionals*. (pp. 299–321). Malvern, PA: HMP Communications.

Lavery, L. A., Armstrong, D. G., Peters, E. J., et al. (2007). Probe-to-bone test for diagnosing diabetic foot osteomyelitis: Reliable or relic? *Diabetes Care, 30*(2), 270–274.

Leaper, D. J., & Durani, P. (2008). Topical antimicrobial therapy of chronic wounds healing by secondary intention using iodine products. *International Wound Journal, 5*(2), 361–368.

Lee, P. C., Turnidge, J., & McDonald, P. J. (1985). Fine-needle aspiration biopsy in diagnosis of soft tissue infections. *Journal of Clinical Microbiology, 22*(1), 80–83.

Levine, N. S., Lindberg, R. B., Mason, A. D., Jr., et al. (1976). The quantitative swab culture and smear: A quick, simple method for determining the number of viable aerobic bacteria on open wounds. *Journal of Trauma, 16*(2), 89–94.

Lineaweaver, W., Howard, R., Soucy, D., et al. (1985a). Topical antimicrobial toxicity. *Archives of Surgery, 120*(3), 267–270.

Lineaweaver, W., McMorris, S., Soucy, D., et al. (1985b). Cellular and bacterial toxicities of topical antimicrobials. *Plastic and Reconstructive Surgery, 75*(3), 394–396.

Lipsky, B. A., & Hoey, C. (2009). Topical antimicrobial therapy for treating chronic wounds. *Clinical Infectious Diseases, 49*(10), 1541–1549.

Maillard, J. Y., & Denyer, S. P. (2006). Focus on silver. *EWMA Journal, 6*, 5–7.

Malmsjo, M., & Ingemansson, R. (2011). Effects of green foam, black foam, and gauze on contraction, blood flow and pressure delivery to the wound bed in negative pressure wound therapy. *Journal of Plastic, Reconstructive and Aesthetic Surgery, 64*, e289–e296.

Martin, L. K., & Drosou, A. (2005). Wound microbiology and the use of antibacterial agents. In A. F. Falabella & R. S. Krisner (Eds.), *Wound healing* (pp. 83–101). Boca Raton, FL: Taylor & Francis Group.

Meberg, A., & Schoyen, R. (1990). Hydrophobic material in routine umbilical cord care and prevention of infections in newborn infants. *Scandinavian Journal of Infectious Diseases, 22*(6), 729–733.

Mertz, P. M., Oliveira-Gandia, M. F., & Davis, S. C. (1999). The evaluation of a cadexomer iodine wound dressing on methicillin resistant *Staphylococcus aureus* (MRSA) in acute wounds. *Dermatologic Surgery, 25*(2), 89–93.

Moore, K., & Gray, D. (2007). Using PHMB antimicrobial to prevent wound infection. *Wounds UK, 3*, 96–102.

Mullder, G. D., Cavorsi, J. P., & Lee, D. K. (2007). Polyhexamethylene biguanide (PHMB): An addendum to current topical antimicrobials. *Wounds, 19*, 173–182.

Namias, N. (2003). Honey in the management of infections. *Surgical Infections (Larchmt), 4*(2), 219–226.

National Pressure Ulcer Advisory Panel and Pan Pacific Pressure Injury Alliance. Prevention and Treatment of Pressure Ulcers: Quick Reference Guide. Haesler, E. 2014. Perth, Australia, Cambridge Media.

Oh, K. J., Park, K. H., Kim, S. N., et al. (2011). Predictive value of intra-amniotic and serum markers for inflammatory lesions of preterm placenta. *Placenta, 32*(10), 732–736.

Percival, S. L., Woods, E., Nutekpor, M., et al. (2008). Prevalence of silver resistance in bacteria isolated from diabetic foot ulcers and efficacy of silver-containing wound dressings. *Ostomy/Wound Management, 54*(3), 30–40.

Phillips, P. L., Yang, Q., Davis, S., et al. (2013). Antimicrobial dressing efficacy against mature *Pseudomonas aeruginosa* biofilm on porcine skin explants. *International Wound Journal*. doi: 10.1111/iwj.12142.

Pieper, B. (2009). Honey-based dressings and wound care: An option for care in the United States. *Journal of Wound, Ostomy, and Continence Nursing, 36*(1), 60–66.

Plankton and Planktonic Bacteria, World of Microbiology and Immunology. Accessed at: http://www.encyclopedia.com/doc/1G2-3409800448.html. Accessed August 31, 2014.

Poon, V. K., & Burd A. (2004). In vitro cytotoxicity of silver: Implication for clinical wound care. *Burns, 30*(2), 140–147.

Probst, A., & Steinenberg, K. A. (2014). Reutlingen. Chronic arterial leg ulcer with MRSA. Case Report 6. BSN Medical.

Robson, M. C., Cooper, D. M., Aslam, R., et al. (2006). Guidelines for the treatment of venous ulcers. *Wound Repair and Regeneration, 14*(6), 649–662.

Robson, M. C., & Krizek T. J. (1973). Predicting skin graft survival. *Journal of Trauma, 13*(3), 213–217.

Robson, M. C. (1997). Wound infection. A failure of wound healing caused by an imbalance of bacteria. *Surgical Clinics of North America, 77*(3), 637–650.

Sauer, K., Camper, A. K., Ehrlich, G. D., et al. (2002). *Pseudomonas aeruginosa* displays multiple phenotypes during development as a biofilm. *Journal of Bacteriology, 184*(4), 1140–1154.

Schultz, G. S., Sibbald, R. G., Falanga, V., et al. (2003). Wound bed preparation: A systematic approach to wound management. *Wound Repair and Regeneration, 11*(Suppl 1), S1–S28.

Serena, T., Robson, M. C., & Cooper, G. J. (2006). Lack of reliability of clinic/visual assessment of chronic wound infection: The incidence of biopsy-proven infection in venous leg ulcers. *Wounds, 18*, 197–202.

Steed, D. L., Attinger, C., Colaizzi, T., et al. (2006). Guidelines for the treatment of diabetic ulcers. *Wound Repair and Regeneration, 14*(6), 680–692.

Steinberg, J. S., & Warren, J. S. (2007). Point-counter point: Probe to bone: Is it the best test for osteomyelitis? *Podiatry Today, 20*, 50–54.

Stoodley, P., Sauer, K., Davies, D., et al. (2002). Biofilms as complex differentiated communities. *Annual Review of Microbiology, 56*, 187–209.

Stotts, N. A. (2004). Wound infection: Diagnosis and management. In M. J. Morrison, L. G. Ovington, & K. Wilkie (Eds.), *Chronic wound care: A problem-based learning approach* (pp. 101–116). St. Louis, MO: Mosby.

Sussman, C., & Bates-Jensen, B. M. (2012). Skin and soft tissue anatomy and wound healing physiology. In C Sussman. & B. M. Bates-Jensen (Eds.), *Wound care: A collaborative practice manual for health professionals*. Philadelphia, PA: Lippincott Williams & Wilkins.

The Gram Stain. (2014). Available at: http://www.ncl.ac.uk/dental/oralbiol/oralenv/tutorials/gramstain.htm. Accessed August 31, 2014.

Treadwell, T. A. (2011). Children and wounds. *Wounds, 23*(11).

Treadwell, T. A., Fuentes, M. L., Walker, D. (2008). Treatment of second degree burns with dehydrated, decellularized amniotic membrane (biovance) vs. a silver dressing (acticoat). *Wound Repair and Regeneration, 16*, A39.

Trengove, N. J., Stacey M. C., McGechie D. F., et al. (1996). Qualitative bacteriology and leg ulcer healing. *Journal of Wound Care, 5*(6), 277–280.

von Hallern, B., & Lang, F. (2005). Cutimed Sorbact proved its practical value as an antibacterial dressing? Medizin Praxis, 8–11.

Watret, L., & McLean, A. (2014). Cleansing diabetic foot wounds: Tap water or saline? *Wounds International, 5*, 1–5.

Weir, D., & Blakely, M. (2011). Case review of the clinical use of an antimicrobial PVA foam dressing. Poster Presentation: Clinical Symposium for Advances in Skin and Wound Care. September 9–11, 2011; Washington, D.C. Available from: www.hollisterwoundcare.com/files/pdfs/posters/HWC%20Weir%20Hydrofera%20Blue%20Poster.pdf

Weir, D., & Brindel, T. (2015). Wound dressings. In R. Hamm, (Ed.), *Text and Atlas of Wound Diagnosis and Treatment.* Burr Ridge, IL: McGraw Hill.

White, J., & Cutting, K. (2006a). Exploring the effects of silver in wound management—What is optimal? *Wounds, 18*, 307–314.

White, R. J., & Cutting, K. F. (2006b). Critical colonization—The concept under scrutiny. *Ostomy/Wound Management, 52*, 50–56.

Whitney, J., Phillips, L., Aslam, R., et al. (2006). Guidelines for the treatment of pressure ulcers. *Wound Repair and Regeneration, 14*(6), 663–679.

Wikipedia. (2014). Available at: http://en.wikipedia.org/wiki/Gram staining. Accessed August 31, 2014.

Xavier, J. B., & Foster, K. R. (2007). Cooperation and conflict in microbial biofilms. *Proceedings of the National Academy of Sciences of the United States of America, 104*(3), 876–881.

QUESTIONS

1. Which statement accurately describes the relationship between skin and microorganisms?
   A. The dry keratinized cells on the surface create a physical barrier to penetration by microorganisms.
   B. The keratinocytes bind and inactivate pathogens.
   C. The normally alkalinic pH produced by the production of sebum by the sebaceous glands creates a hostile environment to microbial growth.
   D. Sweat promotes microorganism growth due to its low pH and high sodium concentrations.

2. The wound care nurse assesses a patient for factors that may delay wound healing. Which of the following is a local factor to consider?
   A. Poorly controlled diabetes
   B. Immunosuppressive drugs
   C. Alcohol and/or tobacco use
   D. Necrotic tissue or foreign bodies

3. The wound care nurse assessing a patient's wound determines that the wound is infected. What is a clinical indicator of this adverse condition?
   A. Reduction of wound dimensions
   B. A plateau in the wound's healing trajectory
   C. Decreasing wound exudate
   D. The continued development of granulation tissue

4. The wound care nurse is performing a wound culture on an infected pressure ulcer. Antibiotic treatment should be initiated for even one of the following:
   A. *Pseudomonas aeruginosa*
   B. Beta-hemolytic *Streptococcus*
   C. *S. aureus*
   D. *Escherichia coli*

5. A wound care nurse orders a culture of a patient wound. A wound culture is performed to:
   A. Determine the stage of healing
   B. Refer the patient for surgical debridement
   C. Determine the type of antibiotic to be used
   D. Determine the wound dressing to be used

6. The practitioner is obtaining a wound culture using the swab technique. When performing this technique, the practitioner would:
   A. Saturate the swab with purulent fluid
   B. Cleanse the wound with antimicrobial cleanser prior to obtaining the culture.
   C. Move the swab in a circular pattern around the perimeter of the wound.
   D. Identify a 1-square cm area of wound free from necrotic tissue to obtain swab specimen.

7. The wound care nurse is assessing wound culture results. Which statement accurately describes a possible finding and its relevancy?
   A. Only biofilm communities are typically detected by standard culture techniques; detection of planktonic bacterial requires additional samples.
   B. A high percentage of all the bacterial species that are present in a chronic wound bed are typically detected by standard aerobic agar plating techniques.
   C. Bacteria are identified by growing bacterial cultures in the lab using the DNA from the bacteria itself.
   D. The MIC identifies the lowest concentration of an antibiotic that inhibits or reduces bacterial growth.

8. For which condition does the "probe to bone" test have a high negative predictive value for osteomyelitis?
   A. Deep nonhealing pressure ulcers
   B. Diabetic foot ulcers
   C. Brain tumors
   D. Cancer of the long bones in children

9. The wound care nurse is planning care for a patient with a partial-thickness pressure wound. What principle of wound cleansing would the nurse incorporate into the plan?
   A. Wounds should be cleansed before debridement but not after debridement.
   B. Wounds should be cleansed with antimicrobial cleanser if the wound is accidentally contaminated.
   C. Wounds should be cleansed at each dressing change with a nonirritating, nontoxic solution.
   D. For most clinical situations, wound cleansing has been replaced by wound disinfection.

10. The wound care nurse is using methylene blue/gentian violet impregnated foam as a wound filler. What is the *unique* advantage of this line of products?
   A. Compatibility with enzymatic agents containing collagenase
   B. Antimicrobial effects
   C. Increased inflammatory response due to released toxins in wound bed
   D. Physically binding and removing bacteria as opposed to killing them

ANSWERS: 1.**A**, 2.**D**, 3.**B**, 4.**B**, 5.**C**, 6.**D**, 7.**D**, 8.**B**, 9.**C**, 10.**A**

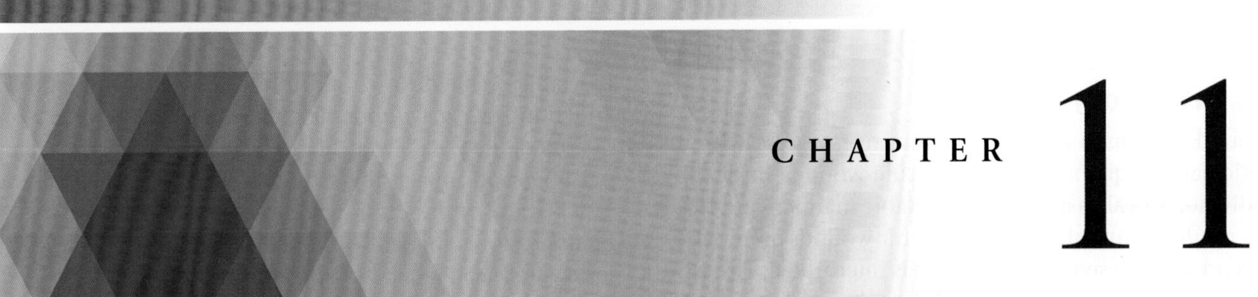

CHAPTER 11

Refractory Wounds

Assessment and Management

Debra S. Netsch

OBJECTIVES

1. Use data from serial wound assessments to identify wound deterioration or failure to progress.
2. Discuss potential causes for failure to heal and implications for assessment and management.
3. Identify indications and guidelines for use of adjunctive therapies, referrals for further evaluation, or medical–surgical intervention.
4. Describe mechanism of action, indications and contraindications, and guidelines for use of each of the following: MMP inhibitors; matrix dressings; growth factors; bioengineered/biologic dressings; negative pressure wound therapy (NPWT); and flaps and grafts.

Topic Outline

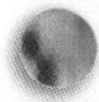 **Introduction**

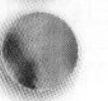 **Refractory Wounds**

- Definition of Refractory Wound
- Factors Resulting in Nonhealing Wounds
  - Inability or Failure to Correct Etiologic Factors
  - Imbalance in Systemic Factors Affecting Repair
  - Local Factors Preventing Repair (Iatrogenic Factors)
  - Adherence Factors
  - Imbalance in Molecular Microenvironment

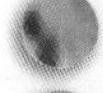 **Assessment of the Nonhealing Wound**

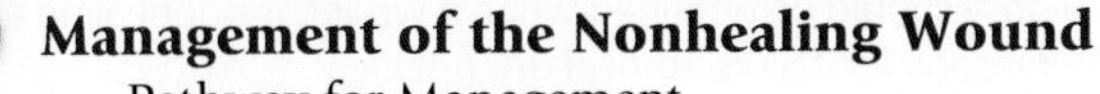 **Management of the Nonhealing Wound**

- Pathway for Management
  - Control or Elimination of Causative Factors
  - Biopsy
  - Goal Verification/Adherence Factors
  - Systemic Support for Healing
  - Optimal Local Wound Care
- Active Wound Therapies
  - MMP Inhibitors
  - Matrix Dressings (Acellular Scaffold Dressings)
  - Bioengineered Skin Substitutes (Cellular Dressings)
  - Growth Factors
  - Negative Pressure Wound Therapy
  - Hyperbaric Oxygen Therapy
  - Electrical Stimulation (E-stim)
  - Ultrasonic Mist (Low-Frequency Noncontact, Nonthermal Ultrasound)
  - Flaps and Grafts

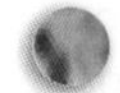 **Indications for Referrals**

- Exemplars

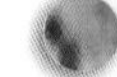 **Conclusion**

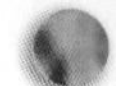 Introduction

Throughout this text, the following pathway has been described for effective wound management: (1) identification and correction of etiologic factors; (2) systemic support for healing; and (3) evidence-based and individualized topical therapy. As noted, the majority of wounds heal when this pathway is followed consistently; however, a significant minority will plateau. This chapter will cover the assessment and management of these refractory wounds, with a focus on active wound therapies.

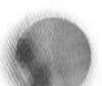

Refractory Wounds

Wound healing is a complex interactive process with an anticipated sequence of events. Acute wounds in healthy individuals heal in a timely predictable manner, and healing results in durable closure. Chronic wounds occur when this predictable sequence of events is interrupted. The term refractory or recalcitrant wound describes a chronic nonhealing or difficult-to-manage wound that does not progress toward healing or is stagnant (Moore et al., 2006; Rolstad & Nix, 2007; Seaman, 2000). Chronic or refractory wound terminology also applies to a frequently recurrent wound. In other words, the wound fails to heal in a timely manner or recurs despite appropriate management (Fonder et al., 2008; Gray & Ratliff, 2006; Lazarus et al., 1994). The WHS defines a recalcitrant wound as one that "fails to proceed through an orderly and timely process to produce anatomical and functional integrity or proceeded through the repair process without establishing a sustained anatomic and functional result" (WHS, 2006). The term refractory or nonhealing wound will be used throughout this chapter to avoid confusion.

CLINICAL PEARL

Acute wounds in healthy individuals heal in a timely predictable manner, with durable closure—chronic wounds occur when this predictable sequence of events is interrupted.

Definition of Refractory Wound

A significant minority of chronic wounds do not respond normally to treatment. A wound is considered refractory if there has not been improvement within 2 to 4 weeks of comprehensive evidence-based therapy or there is no expected and predicted reduction in size of the wound in an established period of time (e.g., 50% reduction in size of diabetic neuropathic ulcers in 4 weeks) (Doughty & Sparks-DeFriese, 2012; Li et al., 2007). Wound size and duration are predictive factors for wound healing outcomes and wound healing time; more specifically, data indicate that the percentage of healing at 3 to 4 weeks is a good predictor of healing outcomes (Rolstad & Nix, 2007; Sussman & Bates-Jensen, 2007).

CLINICAL PEARL

A wound is considered refractory if there has not been improvement within 2 to 4 weeks of comprehensive evidence-based therapy, or there is not the expected and predicted reduction in wound size within an established period of time.

Refractory wounds represent a significant worldwide health problem, afflicting approximately 5 to 7 million per year in the United States alone. The physical and psychological burden is substantial; individuals with nonhealing wounds experience significant morbidity (and even mortality) related to wound infections and amputations, and nonhealing wounds also have a negative effect on quality of life (Asadi et al., 2014). Finally, there is substantial financial impact; the estimated annual cost of care is $20 billion, with additional costs related to treatment of complications, missed work, and assisted living and long-term care (Asadi et al., 2014; Samson et al., 2004).

Refractory wounds are most commonly those that develop as a result of a chronic condition; 90% of all nonhealing wounds are classified as venous ulcers, diabetic neuropathic ulcers, or pressure ulcers. Not surprisingly, refractory wounds are often multifactorial in nature.

Factors Resulting in Nonhealing Wounds

Effective management of a nonhealing wound begins with identification and correction of the factors impairing or delaying repair. These factors fall into four broad categories: inability (or failure) to correct etiologic factors; imbalance in one or more of the multiple systemic factors affecting repair; local factors delaying or preventing repair; and/or imbalance in the molecular environment governing the repair process. Patient adherence factors can adversely affect all aspects of comprehensive management; patient adherence is critical to correction or amelioration of causative factors (e.g., off loading), to systemic support for wound healing (e.g., tight glycemic control or smoking cessation), and to local (topical) wound care. However, in a number of situations, etiologic factors have been controlled, and both systemic and local wound conditions have been established that support repair; yet the wound fails to heal. In this case, the reason for failure to heal is thought to be an imbalance in the molecular environment and structures controlling the repair process.

CLINICAL PEARL

Ninety percent of all nonhealing wounds are classified as venous ulcers, diabetic neuropathic ulcers, or pressure ulcers.

Inability or Failure to Correct Etiologic Factors

In some cases, the ulcer fails to heal because the cycle of injury has not been effectively interrupted, for example, inconsistent offloading of a plantar surface neuropathic ulcer or pressure ulcer or nonadherence to compression and elevation for a venous ulcer. Thus, the wound care team must critically reevaluate the wound and the management plan to assure accurate identification *and treatment* of the causative factors; in addition, a biopsy should be done whenever the wound is nonhealing and the reason for failure to heal is not clear.

CLINICAL PEARL

A biopsy should be obtained when a wound is nonhealing and the reasons for failure to heal are not clear.

Imbalance in Systemic Factors Affecting Repair

Systemic factors affecting repair can be divided into *intrinsic* and *extrinsic* factors; each of the common factors will be briefly discussed here and is addressed in greater depth in other chapters (Fig. 11-1) (Doughty & Sparks-DeFriese, 2012; Rolstad & Nix, 2007; Seaman, 2000; Sussman & Bates-Jensen, 2007).

Intrinsic Factors

Intrinsic (systemic) factors are the patient's comorbidities and physiologic conditions impacting wound healing. These include advanced age, poor nutritional status, chronic diseases (such as diabetes and renal disease), immunosuppression, reduced perfusion and oxygenation, and neurologically impaired skin.

Age

The elderly are at increased risk of skin breakdown (due to thinning of the epidermis, reduced barrier function, and dermal atrophy). In addition, the elderly are at risk for impaired healing; the negative effects of aging are compounded by the comorbidities that are common in the elderly. The diminished proliferative process includes a delayed cellular response to injury, delayed collagen deposition, and reduced tensile strength. The increased prevalence of chronic disease among the elderly contributes to recognition of age as a cofactor for impaired healing (Harding et al., 2005; Seaman, 2000; Sussman & Bates-Jensen, 2007).

Chronic Disease

Chronic diseases involving the cardiopulmonary system adversely affect the oxygen transport pathway, reducing delivery of oxygen to the tissues and removal of carbon dioxide, both of which are required for healing.

Persons with diabetes are also at risk for impaired healing; high glucose levels impair leukocyte function, thus increasing the risk of infection, and also have a negative impact on collagen synthesis, tensile strength, and keratinocyte migration. In addition, growth factors and growth factor receptor sites appear to be reduced. Finally, microvascular and neuropathic disease are common, and both negatively impact healing.

Perfusion and Oxygenation

Adequate perfusion and oxygenation are essential for wound healing. Inadequate perfusion results in failure to heal, and perfusion and oxygenation are compromised by many chronic disease processes, including cardiovascular, pulmonary, and renal diseases. Any condition causing hypovolemia reduces transportation of oxygen and nutrients to the tissues and removal of waste products, and prolonged hypovolemia impairs collagen production and compromises leukocyte function. Overcorrection of hypovolemia can lead to cardiac overload, which further reduces perfusion and oxygenation (Doughty & Sparks-DeFriese, 2012; Stotts et al., 2014; Sussman & Bates-Jensen, 2007).

Immunosuppression

Patients with immunosuppressive conditions (e.g., patients with cancer, human immunodeficiency virus [HIV] infection, and diabetes and those undergoing corticosteroid therapy or chemotherapy) are at risk for poor wound healing due to impairment of the initial inflammatory response required for healing (Doughty & Sparks-DeFriese, 2012; Sussman & Bates-Jensen, 2007).

Neurological Impairment

Patients with spinal cord injuries are known to have delayed healing below the level of the injury, due to changes in perfusion and persistent inflammation, among other factors (see Chapter 15). In addition, these individuals are high risk for pressure ulcer development due to sensory loss, immobility, and altered weight bearing (Doughty & Sparks-DeFriese, 2012; Sussman & Bates-Jensen, 2007).

Extrinsic Factors

Extrinsic factors include external or environmental sources that disrupt the wound healing process. These extrinsic factors include medications, malnutrition, irradiation and chemotherapy, psychophysiologic stress, and wound bioburden and infection (refer to Fig. 11-1).

Intrinsic	Extrinsic	Iatrogenic	Adherence
• Age • Chronic disease • Perfusion & oxygenation • Immunosuppression • Neurologically impaired skin	• Medications • Nutrition • Irradiation & chemotherapy • Psychophysiologic stress • Wound bioburden & infection	• Local ischemia • Inappropriate wound care • Trauma • Wound extent & duration	• Psychosocial issues • Financial impact • Life commitments • Comprehension • Accessibility • Differing goals

FIGURE 11-1. Cofactors impacting nonhealing. (Modified from Sussman, C., & Bates-Jenson, B. (2007). Wound healing physiology: Acute and chronic. In C. Sussman, & B. Bates-Jensen (Eds.), *Wound care: A collaborative practice manual for health professionals* (3rd ed.). Baltimore, MD: Lippincott Williams & Wilkins, Table 2-5, pg 43; additional information: Nix, D., & Peirce, B. (2012). Noncompliance, nonadherence, or barriers to a sustainable plan? In R. Bryant & D. Nix (Eds.), *Acute & chronic wounds: Current management concepts* (4th ed., pp. 408–415). St Louis, MO: Elsevier-Mosby; Rolstad, B., & Nix, D. (2007). Management of wound recalcitrance and deterioration. In D. L. Krasner, G. T. Rodeheaver, & R. G. Sibbald (Eds.). *Chronic wound care: A clinical source book for healthcare professionals* (4th ed., pp. 743–750). Malvern, PA: HMP Communications.)

Medications

Many individuals with chronic wounds take multiple medications to treat chronic conditions; some of these medications negatively impact wound healing. For example, platelet activation is a critical "first step" along the wound healing pathway and can be disrupted by anticoagulant medications (warfarin, heparin, etc.), antiplatelet medications (clopidogrel, salicylates, aspirin, etc.), and nonsteroidal anti-inflammatory medications (cyclooxygenase [COX-2] inhibitors, ibuprofen, naproxen, etc.). Steroids are another class of medications that adversely affect all phases of wound healing. Many other medication classes also disrupt wound healing including immunosuppressive agents, antiprostaglandins, and opioids including morphine (Martin et al., 2010; Karukonda et al., 2000).

CLINICAL PEARL

Many medications have the unintended effect of impairing wound healing; medications with an adverse effect on repair include anticoagulants, antiplatelets, anti-inflammatory agents, steroids, chemotherapeutic agents, antiprostaglandins, and opioids.

Nutrition

Malnutrition, especially protein and calorie malnutrition, is well known to alter wound healing; micronutrient deficiencies can also adversely affect repair (see Chapter 6). Thus, nutritional management must include attention to both macronutrient and micronutrient intake.

Irradiation and Chemotherapy

Radiation therapy interferes with wound healing for years after treatment, due to persistent damage to the vessels and the proliferative cells (fibroblasts) in the treatment area. The end result of radiation therapy is tissue ischemia and compromised proliferative processes in the irradiated field. Chemotherapy interrupts the cell cycle for proliferative cells, thus profoundly and adversely affecting the tissue repair process. The severity and duration of the negative impact of chemotherapy depends on the dose and duration of therapy. In general, the wound care goal for a patient receiving radiation or chemotherapy is maintenance until therapy is complete.

Psychophysiologic Stress

Stress and depression release hormones that negatively affect immune function. Cortisol levels are increased during times of stress, and cortisol is known to adversely affect cytokine production and fibroblast proliferation; cortisol is also associated with increased matrix degradation. Finally, cortisol can disrupt the growth hormone–somatomedin system, and this is surmised to cause poor healing outcomes. Interestingly, stress management strategies such as biofeedback, sleep, positive imagery, hypnosis, and exercise have all been associated with improved healing outcomes (Doughty & Sparks-DeFriese, 2012; Stotts et al., 2014; Sussman & Bates-Jensen, 2007).

Wound Bioburden and Infection

Bacteria in the wound compete with fibroblasts for the nutrients and oxygen essential to extracellular matrix (ECM) formation. In addition, the bacteria release byproducts deleterious to the repair process. Excessive bioburden (critical colonization) can also result in biofilm formation, which further impairs healing and increases the risk for invasive infection. Thus, effective wound management must include ongoing assessment and management of bioburden, and antimicrobial dressings are sometimes used as a "first step" intervention for a poorly healing or plateaued wound (see Chapter 10) (Gray & Ratliff, 2006; Stotts et al., 2014; Sussman & Bates-Jensen, 2007).

CLINICAL PEARL

Antimicrobial dressings are sometimes used as a "first step" intervention for a poorly healing or plateaued wound.

Local Factors Preventing Repair (Iatrogenic Factors)

Iatrogenic factors are treatment-related factors that compromise wound healing, such as inappropriate wound care and trauma to the wound bed.

Inappropriate Wound Care

Appropriate wound management and topical therapy requires clear understanding of the wound healing process and available products and appropriate utilization of dressings and therapies to promote repair. The goal is to establish and maintain a clean moist wound bed; products that are appropriate for highly exudative wounds would be very *in*appropriate for minimally exudative wounds. Inappropriate topical therapy can lead to disruption of the wound healing trajectory. For example, misuse of topical antiseptics can lead to cytotoxicity, and either overhydration or desiccation of the wound bed compromises function of the cells essential to repair.

Trauma

Trauma to the wound bed and periwound area occurs frequently due to inappropriate approaches to wound debridement, improper removal of dressings, excessively high-pressure irrigation, etc. Trauma impedes wound healing and leads to increased susceptibility for wound infection.

Adherence Factors

Factors affecting adherence include much more than the presence or lack of motivation. Many aspects of living with a chronic wound impact on the patient's ability to actively and effectively contribute to the management plan, including psychosocial issues, financial impact, life commitments, comprehension, accessibility to care, and ability to carry out critical aspects of care. Effective wound outcomes require a patient-centered approach and the ability to collaborate with the patient and caregivers to establish (and modify) the wound management plan based on wound status and patient concerns and priorities. Adherence is related to the ability of the person with the wound to participate in and carry out the treatment plan. Adherence can be achieved only when the individual is an active participant in formulating the plan of care in a safe open environment.

CLINICAL PEARL

Effective wound outcomes require a patient-centered approach and the ability to collaborate with the patient and caregivers to establish (and modify) the wound management plan based on wound status and patient concerns and priorities.

Financial Impact

Management of refractory wounds has a negative financial impact that is both societal and personal. Missed work, product costs, medication costs, and the impact of underinsurance or lack of insurance all impact the ability to provide or obtain proper wound management.

Life Commitments

Life commitments such as caring for family members, household chores, attending family functions, and providing for the family may result in competing priorities that disrupt the treatment plan.

Comprehension

Comprehension of the treatment plan, including causative and corrective factors and the consequences of adherence or nonadherence on healing, is one of the factors most critical to adherence; thus, the wound care nurse must consistently work with the patient and family to assure that they understand treatment options and the impact of adherence or nonadherence on outcomes. Factors impacting on comprehension include the patient's and family's ability to learn and comprehend and the wound nurse's ability to explain at a level the patient and family can understand. As explained in Chapter 5, patient adherence is primarily determined by his/her perception of the benefits and disadvantages of the behaviors they are being asked to adopt. The level of comprehension needs to be reassessed at each visit; there should also be clear discussion of patient goals.

Psychosocial Aspects

Psychosocial aspects including beliefs, attitudes, expectations, and cultural issues are factors that affect adherence and that may necessitate adjustments to the management plan.

Accessibility and Ability

The availability and accessibility of wound care products and wound care expertise have an obvious impact on adherence. Thus, the wound care team must be holistic in their approach to wound care and must do everything possible to assist the client to obtain the necessary supplies and access to care.

Differing Goals

Goal setting is essential to adherence. Healing is not always the appropriate goal; when healing *is* the goal, it is important to clearly identify interventions that are the responsibility of the health care team (e.g., selection of appropriate wound therapies) and interventions that are the responsibility of the patient and caregivers (e.g., pressure relief/offloading and tight glycemic control). Once an appropriate goal has been established and agreed upon, care guidelines can be established. The establishment and verification of the goal and care plan related to wound care is vital to patient and caregiver adherence (Nix & Peirce, 2012; Rolstad & Nix, 2007).

Imbalance in Molecular Microenvironment

There are significant differences in the molecular environment of healing wounds as opposed to nonhealing wounds. Normal wound healing is characterized by a balanced interaction among inflammatory and proliferative factors and by steady progression of the wound through the repair process, whereas chronic wounds are characterized by a proinflammatory environment and failure of the wound to progress normally. Specifically, chronic (nonhealing) wounds exhibit a high level of proteases (matrix metalloproteases, or MMPs), which degrade the matrix proteins and growth factors essential for healing (**Table 11-1**). In addition, nonhealing wounds frequently have high numbers of proliferative cells (such as fibroblasts) that are senescent; these cells are unable to reproduce and thus less able to contribute to repair (Doughty & Sparks-DeFriese, 2012; Lobmann et al., 2005).

CLINICAL PEARL

Chronic wounds are characterized by a proinflammatory environment that contributes to failure to heal.

TABLE 11-1 Characteristics of Acute Versus Chronic Wounds

Characteristics	Healing Wounds	Chronic Wounds
Proliferative cellular activity	High	Low
Inflammatory cytokines	Low	High
Protease levels	Low	High
Growth factors	High	Low
Cell response to growth factors	Mitotically competent	Senescent

Compiled from Doughty, D., & Sparks-DeFriese, B. (2012). Wound-healing physiology. In R. Bryant & D. Nix (Eds.), *Acute & chronic wounds: Current management concepts* (4th ed., pp. 63–82). St Louis, MO: Elsevier-Mosby; Lobmann, R., Schultz, G., & Lehnert, H. (2005). Proteases and the diabetic foot syndrome: Mechanisms & therapeutic implications. *Diabetes Care*, *28*(2), 462–471; Trengove, N., Stacey, M., Maculey, S., et al. (1999). Analysis of the acute and chronic wound environments: The role of proteases and their inhibitors. *Wound Repair and Regeneration*, *7*, 442–452.

With normal repair, the ECM provides a scaffold for migrating cells and also stores the growth factors controlling the repair process. A healthy ECM is required for cell attachment and migration and for neoangiogenesis and collagen synthesis and/or epithelial resurfacing, as described in Chapter 2. The high concentrations of proteases (MMPs) and disproportionately high ratio of MMPs to TIMPs (tissue inhibitors of matrix metalloproteases) in chronic wounds may contribute to ECM destruction and to degradation of growth factors and growth factor receptors (Trengove et al., 1999). While the high levels of proteases are a confirmed characteristic of chronic wounds, it is not yet known whether the imbalance in inflammatory and proliferative factors is the *causative factor* for wound chronicity or the *result* of chronicity. In other words, do the high levels of inflammatory proteases *cause* the wound to become refractory to healing, or are the high levels of inflammatory proteases simply an indicator (marker) of the proinflammatory environment caused by some other factors associated with wound chronicity (Vowden, 2011)?

CLINICAL PEARL

While high levels of proteases (MMPs) are a confirmed characteristic of chronic wounds, it is not yet known whether the proinflammatory state is the causative factor for wound chronicity or the result of chronicity.

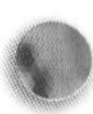

Assessment of the Nonhealing Wound

Effective management of a nonhealing wound requires a knowledgeable wound care clinician and consistent serial assessments. The first goal is prompt detection of a plateau or deterioration in wound status (Fig. 11-2). As stated throughout this text, a wound that deteriorates or fails to demonstrate measurable progress in 2 to 4 weeks despite appropriate comprehensive care is considered to be refractory. Deterioration is typically identified quickly, while failure to progress (a plateau) is more insidious and easily overlooked. Iatrogenic factors (lack of follow-up, multiple different providers, inconsistent documentation, or insufficient understanding of wound healing and wound care) may contribute to delayed recognition of a refractory wound, resulting in ineffective treatment for prolonged periods of time (Rolstad & Nix, 2007).

Lack of progress or deterioration should first prompt a comprehensive reassessment of the patient, wound, and management plan to assure that there is no undiagnosed pathology or inappropriately managed cofactors. Commonly, these wounds have been previously evaluated and treated with a narrow focus on the wound alone. A thorough history and physical assessment are key in distinguishing whether the wound deterioration or plateau is the result of (1) misdiagnosis, (2) uncontrolled associated cofactors, (3) inappropriate wound management, or (4) any combination of these (Harding, 2000; Rolstad & Nix, 2007; Seaman, 2000). Any gaps in the management plan should be immediately corrected.

CLINICAL PEARL

Failure of a wound to progress (or sudden deterioration) should prompt a comprehensive reassessment of the patient, wound, and management plan to rule out undiagnosed pathology, inadequately managed cofactors, or inappropriate wound management.

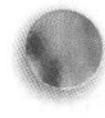

Management of the Nonhealing Wound

Unfortunately, correction of all known etiologic and contributing factors may be insufficient to correct a negative healing trajectory for a chronic wound; the wound may remain refractory despite best efforts due to changes in the microenvironment that create chronicity and prevent repair. In this case, the focus of topical therapy will need

Refractory Wound Criteria

Wound Characteristics
- undermining
- tunneling
- extensive necrotic tissue
- persistent inflammation
- senescent cells

Host Burden
- extensive wounding
- multiple wounds
- prolonged wound duration
- infection & high bioburden

Healing Risk Factors
- diabetes
- vascular disease
- immunocompromise
- hypovolemia

Inadequate Healing Progress
- Full thickness wounds: Fail to improve with appropriate treatment in 2–4 weeks.
- Partial thickness wounds: Fail to improve in 1–2 weeks

FIGURE 11-2. Refractory wound criteria. (Modified with permission from Trovato, M., et al. (2007). Management of the wound environment with advanced therapies. In C. Sussman & B. Bates-Jensen (Eds.), *Wound care: A collaborative practice manual for health professionals* (3rd ed.). Baltimore, MD: Lippincott Williams & Wilkins.)

to shift from passive support for wound healing to active management of the stalled repair process.

At present, there are no diagnostic tests readily available in the United States that confirm or specify the abnormalities in the molecular environment causing the failure to heal, though a point of care test for abnormally high MMP levels has been developed and is expected to become available very soon.

Pathway for Management

Refractory wound management presents a clinical challenge. The three principles of wound care are (1) control or eliminate causative factors, (2) support the host to reduce existing and potential cofactors, and (3) optimize the microwound environment or physiologic wound environment (Rolstad et al., 2012). This framework provides the premise of the pathway for management discussed in this chapter. Each of these principles is discussed as an overview from the perspective of refractory wounds with in-depth discussion in other chapters of this book.

Control or Elimination of Causative Factors

The critical first step in effective wound management is accurate identification and correction of the causative factors. For example, a venous ulcer requires compression and/or elevation to control the underlying venous insufficiency *in addition to* topical therapy to provide moisture balance; topical therapy alone will not promote healing. As noted, management of etiologic factors requires accurate diagnosis on the part of the provider but also requires patient adherence to the prescribed management plan.

Identification and correction of etiologic factors is not easy, and misdiagnosis of primary etiology or contributing cofactors is common. A systematic approach to wound care is promoted by the use of evidence-based guidelines and algorithms such as those created by the Wound Ostomy Continence Nurses' Society (WOCN) or the Wound Healing Society (WHS). However, these guidelines are specific to the type of ulcer; thus, the wound team must first determine wound etiology and must then assure comprehensive and evidence-based management of the etiologic factors, contributing comorbid conditions, and the wound itself using evidence-based guidelines. For example, if a wound is diagnosed as a venous ulcer, then the guidelines pertaining to venous ulcers are instituted. When the ulcer is not responding according to anticipated time frames or normal sequence of healing, then it behooves the provider(s) to reassess the cause or etiology and cofactors. For example, if a vasculitic ulcer is diagnosed as a venous ulcer and managed as a venous ulcer with no treatment of the vasculitis, the wound will not heal until the correct diagnosis is made and the management plan corrected. Even if the primary etiology has been accurately identified, it is common for providers to miss significant confounding factors such as medications. For example, there are documented cases where failure to heal a venous ulcer was due to medication (hydroxyurea) prescribed for treatment of polycythemia vera. Once the hematologist discontinued or changed the medication, the wound healed quickly. Thus, the first step in management of a refractory wound is reassessment of etiologic and contributing factors by a multidisciplinary team (Rolstad & Nix, 2007; Stotts et al., 2014).

CLINICAL PEARL

Misdiagnosis of wound etiology or contributing cofactors is common.

Biopsy

The etiologic factors can change due to wound chronicity; thus, a biopsy is indicated whenever a wound fails to heal and the reasons are unclear. A Marjolin ulcer exemplifies transformation from a chronic wound to a malignancy. Malignant transformation occurs in 1.7% of chronic wounds, and refractory wounds are at high risk for transformation to malignancy. Any suspicion of malignant transformation necessitates biopsy at multiple sites and depths of the wound. Rebiopsy is warranted if the wound does not respond to appropriate treatment (Bryant, 2012). The WHS treatment guidelines for venous ulcers recommend biopsies for histology if the leg ulcer worsens in size and symptoms or does not improve over 4 weeks of appropriate treatment (WHS, 2006).

CLINICAL PEARL

Chronic wounds can deteriorate into malignancy; thus, a biopsy should always be obtained when a wound fails to progress despite appropriate management.

Goal Verification/Adherence Factors

The goal of wound care needs to be discussed, agreed upon, and stated. If goals are not agreed upon, then interventions cannot match, and this can cause failure to heal. Mutual goal setting requires open communication with the patient as the center of the care plan. An exemplar of mutual goal setting would be a paraplegic patient with an ischial pressure ulcer; the wound team may be focused on healing, while the patient's primary goal may be to remain active, up in the wheelchair, and enjoying life. In this case, the goals are misaligned; the wound team is focused on healing while the patient may be content with maintenance. Many providers would note this as an adherence cofactor, but the primary issue is failure to openly communicate and to come to agreement as to goals (Leaper et al., 2012; Nix & Peirce, 2012; Rolstad & Nix, 2007).

Systemic Support for Healing

Wound healing is a systemic phenomenon; thus, support of the host is essential to optimize treatment outcomes. Dressings alone will not heal the wound without support of the host and management of critical cofactors. Glycemic control, nutritional management, adequate hydration, edema reduction, adequate perfusion, and control of comorbidities all are aspects of systemic support that are critical to positive outcomes (Gray & Ratliff, 2006; Rolstad et al., 2012). Support for the host seems logical but is difficult if cofactors are not identified or if management of comorbid conditions conflicts with goals of wound care; for example, wound healing requires adequate protein intake, but low-protein diets are a key management factor for patients in renal failure.

Optimal Local Wound Care

Topical management or wound bed preparation is achieved through topical therapy (wound cleansing and dressing selection), with the goal of establishing a physiologic wound environment that supports healing. The key characteristics of the physiologic wound environment are adequate moisture balance, temperature control, pH regulation, and control of bioburden (Rolstad et al., 2012). The acronym of TIME (Tissue management, Inflammation and infection control, Moisture balance, Epithelial [edge] advancement) provides a quick reference to the key principles of wound bed preparation and a guideline for assessment of wound management and wound status (EWMA, 2004; Leaper et al., 2012). Some authors suggest that the TIME acronym could be redefined as an acronym for overall wound management: Treatment: appropriate treatment plan is in place based upon the original TIME principles; Implementation: mutually agreed-upon treatment plan is initiated and consistently implemented for optimal healing; Monitoring: provide detection of local or systemic adverse reactions and ensure sound clinical practice and appropriate product selection; Evaluation: all treatments are regularly and objectively evaluated with evaluation tools such as wound healing assessment scales, validated pain assessment tool, quality-of-life scores, etc. (Leaper et al., 2012).

Active Wound Therapies

Novel approaches to refractory wound management have been and continue to be developed (active wound therapies) to improve treatment outcomes. Active wound therapies are designed to correct the molecular imbalances characteristic of the refractory wound and to actively stimulate the repair process (Asadi et al., 2014).

CLINICAL PEARL

Active wound therapies are designed to correct the molecular imbalances characteristic of the refractory wound and to actively stimulate the repair process.

Active wound therapies are indicated for refractory wounds and are not indicated for routine management of an appropriately healing wound. The criteria for implementation of active wound therapies have not been well defined; however, their use is well established in wounds that have plateaued or deteriorated despite appropriate comprehensive therapy when the goal is healing. Selected therapies may also be utilized for wounds that are very unlikely to heal in a timely manner with routine care (Fig. 11-3) (Houghton & Campbell, 2007; Trovato et al., 2007).

Appropriate use of active wound therapies requires the provider to understand the mechanisms of action, indications, and contraindications for each of the therapies; additional issues to be addressed include reimbursement guidelines, qualifications of the provider providing the active wound therapy, and availability of the product/therapy (Houghton & Campbell, 2007).

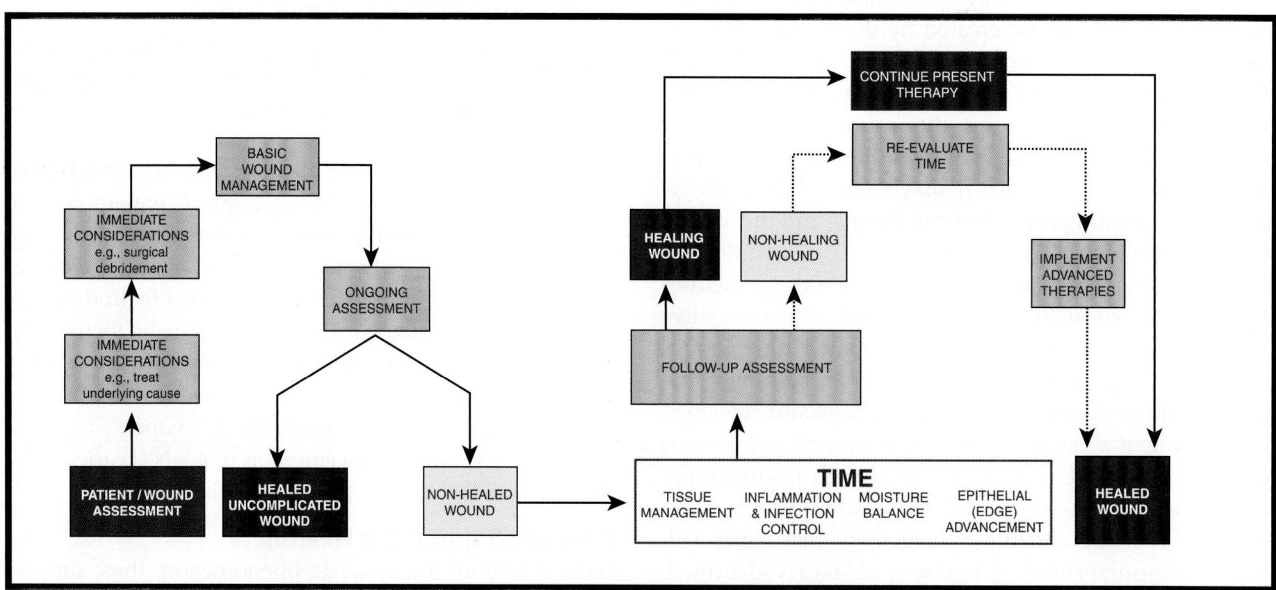

FIGURE 11-3. Decision tree for wound management and implementation of advanced therapies. Reprinted with permission from European Wound Management Association (EWMA). (2004). *Position Document: Wound bed preparation in practice* (p. 4). London, UK: MEP Ltd. http://ewma.org/fileadmin/user_upload/EWMA/pdf/Position_Documents/2004/pos_doc_English_final_04.pdf. Copyright © Medical Education Partnership Ltd., 2004. All rights reserved.

Each of the currently available active wound therapies will be briefly discussed in terms of mechanism of action, guidelines for use, and current evidence base.

MMP Inhibitors

There are several dressings now available that act to reduce the levels of MMPs in the wound bed.

Mechanism of Action

MMPs are essential in all phases of normal wound healing and comprise a large and diverse group of molecules, some of which are proinflammatory and some of which support proliferation and oppose inflammation. The proinflammatory MMPs are particularly important during the inflammatory and remodeling phases of repair, because they act as natural enzymes to support the breakdown of necrotic tissue. Normal wound healing is characterized by high levels of these proinflammatory MMPs during early inflammation with a marked reduction in levels as the wound transitions out of the inflammatory phase and into the proliferative phase. In contrast, as noted, chronic wounds are characterized by persistent high levels of MMPs and persistent inflammation despite the absence of necrotic tissue or infection. Elevated levels of MMP proteases and reduced levels of MMP inhibitors create or contribute to the imbalance found in chronic wounds. The topical application of dressings that provide a gelatin substrate for MMPs (MMP inhibitors) in high concentrations has been shown to reduce the levels of MMPs in the wound bed; the MMPs are attracted to and bound by the ORC (oxidized regenerated cellulose). There are also dressings available that act to down-regulate production of MMPs. Once point-of-care testing for elevated protease levels becomes available, the clinician will be able to make definitive decisions regarding appropriate use of these dressings; in the meantime, use of dressings that modulate MMP activity is a very reasonable "first step" in the management of a nonhealing wound (Lobmann et al., 2005).

> **CLINICAL PEARL**
>
> Once point-of-care testing for elevated MMP levels becomes available, clinicians will be able to make definitive decisions regarding use of these dressings; in the meantime, use of dressings that bind MMPs is a reasonable "first step" in the management of nonhealing wounds.

Guidelines for Use

The wound should be cleansed, and the dressing should then be applied to the viable wound bed; if the wound bed is dry, the dressing should be moistened with a small amount of saline. An appropriate secondary dressing should then be applied. Dressing change frequency is based on volume of exudate, but is typically every 2 to 3 days (Cullen & Ivins, 2010).

Current Evidence

Cullen and colleagues reported that treatment with a protease inhibitor dressing significantly reduced elastase and plasmin activity in the wound bed. Lobmann and colleagues (2005) found that use of these dressings was associated with increased numbers of healed ulcers and reduced time to healing in patients with diabetic foot ulcers and venous ulcers (Lobmann et al., 2005). Many randomized controlled trials (RCTs) have been done that show statistically significant improvement in healing rates with use of these dressings for venous ulcers, diabetic ulcers, and pressure ulcers (Cullen & Ivins, 2010).

Cost Considerations

These dressings are more expensive than standard moisture retentive dressings, but much less costly than other active wound therapies, and for many patients, the cost of the dressing is covered by insurance. Consideration should be given to the benefit versus cost, but the clinician should remember that, when the goal is healing, it is much more cost-effective to use a more expensive therapy that promotes repair than to use a less expensive therapy that does *not* promote healing.

Matrix Dressings (Acellular Scaffold Dressings)

Acellular products (ECM scaffolds) are nonliving products derived from allogeneic, xenographic, biosynthetic, or synthetic materials; because there are no living cells, these products do not cause an antigen–antibody response.

Mechanism of Action

A healthy wound bed is required for healing, because the cells responsible for repair (e.g., fibroblasts and keratinocytes) must be able to attach to the wound bed in order to migrate and carry out repair processes. When the existing wound bed does not support attachment and migration, wound healing does not occur. Use of ECM dressings is postulated to provide a scaffold for attachment and migration of host cells (keratinocytes, fibroblasts, and endothelial cells), thus supporting neoangiogenesis, collagen synthesis, and reepithelialization. As the new ECM is developed, the matrix dressing undergoes controlled degradation.

> **CLINICAL PEARL**
>
> Matrix dressings provide a scaffold for migration and attachment of fibroblasts, endothelial cells, and keratinocytes, thus supporting granulation tissue formation and epithelial resurfacing.

Guidelines for Use

All measures to address etiologic factors must be continued as well as measures for systemic support of wound healing. Matrix dressings should be applied to clean, noninfected, debrided wounds. Manufacturers' guidelines must be followed for application; in general, the dressing should be sized slightly larger than the wound and anchored to the wound bed, followed by an appropriate secondary dressing. Matrix dressings can be used for a wide variety of chronic wounds, including pressure ulcers, nonhealing surgical wounds, venous leg ulcers, and diabetic foot ulcers (Harding et al., 2010).

Current Evidence

There are multiple ECM dressings available; there is little evidence for use of some and RCT evidence supporting use of others. An RCT of one of the most widely available products showed 55% of 120 patients with venous ulcers healed at 12 weeks compared to 34% in the control group ($p < 0.02$) (Mostow et al., 2005).

Cost Considerations

These dressings are more costly than standard moist wound healing products and MMP inhibitors, but less expensive than cellular skin substitutes. There is an application procedure fee that is generally covered by insurance; prior authorization is recommended (AHRQ, 2012; Seaman, 2012), and the wound care nurse should collaborate with the reimbursement experts in her/his agency to assure that all documentation and coverage guidelines are being followed.

Bioengineered Skin Substitutes (Cellular Dressings)

Cellular skin substitutes contain living cells embedded in a bioabsorbable matrix; selected products may use autologous cells (cells donated by the individual) but most involve allogeneic cells obtained from neonatal foreskin or amniotic membrane, which have limited antigenicity (Sheikh et al., 2010). These skin substitutes can be epidermal, dermal, or bilayer (both the epidermal and dermal layers).

Mechanism of Action

Allogeneic skin substitutes deliver healthy living cells to the chronic wound where they secrete growth factors and ECM proteins to stimulate wound repair; because the cells are embedded in a bioabsorbable matrix, these products also provide a scaffold for migration and attachment of host cells. Dermal skin substitutes can be used on wounds with depth; in contrast, the bilayered skin substitutes function as a nonsurgical skin graft and are appropriate for use only on shallow/superficial wounds that are well vascularized and free of necrotic tissue and infection.

CLINICAL PEARL

Bioengineered skin substitutes provide both a scaffold for cell migration and healthy cells to support repair; cells are typically harvested from neonatal foreskin or amniotic membrane, so there is limited antigenic activity.

Guidelines for Use

These products are intended as adjunct therapy and must be used as one component of a comprehensive wound management program, in conjunction with measures to address wound etiology and systemic support. The specific product must be prepared and applied in strict adherence to the manufacturer's recommendations. For example, dermal substitutes typically require thawing according to very specific protocols, with immediate application to the wound bed following thawing. Bilayered skin substitutes must be meshed prior to application (to permit drainage of exudate), and it is critical to apply the product *dermal side down*. The skin substitute is anchored and covered with an appropriate secondary dressing. Frequency of secondary dressing change is based on volume of exudate; frequency of reapplication of the cellular dressing is based on wound status and response, but must be consistent with the manufacturer's recommendation, evidence-based protocols, and third-party reimbursement.

CLINICAL PEARL

Bioengineered skin substitutes are expensive; thus, they must be used appropriately (i.e., application according to manufacturers' guidelines to a wound bed that is viable, free of infection, and well perfused).

Current Evidence

Numerous studies are available that address the efficacy of specific skin substitutes in the management of particular wounds; however, of the 57 skin substitute and a cellular matrix products identified in the Agency for Healthcare Research and Quality (AHRQ) report, only 7 had been studied in RCTs. The seven products studied in RCTs included Apligraf, Dermagraft, Graftjacket acellular matrix, TheraSkin, Hyalograft 3D autograft/LasersSkin (Halomatrix), Oasis wound matrix, and Talymed poly-*N*-acetyl glucosamine. All of the skin substitutes evaluated in RCTs were associated with improved healing outcomes as compared to control groups (who were managed with a variety of moist wound healing dressings, e.g., saline-moistened dressings and petrolatum-impregnated dressings); however, the strength of the evidence for these studies was reported as low to medium, and generalization of findings is not possible due to the different properties and components of each product (AHRQ, 2012). Thus, more data are needed before definitive recommendations can be made for use of these products.

Cost Considerations

Skin substitutes are costly, and there is significant product wasted with each application; thus, it is critical to assure that the product selected for use has demonstrated effectiveness with the type of wound for which it is being used. In addition, the wound nurse must assure that the wound is ready for the advanced therapy product, that is, free of necrotic tissue and infection, and well vascularized. Finally, it is essential to assure that the patient has the ability to heal from a systemic and etiologic perspective. Insurance prior authorization for skin substitutes is recommended (AHRQ, 2012; Seaman, 2012).

Growth Factors

Chronic wound fluid has low concentrations of several growth factors, and normal concentrations and combinations of growth factors are known to be essential to repair. It has been postulated that topical application of exogenous growth factors might rectify the growth factor deficiency and promote healing. Initial experience with autologous growth factors (obtained by drawing the patient's blood, treating the platelets to cause release of growth factors, and then applying the growth factors to the wound) did show promise. Currently, there is a commercially available gel with exogenous growth factors produced by recombinant DNA technology; specifically, the B chain of the platelet-derived growth factor (PDGF) gene has been inserted into yeast to produce the growth factor, which is incorporated into a gel. There is also a therapy that involves production of platelet-rich plasma gel by drawing and treating the patient's blood to generate the plasma gel. It is surmised that, in the future, different combinations and concentrations of growth factors may be applied to different types of chronic wounds at different phases of healing.

Mechanism of Action

The recombinant PDGF has the same mechanisms of action as endogenous PDGF (or PDGF in platelet-rich plasma gel): the ability to control migration of cells needed for repair through chemoattraction; the ability to promote proliferation of the cells needed for repair; and the ability to stimulate cellular activities required for granulation tissue formation and epithelial migration. The limitation of current growth factor therapy is the fact that it provides only one type of growth factor, when a healing wound is characterized by a constantly changing "mix" of growth factors and concentrations. However, the use of recombinant PDGF or platelet-rich plasma gel does replicate the growth factors released during the initial phase of healing in an acute wound.

Guidelines for Use

The currently available growth factor (becaplermin gel) is approved for use only with nonhealing diabetic foot ulcers that are free of necrotic tissue and infection and effectively offloaded. It has not been approved for venous ulcers or pressure ulcer use. A layer of gel should be applied to the wound base and covered with a saline-moistened gauze; the manufacturer recommends removing the gel after 12 hours and replacing with moist saline gauze, but common practice involves a daily dressing change with the gel and damp saline gauze. If the wound fails to show measurable progress within 2 weeks (or when a tube has been used), or if wound size does not decrease by 30% in 10 weeks, therapy should be discontinued. Platelet-rich plasma gel has been used with a variety of nonhealing wounds, and studies are currently ongoing to determine wounds most likely to respond to this therapy and best protocols for use.

> **CLINICAL PEARL**
>
> The growth factor that is currently available commercially (becaplermin gel) is approved for use only with diabetic foot ulcers that are viable, uninfected, and effectively offloaded.

Precautions and Contraindications

Becaplermin gel is contraindicated in patients with known hypersensitivity to any product components or known neoplasms at the application site. A rash at the application site occurs in 2% of patients treated. Safety in pregnancy has not been determined, and a black box warning has been issued regarding increased risk of cancer with use of three or more tubes.

Current Evidence

Multiple clinical studies of diabetic foot ulcers treated with recombinant PDGF showed improved healing rates and reduced time to healing. Smiell and colleagues (1999) reported full healing of wounds treated with PDGF at a rate of 39% higher than those treated with placebo ($p < 0.007$), (becaplermin package insert, 2008; Lobmann et al., 2005; Smiell et al., 1999; Trovato et al., 2007). A meta-analysis of 21 studies comparing chronic or acute wounds treated with PRP to those treated with saline-moistened gauze, Bacitracin, or Vaseline gauze revealed significant reduction in wound area/volume (or complete wound closure) and reduced incidence of complications such as infection among the wounds treated with PRP (Carter et al., 2011).

Cost Considerations

The recombinant DNA gel product is costly, but frequently covered by third-party payers. In addition, significant differences in cost can exist between pharmacies. The platelet-rich plasma therapy is also covered by some third-party payers.

Negative Pressure Wound Therapy

NPWT is one of the most commonly used active wound therapies. It involves lightly filling the wound and any tunnels or undermined areas with gauze or foam and then applying subatmospheric (negative) pressure to the wound through suction at controlled levels. There are a number of different NPWT systems, some of which are gauze based and some of which are foam based; some are designed for acute care settings, with multiple therapy options including intermittent wound irrigation, while others are simple "peel and stick" systems designed for closed surgical incisions or for outpatient care.

Mechanism of Action

Controlled subatmospheric pressure is utilized to enhance moist wound healing. Primary effects demonstrated in multiple in vivo studies include the following: (1) elimination of chronic wound exudate, which is known to impair healing; (2) maintenance of a moist wound surface; (3) reduction in edema, with resultant improvement in perfusion; (4) macrodeformation (traction on the sides of the wound), which promotes wound contraction; and

(5) microdeformation and mechanical stretch on the cells in the wound bed, which changes cell shape and activates intracellular processes that promote healing. Clinically, these cellular effects are manifested as increased angiogenesis and granulation tissue formation and reduction in bacterial bioburden.

CLINICAL PEARL

NPWT "works" by eliminating edema (thus improving perfusion), eliminating exudate while maintaining a moist wound surface, and activating intracellular processes that promote healing (through deformation, or "stretch").

Guidelines for Use

NPWT is indicated only when the goal is wound healing, the wound bed has minimal or no necrotic tissue, and bacterial loads are under control. All other elements of care must be continued (control of etiologic factors and systemic support for healing). Each type of NPWT system has its own nuances, and use and application must be consistent with manufacturers' guidelines. The application process usually involves the following: wound cleansing; protection of the periwound skin with a liquid barrier film and/or transparent adhesive drape; application of appropriate gauze or foam to the wound bed; application of the transparent adhesive dressing to cover the wound; and application of negative pressure via suction catheters or a negative pressure control pad applied to a cutout area of the cover drape. The negative pressure settings should be individualized for the patient and goals of therapy; options include intermittent versus continuous suction and varied levels of negative pressure. Faster granulation has been demonstrated when intermittent suction is used as opposed to continuous; however, continuous suction may be needed for exudate control and pain management and is the standard of care when negative pressure is used to promote fistula closure. The guidelines for levels of negative suction vary based on the manufacturer. Additional considerations include type of foam to be used (when using a foam-based system) and the potential need for a contact layer to reduce tissue trauma, bleeding, and pain with dressing changes. For example, manufacturers providing foam-based systems frequently provide both an open cell reticulated foam (standard care product) and a soft "white" hydrophilic foam. The open cell foam has been associated with faster formation of granulation tissue, but also with increased risk of tissue trauma, bleeding, and pain with removal, due to the fact that the tissue becomes adherent to the open cell foam. In contrast, the hydrophilic foam prevents tissue ingrowth and is frequently the "foam of choice" for the layer in contact with the wound bed. If a hydrophilic foam is not available, a contact layer (impregnated porous gauze or silicone adhesive contact layer) can be placed in the wound bed prior to application of the open cell foam; this protects the structures in the wound bed by preventing adherence, without interfering with the negative pressure therapy.

CLINICAL PEARL

NPWT is indicated only when the goal is wound healing, the wound bed is viable (or there is minimal necrotic tissue), and any infection is being treated.

Dressings are typically changed every 48 to 72 hours.

The wound nurse must educate her/his staff on the appropriate use of NPWT, "troubleshooting" guidelines, and the importance of removing the dressing any time therapy cannot be reestablished within a 2-hour time period. (The staff must understand that, when suction is lost, there is no mechanism for exudate control; allowing the dressing to remain in place without suction for exudate control significantly increases the risk of wound infection.)

NPWT is intended for short-term use to establish a healthy bed of granulation tissue; once this goal has been met, most patients can be transitioned to moist wound healing. NPWT should be promptly discontinued when there is a plateau in response or any deterioration.

CLINICAL PEARL

The most common complications of NPWT are bleeding, pain, and tissue trauma; the risk of complications can be significantly reduced through use of the hydrophilic foam or a nonadherent contact layer dressing in the base of the wound (to prevent tissue adherence).

Contraindications

There are many contraindications to negative pressure therapy, including untreated osteomyelitis, necrotic tissue, exposed blood vessels, exposed organs, nonenteric or unexplored fistulas, and malignancy in the wound. NPWT is also usually contraindicated for use in wounds where the goal of care is comfort or maintenance. The wound nurse should review specific manufacturers' guidelines for the system used in her/his setting and should develop protocols that assure adherence to those guidelines. The wound nurse should also be aware that the FDA has issued an alert to clinicians regarding appropriate use of NPWT; 6 deaths and 77 injuries have been reported to the FDA, due to bleeding and tissue trauma (FDA, 2014).

Current Evidence

The evidence base for use of NPWT includes substantial clinical anecdotal reports and case series reports and limited poor quality studies that collectively support efficacy. More research is needed to support the extensive use of NPWT and/or to clarify indications and contraindications for its use. Many best practice clinical guidelines (WOCN, WHS, etc.) recommend use of NPWT, based primarily on expert opinion.

CLINICAL PEARL

NPWT should be discontinued when there is a plateau in response or deterioration.

Cost Considerations

Use of NPWT systems is costly; thus, appropriate utilization and prior authorization from third-party payers is recommended (AHRQ, 2009; Netsch, 2012; Smith et al., 2014).

Hyperbaric Oxygen Therapy

Hyperbaric oxygen therapy (HBOT) is the systemic administration of oxygen delivered under pressure (atmospheric pressure >1 atmosphere absolute). Specifically, the patient is placed in a pressurized chamber and is then administered 100% oxygen.

Mechanism of Action

Normally, almost all oxygen delivered to the tissues is attached to the hemoglobin molecule on the red blood cell; thus, tissue oxygenation is normally totally dependent on normal perfusion and blood vessels of sufficient patency to permit unimpeded passage of RBCs. Breathing oxygen under pressure significantly increases the amount of oxygen dissolved in the plasma, which provides increased delivery of oxygen to the tissues. Adequate oxygen levels are essential for all phases of healing and for control of bacterial burden; thus, the ability to increase oxygen delivery to the tissues is of potential benefit to patients with compromised perfusion due to vascular disease or prior radiation and to those with complex infections.

Guidelines for Use

HBOT should be considered when wound healing is compromised by severe infection or impaired tissue perfusion. The wound nurse should be aware that HBOT is likely to be of benefit when a wound is ischemic but viable (e.g., the patient with peripheral arterial disease and low ABI but a pale viable wound bed); however, HBOT is *not* of benefit when the wound is already necrotic (e.g., dry gangrene) because it works by delivering oxygenated plasma and necrotic wounds have no plasma flow. Thus, HBOT should be considered as adjunct therapy for limb-threatening wounds caused by diabetes and/or vascular insufficiency. HBO reduces edema by meeting the tissues' oxygen needs, thereby inducing vasoconstriction; this further improves tissue oxygenation. HBO may contribute to resolution of osteomyelitis by providing increased oxygen to the bone, thus improving leukocyte activity. HBOT may also promote healing of grafts and flaps by reducing edema and improving oxygenation.

> **CLINICAL PEARL**
>
> HBOT should be considered when wound healing is compromised by inadequate tissue perfusion or by severe infection.

The wound nurse should therefore refer patients who may benefit from HBO for evaluation; the HBOT center will evaluate the patient to rule out contraindications and can also conduct preliminary testing to determine probability that the patient will benefit. There are a number of absolute or relative contraindications to HBOT, including advanced lung disease, ear disorders that place the patient at risk for barotrauma, selected medications, and claustrophobia. Testing to determine likelihood of effectiveness includes an oxygen challenge test; baseline $TcPO_2$ levels are obtained and then repeated following administration of oxygen via nasal cannula or mask, and significant improvement in tissue oxygen levels suggests that HBOT will be of benefit.

Current Evidence

Boykin and Baylis (2007) reported enhanced nitric oxide levels in diabetic foot ulcers following treatment with HBOT, and a systematic review of RCTs involving HBOT revealed reduced rates of major amputations for diabetic foot ulcers (Kranke et al., 2004). In a review by Gray and Ratliff (2006), HBOT was associated with demonstrated benefit in treatment of diabetic foot ulcers; in contrast, HBOT was of no benefit in treatment of pressure ulcers and venous ulcers.

Cost Considerations

HBO therapy is covered by insurance for specific conditions. Insurance prior authorization is recommended (Broussard, 2012).

Electrical Stimulation (E-stim)

Electrical stimulation has been used in a variety of settings and for a variety of wounds and has in general been found to support healing.

Mechanism of Action

Various types of electrical current can be delivered to the wound and periwound tissues to support wound healing. The most commonly used type is high-voltage pulsed current (HVPC). E-stim is thought to "work" by reducing edema, increasing perfusion, and promoting migration of the cells critical to repair.

Guidelines for Use

E-stim is a nonspecific stimulus for repair that can be used for multiple types of chronic wounds. Wounds are typically treated 3 to 7 times a week for 8 to 12 weeks. If there is no evidence of progress within 10 to 14 days, therapy should be reevaluated. While best practice guidelines recommend consideration of electrical stimulation for nonhealing wounds (WOCN, NPUAP-EPUAP), this therapy is not yet FDA approved for use in wound care (though it is approved for pain and edema management) (FDA, 2014; Isseroff & Dahle, 2012). Electrical stimulation is best provided in conjunction with a physical therapist, as they have the expertise to assure optimal use of this modality.

> **CLINICAL PEARL**
>
> Electrical stimulation is best provided in conjunction with a physical therapist, as they have the expertise to assure optimal use of this treatment modality.

Current Evidence

Studies indicate improved blood flow and enhanced resistance to infection in refractory wounds treated with electrical stimulation. Wolcott and colleagues (1969) evaluated the use of E-stim with ischemic nonhealing wounds and found that wounds treated with standard care and electrical stimulation demonstrated a healing rate of 30%, as compared to 14.7% for wounds managed with standard care alone. Carley and Wainapel (1985) evaluated the effects of E-stim on sacral and lower extremity wounds of varying etiology and found that wounds treated with electrical stimulation healed at a rate of 1.5 to 2.5 times that of the control (no E-stim) group. A similar study of Stages II and III pressure ulcers found a statistically significant increase in the rate of healing ($p < 0.0001$) for wounds in the E-stim group (Wood et al., 1993).

Cost Considerations

Cost is typically covered by insurance through physical therapy application; prior authorization of insurance coverage is recommended (Frantz, 2012; Unger, 2007).

Ultrasonic Mist (Low-Frequency Noncontact, Nonthermal Ultrasound)

Low-frequency noncontact ultrasound has been used as a method of debridement and as a nonspecific stimulus to repair.

Mechanism of Action

Low-frequency noncontact, nonthermal ultrasound utilizes acoustic/sound energy to deliver ultrasound energy through saline mist to the wound bed and periwound tissue. Current evidence suggests that this therapy may augment wound healing through some combination of the following: enhanced debridement of necrotic tissue through enzymatic and fibrinolytic activity, reduced bacterial counts and biofilm production, increased fibroblast migration, and improved blood flow.

CLINICAL PEARL

Low-frequency noncontact, nonthermal ultrasound may promote healing through enhanced fibrinolytic activity, reduced bacterial counts, and improved blood flow.

Guidelines for Use

This therapy is indicated for refractory wounds and burns, with ongoing monitoring to assure effectiveness.

Current Evidence

A retrospective observational study comparing 163 patients with vascular wounds treated with ultrasound + standard care to 47 patients treated with standard care alone revealed significantly higher healing rates among the ultrasound group (53% vs. 32%; $p = 0.009$) (Kavros et al., 2008). Driver and colleagues (2011) conducted a meta-analysis of eight studies involving 444 patients with a variety of chronic wounds with similar findings, that is, higher healing rates among the patients treated with low-frequency noncontact, nonthermal ultrasound. Anecdotal reports also note reduced pain and exudate, and this therapy has been reported to be of benefit in the management of patients with suspected deep tissue injury (sDTI).

Cost Considerations

In the outpatient setting, this therapy may be covered under a debridement code (Unger, 2007).

Flaps and Grafts

In selected refractory wounds, surgical closure may be required. This usually involves either a split-thickness skin graft or a myocutaneous flap procedure. Split-thickness skin grafts are appropriate only for burn care (see Chapter 30) and for shallow/superficial wounds with a healthy well-vascularized wound bed; the principles of management include post-op immobilization of the graft site, use of a bolster dressing or NPWT to maintain close contact between the graft and the underlying wound bed, and prevention of infection (see Chapter 30). Myocutaneous flaps are generally reserved for large defects overlying bony prominences in nonambulatory patients with good potential for healing, such as a wheelchair-bound spinal cord–injured patient with an ischial ulcer. Management priorities include establishment of a healthy granulating wound bed prior to surgery, assurance of adequate nutritional status and systemic support for healing, and protection and close monitoring of the flap to prevent complications due to ischemia, venous congestion, or exposure to pressure and shear (see Chapter 15) (Kane, 2014).

CLINICAL PEARL

Split-thickness skin grafts are appropriate only for management of burns and well-vascularized superficial wounds; post-op management should be focused on maintenance of close adherence between the graft and the underlying wound bed.

Indications for Referrals

A team approach is necessary for refractory wound management. A referral network is not built overnight and takes a conscious effort to find other providers with complementary skills. Referrals are essential whenever the etiology is unclear or specific therapies are required to correct the etiologic factors (such as revascularization or offloading with a boot), medical or nutritional intervention is needed to assure potential for healing, or medical or surgical intervention is needed for wound closure. The wound nurse needs to capitalize on the expertise of other providers to assure optimal outcomes for her/his patients and needs to appreciate the knowledge and skills brought to the table by other disciplines.

Exemplars

Refractory wounds are associated with depression. When depression is suspected, the patient should be referred to their primary care provider or psychiatrist.

Arterial insufficiency impacts wound care. If pulses are not palpable or noninvasive arterial testing suggests arterial insufficiency, a vascular consult is indicated.

A patient with bilateral Stage IV ischial pressure ulcers may require multiple referrals, including the following: seating specialist for evaluation and adjustment of wheelchair and cushion; nutritionist consult to determine caloric and metabolic needs; referral to a plastic surgeon to determine if surgical intervention is an option; and referral to home health care to assist with dressing changes and holistic management.

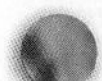

Conclusion

Refractory wounds are complex and require comprehensive assessment to determine probable cause for failure to heal; interventions are then based on assessment data. Key interventions include reassessment of causative and contributing factors and biopsy whenever the etiology is unclear or there is any suspicion of malignant deterioration; evaluation of all systemic factors and comorbid conditions affecting repair; reevaluation of topical therapy to assure appropriate moisture management and control of bacterial loads; and implementation of active wound therapies for wounds determined to be nonhealing despite appropriate comprehensive wound care. While development of active wound therapies is in its infancy, there are a number of options available, including protease-inhibiting dressings, matrix dressings, bioengineered skin substitutes, NPWT, and hyperbaric oxygen therapy. The wound nurse must "match" the evidence regarding the therapy to the specific wound and must remain current in regard to new therapies being developed.

REFERENCES

AHRQ (Agency for Healthcare Research and Quality). (2009). *Technology assessment: Negative pressure wound therapy devices.* Rockville, MD: AHRQ (Agency for Healthcare Research and Quality).

AHRQ (Agency for Healthcare Research and Quality). (2012). *Technology assessment: Skin substitutes for treating chronic wounds.* Rockville, MD: AHRQ (Agency for Healthcare Research and Quality).

Asadi, M., Alamdari, D. H., Rahimi, H. R., et al. (2014). Treatment of life-threatening wounds with a combination of allogeneic platelet-rich plasma, fibrin glue and collagen matrix, and a literature review. *Experimental and Therapeutic Medicine, 8*, 423–429.

Boykin, J. V., Jr., & Baylis, C. (2007). Hyperbaric oxygen therapy mediates increased nitric oxide production associated with wound healing: A preliminary study. *Advances in Skin and Wound Care, 20*(7), 382–388.

Broussard, C. (2012). Hyperbaric oxygenation. In R. Bryant, & D. Nix (Eds.), *Acute & chronic wounds: Current management concepts* (4th ed., pp. 345–352). St Louis, MO: Elsevier-Mosby.

Bryant, R. (2012). Intrinsic diseases and uncommon cutaneous wounds. In R. Bryant & D. Nix (Eds.), *Acute & chronic wounds: Current management concepts* (4th ed., pp. 417–433). St Louis, MO: Elsevier-Mosby.

Carley, P. J., & Wainapel, S. F. (1985). Electrotherapy for acceleration of wound healing: Low intensity direct current. *Archives of Physical Medicine and Rehabilitation, 66*(7), 443–446.

Carter, M. J., Fylling, C. P., & Parnell, L. K. (2011). Use of platelet rich plasma gel on wound healing: A systematic review and meta-analysis. *ePlasty, 11*, e38.

Cullen, B., & Ivins, N. (2010). Promogran and promogran prisma: Made easy. *Wounds International, 1*(3), 1–6.

Doughty, D., & Sparks-DeFriese, B. (2012). Wound-healing physiology. In R. Bryant & D. Nix (Eds.), *Acute & chronic wounds: Current management concepts* (4th ed., pp. 63–82). St Louis, MO: Elsevier-Mosby.

Driver, V. R., Yao, M., & Miller, C. J. (2011). Noncontact low-frequency ultrasound therapy in the treatment of chronic wounds: A meta-analysis. *Wound Repair and Regeneration, 19*(4), 475–480.

European Wound Management Association (EWMA). (2004). *Position Document: Wound bed preparation in practice.* London, UK: MEP Ltd.

Fonder, M., Lazarus, G., Cowan, D., et al. (2008). Treating the chronic wound: A practical approach to the care of nonhealing wounds and wound care dressings. *Journal of American Academy of Dermatology, 58*(2), 185–206.

Frantz, R. (2012). Electrical stimulation. In R. Bryant & D. Nix (Eds.), *Acute & chronic wounds: Current management concepts* (4th ed., pp. 353–359). St Louis, MO: Elsevier-Mosby.

Gray, M., & Ratliff, C. (2006). Is HBO therapy effective for the management of chronic wounds? *JWOCN, 33*, 21–25.

Harding, K. (2000). Nonhealing wounds: recalcitrant, chronic, or not understood? *Ostomy Wound Management, 46*(1A Suppl), 4S–7S.

Harding, K., Moore, K. & Phillips, T. (2005). Wound chronicity and fibroblast senescence—Implications for treatment. *International Wound Journal, 2*, 364–368.

Harding, K., Kirsner, R., Lee, D., et al. (2010). *International consensus. Acellular matrices for the treatment of wounds. An expert working group review.* London, UK: Wounds International.

Houghton, P. & Campbell, K. (2007). Therapeutic modalities in the treatment of chronic recalcitrant wounds. In D. L. Krasner, G. T. Rodeheaver, & R. G. Sibbald (Eds.), *Chronic wound care: A clinical source book for healthcare professionals* (4th ed., pp. 403–415). Malvern, PA: HMP Communications.

Isseroff, R. R., & Dahle, S. E. (2012). Electrostimulation therapy and wound healing: Where are we now? *Advances in Wound Care, 1*(6), 238–243.

Kane, D. P. (2014). Surgical repair in advanced wound caring. In D. L. Krasner (Ed.), *Chronic wound care: The essentials* (pp. 279–291). Malvern, PA: HMP Communications.

Karukonda, S. R., Flynn, T. C., Boh, E. E., et al. (2000). The effects of drugs on wound healing—Part II. Specific classes of drugs and their effect on healing wounds. *International Journal of Dermatology, 39*, 321–333.

Kavros, S. J., Liedl, D. A., Boon, A. J., et al. (2008). Expedited wound healing with noncontact, low-frequency ultrasound therapy in chronic wounds: A retrospective analysis. *Advances in Skin and Wound Care, 21*(9), 416–423.

Kranke, P., Bennett, M., Roeckl-Wiedmann, I., et al. (2004). Hyperbaric oxygen therapy for chronic wounds. *Cochrane Database of Systematic Reviews, 1*, CD004123.

Lazarus, G., Cooper, D., Knighton, D., et al. (1994). Definitions and guidelines for assessment of wounds and evaluation of healing. *Wound Repair and Regeneration, 2*, 165–170.

Leaper, D., Schultz, G., Carville, K., et al. (2012). Extending the TIME concept: What have we learned in the past 10 years? *International Wound Journal, 9*(Suppl 2), 1–19.

Li, J., Chen, J., Kirsner, R. (2007). Pathophysiology of acute wound healing. *Clinics in Dermatology, 25*(1), 9–18.

Lobmann, R., Schultz, G., & Lehnert, H. (2005) Proteases and the diabetic foot syndrome: Mechanisms & therapeutic implications. *Diabetes Care, 28*(2), 462–471.

Martin, J., Koodie, L., Krishnan, A., et al. (2010). Immunopathy and infectious diseases: Chronic morphine administration delays wound healing by inhibiting immune cell recruitment to the wound site. *American Journal of Pathology, 176*(2), 786–799.

Moore, K., McCallion, R., Searle, R., et al. (2006). Prediction and monitoring the therapeutic response of chronic dermal wounds. *International Wound Journal, 3*, 89–96.

Mostow, E. N., et al. (2005). Effectiveness of an extracellular matrix graft (Oasis wound matrix) in the treatment of chronic leg ulcers: A randomized clinical trial. *Journal of Vascular Surgery, 41*, 837–843.

Netsch, D. (2012). Negative pressure wound therapy. In R. Bryant & D. Nix (Eds.), *Acute & chronic wounds: Current management concepts* (4th ed., pp. 337–344). St Louis, MO: Elsevier-Mosby.

Nix, D., & Peirce, B. (2012). Noncompliance, nonadherence, or barriers to a sustainable plan? In R. Bryant & D. Nix (Eds.), *Acute & chronic wounds: Current management concepts* (4th ed., pp. 408–415). St Louis, MO: Elsevier-Mosby.

Rolstad, B. & Nix, D. (2007). Management of wound recalcitrance and deterioration. In D. L. Krasner, G. T. Rodeheaver, & R. G. Sibbald (Eds.), *Chronic wound care: A clinical source book for healthcare professionals* (4th ed., pp. 743–750). Malvern, PA: HMP Communications.

Rolstad, B., Bryant, R., & Nix, D. (2012). Topical management. In R. Bryant & D. Nix (Eds.), *Acute & chronic wounds: Current management concepts* (4th ed., pp. 289–306). St Louis, MO: Elsevier-Mosby.

Samson, D., Lefevre, F., & Aronson, N. (2004). Wound-healing technologies: Low-level laser and vacuum-assisted closure. In *Evidence report/technology assessment (number 111)*. Washington, DC: Agency for Healthcare Research and Quality (AHRQ).

Seaman, S. (2000). Considerations for the global assessment and treatment of patients with recalcitrant wounds. *Ostomy Wound Management, 46*(1A Suppl), 10S–29S.

Seaman, S. (2012). Skin substitutes and extracellular matrix scaffolds. In R. Bryant & D. Nix (Eds.), *Acute & chronic wounds: Current management concepts* (4th ed., pp. 308–323). St Louis, MO: Elsevier-Mosby.

Sheikh, S. S., Sheikh, S. S., & Fetterolf, D. E. (2014). Use of dehydrated human amniotic membrane allografts to promote healing in patients with refractory non healing wounds. *International Wound Journal, 11*(6), 711–717. doi:10.1111/iwj.12035.

Smiell, J. M., Wieman, T. J., Steed, D. L., et al. (1999). Efficacy and safety of becaplermin (recombinant human platelet-derived growth factor-BB) in patients with non-healing, lower extremity diabetic ulcers: A combined analysis of four randomized studies. *Wound Repair and Regeneration, 7*, 335–346.

Smith, A., Whittington, K., Frykberg, R., et al. (2014). Negative pressure wound therapy. In: D. L. Krasner (Ed.), *Chronic wound care: The essentials* (pp. 195–223). Malvern, PA: HMP Communications.

Stotts, N. A., Wipke-Tevis, D. D., & Hopf, H. W. (2014). Cofactors in impaired wound healing. In: D. L. Krasner (Ed.), *Chronic wound care: The essentials* (pp. 79–86). Malvern, PA: HMP Communications.

Sussman, C., & Bates-Jensen, B. (2007). Wound healing physiology: Acute and chronic. In C. Sussman, & B. Bates-Jensen (Eds.), *Wound care: A collaborative practice manual for health professionals* (3rd ed., pp. 21–42). Baltimore, MD: Lippincott Williams & Wilkins.

Trengove, N., Stacey, M., Maculey, S., et al. (1999). Analysis of the acute and chronic wound environments: The role of proteases and their inhibitors. *Wound Repair and Regeneration, 7*, 442–452.

Trovato, M., Granick, M., Tomaselli, N., et al. (2007). Management of the wound environment with advanced therapies. In C. Sussman, & B. Bates-Jensen (Eds.), *Wound care: A collaborative practice manual for health professionals* (3rd ed., pp. 268–277). Baltimore, MD: Lippincott Williams & Wilkins.

Unger, P. (2007). The physical therapist's role in wound management. In D. L. Krasner, G. T. Rodeheaver, R. G. Sibbald (Eds.), *Chronic wound care: A clinical source book for healthcare professionals* (4th ed., pp. 381–388). Malvern, PA: HMP Communications.

Vowden, P. (2011). Hard-to-heal wounds: Made easy. *Wounds International, 2*(4).

Wolcott, L. E., Wheeler, P. C., Hardwicke, H. M., et al. (1969). Accelerated healing of skin ulcer by electrotherapy: Preliminary clinical results. *Southern Medical Journal, 62*(7), 795–801.

Wood, J. M, Evans, P. E., Schallreuter, K. U., et al. (1993). Multicenter study on the use of pulsed low-intensity direct current for healing chronic stage II and stage III decubitus ulcers. *Archives of Dermatology, 129*(8), 999–1009.

Wound healing society (WHS). (2006). Guidelines for the treatment of venous ulcers. *Wound Repair and Regeneration, 14*, 649–662.

Food and Drug Administration (FDA). E Stim Devices. Retrieved November 1, 2014, from http://www.accessdata.fda.gov/scripts/cdrh/devicesatfda/index.cfm

Food and Drug Administration (FDA). Negative pressure wound therapy (NPWT): Preliminary public health notice. Retrieved July 1, 2014, from http://www.fda.gov/Safety/MedWatch/SafetyInformation/SafetyAlertsforHumanMedicalProducts/ucm190704.htm

QUESTIONS

1. The wound care nurse is assessing a patient with a diabetic neuropathic ulcer. What criteria must exist for the wound to be considered refractory?
   A. There is no improvement in the wound in 1 week.
   B. There is no reduction in the size of the wound in 2 to 4 weeks despite appropriate management.
   C. The wound becomes infected after 1 week of management.
   D. The wound heals in a timely predictable manner with durable closure.

2. A wound care nurse is assessing a patient with a pressure ulcer that is nonhealing without a clear reason for the failure to heal. What would most likely be the nurse's next action?
   A. Order a CAT scan.
   B. Order debridement.
   C. Switch to a different absorptive moist wound healing dressing.
   D. Order a biopsy.

3. Which of the following is an extrinsic factor affecting wound repair?
   A. Patient comorbidities
   B. Patient age
   C. Medications
   D. Perfusion and oxygenation

4. Which medication places a patient at greater risk for delayed wound healing?
   A. Antiplatelet medication
   B. Insulin
   C. Antidepressants
   D. Human growth factor

5. What is the wound care goal for a patient who is receiving radiation to treat cancer?
   A. Maintenance
   B. Topical therapy
   C. Pharmacological therapy
   D. Identification of etiologic factors

6. What is one effect of psychophysiologic stress on wound healing?
   A. Bacteria form that release by-products deleterious to the wound repair process.
   B. Stress causes persistent damage to the proliferative cells in the wound.
   C. Increased cortisol levels adversely affect cytokine production.
   D. Biofilm formation occurs, impairing wound healing.

7. Which characteristic of nonhealing wounds is responsible for degrading the matrix proteins and growth factors essential for healing?
   A. Low ratio of matrix metalloproteases (MMPs) to tissue inhibitors of matrix metalloproteases (TIMPs)
   B. High levels of matrix metalloproteases (MMPs), which degrade the matrix proteins and growth factors essential for healing
   C. A balanced interaction among inflammatory and proliferative factors and slowing progression of the wound through the repair process
   D. Excessive bioburden (critical colonization) resulting in biofilm formation, increasing the risk for infection

8. What is the critical first step in effective wound management?
   A. Initiation of topical wound therapy
   B. Goal verification and assessment of adherence factors
   C. Initiation of pharmacological therapy
   D. Accurate identification and correction of the causative factors

9. The wound care nurse recommends active wound therapy to treat a refractory wound. What is the goal of this therapy?
   A. Correct the molecular imbalances in the wound
   B. Increase the levels of MMPs in the wound bed
   C. Reduce the levels of MMP inhibitors
   D. Increase elastase and plasmin activity in the wound bed

10. The wound care nurse recommends a bioengineered skin substitute to treat a venous ulcer that has progressed to refractory wound stage. What is a therapeutic effect of this type of cellular dressing?
    A. Provides a scaffold for cell migration
    B. Reduces the level of biofilms in the wound
    C. Promotes an antigen–antibody response
    D. Reduces elastase and plasmin activity in the wound bed

11. For which patient would the wound care nurse recommend the growth factor becaplermin gel as therapy?
    A. A patient with an infected incisional wound
    B. A patient with a pressure ulcer on the back of the head
    C. A patient with a nonhealing diabetic foot ulcer
    D. A patient with a nonhealing stab wound

12. What is one of the criteria that must be met to consider negative pressure wound therapy (NPWT)?
    A. The goal of wound healing is maintenance.
    B. The wound bed has a high level of necrotic tissue.
    C. Any infection in the wound bed is being treated.
    D. There is a malignancy in the wound.

13. For which patient would the wound care nurse most likely recommend hyperbaric oxygenation therapy (HBOT)?
    A. A patient who has a comorbid malignancy
    B. A patient whose wound healing is compromised by inadequate tissue perfusion
    C. A patient who has a viable wound bed not responding to NPWT
    D. A wheelchair-bound patient with an ischial ulcer

ANSWERS: 1.**B**, 2.**D**, 3.**C**, 4.**A**, 5.**A**, 6.**C**, 7.**B**, 8.**D**, 9.**A**, 10.**A**, 11.**C**, 12.**C**, 13.**B**

CHAPTER 12

Skin and Wound Care for Neonatal and Pediatric Populations

Carolyn Lund and Charleen Singh

OBJECTIVES

1. Describe the anatomy and physiology of the skin and soft tissue, changes across the lifespan, and implications for maintenance of skin health.
2. Describe the pathology, assessment, and management of wounds unique to the neonatal and pediatric populations.

Topic Outline

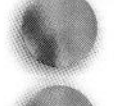

Introduction

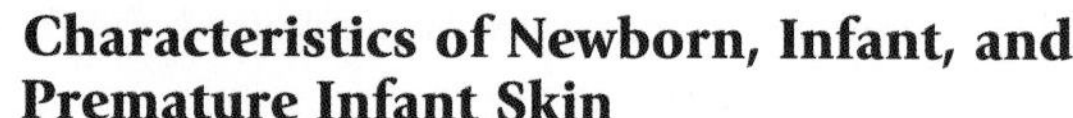

Characteristics of Newborn, Infant, and Premature Infant Skin

- Stratum Corneum and Epidermis
- Dermis
- Skin pH
- Risk of Toxicity from Topical Agents

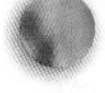

Skin Assessment and Risk Factors for Skin Breakdown

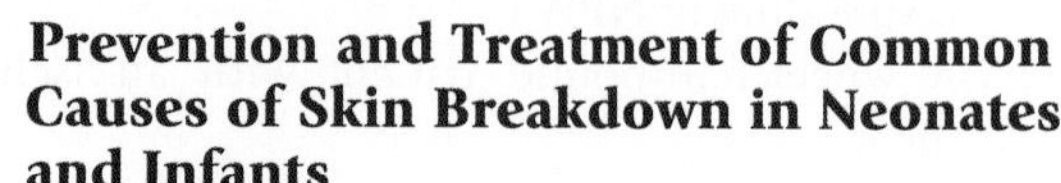

Prevention and Treatment of Common Causes of Skin Breakdown in Neonates and Infants

- Damage Due to Skin Disinfectants
- Adhesive-Related Skin Injury
  - Adhesive Removers
  - Tackifiers
  - Barrier Products
  - Preventive Measures
- Intravenous Extravasations
  - Prevention
  - Management
  - Wound Care
- Diaper Dermatitis
  - Prevention
  - Treatment
  - Candidiasis

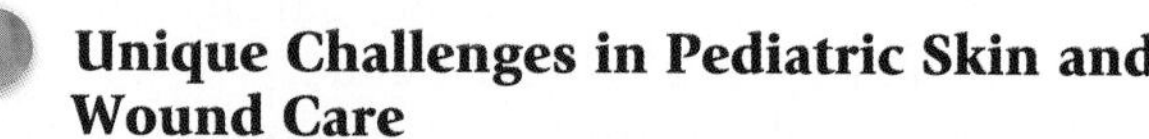

Unique Challenges in Pediatric Skin and Wound Care

- Physiology Pediatric Skin and Wound Healing
  - Scar Appearance
  - Impact of Developmental Stage
- Common Challenge: Conflicting Plans of Care
  - Description of Clinical Situation
  - Wound Care Nurse Response
  - Discussion
- Common Clinical Challenge: Multiple Comparable Plans That Appear to Be Conflicting
  - Description of Clinical Situation
  - Wound Care Nurse Response
  - Discussion
- Common Clinical Challenge: Resistance/Nonadherence
  - Description of Current Clinical Situation (the Little Girl Who Said "I Won't Oh No I Won't")
  - Wound Care Nurse Response
  - Discussion
- Common Clinical Challenge: Concern About Wound Appearance and Scarring
  - Description of Clinical Situation
  - Wound Care Nurse Response
  - Discussion

Skin Disorders Commonly Seen in the Pediatric Population

- Atopic Dermatitis
  - Management
  - Description of Clinical Scenario
  - Wound Care Nurse Response

Introduction

Skin and wound care for neonates, infants, and children requires an understanding of skin characteristics unique to these populations. This is particularly true of neonates in the newborn intensive care unit (NICU), who present particular challenges for nurses who care for them. Daily skin care practices such as antimicrobial skin disinfection and adhesive removal place these newborns at risk for skin trauma and/or loss of normal skin barrier function. Infants in the NICU who were born prematurely, are critically ill, or require surgery are at especially high risk for these types of injury. Other causes of skin damage include intravenous extravasation of irritating substances such as calcium gluconate, diaper dermatitis, and pressure ulcers, most of which are related to use of medical devices (e.g., continuous positive airway nasal prongs and masks [NCPAP], electroencephalogram [EEG] electrodes, intravenous hubs, and pulse oximeter sensors).

An understanding of the unique anatomic and physiologic differences in premature, full-term newborn, and young infant skin is fundamental to providing effective care to these populations.

Characteristics of Newborn, Infant, and Premature Infant Skin

Newborn skin undergoes an adaptation process during the transition from the aquatic environment of the uterus to the aerobic environment after birth. The skin assists in thermoregulation, serves as a barrier against toxins and microorganisms, is a reservoir for fat storage and insulation, and is a primary interface for tactile sensation and communication.

Stratum Corneum and Epidermis

The stratum corneum, which provides the important barrier function of the skin, contains 10 to 20 layers in the adult and in the full-term newborn. Although full-term newborns have been shown to have skin barrier function comparable to that of adult skin as indicated by transepidermal water loss (TEWL) (Yosipovitch et al., 2000), there is now some evidence that the stratum corneum does not function as well as adult skin during the first year of life (Nikolovski et al., 2008); in addition, infant skin is 30% thinner than adult skin (Stamatas et al., 2011). Furthermore, the basal layer of the epidermis is 20% thinner than that of the adult, and the keratinocytes in this layer have a higher cell turnover rate, which may account for the faster wound healing that has been observed in neonates.

The premature infant has far fewer cell layers in the stratum corneum, with the specific number determined by gestational age. At <30 weeks of gestation, there may be as few as two or three layers (Holbrook, 1982), and the extremely premature infant (23 to 24 weeks of gestation) has almost no stratum corneum and negligible barrier function (Agren et al., 1998). The deficient stratum corneum results in excessive fluid and evaporative heat losses during the first weeks of life, leading to increased risk of dehydration and significant alterations in electrolyte levels, such as hypernatremia (Bhatia, 2006). Techniques used to reduce these losses include the use of polyethylene coverings immediately after delivery (Bissinger & Annibale, 2010; Knobel et al., 2005; Vohra, 2004) and use of high levels of relative humidity (>70% RH) in incubators (Gaylord et al., 2001; Kim et al., 2010). Topical treatments such as the application of transparent adhesive dressings (Bhandari et al., 2005; Mancini et al., 1994) and use of topical ointments and skin protectants have been described in small studies (Beeram et al., 2006; Brandon et al., 2010) but remain controversial due to concerns for infection (Edwards et al., 2004).

Maturation of the skin barrier, particularly for infants of 23 to 25 weeks of gestation, occurs over time (Agren et al., 1998; Sedin et al., 1985), with evidence of mature barrier function delayed until about 30 to 32 weeks of postconceptional age (Kalia et al., 1998).

Dermis

The dermis of the full-term newborn is thinner, and not as well developed as the adult dermis. The collagen and elastin fibers are shorter and less dense, and the reticular layer of the dermis is absent, which makes the skin feel very soft. There are reduced total lipid levels and fewer sebaceous glands in the dermal layer in infancy (Stamatas et al., 2011).

Premature and newborn infants exhibit decreased cohesion between the epidermis and dermis, which places them at risk for skin injury from removal of medical adhesives. When extremely aggressive adhesives are used, the bond between the adhesive and epidermis may be stronger than that between the epidermis and dermis, resulting in stripping of the epidermal layer and loss of or significantly diminished skin barrier function (Lund et al., 1997).

Skin pH

Skin is normally characterized by an acidic pH, due to a number of chemical and biologic processes involving the stratum corneum. This "acid mantle" of the skin (pH < 5) has been documented extensively in children and adults.

The acidic skin surface contributes to the immune function of the stratum corneum by inhibiting the growth of pathogenic microorganisms and supporting the proliferation of commensal, or "healthy," bacteria on the skin (Larson & Dinulos, 2005; Visscher et al., 2011).

Full-term newborns are born with an alkaline skin surface (pH > 6.0), but within the first 4 days after birth, the pH falls to <5.0 (Behrendt & Green, 1971). In a study comparing full-term newborns to adults, the mean pH of the newborn skin measured 7.08 on the first day of life, as compared to 5.7 for adult skin pH (Yosipovitch et al., 2000). Skin surface pH in premature infants of varying gestational ages has been reported to be >6 on the first day of life; however, it decreases to 5.5 by the end of the first week and 5.1 by the end of the first month (Fox et al., 1998). Bathing and other topical treatments transiently alter skin pH (Gfatter et al., 1997), and diapered skin has a higher pH due to the combined effects of urine contact and occlusion (Visscher et al., 2002). The higher pH of diapered skin reduces the barrier function of the stratum corneum, rendering it more susceptible to mechanical damage from friction (Visscher et al., 2011).

Risk of Toxicity from Topical Agents

Toxicity from topically applied substances has been reported in numerous case reports due to the increased permeability of both preterm and full-term newborn skin. This is due to a number of factors including the fact that newborn skin is 20% to 40% thinner than adult skin and the ratio of body surface to weight is nearly five times greater in newborns than in older children and adults, which places newborns at increased risk for percutaneous absorption and toxicity. Examples of toxicity from percutaneous absorption include encephalopathy and death among premature infants bathed with hexachlorophene, and alterations in iodine levels and thyroid function related to routine use of povidone–iodine in intensive care nurseries (Linder et al., 1997, Mancini, 2004; Parravicini et al., 1996; Siegfried, 2008; Smerdely et al., 1989).

CLINICAL PEARL

The skin of premature infants and neonates is very permeable; therefore, the wound nurse must assure that topical agents are approved for use in this population.

Skin Assessment and Risk Factors for Skin Breakdown

In the NICU, a thorough examination of all skin surfaces should be done once or twice daily to monitor skin integrity. Early signs such as skin abrasions or small excoriations may call for either diagnostic or treatment procedures. A scoring tool can be used to objectively document skin status; for example, the Neonatal Skin Condition Score (NSCS) was used in the Association of Women's Health, Obstetric and Neonatal Nurses (AWHONN)/National Association of Neonatal Nurses (NANN) research-based practice project, has been extensively used in both premature and full-term infants, and has established validity and reliability (Lund & Osborne, 2004). This scoring system can be integrated into skin care protocols to identify neonates with excessive dryness, erythema, or skin breakdown. The Braden Q is commonly used to assess risk for pressure ulcers in the infant population but does not assess risk for device-related pressure ulcers, which are the most common type of pressure ulcers in this population. When ischemic pressure ulcers are encountered, they generally involve critically ill, ventilated infants who cannot be moved or turned easily, such as those who require high-frequency ventilation or undergo long surgical procedures. The occiput of the infant's head is often the location of these pressure ulcers, as the head is large and heavy in a newborn or young infant, compared to the rest of their body. Measures to prevent occipital pressure ulcers include the use of gel pillows or mattresses, and frequent repositioning using a two-person approach; the second care provider maintains position of the endotracheal tube (ET) during the turning procedure.

Every newborn and infant in the NICU is at risk for skin damage, including chemical burns from skin disinfectants, medical adhesive–related skin injuries (MARSI), diaper dermatitis, and intravenous extravasations. Evidence-based recommendations for preventing and treating skin breakdown, maintaining barrier function of the immature skin, and promoting skin integrity are integrated into a skin care guideline for neonatal nurses, which is available through the Association of Women's Health, Obstetric and Neonatal Nursing (2013). In the next section, issues related to skin disinfection, medical adhesives, intravenous extravasation, and diaper dermatitis are discussed for the NICU patient.

Prevention and Treatment of Common Causes of Skin Breakdown in Neonates and Infants

Damage Due to Skin Disinfectants

Decontamination of the skin prior to invasive procedures such as venipuncture and placement of umbilical catheters and chest tubes is common practice in NICUs. However, there are anecdotal reports of skin injury involving blistering, burns, and sloughing following use of disinfectants with isopropyl alcohol or chlorhexidine gluconate (CHG) in premature infants (Andersen et al., 2005; Harpin & Rutter, 1982; Kutsch & Ottinger, 2014; Linder et al., 2004; Mannan et al., 2007; Reynolds et al., 2005; Sardesai et al., 2011; Schick & Milstein, 1981).

Although a number of studies support the efficacy of chlorhexidine-containing solutions in preventing

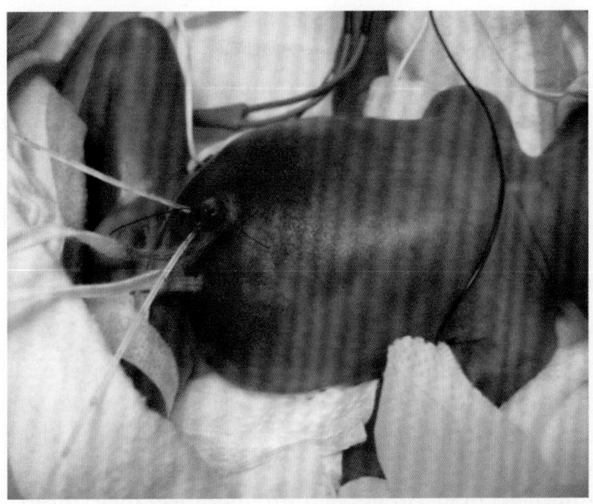
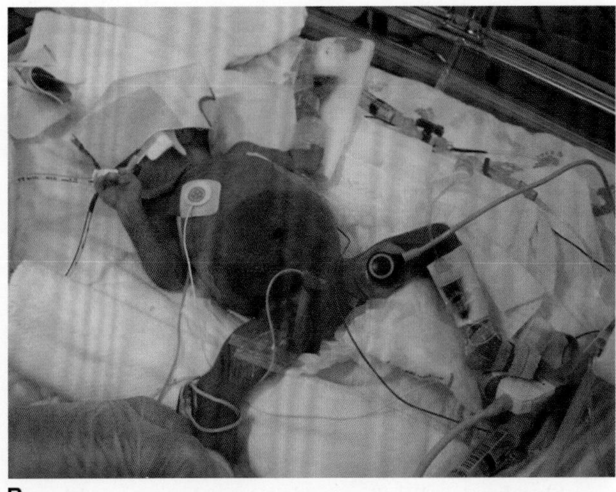

FIGURE 12-1. **A, B.** Chemical burns in two very low birth weight infants from disinfectant containing 2% chlorhexidine gluconate and 70% isopropyl alcohol.

colonization and infection of peripheral intravenous catheters in neonates (Chaiyakunapruk et al., 2002; Garland et al., 1995), large studies to determine the best disinfectant for use in this population are not available. CHG is currently available in the United States as a 2% aqueous solution in 4-ounce bottles, as a tincture of 2% or 3.15% CHG in 70% isopropyl alcohol in single-use packages, and as a wipe containing 0.5% CHG in 70% isopropyl alcohol. According to FDA regulations, chlorhexidine–isopropyl products are now labeled "use with care in premature infants or infants <2 months of age. These products may cause skin irritation or chemical burns" (FDA, 2012). While CHG–alcohol products are commonly used for skin disinfection prior to invasive procedures, the nurse must be aware that the combination (CHG and isopropyl alcohol) has a significant potential for skin injury in very low birth weight (VLBW) infants and cannot be recommended for use in these patients (Fig. 12-1).

In addition to use in skin disinfection prior to invasive procedures, CHG products are commonly used for daily bathing in critical care units and have been shown to decrease infections in pediatric intensive care unit patients >2 months of age (Milstone et al., 2013); however, this practice has not been studied in NICU patients, and there is the potential for toxicity with repeated full body exposure to chlorhexidine. Further study is needed regarding the antimicrobial benefits, the duration of effect, and the potential risks, especially in the NICU population. For example, Da Cunha et al. (2008) found that bathing full-term neonates with CHG reduced skin colonization in some areas, such as the axilla, but not in the groin, and Sankar et al. (2009) found that bathing premature infants with CHG reduced skin colonization only transiently. Concerns have also been raised about the potentially negative effect of CHG on normal skin colonization.

Adhesive-Related Skin Injury

One of the most common practices in the NICU is the application and removal of adhesives that secure ET tubes, IV devices, and monitoring probes and electrodes. An evidence-based practice project involving 2,820 premature and term newborns found that adhesives were the primary cause of skin breakdown among NICU patients (Lund et al., 2001). Changes in TEWL and skin barrier function are seen in adults after 10 consecutive removals of adhesive tape; these changes occur after only one removal of plastic perforated tape in neonates (Lund et al., 1997). Types of damage from adhesive removal include epidermal stripping, tearing, maceration, tension blisters, chemical irritation, sensitization, and folliculitis (Hoath & Narendran, 2000; McNichol et al., 2013) (Fig. 12-2).

Adhesive Removers

Adhesive removers are sometimes used to prevent discomfort and skin disruption from adhesive removal. There are three categories of adhesive removers: alcohol/organic-based solvents, oil-based solvents, and silicone-

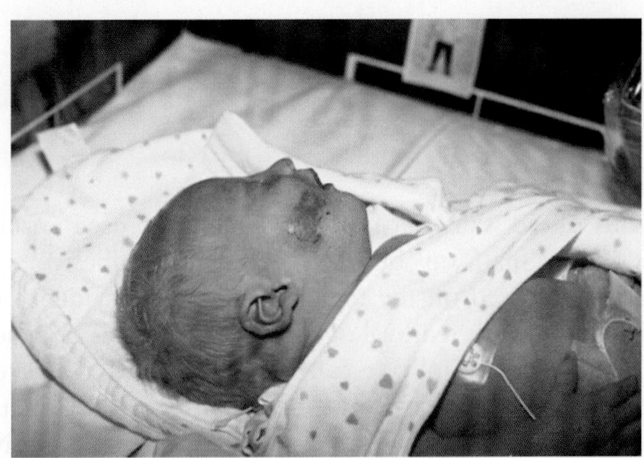

FIGURE 12-2. Example of epidermal stripping from medical adhesive removal in premature infant.

based removers (Black, 2007). The alcohol/organic-based removers contain hydrocarbon derivatives or petroleum distillates that have potential or proven toxicities. This is of particular concern with premature infants, due to their underdeveloped stratum corneum, increased skin permeability, larger surface area/body weight ratio, and immature hepatic and renal function. As evidence of the potential for severe damage, there is a case report of toxic epidermal necrosis in a premature infant resulting from the use of a solvent in this category (Ittmann, 1993). Mineral oil, petrolatum, and citrus-based products may be helpful in removing adhesives but should not be used if the site must be used again for reapplication of adhesives, such as with the retaping of an ET tube. Silicone-based removers form an interposing layer between adhesive and skin, evaporate readily after application, and do not leave a residue (Black, 2007); thus, they have been advocated for patients with extremely fragile skin, such as infants with epidermolysis bullosa (Stephen-Haynes, 2008). Further studies with silicone-based removers are needed to assure appropriateness of these products with the NICU population. Other approaches to prevention of MARSI include removing adhesives with water-soaked cotton balls, and gently pulling the adhesive parallel to the skin surface rather than straight up at a 90-degree angle (Lund & Tucker, 2003).

Tackifiers

Skin-bonding agents, or "tackifiers," promote adherence; examples of these products include tincture of benzoin and Mastisol. Unfortunately, they may create a bond between the adhesive and epidermis that is stronger than the fragile cohesion of the epidermis to the dermis; when the adhesive is removed, epidermal stripping may result. Skin barrier films that are silicone based and alcohol free are reported to reduce skin trauma from repeated adhesive removal (Black, 2007). The use of a skin protectant underneath the tape used to secure intravenous lines in newborns provided skin protection (Irving, 2001) and reduced TEWL (Brandon et al., 2010).

CLINICAL PEARL

Neonates and premature infants are at high risk for skin tears; nurses should avoid use of tape when possible and should consider use of tapes with "gentle adhesives."

Barrier Products

Hydrocolloid skin barriers are sometimes used in the NICU as a "platform" between the skin and adhesive; this practice is based on the reduction in visible evidence of skin trauma with removal of the hydrocolloid as opposed to tape removal (Dollison & Beckstrand, 1995). However, a controlled trial of a hydrocolloid barrier (HolliHesive), plastic tape (Transpore), and a hydrophilic gel adhesive found that significant skin disruption, as measured by TEWL and visual inspection, occurred with removal of both the hydrocolloid barrier and plastic tape (Lund et al., 1997). Significant changes were measured after a single adhesive application and removal in all three weight groups studied (<1,000 g, 1,001 to 1,500 g, and >1,501 g), indicating that even large neonates are at risk for skin injury from tape removal. Despite this finding, hydrocolloid adhesive products continue to be used in the NICU because they mold well to curved surfaces and adhere even with moisture.

Preventive Measures

Prevention of skin trauma from adhesive removal includes minimizing tape use when possible by using smaller pieces, backing the adhesive with cotton, and delaying tape removal until adherence is reduced. Hydrocolloid adhesives may prove helpful, because they mold and adhere well to body contours and often attach better in moist conditions; however, as noted above, these products can also cause skin damage and should be used with caution. The use of soft wraps to secure pulse oximeter probes and hydrogel electrocardiogram electrodes is an excellent strategy when feasible. Silicone-based adhesive products have been shown to improve adherence to wounds and to reduce discomfort with removal (Dykes et al., 2001; Gotschall et al., 1998). Silicone tapes, the newest class of adhesives, are very gentle to the skin but do not adhere well to plastic materials and cannot be used to secure critical tubes and appliances (McNichol et al., 2013); however, they may prove beneficial if developed for other adhesive products in neonates, such as electrodes or sensors.

Intravenous Extravasations

Extravasation injuries can be serious in the neonatal population; thus, every effort must be made to prevent extravasation, and any injury that does occur must be promptly detected and treated.

Prevention

Prevention of tissue injury from IV extravasations includes securing IV devices with transparent dressings or plastic tape so that the insertion site is clearly visible and observing the site with appropriate documentation every hour. If the IV device is placed in a limb, the tape securing the arm or leg to the rigid board should be placed loosely over the joint (such as the elbow or knee) and not over the skin directly above the insertion site. This allows any extravasated fluid and medications to diffuse over a larger surface rather than being concentrated and confined to a small, constricted area, which can result in greater tissue injury. An alternative approach that is being used by some NICUs with success is to eliminate use of the rigid board. Using central venous lines (such as percutaneously inserted central venous catheters) to infuse highly irritating solutions and medications is also recommended. In addition, many nurseries limit the glucose concentrations in peripheral lines to 12.5% and the amino acid concentrations to 2%. Use of peripheral veins for infusion of calcium-containing intravenous fluids is debatable as calcium is extremely irritating to the intima of the vein. In some NICUs, calcium solutions are never infused continuously through a peripheral vein; when used, the concentration of calcium gluconate should be limited to 200 mg/100 mL.

CLINICAL PEARL

Extravasation injuries are common in neonates—prompt recognition and treatment are essential in minimizing tissue damage and tissue loss.

Management

If IV fluid has extravasated into surrounding tissue, the IV device should be removed and the extremity elevated (Fig. 12-3). Use of moisture, heat, or cold is not recommended because the tissue is vulnerable at this point to further injury. Hyaluronidase (Amphadase, Vitrase, Hylenex) can be extremely helpful if administered shortly after the extravasation is identified. This medication is an enzyme that breaks down the interstitial barrier and allows the extravasated fluid to diffuse over a larger area, thus preventing or limiting tissue necrosis (Beaulieu, 2012). The dose of hyaluronidase is 15 to 20 units diluted to 1 mL. It is administered via subcutaneous injections at five points around the periphery of the extravasation site and ideally is administered within 1 to 2 hours of the extravasation. Extravasations for which hyaluronidase may be helpful include those with evidence of blanching, discoloration, or blistering and extravasations involving hypertonic or calcium-containing solutions, even if the site appears relatively undisturbed. The use of an extravasation scale for treatment of IV extravasations may improve communication and consistency in providing appropriate immediate care (Amjad et al., 2011; Simona, 2012).

Calcium-containing solutions may cause deep tissue injury even when the epidermal tissues are not involved. In addition to hyaluronidase administration, creating multiple puncture holes over the area of swelling and gently palpating the involved area, or simply allowing the extravasated fluid to leak out, can promote removal of the infiltrate and reduce the risk of tissue necrosis (Chandavasu et al., 1986; Sawatzky-Dicksson & Bodnaryk, 2006). Saline washout is another technique described to facilitate the removal of extravasated irritants from tissues surrounding an IV site (Casanova et al., 2001; Davies et al., 1994).

Hyaluronidase is not recommended in the extravasation of vasoconstrictive medications such as dopamine, because it may extend the area of vasoconstriction. Phentolamine (Regitine) is used in this case, because it directly counteracts the action of dopamine. The method of delivery is the same as for hyaluronidase, with the total dose (0.5 mg) diluted to 1 mL, and injected in five sites subcutaneously around the periphery of the extravasation (Thigpen, 2007).

Wound Care

When tissue injury occurs after extravasation, moist wound-healing principles are utilized to promote healing without scarring. One approach with multiple anecdotal reports of success involves a generous application of amorphous hydrogel to the site, followed by placement of the extremity into a plastic bag, the so-called "bag/boot" method. This technique is also beneficial for 12 to 24 hours following hyaluronidase injections and establishment of multiple punctures for drainage of the extravasated fluid, as it promotes the ongoing drainage of the irritating vesicant. In most cases, major tissue loss and the need for skin grafts can be prevented by the use of appropriate wound-healing techniques. However, in the most severe cases involving compartment syndrome to the extremity or deep-tissue necrosis, a plastic surgery consultation may be necessary.

Diaper Dermatitis

A common skin disruption that occurs in neonates and infants is diaper dermatitis. There are a number of factors that contribute to the development and severity of diaper dermatitis, but the condition of the skin at baseline

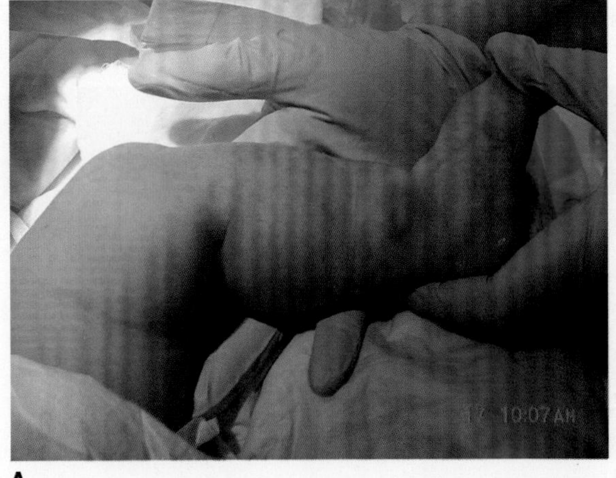

A

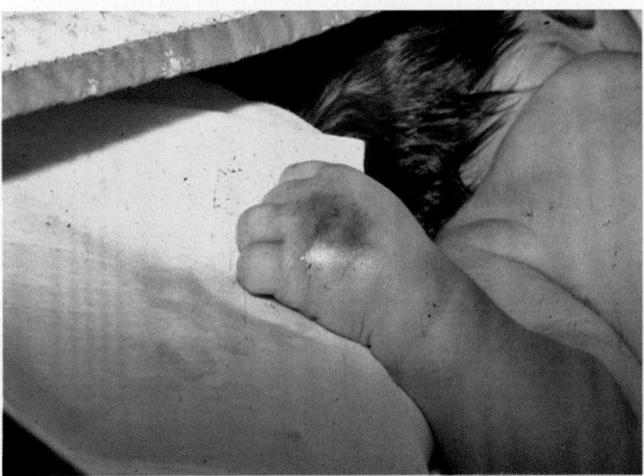

B

FIGURE 12-3. **A, B.** Intravenous extravasation that will require immediate intervention to prevent wound.

is a major determinant in the progression of skin injury. Review articles provide an excellent background for current evidence-based care in the prevention and treatment of diaper dermatitis (Adam, 2008; Heimall et al., 2012).

The pathogenesis of diaper dermatitis involves maceration, compounded by friction injury and/or damage from microbial invasion or enzymatic activity. Skin that is moist and macerated becomes more permeable and susceptible to injury because wetness increases friction. In addition, moisture-laden skin is associated with higher levels of microorganisms as compared to dry skin. Another contributing factor to skin injury is the effect of an alkaline skin pH. The normal skin pH is acidic, ranging between 4.0 and 5.5; however, occluded and macerated skin is typically alkaline (Visscher et al., 2000; Visscher et al., 2002). When the skin pH is more alkaline, there is increased vulnerability to injury and penetration by microorganisms. In addition, an alkaline pH stimulates fecal enzyme activity; stool contains both proteases and lipases, which, when activated, can cause significant damage to the protein and fat components of the skin. This enzymatic damage is responsible for much of the contact irritant diaper dermatitis commonly seen in clinical practice.

Prevention

Strategies for preventing diaper dermatitis include maintaining a dry and acidic skin surface. Frequent diaper changes are recommended, especially in the newborn period. Superabsorbent gelled diapers with breathable covers have been shown to keep the skin surface dryer by "wicking" the moisture away from the skin and separating urine from feces (Kosemund, 2009; Lin et al., 2005; Nield & Kamat, 2007; Rai et al., 2009; Scheinfeld, 2005). The routine use of petrolatum-based ointments may prevent the progression to diaper dermatitis in neonates and infants at risk, such as those with watery stools from opiate withdrawal or malabsorption. Use of powders is discouraged because of the risk of inhalation of particles into the respiratory tract.

Treatment

Once skin injury from diaper dermatitis has occurred, protecting the damaged skin to prevent reinjury is the primary goal of treatment (Fig. 12-4). Topical treatment for diaper dermatitis involves ointments and creams containing a variety of ingredients such as zinc oxide and petrolatum (Heimall, 2012). Generous application of protective skin barriers that contain zinc oxide can prevent further injury while allowing the skin to heal. Once denudation occurs, keeping the skin open to air is not an effective strategy; the damaged tissue requires a moist surface for healing, and leaving the damaged surface open to air provides no protection against exposure to stool during recurrent diarrheal episodes. All caregivers must be taught that it is not necessary or desirable to completely remove the skin barrier ointment with each diaper change, because this causes additional trauma that disrupts healing tissue. Instead, the caregiver should remove the layers of ointment soiled with stool and should reapply the barrier generously to the affected areas with each diaper change. Another class of barrier products are liquid silicone-based and alcohol-free barrier films, which are designed to repel moisture and protect the skin from irritants (Heimall, 2012); these products are FDA approved for use in infants >28 days of age but are frequently used "off-label" and have been beneficial when used on neonatal ostomy patients.

Candidiasis

Candida albicans can also be a contributing factor to diaper dermatitis. The yeast rash presents as a brightly erythematous, sharply marginated dermatitis that involves the inguinal folds as well as the buttocks, thighs, and genitalia, typically with characteristic "satellite" lesions (Fig. 12-5). Treatment with an antifungal ointment or cream is necessary. Antifungal preparations include Mycostatin, miconazole, clotrimazole, and ketoconazole in ointment or cream forms; ointments are preferable to coat the skin and repel moisture. If the dermatitis involves both a fungal rash and denudation due to contact irritant dermatitis, it may be necessary to layer the ointment with the antifungal preparation; in this case, Mycostatin or miconazole powder can be dusted onto the area, followed by application of an alcohol-free skin protectant to "seal" the powder onto the skin surface, followed by a generous application of a skin barrier cream such as zinc oxide or pectin paste.

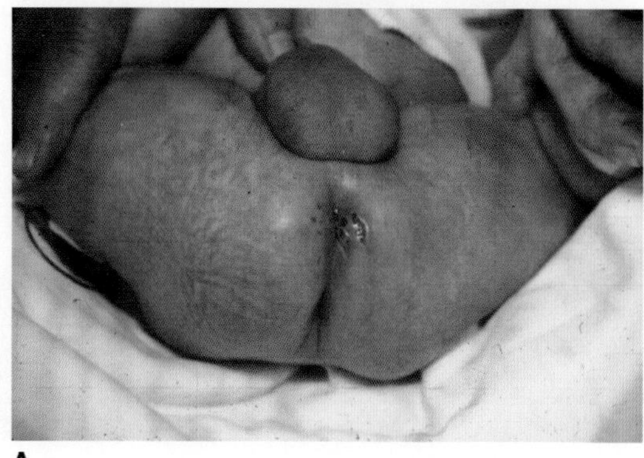
A

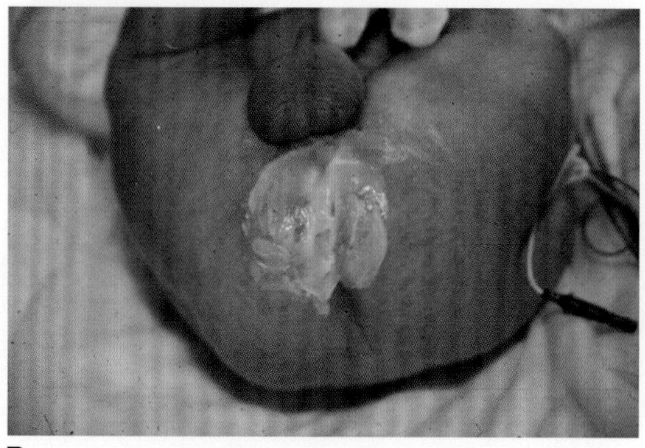
B

FIGURE 12-4. **A, B.** Contact irritant diaper dermatitis and use of effective topical barrier to prevent reinjury.

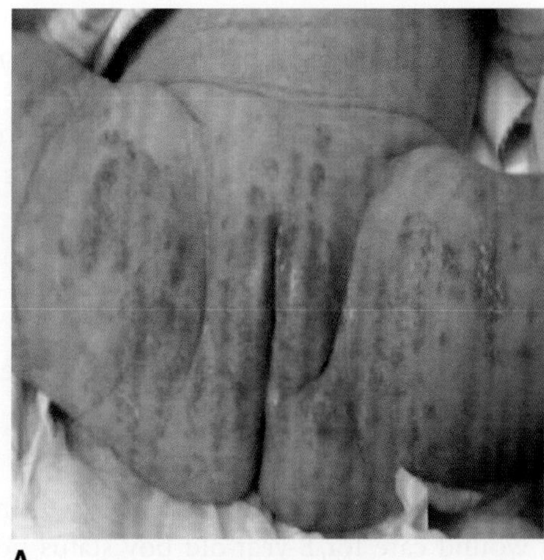

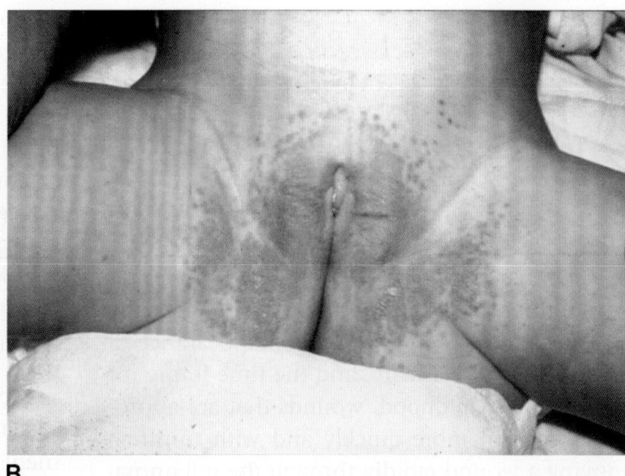

A **B**

FIGURE 12-5. A, B. Examples of diaper dermatitis caused by *Candida albicans*.

Occasionally, infants may experience extremely severe diaper dermatitis from intestinal malabsorption syndromes, opiate withdrawal, or constant dribbling of stool due to compromised sphincter function (e.g., infants with myelomeningocele or those undergoing a "pull-through" procedure for Hirschsprung's disease or anorectal atresia). In the case of malabsorption, there is rapid transit through the small intestine; this results in a complex clinical situation that includes abnormally alkaline stool, increased stool volume, higher levels of activated enzymes, and undigested carbohydrates and fats. Infants with malabsorption syndromes are at risk for nutritional deficiencies and dehydration in addition to severe diaper dermatitis and require thorough medical evaluation.

While optimal nutritional therapy is being addressed with special diets or parenteral nutrition, skin protection from injury should be initiated. Products that contain carboxymethylcellulose, petrolatum, and zinc oxide without alcohol, such as Ilex, may provide a sturdier barrier for these infants than zinc oxide alone. The skin should be thoroughly but gently cleansed followed by a very thick application of the barrier paste; the barrier paste is then covered by a greasy ointment such as petrolatum to prevent adherence of the barrier paste to the diaper. When the infant has a stool, it is not necessary to completely remove the barrier paste; the stool can be gently wiped away before reapplying the thick paste barrier. The skin will heal under this protective covering as long as it is protected from reinjury. Another approach that is described is the "crusting" technique; pectin-based powder is dusted onto the skin followed by application of a silicone-based liquid skin barrier (Gray, 2007; Heimall, 2012).

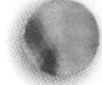 Unique Challenges in Pediatric Skin and Wound Care

The wound care practitioner has a unique role in the pediatric setting. The role is diverse and challenging, because the wound care practitioner is frequently expected to serve as a liaison between various disciplines and the child and family, and must be able to identify the commonalities in goals and practices in order to develop a wound care plan that is acceptable to all involved. The wound care practitioner in pediatrics needs to become familiar with the multiple providers and their preferred methods of management for surgical sites and wounds and must be able to "speak their language" while promoting evidence-based practice and advocating for the parents and child. Thus, communication and collaboration skills are just as important as wound care skills in meeting the needs of the pediatric population, and an initial focus of role development for the wound care nurse new to the setting is development of collaborative relationships with other members of the multidisciplinary team. In developing a plan of care for the pediatric patient, the nurse must consider three questions: (1) Is this plan consistent with evidence-based recommendations for promotion of wound healing? (2) Does this plan work for the caregiver? (3) Does this plan work for the child and parents?

The wound care nurse must also realize that, in many situations, the wound is a complication of a primary diagnosis or a surgical procedure, which means the child and family may have multiple issues and challenges to address in addition to the wound. This means that their tolerance for discussion of multiple ideas and plans of care is likely to be very limited! Parents frequently report that they are hearing conflicting messages regarding wound care and what to expect, which makes them wonder if anyone really knows what they are doing; it is the responsibility of the wound care practitioner to explain to the parents the common principles underlying all recommendations and to work with the entire team to develop a plan that works for the parents and the child. It is also important to acknowledge that wound care can be challenging and to use available resources and strategies (such as the child life specialist and premedication) to facilitate dressing changes and wound management at home; these approaches support family-centered care.

CLINICAL PEARL

Wound care for the pediatric patient must be evidence based but must also be acceptable and feasible for the child and parent.

Physiology Pediatric Skin and Wound Healing

Throughout childhood the skin continues to change as the child grows; these changes involve general appearance of the skin, its texture and elasticity, and the time frame for healing. During early childhood, wounds that are appropriately managed heal more quickly and with minimal scarring; moving a wound rapidly through the inflammatory phase (by eliminating necrotic tissue and controlling bacterial loads) is an important strategy for minimizing scarring (Nick et al., 2010). Scars acquired in early childhood fade, stretch, and become less obvious in later years (Nick et al., 2010). The wound care nurse must be able to explain the basic healing process in simple terms and must also be able to address concerns regarding both short-term and long-term outcomes and expectations (e.g., wound healing and wound management short term and scar appearance long term).

Scar Appearance

As noted, a concern for all parents is the potential impact of the wound and eventual scar on the child's body image and the appearance of the healed wound and scar. The wound care clinician should be prepared to discuss wound-healing outcomes and options for scar management. If there is a history of keloid formation, the family should be provided with options for future management including referral to plastic surgery.

Impact of Developmental Stage

Pediatric skin and wound care must be provided within the framework of overall growth and development, with particular attention to differences in skin condition, activity levels, and perspiration. Dressing options frequently vary based on the age and development of a child. For example, a toddler who has soft supple skin will benefit from a silicone-based dressing or a dressing that has a 5-day wear time, whereas a teenager who is prone to sweating may need a dressing with greater adhesion and more resistance to moisture and activity.

For the new pediatric wound care practitioner, it is beneficial to be familiar with common skin conditions of childhood. The pediatric wound care practitioner may not be directly responsible for management of these conditions; however, she or he will frequently be responsible for facilitating and coordinating care and may also be asked to provide input as to care options. In addition, the pediatric wound care nurse is frequently asked to provide "interim recommendations" for wound management until consults can be placed and responded to, and the wound care nurse may be asked to provide wound care support to a variety of medical and surgical services.

In the next section, case scenarios are utilized to highlight common challenges faced by the pediatric wound care nurse.

Common Challenge: Conflicting Plans of Care

Conflicting plans of care are a common challenge, as will be illustrated by the following example.

Description of Clinical Situation

Wound care nurse consulted for assistance with management of wound care for 8-year-old boy status post traumatic injury requiring negative pressure wound therapy (NPWT) for abdominal wound with multiple fistulas. Current issues include the following: the NPWT system leaks every few hours with dislodgement of dressings, multiple different plans have been suggested by different services and practitioners to manage the drainage, and the family, child, and staff are visibly upset.

Wound Care Nurse Response

The wound care nurse identified the following goals: (1) assess the current system to determine the reasons for leakage and system failure, (2) consult and collaborate with the various care services and practitioners to develop a management plan acceptable to all, (3) communicate plan to the primary service and provider via verbal and written communication, (4) provide clinical assistance to the staff in implementation of the plan, and (5) educate the child and family on the management plan.

Discussion

In this case, all team members had the same goal but there were multiple opinions as to how to meet that goal. The wound care nurse assessed the current management approach and identified areas of consistent failure; she then used her knowledge of current innovative strategies for management of abdominal wounds with multiple fistulas to suggest a different approach and supported her recommendation with evidence-based literature and illustrations as well as clinical demonstration and support to the staff (Brindle, 2009). She was then able to talk with the family and child to explain that everyone was trying to solve the same problem and to assure the family and child that the entire team would work together and with them to assure an effective management plan prior to discharge (Figs. 12-6 and 12-7).

Common Clinical Challenge: Multiple Comparable Plans That Appear to Be Conflicting

In many situations, there are multiple proposed plans of care that appear to be conflicting but are based on the same underlying principles of care. In this case, the

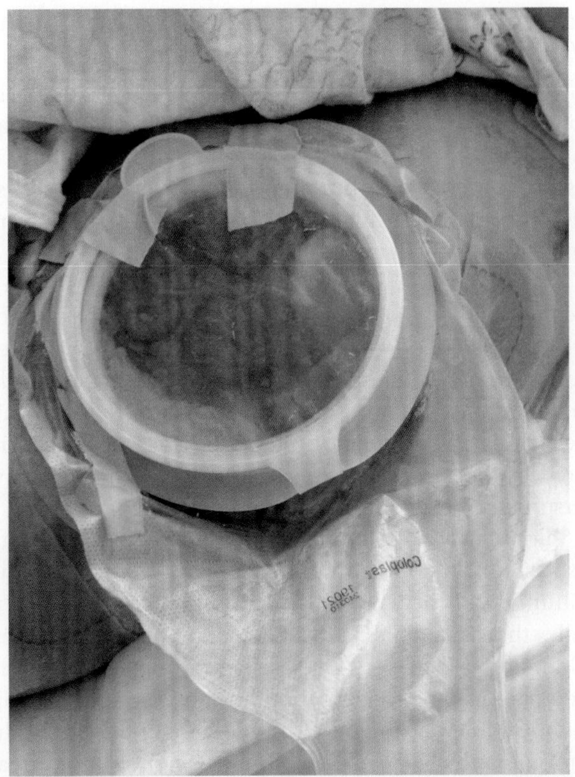

FIGURE 12-6. Post-op pouching system used to manage fistula drainage in a small child.

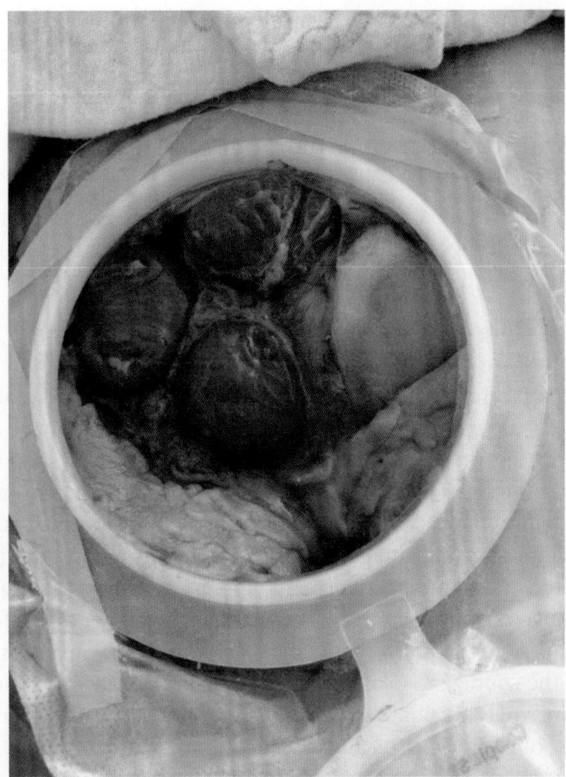

FIGURE 12-7. Use of post-op pouch to manage fistulas when fistula management system and NPWT are ineffective.

wound care nurse is challenged to identify the central principles that are common to all plans *and* to evidence-based management of the problem, to synthesize the various suggestions into a comprehensive and simplified plan, and to bring the various clinicians together in support of the plan. This requires the wound nurse to have positive working relationships with all involved practitioners, to be current in terms of concepts and supplies, and to be able to explain to all involved how the recommended plan and products are compatible with their recommendations.

Description of Clinical Situation

Wound care nurse is consulted regarding the management of a 15-year-old boy with a rheumatology diagnosis who has pea-sized full-thickness wounds on the extremities; the wounds have been slow to heal, and there are areas of slough in the wound bed. At present, there are wound care recommendations from dermatology, plastic surgery, general surgery, and an outside consultant that all appear to be different; the wound care nurse finds multiple supplies at the bedside, and the parents, patient, and staff all voice concerns and confusion. Currently recommended care plans include the following: Burrow's solution to dry the wounds, followed by moist gauze packing (dermatology); irrigate with N/S twice daily, pack with nonwoven strip gauze, and cover with bordered foam dressing (plastic surgery); irrigate with N/S twice daily, pack with nonwoven strip gauze, and cover (surgery); and irrigate with Dakin's twice daily, pack with nonwoven strip gauze, and cover with gauze and tape.

Wound Care Nurse Response

The wound care nurse identified the following goals: (1) discuss with the care team the goals for healing; (2) review the patient's record to identify any impediments to healing; (3) identify commonalities between the recommended treatment plans for cleansing, packing, and covering the wound, within the framework of evidence-based wound care; (4) identify the patient's and family's preferences in regard to wound care (which care regimen do they prefer, and why?)

Discussion

The discussion with the care team revealed that the goal was wound healing, with identified subgoals that included establishment of a clean wound bed, prevention of infection, and promotion of granulation tissue. The commonalities among the care orders were routine cleansing, use of a packing agent to fill the shallow craters, and covering the wound to prevent trauma and bacterial invasion; some included use of agents to inhibit bacterial growth. The patient wanted a dressing that was easy to apply and did not cause pain with removal; he preferred daily as opposed to twice-daily dressing changes. Based on all of these considerations, and with the goal of promoting healing, the wound nurse recommended the following: daily dressing changes, clean wounds with normal saline, fill craters lightly with medical-grade honey–based calcium alginate (to promote autolysis, inhibit bacterial growth, and provide exudate control), and cover with foam border dressing.

Common Clinical Challenge: Resistance/ Nonadherence

In some situations, the child is totally resistant to the care plan, and the parents have a hard time forcing the issue; thus, wound care is not consistently done.

Description of Current Clinical Situation (the Little Girl Who Said "I Won't Oh No I Won't")

Wound care nurse consulted regarding the management of a 3-year-old girl who was status post incision and drainage of an abscess on the chest wall; wound is nonhealing despite IV antibiotics given through PICC line. Current plan requires dressing changes three times daily with wet-to-dry gauze packing covered with gauze and tape. Parents report that the child is "screaming, crying, and yelling" with every dressing change, requiring them and her nanny to hold her down for the dressing change, which they do when they can muster up the courage to deal with the screaming and yelling. They admit that most days the dressing does not get changed, and they often find her picking or scratching at the dressing.

Wound Care Nurse Response

The wound care nurse identified the following goals: (1) determine child's specific concerns about wound care and the frequency of dressing change she would find acceptable; (2) determine parents' goals for care; (3) develop a wound care plan that promotes healing and protects wound from trauma and bacterial invasion, while minimizing barriers and resistance to care; and (4) achieve support for modified care plan.

Discussion

The identified barriers to wound care included pain with dressing removal and the frequency of dressing changes. The parents' primary goal was to promote wound healing, but they stated that they could not force their child to go through a painful procedure three times a day if there were any alternatives. The wound care nurse recommended the following: change dressing every 3 days as opposed to three times daily; use honey–based calcium alginate dressing to the wound bed to absorb drainage, maintain a moist surface, and provide atraumatic removal; cover with silicone adhesive–bordered foam dressing to minimize pain with removal; and use silicone-based adhesive remover to further reduce discomfort with dressing removal. Use of the honey-based alginate dressing provided antimicrobial effects and better exudate control than gauze, and the foam cover dressing provided further absorption as well as protection against bacterial invasion. The silicone adhesive and silicone adhesive remover almost totally eliminated the discomfort related to dressing removal. The child was also allowed to call "time out" during the dressing change procedure.

Common Clinical Challenge: Concern about Wound Appearance and Scarring

The pediatric wound care nurse has to be cognizant of the potential impact of a wound on the child's body image and should give the child or teenager an opportunity to discuss concerns regarding the wound, the healing process, and outcomes, particularly scar formation. These issues are typically of particular concern for teenagers.

A very common wound in the adolescent population is the pilonidal cyst, which is a cyst that involves the hair follicles and sebaceous glands in the natal cleft. The cyst presents clinically as an abscess at the superior aspect of the natal cleft; there may be additional circular wounds within the cleft itself. Pilonidal cyst development is typically triggered by hormonal changes, hair growth, and excessive perspiration related to activity and heat.

Pilonidal cysts occur in 26 per 100,000 people and are associated with a major negative impact on quality of life (Ghnnam & Hafez, 2011). They occur more commonly in males than in females, and 11% reoccur following surgery (Ghnnam & Hafez, 2011). Teenagers often delay telling their parents or caregivers about the abscess until the pain is unbearable or a friend encourages them to seek health care guidance. For smaller pilonidal cysts, simple treatment measures may be effective and sufficient: removing all hair from the area, sitz bath soaks and good hygiene, and appropriate topical therapy (absorption of exudate, maintenance of a moist surface, separation of the two sides of the natal cleft, and avoidance of pressure and trauma) (Ghnnam & Hafez, 2011). However, in many cases, surgical incision and drainage is required, and the wound is either left open to heal through secondary intention or closed by a flap procedure.

When incision and drainage is required, the surgical incision begins at the superior aspect of the natal cleft and down into the cleft (Ghnnam & Hafez, 2011). The pediatric wound care nurse needs to be sensitive to the effect of the healing and scarring process on the adolescent's body image. The top of the natal cleft is the area where bikini bottoms and swim trunks typically rest. In addition, scarring in this area can impact the individual's comfort with sexual intimacy. Reassuring the teenager that the team will do everything possible to minimize scarring and discomfort is therefore a critical aspect of wound management. These patients may be referred to tertiary pediatric centers for wound care following surgery complicated by impaired wound healing.

Description of Clinical Situation

Wound nurse consulted regarding management of pilonidal cyst wound. The patient is a 17-year-old male who states "my mom will drive for hours to get us here if you can heal this wound." States he has had two operations over the past 18 months and a nonhealing wound for 12 months; he has stopped participating in sports, has missed many classes in his senior year, and is at risk for not graduating with his class. On assessment, the wound measures 10 × 6 cm with variable depth; he is currently managing the wound with gauze dressings and states he has also used some collagen dressings. He is very concerned about odor and leakage and does not go to school on hot days due to those issues.

Wound Care Nurse Response

The wound care nurse determined the following goals: (1) conduct a comprehensive assessment to identify any systemic barriers to healing (e.g., undiagnosed diabetes, anemia, smoking, insufficient protein intake); (2) assess for hair growth and review current hygienic care and wound care; (3) develop a management plan that is feasible for the patient and supporting individuals and that provides hair removal, exudate control, a moist wound surface, and separation of the sides of the wound and that does not add bulk or abrasive force; (4) assure availability of surgery for consultation if needed; and (5) collaborate with primary provider on wound care.

Discussion

The wound nurse talked with the patient and his mother and found them both to be highly motivated; both stated they would prefer to avoid a repeat surgery if possible. The wound nurse recommended the following as initial therapy:

(1) Exfoliate hair from wound margins using waxing strips, and tweeze out any hairs encroaching on the wound surface; (2) shower after dressing removal to thoroughly cleanse the area; (3) apply a low-profile antimicrobial absorptive dressing to the wound base (e.g., silver-based hydrofiber or alginate, or medical-grade honey–based gel); and (4) cover with thin silicone adhesive dressing (either silicone adhesive foam or silicone adhesive transfer dressing). Consider use of a thin strip of wicking fabric over the dressing at the superior aspect of the cleft. The wound nurse taught the patient and his mother the critical aspects of daily wound care, emphasized the importance of a thin dressing that allowed the buttocks to close appropriately while also providing separation and elimination of frictional forces, and offered him the option to come to clinic daily for dressing changes until he felt comfortable doing the dressing himself. She also discussed the importance of adequate protein intake and pressure reduction and provided the patient with a list of high-protein foods and a foam cushion. Finally, she discussed the option to use NPWT if the wound did not respond to the initial protocol. (If NPWT is used, the caregiver must size the foam to be slightly smaller than the diameter of the wound.)

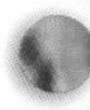

Skin Disorders Commonly Seen in the Pediatric Population

Atopic Dermatitis

Atopic dermatitis is commonly known as eczema and is a chronic inflammatory disease (Janmohamed et al., 2014) that occurs in children but often persists into adulthood. The classic symptoms include skin dryness, erythema, intense pruritis, weeping, and crusting, all of which impact quality of life (Janmohamed et al., 2014). The lichenification process can also cause disfigurement, which impacts on body image. The goal of treatment is not cure but elimination of triggers and symptom management (Janmohamed et al., 2014).

Management

Eczema is a challenging disease that requires a multidimensional approach. The five main principles underlying topical therapy include: maintaining the pH balance of the skin, restoring and maintaining skin hydration through use of humectant and emollients, minimizing exacerbating factors, providing patient education, and assuring appropriate pharmacological treatment (Visser, 2014).

The wound care nurse can comanage the child with a dermatologist or can choose to manage the child independently within limitations imposed by her or his scope of practice and knowledge level. Open eczematous lesions are at risk for bacterial, viral, and dermatophyte infections, which are manifest by extending or intense erythema, tenderness to touch, increased drainage, or odor. A punched out appearance and hemorrhagic vesicles are indicative of a secondary herpes simplex infection that requires immediate systemic treatment. Initial treatment should include a systemic antiviral, a broad-spectrum antibacterial, an antimicrobial dressing, and close monitoring. Initial treatment with a broad-spectrum antibacterial in addition to the antiviral ensures that a staph infection which is masked is not left untreated. Identification of exacerbating factors is crucial for minimizing flares; triggering factors commonly include food allergies, heat, and humidity. Given the correlation between food allergies and eczema, consultation with an allergist is extremely helpful for most children to identify which food or items in the environment are triggers.

The wound care clinician should develop a therapeutic relationship with the child and family. Education should emphasize skin hygiene, identification and avoidance of irritants, and the routine use of emollients and humectants to maintain soft supple skin. The wound care clinician is in a unique position to provide ongoing education and support for the child and family.

Description of Clinical Scenario

Wound nurse consulted for care of 9-year-old girl with extensive eczema involving her face, neck, and arms who is shy, good at school, and has been dealing with eczema since she was 3 years old. The patient has been admitted to rule out bacterial, viral, and/or dermatophyte infection secondary to lesions from eczema; transported from outside facility with wet dressings over her arms and neck that are to be kept moist at all times. The child states that the dressings made her sad and made her feel like she could not go to school and she loved school. She also stated that she didn't think her skin condition would ever change.

Wound Care Nurse Response

The wound care nurse established the following goals: (1) establish a trusting relationship with the child and family; (2) obtain a history of previously used products and current skin care routine; (3) identify a dressing that meets the goals of care and allows the child to return to school; and (4) educate the child and family regarding eczema management.

The wound nurse talked with the patient and family regarding low-profile dressings that are easy to conceal and showed them samples of a medical-grade honey alginate dressing that could be applied directly to the open wounds and covered with a light silicone adhesive foam or wicking fabric secured with stretch net; these dressings could be changed daily with minimal or no discomfort, could be easily concealed under long sleeve clothing, and would keep her clothing dry. The wound nurse also emphasized the importance of maintaining skin pH using a pH-balanced cleanser with an antimicrobial agent followed by daily use of a dimethicone 6% moisturizer (e.g., Sween 24 by Coloplast) (Figs. 12-8 to 12-13).

Contact Dermatitis

Contact dermatitis is inflammation of the dermis and epidermis, which has been triggered by a substance that came in contact with the skin surface. There are two broad categories of contact dermatitis: irritant dermatitis and allergic dermatitis. Irritant contact dermatitis may involve either diaper dermatitis or dermatitis involving intact dry skin. Diaper dermatitis is common in children of all ages who require diapering (even short term) for incontinence. During an acute illness requiring antibiotics, stool pH

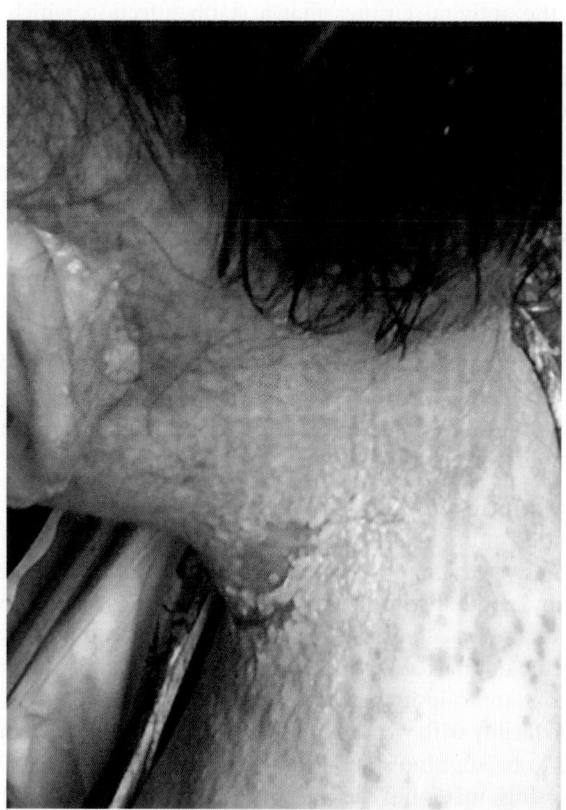

FIGURE 12-8. A young girl with severe eczema on initial presentation to OR.

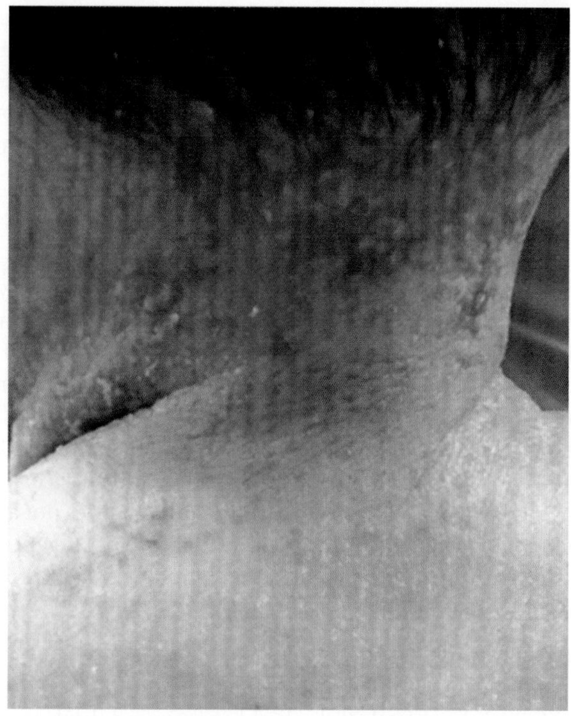

FIGURE 12-9. Response to treatment that included antivirals, antibiotics, medical-grade honey to open lesions; daily cleansing with pH-balanced cleanser; and moisturizing with 6% dimethicone.

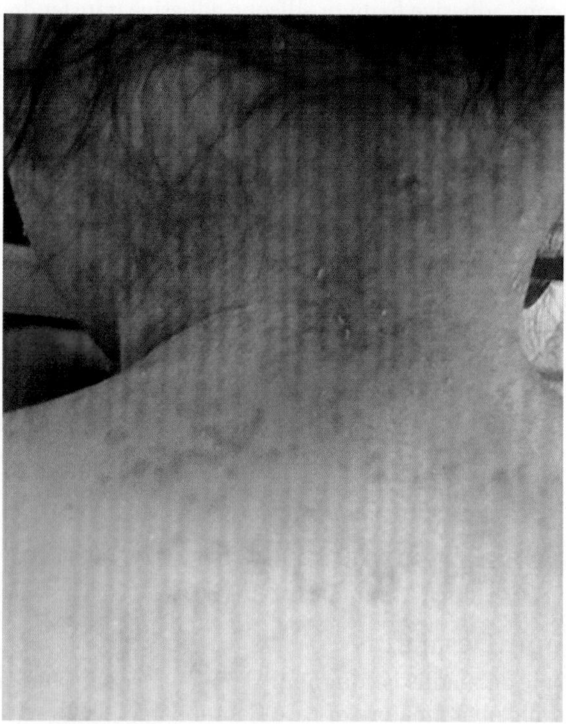

FIGURE 12-10. Skin at the time of discharge.

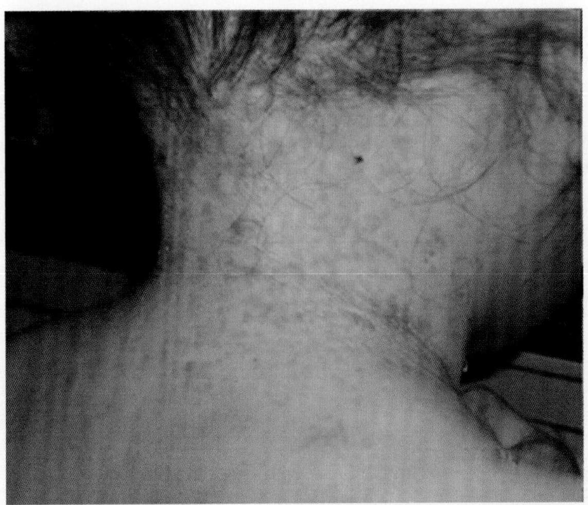

FIGURE 12-11. Skin showing progressive healing.

frequently changes, which makes it highly irritating to the skin. Prevention includes application of a thin clear skin barrier with all diapered children during an acute illness, either a petrolatum-based ointment or a liquid barrier film. If the diaper dermatitis involves a fungal infection, the child should be treated with an antifungal agent, as discussed earlier in this chapter. The wound care nurse should be aware that there are multiple strands of *C. albicans* and not all are responsive to nystatin; if the child with a fungal rash fails to respond to nystatin, she or he should be treated with a broad-spectrum antifungal such as miconazole (Fridkin & Jarvis, 1996). The wound nurse should also realize that fungal rashes developing following broad-spectrum intravenous antibiotic therapy are more likely to be resistant to nystatin than those developing following milder oral agents (Fridkin & Jarvis, 1996). There is extensive research ongoing into treatment for resistant fungal infections (Vandeputte et al., 2012). The wound nurse should always query patients in regard to recent antibiotic therapy and continence status. In the interest of avoiding polypharmacy at the bedside and simplifying skin care routines, a combined barrier and antifungal ointment is

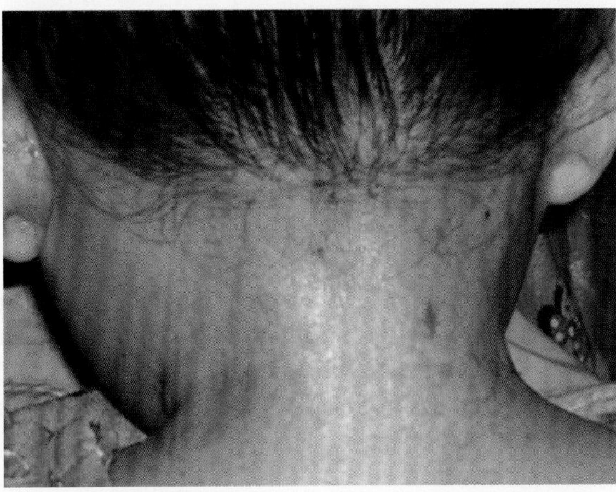

FIGURE 12-12. Skin showing progressive healing.

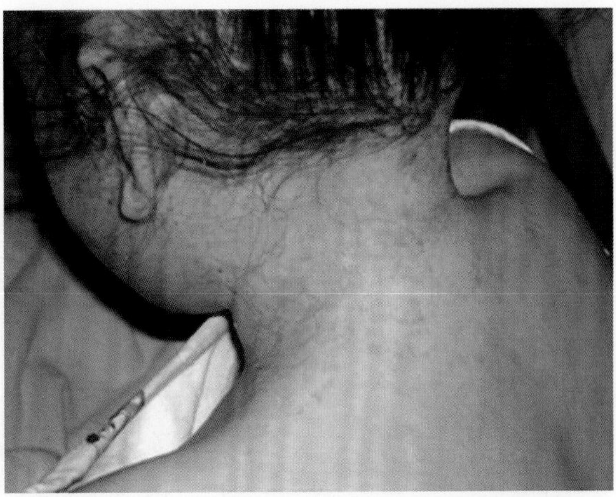

FIGURE 12-13. Skin showing progressive healing.

frequently recommended for children who are incontinent and who present with a fungal rash. Prompt treatment of diaper dermatitis is important in order to prevent denudation, which increases the risk for Candida invasion of the skin, soft tissue, and even blood (Fridkin & Jarvis, 1996).

Algorithms are an effective tool for improving standards of care and outcomes. See Figure 12-14 for a sample algorithm addressing prevention and management of diaper dermatitis.

CLINICAL PEARL

Algorithms are an effective tool for improving standards of care and outcomes.

Epidermolysis Bullosa

Epidermolysis bullosa (EB) is a rare skin condition affecting the junction between the epidermis and dermis, with an incidence of 1/50,000 live births or 50 in 1 million live births. There are three main types of EB: epidermolysis bullosa simplex, junctional epidermolysis bullosa, and dystrophic epidermolysis bullosa. Epidermolysis bullosa simplex accounts for 92% of all cases and is autosomal dominant; junctional is autosomal recessive and rare, accounting for only 1% to 2% of the cases. Dystrophic EB can be either dominant or recessive and accounts for approximately 5% to 6% of cases. EB simplex typically affects the hands and feet and is the simplest form of EB. During the first year of life, the infant may experience blistering over the arms and legs; fortunately, toward the end of the first year of life, the blistering becomes limited to the hands and feet. Autosomal recessive EB is the severest form of EB; these infants have blisters present at birth caused by the friction experienced during delivery. The mucous membranes and lining of the gastrointestinal tract are also involved, which makes feeding difficult. The child often suffers from calorie deficiencies due to the combined problems of impaired intake and increased caloric demands related to wound healing (Thompson et al., 2014).

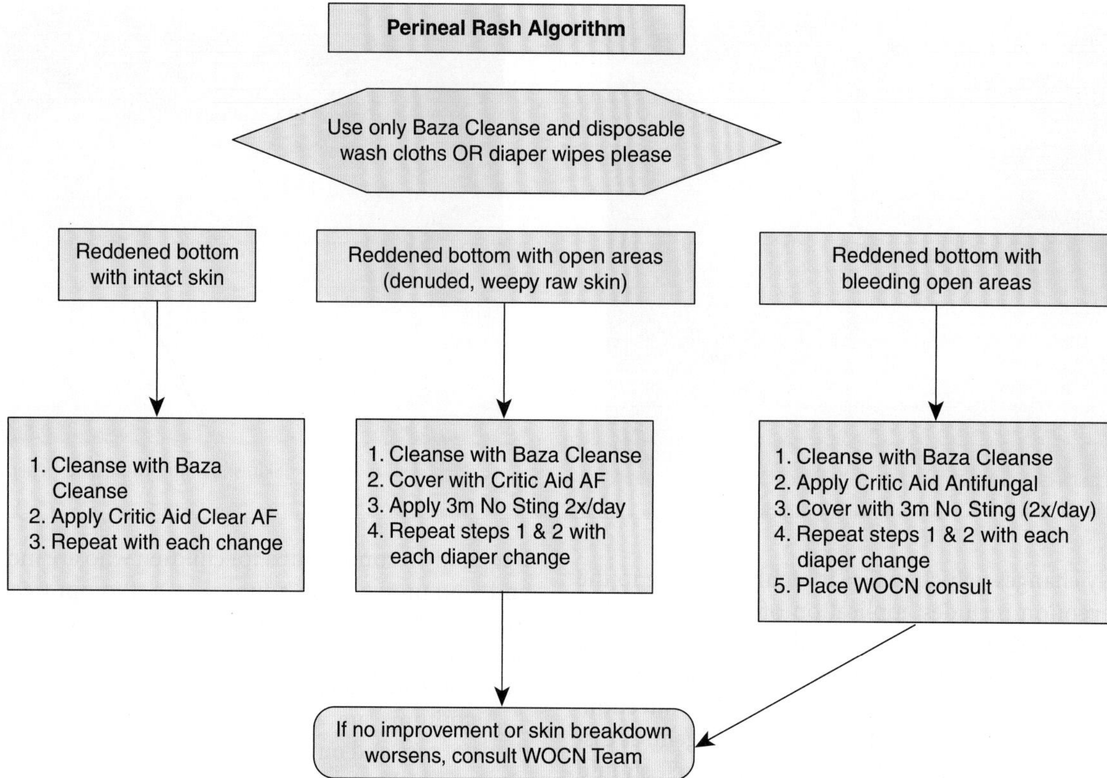

FIGURE 12-14. Sample perineal rash algorithm used housewide at Stanford Children's Hospital.

Management

EB is diagnosed in infancy, often within the first few weeks of life. EB is initially managed in the neonatal intensive care unit; thus, the neonatal intensive care unit must have a policy for management of these infants and their lesions. The child will be managed by dermatology and the neonatologist; however, the pediatric wound care nurse can assist with initiation of treatment, education of the parents, and case management (e.g., by ordering supplies).

The pediatric wound care nurse can also support the families during adjustment to the unexpected and devastating diagnosis by connecting them to the Debra foundation (debra.org, 2014). The families are often not expecting a diagnosis of EB and need support not only in adjusting to the diagnosis but also in preparing to bring the baby home (debra.org, 2014). The baby diagnosed with EB needs to be protected from friction; even light pressure and friction caused by hugging and kissing can result in blisters. Thus, adjustment to the diagnosis includes changing perceptions regarding good parenting behaviors and how to include the extended family (debra.org, 2014). Providing ongoing support prior to and following discharge home should be a team approach that includes social work, case management, dermatology, and wound care (debra.org, 2014). There is ongoing research in wound healing for children with EB; evolving treatment strategies include gene therapy and advanced topical therapy (Cutlar et al., 2014).

Older children who have lived their entire lives with EB will have an established routine for dressing changes and preferences regarding dressings (debra.org, 2014). Children with EB will also easily verbalize what they can and cannot do. The pediatric wound care nurse needs to involve the child and follow his or her lead in dressing changes and activity.

Topical Therapy

Only nonadhesive dressings or those with gentle adhesive technology should be used in direct contact with the child. Moisturizers should be used in generous amounts to prevent friction and blister formation. Low-friction antimicrobial linens should be strongly recommended for routine use (NPUAP, 2014). Blisters should be drained immediately to prevent enlargement. Central lines if needed should be tunneled and then secured with a single stitch. Special considerations in the OR include avoiding use of tapes directly on the skin. ET tubes should be secured with a mask placed behind the child's head with the ties then secured around the ET tube (Figs. 12-15 to 12-18).

The dressing regimen for an individual child is created in conjunction with dermatology and modified over time to reflect the child's growth and changes in activity. The child is continually monitored for sepsis, and the parents are given instructions as to signs of wound infection and proper response, as well as daily skin and wound care and blister management.

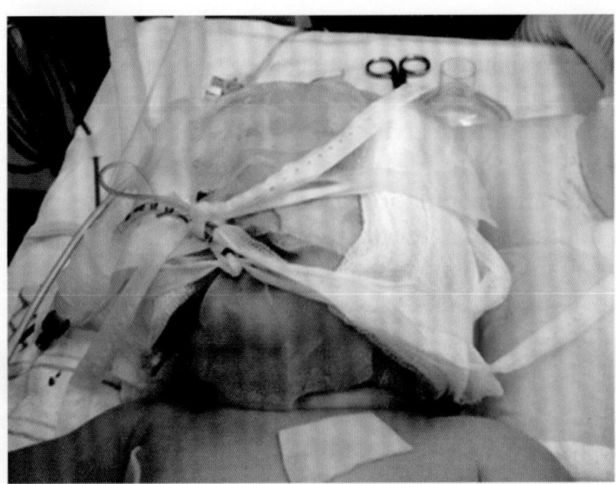

FIGURE 12-15. Method for securing ET tube for a child with EB.The face is protected with petrolatum and nonadhesive contact layer; surgical mask is placed behind the child's head, and ties are used to secure ETT. Gauze is used to pad and protect the skin under ties.

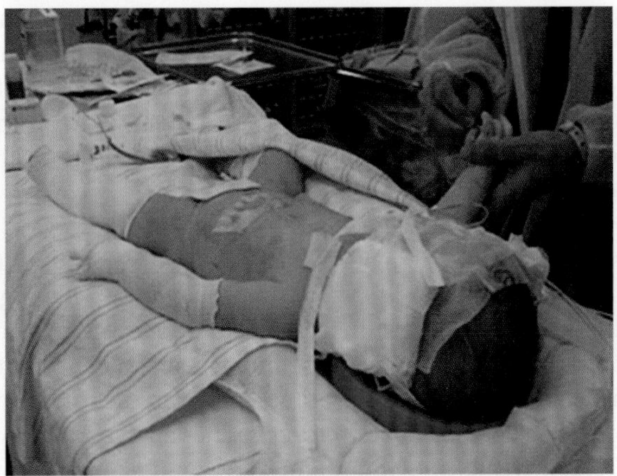

FIGURE 12-16. Placement of child with EB in OR. Warming blanket covered with soft blanket that is placed directly beneath the child, the head is cushioned, and extremity dressings remain in place.

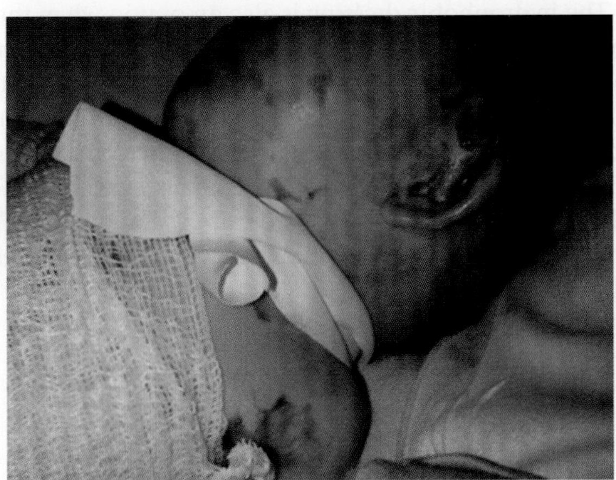

FIGURE 12-17. Placement of child with EB post-op. Dressings are secured over open lesions; moisture wicking fabric is in skin folds; the child is resting on fluidized air positioner covered with soft cloth.

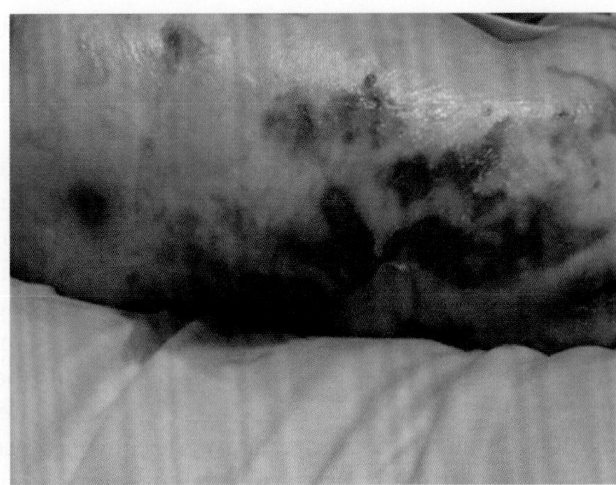

FIGURE 12-18. A child with EB: open blisters on the lower back.

Reperfusion Injury

Reperfusion injury is seen after periods of extreme ischemia. Irreversible tissue damage can occur within 3 hours of extreme ischemia (Blaisdell, 2002); the thrombotic and inflammatory responses associated with reperfusion injury begin after the ischemia has been corrected. The tissue damage associated with reperfusion injury may be uniform (as if a tourniquet was applied) or may be patchy (Blaisdell, 2002). The injury often involves the tips of the ears, fingers, nose, or toes. The extent of reperfusion injury will depend on the duration of the ischemia and level of damage to collateral vessels (Blaisdell, 2002). Once the blood flow and blood pressure are normalized and stabilized, the reperfusion injury becomes evident. Reperfusion injury is a complicated pathologic process with the potential for devastating consequences including amputation. Smaller areas of ischemic damage may be managed with advanced wound care (Mohr et al., 2014).

Wound Care for the Pediatric Population

Pediatric wound care is based on the principles of wound care and topical therapy addressed in previous chapters in this text, with modifications based on issues related to child development. Families and caregivers providing or assisting with wound care must be involved in the plan of care to promote family-centered care and compliance. Families and caregivers need to be encouraged to practice the wound care and dressing change with the support of clinicians as often as possible while in the acute care setting. Topical therapy should be simplified as much as possible, nonthreatening to the child, and supportive of concerns related to body image.

Dressing Selection

Low-profile dressings that do not interfere with the normal activities of the child are excellent choices. For example, a dressing should, whenever possible, allow older infants to explore their hands and feet and should support crawling and learning to stand. Likewise, the dressing for a toddler should allow play activities. The older child should be encouraged to discuss what they want from a dressing. Topical therapy should always be designed to minimize pain and discomfort; key strategies include use of dressings with gentle adhesives, such as silicone, and advanced wound dressings that reduce dressing change frequency. Options for advanced dressings that do not require daily dressing changes include foam dressings, silver-impregnated dressings, calcium alginate dressings (plain, silver impregnated, or impregnated with leptospermum honey), Hydrofiber dressings (plain or silver impregnated), glycerine-based gel dressings, and silicone-based contact layer dressings. Using appropriate primary and secondary dressings can reduce dressing changes to every few days or weekly.

Advanced dressings should be considered as first-line dressings in pediatrics in order to promote healing while minimizing pain and trauma. One of the newer dressings of particular benefit in the pediatric setting is leptospermum honey–based dressings. The leptospermum honey increases the osmotic pressure in the wound bed, thus providing a moist surface that also promotes autolysis (Weissenstein et al., 2014). Creating a chart for dressing selection that includes a picture of the product, indications for use, directions for use, and special considerations can assure appropriate selection and utilization of dressings by staff throughout the agency (Fig. 12-19).

Negative Pressure Wound Therapy

NPWT is an "active wound therapy" that is commonly recommended for nonhealing wounds, and pediatric wound care nurses are frequently asked about safety of use in this population (Rentea et al., 2013). Small studies have demonstrated safe use in children >1 year of age, and a larger retrospective study demonstrated safe use in 290 pediatric cases (Rentea et al., 2013). However, there are increasing data that support the use of NPWT in infants younger than 1 year of age. Stoffan et al. (2012) reported safe use of NPWT in neonates and infants; they reviewed cases over a 10-year period of time in which NPWT was used in infants. Most authors recommend beginning NPWT at low levels of pressure for small infants (e.g., –50 to –75 mm Hg) and gradually increasing for older infants and toddlers (Rentea et al., 2013; Stoffan et al., 2012). Anecdotally, pediatric surgeons have reported good outcomes when the pressure was kept close to the child's mean arterial pressure; pressure limits of –50 to –75 mm Hg are recommended for hemodynamically unstable children. For all children, the NPWT should be managed by an interdisciplinary team, which should include (at a minimum) members from the surgical service, the wound care nurse, and child life therapy. Principles underlying effective use of NPWT in the pediatric population are essentially the same as those for adults, with a few additional considerations related to pain management.

CLINICAL PEARL

NPWT can be safely used in neonatal and pediatric populations with modifications and careful monitoring.

To reduce trauma, bleeding, and pain during dressing changes, the wound nurse should implement measures to prevent tissue adherence and growth into the wound vacuum sponge. Use of a contact layer between the wound bed and the sponge is a simple and effective way to prevent adherence and ingrowth; options for contact layer include a silicone fenestrated dressing, emollient-impregnated dressing, and ionic silver fenestrated dressing. Use of a contact layer also minimizes the effort required to remove the sponge from the wound bed and reduces the overall dressing change time.

Measures to prevent sponge adherence to organs is also an essential element of care when NPWT is used for wounds with exposed organs in the wound bed; organ adherence could result in organ perforation, fistula formation, or massive bleeding with sponge removal. The hydrophobic white sponge can be used in conjunction with a contact layer to effectively prevent adherence and ingrowth of organ tissue into the foam. The wound nurse should collaborate with clinical nurse specialist and physician groups to educate all involved staff regarding safe use of NPWT in the pediatric population and should also assure that policies and procedures regarding NPWT are current and evidence based.

The hydrophobic dressing is also an option when there is uneven healing and differing rates of granulation within the wound bed. Areas of more exuberant granulation tissue can be covered with the hydrophobic dressing to provide slower granulation, and the areas where granulation is less active can be covered with a contact layer and open cell reticulated (black) foam to optimize granulation. The wound care nurse should assess the wound at each dressing change; when the rate of granulation throughout the

<table>
<tr><td>Medi-Honey 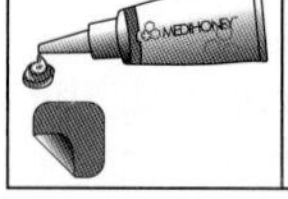</td><td>Made from Active Leptospermum Honey in New Zealand. Packaged in Canada. Created by Derma Science. Balances the wound bed pH, brings moisture to the wound bed, and creates an antimicrobial environment.</td><td>Used for deep and shallow wounds. Can be used in draining wounds with the alginate format. Tube format can be used to coat a wound or a filler dressing.</td><td>Can be left in place up to 3 days or longer depending on the dressing.</td><td>Available as an all in one dressing or a primary dressing which needs a cover.</td><td>No known contraindications</td><td>Debrides wounds while healing which minimizes open wound bed time. Improves wound healing times. Consult WOCN</td></tr>
</table>

FIGURE 12-19. Example of product reference guide for staff; can be incorporated into wound care policies and procedures.

wound bed is comparable, the entire wound can be managed with a contact layer and reticulated foam.

Another measure to reduce pain associated with NPWT is to utilize the continuous setting as opposed to intermittent setting on the vacuum pump. When the pump is in intermittent mode, the cyclical contraction and relaxation of the foam is likely to be perceived as pain. Use of the continuous setting reduces the need for pain medication during therapy; typically, analgesics can be limited to premedication just prior to dressing changes. For younger children and children with very difficult and painful wounds, it may be necessary to do the NPWT dressing changes in an ambulatory procedure unit with sedation managed by anesthesiology.

The time frame for NPWT ranges from 1 week to several weeks, depending on the size and location of the wound. If therapy is prolonged for more than 2 weeks, the plan of care should be discussed with the child and family to ensure minimal disruption of school and related activities.

All caregivers should be taught to carefully monitor the drainage collected in the NPWT canister. The volume of drainage will vary based on the wound type and stage of healing; there is normally a progressive reduction in the volume of drainage as the wound progresses. If the volume of drainage suddenly increases (or remains unexpectedly high), further evaluation is needed to rule out any complications; surgical evaluation may be needed. Any sanguineous drainage (or a change from serous to sanguineous drainage) should be monitored closely; sanguineous drainage exceeding 5% of the child's blood volume should be explored immediately (Rentea et al., 2013). (There have been anecdotal reports of vascular anomalies or vessels bleeding into the dressing requiring blood transfusions.) The amount of sanguineous drainage should be discussed with the collaborating surgical service and documented.

A sudden increase in volume of drainage accompanied by a change in drainage color must be evaluated to ensure no fistulas have developed between the wound bed and underlying organs or the lymphatic system. Pale yellow thin exudate usually requires radiologic evaluation to ensure that no communication has developed between the lymphatic system or the bladder depending on the location of the NPWT. There is a higher risk of fistula development when NPWT is used inappropriately and/or with poor technique.

In summary, NPWT is a valuable adjunctive therapy in wound management but must be utilized appropriately and cautiously to prevent complications The pediatric wound care nurse should provide support to the surgical service and nursing staff in decision making regarding indications and contraindications to use, appropriate settings, and use of appropriate contact layers. In addition, the wound care nurse must establish appropriate policies and procedures and must educate all caregivers regarding problem solving and monitoring of patients receiving NPWT.

Biologic Dressings

Biologic dressings have a role in pediatric wound care and should be considered as an option for challenging wounds or simple wounds in patients with complicated systemic disease processes.

The role of the pediatric wound care practitioner includes recommendations for use of biologic dressings in situations where there is delayed healing, assuring that the wound bed is ready for a biologic dressing, and critically reviewing all systemic factors to assure that there are no known impediments to healing.

Prevention of Skin Breakdown

A key responsibility of the pediatric wound care nurse is maintenance of skin integrity for children. All products used in skin and wound care should be approved for use in children. Silicone- or gel-based adhesive products should be the gold standard in pediatric care to minimize skin trauma and pain from adhesives. Any medical devices should be used with caution to minimize the risk of skin damage; specifically, thin adhesive foam or hydrocolloid dressings should be used under the device to provide padding, and the adhesive in direct contact with the skin should be skin friendly (e.g., silicone or gel based). In situations in which use of a protective dressing is not feasible, the device should be routinely repositioned every 8 hours and skin integrity should be assessed every 4 hours. All dressing and adhesive products should be removed with adhesive remover that is silicone based to promote skin integrity and reduce the risk of adhesive trauma.

All support surfaces in a pediatric care setting should provide even pressure redistribution; surfaces may be foam based, gel based, or air based. Positioners should be utilized for off-loading and to support natural alignment. Techniques to protect and float at risk areas (e.g., ears, elbows, heels, and occiput) include creation of wells in fluidized positioners or strategic placement of off-loading cushions.

The pediatric wound care practitioner should collaborate with staff and leadership in his or her agency to ensure best practices for pressure ulcer prevention. An important aspect of pressure ulcer prevention is prompt identification of at-risk patients through routine use of a pressure ulcer risk assessment tool. Currently, there are three validated tools for assessing pressure ulcer risk in the pediatric population (Anthony et al., 2010): Braden Q, Garvin, and Glamorgan. The most widely used tool for children aged 1 to 21 years is the Braden Q (Noonan et al., 2011). Any child determined to be at risk should be immediately placed on a prevention protocol that includes appropriate support surfaces and repositioning devices as well as routine turning and positioning. Most pediatric hospitals participate in initiatives to collect data on outcomes and risk assessments, which allow each agency to compare their outcomes with comparable facilities; use of a validated risk assessment tool is a criterion for participation in these national initiatives (CALNOC, 2014).

Key responsibilities of the wound care nurse in pressure ulcer prevention include maintenance of current evidence-based protocols for risk assessment and prevention; collaboration with purchasing and value analysis committee to assure appropriate support surfaces, positioners, and skin care products; collaboration with clinical nurse educators and staff to keep staff current in risk assessment and pressure ulcer prevention; and implementation of programs to educate and engage parents in pressure ulcer prevention.

Conclusion

The pediatric wound care nurse plays a critical role in skin protection and wound care for the neonatal and pediatric population. Major responsibilities include selection of products shown to be safe and effective in this population; protocol development and staff education regarding prevention of pressure ulcers, medical device–related injuries, skin tears, and extravasation injuries; and individualized wound care that is both evidence based and family oriented.

REFERENCES

Adam, R. (2008). Skin care of the diaper area. *Pediatric Dermatology, 25*(4), 427–433.

Agren, J., Sjors, G., & Sedin G. (1998). Transepidermal water loss in infants born at 24 and 25 weeks of estation. *Acta Paediatrica, 87*, 1185–1190.

Amjad, I., Murphy, T., Nylander-Housholder, L., et al. (2011). A new approach to management of intravenous infiltration in pediatric patients: Pathophysiology, classification, and treatment. *Journal of Infusion Nursing, 34*,242–249.

Andersen, C., Hart, J., Vemgal, P., et al. (2005). Prospective evaluation of a multi-factorial strategy on the impact of nosocomial infection in very low birth weight infants. *Journal of Hospital Infection, 61*, 162–167.

Anthony, D., Willock, J., & Baharestani, M. (2010). A comparison of Braden Q, Garvin and Glamorgan risk assessment scales in paediatrics. *Journal of Tissue Viability, 19*(3), 98–105.

Association of Women's Health, Obstetric and Neonatal Nurses. (2013). *Evidence-based clinical practice guideline: Neonatal skin care* (3rd ed.). Washington, DC: Association of Women's Health, Obstetric and Neonatal Nurses.

Beaulieu, M. J. (2012). Hyaluronidase for extravasation management. *Neonatal Network, 31*(6), 413–418.

Beeram, M., Olvera, R., Krauss, D., et al. (2006). Effects of topical emollient therapy on infants at or less than 27 weeks' gestation. *Journal of the National Medical Association, 98*(2), 261–264.

Behrendt, H., & Green, M. 1971. *Patterns of skin pH from birth through adolescence*. Springfield, IL: Charles C Thomas.

Bhandari, V., Brodsky, N., & Porat, R. (2005). Improved outcome of extremely low birth weight infants with tegaderm application to skin. *Journal of Perinatology, 25*, 276–281.

Bhatia, J. (2006). Fluid and electrolyte management in the very low birth weight neonate. *Journal of Perinatology, 26*(Suppl 1), S19–S21.

Bissinger, R., & Annibale, D. (2010). Thermoregulation in very low birth weight infants during the golden hour: Results and implications. *Advances in Neonatal Care, 10*, 230–238.

Black, P. (2007). Peristomal skin care: An overview of available products. *British Journal of Nursing, 16*(17), 1048, 1050, 1052–1054 passim.

Blaisdell, F. W. (2002). The pathophysiology of skeletal muscle ischemia and the reperfusion syndrome: A review. *Vascular, 10*(6), 620–630.

Brandon, D. H., Coe, K., Hudson-Barr, D., et al. (2010). Effectiveness of no-sting skin protectant and Aquaphor on water loss and skin integrity in premature infants. *Journal of Perinatology, 30*(6), 414–419.

Brindle, C. T., & Blankenship, J. (2009). Management of complex abdominal wounds with small bowel isolation technique and exudate control to improve outcomes. *Journal of Wound Ostomy Continence Nursing, 36*(4), 396–403.

CALNOC. (2014). Overview of CALNOC. http://www.calnoc.org/

Casanova, D., Bardot, J., & Magalon, G. (2001). Emergency treatment of accidental infusion leakage in the newborn: Report of 14 cases. *British Journal of Plastic Surgery, 54*, 396–399.

Chaiyakunapruk, N., Veenstra D. L., Lipsky, B. A., et al. (2002). Chlorhexidine compared with povidone-iodine solution for vascular catheter-site care: A meta-analysis. *Annals of Internal Medicine, 136*, 792–801.

Chandavasu, O., Garrow, E., Valsa, V., et al. (1986). A new method for the prevention of skin sloughs and necrosis secondary to intravenous infiltration. *American Journal of Perinatology, 3*, 4–5.

Cutlar, L., Greiser, U., & Wang, W. (2014). Gene therapy: Pursuing restoration of dermal adhesion in recessive dystrophic epidermolysis bullosa. *Experimental Dermatology, 23*(1), 1–6.

Da Cunha, M. L., Procianoy, R. S., Franceschini, D. T., et al. (2008). Effect of the first bath with chlorhexidine on skin colonization with Staphylococcus aureus in normal healthy term newborns. *Scandinavian Journal of Infectious Diseases, 40*(8), 615–620.

Davies, J., Gault, D., & Buchdahl, R. (1994). Preventing the scars of neonatal intensive care. *Archives of Disease in Childhood - Fetal and Neonatal Edition, 70*, F50–F51.

Debra: The Dystrophic Epidermolysis Eullosa Research and Association of America. 2014. http://www.debra.org/

Dollison, E., & Beckstrand, J. (1995). Adhesive tape vs. pectin-based barrier use in preterm infants. *Neonatal Network, 14*, 35–39.

Dykes, P. J., Heggie, R., & Hill, S. A. (2001). Effects of adhesive dressings on the stratum corneum of the skin. *Journal of Wound Care, 10*, 7–10.

Edwards, W., Conner, J., & Soll, R. (2004). The effect of prophylactic ointment therapy on nosocomial sepsis rates and skin integrity in infants of birth weights 501–1000 grams. *Pediatrics, 113*, 1195–1203.

Fox, C., Nelson, O., & Wareham, J. (1998). The timing of skin acidification in very low birth weight infants. *Journal of Perinatology, 18*(4), 272–275.

Fridkin, S. K., & Jarvis, W. R. (1996). Epidemiology of nosocomial fungal infections. *Clinical Microbiology Reviews, 9*(4), 499–511.

Garland, J., Buck, R., & Maloney, P. (1995). Comparison of 10% povidone-iodine and 0.5% chlorhexidine gluconate for the prevention of peripheral intravenous catheter colonization in neonates: A prospective trial. *Pediatric Infectious Disease Journal, 14*, 510–516.

Gaylord, M., Wright, K., Lorch, K., et al. (2001). Improved fluid management utilizing humidified incubators in extremely low birth weight infants. *Journal of Perinatology, 21*, 438–443.

Gfatter, R., Hack, P., & Braun, F. (1997). Effects of soap and detergents on skin surface pH, stratum corneum hydration and fat content in infants. *Dermatology, 195*, 258–262.

Ghnnam W. M., & Hafez, D. M. (2011). Laser hair removal as adjunct to surgery for pilonidal sinus: Our initial experience. *Journal of Cutaneous and Aesthetic Surgery, 4* (3), 192.

Gotschall, C. S., Morrison, M., & Eichelberger, M. (1998). Prospective, randomized study of the efficacy of Mepitel on children with partial-thickness scalds. *Journal of Burn Care and Rehabilitation, 19*, 279–283.

Gray, M. (2007). Incontinence-related skin damage: Essential knowledge. *Ostomy and Wound Management, 53*, 28–32.

Harpin, V., & Rutter, N. (1982). Percutaneous alcohol absorption and skin necrosis in a preterm infant. *Archives of Disease in Childhood, 57*, 825.

Heimall, L. M., Storey, B., Stellar, J. J., et al. (2012). Beginning at the bottom: Evidence-based care of diaper dermatitis. *MCN. The American Journal of Maternal Child Nursing, 37*(1), 10–16.

Hoath, S., & Narendran, V. (2000). Adhesives and emollients in the preterm infant. *Seminars in Neonatology, 5*, 112–119.

Hoath, S., & Pickins, W. L. (2003). The biology and role of vernix. In S. Hoath. & H. Maibach (Eds.), *Neonatal skin: Structure and function* (2nd ed.). New York, NY: Marcel Dekker Inc.

Holbrook, K. A. (1982). A histological comparison of infant and adult skin. In H. I. Maibach & E. K. Boisits (Eds.), *Neonatal skin: Structure and function*. New York, NY: Marcel Dekker, Inc.

Irving, V. (2001). Reducing the risk of epidermal stripping in the neonatal population: An evaluation of an alcohol free barrier film. *Journal of Neonatal Nursing, 7*, 5–8.

Ittmann, P., & Bozynski, M. (1993). Toxic epidermal necrolysis in a newborn infant after exposure to adhesive removal. *Journal of Perinatology, 13*(6), 476–477.

Janmohamed, S. R., Oranje, A. P., Devillers, A. C., et al. (2014). The proactive wet-wrap method with diluted corticosteroids versus emollients in children with atopic dermatitis: A prospective, randomized, double-blind, placebo-controlled trial. *Journal of the American Academy of Dermatology, 70*(6), 1076–1082.

Kalia, Y., Nonato, L., Lund, C., et al. (1998). Development of the skin barrier function in premature infants. *Journal of Investigative Dermatology, 111*, 320–326.

Kim, S., Lee, E., Chen, J., et al. (2010). Improved care and growth outcomes by using humidified hybrid incubators in very preterm infants. *Pediatrics, 125*(1), e137–e145.

Knobel, R., Simmer, J., & Holbert, D. (2005). Heat loss prevention for preterm infants in the delivery room. *Journal of Perinatology, 25*, 304–308.

Kosemund, K., Schlatter, H., Ochsenhirt, J., et al. (2009). Safety evaluation of superabsorbent baby diapers. *Regulatory Toxicology and Pharmacology, 53*(2), 81–89.

Kutsch, J., & Ottinger, D. (2014). Neonatal skin and chlorhexidine: A burning experience. *Neonatal Network, 33*, 19–23.

Larson, A. A., & Dinulos, J. G. (2005). Cutaneous bacterial infections in the newborn. *Current Opinion in Pediatrics, 17*, 481–485.

Lin, R., Tinkle, L., & Janniger, C. (2005). Skin care of the healthy newborn. *Cutis, 75*, 25–30.

Linder, N., Davidovich, N., Reichman, B., et al. (1997). Topical iodine-containing antiseptics and subclinical hypothyroidism in preterm infants. *Journal of Pediatrics, 131*, 434–439.

Linder, N., Prince, S., Barzilai, A., et al. (2004). Disinfection with 10% povidone-iodine versus 0.5% chlorhexidine gloconate in 70% isopropanol in the neonatal intensive care unit. *Acta Paediatrica, 93*, 205–210.

Lund, C., Nonato, L., Kuller, J., et al. (1997). Disruption of barrier function in neonatal skin associated with adhesive removal. *Journal of Pediatrics, 131*, 367–372.

Lund, C. H., & Osborne, J. W. (2004). Validity and reliability of the neonatal skin condition score. *Journal of Obstetric, Gynecologic, and Neonatal Nursing, 33*, 320–327.

Lund, C., Osborne, J., Kuller, J., et al. (2001). Neonatal skin care: Clinical outcomes of the AWHONN/NANN evidence-based clinical practice guideline. *Journal of Obstetric, Gynecologic, and Neonatal Nursing, 30*, 41–51.

Lund, C, & Tucker, J. (2003). Adhesion and newborn skin. In S. B. Hoath & H. I. Maibach (Eds.), *Neonatal skin: Structure and function* (2nd ed., pp. 299–324). New York, NY: Marcel Dekker.

Mancini, A. (2004). Skin. *Pediatrics, 113*(4 Suppl), 1114–1119.

Mancini, A., Sookdeo-Drost, S., Madison, K., et al. (1994). Semipermeable dressings improve epidermal barrier function in premature infants. *Pediatric Research, 36*, 306–314.

Mannan, K., Chow, P., Lissauer, T., et al. (2007). Mistaken identity of skin cleansing solution leading to extensive chemical burns in an extremely preterm infant. *Acta Paediatrica, 96*(10), 1536–1537.

McNichol, L., Lund, C., Rosen, T., et al. (2013). Medical adhesives and patient safety: State of the science. *Journal of Wound, Ostomy and Continence Nursing, 40*, 365–380.

Milstone, A. M., Elward, A., Song, X., et al. (2013). Daily chlorhexidine bathing to reduce bacteraemia in critically ill children: A multicenter, cluster-randomised, crossover trial. *Lancet, 381*, 1099–1106.

Mohr, L. D., Reyna, R., & Amaya, R. (2014). Neonatal case studies using active leptospermum honey. *Journal of Wound Ostomy and Continence Nursing, 41*(3), 213–218.

National Presssure Ulcer Advisory Panel, European Pressure Ulcer Advisory Panel, and Pan Pacific Pressure Injury Alliance. (2014). In E. Haesler (Ed.), *Prevention and treatment of pressure ulcers: Clinical practice guideline*. Perth, Australia: Cambridge Media.

Nick, O., Anthony, M., Adam, B., et al. (2010). Therapeutic improvement of scarring: Mechanisms of scarless and scar-forming healing and approaches to the discovery of new treatments. *Dermatology Research and Practice.* doi: 10.1155/2010/405262

Nield, L., & Kamat, D. (2007). Prevention, diagnosis, and management of diaper dermatitits. *Clinical Pediatrics, 46*, 480–486.

Nikolovski, J., Stamatas, G. N., Kollias, N., et al. (2008). Barrier function and water-holding and transport properties of infant stratum corneum are different from adult and continue to develop through the first year of life. *Journal of Investigative Dermatology, 128*, 1728–1736.

Noonan, C., Quigley, S., & Curley, M. A. (2011). Using the Braden Q Scale to predict pressure ulcer risk in pediatric patients. *Journal of Pediatric Nursing, 26*(6), 566–575.

Parravicini, E., Fontana, C., Paterlini, G., et al. (1996). Iodine, thyroid function, and very low birth weight infants. *Pediatrics, 98*, 730–734.

Rai, P., Lee, B., Liu, T., et al. (2009). Safety evaluation of disposable baby diapers using principles of quantitative risk assessment. *Journal of Toxicology and Environmental Health, Part A, 72*, 1262–1271.

Rentea, R. M., Somers, K. K., Cassidy, L., et al. (2013). Negative pressure wound therapy in infants and children: A single-institution experience. *Journal of Surgical Research, 184*(1), 658–664.

Reynolds, P. R., Banerjee, S., Meek, J. H. (2005). Alcohol burns in extremely low birthweight infants: Still occurring. *Archives of Disease in Childhood - Fetal and Neonatal Edition, 90*, F10.

Sankar, M. J., Paul, V. K., Kapil, A., et al. (2009). Does skin cleansing with chlorhexidine affect skin condition, temperature and colonization in hospitalized preterm low birth weight infants? A randomized clinical trial. *Journal of Perinatology, 29*, 795–801.

Sardesai, S. R., Kornacka, M. K., Walas, W., et al. (2011). Iatrogenic skin injury in the neonatal intensive care unit. *The Journal of Maternal-Fetal & Neonatal Medicine, 24*(2), 197–203.

Sawatzky-Dicksson, D., & Bodnaryk, K. (2006). Neonatal intravenous extravasation injuries: Evaluation of a wound care protocol. *Neonatal Network, 25*, 13–19.

Scheinfeld, N. (2005). Diaper dermatitits. A review and brief survey of eruptions of the diaper area. *Journal of Clinical Dermatology, 6*, 273–281.

Schick, J. B., & Milstein, J. M. (1981). Burn hazard of isopropyl alcohol in the neonate. *Pediatrics, 68*, 587–588.

Sedin, G., Hammarlund, K., Nilsson, G., et al. (1985). Measurements of transepidermal water loss in newborn infants. *Clinics in Perinatology, 12*, 79–99.

Siegfried, E. (2008). Neonatal slin care and toxicology (chapter 5). In L. Eichenfield., I. Frieden., & N. Esterly (Eds.), *Textbook of neonatal dermatology*. Philadelphia, PA: W. B. Saunders Co.

Simona, R. (2012). A pediatric peripheral intravenous infiltration assessment tool. *Journal of Infusion Nursing, 35*, 243–248.

Smerdely, P., Lim, A., Boyages, S., et al. (1989). Topical iodine-containing antiseptics and neonatal hypothyroidism in very-low-birth weight infants. *Lancet, 16*, 661–664.

Stamatas, G. N., Nikolovski, J., Mack, M., et al. (2011). Infant skin physiology and development during the first years of life: A review of recent findings based on in vivo studies. *International Journal of Cosmetic Science, 33*(1), 17–24.

Stephen-Haynes, J. (2008). Skin integrity and silicone: Appeel "no-sting" medical adhesive remover. *British Journal of Nursing, 17*(12), 792–795.

Stoffan, A. P., Ricca, R., Lien, C., et al. (2012). Use of negative pressure wound therapy for abdominal wounds in neonates and infants. *Journal of Pediatric Surgery, 47*(8), 1555-1559.

Thigpen, J. (2007). Peripheral intravenous extravasation: Nursing procedure for initial treatment. *Neonatal Network, 26*, 379–384.

Thompson, K. L., Leu, M. G., Drummond, K. L., et al. (2014). Nutrition interventions to optimize pediatric wound healing an evidence-based clinical pathway. *Nutrition in Clinical Practice, 29*, 473.

United States Food & Drug Administration. (2012). *2% chlorhexidine gluconate (CHG); Safety labeling changes approved by FDA Center for Drug Evaluation and Research (CDER)*. Silver Spring, MD: FDA.

Vandeputte, P., Ferrari, S., & Coste, T. (2012). Antifungal resistance and new strategies to control fungal infections. *International Journal of Microbiology*, (12). doi: 10.1155/2012/71368

Visscher, M. O., Chatterjee, R., Ebel, J., et al. (2002). Biomedical assessment and instrumental evaluation of healthy infant skin. *Pediatric Dermatology, 19*, 473–482.

Visscher, M. O., Chatterjee, R., Munson, K. A., et al. (2000). Changes in diapered and nondiapered infant skin over the first month of life. *Pediatric Dermatology, 17*, 45–51.

Visscher, M. O., Utturkar, R., Pickens, W. L., et al. (2011). Neonatal skin maturation—vernix caseosa and free amino acids. *Pediatric Dermatology, 28*, 122–132.

Visser, W. I. (2014). Non-pharmacological management of atopic dermatitis, including emollients. *Current Allergy and Clinical Immunology, 27*(2), 88.

Vohra, S., Roberts, R.S., Zhang, B., et al. (2004). Heat loss prevention in the delivery room: A randomized controlled trial of polyethylene occlusive skin wrapping in very preterm infants. *Journal of Pediatrics, 145*(6), 750–753.

Weissenstein, A., Luchter, E., & Bittmann, S. (2014). Medical honey and its role in paediatric patients. *British Journal of Nursing, 23*(6 Suppl), S30–S34.

Yosipovitch, G., Maayan-Metzger, A., Merlob, P. P., et al. (2000). Skin barrier properties in different body areas in neonates. *Pediatrics 106*, 105, 2000.

QUESTIONS

1. The wound care nurse must pay special attention to the skin of a neonate. What is a characteristic of a newborn's skin that makes it more fragile?
- A. For the first year, the stratum corneum does not function as well as adult skin.
- B. The basement layer of the epidermis has not yet formed.
- C. The keratinocytes in the basal layer have a slower turnover rate.
- D. The dermis of the neonate is thicker than that of the adult.

2. Neonates in the NICU are at greatest risk for pressure ulcer development related to:
- A. Shear forces
- B. Device-related pressure
- C. Adhesive-related wounds
- D. Ischemic pressure

3. The wound care nurse is managing the care of neonates in an NICU. Which intervention is a recommended prevention/treatment measure for this population?
- A. Neonates in the NICU should be bathed with a chlorhexidine gluconate product daily.
- B. Silicone-based adhesive removers should be used for neonates with extremely fragile skin.
- C. IV devices should be secured with transparent dressings or plastic tape and observed with documentation every 3 hours.
- D. If extravasation occurs at an IV line, the device should be removed and a cold compress should be applied to the area.

4. The wound nurse is caring for a neonate whose IV fluid has extravasated into the surrounding tissue. The nurse administered hyaluronidase shortly after the extravasation was identified. Which step of this procedure was performed correctly?
- A. The nurse administers hyaluronidase via an intradermal injection.
- B. The nurse injects hyaluronidase directly into the venipuncture site.
- C. Ideally, the nurse administers hyaluronidase within 24 hours of extravasation.
- D. The nurse administers 15 units of hyaluronidase diluted to 1 mL.

5. The wound care nurse is teaching the parents of a neonate how to prevent and treat diaper rash. What teaching point is a recommended intervention?
- A. Avoid using topical treatments containing zinc oxide and petrolatum.
- B. Once denudation occurs, keep the skin open to air.
- C. Do not remove skin barrier ointment completely with each diaper change.
- D. Use baby powder on damaged skin to keep the area moisture free.

6. In which age group would the wound care nurse be most likely to document a pilonidal cyst?
- A. Neonates
- B. Toddlers
- C. School-age children
- D. Adolescents

7. The wound care nurse is caring for an adolescent with atopic dermatitis. What should be the emphasis of education for this patient?
A. Skin hygiene and use of emollients
B. Exfoliating hair from the area
C. Frequent dressing changes
D. Nutritional counseling

8. The wound care nurse is planning care for patients on a pediatric unit. Which intervention does NOT follow recommended guidelines for pediatric wound care?
A. Using low-profile dressings to protect skin from childhood activities
B. Using dressings that require daily dressing changes whenever possible
C. Using advanced dressings as first-line dressings
D. Involving caregivers assisting or providing wound care in plan of care

9. The wound care nurse is recommending a dressing for a pediatric patient whose pressure ulcer is healing unevenly with differing rates of granulation within the wound bed. What type of dressing used in conjunction with negative pressure wound therapy (NPWT) would be the best choice for this patient?
A. Hydrophobic dressing
B. Silicon fenestrated dressing
C. Emollient-impregnated dressing
D. Ionic silver fenestrated dressing

10. A key responsibility of the pediatric wound care nurse is to maintain skin integrity for children. What intervention is recommended to prevent skin breakdown for this population?
A. Using aggressive adhesive products to reduce dressing change frequency
B. Placing thin adhesive foam under any medical devices used
C. Removing all adhesive products with alcohol-based adhesive remover
D. Using circular donut devices to off-load the occipital area

ANSWERS: 1.**A**, 2.**B**, 3.**B**, 4.**D**, 5.**C**, 6.**D**, 7.**A**, 8.**B**, 9.**A**, 10.**B**

CHAPTER 13

Skin and Wound Care for the Geriatric Population

Bonny Flemister

OBJECTIVES

1. Describe the anatomy and physiology of the skin and soft tissue, changes across the lifespan, and implications for management of skin health.
2. Describe skin conditions and lesions that are common among the elderly and implications for the skin and wound care nurse.
3. Discuss the role of the skin and wound care nurse in prevention and management of the following: delirium, elder abuse, malnutrition, and polypharmacy.

Topic Outline

Introduction

Longer lifespans and aging baby boomers will combine to double the population of Americans aged 65 years or older in the next 25 years (to about 72 million); by 2030, older adults will constitute about 20% of the U.S. population. As a result of our aging population, the leading causes of death have shifted over the last 100 years from acute illness and infection to degenerative illness and chronic conditions, many of which involve skin and wound conditions (Centers for Disease Control and Prevention, 2013).

CLINICAL PEARL

By 2030, older adults will constitute 20% of the U.S. population.

The older (senescent) individual is at risk for conditions other than those captured by medical diagnoses. The term "geriatric syndrome" is used to capture those clinical conditions in older persons that do not fit into discrete disease categories and cannot be treated with the traditional medical model. Geriatric conditions such as pressure ulcers, incontinence, polypharmacy, delirium, and malnutrition often fall outside the medical disease models that now govern much of health care. These conditions are within the scope of practice for the wound care nurse, and skin and wound care for the older individual must include assessment for and attention to these potential comorbid conditions (Inouye et al., 2007).

Age-Related Changes in Skin and Wound Healing

Skin is a renewable tissue, and normal function of proliferative cells (epithelial cells, fibroblasts, and endothelial cells) plays a vital role in maintenance of skin integrity throughout life (Fig. 13-1). Unfortunately, endogenous and exogenous changes associated with aging cause a reduction in the proliferative ability of these cells, with eventual progression to senescence.

Cellular Senescence

Senescence is a term used interchangeably with aging, and describes cells that remain viable but no longer continue the process of mitosis (reproduction). The hallmark of senescent cells is their inability to initiate DNA replication and subsequent cell division; they have lost the ability to progress through the cell cycle. Senescence is different than apoptosis, which signifies cell death programmed within the cell's DNA (cell self-destruction). One example of apoptosis is the normal cell cycle for keratinocytes, in which the migrating keratinocyte loses its DNA and becomes filled with keratin, and the mature keratinocyte is shed from the skin surface as new keratinocytes arrive to take its place. This normal apoptosis maintains the structural integrity and homeostatic function of the epidermis. Interestingly, extreme physiologic stress can cause premature senescence or apoptosis of normally proliferating cells. Research indicates that proliferating cells respond to extreme stress in one of three ways: (1) complete recovery with the ability to continue subsequent cell cycles, (2) senescence, or (3) apoptosis (Campisi & d'Adda di Fagagna, 2007).

CLINICAL PEARL

Senescence refers to cells that no longer have the ability to reproduce; apoptosis refers to programmed cell death.

Chronological aging results from the passage of time alone, and there are a number of changes in cell biology associated with aging. For example, clinical manifestations of aging are the result of cumulative cellular damage and mutations in cellular DNA, and it is well documented that DNA damage and mutations increase with age while the cells' capacity to repair such damage decreases every year. In addition, cells seem to have a genetically determined reproductive lifespan involving the number of telomeres. Telomeres are lengths of duplicate DNA pairs located at the end of chromosomes, and with each DNA replication, one base pair of telomeric DNA is lost. Over time, the loss of telomeres results in cellular senescence (the inability to reproduce) or in spontaneous cellular death (apoptosis).

Altered Fibroblast Function

Fibroblasts are critical to maintenance of normal dermal structure and to wound healing; thus, it is important to consider changes in fibroblast function associated with aging (Yaar, 2006). One change is progressive loss of fibroblasts and reduced proliferative capacity of the remaining fibroblasts, due in part to changes in telomeric DNA; even under normal conditions, fibroblasts lose 30% of telomere length during adulthood (Yaar, 2006). Allsopp and colleagues (1992) observed that telomere length predicts replicative capacity of human fibroblasts. Older-aged subjects had cell strains with shorter telomeres that underwent significantly fewer doublings than younger subjects' cells, which had longer telomeres and more ability to replicate. The study also showed that fibroblasts from Hutchinson-Gilford progeria subjects had short telomeres, consistent with reduced division potential. Some investigators speculate that gender-specific differences in longevity are at least in part due to hormonal regulation of telomere function (Emmerson & Hardman, 2012).

Aging results in reduced levels of signaling molecules (cytokines and chemokines) and in levels of receptors for these molecules. Specific changes include reduced expression and receptors for the interleukin-1 cytokine family, which affects immune function and the inflammatory

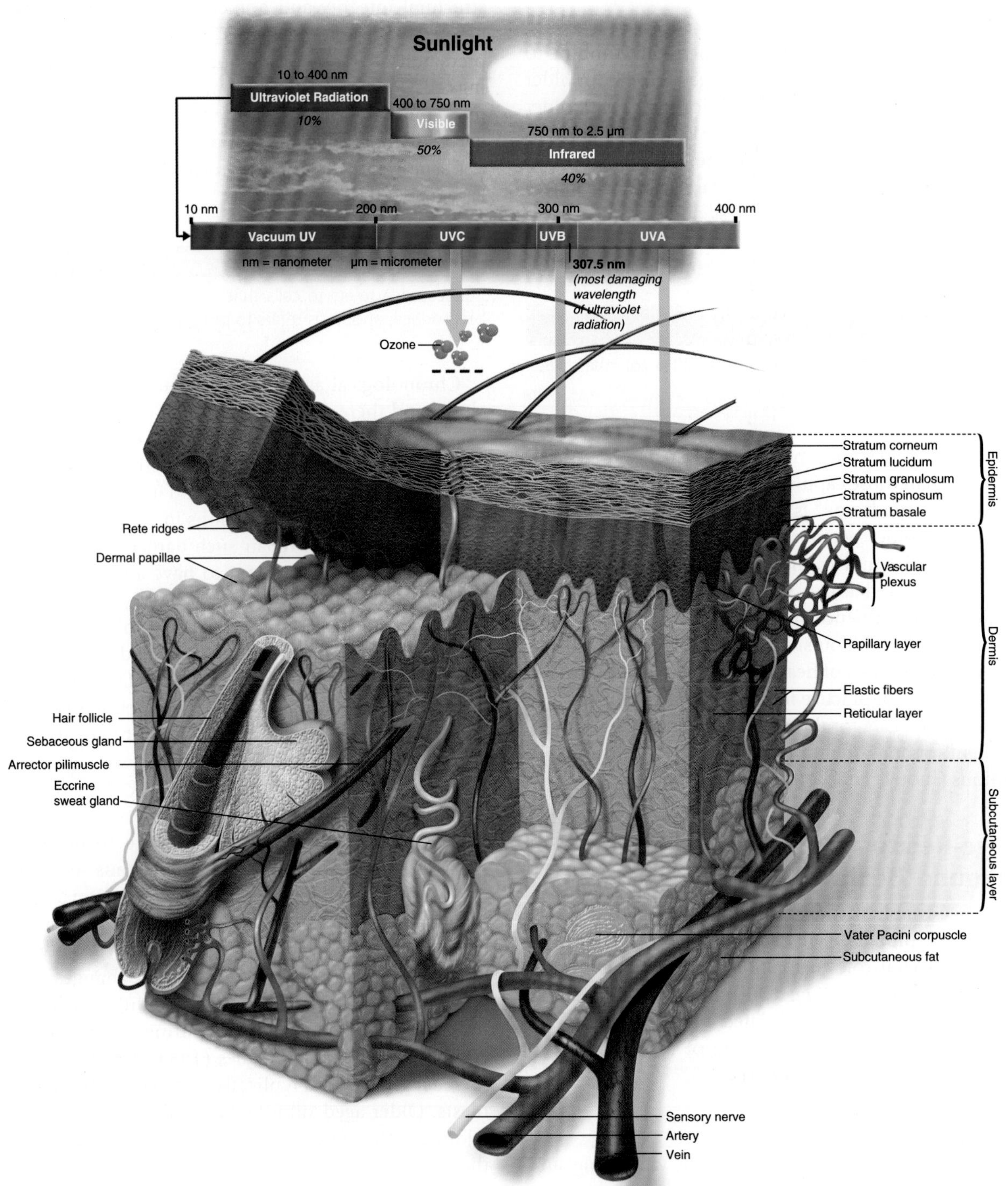

FIGURE 13-1. Skin cross section with UV rays labeled.

response, and reduced fibroblast receptors for growth factors and hormones, such as epidermal growth factor and platelet-derived growth factors (PDGFs) (Allsopp et al., 1992). These changes result in dermal atrophy and in prolongation of the time required for collagen synthesis and extracellular matrix production. Specific changes include progressive deterioration of dermal elastin and progressive disorganization and thinning of dermal collagen, resulting in diminished dermal strength and elasticity (Yaar, 2006).

CLINICAL PEARL

Changes in fibroblast function associated with aging result in dermal atrophy and in prolongation of the time required for collagen synthesis.

Reduced Inflammatory Response

There are also changes in the inflammatory phase of wound repair and in the body's ability to recognize and destroy pathogens and malignant cells. For example, cytokines and chemokines (such as the interleukin-1 family) are signaling and receptor molecules that initiate and control the inflammatory process, and aging is associated with declining levels of these molecules. In addition, autoimmune conditions are associated with reduced levels of cytokines, and these conditions are more common in the elderly. There is also decreased production of mast cells, and these cells are thought to act as sentinels for early infection and early recognition of pathogens. Furthermore, there is atrophy of the cutaneous vasculature, resulting in reduced perfusion even in healthy older adults. This compromises delivery of immune cells to the skin, which is important because the innate lymphoid cells and T cells that seed the tissue early in development cannot replicate in situ to maintain their numbers.

CLINICAL PEARL

The elderly are less able to mount an appropriate inflammatory response and thus are at risk for infection and delayed wound healing.

Altered Melanocyte Function

Finally, there is a change in the distribution and number of melanocytes (10% to 40% reduction in numbers per decade); the melanocytes may also deteriorate or lose the normal contact and interaction with epidermal cells. The most obvious impact is loss of normal pigmentation to the skin and hair ("age spots" and graying of the hair). This is significant because unprotected exposure to ultraviolet (UV) light can interfere with the Langerhans cells' ability to eradicate carcinogenic cells (Farage et al., 2008).

Reduced Vitamin D Production

Another change that may affect the individual's health is a decline in vitamin D production and vitamin D receptors.

Reduced Sensory Function

In addition to changes in the skin that render the individual more vulnerable to cutaneous infections and malignancies, there are changes in the skin's nervous system that adversely affect the person's ability to recognize and respond appropriately to warning signs of impending damage. For example, there is a 30% reduction in nerve receptors in the skin and there is also a reduction in production of neurotransmitters; this means that an elderly patient is less aware of pain, pressure, and exposure to heat and cold, even if he or she is alert and oriented. This is one reason the elderly are at increased risk for pressure ulcers, burns, and frostbite.

CLINICAL PEARL

The elderly have reduced sensory function, which means they may not sense impending damage from unrelieved pressure or thermal trauma, even if they are alert and oriented.

Thinning of Adipose Layer

While this discussion has focused on the layers and structures of the skin itself, it should be noted that the subcutaneous (adipose) tissue also undergoes changes with aging, most notably thinning and reduced perfusion.

In summary, the aging process is responsible for a number of changes in cellular DNA that influence cellular activity and the capacity for reproduction as well as the ability to "self-protect." These changes lead to deviant cellular responses that may adversely affect maintenance of normal skin and the ability to heal (Yaar, 2006). While it is the visible signs of aging that sometimes create the most concern, it is the underlying histological changes that are most likely to interfere with normal healing. This chapter addresses implications for skin and wound care in the older adult.

Impact of Ethnicity

Wound care nurses care for individuals of all ethnicities; thus, the wound care nurse needs to be knowledgeable regarding the impact of ethnicity on skin structure and function. The evident differences relate to the melanin cells and ceramides in the epidermis. While our understanding of ethnic skin differences remains incomplete, it is known that darkly pigmented skin retains a younger appearance with less visible signs of aging than lightly pigmented skin; this may be due to greater protection against photoaging afforded by the increased activity of skin melanocytes. (However, skin of all ethnicities is eventually affected by photoaging.) Darker skin demonstrates greater intercellular cohesion and higher ceramide levels, which helps to explain their lower incidence of skin tears. Considering that people of darker skin tones constitute most of the world's population, it is evident that we need more research into ethnic skin differences and the implications for skin care (Rawlings, 2006).

Impact of Estrogen

In recent years, there have been numerous studies on the influence of hormones such as estrogen on wound healing. Estrogen influences the function of all major organ systems within the body, and skin is the largest nonreproductive target due to estrogen receptors located in the skin. Current evidence indicates that estrogen levels have a significant effect on both skin health and normal repair.

Estrogen and Skin Health

The effects of estrogen on skin health are well known and documented by the effects of transdermal estrogen application: enhanced keratinocyte proliferation, resulting in thickening of the epidermis; increased production of skin lipids, which enhances the softness and the barrier function of the skin; improved skin hydration, due in part to increased lipid production; and increased skin elasticity (Archer, 2012; Gilliver et al., 2007; Hall & Phillips, 2005; Shu & Maibach, 2011). The increase in skin thickness and skin lipids seems to be of particular importance. Aging skin is characterized by a progressive decline in skin thickness, due primarily to atrophic changes affecting the dermis; these changes include a reduction in fibroblasts, which results in reduced production of dermal collagen, elastin, and proteoglycans (Archer, 2012). Collagen loss per postmenopausal year is estimated to be 2.1%, independent of a woman's age; this is accompanied by a 1.1% decline in skin thickness per postmenopausal year (Archer, 2012). The combined effects of skin aging and loss of estrogen can result in loss of as much as 30% of the dermal collagen in the first 5 years after menopause. Estrogen may reduce the rate of collagen loss, because estrogen has been shown to increase fibroblast proliferation and collagen production. In addition, estrogen can reduce the levels of tissue-degrading matrix metalloproteinases in the connective tissue (Shu & Maibach, 2011).

Skin oils have a major impact both on skin texture and softness and on the barrier function of the skin (because skin oils are responsible for "filling the gap" between skin cells to create an intact barrier that prevents water loss and also prevents penetration by irritants and pathogens) (Pappas, 2009). The production of these skin oils (e.g., sebum) declines after menopause; however, hormone replacement therapy (HRT) has been shown to increase production by 35% as compared to women not receiving HRT (Archer, 2012). Data from the first U.S. National Health and Nutrition Examination Survey (NHANES I), a large population-based cohort study, concluded that noncontraceptive estrogen use significantly reduced skin dryness (Dunn et al., 1997).

Estrogen in Wound Healing

Estrogen may also impact on wound healing. For example, estrogen may help to modulate the inflammatory response in open wounds. Recent studies have highlighted the role of a prolonged inflammatory response, up-regulated protease activity, and reduced matrix deposition in age-related impaired healing (Gilliver et al., 2007), and high neutrophil counts have been demonstrated in the wounds of elderly patients. However, estrogen has been shown to decrease neutrophil chemotaxis and adhesion, thereby reducing the inflammatory response and allowing for improved matrix formation (Ashcroft et al., 1999; Shu & Maibach, 2011). These findings are supported by in vivo human studies demonstrating that application of topical estrogen significantly reduced the number of neutrophils at the wound site, as compared with placebo treatment (Shu & Maibach, 2011).

CLINICAL PEARL

Estrogen is known to affect skin health and skin softness, and emerging evidence suggests that estrogen may also impact significantly on wound healing.

Estrogen may also enhance the processes involved in granulation tissue formation, such as neoangiogenesis and collagen synthesis. There is some evidence that estrogen has a direct effect on the endothelial cells responsible for new vessel formation (Gilliver et al., 2007). It is these newly formed vessels in the granulation tissue that transport the oxygen and nutrients required for healing (Shu & Maibach, 2011; Xin et al., 2009). Estrogen is also known to affect the proliferative phase of wound healing by influencing the cells critical to synthesis of new tissue, including fibroblasts and keratinocytes (Gilliver et al., 2007). In addition, estrogen stimulates the expression of PDGF by monocytes and macrophages, which contributes to the overall regulation of wound-healing processes (Gilliver et al., 2007). The potential positive effects of estrogen on wound healing are supported by results of a randomized double-blind study by Ashcroft et al. (1997) that showed improved wound healing in females treated with systemic estrogen, as well as a reduced incidence of chronic wounds in women receiving estrogen replacement therapy. Similarly, Margolis documented a 30% to 40% reduction in the incidence of venous or pressure ulcers among 44,195 randomly selected elderly women aged 65 to 95 years who received HRT (Margolis, 2002).

The role of estrogen in wound healing is complex and not fully understood, though current evidence supports its role in promotion of wound healing and prevention of chronic wounds. However, much of the evidence is controversial. In light of recent data regarding long-term use of estrogen supplementation, the risk-to-benefit ratio of this therapy needs to be carefully weighed (Hall & Phillips, 2005).

Impact of pH

For nearly 100 years, an "acid mantle" has been considered a characteristic of healthy skin; specifically, pH has been shown to be a key factor in maintenance of an intact barrier, the integrity and hydration of the stratum corneum (SC), and added protection against microbes (Ali & Yosipovitch, 2013).

The optimal skin pH is approximately 5.4, with a range of 4 to 6; in addition to being hostile to invading organisms, this pH level promotes the function of key enzymes that promote skin health and normal barrier function. The pH of the SC regulates at least three epidermal functions: antimicrobial resistance, normal permeability and resistance to penetration by irritant substances, and skin integrity and cohesion. Normally, this pH is maintained by the skin lipids and sweat produced by the sebaceous and sweat glands; in addition, the organisms normally found on the skin (e.g., *Staphylococcus epidermidis*) contribute to the acidic pH by breaking down the fatty acids (Ansari, 2014). This finding suggests that the normal resident bacteria contribute to skin health and to maintenance of an acidic pH, which has implications for routine skin care and for use of antimicrobial cleansers (Blaak et al., 2011).

Aging can adversely affect skin pH, thus adversely affecting skin health. This is due in part to reduced numbers and activity of the sebaceous and sweat glands, which results in reduced production of the skin lipids and sweat that help to maintain acidic pH.

It is well documented that skin pH rises with aging, beginning as early as age 50 and rising significantly by age 70 and beyond. Studies consistently demonstrate significantly higher skin pH in the elderly (67 to 95 years, mean age 81) as compared to younger individuals. The rising pH reduces the integrity of the skin barrier and also supports the growth of pathogens; normal skin flora appears to thrive in an acidic environment, while pathogens grow best in a neutral or alkaline environment. In addition, an acidic pH seems to promote attachment of the resident bacteria to the skin, while an alkaline pH promotes shedding of the "good" bacteria from the skin (Ansari, 2014).

CLINICAL PEARL

Skin pH rises with aging, thus compromising skin health and barrier function; this is due in part to reduced activity of the sebaceous and sweat glands.

Maintaining Skin Health

Studies show that between 70% and 85% of elderly individuals suffer from skin problems (xerosis, pruritus) and skin diseases (contact dermatitis, other eczema, candidiasis); these data strongly suggest a correlation between overall health of the skin (including pH) and the skin conditions commonly found in the elderly. In addition, the rising pH of the skin, along with thinning of the epidermal layer and reduced cohesion between the epidermis and dermis, results in reduced resistance to minor trauma such as tape trauma. Thus, medical adhesive–related skin injury (MARSI) is commonly seen in the elderly. Clearly, one priority in management of the elderly individual is maintenance of skin health; thus, the wound care nurse must carefully evaluate both skin care products and skin care practices in her or his setting. Particular attention should be given to agents used for general cleansing and for perineal cleansing following incontinent episodes; products should be selected that promote/maintain an acidic pH and that do not require rinsing. Unnecessary use of antimicrobial agents should be avoided, since normal skin flora help to maintain skin health and acidity. The wound nurse should also consider the type of bathing cloth used; soft disposable wipes are preferable, and abrasive cloths and scrubbing technique should be strictly avoided. Finally, routine use of emollients helps to maintain skin softness and an intact barrier; this is discussed further in the section on management of xerosis and pruritis (White-Chu & Reddy, 2011).

Other factors affecting overall skin health include temperature, humidity, and overall hydration; high temperatures increase evaporative loss as does an environment with low humidity, and systemic hydration affects hydration of the skin. Therefore, the wound nurse should promote adequate fluid intake for any elderly patient and should recommend bathing with water that is warm but not hot.

Photoaging

Changes in the skin associated with aging are due to a combination of intrinsic and extrinsic factors. Intrinsic factors are typically unalterable and include the normal aging process and related changes in the DNA of skin cells. Extrinsic factors include lifestyle, environment, pollution, exposure to nicotine, exposure to UV light, diet, and hydration. Medications may also affect the skin; for example, drugs to lower cholesterol may cause abnormal desquamation of the skin (Farage et al., 2008, 2009).

The most damaging extrinsic factors are smoking and photodamage caused by exposure to UV light. It is estimated that up to 90% of visible skin aging is the effect of sunlight. It was once thought that sun only affected the epidermis, but it is now known that both UVA and UVB rays penetrate to the dermis and contribute to the chronic skin damage associated with photoaging. The changes in the dermis include degradation of collagen and impaired deposition of elastin. With severe damage, the dermis becomes a mess of tangled elastic fibers and tightly packed collagen. The damaged dermal tissue is unable to maintain normal vasculature, and photoaged skin demonstrates reduced perfusion. Sun-damaged skin is also less able to mount a normal inflammatory response to injury. In addition to causing significant damage to both the epidermis and dermis and accelerating the visible signs of aging, photodamage also increases the risk of cutaneous neoplasms. This is because UV light damages genetic material through replication errors and the creation of free radicals. In addition, UV light interferes with enzymatic activities required for repair of damaged DNA and compromises the function of Langerhans cells, which are responsible for the eradication of carcinogenic cells (Farage et al., 2008). Thus, the wound care clinician should be alert to patient history and physical findings consistent with high levels of UV exposure and should be cognizant of the increased risk for all forms of skin cancer in these individuals. In addition, the wound care nurse should educate the patient regarding the importance of routine dermatologic checkups and prompt reporting of any lesion that is increasing in size or atypical in appearance. All elderly individuals should be encouraged to use sunscreen routinely and to wear light long-sleeved clothing and broad-brimmed hats when outside. In addition, elderly individuals should be counseled to wear sunglasses on a routine basis for protection against cataract formation as well as protection of the eyelids against skin malignancy.

CLINICAL PEARL

Sun exposure and cigarette smoking are the most significant extrinsic factors contributing to skin aging and skin damage.

Xerosis and Pruritis

Xerosis is a broad term used to denote abnormal dryness of mucous membranes, skin, and/or eyes; xerosis cutis is a more specific term that is the preferred medical term for abnormally dry skin. However, in clinical practice, the term xerosis is typically used to indicate very dry skin. Pruritus or itch is the unpleasant skin sensation that provokes the urge to scratch; pruritis frequently accompanies xerosis, and the term xerosis is sometimes used incorrectly to denote chronic itching. Xerosis is the cause of 40% of pruritus in the elderly and is found in an estimated 58% of nursing home residents and 85% of individuals >70 years of age (Chang et al., 2013a). While underlying systemic disease is a common cause of xerosis, the elderly often have emotional or psychological stress that intensifies the itching. It is important for the clinician to remember that aging involves a series of losses and that emotional stress can exacerbate symptoms such as pain and itch.

Xerosis accompanied by intense itching and repetitive scratching can result in secondary lesions with a cracked porcelain pattern or linear fissures, particularly on the lower legs. In some cases, fissures penetrate into the dermis, disrupting capillaries and causing bleeding (Farage et al., 2009).

Pathology

Xerosis is due in part to reduced production of the sebum and skin lipids that are the skin's natural moisturizers. The end result is increased dryness and flaking of the skin and compromised barrier function (White-Chu & Reddy, 2011). Medications can also play a role in xerosis. Systemic as well as topical agents should be reviewed, as polypharmacy is prevalent in the elderly and there are numerous medications that could cause or contribute to xerosis. These include antibacterials, diuretics, NSAIDs, calcium channel antagonists (Farage et al., 2009), hypercholesterolemic agents, antiandrogens, cimetidine, opioids, and angiotensin-converting enzyme inhibitors (White-Chu & Reddy, 2011). The patient should also be assessed for common comorbid conditions associated with xerosis and pruritis: liver failure, renal insufficiency, neuropathy, or malignancy (Chang et al., 2013a).

CLINICAL PEARL

Xerosis (dry skin) and pruritis (itching) are common in the elderly due to reduced production of sebum and skin lipids. Thus, routine use of moisturizers is a critical element of care.

Management

The first steps in managing xerosis in the aging patient are rehydration of the skin followed by application of an agent to seal in the hydration (Fig. 13-2). Specific measures include changing bathing schedules and routine application of emollients. Common recommendations for treatment of dry skin include the following: reduce frequency of bathing and use lukewarm (not hot) water; limit showering or bathing to <5 minutes; minimize use of nonirritating, moisturizing soap (apply only to hair-bearing or soiled areas); and apply cream or ointment-type moisturizer of choice to the skin while still damp (Chang et al., 2013b; LeBlanc & Baranoski, 2009; White-Chu & Reddy, 2011). Although traditional recommendations include restricted bathing, some authors point out that immersion in water is actually needed to rehydrate the stratum corneum (SC) and suggest that the best approach is to provide at least 10 minutes of immersion in tepid water; these authors agree with minimal use of soaps and stipulate that a better approach is use of a gentle nonirritating cleanser (e.g., a moisturizing foam cleanser or shower gel). They also emphasize the need for generous application of moisturizers immediately following the bath; the moisturizer provides lipids to fill the gaps between the keratinocytes, helping to maintain an intact barrier and reduce flaking (Farage et al., 2009; White-Chu & Reddy, 2011).

As noted, moisturizers are a critical aspect of treatment for xerosis and pruritis and typically should be applied at least twice a day. While there is agreement that effective moisturizers are critical to management of xerosis and pruritis, there is very little agreement as to which products are best. There are two major types of moisturizers: emollients and humectants.

Emollients

Emollients are designed to penetrate the SC, to fill the gaps between the skin cells, and to retard water loss; they

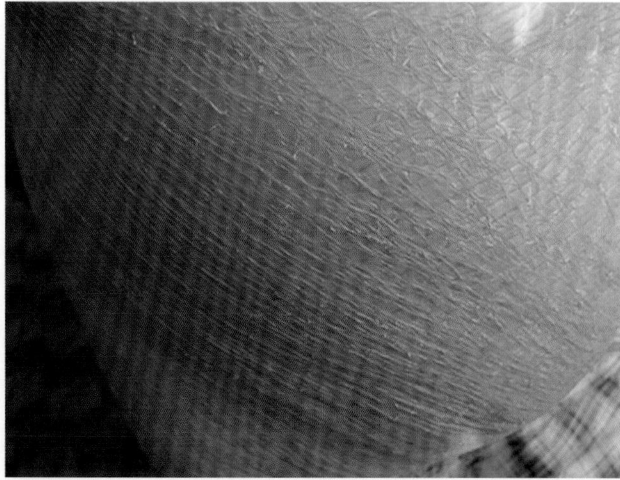

FIGURE 13-2. Xerosis. Minimal dryness, manifested by the slightest fine scaling.

are available in a wide variety of commercial products (creams, lotions, ointments) and are appropriate for both normal and fragile skin.

Humectants

In contrast, humectants are designed to attract and hold water within the SC and to promote desloughing of thick dry skin; common ingredients are urea compounds and alpha-hydroxy acids (AHAs). One potential advantage of humectants containing lactic acid or AHAs (e.g., ammonium lactate 12% lotion) is the acidic pH, which can help restore normal skin pH in addition to promoting keratolysis of hyperkeratotic skin. However, if the skin is fissured or cracked, stinging and irritation might limit AHA usage (Chang et al., 2013a). In addition, humectants are not appropriate for use on overhydrated or thin fragile skin (because humectants attract water and promote desloughing).

CLINICAL PEARL

Humectants are designed to attract water and to "deslough" dry rough skin; these agents are inappropriate for overhydrated or thin fragile skin.

While the ideal emollient would also be acidic, information regarding the pH of available moisturizers is not readily accessible (Shi, Tran, & Lio, 2012). In a recent study, investigators measured the pH of several moisturizers commonly used in the United States and found that some had quite alkaline pH levels. While there are guidelines for appropriate use of emollients versus humectants, there is little evidence that any one emollient or any one humectant is better than another, though it is recognized that commercially available skin creams vary in their ability to retain moisture in the skin (Young & Chakravarthy, 2014). Thus, decisions at present should be based at least in part on the patient's preference and the cost involved.

One potential problem with use of emollient products is the potential for contact dermatitis; selected emollients include a number of common skin sensitizers (e.g., balsam of Peru, lanolin, propylene glycol, parabens, formaldehyde, fragrance, vitamin E, aloe vera, and antibiotics) (White-Chu & Reddy, 2011), and contact dermatitis is common in the elderly. Therefore, an irritant or allergen in the topical agent should be considered whenever symptoms worsen with therapy. Patch testing or switching to another emollient with different ingredients may be helpful (White-Chu & Reddy, 2011).

Age-Related Skin Lesions

Many patients and providers do not differentiate between skin changes caused by photoaging and those caused by chronologic aging; they simply attribute any skin changes to "old age." In reality, the effects of photoaging are superimposed on intrinsic (chronologic) aging. Older individuals who have also been exposed to UV light are at increased risk for the skin changes typically attributed to aging, and the lesions may occur at an earlier age in these individuals. The following conditions are frequently seen by the wound nurse.

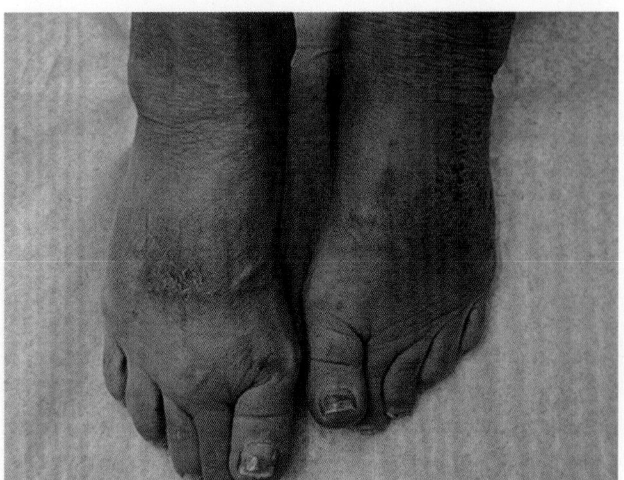

FIGURE 13-3. Shoe allergic contact dermatitis.

Contact Dermatitis

Contact dermatitis occurs in as many as 11% of the older population; it is more common in women (Farage et al., 2009). The higher incidence may be due in part to the fact that the elderly have had years of exposure and sensitization to potential allergens (Fig. 13-3). The sensitivity reaction may be delayed in the older individual due to a reduction in Langerhans cells and vascular response, but it typically manifests within 24 hours of exposure. The most common offenders are topical medications or their inactive ingredients; for example, up to 81% of patients treated for chronic leg ulcers exhibit allergic reactions to topical products (Farage et al., 2009). Thus, the clinician should limit use of topical products to those that are essential, should be alert to products containing common sensitizing agents, and should consider patch testing high-risk patients such as those with ulcers or dermatitis involving the lower extremities.

Seborrheic Dermatitis

Seborrheic dermatitis is a chronic inflammation involving lipid-rich areas of the body, which affects approximately 31% of the geriatric population. Common sites of involvement are areas with numerous sebaceous glands, such as the eyebrows, paranasal area, scalp, axillae, and groin. The pathology is thought to involve an abnormal response to yeast organisms normally found on the skin. The lesions typically present as areas of yellow or white scaling;

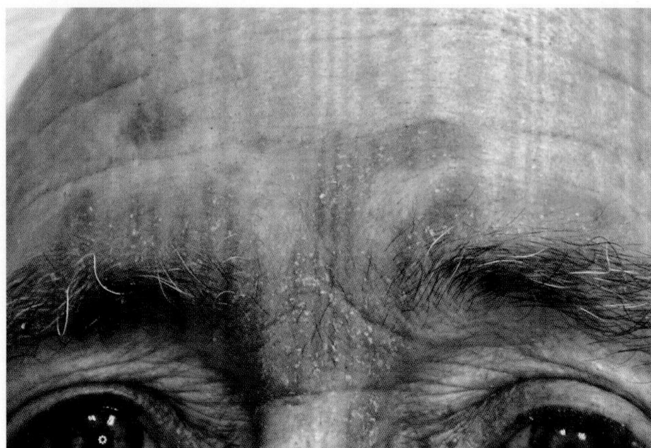

FIGURE 13-4. Seborrheic dermatitis on the glabellar region.

the underlying skin may be erythematous (Fig. 13-4). Treatment is usually topical, and therapies include anti-inflammatory preparations (e.g., corticosteroids or calcineurin inhibitors), keratolytic agents (e.g., pyrithione zinc, sulfur, coal tar, salicylic acid), and antifungal medications (e.g., ketoconazole). The medication is usually administered as a medicated shampoo. The shampoo should be lathered abundantly, rubbed into the scalp and affected areas, and left on for approximately 5 minutes before rinsing. Twice-weekly application is usually recommended (Farage et al., 2009).

Infections

Skin and soft tissue infections (SSTIs) have become the second most common type of infection among persons residing in long-term care facilities (Kish et al., 2010). This may be due in part to cellular senescence, which leads to thinning of the epidermis and a compromised epidermal barrier; defects in the barrier permit penetration by pathogens. In addition, there is a 40% reduction in mast cells and an almost 50% reduction in intradermal macrophages and Langerhans cells, the cells responsible for cellular immunity and for identification and destruction of pathogens. Furthermore, there is a reduction in the number and activity of the sweat glands, and sweat normally provides antimicrobial activity against a variety of pathogenic microorganisms (White-Chu & Reddy, 2011). Finally, the dry skin commonly found in the elderly is associated with itching and scratching, and the subsequent microabrasions set the stage for invasion by pathogens.

CLINICAL PEARL

SSTIs are the second most common type of infection among individuals living in long-term care facilities.

Candidiasis

Cutaneous fungal infection is one of the most common skin diseases in the elderly, due to alterations in barrier function of the skin (Fig. 13-5) (Chang et al., 2013a). Risk is further increased by exposure to moisture (as occurs with diaphoresis and incontinence) and antibiotic administration, as well as poorly controlled diabetes (Ali & Yosipovitch, 2013; Chang et al., 2013a). Fungal infections caused by yeast organisms (such as *Candida albicans*) typically present as a tender and pruritic maculopapular rash that is confluent in the center with distinct border lesions; in contrast, infections caused by tinea organisms are characterized by a rash that is most intense at the periphery, with central clearing (Chang et al., 2013a). Diagnosis is usually made on the basis of clinical presentation but can be confirmed by skin scrapings examined under a microscope; treatment involves an antifungal agent. The specific treatment depends on the location and severity of infection. Skin infections usually respond to medicated creams. Medicated suppositories may be used to treat vaginal yeast infections. Thrush may be treated with a medicated mouthwash or lozenges that dissolve in the mouth. Severe infections or infections in someone with a compromised immune system may be treated with oral antifungal medications.

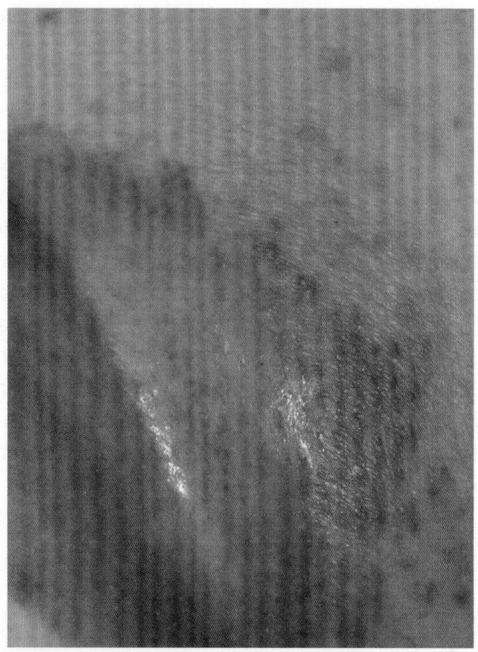

FIGURE 13-5. Cutaneous candidiasis classically produces red plaques with peripheral pustules and satellite lesions.

Herpes Zoster

Aging also increases the risk for herpes zoster (shingles), which is caused by reactivation of the varicella virus (VZV); the virus lies dormant in the major sensory ganglia following primary infection earlier in life (Fig. 13-6). One factor that increases the risk for herpes zoster in the elderly is the substantial reduction in the number of Langerhans cells in all layers of the epidermis; Langerhans cells are

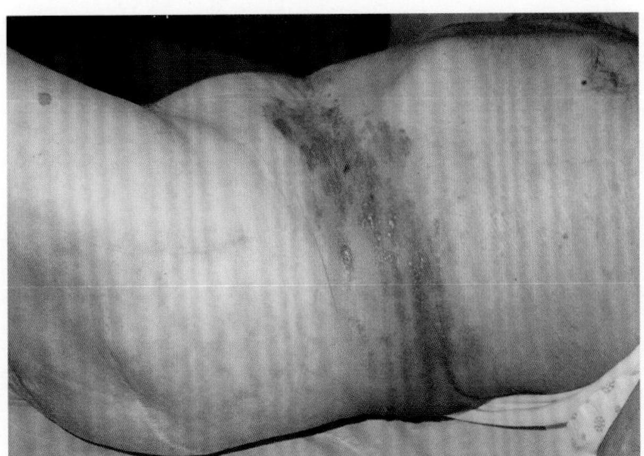

FIGURE 13-6. Herpes zoster: Cutaneous findings that typically appear unilaterally, stopping abruptly at the midline of the limit of sensory coverage of the involved dermatome.

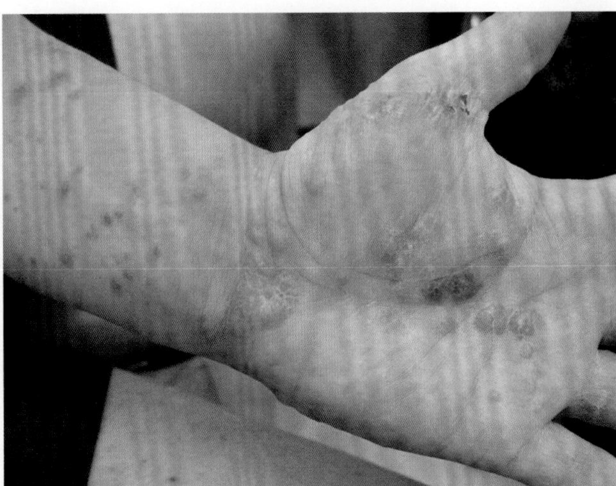

FIGURE 13-7. Scabies: Caused by a burrowing mite, which produces severe, intensely itching lesions in the area of its burrows.

equipped to destroy incoming viruses. VZV often presents with prodromal pain, itching or burning, or a sharp stabbing pain that occurs before the onset of rash. Depending on the affected dermatome, prodromal pain may be misdiagnosed as myocardial infarction, appendicitis, or a gallbladder or kidney stone attack (Weinberg, Vafaie, & Scheinfeld, 2004). Acute herpes zoster typically manifests as acute pain accompanied by a vesicular rash that follows the path of the involved dermatome; the pain persists until the rash subsides and sometimes past that point (Chang et al., 2013a).

Complications can include pain, lasting for months or even years after the disappearance of the rash; this is known as postherpetic neuralgia (PHN). Approximately half of all zoster patients will experience PHN persisting at least 120 days after rash onset (Chang et al., 2013a). Another very serious complication is blindness, which can occur if the involved dermatome involves the optic nerve; thus, any patient with facial lesions requires prompt referral to ophthalmology. Management of zoster requires early administration of systemic antiviral agents, which are designed to reduce viral replication and thereby to reduce nerve damage, inflammation, and duration and severity of pain. Early and consistent pain management, in addition to proper skin care, moist wound healing, and colloidal oatmeal baths, is essential to the prevention of PHN (Weinberg et al., 2004).

CLINICAL PEARL

Aging increases the risk for herpes zoster, which is acutely painful and can result in PHN; there is a vaccine available but few eligible individuals receive the vaccine.

Scabies

Scabies is common among residents in nursing homes and extended care facilities in the United States (Fig. 13-7). It is caused by a mite that burrows under the skin; superficial burrows are typically seen on the hands (particularly the finger webs), wrists, extensor surfaces of the elbows and knees, back, buttocks, and external genitalia (the face and scalp are usually spared). It is characterized by intense itching, especially at night; this results in scratching and excoriations that make it difficult to distinguish from other pruritic skin conditions. Scabies can be problematic among residents in nursing home facilities, spreading rapidly and persistently by cross transmission. It is spread by direct skin contact and is exceptionally contagious, being passed easily from patient to patient and patient to staff (Kish et al., 2010). Scabies should always be included in the differential assessment of any acutely pruritic skin condition. Accurate diagnosis can be difficult because it requires visualization of the mites or eggs from a skin scraping; thus, sometimes the decision is made to treat empirically with topical or systemic scabicidal agents. In addition, treatment must include meticulous attention to laundering of clothing and bedding.

CLINICAL PEARL

Scabies is common in long-term care facilities and is extremely contagious; it should be included in the differential assessment of any pruritic rash.

Benign and Malignant Lesions

In addition to inflammatory and infectious lesions, the elderly are at risk for a number of benign skin conditions and a range of skin malignancies. The pathology, presentation, and management of these lesions are covered in **Table 13-1** and Figure 13-8. Common anatomic locations for the various lesions are displayed in Figure 13-9.

TABLE 13-1 Benign and Malignant Lesions Common in the Elderly

Type of Lesion	Features	Photoaging	Location	Example	Treatment
Acrochordon (skin tag)	Papilloma; soft, pedunculated papilloma is typical of a fibroepithelial polyp	No	Neck, axilla, trunk	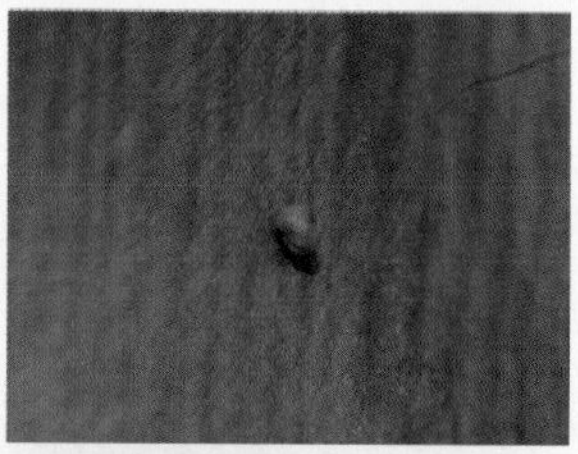	Electrocautery or scalpel
Lentigo (liver spots)	Macule with various colors, from light tan to black. Round or oval; flat or slightly elevated	Yes	Anywhere on the body	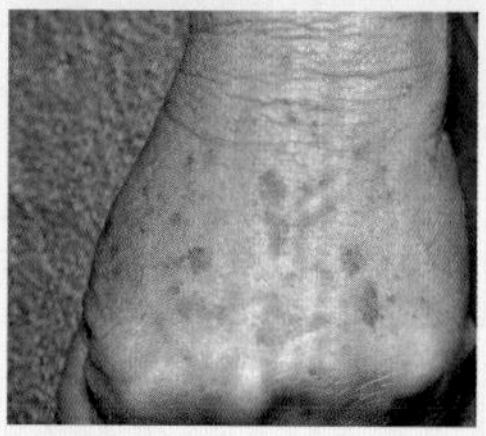	Prescription-strength retinol and hydroquinone (HC) cream, microdermabrasion, chemical peels, chemical spot treatments, laser treatments, and light therapy to lighten
Solar elastosis (dermatoheliosis)	Abnormal accumulation of elastin within the dermis; appears as thickened, dry, wrinkled skin	Yes	Sun-exposed skin	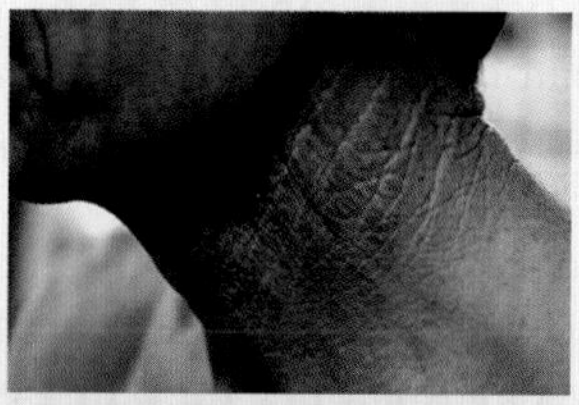	Treatment usually ineffective; minimize sun exposure; sunscreen
Seborrheic keratosis	Elevated sharply defined edge; color varies from light brown to black; warty scale that crumbles; can sometimes be scratched away but looks attached	No	Face, arms, back, and trunk Can be irritated or traumatized depending on the location	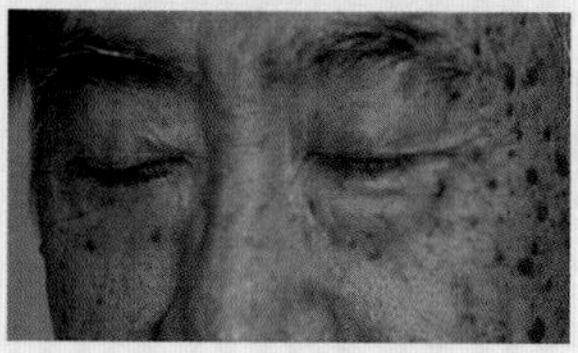	Most often confused with malignant melanoma by clinicians who are not dermatologists. Usually not precancerous but needs to be evaluated to determine if precancerous
Actinic keratosis	Small, rough, poorly demarcated lesion. Seldom larger than 1 cm. May develop a white rough surface scale	Yes; cumulative long-term sun exposure	Head, neck, forearms, and hands. Difficult to see on the lips	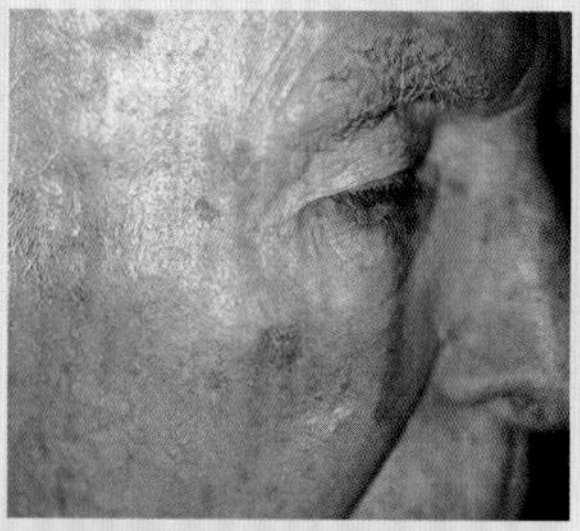	Benign lesions that may give rise to squamous cell carcinoma (if unsure, biopsy)
Squamous cell carcinoma	Opaque nodule or red nodule; rough, scaly, sometimes ulcerated. Crusting usually present	Yes	Sun-exposed areas; usually head and neck	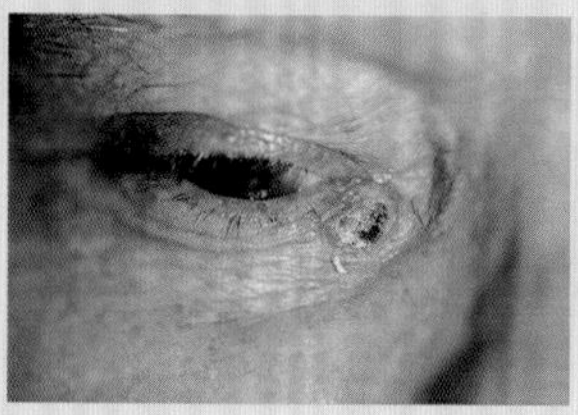	Can metastasize Refer for biopsy

TABLE 13-1 Benign and Malignant Lesions Common in the Elderly (*Continued*)

Type of Lesion	Features	Photoaging	Location	Example	Treatment
Basal cell	Raised, pearly edges; may be more pigmented in patients with darker skin	Yes	Sun-exposed areas; usually head and neck		Refer for biopsy
Melanoma	A asymmetry B border irregularity C color variations D diameter E evolving lesion See below	Yes	Men upper back, women upper back and lower legs		Refer for biopsy

Partial-Thickness Wound Healing

Elderly skin is in a progressive state of decline and is therefore more susceptible to damage from friction, MARSI, and moisture-associated skin damage (MASD). See Chapter 17 for further discussion of common "top–down" injuries.

In addition to increased risk for partial-thickness skin loss, the time required for healing is frequently prolonged, even when the wound is relatively superficial. This is because aging keratinocytes have reduced proliferative capacity and reduced ability to produce cytokines and other molecules critical to cell–cell communication. This compromise in keratinocyte function may be due in part to the marked reduction in Langerhans cells; there is considerable evidence that Langerhans cells regulate the function, differentiation, and proliferation of epidermal keratinocytes.

CLINICAL PEARL

Partial-thickness wound healing is frequently prolonged in the elderly, due to reduced keratinocyte proliferative capacity and reduced cell-to-cell communication.

There are also marked changes in the basement membrane (junction between the epidermis and dermis) that contribute to the elderly individual's risk for skin tears and for delayed partial-thickness healing. The basement membrane is not a true membrane; it is in fact composed of thin layers of specialized extracellular matrix that become less organized with aging. This area is normally characterized by the interlocking dermal papillae and epidermal rete pegs. With age, the matrix dermal papillae flatten and the interlocking configuration is lost, resulting in reduced epidermal tensile strength and increased risk for skin tears and MARSI. (See Chapter 17 for an in-depth discussion of MARSI and skin tears.)

While there are changes in the epidermis and basement membrane associated with aging, it is the dermis that sustains the greatest structural and atrophic changes. These changes include a loss of fibroblasts and a doubling of replication time for the remaining fibroblasts; this causes reduced production of dermal collagen, elastin, and proteoglycans and a significant increase in the time required for repair of dermal damage (Farage et al., 2009).

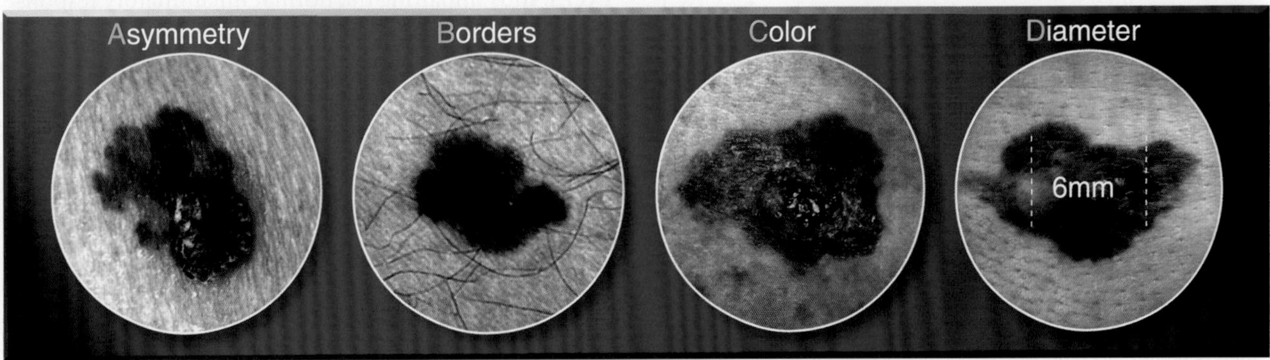

FIGURE 13-8. The ABCD's of malignant melanoma.

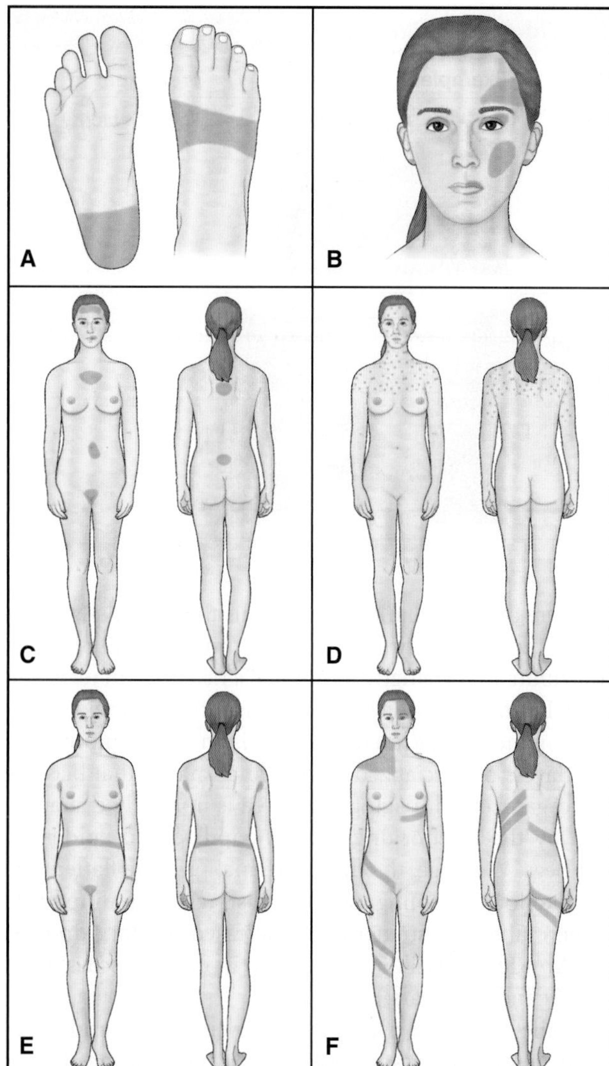

FIGURE 13-9. Anatomic distribution of common skin disorders. **A.** Contact dermatitis (shoes). **B.** Contact dermatitis (cosmetics, perfumes, earrings). **C.** Seborrheic dermatitis. **D.** Acne. **E.** Scabies. **F.** Herpes zoster (shingles).

Reduced blood flow is another characteristic of aging skin that negatively impacts on healing. There is a 30% decrease in the cross-sectional area of dermal venules in older skin and a 60% decrease in basal and peak cutaneous blood flow (Archer, 2012). These vascular changes render the elderly more susceptible to pressure ulcers and vascular ulcers and also compromise their ability to effect skin repair.

Despite the vulnerability of the older patient's skin, partial-thickness wounds will heal by regeneration as long as the cause can be eliminated and the wound surface is kept clean and moist.

CLINICAL PEARL

Despite changes in proliferative capacity, partial-thickness wounds in the elderly will heal so long as causative factors are eliminated and the wound surface is kept clean and moist.

Full-Thickness Wound Healing

Chapters 2 and 18 provide foundational information regarding the pathology of full-thickness injury and the processes involved in full-thickness wound healing. This section addresses aspects of healing unique to the elderly.

As explained in Chapter 2, the primary processes involved in full-thickness repair include hemostasis (acute wounds), inflammation, proliferation of new tissue (granulation tissue formation), contraction (in open wounds), and epithelial resurfacing. There are changes unique to aging that affect each of these processes.

Hemostasis (Acute Wounds Only)

Platelet aggregation and adherence to the endothelium is enhanced in aged subjects. In addition, there is increased degranulation of platelets and release of growth factors (TGF-β, TGF-α, and PDGF) (Gosain & DiPietro, 2004).

Inflammation

The inflammatory phase is critical to repair and is dependent on normal numbers and function of neutrophils and macrophages, with macrophages playing the more important role. Unfortunately, aging is associated with reduced numbers of macrophages, which at least partially explains the diminished inflammatory response that is typically seen. In addition, the reduced numbers of mast cells, B lymphocytes, and T cells compromises the ability to manage bacterial loads. Finally, changes in capillary permeability limit neutrophil migration into the wound bed. The end result is a prolonged inflammatory phase and increased risk of infection; frequently, the wound nurse must supplement the reduced inflammatory response through use of debridement and antimicrobial agents.

A recent study by Jiang et al. (2012) provides additional insight into the ways in which the normal inflammatory response may be altered in the elderly; they measured the levels of two different proteins in full-thickness (stage III) pressure ulcers. The first protein (Bax protein) is known to induce suicide (apoptosis) in T cells, thus impairing the normal inflammatory response. The second protein (Bcl-2) is found in healthy skin and inhibits cell death (apoptosis). Samples were taken from the surrounding skin, the wound edge, and the necrotic center. These investigators found that the number of Bax cells progressively increased from the wound edge to the necrotic center of the wound, while the Bcl-2 cells were significantly lower in the center with increasingly higher numbers at the skin edge. They concluded that an imbalance between apoptotic and proliferative cells contributed to impaired healing. This is important because the percentages of senescent and apoptotic cells is higher in the elderly, as previously discussed.

Proliferative Phase

All aspects of the proliferative phase are compromised to some extent in the elderly: angiogenesis, collagen synthesis, contraction, and epithelial resurfacing. The two factors that seem to have the greatest negative impact on granulation tissue formation (angiogenesis and collagen synthesis) are impaired perfusion and diminished fibroblast function. Adequate perfusion is critical to all phases of healing, including granulation tissue formation, and, as already discussed, aging is associated with a "normal" reduction in blood flow to the soft tissues; this means that, even under the best of conditions, the rate of granulation tissue formation will be reduced in the elderly. If the individual with the wound also suffers from macrovascular and/or microvascular disease, the delay may be significant or healing may be impossible. Thus, assessment of perfusion status is of vital importance, and the wound nurse must do everything possible to optimize perfusion in the elderly.

Fibroblasts are the cells responsible for synthesis of collagen and other connective tissue proteins, but the cellular senescence associated with aging reduces the number of proliferative fibroblasts and their response to growth factors. This results in a prolonged time frame for collagen synthesis; in addition, the collagen may be of poor quality (Chang et al., 2013a).

As explained in Chapter 2, contraction of newly formed extracellular matrix proteins can significantly reduce the time to healing by reducing the size of the defect. Contraction is impaired in the elderly, possibly due to reduced numbers of myofibroblasts, which are derived from fibroblasts and essential for contraction.

The final step in the proliferative phase for open wounds is epithelial resurfacing, which can be impaired by a number of factors. First of all, the rate of keratinocyte proliferation is reduced in the elderly. Secondly, keratinocytes require a healthy wound bed (normal extracellular matrix) in order to migrate and attach; if collagen synthesis is impaired, the defective new tissue inhibits epithelial migration and resurfacing. Thirdly, macrophages normally produce substances that promote keratinocyte proliferation (such as ceramides), and macrophage numbers are diminished in the elderly (Seyfarth et al., 2011). Finally, age-related stress can result in increased production of cortisol, glucocorticoids, and epinephrine, and epidermal cells can serve as an extra-adrenal source of both epinephrine and cortisol; this has been linked to impaired healing in experimental models (Stojadinovic et al., 2012).

Remodeling (Maturation)

During the maturation phase, the early "provisional" (type III) collagen is replaced with mature (type I) collagen, which is essential to development of tensile strength. (The early type III collagen lacks tensile strength.) This involves the dual processes of breakdown of the early collagen and synthesis of the mature collagen. The elderly are at risk for defective remodeling that results in failure to develop tensile strength; this may be due in part to compromised fibroblast function and in part to comorbidities affecting tissue oxygenation and nutritional status. In some situations, the rate of collagen breakdown exceeds the rate of collagen synthesis, creating increased risk for breakdown of the newly closed wound. The wound nurse needs to be aware that full-thickness wounds are at risk even after they have closed. Since full-thickness wounds "heal" by replacing the lost tissue with scar tissue, they never return to the original state of health or tensile strength. At best, a closed full-thickness wound attains 80% of original tensile strength; thus, they are always at risk for repeat breakdown.

CLINICAL PEARL

Multiple factors increase the risk for impaired full-thickness wound healing in the elderly, including reduced proliferation and activity of endothelial cells, fibroblasts, and keratinocytes, reduced perfusion, and any comorbidities; however, most elderly retain the capacity to heal so long as management is comprehensive and appropriate.

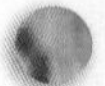

Elder Abuse

In one study of 5,777 subjects aged 60 years or older, 1 in 10 respondents reported emotional, physical, or sexual mistreatment or neglect in the previous year (Acierno et al., 2010). If those statistics are extrapolated to the entire elderly population, it suggests that there are 2 to 5 million victims of elder abuse per year in the United States. In addition to these forms of abuse, elders are frequently the victims of exploitation (the illegal taking, misuse, or concealment of funds, property, or assets of a vulnerable adult). Statistics also suggest that, for every report of abuse, 23.5 cases go unreported, possibly because the elder may be unable to report the abuse and health care providers do not always recognize signs and symptoms of abuse. Wound care nurses are frontline staff who are frequently involved in the care of vulnerable elderly individuals; thus, they can play an important role in identification and reporting of suspected abuse. The cutaneous signs of elder physical abuse are purpura and petechiae, wounds in various stages of healing, multiple difficult-to-explain scars, defensive wounds, bilateral or parallel injuries on the extremities indicating restraint, severe incontinence-associated dermatitis (IAD), and pressure ulcers.

Timely and appropriate intervention is required in cases of suspected elder abuse. While the reporting rate is higher in nursing homes, it is in the home and the community where most elder abuse occurs (Chang et al., 2013b). It is the responsibility of every nurse to

1. Develop an awareness of elder abuse and neglect
2. Recognize the signs and symptoms of elder abuse

3. Learn how to appropriately and comfortably talk with possible victims
4. Identify resources for reporting suspected abuse and neglect

http://www.centeronelderabuse.org/docs/intro-to-elder-abuse-for-undergrad-nurses.slides.pdf

CLINICAL PEARL

Elder abuse is extremely common; thus, the wound nurse needs to be alert to any indicators of abuse and should know that prompt reporting of any suspected abuse is now a legal mandate.

Signs of elder abuse are sometimes subtle, and the nurse needs to remember that it is not necessary to substantiate the abuse before reporting. The nurse also needs to know that reporting suspected abuse is now a legal mandate.

 Delirium

Intact cognition plays a critical role in an individual's ability to recognize and appropriately respond to ischemic discomfort; thus, cognitive impairment is a potential risk factor for pressure ulcer development. There are a number of conditions that can adversely affect cognitive function in the elderly; they are at increased risk for dementia, for delirium, and for delirium superimposed on dementia. It is essential for the wound care clinician to be knowledgeable regarding conditions commonly impacting on cognitive function and the implications for prevention, recognition, and management (Popeo, 2011).

Dementia is recognized as a chronic, progressive, or persistent disorder of the mental processes caused by brain disease or injury and marked by memory disorders, personality changes, and impaired reasoning. In contrast, delirium is defined as an acutely altered and fluctuating mental status with features of inattention and altered level of consciousness. The DSM-IV-TR defines delirium as a "disturbance of consciousness and a change in cognition that develop over a short period of time" (American Psychiatric Association, 2000; 4th ed., text review.; DSM-IV-TR). While delirium can occur in all age groups, it occurs more frequently in the elderly (Robinson et al., 2009; Rudolph & Marcantonio, 2011). A critical difference between dementia and delirium is the fact that delirium is reversible, whereas dementia is *not* reversible. However, it is important to realize that the patient with dementia can develop a superimposed delirium that causes a sudden and rapid deterioration in mental status; once the causative factors for the delirium have been identified and corrected, the patient's mental status returns to baseline. It is also important to realize that patients are sometimes "labeled" as having dementia or "Alzheimer's," even though no workup has ever been done. It is therefore critically important to refer any patient with cognitive impairment of unknown origin for evaluation, since some conditions resulting in "dementia" are actually treatable (e.g., normal pressure hydrocephalus).

While delirium is a very common syndrome, it is frequently missed. One difficulty is the fact that delirium has a number of different clinical presentations. Hyperactive delirium is rare but more easily recognized because its symptoms of restlessness, irritability, antagonism, or agitation are more easily identified. However, the majority of patients (over 70%) present with hypoactive delirium, with less obvious symptoms of lethargy, decreased alertness, and poor motivation. In 29% of cases, the clinical presentation involves a combination of hyperactive and hypoactive symptoms (Marcantonio et al., 2002).

Postoperative delirium (POD) typically occurs between 1 and 3 days postoperatively, and the etiology remains unclear (Bryson & Wyand, 2006). These patients often emerge from anesthesia smoothly and may be lucid in the postanesthesia care unit. However, after this initial lucid interval, the patient develops the classic fluctuating mental status, most commonly between postoperative days 1 and 3 (Chang et al., 2013b; Deiner & Silverstein, 2009). Benzodiazepines have significant effect on cognition and may precipitate delirium. While polypharmacy and opioids may precipitate delirium, uncontrolled pain may also precipitate dealirium. The practice of prophylaxis with antipsychotics should be avoided at present due to increased risk of death, delirium, and complications in older patients attributed to this class of drugs (Morimoto et al., 2009; Rudolph & Marcantonio, 2011; Yang et al., 2011).

Risk Factors

The most common independent risk factor for delirium is preexisting dementia, which is associated with up to two thirds of all cases of delirium (Fong et al., 2009; Robinson et al., 2009). Additional risk factors include preoperative physical impairment or altered functional status, preoperative depression, long history of alcohol abuse (Morimoto et al., 2009; Rudolph & Marcantonio, 2011), low educational level (Szokol, 2010), inadequately managed postoperative pain (Leung et al., 2009), comorbidities, psychopathology, impaired vision or hearing, psychotropic drugs, increased age, greater duration of anesthesia, a second operation, and postoperative respiratory infection (Szokol, 2010).

Of importance to wound care nurses, patients with delirium were three times more likely than patients who did not experience delirium to develop a wound infection during hospitalization (Redelmeier et al., 2008).

Assessment and Recognition

Even well-intentioned staff frequently fail to assess cognitive status, despite the fact that delirium affects an estimated 14% to 56% of all hospitalized elderly patients and significantly increases the risk of complications (e.g., decreased oral intake, pressure ulcers, aspiration, and pulmonary emboli) and the likelihood of discharge to a long-term care facility (Chen et al., 2011; Rudolph & Marcantonio, 2011). Therefore, validated assessment tools (e.g., Mini–Mental Status Exam, MMSE) should be used to assess cognition whenever there are any concerns regarding delirium (Yang et al., 2011).

CLINICAL PEARL

Delirium affects 14% to 56% of all hospitalized elderly; at least 30% to 40% of these cases are preventable through measures such as judicious use of pain medications, measures to improve sleep, and maintenance of fluid and electrolyte balance, glycemic control, and oxygenation.

Prevention and Intervention

An estimated 30% to 40% of cases of delirium are preventable, and prevention is the most effective strategy for minimizing the occurrence of delirium and its adverse outcomes (Fong et al., 2009; Siddiqi et al., 2007). There are two basic interventions for delirium prevention and management: nonpharmacological and pharmacological. Nonpharmacologic strategies include environmental measures to optimize sleep, maintenance of fluid and electrolyte balance, glycemic control, prevention of hypoxia, infection prevention, judicious use of pain medication, avoidance of prophylactic use of psychoactive medications, and reorientation when indicated.

Educational programs should be implemented that increase clinicians' awareness of effective preventive measures, early recognition, and both nonpharmacologic and pharmacologic strategies for management of delirium.

Implications

Wound care nurses interact with the family and patient to assess for skin problems, determine risk for pressure ulcers, and develop an individualized treatment plan. If the patient has unrecognized delirium, the plan cannot effectively address the needs of the patient, family, or caregivers. Therefore, wound care nurses must become knowledgeable regarding basic cognitive assessment and must modify their management plans based on assessment findings.

Malnutrition

Chapter 6 addresses nutritional needs for wound healing and implications for assessment and intervention. Nutritional management is of particular importance to the wound nurse caring for an elderly patient, and most especially an institutionalized elder, because undernutrition and protein–energy malnutrition are seen at an alarmingly high rate in the institutionalized elderly. The combination of immunosenescence, loss of mobility, and loss of soft tissue and muscle increases the risk of pressure ulcers by 74%. Harris and Fraser (2004) identified the following as factors that delay healing and increase the risk of pressure ulcer development in the elderly (Box 13-1). Practical and sensible suggestions for long-term care would include making restrictive diets more liberal, encouraging family and friends to bring foods from home, making adjustments for favorite foods, and referrals to speech pathologist for suspected swallowing problems.

BOX 13-1. Risk Factors for Malnutrition, Delayed Healing and Increased Risk of Pressure Ulcers in Elderly

- Dependency on others for help with eating
  - Impaired cognition and/or communication
  - Poor positioning
  - Frequent acute illnesses with nausea, vomiting, and/or diarrhea
  - Medications that decrease appetite or increase nutrient losses
  - Polypharmacy: Medications that decrease appetite or increase nutrient losses
  - Decreased thirst response, decreased ability to concentrate urine
  - Psychosocial factors such as isolation and depression
  - Intentional fluid restriction because of fear of incontinence or choking (dysphagia)
- Monotony of diet
- Higher nutrient density requirements along with the demands of age, illness, and disease on the body

CLINICAL PEARL

Simple measures to improve nutrient intake among the elderly include liberalization of diets, encouraging friends and family to bring food from home, and prompt referral to speech pathology for suspected swallowing problems.

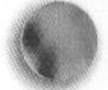

Polypharmacy

At the time of this publication, individuals aged 65 years and older account for approximately 13% of the U.S. population, yet they consume at least a third of all prescription medicines. Nearly half (40%) are taking more than five drugs (Yang et al., 2011). Residents in nursing homes who are prescribed fewer than five drugs are almost nonexistent. Polypharmacy among the elderly is increasing, is a common cause of admission to the hospital, and is also an important cause of morbidity and death.

Polypharmacy can be defined as: (1) unintentionally prescribing too many medications (traditionally defined as more than four), (2) taking medications with duplicate mechanisms of action, or (3) inadvertently adding medications that interact with others. The truth remains that 10% of hospital admissions are related to adverse drug reactions (ADRs). According to multivariate analysis, it is not the patients' age alone that predicts adverse drug events; it is the total number of medications they take or the extent of their comorbid conditions (Endo et al., 2013).

Many duplications and potential interactions occur as a result of multiple transitions among various providers and care settings, with each discharging and admitting provider writing medication orders that may not be adequately reviewed for duplicate effects or potential interactions. Polypharmacy also increases the risk of drug-induced autoimmune cutaneous disease (Milgrom & Huang, 2014); skin reactions account for 7.9% of adverse events. Interestingly, females have a 1.5- to 1.7-fold greater risk of developing an ADR, including adverse skin reactions, as compared to males (Rademaker, 2001).

Advanced practice nurses (APRNs) are frequently asked to assess and manage elderly individuals with dermatologic conditions, but there is limited evidence-based guidance for either topical or systemic medications in this population (primarily because most clinical trials exclude older patients). Until such evidence becomes available, the APRN must utilize the following physiologic principles when prescribing: (1) thinning of the skin and compromise of the barrier function means that topical agents will be absorbed more effectively; (2) changes in distribution of the adipose tissue and reduced muscle mass can also affect drug absorption; and (3) alterations in renal and hepatic function can render the elder more susceptible to drug toxicity. These aspects of pharmacokinetics are typically not emphasized in drug labeling and dosing recommendations. The APRN must also be aware that the most common drug-to-drug interactions occur with nonprescription medications; it is therefore essential to carefully review all medications including over-the-counter (OTC) medication and integrative therapies such as herbs and alternative "natural" products (**Table 13-2**).

TABLE 13-2 Medication Considerations for the Elderly

Drug Category	Considerations for the *Older* Patient	Implications
Antimicrobials	Account for 20% of ADR One out of six hospital admissions	May induce hypoglycemia; has been fatal in elderly patient Trimethoprim/sulfamethoxazole is most common cause of fixed drug eruptions (Patel & Marfatia, 2008) Quinolones: some of the most common causes of antibiotic allergy Monitor with warfarin for increased bleeding
Oral ketoconazole	Frequently prescribed for candidiasis	Concurrent administration of ketoconazole and high-dose statin therapy increases the risk of statin-induced rhabdomyolysis. Statin dose might need to be decreased or temporarily held during the antifungal treatment (Endo et al., 2013). Monitor with warfarin for increased bleeding
Topical glucocorticosteroids	Cutaneous adverse effects occur frequently with prolonged use, and frequently associated with adverse effects, depending on the drug, the vehicle, and the area being treated. The rate of contact sensitization against corticosteroids is considerably higher than generally believed. Reported incidence of infection may be from 16% to 43% ADR often not reported, due to time from application until event. Low potency preferred for elderly fragile skin (Hengge et al., 2006)	Systemic reactions have been reported to follow topical application a. Hyperglycemia b. Glaucoma c. Adrenal insufficiency Effects on wound healing a. Keratinocytes (epidermal atrophy, delayed reepithelialization) b. Fibroblasts (reduced collagen and ground substance, resulting in dermal atrophy and striae) c. Vascular connective tissue (telangiectasia, purpura, easy bruising) d. Impaired angiogenesis (delayed granulation tissue) Most frequent a. Atrophy b. Striae c. Rosacea d. Perioral dermatitis e. Acne f. Purpura g. Suppressed inflammation; increased fungal or bacterial growth h. Mask lesions from herpes simplex, molluscum contagiosum, and scabies infection Lower-frequency dose side effects include a. Hypertrichosis b. Pigmentation alterations c. Exacerbation of skin infections

TABLE 13-2 Medication Considerations for the Elderly (*Continued*)

Drug Category	Considerations for the *Older* Patient	Implications
Systemic glucocorticosteroids	Oral corticosteroid use in the elderly patient should be a last resort after conservative, conventional therapy has failed for specific indications.	Systemic ADR (see Topical) a. Dependence b. Weight gain c. Masking of infection d. Fluid retention e. Worsening or precipitation of hypertension f. Diabetes g. Cataract h. Osteoporosis
Diphenhydramine	In hospital, 24% of diphenhydramine doses were administered inappropriately. Diphenhydramine administration in older hospitalized patients associated with an increased risk of cognitive decline and other adverse effects with a dose–response relationship.	a. Increased risk for delirium b. Increased risk for urinary catheter placement c. Anticholinergic activity; counteracts cholinesterase inhibitors for dementia d. OTC sleep aides contain diphenhydramine (Agostini, 2001)
Oxybutynin and tolterodine	Antimuscarinic (anticholinergic) used for urinary incontinence. Many lack documentation of effects; therefore are not based on RCTs satisfying currently required criteria.	a. May cross blood–brain barrier causing EEG activity changes b. Contribute to delirium c. Constipation d. Dry mouth may decrease food intake e. Dry eyes and blurred vision f. Confusion g. Dizziness h. Falls i. Calcium defects j. Counteract cholinesterase inhibitors for treating Alzheimer's
Diuretics	Not effective or appropriate for venous edema caused by venous insufficiency. Administration of diuretics to these patients is associated with significant risk for dehydration and renal impairment (Reddy et al., 2007).	Extremely low levels of sodium caused by thiazide diuretics have been associated with death and neurologic damage in elderly patients. Thiazides are known to cause cutaneous reactions.

CLINICAL PEARL

Consider an ADR as a potential cause of any new symptom. In this case, it is better to discontinue the problematic drug than to add another drug.

CLINICAL PEARL

Continuity of care is a major challenge in management of elderly patients being discharged from the hospital, because hospital care is managed by hospitalists who do not follow the patient after discharge.

Pain management is a major challenge for the geriatric population (American Geriatric Society, 1998). Pain in the elderly is underreported and undertreated. Twenty-five to fifty percent of community-dwelling elders have pain (Ferrell, 1991), and the documented prevalence of pain in nursing home residents is 45% to 80%. Elderly patients with cancer have daily pain (Ferrell et al., 1995).

While there are a number of pain relievers that are safe for elderly people, careful selection is advised. The risks associated with commonly used analgesics are addressed in Boxes 13-2 and 13-3.

The American Geriatric Society (1998) provides the following recommendations for pain management in the elderly:

- Acetaminophen is the drug of choice for management of mild-to-moderate musculoskeletal pain.
- For chronic pain, acetaminophen should be given routinely.
- NSAIDs should be used with caution.
  - High-dose long-term NSAID use should be avoided.
  - When used for chronic pain, NSAIDs should be given as needed rather than daily or around the clock.
- Opioids can be safely and effectively used in older adults. Start low and go slow, but don't stop (Pautex & Vogt-Ferrier, 2006).

BOX 13-2. Risks Associated with Acetaminophen

Acetaminophen (APAP) is found in over 600 OTC and prescription medicines, and the maximum safe dose is 4,000 mg/d. Many elderly people think these drugs are safe because they are "over the counter."

- In 2009, the FDA recommended changing the maximum single dose to 650 mg (rather than 1,000) and the maximum daily dose to 3,250 mg (rather than 4,000).
- Acetaminophen is the number one cause of acute liver failure.
- Data from five surveillance systems revealed the following statistics related to acetaminophen overdoses from 1990 to 1998 in the United States: 56,000 emergency room visits, 26,000 hospitalizations, and 458 deaths. (Acetaminophen overdose and liver injury—background and options for reducing injury. Food and Drug Administration.) http://www.fda.gov/ohrms/dockets/ac/09/briefing/20
- Acetaminophen should not be used in patients taking warfarin.

CLINICAL PEARL

NSAIDs are the drugs most commonly associated with cutaneous reactions: Ibuprofen was a common cause of erythema multiforme and Stevens-Johnson syndrome (Patel & Marfatia, 2008).

CLINICAL PEARL

80-year-old people have livers and kidneys with 80 years of use.

BOX 13-3. Risks Associated with Nonsteroidal Anti-Inflammatory Drugs (NSAIDs)

- More than 17 million Americans use NSAIDs daily.
- Adverse renal events occur in approximately 1%–5% of all patients using NSAIDs.
- NSAIDs cause significant morbidity and mortality in the elderly.
- NSAIDs may be poorly tolerated by the elderly.
- NSAIDs are highly protein bound.
- Fluid retention can occur and can exacerbate heart failure.
- COX 2 NSAIDS reduce GI and platelet side effects but not renal damage.
- Side effects are dose and duration dependent.
- Greater than 70% of NSAIDS are prescribed as routine dose.
- Ibuprofen (Motrin, Advil, Nuprin, etc.) 2,400 mg/24 hours (q6–8h dosing).
- Gastric, renal, and abnormal platelet function may occur and are usually dose dependent; constipation, confusion, and headaches may be more common in older patients.

In individuals aged 60 years or older, the risk of GI bleeding reaches 3% to 4%; for those with a history of gastrointestinal bleeding, the risk is about 9% ("AGS clinical practice guidelines: the management of chronic pain in older persons," 1998).

Conclusion

Skin and wound care for the elderly presents a number of challenges; the wound nurse must assure appropriate routine care and safe handling to reduce the risk of xerosis, pruritis, and skin tears. In addition, the wound nurse must be knowledgeable about common benign skin conditions and their management and must refer any patient with any evidence of skin malignancy. The wound nurse must recognize the many factors leading to delayed healing in the elderly and the critical importance of comprehensive and evidence-based wound management. Finally, the wound nurse must be alert to geriatric syndromes such as delirium, malnutrition, elder abuse, and polypharmacy and must contribute to prevention and prompt detection of these conditions.

REFERENCES

Acierno, R., Hernandez, M. A., Amstadter, A. B., et al. (2010). Prevalence and correlates of emotional, physical, sexual, and financial abuse and potential neglect in the United States: The National Elder Mistreatment Study. *American Journal of Public Health, 100*(2), 292–297. doi: 10.2105/AJPH.2009.163089

Agostini, J. V., Leo-Summers, L. S., & Inouye, S. (2001). Cognitive and other adverse effects of diphenhydramine use in hospitalized older patients. *Archives of Internal Medicine, 161*(17), 2091–2097.

Ali, S. M., & Yosipovitch, G. (2013). Skin pH: from basic science to basic skin care. *Acta Dermato-Venereologica, 93*(3), 261–267.

Allsopp, R. C., Vaziri, H., Patterson, C., et al. (1992). Telomere length predicts replicative capacity in human fibroblasts. *Proceedings of the National Academy of Sciences of the USA, 89*(21), 10114–10118.

American Geriatric Society. (1998). Clinical practice guidelines: The management of chronic pain in older persons. *Geriatrics, 53* (Suppl 3), S6–S7.

American Psychiatric Association. (2000). *Diagnostic and statistical manual of mental disorders* (4th ed., text review). Washington, DC: American Psychiatric Association.

Ansari, S. A. (2014). Skin pH and skin flora. In A. O. Barel, M. Paye, & H. I. Maibach (Eds.), *Handbook of cosmetic science and technology* (4th ed., pp. 163–174). Boca Raton, FL: CRC Press.

Archer, D. F. (2012). Postmenopausal skin and estrogen. *Gynecological Endocrinology, 28*(Suppl2), 2–6. doi: 10.3109/09513590.2012.705392

Ashcroft, G. S., Dodsworth, J., van Boxtel, E., et al. (1997). Estrogen accelerates cutaneous wound healing associated with an increase in TGF-beta1 levels. *Nature Medicine, 3*(11), 1209–1215.

Ashcroft, G. S., Greenwell-Wild, T., Horan, M. A., et al. (1999). Topical estrogen accelerates cutaneous wound healing in aged humans associated with an altered inflammatory response. *American Journal of Pathology, 155*(4), 1137–1146. doi: 10.1016/S0002-9440(10)65217-0.

Blaak, J., Wohlfart, R., & Schurer, N. (2011). Treatment of aged skin with a pH 4 skin care product normalizes increased skin surface pH and improves barrier function: Results of a pilot study. *Journal of Cosmetics, Dermatological Sciences and Applications, 1*, 50–58.

Bryson, G. L., & Wyand, A. (2006). Evidence-based clinical update: General anesthesia and the risk of delirium and postoperative cognitive dysfunction. *Canadian Journal of Anesthesia, 53*(7), 669–677.

Campisi, J., & d'Adda di Fagagna, F. (2007). Cellular senescence: When bad things happen to good cells. *Nature Reviews Molecular Cell Biology, 8*(9), 729–740. doi: 10.1038/nrm2233.

Centers for Disease Control and Prevention. (2013). *The state of aging and health in America*. Atlanta, GA: Centers for Disease Control and Prevention, US Dept of Health and Human Services.

Chang, A. L., Wong, J. W., Endo, J. O., et al. (2013a). Geriatric dermatology review: Major changes in skin function in older patients and their contribution to common clinical challenges. *Journal of the American Medical Directors Association, 14*(10), 724–730. doi:10.1016/j.jamda.2013.02.014.

Chang, A. L., Wong, J. W., Endo, J. O., et al. (2013b). Geriatric dermatology: Part II. Risk factors and cutaneous signs of elder mistreatment for the dermatologist. *Journal of the American Academy of Dermatology, 68*(4), 533.e1–e10; quiz 543–534. doi: 10.1016/j.jaad.2013.01.001.

Chen, C. C., Chiu, M. J., Chen, S. P., et al. (2011). Patterns of cognitive change in elderly patients during and 6 months after hospitalisation: A prospective cohort study. *International Journal of Nursing Studies, 48*(3), 338–346. doi:10.1016/ j.ijnurstu.2010.03.011.

Deiner, S., & Silverstein, J. H. (2009). Postoperative delirium and cognitive dysfunction. *British Journal of Anaesthesia, 103*(Suppl 1), i41–i46. doi: 10.1093/bja/aep291.

Dunn, L. B., Damesyn, M., Moore, A. A., et al. (1997). Does estrogen prevent skin aging? Results from the First National Health and Nutrition Examination Survey (NHANES I). *Archives of Dermatology, 133*(3), 339–342.

Emmerson, E., & Hardman, M. J. (2012). The role of estrogen deficiency in skin ageing and wound healing. *Biogerontology, 13*(1), 3–20.

Endo, J. O., Wong, J. W., Norman, R. A., et al. (2013). Geriatric dermatology: Part I. Geriatric pharmacology for the dermatologist. *Journal of the American Academy of Dermatology, 68*(4), 521.e1–e10; quiz 531–522. doi: 10.1016/j.jaad.2012.10.063.

Farage, M. A., Miller, K. W., Berardesca, E., et al. (2009). Clinical implications of aging skin: Cutaneous disorders in the elderly. *American Journal of Clinical Dermatology, 10*(2), 73–86. doi: 10.2165/00128071-200910020-00001.

Farage, M. A., Miller, K. W., Elsner, P., et al. (2008). Intrinsic and extrinsic factors in skin ageing: A review. *International Journal of Cosmetic Science, 30*(2), 87–95. doi: 10.1111/j.1468-2494.2007.00415.x.

Ferrell, B. A. (1991). Pain management in elderly people. *Journal of American Geriatrics Society, 39*(1), 64–73.

Ferrell, B. R., Grant, M., Chan, J., et al. (1995). The impact of cancer pain education on family caregivers of elderly patients. *Oncology Nursing Forum, 22*(8), 1211–1218.

Fong, T. G., Tulebaev, S. R., & Inouye, S. K. (2009). Delirium in elderly adults: Diagnosis, prevention and treatment. *Nature Reviews Neurology, 5*(4), 210–220.

Gilliver, S. C., Ashworth, J. J., & Ashcroft, G. S. (2007). The hormonal regulation of cutaneous wound healing. *Clinics in Dermatology, 25*(1), 56–62. doi: 10.1016/j.clindermatol.2006.09.012.

Gosain, A., & DiPietro, L. A. (2004). Aging and wound healing. *World Journal of Surgery, 28*(3), 321–326.

Hall, G., & Phillips, T. J. (2005). Estrogen and skin: The effects of estrogen, menopause, and hormone replacement therapy on the skin. *Journal of the American Academy of Dermatology, 53*(4), 555–568; quiz 569–572. doi: 10.1016/j.jaad.2004.08.039.

Harris, C. L., & Fraser, C. (2004). Malnutrition in the institutionalized elderly: The effects on wound healing. *Ostomy/Wound Management, 50*(10), 54–63.

Hengge, U. R., Ruzicka, T., Schwartz, R. A., et al. (2006). Adverse effects of topical glucocorticosteroids. *Journal of the American Academy of Dermatology,54*(1),1–15;quiz16–18.doi:10.1016/j.jaad.2005.01.010.

Inouye, S. K., Studenski, S., Tinetti, M. E., et al. (2007). Geriatric syndromes: Clinical, research, and policy implications of a core geriatric concept. *Journal of American Geriatrics Society, 55*(5), 780–791.

Jiang, L., Zhang, E., Yang, Y., et al. (2012). Effectiveness of apoptotic factors expressed on the wounds of patients with Stage III pressure ulcers. *Journal of Wound Ostomy Continence Nursing,* 39(4), 391–396.

Kish, T. D., Chang, M. H., & Fung, H. B. (2010). Treatment of skin and soft tissue infections in the elderly: A review. *American Journal of Geriatric Pharmacotherapy, 8*(6), 485–513.

LeBlanc, K., & Baranoski, S. (2009). Prevention and management of skin tears. *Advances in Skin & Wound Care, 22*(7), 325–332.

Leung, J. M., Sands, L. P., Paul, S., et al. (2009). Does postoperative delirium limit the use of patient-controlled analgesia in older surgical patients? *Anesthesiology, 111*(3), 625–631. doi: 10.1097/ALN.0b013e3181acf7e6.

Marcantonio, E., Ta, T., Duthie, E., et al. (2002). Delirium severity and psychomotor types: Their relationship with outcomes after hip fracture repair. *Journal of American Geriatrics Society, 50*(5), 850–857.

Margolis, D. J., Knauss, J., & Bilker, W. (2002). Hormone replacement therapy and prevention of pressure ulcers and venous leg ulcers. *Lancet, 359*(9307), 675–677.

Milgrom, H., & Huang, H. (2014). Allergic disorders at a venerable age: A mini-review. *Gerontology, 60*(2), 99–107. doi: 10.1159/000355307.

Morimoto, Y., Yoshimura, M., Utada, K., et al. (2009). Prediction of postoperative delirium after abdominal surgery in the elderly. *Journal of Anesthesia, 23*(1), 51–56. doi: 10.1007/s00540-008-0688-1.

Pappas, A. (2009). Epidermal surface lipids. *Dermatoendocrinology, 1*(2), 72–76.

Patel, R. M., & Marfatia, Y. S. (2008). Clinical study of cutaneous drug eruptions in 200 patients. *Indian Journal of Dermatology, Venereology and Leprology, 74*(4), 430.

Pautex, S., & Vogt-Ferrier, N. (2006). Management of chronic pain in older persons. *Revue Médicale Suisse, 2*(71), 1629–1630, 1632–1623.

Popeo, D. M. (2011). Delirium in older adults. *Mount Sinai Journal of Medicine, 78*(4), 571–582. doi: 10.1002/msj.20267.

Rademaker, M. (2001). Do women have more adverse drug reactions? *American Journal of Clinical Dermatology, 2*(6), 349–351.

Rawlings, A. V. (2006). Ethnic skin types: are there differences in skin structure and function? *International Journal of Cosmetic Science, 28*(2), 79–93.

Reddy, M., Holroyd-Leduc, J., Cheung, C., et al. (2007). Geriatric principles in the practice of chronic wound care. In D. Krasner, G. T. Rodeheaver, & R. G. Sibbald (Eds.), *Chronic Wound Care: A Clinical Source Book for Healthcare Professionals* (4th ed., pp. 663–768). Malvern, PA: HMP Communications.

Redelmeier, D. A., Thiruchelvam, D., & Daneman, N. (2008). Delirium after elective surgery among elderly patients taking statins. *CMAJ, 179*(7), 645–652. doi: 10.1503/cmaj.080443.

Robinson, T. N., Raeburn, C. D., Tran, Z. V., et al. (2009). Postoperative delirium in the elderly: Risk factors and outcomes. *Annals of Surgery, 249*(1), 173–178. doi: 10.1097/SLA.0b013e31818e4776.

Rudolph, J. L., & Marcantonio, E. R. (2011). Review articles: Postoperative delirium: acute change with long-term implications. *Anesthesia and Analgesia,112*(5),1202–1211.doi:10.1213/ANE.0b013e3182147f6d.

Seyfarth, F., Schliemann, S., Antonov, D., et al. (2011). Teaching interventions in contact dermatitis. *Dermatitis, 22*(1), 8–15.

Shi, V. Y., Tran, K., & Lio, P. A. (2012). A comparison of physiochemical properties of a selection of modern moisturizers: hydrophilic index and pH. *Journal of Drugs and Dermatology, 11*(5), 633–636.

Shu, Y. Y., & Maibach, H. I. (2011). Estrogen and skin: Therapeutic options. *American Journal of Clinical Dermatology, 12*(5), 297–311. doi: 10.2165/11589180-000000000-00000.

Siddiqi, N., Stockdale, R., Britton, A. M., et al. (2007). Interventions for preventing delirium in hospitalised patients. *Cochrane Database of Systematic Reviews,* (2), CD005563. doi: 10.1002/14651858.CD005563.pub2.

Siddiqi, N., Young, J., House, A. O., et al. (2011). Stop Delirium! A complex intervention to prevent delirium in care homes: A mixed-methods feasibility study. *Age and Ageing, 40*(1), 90–98. doi: 10.1093/ageing/afq126.

Stojadinovic, O., Gordon, K., Lebrun, E., et al. (2012). Stress-induced hormones cortisol and epinephrine impair wound epithelialization. *Adv Wound Care, 1*(1), 29–35.

Szokol, J. W. (2010). Postoperative cognitive dysfunction. *Conferencias Magistrales, 33*(Suppl 1), S249–S253.

Weinberg, J. M., Vafaie, J., & Scheinfeld, N. S. (2004). Skin infections in the elderly. *Dermatologic Clinics, 22*(1), 51–61.

White-Chu, E. F., & Reddy, M. (2011). Dry skin in the elderly: Complexities of a common problem. *Clinics in Dermatology, 29*(1), 37–42. doi: 10.1016/j.clindermatol.2010.07.005.

Xin, S., Liu, W., & Cheng, B. (2009). Biological effects of estrogen on capillary vessel formation in wound healing. *Zhongguo Xiu Fu Chong Jian Wai Ke Za Zhi, 23*(12), 1502–1505.

Yaar, M. (2006). Clinical and histological features of intrinsic versus extrinsic skin aging. In B. A. Gilchrest, J. Krutmann (Eds.), *Skin Aging* (1st ed., pp. 198). Germany: Springer.

Yang, R., Wolfson, M., & Lewis, M. C. (2011). Unique aspects of the elderly surgical population: An anesthesiologist's perspective. *Geriatriatric Orthopedic Surgery & Rehabilitation, 2*(2), 56–64. doi: 10.1177/2151458510394606.

Young, D. L., & Chakravarthy, D. (2014). A controlled laboratory comparison of 4 topical skin creams moisturizing capability on human subjects. *Journal of Wound, Ostomy, and Continence Nursing, 41*(2), 168–174. doi: 110.1097/WON.0000000000000011.

QUESTIONS

1. The wound care nurse is assessing patients in a long-term care facility for pressure ulcers. What adverse age-related changes in cell biology may contribute to the development of these wounds?
A. Cell strains with longer telomeres that undergo significantly fewer doublings than younger subjects' cells
B. Progressive increase of fibroblasts and increased proliferative capacity of the remaining fibroblasts
C. Increased inflammatory response due to a decreased production of mast cells
D. Loss of telomeres resulting in cellular senescence or spontaneous cellular death

2. Which age-related skin alteration may interfere with the Langerhans cells' ability to eradicate carcinogenic cells?
A. Reduced melanocyte function
B. Thinning of adipose layer
C. Reduced vitamin D production
D. Altered fibroblast function

3. What age-related alteration, critical to maintenance of normal dermal function, is a common cause of delayed wound healing in the elderly?
A. Altered melanocyte function
B. Thinning of adipose layer
C. Reduced vitamin D production
D. Altered fibroblast function

4. An elderly patient presents with documented symptoms of prodromal pain, itching, and a sharp stabbing pain, followed by a vesicular rash. What skin alteration is most likely the cause of these symptoms?
A. Candidiasis
B. Contact dermatitis
C. Herpes zoster
D. Scabies

5. An elderly patient with a partial-thickness pressure ulcer is experiencing delayed wound healing. What age-related factor may contribute to this condition?
A. Increased keratinocyte proliferative capacity
B. Reduced cell-to-cell communication
C. Increased blood flow
D. Tripling of repetition time for fibroblasts

6. Which statement accurately describes an age-related skin alteration that may delay full-thickness wound healing?
A. There is reduced fibroblast function.
B. An increased degranulation of platelets and release of growth factors and platelet-derived growth factor occurs.
C. There are increased numbers of macrophages, which partially explains the diminished inflammatory response that is typically seen.
D. Age-related stress can result in decreased production of cortisol, glucocorticoids, and epinephrine, which delays wound healing.

7. An elderly patient with a full-thickness wound is experiencing a delayed remodeling phase of wound repair. What is a usual causative factor?
A. Failure to develop tensile strength in the wound
B. Increased perfusion to the wound
C. Increased epithelial migration and resurfacing
D. Increased rate of granulation tissue formation

8. The wound care nurse visiting a patient in a nursing home suspects that the patient is a victim of elder abuse. In this situation the nurse should:
A. Investigate the nursing home staff
B. Substantiate the abuse before reporting to the proper authorities
C. Report the suspected abuse to legal authorities
D. Inform the elder of his or her legal right to report the abuse

9. A patient in a long-term care facility is experiencing a disturbance of consciousness and change in cognition developing over a short period of time. Symptoms include restlessness, irritability, and agitation. What condition would the nurse suspect?
A. Alzheimer's disease
B. Hyperactive delirium
C. Hypoactive delirium
D. Dementia

10. The wound care nurse assesses an elderly patient with delayed wound healing who is being treated with topical glucocorticosteroids for severe eczema. For what systemic reaction would the nurse monitor this patient?
A. Fluid retention
B. Diabetes
C. Cataracts
D. Hyperglycemia

11. A wound care nurse is monitoring a patient who has been prescribed diphenhydramine for insomnia. This patient is at greater risk for:
A. Delirium
B. Hypertension
C. Perioral dermatitis
D. Rhabdomyolysis

12. Which statement accurately describes a recommendation for pain management in the elderly?
A. NSAIDs should be given routinely for chronic pain.
B. Opioids cannot be safely used in older adults.
C. Acetaminophen should be given for mild-to-moderate musculoskeletal pain.
D. High doses of NSAIDs should be given for acute pain.

ANSWERS: 1.**D**, 2.**A**, 3.**D**, 4.**C**, 5.**B**, 6.**A**, 7.**A**, 8.**C**, 9.**B**, 10.**D**, 11.**A**, 12.**C**

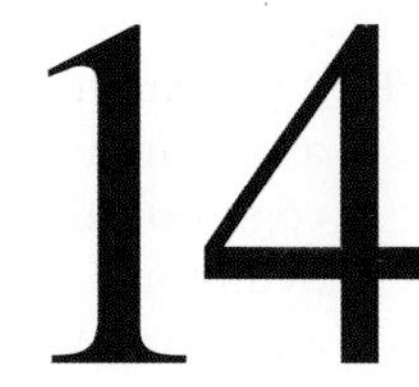

CHAPTER 14

Skin and Wound Care for the Bariatric Population

Susan S. Morello

OBJECTIVES

1. Describe common skin care issues for the bariatric patient, to include measures for prevention and management.
2. Discuss issues related to pressure ulcer prevention among special populations, to include the bariatric patient.
3. Explain why bariatric patients are at increased risk for surgical wound dehiscence and implications for prevention and management.
4. Describe factors to be considered in selection of beds, mattresses, chair cushions, and room equipment for bariatric patients.
5. Discuss psychosocial issues to be addressed when caring for bariatric patients.

Topic Outline

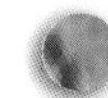 Introduction

The number of morbidly obese individuals is increasing, and skin and wound care for this group presents specific challenges. Those challenges are the focus of this chapter.

Definitions

The CDC (Centers for Disease Control) refers to individuals whose weight exceeds the ranges generally considered healthy for one's height as obese and overweight. The standard unit of measurement used to determine whether an adult is overweight or obese is the Body Mass Index (BMI). BMI is calculated by dividing the individual's weight in kilograms by her/his height in meters squared. A BMI of 25 is considered normal, a BMI of >25 to 29 is considered overweight, and a BMI of >30 meets the definition for obese. Some sources further classify individuals as obese (BMI > 30), severely obese (BMI > 35), morbidly obese (BMI > 40), and super obese (BMI > 50) (Obesity Surgery Dallas, 2014). BMI is considered to be a measurement of risk for adverse health conditions; however, the BMI score does not adjust for factors such as bodybuilding, gender, or ethnic differences, and these factors must be considered when interpreting BMI for an individual. Another method used to calculate an individual's adipose tissue is the Body Adiposity Index (BAI). BAI uses hip width measurement instead of weight, and a different formula for calculation (Bergman et al., 2011). The BAI may provide a more accurate measurement of body adiposity and as such may be a better indicator for adverse health conditions. Research on use of the BAI is ongoing, so at present BMI remains the most consistently used indicator for obesity.

Prevalence

In 1985, the CDC published figures that indicated that the percentage of overweight and obese adults in the United States was increasing. Those early figures revealed that the obese population of the United States was as high as 14% in some areas of the country. Over the next 15 years, the percentages continued to increase. By 2012, the number of obese adults in the United States had risen to the point that the state with the lowest percentage of obese adults (Colorado with 20.5%) had surpassed the 14% high reported in 1985 (CDC, 2014b). According to the Trust for America's Health, the percentage of adults who are overweight or obese has doubled in the past 30 years and is now about 68% (Levi et al., 2013).

The problem of rising obesity rates is not an issue for the United States alone. According to the World Health Organization, at least 35% of the world's adults (those over 20 years of age) are overweight and, in 2008, 10% of men and 14% of women worldwide were classified as obese (World Health Organization, 2014). In addition, obesity is not limited to the adult population. In 2012, the incidence of obesity in children aged 6 to 11 in the United States was nearly 12% and for adolescents aged 12 to 19 nearly 21%. Although there are many programs available to help curb the rising rate of childhood obesity, studies indicate that most children who are overweight and obese carry that weight into adulthood (CDC, 2014a). This is an unfortunate indication that the bariatric patient population will probably continue to rise for many years to come.

CLINICAL PEARL

The prevalence of obesity is rising worldwide, among children as well as adults, and current data indicate that most obese children carry the increased weight into adulthood; this indicates that the bariatric population will probably continue to rise for many years to come.

Health and Fiscal Impact

Regardless of the method used to determine obesity, what is known is that the risk of adverse health conditions increases as obesity increases. In 2013, the American Medical Association classified obesity as a disease, which represented a change from the previous stance that obesity was a life style problem. Although an imbalance between caloric intake and activity (energy expenditure) remains the primary etiologic factor for obesity, it is now recognized that genetic, metabolic, environmental, and other factors also play a role in the development of this disease (Gallagher, 2005). The epidemic of obesity has been identified as the leading cause of death and disability in the United States (Blackett et al., 2011). Hypertension, heart disease, type 2 diabetes, and stroke are just a few of the comorbidities associated with obesity and severe obesity (Beitz, 2014). Often these chronic conditions lead to hospitalization and add to the already-rising costs of health care. In the United States, during 2009, over $150 billion was spent on direct medical costs associated with obesity. In that same year, the indirect costs of obesity (lost work hours, insurance premiums and compensations, and lower wages) totaled $6.4 billion, and obesity related loss of productivity totaled $30 billion (Hoffman, 2013). The numbers are even higher when health care for overweight individuals is included; it is estimated that over $300 billion is spent annually on the health care needs of the obese and overweight population (Blackett et al., 2011). All those dollars reflect the monetary cost of obesity and its related diseases. The greater cost is that of life...more than 100,000 obesity-related deaths occur each year (Schafer & Ferraro, 2007).

CLINICAL PEARL

More than 100,000 obesity-related deaths occur each year.

Skin Care for the Bariatric Patient

Currently, the number of obese and overweight individuals in our hospitals is increasing, and these individuals are admitted with more comorbidities and require longer lengths of stay than the nonbariatric patient (Lowe, 2008; Schafer & Ferraro, 2007). Increased weight, limited mobility, excessive moisture (from increased perspiration), and reduced tissue perfusion and oxygenation all contribute to increased risk for skin injury (Kennedy-Evans et al., 2007; Shipman & Millington, 2011). In addition, the stress and anxiety associated with hospitalization can negatively affect skin integrity. The systemic effects of hormones and cytokines may also play a contributing role in skin breakdown (Guo & de Pieto, 2010). Prevention of skin breakdown and treatment of preexisting skin issues become a primary focus in caring for the obese patient.

Assessment

The first step in prevention is a comprehensive assessment, including history, comorbidities, risk assessment, and thorough inspection of the skin with special attention to pressure point areas. Use of pressure ulcer risk assessment tools such as the Braden scale is extremely useful in determining risk for pressure ulcer development; while the total score provides an overall summary of risk, subscale scores provide invaluable insight into particular risk factors that must be addressed. Although all subscales are important, when evaluating the obese patient, special attention needs to be paid to the areas of moisture, mobility, and friction and shear.

CLINICAL PEARL

When assessing a bariatric patient for pressure ulcer risk status, particular attention should be paid to the areas of moisture, mobility, and friction and shear.

When assessing exposure to moisture, the nurse should carefully examine the skin between body folds, such as under the breasts, under the pannus, and in the perineal area. It is important to be gentle when examining the pannus; the nurse should carefully lift the pannus and should examine both the upper and lower surfaces of the skin at the innermost junction. Lifting a pannus that is extremely heavy may require use of lifting equipment. Often skin folds in the neck, upper arms, legs, ankles, and the gluteal sulcus (gluteal fold) are overlooked. A patient may deny incontinence but still exhibit signs of irritation and moisture damage in the perineal area, which may be due to inadequate cleansing as opposed to incontinence. Thus, visual inspection of the perineal skin is essential; it is not sufficient to simply ask the patient about incontinence.

Asking the patient to turn in bed for skin assessment provides an excellent opportunity to assess how well the patient moves in bed and the adequacy of the current bed. Is the patient able to turn himself? Is there sufficient room in the bed for the patient to turn unassisted or with assistance? Is there need for a trapeze or other mobility equipment? In addition to evaluating the patient, the nurse should also evaluate the need for safe patient handling equipment, transfer and repositioning devices, and bariatric bed and mattress. Although mobility and activity are often separate subscales, when evaluating mobility, the nurse should assess the patient's ability to sit up in bed, move to the side of the bed, and transfer or stand. This last set of maneuvers can be accomplished in reverse if the patient is sitting in a chair at the beginning of the assessment.

CLINICAL PEARL

Asking the patient to turn in bed for skin assessment provides an excellent opportunity to assess the individual for mobility.

Sensory perception may be impaired by medications, fatigue, medical issues, or diminished tissue perfusion and should be assessed routinely (and at least daily). The nurse should be particularly alert to the skin under tubes, compression devices, and other devices that may lead to medical device–related pressure ulcers. Wrinkled sheets, excess linen, and incontinence pads may also contribute to increased pressure and therefore increased risk for skin breakdown. The nurse should determine whether or not the patient senses discomfort related to medical devices or objects that create pressure points.

Accurate assessment of activity is also important and requires the nurse to do more than ask the patient about his/her ability to walk. The obese patient may report he or she has no issues with activity. Patients may state that they are not hampered when they walk, have no difficulty getting around or transferring, and generally need no assistance with these activities. That may or may not be the situation at home. However, they are in an unfamiliar place, often in a room filled with medical equipment and little space to move around, surroundings quite different than those at home. Activity is therefore best evaluated on a day-to-day basis. It is important to ask the patient to transfer from the bed to a chair, to walk to the bathroom, or to ambulate in the room and hall, and to carefully observe the patient during performance of these activities. Part of evaluating activity means determining whether or not activity is self-motivated or primarily motivated by nursing staff. All of the above data contribute to a full and accurate assessment of the patient's activity level.

In addition to an in-depth skin and risk assessment, every bariatric patient should have a complete nutritional assessment to determine if protein, carbohydrate, fluid, and other nutritional requirements for health and healing are being met. Monitoring intake and output for 48 hours is helpful when a nutritional consult is not immediately available.

Factors known to contribute to compromised skin integrity in the bariatric patient include excess weight, moisture issues, reduced tissue perfusion, and comorbidities (Kennedy-Evans et al., 2007). These individuals are at major risk for shear and friction damage due to difficulty in turning and transferring in and out of bed; the risk is increased among those with dry fragile skin or hot wet skin. Bariatric patients are also at risk for skin tears that occur when they bump against the side rails or other equipment, or related to assistance required for moving and transferring. Finally, they are at risk for pressure ulcers due to the excess weight and their difficulty in turning and repositioning themselves. In summary, the majority of bariatric patients are at risk for moisture-associated skin damage (MASD), friction and shear injuries, skin tears, and pressure ulcers, and they require aggressive and comprehensive preventive care to maintain skin integrity (Beitz, 2014; Black et al., 2011; Gray et al., 2011).

CLINICAL PEARL

The majority of bariatric patients are at risk for MASD, friction and shear injuries, skin tears, and pressure ulcers.

Skin and risk assessment should be completed daily for the bariatric patient, even in areas such as rehabilitation units where risk assessment is generally performed on a weekly basis. In critical care areas, skin and risk assessment should be performed more frequently and minimally once every shift for the bariatric patient.

Routine Skin Care

Maintaining the integrity of the skin is primary in prevention of skin breakdown; and maintenance begins with daily skin care. The basic components of skin care should be provided to every patient and include the following: (1) daily inspection, (2) routine cleansing, (3) moisturization, and (4) protection. Patients who are not at risk for skin breakdown and who have no mobility or moisture issues may not require daily inspection unless their at-risk status changes. However, individuals with compromised circulation, moisture problems related to incontinence or diaphoresis, or issues with activity, mobility, or sensory function require daily skin assessment and routine skin care protocols, whether they are at home or in a health care facility. Discharge planning for obese patients should include instructions for daily skin inspection and proper skin care. Because adequate maintenance of skin may be difficult if not impossible for the obese and severely obese individual, discharge planning and education should include individual(s) who are assisting with care of the bariatric patient in the home setting. If the patient receives care from a home health care provider or home aide, instruction for proper skin care should be communicated to those individuals as well.

CLINICAL PEARL

Many obese and severely obese individuals are unable to provide hygienic care independently; thus, discharge instructions regarding skin care should be communicated to assisting individuals as well as the patient.

Full bathing need not be a daily requirement; however, daily cleansing should be provided to the following areas: under the arms (armpits), under the breasts, within all skin folds, and the perineal area. In addition, daily skin care should include any areas with excessive moisture loss or accumulation, for example, weeping legs, arms, or neck. Protecting the pH balance of the skin is important to maintenance of skin integrity; thus, cleansing is ideally done using a pH-balanced liquid soap or skin cleanser or disposable pH-balanced cleansing wipes. Cleansing agents should be free of perfumes and other skin irritants, and the skin should be gently washed without scrubbing; drying should involve patting but not rubbing, which could irritate the skin. A cool hairdryer may also be used to dry the skin, especially in areas that are more difficult to access (Black et al., 2011). Disposable cleansing wipes are generally pH balanced, do not require rinsing, and dry quickly without the use of a towel or hairdryer; they are preferred by many for those reasons.

Hygienic care for the obese patient is no different than for nonbariatric patients with at-risk skin; the same principles for washing and drying apply to both groups. However, care for the bariatric patient must include measures to assure adequate cleansing and drying within all of the skin folds. Because the area within the skin folds remains moist due to perspiration (Gray et al., 2011), these areas should be examined periodically throughout the day and cleaned and dried if moist. In addition, the nurse should use wicking products or absorptive products to keep skin folds dry; specific options will be discussed later in this chapter. Routine cleansing of these areas is also important, in order to eliminate bacteria that could contribute to skin breakdown. Most of the smaller skin folds are easy to access and easy to clean. The larger skin folds on the abdomen (under the pannus) and on the back may require assistance with lifting to enable proper cleaning. To facilitate safe elevation of the pannus, lifting devices should be used. The use of a pannus sling promotes patient comfort and dignity and helps prevent staff injury; slings are available that can be used with either an overhead or a floor lift. If irritation or a wound is present on either surface of the pannus, dressings or medication should be applied prior to removal of the pannus sling.

CLINICAL PEARL

Skin folds represent high-risk areas for the bariatric patient; the skin must be cleansed and dried, and wicking fabrics (or substitutes) should be routinely used to prevent maceration and friction.

In addition to appropriate cleansing, maintenance of skin integrity for the bariatric patient includes routine use of appropriate moisturizers (Beitz, 2014). Moisturizers may contain emollients or humectants or a combination of the two (Black et al., 2011). Humectants attract water to the stratum corneum from the dermis and are indicated for extremely dry rough skin; they are not appropriate for skin folds and areas of trapped moisture. Emollients smooth flaky skin cells (O'Lenick, 2009) by replacing intercellular lipids in the stratum corneum (Black et al., 2011), which helps to maintain the integrity of the skin barrier; these products are appropriate for general use, even on fragile skin that is frequently moist. Like cleansing products, lotions and creams should be free of fragrance and other irritants. They can be applied multiple times during the day to maintain healthy skin. If profuse sweating is present, the skin should be cleansed prior to application of the lotion or cream, and the nurse should assure that the product is nonocclusive; agents containing dimethicone are usually a good choice.

The final step in skin care is protection of skin that is exposed to excessive moisture from urine and/or stool; this involves use of moisture barrier products such as petrolatum-based products or clear plasticizing barrier films. Chapter 17 provides an in-depth discussion of prevention and management of MASD, specifically incontinence-associated dermatitis (IAD) and intertriginous dermatitis (ITD). Thus the discussion in this chapter will be limited to specific considerations for the bariatric patient related to these conditions.

Incontinence-Associated Dermatitis

Prevention of skin damage is always the primary goal. Careful assessment will identify patients at risk for IAD, who require prevention measures beyond normal skin cleansing and moisturizing. Use of ointments containing dimethicone, petrolatum, or zinc oxide applied to the perineal and buttocks areas provides protection from both moisture and chemical irritants. The ointment should be applied after initial cleaning and reapplied after each toileting or incontinence episode. Caregivers need to know that it is not necessary to remove barrier ointment after each toileting or incontinent episode; rather, they should simply wipe away any soiled ointment and replace with additional barrier ointment. A perineal cleanser or wipe should be used to gently remove the ointment once daily in order to inspect the skin.

Routine protection of the perineal area should continue after discharge. Although the bariatric patient may not complain of incontinence, it may be difficult for the bariatric or obese person to properly clean themselves after toileting. The importance of routine cleansing and protection of the skin in the perineal area and buttocks should be discussed with the patient prior to discharge. If self-application of protective ointments is difficult for the individual, she/he can be instructed to use a three-in-one product that provides cleansing, moisturizing, and protection in a disposable wipe. In addition, personal hygiene accessories are available that can assist the patient in cleansing and in application of ointments to the perineal and buttocks areas.

CLINICAL PEARL

Personal hygiene accessories are available that assist the patient to cleanse the perineal area and to provide protective creams and ointments.

Intertriginous Dermatitis (ITD)

Excessive sweating, a more alkaline pH at the surface of the skin, and decreased capillary flow have a detrimental effect on the skin's moisture barrier (Gray et al., 2011). This is even more apparent in the skin folds, especially underneath the pannus and under the breasts. These areas generate and trap moisture, which can result in ITD if appropriate preventive care is not provided. Because it is often difficult for the bariatric individual to adequately clean and dry within the skin folds, these areas can become macerated and can also serve as a breeding ground for bacterial and fungal growth.

Controlling the moisture in skin folds, especially the deep skin folds, is extremely important. The use of absorbent linen (e.g., soft towels, thick cotton athletic socks, or cloth diapers) or soft absorptive pads such as abdominal pads or sanitary pads placed within the skin folds and under the breasts may be helpful. These products absorb the moisture and also separate the skin folds, thus protecting against frictional forces. Absorptive linens and pads should be changed frequently to prevent moisture damage and odor. In addition, it may be necessary to find ways to stabilize the absorptive linen or pad when the patient is out of bed.

There are products that have been made specifically to absorb and wick away moisture (e.g., Interdry, Coloplast, Inc.). This specific type of textile is a polyurethane-coated material impregnated with antimicrobial silver; one end of the fabric sheet should be placed at the base of the fold, and the other end should extend about 4 to 6 inches beyond the fold. This provides for wicking and evaporation of moisture on a continual basis and also provides for separation of the folds and protection against frictional forces. Because the material is a single layer and thin, it generally remains in place when the patient gets out of bed.

If bacterial or fungal infection develops within the folds, appropriate medicated powder or cream should be applied sparingly. While this may address the infection, there is still a need for absorption of excess moisture. Previously discussed measures should be initiated after treatment with medication.

Friction Injury

In addition to prevention of MASD, skin care for the bariatric patient should include measures to prevent friction damage. Friction damage can occur when moist or fragile skin surfaces are exposed to superficial abrasive (rubbing) force, such as when the sides of a skin fold rub against each other. Preventive measures include wicking moisture away from body folds, gentle handling during bathing and positioning, separation of skin folds (with either wicking fabric or absorptive pads or linens), and protective dressings to vulnerable sites, such as use of gentle adhesive foam dressings to the sacrococcygeal area.

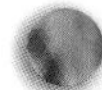 Pressure Ulcer Prevention

Pressure ulcers are addressed in depth in Chapters 18 and 19; however, it is important for all caregivers to recognize that obese individuals are at increased risk for pressure ulcers, when hospitalized and when at home. As noted earlier in this chapter, the skin of the bariatric patient is poorly vascularized, may be dry and fragile, is prone to maceration from excess sweating, and is also exposed to friction and shear, all of which contribute to increased risk for pressure ulcers. Immobility, poor nutrition and inadequate equipment can further add to the risk (Mathison, 2003). In addition, when the obese person's tissues are exposed to pressure, there is a more significant compromise in perfusion due to the greater weight applied to the tissue in contact with the bed or chair; this results in more significant cell deformation and increased likelihood of pressure ulcers and other pressure-related skin injuries (Lowe, 2008). Pressure ulcers generally occur over bony prominences, but atypical pressure ulcers may develop in obese patients at any site where pressure, moisture, friction, and shear are present, for example, within the skin folds, at the neck, upper back, upper medial thigh, flanks, and posterior legs and ankles (Beitz, 2014). This is even more apparent in the critically ill bariatric patient; studies have shown that a critically ill person's chances of acquiring a pressure ulcer are 1.5 times greater when their BMI is between 30 and 39.9. If the BMI is ≥40, there is a threefold increase in risk of pressure ulcer development (Lowe, 2008).

CLINICAL PEARL

Individuals with BMI >30 are at increased risk for pressure ulcer development; individuals with BMI >40 are at three times greater risk than an individual of normal weight.

Pressure ulcer prevention protocols and daily skin and risk reassessment should be initiated on admission. Proper skin care is a major component of prevention and treatment, as are frequent turning and repositioning. Assessment should include routine inspection of the skin under tubes, drains, and other medical devices as these can be an overlooked source of pressure damage.

Selection of the appropriate bed frame and support surface is of critical importance for the bariatric patient (Fig. 14-1). Based on the increasing number and size of bariatric patients, many mattress manufacturers have increased the weight limits for replacement mattresses and bed frames to 500 pounds in order to accommodate the majority of these individuals. However, weight tolerance cannot be the only consideration when selecting a mattress; the girth of the obese person should also be taken into account when making this decision. There must be adequate space on each side of the patient both for patient comfort and to facilitate turning. Although no exact formula exits for the amount of extra space needed, the rule of thumb is 12 to 16 inches total space or 6 to 8 inches on each side of the mattress. Most often this will provide adequate space for the patient to turn unassisted in bed and/or for the staff to assist with safely turning the patient.

CLINICAL PEARL

In determining the need for a bariatric bed, the nurse must consider both patient weight and patient girth.

There are many bed frames and mattresses available for the bariatric patient. When selecting a bariatric bed, the nurse must verify that the weight of the patient falls within the weight limits of the frame and mattress as specified by the manufacturer. The use of a low bed is frequently beneficial since it will allow the bariatric patient assistance in egress from the bed. The wound nurse should assure that guidelines regarding bed selection are readily available to those ordering the equipment. A bed algorithm linking hip width and weight to the appropriate bed is a very useful tool in accomplishing this task.

Once the proper bed has been selected, mattress selection becomes the next important decision. Support surfaces are discussed in Chapter 20 of this text, but a few points about selection of a support surface for a bariatric patient will be considered here. The requirement of a bariatric bed frame does not always necessitate a specialty support surface. Foam and enhanced foam mattresses are available and can be used when mobility, exposure to moisture, sensory status, and level of consciousness are within normal limits. If the patient is at-risk in any of these areas, a therapeutic air support surface should be considered. A low air loss mattress with or without alternating pressure therapy can address moisture issues and provide pressure redistribution to help prevent pressure ulcer occurrence.

If pulmonary or respiratory conditions exist, a mattress with lateral rotation can be provided for the bariatric patient. Although this type of surface provides pulmonary therapy and can be used to assist in turning the patient, it must be remembered that this type of support surface does not provide adequate pressure redistribution for the

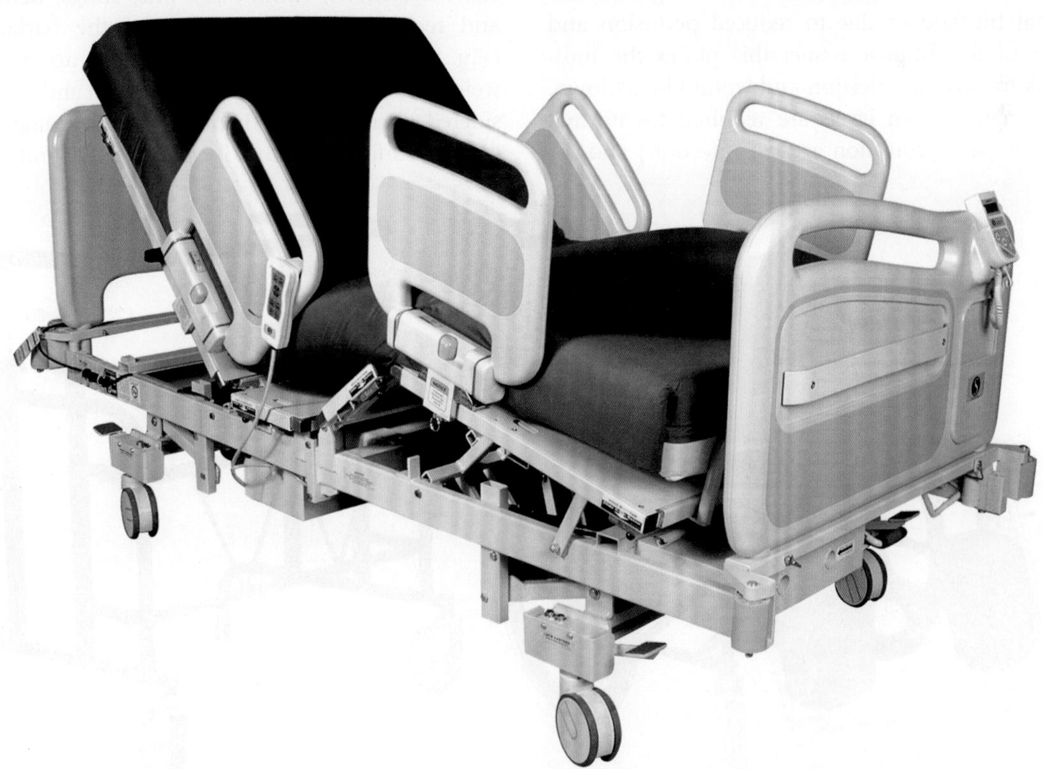

FIGURE 14-1. Bariatric bed. Proper selection of a bed and support surface for the bariatric patient is determined by height, weight, and width of the patient as well as the need for prevention and/or treatment of skin integrity issues. (Reprinted with permission from Sizewise.)

prevention of pressure ulcers. Turning and repositioning are still required. Studies suggest that 18 hours of rotation therapy is necessary per day for adequate pulmonary toileting (Ahrens et al., 2004; Shapiro & Keegan, 1992; Traver et al., 1995). These data suggest that, in most cases, rotation therapy can be interrupted for 30 minutes every 2 to 3 hours for turning and repositioning to help prevent pressure damage.

Pressure ulcer prevention must also include attention to prevention of shear damage, which occurs when the patient slides down in bed. The deep tissue layers move down in response to gravity, while the superficial layers remain adherent to the sheets; the intervening tissue layers undergo shear force, which causes compression of the vessels passing through the soft tissue. Shear damage commonly involves the coccyx and ischial tuberosity areas. The use of protective dressings on the sacral area of at-risk bariatric patients may help to prevent this type of skin and soft tissue injury. In addition, physical therapy can assist the patient in learning how to move in bed and how to transfer properly in order to reduce the risk of shear injury. Use of a trapeze may also assist the bariatric patient with bed mobility and sitting up. Placing the bed in the lowest position and use of a walker can help to reduce friction and shear damage during transfers.

Surgical Wound Dehiscence

Another area of concern when working with the bariatric patient population is the postsurgical complication of wound dehiscence. Bariatric patients are at greater risk for incisional breakdown due to reduced perfusion and oxygenation of the adipose tissue; this places the individual at risk for wound infection and wound breakdown, because adequate oxygen levels are required for normal WBC function (and protection against infection) and for all aspects of wound healing, including collagen synthesis (Kennedy-Evans et al., 2007; Shipman & Millington, 2011). In addition, the increased weight of the abdominal wall creates increased mechanical stress along the incision, further increasing the risk of incisional breakdown (Lowe, 2008).

The nurse must provide ongoing monitoring of the incision for any evidence of infection and/or excess mechanical stress. An abdominal binder may be used to offset the effects of the increased adipose tissue (Lowe, 2008). It is important to assure proper sizing of the abdominal binder; ideally, abdominal girth should be measured prior to surgery in order to have the proper-size abdominal binder available after surgery. Application of the binder postoperatively should be based on physician order and/or facility policy and procedure. Although the use of negative pressure wound therapy (NPWT) has been suggested as one strategy for prevention of wound dehiscence, to date there are no studies demonstrating effectiveness in reducing wound dehiscence (Ingargiola et al., 2013; Payne & Edwards, 2014).

CLINICAL PEARL

Appropriately sized binders may help reduce the risk of incisional dehiscence.

Bariatric Equipment

Standard-sized equipment essentials, for example, walkers, wheelchairs, commodes, lifts, slings, bedside chairs, and recliners, are inadequate for the bariatric patient (Fig. 14-2). These products must also accommodate the weight and width of the bariatric patient and should be considered when ordering a bariatric bed. Including them on the support surface algorithm is encouraged. Family and visitors

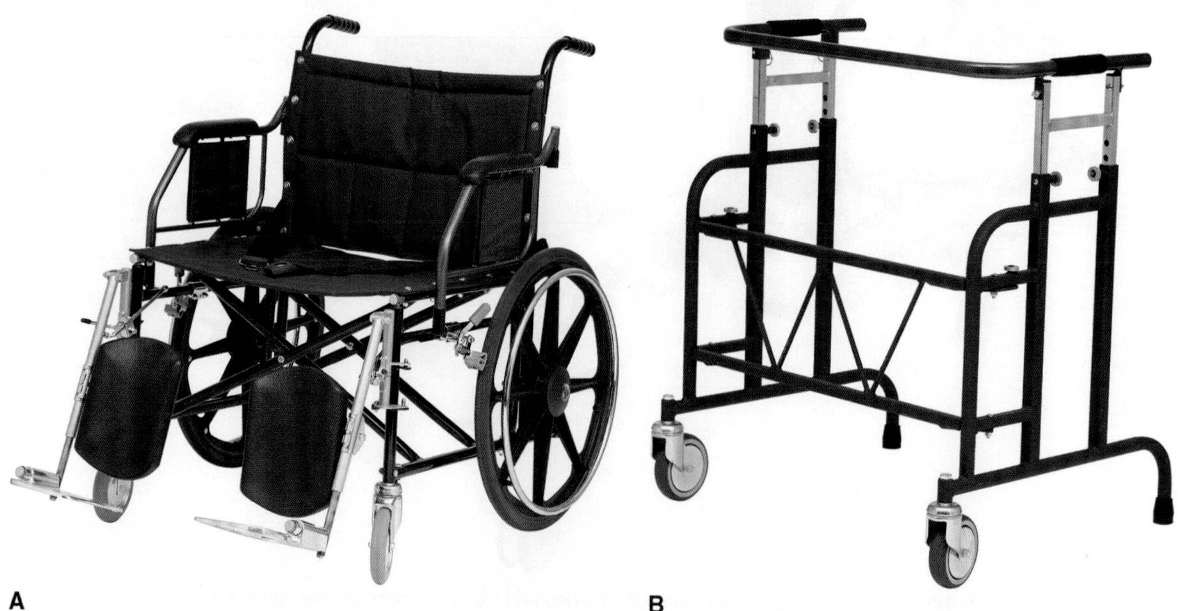

A B

FIGURE 14-2. Wheelchair and walker. When additional mobility equipment is needed for the bariatric patient, equipment must meet the weight capacity of the intended patient and be single-patient use only. (Reprinted with permission of Sizewise.)

may be obese as well, so furniture in the room of the bariatric patient should have extended-capacity weight limits.

Hospital gowns and other clothing needs can be obtained in a variety of larger sizes and should be readily available for the patient. The use of larger bedpans, underpads, tracheostomy ties, catheters, and the like not only contribute to the comfort of the patient but are added protection from pressure injury.

Safe Patient Handling

Many health care facilities have implemented programs to prevent patient and staff injury; this type of program is extremely important when caring for bariatric patients. Wound care requires the staff to turn patients, elevate the limbs, and inspect the interior surfaces of the skin folds, all of which are associated with risk of injury. When one considers that the weight of a person's leg is approximately 16% of their total body weight, it is clear that the simple act of elevating the leg of a bariatric person exceeds the recommended safety limits for weight lifting (Muir & Archer-Heese, 2009) and places all health care workers at risk for injury. This task and many others that are performed on a daily basis mandate that the staff become active participants in workplace safety programs. While it may be more time consuming to obtain staff assistance and proper equipment that is not readily available in the patient's room or in the clinic area, concern for safety of the patient and those involved with the task at hand needs to be foremost in everyone's mind. The use of lifts and specialty slings, for example, pannus and limb slings, can relieve some of the risk (Figs. 14-3 and 14-4).

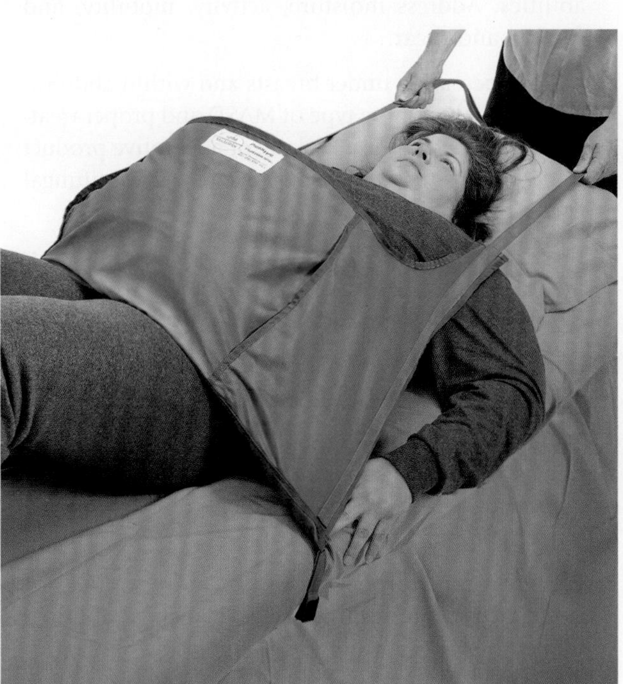

FIGURE 14-3. Pannus sling. Use of pannus sling allows safe elevation of pannus for examination of skin without discomfort to the patient or risk of injury to health care provider. (Reprinted with permission of Alpha Modalities LLC—Sling Specialists in Safe Patient Mobility.)

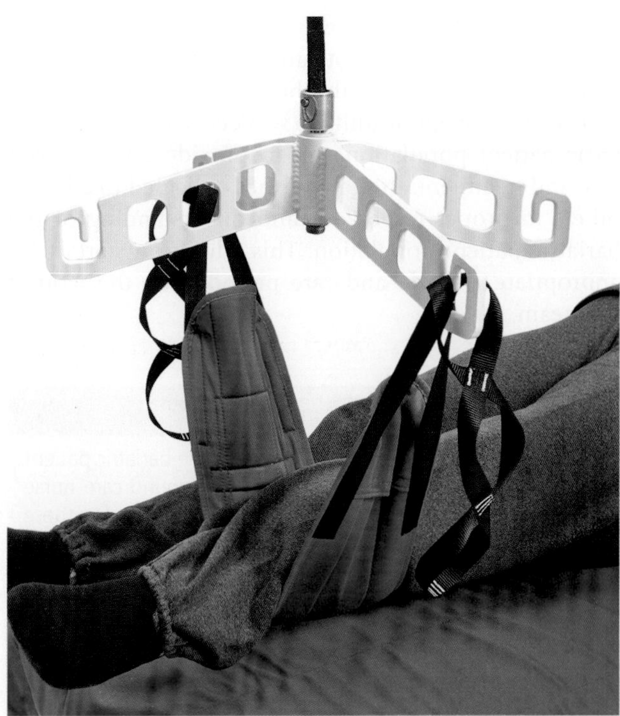

FIGURE 14-4. Limb sling. Limb sling provides safe elevation of an arm or leg for examination or treatment; it enhances comfort for the patient and safety for the health care provider. (Reprinted with permission of Alpha Modalities LLC—Sling Specialists in Safe Patient Mobility.)

Not all at-risk tasks can be eliminated, so staff must learn to rely on the use of equipment to assist with those tasks.

> **CLINICAL PEARL**
>
> Safe patient handling of bariatric patients requires the use of lifts and pannus slings; even lifting the leg of a bariatric patient exceeds safe lifting guidelines.

Bariatric Sensitivity

The increase in the bariatric population in our health care systems is accompanied by an increase in bariatric prejudice. Studies show that health care providers are not exempt from this type of bias (Puhl & Heuer, 2009). Preconceived ideas about the causes of obesity, expectations of noncompliance, and a belief that the obese person lacks motivation have all been identified as contributing factors to insensitivity and prejudice related to the bariatric patient population. Verbiage indicating "large size" or "big boy" is an example of how health care workers refer to bariatric patients and equipment. Obese patients are aware of their size and the prejudice that many health care workers exhibit toward them. They often put off needed care and medical attention for fear of comments and rejection (Payne & Edwards, 2014). Bariatric sensitivity programs are a requirement at many health care facilities and have some effect on the reduction of bariatric bias. The most effective strategy in eradication of weight stigma and bias is the awareness that it exists and the motivation to change ideas and practices that perpetuate this behavior. Wound care providers have the opportunity to work closely with the bariatric patient population and to provide unprejudiced care and treatment; they are further obligated to educate others in proper respect for and understanding of the bariatric patient population. This education starts with appropriate attitude and care provided by the wound care team.

CLINICAL PEARL

Prejudice and bias are significant issues for the bariatric patient and a major barrier to health seeking; the wound care nurse should model respect and sensitivity when caring for these individuals.

Conclusion

Bariatric patients are at greater risk for MASD, friction injury, pressure/shear damage, and incisional dehiscence, due to issues with mobility, activity, and moisture trapping. The wound care nurse must implement an appropriate skin care program with particular attention to moisture management and routine repositioning; this requires separation of body folds for inspection, cleansing, and application of wicking products in addition to routine turning. Strategies to facilitate appropriate skin care and pressure ulcer prevention care include assuring availability and appropriate use of bariatric beds, mattresses, cushions, and positioners. The bariatric patient is also at risk for incisional dehiscence; one strategy for minimizing risk is routine use of a binder. Finally, the wound care nurse must address issues related to bias and must approach the care of these patients with respect and sensitivity.

CASE STUDY

Peggy R. is a 52-year-old obese female admitted to the hospital for complications following cholecystectomy surgery 12 days ago. She was discharged 4 days ago with no significant medical issues. Abdominal wound was intact. She has a history of HTN and DM, which are controlled with medication and diet. Physician orders include blood tests, medications, and nutrition consult, as well as abdominal wound care.

Admission assessment notes the following: Wt. 346 pounds (157 kg), abdominal wound (surgical wound) open and draining, pain level at 8 (on a 1 to 10 pain level scale), BP 157/88, Temp 101.6, Resp. 18.

Skin risk assessment notes the following: Open abdominal wound, Braden Score 18, no apparent pressure areas, open areas under breast and within abdominal fold, erythema present in perianal area, remainder of skin dry and intact.

Plan of action:

1. Evaluate for proper bed and support surface. Consider ordering a bariatric bed with appropriate surface. May be within weight limit for facility bed but consider width of patient in bed and if sufficient space for patient to turn or be turned on surface.
2. Examine Braden subscale scores to determine if patient at risk in any category rather than basing need for prevention only on total score. Braden subscale scores: Sensory Perception 4, Moisture 2, Activity 4, Mobility 3, Nutrition 3, Friction and Shear 2. Initial Braden score based substantially on the patient's responses to questions re: mobility, activity, sensory awareness, nutritional intake, and exposure to moisture. Need to re evaluate risk score based on patient's current condition and actual abilities. Address moisture, activity, mobility, and friction and shear.
3. Assess open areas under breasts and within abdominal fold to determine type of MASD and proper treatment (will need to use wicking or absorptive product under breast and pannus; may need to add antifungal agent if candidiasis present).
4. Assess erythema in perianal area to determine treatment (will probably need moisturizer–moisture barrier combination product)
5. Initiate enhanced skin care regimen to include addressing excess moisture and dry skin.
6. Evaluate need for additional equipment to facilitate safe handling of the patient. If required, order equipment with weight capacity sufficient to accommodate the weight and girth of the patient.
7. Provide wound care that maintains moist wound bed and effective control of exudate; consider abdominal binder to reduce traction on wound edges.

REFERENCES

Ahrens, T., Kollef, M., Stewart, J., et al. (2004). Effect of kinetic therapy on pulmonary complications. *American Journal of Critical Care, 13*(5), 376–382.

Beitz, J. (2014). Providing quality skin and wound care for the bariatric patient: An overview of clinical challenges. *Ostomy Wound Management, 60*(1), 12–21.

Bergman, R., Stefanovski, D., Buchanan, T., et al. (2011). A Better Index of Body Adiposity. Retrieved June 5, 2014 from http://www.ncbi.nlm.nih.gov/pubmed/21372804

Black, J., Gray, M., Bliss, D., et al. (2011). MASD Part 2: Incontinence-associated dermatitis and intertriginous dermatitis. *Journal of Wound, Ostomy, and Continence Nursing, 38*(4), 359–370.

Blackett, A., Gallagher, S., Dugan, S., et al. (2011). Caring for persons with bariatric health care issues. *Journal of Wound, Ostomy, and Continence Nursing, 38*(2), 133–138.

Centers for Disease Control. (2014a). Childhood Obesity Facts. Retrieved June 5, 2014, from: http://www.cdc.gov/healthyyouth/obesity/facts.html

Centers for Disease Control. (2014b). Obesity and Overweight. Retrieved June 5, 2014 from http://www.cdc.gov/obesity/data/adult.html

Gallagher, S. (2005). Overview. *The challenges of caring for the obese patient.* Edgemont, PA: Matrix Medical Communications.

Gray, M., Black, J., Baharestani, M., et al. (2011). MASD Part 1: Overview and pathophysiology. *Journal of Wound, Ostomy and Continence Nursing, 38*, 233–241.

Guo, S., & de Pieto, L. (2010). Factors affecting wound healing. *Journal of Dental Research, 89*(3), 219–229.

Hoffman, B. (2013). The Business of Obesity: What it Costs Us. Retrieved June 7, 2014 from: http://www.forbes.com/sites/bethhoffman/2013/03/22/the-business-of-obesity/

Ingargiola, M., Danalia, L., & Lee, E. (2013, January). Does the Application of Incisional Negative Pressure Therapy to High-risk Wounds Prevent Surgical Site Complications? Retrieved October 11, 2014, from http://www.ncbi.nlm.nih.gov/pubmed/24106562

Kennedy-Evans, K., Henn, T., & Levine, N. (2007). Skin and wound care for the bariatric patient. In *Chronic wound care: a clinical sourcebook for healthcare professionals* (4th ed., pp. 659–699). Malvern, PA: HMP Communications.

Levi, J., Segal, L., Thomas, K., et al. (2013). F as in Fat: How Obesity Threatens America's Future. Retrieved January 14, 2014 from: http://healthyamericans.org/report/108/

Lowe, J. (2008). Skin integrity in critically ill obese patients. *Critical Care Nursing Clinics of North America, 21*(3), 311.

Mathison, C. (2003). Skin and wound care challenges in the hospitalized morbidly obese patient. *Journal of Wound, Ostomy, and Continence Nursing, 30*(2), 78–83.

Muir, M., & Archer-Heese, G. (2009). Essentials of a Bariatric Patient Handling Program. Retrieved July 19, 2014 from: http://www.nursingworld.org/MainMenuCategories/ANAMarketplace/ANAPeriodicals/OJIN/TableofContents/ Vol142009/No1Jan09/Bariatric-Patient-Handling-Program-.html

O'Lenick, A. (2009). Comparatively Speaking: Humectants vs Emollients vs Occlusive Agents. Retrieved July 11, 2014 from: http://www.cosmeticsandtoiletries.com

Obesity Surgery Dallas. (2014). Obesity: BMI Classifications. Retrieved June 5, 2014 from http://www.obesitysurgerydallas.com/bmi.html

Payne, C., & Edwards, D. (2014, January). Application of the Single Use Negative Pressure Wound Therapy Device (PICO) on a Heterogeneous Group of Surgical and Traumatic Wounds. Retrieved October 11, 2014, from http://www.ncbi.nlm.nih.gov/pubmed/24917894

Puhl, R., & Heuer, C. (2009). The stigma of obesity: A review and update. *Obesity, 17*(5), 941–964.

Schafer, M., & Ferraro, K. (2007). Obesity and hospitalization over the adult life course: Does duration of exposure increase use? *Journal of Health and Social Behavior, 48*(4), 434–449.

Shapiro, M., & Keegan, M. (1992). Continuous oscillation therapy for the treatment of pulmonary contusion. *American Surgery, 58*(9), 546–550.

Shipman, A. & Millington, G. (2011). Obesity and the skin. *British Journal of Dermatology, 165*(4), 743–750.

Traver, G., Tyler, M., Hudson, C., et al. (1995). Continuous oscillation: Outcome in critically ill patients. *Journal of Critical Care, 10*(3), 97–103.

World Health Organization. (2014). Overweight: Situation and Trends. Retrieved June 5, 2014 from: http://www.who.int/gho/ncd/risk_factors/overweight_text/en

QUESTIONS

1. A wound care nurse is devising a skin care protocol for bariatric patients. Which intervention would the nurse include?

A. Scrub the skin thoroughly to remove harmful bacteria from perspiration.

B. Make full bathing with antibacterial soap daily requirement.

C. Use liquid bar soap with alkaline pH and a gentle cloth to cleanse the skin.

D. Lift all skin folds; pat dry or use a hair dryer on cool to assure complete drying.

2. A bariatric patient presents with a rash diagnosed as intertriginous dermatitis. In what area of the body is this condition usually found?

A. Perineal area

B. Under the breasts

C. Arms and legs

D. On the scalp

3. A wound care nurse is caring for a patient who is at risk for friction injury. Which of the following is a preventive measure for this type of skin alteration?

A. Separating skin folds with wicking fabric

B. Using powder under skin folds

C. Using moisturizers in skin folds

D. Avoiding the use of adhesive foam dressings

4. For which patient is the risk for pressure ulcers three times greater than the general population?

A. A patient with a body mass index (BMI) less than 30.

B. A patient with a body mass index (BMI) between 30 and 40.

C. A patient with a body mass index (BMI) greater than 40.

D. Body mass index is not an indicator of pressure ulcer risk.

5. The wound care nurse is choosing a bed for a bariatric patient who has orders for bed rest. What guideline would the nurse consider when making the choice?
A. The bed should be raised to accommodate turning and repositioning.
B. A foam mattress is the product of choice for this patient
C. A mattress with a continuous lateral rotation feature is required .
D. There should be 6 to 8 inches of extra space on each side of the patient to accommodate turning in bed.

6. Which area of the body is most prone to shear damage?
A. Back of the head
B. Coccyx
C. Knees
D. Shoulders

7. The wound care nurse measures a bariatric patient's abdominal girth to determine an appropriate abdominal binder size. What complication might this intervention prevent?
A. Pressure ulcers
B. Wound infection
C. MASD
D. Wound dehiscence

8. When choosing equipment for a bariatric patient, the major consideration is:
A. Patient preference
B. Patient and staff safety
C. Cost-effectiveness
D. Patient and staff compliance

9. What is a common reason that bariatric patients may put off needed medical attention?
A. Lack of motivation
B. Lack of financial means
C. Fear of rejection
D. Lack of transportation

10. A wound nurse is implementing a skin care program for a bariatric patient with intertriginous dermatitis. The nurse should pay particular attention to:
A. Routine repositioning
B. Maintaining a moist environment
C. Reduction of calories
D. Odor control

ANSWERS: 1.**D**, 2.**B**, 3.**A**, 4.**C**, 5.**D**, 6.**B**, 7.**D**, 8.**B**, 9.**C**, 10.**D**

CHAPTER 15

Skin and Wound Care for the Spinal Cord–Injured Patient

Laurie M. Rappl and David M. Brienza

OBJECTIVES

1. Describe factors that increase the risk for pressure ulcers among SCI individuals and implications for prevention.
2. Describe factors that negatively impact healing among SCI individuals.
3. Select/recommend appropriate pressure redistribution devices for bed, chair, and heels.
4. Describe guidelines for comprehensive management of a pressure ulcer in an SCI individual.

Topic Outline

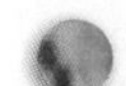 Introduction

People who sustain spinal cord injuries (SCIs) develop pressure ulcers (PUs) at an alarmingly high rate in the days and weeks immediately following their injury and throughout their lifetimes (Brienza & Karg, 2012; Chen et al., 2005). The effects of these wounds go far beyond acute medical complications to negatively impact quality of life and physical, psychological, emotional, and financial status (Krishnan, 2014). In this chapter, we explore the incidence and prevalence of PUs in this population, SCI-specific risk factors, causes of impaired healing, recommendations for preventive care and support surface selection, treatment options, and strategies to reduce recidivism. Most prevention and treatment strategies developed for other high-risk populations also apply to the SCI population; however, there are considerations unique to the neurological deficits associated with SCI that make wheelchair seating and general repositioning critically important for people with SCI.

CLINICAL PEARL

Individuals with SCIs are at high risk for PU development and for impaired healing throughout their lifetimes.

Demographics

Spinal Cord Injury Population

The number of people with SCI is substantial. While statistics for incidence and prevalence of SCI have not been directly determined in the course of the past 30 years, based on extrapolations from several sources, the injury rate is presently estimated to be 40 per million of population, resulting in 11,000 SCI annually in the United States. The estimated number of people living with SCI in the United States is presently above 250,000. This information is an estimate based on extrapolations from several studies and is from the National Spinal Cord Injury Statistics Center (NSCISC) (www.spinalcord.uab.edu). Males presently account for 78% of SCI, down slightly from 81% prior to 1980. The average age at injury has risen from 28.7 years in the 1970s to 38 years since 2000. This trend appears to be at least partially attributable to the aging of the U.S. population. Vehicular crashes constitute the predominant cause, particularly for teens and young adults; the incidence of SCI caused by vehicular accidents declines in the middle-aged population and decreases rapidly with advancing age. Falls constitute the dominant cause of SCI for those above 60 years. The incidence of SCI attributable to violence and sports-related injuries also decreases with advancing age.

Incidence and Prevalence of Pressure Ulcers

PUs are the most common complication of SCI (Regan et al., 2012). An analysis of the National Spinal Cord Injury Database indicates that PUs occur in 33.5% of cases (NSCISC, 2006; Cardenas et al., 2004). The second leading cause of death in individuals with SCI is septicemia (88.6%), which is usually associated with urinary tract infections (UTIs), pneumonia, and/or presence of PUs (NSCISC, 2011). Of the estimated 232,000 to 316,000 individuals with SCI in the United States, up to 85% will develop a PU at some point during their life (Mawson et al., 1988; Richardson & Meyer, 1981; National Spinal Cord Injury Statistical Center, 2011). In addition, PU complications cause up to 60,000 deaths a year, with 7% to 8% of these occurring in persons with SCI (Kynes, 1986).

Differences in incidence and prevalence trends have been noted related to the time postinjury for people with SCI. According to data collected from the Model Spinal Cord Injury Systems, one third of individuals with SCI will develop at least one PU during their initial acute or inpatient rehabilitation stay. Chen and colleagues found the risk of developing a PU to be relatively constant during the first 10 years postinjury (prevalence rate of 11.5% to 14.3% for stage II or higher PUs); however, rates tended to increase 15 years postinjury (prevalence rate of 21.0% for stage II or higher PU) (Chen et al., 1999b). In Italy, Pagliacci and colleagues found that 26.9% of 684 people in 32 rehabilitation centers had one or more PUs upon admission (Pagliacci et al., 2003).

CLINICAL PEARL

One third of SCI patients develop at least one PU during their initial acute or inpatient rehabilitation stay.

Associations between PU risk and neurological level of injury and impairment category have been reported (Brienza & Karg, 2012). Becker and DeLisa noted a higher incidence of PUs in those with complete injury or a higher level of injury (Becker & DeLisa, 1999). Saladin also found an association between severity of injury and increased risk (Saladin & Krause, 2009). Hitzig reported results from a self-reported incidence study where incidence rates for complete tetraplegia and paraplegia were 42.7% and 44.9%, respectively, compared to 20.4% and 20.7% for incomplete tetraplegia and paraplegia, respectively (Hitzig et al., 2008). The 2006 NSCID analysis revealed that those with complete tetraplegia were at highest risk for developing PUs (53.4%), followed by those with complete paraplegia (39%), incomplete tetraplegia (28.7%), and incomplete paraplegia (18.3%) (NSCISC, 2006).

Pressure Ulcer Prevention

The high risk of developing PUs for people with SCI is most commonly attributed to decreased mobility and sensation and physiological changes after SCI, but recent literature suggests that factors such as diabetes and depression are also important (Smith et al., 2008).

Risk Factors

The complete list of potential factors is very long, with more than 200 individual factors mentioned in the literature (Byrne & Salzberg, 1996). Cardiac disease and renal disease have been shown to be associated with increased risk of developing PUs (Salzberg et al., 1998). Those with traumatic injury appear to be at higher risk compared to those with nontraumatic SCIs (McKinley et al., 2002). Males with SCI have a higher risk than females (Chen et al., 1999a). A history of smoking, alcohol or drug use (Krause et al., 2001), medical comorbidities such as diabetes mellitus (Çakmak et al., 2009; Salzberg et al., 1996), impaired oxygenation or hypotension (Wilczweski et al., 2012), and infections such as pneumonia, UTIs, osteomyelitis, and other bacterial infections (Fogerty et al., 2008; Salzberg et al., 1998) have all been shown to increase risk. Dependence on mechanical ventilators (Manzano et al., 2010) and use of steroids (Wilczweski et al., 2012) are additional risk factors. In addition, as is the case for the broader populations of people at risk, moisture and/or urinary and fecal incontinence, hypo/hyperthermia, friction, and shear have been shown to increase risk, especially in acute and intensive care unit patients (Banks et al., 2012; Peerless et al., 1999; Reddy et al., 2006; Salzberg et al., 1996; Stover et al., 1995; Watts et al., 1998; Wilczweski et al., 2012). Compromised nutrition or low serum albumin levels, decreased mobility and sensation, and impaired cognitive function have all been shown to increase risk for people with SCI (Çakmak et al., 2009; Salzberg et al., 1996).

The delivery of oxygen and other nutrients to damaged and at-risk tissue is critical to prevention of PUs and repair of damaged tissue. In SCI, the circulatory system below the level of injury is significantly and adversely affected. Significant changes include reduced blood pressure due to loss of supraspinal control of the vascular bed (Inskip et al., 2009; Teasell et al., 2000) and impaired vascular function (Thijssen et al., 2010).

CLINICAL PEARL

In addition to immobility and inactivity, individuals with SCI are at risk for pressure damage due to impaired blood flow and oxygenation below the level of the injury.

Other physiological changes that affect PU risk relate directly to the mechanical characteristics of the soft tissues and how those mechanical characteristics affect loading and the concentrations of stress and strain in the soft tissues. These changes are particularly relevant to the potential of developing deep tissue injury (DTI). Pathoanatomical and pathophysiological changes occur in the buttocks, as tissues adapt to the chronic sitting and inactivity and to muscular denervation. These changes include bone shape adaptation (loss of cortical bone and flattening of the tips of the ischial tuberosities) as well as muscular atrophy, fat infiltration into muscles, and sometimes muscle spasms (Castro et al., 1999; de Bruin et al., 2000; Gefen, 2014; Giangregorio & McCartney, 2006; Rittweger et al., 2006). These alterations in the weight-bearing structures affect the loading and weight-bearing properties of the internal tissues. The mechanical loading properties around these anatomical interfaces have a critical effect on the risk of DTI. The biomechanical interaction is person specific and influenced by individual anatomy, tissue mechanics, and the body–support interfaces such as cushion and mattresses (Agam & Gefen, 2008; Gefen, 2008; Levy et al., 2014; Linder-Ganz & Gefen, 2009; Linder-Ganz et al., 2008; Portnoy et al., 2011).

CLINICAL PEARL

Muscle atrophy and changes in the shape of the bony prominences adversely affect normal weight bearing and tissue loading in the SCI individual.

Risk Assessment

The most commonly used and studied risk assessment scales (Braden Scale [Bergstrom et al., 1987], Norton Scale [Norton, 1980], and Waterlow Scale [Kottner et al., 2009]) have not been validated for people with SCI and are likely not completely appropriate given the population's unique combination of risk factors. Mortenson and colleagues undertook a systematic review of risk assessment scales for use in an SCI population (Mortenson & Miller, 2007). Seven scales (Abruzzese, Braden, Gosnell, Norton, SCIPUS, SCIPUS-A, and Waterlow) were evaluated. Of the seven scales reviewed, concurrent validity was assessed for only three of the scales, the Norton Scale, Waterlow Scale, and Braden Scale. For reasons including reliability, validity, administrator burden, and respondent burden, each of these three scales was determined to have poor to adequate predictive validity for the SCI population.

Salzberg attempted to develop a risk assessment scale for people with SCI, *The Pressure Ulcer Assessment Scale for the Spinal Cord Injured* (Salzberg Scale). This scale is composed of 15 risk factors: level of activity; degree of mobility; completeness of SCI; urinary incontinence; diagnosis of autonomic dysreflexia (AD); age; comorbidities such as those pertaining to cardiac, pulmonary, and renal pathophysiology; level of cognition; diagnosis of diabetes; history of cigarette smoking; residency; and diagnosis of hypoalbuminemia and anemia (Byrne & Salzberg, 1996). However, this scale has not been validated and has yet to be recommended for use pending completion of further psychometric evaluation (CfSCMCP Guidelines, 2001). The Salzberg Scale was included in the evaluation undertaken by Mortenson, but despite its higher sensitivity (74.7%) and specificity (56.6%) scores, it could not be deemed the best assessment tool since it has not been validated. Mortenson recommended the use of either the Braden Scale or Waterlow Scale, despite their apparent lack of content validity for the SCI population. He based this recommendation on the similar performance and closeness to the Salzberg Scale scoring associated with these tools and on their performance on psychometric evaluation.

Preventive Measures

Because the causes of PUs include biological, behavioral, and social factors, prevention and patient education must address all of these issues. The person with an SCI has to become aware of body systems that normally require no thought at all. The range of new things the person must learn to do and monitor can be overwhelming, especially in the acute phases of SCI. Thus, emotional support is a critical aspect of management and must extend well beyond the acute phase. Support involves much more than verbal instruction and pointing out negative behaviors; encouragement, assistance with problem solving, and advocacy are essential strategies in helping the patient to successfully incorporate the new lifestyle and behaviors.

Prevention has to become a lifestyle, incorporating not only the interventions and behaviors discussed below but, more broadly, an awareness of the body and self-respect; a belief that personal health is important and can be achieved; adjustment of social environments; acquiring needed attendant care, equipment, and transportation; readiness for change; and self-efficacy. Many team members play a role in assisting the person with an SCI to become self-sufficient in PU prevention. Medicine, nursing, and physical and occupational therapy are givens, as well as certified durable medical equipment and seating specialists. Social workers, psychologists, and nutritionists may be required as well. Skill in the areas of counseling, problem solving, and motivational interviewing may be helpful.

CLINICAL PEARL

Effective PU prevention requires multiple lifestyle adaptations and a 24 hours a day/7 days a week commitment that is very difficult to maintain long term; thus, multidisciplinary patient-focused care and counseling is essential.

There are a number of resources available to both clinicians and patients in the area of PU prevention. The Paralyzed Veterans of America (PVA) and the Consortium for Spinal Cord Medicine have published a very complete Clinical Practice Guideline "Pressure Ulcer Prevention and Treatment Following Spinal Cord Injury." The Consortium began an update of this extensive monograph in 2014. All monographs written or sponsored by the PVA are available free of charge from the PVA (CfSCMCP Guidelines, 2001).

The SCIRE (Spinal Cord Injury Rehabilitation Evidence) project is a collaborative effort involving Canadian researchers, clinicians, scientists and consumers, health centers, and universities. The project involves review and rating of articles on a wide variety of topics related to SCI, including PU prevention and treatment. Since it is ongoing and free, it is worth bookmarking the Web site (www.scireproject.com) and referencing for quality information.

In addition, the University of Alabama School of Medicine Department of Physical Medicine and Rehabilitation has an extensive list of very helpful brochures, articles, and "how to" videos designed to teach patients self-care, specifically in regard to prevention of PUs (UAB et al., 2014). Many commonly recommended preventive interventions, especially those involving patient behaviors, have only poor-to-moderate quality of evidence supporting their usefulness in preventing PUs. Therefore, at this time, prevention must be guided by expert opinion (Guihan & Bombardier, 2012). Despite the lack of objective evidence, behavioral strategies are consistently regarded as essential to good health and positive outcomes; therefore, prevention practices should continue to be taught, reinforced, and supported.

Patient education must fit the patient's learning style and be tailored to the unique needs and constraints of that patient. Individualizing the material and the recommended interventions has been shown to improve effectiveness (Vaishampayan, 2011).

Activity/Mobility/Transfers

This aspect of prevention includes all types of activity, from self-repositioning in bed to quality of transfers to general mobility. People should be encouraged to move as often as possible and should be provided the means to be as independent in repositioning as possible. This may entail use of an overhead trapeze or side rail bars when in bed, a firmer mattress, wheelchair modifications, and cushion choices. The more independent and mobile a person is, the more likely they are to effectively and routinely off-load bony prominences. In addition, mobility and activity improve overall health, increasing resistance to PUs.

Transfers are the first skill learned after an SCI and are a major source of tissue trauma due to inconsistencies in technique and challenging surfaces and situations. All individuals need to be taught and encouraged to do "clean" transfers (i.e., transfers that avoid sliding or bumping against objects such as wheels, skirt guards, toilet seats, or shower bench edges). Gentle landings on the intended surface are encouraged because initial contact with the seat puts very high tissue loads on the skin and at the edges of any scars, as opposed to the slow and constant rate at which fat loads (Levy, 2013). Sliding boards can be particularly dangerous to the skin and tissue, because sliding of the body against the hard transfer board can cause shearing. DeJong et al. (2014) studied the factors associated with risk of PU development while in acute rehabilitation, and one of the two variables most predictive of PU development was the need for at least moderate assistance to perform a transfer on admission. Gaining as much independence as possible is a key goal in rehabilitation. If the persons are unable to self-transfer, they need to know how to properly educate an assistant or attendant to transfer them safely.

CLINICAL PEARL

Transfers are a major source of tissue trauma; individuals must be assisted and taught to do "clean" transfers.

Unweighting Bony Prominences

Excessive weight on bony prominences is a prime cause of PUs. The person without protective sensation has to become aware of bony prominences that are sustaining pressure when in bed, in a wheelchair, on a sliding board, or in a standing frame. When in bed, the person needs to pay attention to length of time in one position and needs to know how and be able to shift his or her weight to alternate positions. Frequent position changes are recommended, and unweighting the posterior surface of the body is advised if at all possible; sleeping in the prone position is optimal, and a variety of side-lying positions is recommended for those who are unable to sleep in the prone position. Physical or occupational therapy may be able to assist with ideas for positioning and assistive devices such as wedges and molded pillows that can help maintain off-loaded positions. This should be considered no matter what support surface is being used; no support surface can protect the tissue as effectively as positioning off of the bony prominence.

Weight Shifts

Weight shifts in the sitting position involve changing body posture to significantly reduce pressure over the ischial/sacral area. Most rehabilitation programs teach a complete unweighting, which involves lifting the body off the seat cushion using the armrests or wheels for leverage ("push-up"). Unweighting is meant to restore blood flow to areas that are ischemic due to closure of the capillaries, with the goal of returning the transcutaneous partial pressure of oxygen ($TcPO_2$) to unloaded levels.

Bader (1990) determined that full recovery of tissue perfusion could not be achieved in <2 minutes. More than 20 years later, Coggrave & Rose (2003) calculated that the mean duration of a weight shift required to return transcutaneous partial pressure of oxygen ($TcPO_2$) to unloaded levels following upright sitting was 1 minute 51 seconds (range = 42 to 210 seconds). The duration of off-weighting required to restore transcutaneous oxygen levels to normal is much longer than the time frame commonly recommended for push-ups (most clinicians and guidelines recommend 30- to 60-second push-ups every 15 to 30 minutes). In addition, push-ups are difficult to accomplish and difficult to maintain for even one full minute for most individuals, let alone at the recommended frequencies. Not surprisingly, Guihan & Bombardier (2012) found that only about 50% of people with SCI perform regular pressure relief maneuvers. Alternative means of reducing pressures such as forward leaning with the elbows or chest on the knees, side leaning with the shoulder and elbow over the wheel or further, and tilting the seat-and-back unit to > 65 degrees for 1 minute have been shown to result in major reductions in ischial interface pressures and significant increases in buttock blood flow and $TcPO_2$ (Coggrave & Rose, 2003; Makhsous et al., 2007; Sonenblum & Sprigle, 2011; Sprigle & Sonenblum, 2011). The specific frequency of weight shifts required to reduce PU incidence has not been determined, but we do know that excessive pressure on any part of the body must be relieved periodically to restore normal hemodynamic and $TcPO_2$ levels. Any relief of pressure is beneficial.

CLINICAL PEARL

Current evidence suggests that the commonly recommended "wheelchair push-ups" must be maintained for 2 minutes to effectively restore perfusion—which is not possible for most individuals. Alternative approaches to off-loading must be explored with the individual.

Substance Abuse Avoidance

Tobacco, street drugs, and excessive alcohol are known to cause tissue changes that increase susceptibility to tissue breakdown and to inhibition of wound healing. In addition, substance abuse may reflect a lifestyle that is not conducive to good health or social adaptation. Substance abuse has a negative effect on psychosocial adaptation to disability and further compromises the ability to carry out PU prevention measures. Therefore, the clinician should provide education and counseling regarding smoking cessation, drug avoidance, and moderation in alcohol use.

Skin Checks

Most rehabilitation programs teach at least once daily visual examination of all bony prominences, especially the sitting surfaces of the sacrum, coccyx, ischials, and posterior femurs. This can be done by a caregiver or attendant or with the use of a mirror or cell phone camera. Any changes in skin integrity or color should be noted. Reddened areas that do not return to normal color after unweighting for a minimum of 1 hour require immediate response and intervention.

However, visual inspection alone is not enough. Most PUs on persons with SCI begin in the subdermal tissues because these tissues are more susceptible than the skin to ischemic damage. This explains the deep and undermined wounds seen so often on those with SCI, and the phenomenon of the PU "just appearing" 1 day with no visible warning; the damage was taking place in the deep tissues and produced no visible changes in the skin, so the problem was undetected and unaddressed. It is therefore important for the SCI individual (and/or caregiver) to use palpation as well as visual inspection. They need to become familiar with the normal texture of their tissue; they can then be taught to gently pinch the skin and tissues to detect any changes in integrity (much like the premise of breast self-examinations, where the woman is taught to palpate the tissues on a routine basis and to assess for any changes over time). Changes may be noted as areas of firmness, softness, or mushiness in comparison to the surrounding tissue or as a cyst-like ball. The area may also feel warm to the touch as compared to the contralateral side or the upper leg.

Immediacy of action is essential when an ulcer is detected or suspected. Any of the tissue changes described above are causes for concern. Help should be sought immediately as prompt intervention for early damage increases the probability that the damage can be limited and that conservative management will be effective in restoring tissue integrity.

> **CLINICAL PEARL**
>
> A key component of care and education is careful skin inspection at least daily with immediate response to areas of discoloration that do not resolve within an hour.

Hygiene

Daily bathing is not necessary, nor always feasible due to the possible need for attendant care to accomplish. The best approach to cleansing is to use pH-balanced no-rinse cleansers; baby wipes can be used for perineal cleansing. Strong alkaline soaps and cleansers should not be used on a regular basis because they strip the skin of the protective acid mantle formed by the normal skin secretions of sweat and sebum. The normal skin pH is 4 to 5.5, and this normal acidity protects against bacterial or fungal overgrowth and contributes to skin health.

Management of Bowel and Bladder Incontinence

Bladder incontinence can keep the skin in the vulnerable ischial area constantly "wet," which makes it more susceptible to breakdown. Fecal contamination of the skin further increases the risk of skin breakdown, due to the enzymes and bacteria in the stool. Bowel and bladder incontinence is anecdotally regarded as more debilitating than the inability to walk. Thus, establishment of an effective bladder and bowel management program is as essential to skin health as it is to psychosocial adaptation.

Nutrition

Proper nutrition levels and healthy eating patterns are essential for optimum health. The constant state of inflammation present in chronic SCI has been linked to reduced albumin and hematocrit levels. Salzburg et al., (1998) identified two nutritional parameters as indicators of increased risk for breakdown: albumin < 3.4 or total protein < 6.4 and hematocrit < 36% or hemoglobin < 12.0. These data further underscore the importance of a healthy diet and normal weight for the SCI person. An added challenge to maintenance of normal weight is the fact that many people with SCI live a relatively sedentary lifestyle; the resulting tendency to weight gain is further compounded by poor eating habits. In addition, there is a natural increase in visceral adipose tissue after the SCI. Thus, ongoing attention to a nutritious diet and to weight control is another factor that must be consciously addressed by the SCI person.

Management of Systemic Comorbidities

As with the general population, many persons with SCI are dealing with multiple medical comorbidities including diabetes, pulmonary disease, cardiac disease, and renal failure, and any comorbidities add to the constant demands related to the SCI. The natural increase in visceral adipose tissue noted above increases the SCI individual's susceptibility to development of all of these comorbidities. Those with SCI are at 1.4- and 2-fold higher risk of mortality from diabetes and congestive heart failure, respectively, than are able-bodied persons (Edwards et al., 2008). Any coexisting condition affects overall health and can increase the risk for PU development. Effective management of all comorbid conditions is an important component of a comprehensive PU prevention strategy.

Autonomic dysreflexia or hyperreflexia refers to overactivity of the sympathetic nervous system, usually in response to a noxious stimulus below the level of injury. The parasympathetic system is unable to counter the sympathetic stimulation due to the interruption of nerve fibers and signals through the spinal cord. Triggering stimuli can include the beginning stages of a PU, an overfilled bladder, an infection, or an injury that would ordinarily cause significant pain in sensate areas of the body. AD is usually experienced only by persons with injuries above T5. Dysreflexia manifests as sudden hypertension, pounding headache, sweating, flushing or blotching of the skin, and nausea. AD is considered a medical emergency and must be dealt with immediately by finding the cause of the stimulus and correcting or addressing it. AD can be considered an aggressive form of protective sensation if there is awareness that it indicates a harmful condition occurring in insensate areas of the body.

> **CLINICAL PEARL**
>
> Skin damage can trigger AD in the individual with an SCI above the level of T5; this is a medical emergency.

Impaired cognitive function will affect the person's ability to carry out all of the prevention strategies required. While most individuals with SCI have normal cognition, the clinician must always be alert to indicators of cognitive impairment and, if noted, should conduct a cognitive assessment. For the SCI person who does have cognitive impairment, it is essential to provide instruction and guidance regarding prevention strategies in a way that the person can understand, internalize, and act upon.

Spasticity Management

Spasticity causes uncontrollable movements of the body and is a common complication of SCI. The movement can be as limited as a bouncing leg that rubs against part of the wheelchair or as extensive as full body extension or flexion. Spasticity can prevent maintenance of an upright posture, put the limbs at risk for injury, or be so difficult to manage that the person is not able to focus any attention on other issues, such as PU prevention (McKinley et al., 1999). Thus, the care team must work together with the person to ensure effective management of spasticity.

Maintenance of Durable Medical Equipment

Prescribed equipment must be maintained in order to perform as intended. There has to be personal responsibility and accountability for the proper functioning of all durable medical equipment. A malfunctioning or worn out seat cushion can be dangerous not just because it has lost its protective properties but also because the user believes he or she is protected because "I'm sitting on my cushion."

The seat cushion and the wheelchair work as a unit to protect the patient and provide mobility. The importance of a properly selected and maintained wheelchair and seat cushion is reflected by the fact that 47% of all PUs occur over the ischial tuberosities and sacrum (Bogie et al., 1995).

Assistive technology is the term given to durable medical equipment that helps provide accommodation to a disability, including wheelchairs, seat cushions, environmental controls, and a variety of other devices. There are a large number and variety of devices available, and effective use requires a clear understanding of the indications, contraindications, and utilization guidelines for each. Fortunately, there are certified specialists (assistive technology professionals, or ATPs) who possess the in-depth knowledge to effectively match products and individuals. It is extremely beneficial for any person with an SCI to be seen by an ATP in order to be evaluated and fitted to the equipment that affords that individual the most protection and function. The certification is administered by the Rehabilitation Engineering Society of North America, or RESNA. ATPs can be found through the search feature on the Web site (www. Resna.org).

Most centers that specialize in SCI have specialized seating clinics that provide a comprehensive evaluation, including range of motion, mobility, pressure mapping, equipment trials, education in maintenance and usage, repairs, equipment prescription, options, and reimbursement. These specialized clinics have been shown to reduce the incidence of PUs and readmission rates of persons with recurrent PUs (Kennedy et al., 2003).

Seat cushions are a primary intervention for both prevention and treatment of PUs. The primary mechanism of action is redistribution of *pressure* off of the prominent and vulnerable ischial tuberosities, with the goal of reducing tissue interface pressures and thereby minimizing tissue damage. Cushions can also help to reduce *shearing forces*, the opposing forces that cause the soft tissue layers to slide against one another when the skin is pulled in one direction and the skeleton (bone) and muscle pulls in the opposite direction. Shaped cushions can help to maintain an upright sitting *position* to reduce the sliding that can cause shearing. This upright position improves function and movement and keeps the body structurally aligned. Lastly, some cushions address *heat and moisture* buildup, thus improving skin health and resistance to damage.

In addition to these therapeutic considerations, there are practical issues that should be considered. For example, flatter cushions facilitate dressing because pants can be pulled up and down easily. Flatter cushions are also easier to transfer onto as they do not have higher outer edges that require a bigger lift. Cushions should be easy to keep clean as incontinence is a comorbidity for many wheelchair users. Ease of maintenance has to be considered because if the cushion is not maintained, it can lose its cushioning and protective properties and put the user at risk.

CLINICAL PEARL

A correctly sized wheelchair and an optimal pressure redistribution cushion are critical components of an effective PU prevention program; the individual with an SCI should be referred to a seating clinic or ATP.

Tissue deformation occurs when the soft tissues are compressed by the bony prominences internally and a hard or firm surface externally. The deformation causes internal stresses, compression of capillaries, prevention of blood and lymph flow and waste removal, and cellular damage or death. Managing this deformation is key to maintaining healthy tissue (Sprigle & Sonenblum, 2011). Deformation is reduced when the cushion provides immersion of the ischials and pelvis into the cushion but also provides sufficient support to prevent bottoming out. The cushion should effectively envelop (conform to) the skeleton, thereby spreading interface pressure across the whole seating surface. Alternatively, some cushions completely eliminate pressure under the ischials and spread all of the pressure to the rest of the sitting surface of the body.

Standards have been developed to measure the ability of a cushion to immerse and conform to the bony prominences to protect the ischials. While these standards are not based on clinical outcomes in regard to PU prevention, they are an objective way to compare cushions against a standard cushion and in relation to each other. These standards have been used to group cushions into codes for Medicare coverage. The four groups of codes are (1) general use, (2) skin protection, (3) positioning, and (4) skin protection and positioning. In comparing the criteria, each subsequent group (from 1 to 4) has increasingly difficult standards to meet and in general are increasingly complex in design. Some of the criteria include depth when loaded using a standard loading device, deflection when overloaded, and peak interface pressures at the ischial tuberosities compared to a standard reference cushion. The positioning cushions are required to have structural features such as supports around the medial and lateral thighs or a ridge in front of the ischials to prevent forward migration (Noridian—Medicare Pricing, Data Analysis and Coding [PDAC], 2014).

Interface pressures are used to compare devices and are sometimes used in clinical practice to evaluate seat cushion efficacy for specific patients. To measure interface pressures, a mat that contains hundreds of pressure sensors is placed between the person and the seat cushion and connected to a computer screen. This provides a visual display of interface pressures across the entire seating surface. (Pressure distribution can be displayed in numbers or colors, with either approach clearly indicating points of higher pressure.) These data can then be used to modify the equipment as needed and/or to select the best cushion for a particular patient.

Shearing may be as destructive to tissues as pressure but is more difficult to understand and to measure (see Chapters 16 and 18). Shearing occurs when tissues move in horizontal planes or across each other and across bony prominences, in contrast to interface or direct pressures, which are exerted perpendicularly onto the soft tissue and bony prominence. As tissues are moved horizontally across each other, they exert tearing forces on each other and between each other. Shearing is thought to be the causative factor for the undermining that is typical of PUs on those with SCI. Support surfaces that move with body movement may reduce shearing by absorbing the horizontal movement.

Types of Cushions

There are hundreds of cushions on the market, ranging from simple foam slabs to air- or gel-filled bladders to powered alternating pressure seat cushions. General descriptors for each type of cushion are as follows:

Foam

Foam is made in a chemical process that can be manipulated to produce various levels of density, stiffness, conformability, and memory. Foams are measured by the indentation load deflection or the ILD, the ability of the foam to permit a disc of standard weight to indent the mattress by 25% or 65% of its standard thickness. Foams are usually layered to provide support in the lower levels and softness for immersion in the upper levels. Foams can be shaped, are lightweight, and facilitate transfers and dressing. However, the time frame for which they are effective (performance life) may be shorter, and their ability to effectively envelop (conform to) the body may be limited.

Air

There are simple air cushions made of a single chamber or more complex ones made with multiple cells that offer better immersion and envelopment. Air cushions provide less stability when the person is moving or leaning and require maintenance to prevent holes and to detect slow leaks. They can also make transfers and dressing more difficult due to instability.

Gel

No standards have been developed to help the clinician or buyer compare gels to each other or to predetermine what kind of gel is being used. Gels depend on flowability to conform to the body, a property called viscosity. Low-viscosity gels are more syrup-like and flow easily but may bottom out unless they are contained in a limiting and thick-walled bladder, which limits the flow but increases the interface pressure. Moderate-viscosity gels that are paste-like have a slower flow rate and are more conformable; they are more appropriate for use in the SCI population. High-viscosity gels have no flow properties at all and therefore have little to offer in terms of immersion and envelopment. They are not used for SCI individuals as full-time wheelchair cushions but may be used for short-term use such as in cars or on shower benches. Gel cushions can be heavy and can retain heat and moisture next to the skin.

Dynamic

Powered cushions that automatically change pressures at regular intervals are available. A small study showed that one of these cushions relieved pressure enough to provide complete recovery of tissue perfusion and also demonstrated slower vascular recovery among individuals with SCI as opposed to controls (Makhsous et al., 2007). These are promising data, but more study is needed. In addition, cost and maintenance of these products needs to be considered.

CLINICAL PEARL

The field of durable medical equipment is increasingly complex; an assistive technology provider (ATP) can provide invaluable guidance in selection of the best equipment for a specific individual.

Telemedicine

Telemedicine may be a valuable modality for monitoring patients' skin, providing encouragement and instruction, and treating and preventing PUs. Many people live long distances from a center or clinician specializing in SCI care, and transportation difficulties or the need to remain off-weighted in bed prevent timely assessment and treatment. Consultation using cell phone cameras, tablet computers, Skype, and open market purchased cameras and computers are helping to connect clinicians and patients in the best place for care—the home (Mathewson et al., 1999). Caregivers can be educated, recommendations made for ulcer care, and encouragement provided for prevention measures, all in the setting where these activities have to happen.

Measures to Reduce Recidivism

Jones et al. (2003) studied the effects of various approaches to positive reinforcement for prevention of recurrent ulcers. They found that the addition of monetary rewards for ulcer prevention or improvement led to positive results. They concluded that PU recurrence may be linked to insufficient positive consequences for prevention as well as to insufficient negative consequences (pain) for failure to adhere to prevention interventions.

Community Support for Prevention

Prevention has to become a lifestyle, incorporating the interventions and behaviors discussed above.

Incorporating body awareness, self-respect, a belief in success, and self-efficacy and readiness to change are less tangible but just as important. Social support may be needed to acquire needed attendant care, equipment and transportation, and reasonable living accommodations. Community- and home-based programs have been and continue to be attempted in order to support persons with SCI in making the wide range of physical, social, and psychological adjustments required for a "prevention lifestyle." These have included regular phone support, telehealth, monetary incentives to remain ulcer free, supportive social networks, and psychological assistance. The complexity of these programs and difficulties in implementation have hampered clear measurement of outcomes. One such program, the Lifestyle Redesign Pressure Ulcer Prevention Program (LR-PUP), is an innovative, comprehensive, and complex program in the underserved areas of Los Angeles. The program entails both facility visits by the patients and home visits by the clinicians. The organizers have encountered significant challenges in the early stages and have had to make major modifications including increased staffing and training, which underscores the complexity of PU prevention in this physically and psychosocially complex patient population. This randomized controlled trial is ongoing, and the investigators hope to be able to demonstrate positive outcomes as well as cost savings related to ulcers prevented (Clark et al., 2014; Vaishampayan et al., 2011).

Increased Risk for Impaired Healing

The high recidivism rates noted earlier and the notoriously slow rate of healing for PUs in SCI patients have led many clinicians and researchers to question whether there are physiological factors at play in addition to the obvious factors: lack of protective sensation, possible patient behaviors that compromise healing, and the reduced tensile strength of scar tissue. As a result, there have been a number of studies focused on the metabolic and physiological differences in the skin above and below the level of the SCI lesion; these studies are enhancing our understanding of the potential deficits in the repair process affecting SCI individuals. Rappl (2008) summarized these differences with respect to the wound-healing cascade and the ways in which SCI impairs the normal processes involved in wound repair; these differences are outlined in **Table 15-1** and are grouped according to the major physiologic category. This helps the clinician to conceptualize the deficit within the framework of the wound-healing cascade and to see how the deficit might impair wound healing. Any one of the deficits shown in **Table 15-1** would impact wound healing, but when taken together, the impact is seen to be extensive and adds clarity to the frustrations encountered in clinical practice. This summary also helps to explain why modalities and treatments that seem to be effective in management of other types of wounds are less effective with SCI wounds.

TABLE 15-1 Factors Leading to Impaired Healing

Vascular Changes
- Abnormal vascular response
- Reduced density of adrenergic receptors
- Decreased blood flow
- Decreased blood pressure
- Decreased blood supply

End Result: Reduced $TcPO_2$ levels (five times lower than levels in innervated tissues)

Decreased collagen and collagen precursors
- Increased collagen catabolism
- Increase in urinary excretion of glycosaminoglycans (GAGs)
- Decreased concentration of amino acids
- Decrease in levels of enzymes involved in biosynthesis

Reduced quality of collagen
- Decrease in proportion of type I to type III collagen

Impaired fibroblast activity
- Decreased fibronectin, a glycoprotein

Constant inflammatory state

Vascular Changes

Intuitively, there is reduced perfusion below the level of injury due to lack of active movement in the lower extremities. However, the deficits listed in **Table 15-1** indicate more profound problems. The SCI interrupts the spinal vasomotor pathway, specifically the input from sympathetic system that arises in the thoracic and lumbar spine. The counterbalancing parasympathetic nerves originate from the cranial nerves and the sacral area and are not affected by the SCI (Claus-Walker et al., 1977; Guttmann, 1976). This impairment in sympathetic stimulation leads to a loss of tone in the vascular bed, generalized vasodilation, and decreased vascular resistance, which results in decreased blood pressure and diminished blood flow. The loss of sympathetic innervation causes a reduction in the density of both alpha- and beta-adrenergic receptors, which explains the abnormal vascular reactions and tendency toward vasodilation. Vasodilation results in decreased blood pressure, which adversely affects perfusion of the tissues in a given area.

Makshous found that, compared to controls, persons with SCI had a significantly slower rate of reperfusion of tissues following unweighting (Makhsous et al., 2007). Bogie et al. (1995) found that subjects with SCIs below T6 showed a progressive loss in ability to maintain blood flow in the sitting position, indicating that paraplegics are at higher risk than tetraplegics. These findings suggest an altered or slowed blood flow response to pressure, which can lead to tissue damage since diminished tissue perfusion limits the delivery of nutrients, enzymes, and oxygen to the tissues. A normal inflammatory response depends on vasodilation to bring blood and the cells needed for wound healing to the wound site. This response is most likely impaired in the SCI individual since there is chronic vasodilation throughout the entire lower body and loss of the ability to regulate blood flow in response to metabolic demands.

Decreased Transcutaneous Oxygen Levels

Several studies from the 1990s provide comparable findings in terms of transcutaneous oxygen levels ($TcPO_2$) in SCI patients; specifically, they found $TcPO_2$ levels to be up to five times lower below the level of injury than above (Bogie et al., 1995; Lindan, 1961; Mawson et al., 1993; Patterson et al., 1993). This is significant because oxygen is needed at all points in the wound-healing cascade. Keratinocytes require O_2 for building epithelium, and fibroblasts need oxygen to synthesize collagen. In addition, oxygen is needed for phagocytosis and prevention of infection and to meet the metabolic demands of the tissue. The hypoxia normally found within the wound (as compared to the surrounding tissue) stimulates angiogenesis and collagen synthesis. Both of these responses may be impaired by the reduced oxygen gradient between the healthy (unwounded) tissue and the wound.

Decreased Collagen, Extracellular Matrix, and Their Precursors

Collagen is degraded or catabolized in denervated, insensate tissues (Claus-Walker et al., 1977), as evidenced by increased excretion of collagen catabolites and glycosaminoglycans (GAGs) in the urine of persons with SCI. Those on bed rest are extremely vulnerable, excreting three to four times more than an ambulatory adult. Tissue biopsies taken from the edges of PUs in quadriplegic patients reveal very low levels of collagen fibers (Hunter & Rajan, 1971). This is extremely important, because collagen is the primary component of the new extracellular matrix that must be created to fill the defect. Collagen also attracts leukocytes, macrophages, and monocytes for wound cleansing and fibroblasts for tissue building.

In addition to the ongoing breakdown and excretion of collagen in SCI patients, the tissues below the level of the lesion have been found deficient in at least some of the amino acids and enzymes needed to synthesize collagen (Claus-Walker et al., 1977; Rodriguez & Claus-Walker, 1988). Without all of the necessary resources for production of normal collagen, the body can make only defective collagen fibrils, which results in a weakened extracellular matrix.

Poor-Quality Collagen

As explained in Chapter 2, the early extracellular matrix is composed primarily of type III collagen, which has very minimal tensile strength; this is gradually converted to type I collagen during the maturation phase, which provides tensile strength. SCI tissues below the level of injury have been shown to have a greater proportion of type III to type I (Rodriguez & Markowski, 1995). This means the "healed" ulcer has poor tensile strength, which may be one of the causative factors in PU recurrence.

Decreased Fibronectin

SCI patients with poorly healing wounds were found to have a significantly lower concentration of fibronectin, a large glycoprotein with many functions (Vaziri et al., 1992). Fibronectin facilitates phagocytosis; promotes neovascular growth; promotes fibroblast migration, attachment, and proliferation; and supports the production of collagen. Fibronectin is also part of the scaffold for the new extracellular matrix. In addition to the decreased levels of fibronectin in SCI tissues, Cruse et al. (2002) found reduced adhesion or binding capacities among lymphocytes, impaired cellular interaction, and a lack of structural and functional protein in the extracellular matrix.

Constant Inflammatory State

Persons with chronic SCI show serologic evidence of a systemic inflammatory state as evidenced by increased C-reactive protein (CRP) levels (Edwards et al., 2008; Frost et al., 2005); this was found to be true whether or not the individual was symptomatic. Frost found the inflammatory state to be particularly significant in those with indwelling catheters and existing PUs. Increased CRP was also correlated with lower albumin and hemoglobin levels (Frost et al., 2005), Edwards found that CRP in those with SCI was nearly double that of matched non-SCI subjects. He also found that the level of visceral adipose tissue was 58% higher and total adipose tissue was 26% higher in those with SCI compared to those without SCI. Adipose tissue produces and releases proinflammatory molecules that have been implicated in many health problems including diabetes and cardiovascular disease (Fantuzzi, 2005). This inflammatory state negatively affects the health of the entire body.

CLINICAL PEARL

There are many physiological changes that occur as a result of an SCI that contribute to delayed healing despite appropriate management: these include reduced perfusion, reduced synthesis of collagen and fibronectin, and persistent inflammation.

Management Guidelines Specific to SCI Population

PUs in persons with SCI are frequently large, deep, and undermined and are notoriously difficult to heal. This may be due in part to the multiple physiological changes that occur as a result of the SCI, the alterations in the cells and processes involved in repair, and the difficulties in keeping these wounds off-loaded. Evidence used to justify treatment options should be generated by studies involving persons with SCI because, as previously discussed, tissues in SCI are different from tissues in non-SCI individuals. Effective management begins with the basic principles discussed throughout this text: off-loading of the involved area; attention to systemic factors such as nutritional status, glycemic control, and tobacco cessation; and topical therapy to establish a clean wound bed, control bacterial loads, and promote healing. Since repair in the SCI individual is frequently impaired, advanced wound therapies are frequently required to provide scaffolding for migrating cells and to promote granulation tissue formation. Conservative healing by secondary intention is generally preferable to invasive surgery.

The SCIRE (Spinal Cord Injury Rehabilitation Evidence) project reviews PU treatment articles on an ongoing basis and posts the newest information on their Web site (www.scireproject.com). SCIRE 3.0 (2009) is referenced in the following discussion as the first author, Regan.

Off-loading

Reducing or eliminating pressure to the wound is always the first treatment priority in PU healing. Since PUs most often occur on the ischials and sacrum/coccyx in those with SCI (Biglari et al., 2013), this means extended periods of bed rest. This forced immobility is extremely difficult to carry out. The person on bed rest usually cannot work, cannot take care of themselves or anyone else, and cannot take care of a household. There is virtually no social life, little mental stimulation, and no physical exercise. The person on bed rest does not burn enough calories to cause hunger so nutritional intake frequently fails to meet minimal requirements and is insufficient to support healing. In addition, prolonged bed rest results in other negative outcomes that compromise health and quality of life: these include pain, stiffness, contractures, and deconditioning, and possibly a disruption in established bowel and bladder management programs and internal organ function. Because the individual's lifestyle is completely interrupted by bed rest, psychological changes occur and depression is common. These sequelae of immobility are real and must be addressed; clinicians must remember that bed rest negatively impacts every aspect of the individual's life, while the benefits are somewhat abstract. In most cases, the person cannot see the ulcer, and the ulcer does not usually cause pain or other symptoms that would make it "real" and that would encourage off-loading. Without pain as a clear negative consequence to sitting, the person must decide to stay in bed and endure the trials listed above. It is not surprising that patients become "noncompliant" to bed rest recommendations.

Some programs (e.g., Rehab Station in Stockholm, Sweden) now allow limited sitting, up to 1 hour three times per day, with the goals of increasing compliance, decreasing emotional depression caused by isolation and inactivity, and minimizing the pulmonary complications to which those with SCI are particularly vulnerable. Their data indicate that wounds will heal with limited sitting in a safe cushion environment, so long as there is a comprehensive wound care program that includes appropriate positioning in bed, bowel/bladder management, and wound management and stimulation. The trade-off of a small amount of limited sitting may be enough to offset the huge negative consequences of bed rest.

CLINICAL PEARL

Complete bed rest is socially, psychologically, and physically debilitating. Limited sitting with appropriate use of pressure redistribution cushions may support healing while offsetting the very negative consequences of bed rest.

Electrical Stimulation (E-stim)

E-stim has been studied more than any other modality for healing PUs in those with SCI. E-stim for wound healing has been studied since the 1940s, but we still lack a clear understanding of the mechanism of action. E-stim has been credited with reducing infection, increasing perfusion, and accelerating wound healing (Thakral et al., 2013). There is evidence that e-stim increases collagen synthesis and wound tensile strength, increases the rate of wound epithelialization, and increases oxygen delivery and bactericidal activity. It is believed that e-stim imitates or enhances the natural electrical current that occurs in the body; when applied to injured tissues, e-stim increases migration of neutrophils and macrophages into the wound bed and stimulates fibroblast activity.

There are many different ways to deliver e-stim including direct current (DC), alternating current (AC), high-voltage pulsed current (HVPC), and low-intensity direct current (LIDC). The parameters of the stimulation (wave form, pulse, frequency, phase duration, and voltage) also vary, as does placement of the electrodes around the wound and use of positive versus negative polarity. It has even been proposed that optimal parameters for the e-stim and for electrode placement may vary depending on the phase of wound healing and wound characteristics. Frequency of application and total time of treatment per day and week also vary. Despite all of these variations in the e-stim applied, literature has consistently shown benefits to wound healing.

In a systematic review on e-stim for prevention or for treatment of wounds in SCI individuals, Liu and colleagues (Lui, 2013) reviewed randomized controlled trials (RCTs), non-RCTs, prospective cohort studies, case series, case–controls, and case reports. Of the 11 studies reviewed, 6 were RCTs. All 11 studies showed enhanced PU healing. The authors concluded that the combined evidence provided by studies done to date meets the criteria for limited grade 1 evidence.

The types of e-stim used in the six RCTs illustrates the variety in e-stim delivery. Griffin and colleagues studied HVPC on pelvic PUs (Griffin et al., 1991), and Stefanovska and colleagues found that low-frequency pulsed AC current provided better results than DC (Stefanovska et al., 1993). Baker and colleagues demonstrated that asymmetric biphasic stimulation was best for wound healing and that adding symmetric biphasic stimulation to healing wounds improved the healing rate over no stimulation (Baker et al., 1996). Adegoke and Badmos used interrupted DC current compared to sham, Salzberg used a pulsed electromagnetic field versus control, and Houghton and colleagues used HVPC with standard wound care versus standard wound care with no HVPC (Adegoke & Badmos, 2001). All reported improved results when e-stim was used, regardless of the method for delivery of that stimulation.

Negative Pressure Wound Therapy

While negative pressure wound therapy (NPWT) is widely used for treating PUs, especially deep and highly exudative ulcers, there are few studies examining the effects in SCI individuals. Despite this, NPWT is frequently used and is always noted as a treatment for SCI PUs in articles describing management of these wounds. Benefits include dressing changes every 2 to 3 days rather than daily and better management of exudate as compared to absorbent dressings. The firmness of the foam or gauze within the wound when the suction is applied can become a pressure point, as can the tubing connecting the wound insert material to the pump. Since the majority of SCI wounds are on the sitting surfaces of the body, this can lead to new PUs unless the clinician uses the bridging technique to assure that the pressure control pad and tubing are placed over non–weight-bearing surfaces.

Ho and colleagues compared wound healing in 33 wounds managed with NPWT and 53 wounds managed with "standard wound care" (Ho et al., 2010). Standard wound care included pressure relief, debridement, dressing changes to ensure moist wound healing, biophysical modalities such as hydrotherapy, and wound cleansing with each dressing change. The most common therapies used were chemical debridement, antimicrobials, cleansing solutions, wound fillers, contact layers, hydrogels and hydrocolloids, foams, alginates, and mechanical debridement. They found no significant difference in healing rates as evidenced by reduction in wound surface area between the two groups. They did find that patients managed with NPWT who healed had significantly higher albumin levels as compared to patients who did not heal with NPWT (3.3 ± 0.5 vs. 2.9 ± 0.4; $p < 0.5$). There was no difference in albumin levels between healers and nonhealers in the group that did not receive NPWT. They concluded that nutrition seems to be an important factor in success with NPWT and hypothesized that the NPWT may have contributed to the lower albumin levels.

deLaat analyzed outcomes for the SCI subgroup in a prospective RCT designed to evaluate the impact of NPWT for "difficult-to-treat wounds." Their results showed that the SCI group had the same outcomes as the entire study group; wounds managed with NPWT healed twice as fast as those managed with sodium hypochlorite (deLaat, 2011).

Anecdotally, the tissue resulting from NPWT is being reported as less vascular than normal scar tissue (Ennis, 2013), which could increase the risk for recurrent breakdown; however, more study is needed to verify these results and the implications.

Ultraviolet C (UVC)

Ultraviolet light is easy to apply, and UVC has been shown to be effective against multidrug-resistant microorganisms including MRSA and VRE (Conner-Kerr et al., 1998; Dai et al., 2012). In 2013, Nussbaum studied the effects of UVC in management of stage 2, 3, and 4 PUs in SCI. The only statistically significant benefit was found with stage 2 wounds. In 1994, this same author found that UVC along with ultrasound and good nursing care was associated with better healing outcomes than laser or good nursing care alone (Nussbaum, 1994). Decreasing bioburden is a basic tenet of modern wound care and has been shown to be critical to creation of a wound environment conducive to new tissue growth. Further research is needed to determine whether UVC can effectively control bioburden without interfering with healing; if so, UVC could potentially replace antiseptic agents that are frequently used to control bioburden but are known to be cytotoxic in stronger concentrations.

Platelet-Rich Plasma (PRP) and PRP Gel

Two studies have evaluated PRP in management of SCI wounds, though each study used a different formulation. Scevola (2010) conducted a prospective randomized trial involving 13 patients with 16 stage III or IV PUs comparing the use of a high-concentration cryopreserved PRP against standard protocol, which included iodoform packing, sodium/alginate foam dressing, or NPWT. In this study, the PRP group had a statistically significant faster time to granulation ($p = 0.025$), indicating that the PRP promoted faster healing as compared to the non-PRP group. At the end of the study, no statistically significant difference was found in volume reduction between the two groups ($p = 0.76$), and all wounds showed significant volume reduction compared to the start of the study ($p < 0.001$). The second study involved the use of a low concentration, nonfrozen PRP in a case series of 20 wounds on 20 patients; wound volume, area, undermining, and tunneling were measured over time. In this study, wound volume (baseline 53.4 cm^3) was reduced by 56% in 3.4 weeks with four treatments; all figures are averages (Rappl, 2011).

Other modalities such as Medihoney and ultrasound-guided debridement have been reported to be beneficial for SCI wounds, but further research is needed (Biglari et al., 2011; Hill, 2012). The SCIRE project is a good resource for current publications on PU treatment (SCIREproject.com).

CLINICAL PEARL

Advanced wound therapies such as electrical stimulation or platelet-rich plasma gel may be needed to promote healing. Data to date do not support NPWT as being more effective than other advanced therapies in this population.

Tools commonly used to monitor PU healing, such as the PUSH Tool and the BWAT, are not the best tool for evaluation of healing in SCI individuals. They lack established validity, reliability, and sensitivity for persons with SCI; they are designed mainly for use with older populations; and they omit clinical characteristics unique to PUs in persons with SCI (Thomason et al., 2014). The Spinal

Cord Impairment Pressure Ulcer Monitoring Tool (SCI-PUMT) has been developed and validated and is recommended for use in SCI wounds.

Skin or Tissue Flap Surgery

Surgical management to close large or nonhealing PUs involves one of a variety of procedures collectively called "flap" surgeries. These entail creating a "flap" from adjacent tissues that can include skin, fat, muscle, and perfusing blood vessels. This flap of tissue is advanced or rotated over the ulcer site to close the deficit with tissue that is well vascularized rather than the relatively avascular scar tissue that can take months to develop. Benefits to the patient are speed of closure, elimination of dead space, improved vascularity, and weight-bearing tissue that is more resistant to pressure, shearing, and damage. However, flap surgeries are major surgeries and can entail hours under anesthesia. They carry the same health risks as other major surgeries and are not to be entered into lightly.

Skin or tissue flaps are done less frequently now than in the past. Conservative management is considered preferable, especially with the advent of many advanced modalities not previously available. Patients should be thoroughly screened prior to surgery to maximize the chance of success. Flaps are expensive in direct surgical costs, extensive care postsurgically, and in life interruption for the patient. In addition, there is a relatively high rate of complications; Biglari et al. (2013) recently reported a 21% complication rate out of 421 skin flaps. The most common complication was suture line dehiscence (31%) followed by infection (25.2%), hematoma (19.5%), partial necrosis (13.7%), and total flap necrosis (10.3%).

Flap surgeries can create major changes to the anatomy. In addition, it can be difficult to find plastic surgeons who have expertise in flap surgery and flap management. Patient health and the quality of the transposed tissue must be optimal, and the patient must take responsibility for maintaining a healthy lifestyle and for following acute and long-term postflap protocols. The behaviors that contributed to the wound must be modified or the wound will simply reoccur. A strong social support network is necessary to comply with the long periods of immobility and subsequent limited mobility during return to life postsurgically. If these criteria cannot be met, the patient is not a candidate and faces the long road of closure by secondary intention.

Postflap care is critical to promote healing and to minimize complications such as dehiscence, flap failure, or reoccurrence of the wound. The flap must be closely monitored for ischemic changes (pallor or cyanosis and coolness); such changes must be promptly reported to the surgeon so that perfusion can be restored (e.g., via embolectomy). It is equally important to monitor the flap for venous congestion, which is evidenced by increasing warmth and edema as well as deep discoloration; failure to manage the venous congestion can cause eventual ischemia and flap loss. NPWT is commonly used postflap to minimize edema and promote perfusion; leech therapy is also sometimes used to manage acute venous congestion. Effective off-loading of the flap is another critical intervention; patients have to off-load the surgical site entirely for up to 6 weeks and are usually placed on specialty support surfaces to minimize the risk of developing other PUs. High air loss (air fluidized) surfaces were considered "standard of care" for many years but presented many challenges: high rental costs, difficulty for the clinician in providing care for patients in these beds, and the extreme physical discomfort and accompanying personality changes caused by the lack of physical support. As a result, many agencies and clinicians now utilize other advanced surfaces, such as low air loss and/or alternating pressure, with the specific surface dependent on protocols and patient criteria (Fleck et al., 2010). A more stable mattress surface enhances self-bed mobility and facilitates position changes, and stability of the mattress edges enhances transfers during the rehabilitation/readjustment to sitting phase. If the patient is positioned off of the surgery site, the mattress will be helping to prevent other PUs and not interfering with the healing of the surgery site.

CLINICAL PEARL

The patient undergoing myocutaneous flap surgery requires meticulous postoperative care: consistent high level pressure and shear reduction, nutritional support, and monitoring for indicators of flap ischemia or congestion.

Acute post-op care includes assistance in bed mobility and positioning, bowel and bladder management, range of motion and resistive exercise. It is universally recommended that sitting begin 3 to 6 weeks after surgery. At Shepherd Center, Atlanta, Georgia, massage of the surgical site and stretching of the tissues beyond 90-degree hip flexion are begun 2 to 3 weeks post-op. After approximately 1 week of massage and stretching, sitting is resumed in staged increments of an additional ½ to 1 hour each day. Patients are instructed in safe transfer techniques and are taught to avoid stretching the buttocks tissues by limiting hip flexion and avoiding toilet seats for 6 months postflap (Hill, 2012). It is essential to evaluate the individual's home seating surface and sleeping surface and to assure that they provide optimal pressure redistribution; it is also essential to talk openly with the person about off-loading techniques when up in the chair and the critical importance of adherence to these techniques. Home instruction and education is critically important to arm the patient with as much inspiration as possible to avoid a recurrence in the future.

Conclusion

Wounds in persons with SCI are quick to develop, agonizingly slow to heal, and prone to complications, undermining, and depth. The effects of these wounds go far beyond acute medical complications to negatively impact physical, psychological, emotional, and financial status and quality of life. Physiological changes that occur due to the SCI render the tissues below the level of injury markedly different from innervated tissues and slower to respond to wound-healing modalities. Care of these wounds involves wound-healing modalities as well as encouragement in maintaining healthy lifestyle practices specific to the SCI. A comprehensive plan of care including emotional and social support and advocacy may be necessary to achieve wound healing.

CASE STUDY

Sheila is a 45-year-old woman with a 26-year history of SCI at T12. She presents with a PU on her right ischium of 1-year duration. She reports two previous wounds on this same location over the past 19 years. The ischium is especially pointed in shape compared to the left ischium. Sheila is a college-educated woman, well nourished, and appears within normal ranges for her height and weight. She is a nonsmoker and drinks on occasion. She is on no prescription medications and is nondiabetic.

She has been addressing the wound at home with samples of advanced dressings given her by nurse friends and consulting with her primary physician who is an internal medicine specialist. Over the year, she has voluntarily increased her bed rest time while trying to maintain a full-time job. Her employer has allowed her to limit her in office time and increase time working from home. Despite this, the wound increased in size over the year, although not quite reaching bone.

The size of the wound eventually caused Sheila to go on full-time bed rest and to seek further medical attention. Without a wound center or an SCI center in her city, her primary care physician referred her to a local plastic surgeon who was reported to have the best skills and bedside manner in doing the few flap surgeries required in the area per year. Sheila wanted to avoid flap surgery at any cost, and this plastic surgeon also stepped carefully into flaps. He did two serial debridements and prescribed bed rest and various new advanced dressings over 1 month. The wound did not show improvement after this treatment; in fact, it worsened.

She asked her primary doctor to refer her to the wound care center in a neighboring city, even though they specialized in diabetic and vascular wounds and HBO and reportedly did not see many SCI patients. Luckily, the director of the wound center is an infectious disease specialist who diagnosed osteomyelitis and placed her on IV antibiotics for 6 weeks. She prescribed NPWT, which was applied for several weeks. The wound responded for 3 weeks and then stalled at approximately 4 cm × 4 cm × 2 cm deep. The plastic surgeon at this wound care center recommended flap surgery, but his post-op protocol of 6 weeks on air-fluidized support surface, and then a graduated sitting program working up to full day sitting over 3 months was too slow for Sheila.

Sheila asked the center to try a low concentration form of PRP. The first application including 5 days of bed rest resulted in significant visual wound healing. The wound closed completely within 1 month and successive weekly applications of the PRP.

This wound reopened 5 years later. Sheila was referred to the new local wound care center that specialized in vascular and diabetic wounds. Tentative debridements and various advanced dressings were tried, as well as NPWT. The previous plastic surgeon again did a deep debridement and continued the NPWT, with slow results. The low concentration PRP was also tried, with minimal results. Eventually, a secondary diagnosis of osteomyelitis was made. Sheila consulted with a plastic surgeon who had serviced a nationally recognized SCI center within a 3-hour drive of her home. He recommended a "small flap" procedure with debridement of the osteomyelitic bone and an aggressive rehabilitation program post-op. The 45-minute surgery was performed at a hospital adjacent to the SCI center, and Sheila was placed on complete bed rest for 2 weeks on a foam mattress, repositioning with low-to-moderate nursing assistance at frequent time intervals and limiting hip flexion to <60 degrees. Within 3 weeks of the surgery, PT was ordered to begin scar massage and stretching to 100 degrees of hip flexion. After 5 days of this treatment, sitting began with 1 hour morning and afternoon, increasing by 30-minute increments each day for each sitting session. The hospital seating clinic advised no changes to sitting posture in her wheelchair but did advise use of a 4-inch-thick multicelled air cushion. At the end of 1 week, Sheila was sent home with instructions to continue the slow return to sitting and to follow a lengthy list of cautions aimed at limiting stress to the newly formed scar tissue for 6 months. These limitations included no hip flexion past 110 degrees, no sitting on a toilet or toilet-type shower seat, no sliding boards, and never sitting without a cushion among many others. Sheila tried the air cushion but found it too difficult for dressing, transfers, and sitting stability and gradually returned to her original customized foam cushion with ischial cut out. Sheila returned to work shortly after hospital discharge gradually increasing from part time to full time, while followed the stress-limitation directions diligently for nearly 6 months.

She remains ulcer free 3 years later.

REFERENCES

Adegoke, B., & Badmos, K. (2001). Acceleration of pressure ulcer healing in spinal cord injured patients using interrupted direct current. *African Journal of Medicine and Medical Sciences, 30*(3), 195–197.

Agam, L., & Gefen, A. (2008). Toward real-time detection of deep tissue injury risk in wheelchair users using Hertz contact theory. *Journal of Rehabilitation Research and Development, 45*(4), 537–550.

Bader, D. L. (1990). The recovery characteristics of soft tissues following repeated loading. *Journal of Rehabilitation Research and Development, 27*(2), 141–150.

Baker, L. L., Rubayi, S., Villar, F., et al. (1996). Effect of electrical stimulation waveform on healing of ulcers in human beings with spinal cord injury. *Wound Repair and Regeneration, 4*(1), 21–28.

Banks, M., Graves, N., Bauer, J., et al. (2012). Cost effectiveness of nutrition support in the prevention of pressure ulcer in hospitals. *European Journal of Clinical Nutrition, 67*, 42–46.

Becker, B. E., & DeLisa, J. A. (1999). Model spinal cord injury system trends, and implications for the future. *Archives of Physical Medication and Rehabilitation, 80*(11), 1514–1521.

Bergstrom, N., Braden, B. J., Laguzza, A., et al. (1987). The Braden Scale for predicting pressure sore risk. *Nursing Research, 36*(4), 205–210.

Biglari, B., Vd Linden, P., Simon, A., et al. (2011). Use of Medihoney as a non-surgical therapy for chronic pressure ulcers in patients with spinal cord injury. *Spinal Cord, 50*(2), 165–169.

Biglari, B., Büchler, A., Reitzel, T., et al. (2013). A retrospective study on flap complications after pressure ulcer surgery in spinal cord-injured patients. *Spinal Cord, 52*(1), 80–83.

Bogie, K., Nuseibeh, I., & Bader, D. (1995). Early progressive changes in tissue viability in the seated spinal cord injured subject. *Spinal Cord, 33*(3), 141–147.

Brienza, D., & Karg, P. (2012). Pressure ulcers in people with spinal cord injury. In *Pressure ulcers in America: prevalence, incidence, and implications for the future* (2nd ed., pp. 107–112), Washington, DC: National Pressure Ulcer Advisory Panel.

Byrne, D., & Salzberg, C. (1996). Major risk factors for pressure ulcers in the spinal cord disabled: A literature review. *Spinal Cord, 34*(5), 255–263.

Çakmak, S. K., Gül, Ü., Özer, S., et al. (2009). Risk factors for pressure ulcers. *Advances in Skin and Wound Care, 22*(9), 412–415.

Cardenas, D. D., Hoffman, J. M., Kirshblum, S., et al. (2004). Etiology and incidence of rehospitalization after traumatic spinal cord injury: A multicenter analysis. *Archives of Physical Medication and Rehabilitation, 85*(11), 1757–1763.

Castro, M., Apple Jr, D., Staron, R., et al. (1999). Influence of complete spinal cord injury on skeletal muscle within 6 month of injury. *Journal of Applied Physics, 86*, 350–358.

CfSCMCP Guidelines. (2001). Pressure ulcer prevention and treatment following spinal cord injury: A clinical practice guideline for health-care professionals. *The Journal of Spinal Cord Medicine, 24*, S40.

Chen, D., Apple Jr, D. F., Hudson, L. M., et al. (1999a). Medical complications during acute rehabilitation following spinal cord injury—current experience of the Model Systems. *Archives of Physical Medicine and Rehabilitation, 80*(11), 1397.

Chen, D., Apple Jr, D. F., Hudson, L. M., et al. (1999b). Medical complications during acute rehabilitation following spinal cord injury—current experience of the Model Systems. *Archives of Physical Medicine and Rehabilitation, 80*(11), 1397–1401.

Chen, Y., Devivo, M. J., & Jackson, A. B. (2005). Pressure ulcer prevalence in people with spinal cord injury: Age-period-duration effects. *Archives of Physical Medicine and Rehabilitation, 86*(6), 1208–1213.

Clark, F., Pyatak, E. A., Carlson, M., et al. (2014). Implementing trials of complex interventions in community settings: The USC–Rancho Los Amigos Pressure Ulcer Prevention Study (PUPS). *Clinical Trials, 11*(2), 218–229, doi: 1740774514521904.

Claus-Walker, J., Singh, J., Leach, C., et al. (1977). The urinary excretion of collagen degradation products by quadriplegic patients and during weightlessness. *The Journal of Bone and Joint Surgery, 59*(2), 209–212.

Coggrave, M., & Rose, L. (2003). A specialist seating assessment clinic: Changing pressure relief practice. *Spinal Cord, 41*(12), 692–695.

Conner-Kerr, T., Sullivan, P., Gaillard, J., et al. (1998). The effects of ultraviolet radiation on antibiotic-resistant bacteria in vitro. *Ostomy/Wound Management, 44*(10), 50–56.

Cruse, J., Wang, H., Lewis, R., et al. (2002). Cellular and molecular alterations in spinal cord injury patients with pressure ulcers: A preliminary report. *Experimental and Molecular Pathology, 72*(2), 124–131.

Dai, T., Vrahas, M. S., Murray, C. K., et al. (2012). Ultraviolet C irradiation: An alternative antimicrobial approach to localized infections? *Expert Review of Anti-Infective Therapy, 10*(2), 185–195.

de Bruin, E., Herzog, R., Rozendal, R., et al. (2000). Estimation of geometric properties of cortical bone in spinal cord injury. *Archives of Physical Medicine and Rehabilitation, 81*, 150–156.

de Laat, E. H., van den Boogaard, M. H., Spauwen, P. H., et al. (2011). Faster wound healing with topical negative pressure therapy in difficult-to-heal wounds: A prospective randomized controlled trial. *Annals of Plastic Surgery, 67*(6), 626–631.

DeJong, G., Hsieh, C., Brown, P., et al. (2014). Factors associated with pressure ulcer development in spinal cord injury rehabilitation. *American Journal of Physical Medicine and Rehabilitation, 93*(11), 971–986.

Edwards, L. A., Bugaresti, J. M., & Buchholz, A. C. (2008). Visceral adipose tissue and the ratio of visceral to subcutaneous adipose tissue are greater in adults with than in those without spinal cord injury, despite matching waist circumferences. *The American Journal of Clinical Nutrition, 87*(3), 600–607.

Ennis, W. (2013). Cell and tissue therapy. *Paper presented at the Symposium on Advanced Wound Care Spring, Denver, CO.*

Fantuzzi, G. (2005). Adipose tissue, adipokines, and inflammation. *Journal of Allergy and Clinical Immunology, 115*(5), 911–919.

Fleck, C. A., Rappl, L. M., Simman, R., et al. (2010). Use of alternatives to air-fluidized support surfaces in the care of complex wounds in postflap and postgraft patients. *The Journal of the American College of Certified Wound Specialists, 2*(1), 4–8.

Fogerty, M. D., Abumrad, N. N., Nanney, L., et al. (2008). Risk factors for pressure ulcers in acute care hospitals. *Wound Repair and Regeneration, 16*(1), 11–18.

Frost, F., Roach, M. J., Kushner, I., et al. (2005). Inflammatory C-reactive protein and cytokine levels in asymptomatic people with chronic spinal cord injury. *Archives of Physical Medicine and Rehabilitation, 86*(2), 312–317.

Gefen, A. (2008). The Compression Intensity Index: A practical anatomical estimate of the biomechanical risk for a deep tissue injury. *Technology and Health Care, 16*(2), 141–149.

Gefen, A. (2014). Tissue changes in patients following spinal cord injury and implications for wheelchair cushions and tissue loading: A literature review. *Ostomy Wound Management, 60*(2), 34–45.

Giangregorio, L., & McCartney, N. (2006). Bone loss and muscle atrophy in spinal cord injury: Epidemiology, fracture prediction, and rehabilitation strategies. *The Journal of Spinal Cord Medicine, 29*, 489–500.

Griffin, J. W., Tooms, R. E., Mendius, R. A., et al. (1991). Efficacy of high voltage pulsed current for healing of pressure ulcers in patients with spinal cord injury. *Physical Therapy, 71*(6), 433–442.

Guihan, M., & Bombardier, C. H. (2012). Potentially modifiable risk factors among veterans with spinal cord injury hospitalized for severe pressure ulcers: a descriptive study. *Journal of Spinal Cord Medicine, 35*(4), 240–250.

Guttmann, L. (1976). *Spinal cord injuries: comprehensive management and research* (vol.6), Oxford, England: Blackwell Scientific Publications.

Hill, J. (2012). Postoperative flap management at Shepherd Center. *Rehabilitation and Management, 25*(7), 18–21.

Hitzig, S. L., Tonack, M., Campbell, K. A., et al. (2008). Secondary health complications in an aging Canadian spinal cord injury sample. *American Journal of Physical Medicine and Rehabilitation, 87*(7), 545–555, doi: 10.1097/PHM.0b013e31817c16d610.1097/PHM.0b013e31817c16d6.

Ho, C. H., Powell, H. L., Collins, J. F., et al. (2010). Poor nutrition is a relative contraindication to negative pressure wound therapy for pressure ulcers: Preliminary observations in patients with spinal cord injury. *Advances in Skin and Wound Care, 23*(11), 508–516.

Hunter, T., & Rajan, K. (1971). The role of ascorbic acid in the pathogenesis and treatment of pressure sores. *Spinal Cord, 8*(4), 211–216.

Inskip, J. A., Ramer, L. M., Ramer, M. S., et al. (2009). Autonomic assessment of animals with spinal cord injury: Tools, techniques and translation. *Spinal Cord, 47*, 2–35.

Jones, M., Mathewson, C., Adkins, V., et al. (2003). Use of behavioral contingencies to promote prevention of recurrent pressure ulcers. *Archives of Physical Medicine & Rehabilitation, 84*(6), 796–802.

Kennedy, P., Berry, C., Coggrave, M., et al. (2003). The effect of a specialist seating assessment clinic on the skin management of individuals with spinal cord injury. *Journal of Tissue Viability, 13*(3), 122–125.

Kottner, J., Dassen, T., & Tannen, A. (2009). Inter- and intrarater reliability of the Waterlow pressure sore risk scale: A systematic review. *International Journal of Nursing Studies, 46*(3), 369–379, doi: 10.1016/j.ijnurstu.2008.09.01010.1016/j.ijnurstu.2008.09.010.

Krause, J. S., Vines, C. L., Farley, T. L., et al. (2001). An exploratory study of pressure ulcers after spinal cord injury: Relationship to protective behaviors and risk factors. *Archives of Physical Medicine and Rehabilitation, 82*(1), 107–113.

Krishnan, S. (2014). *Factors associated with occurrence and early detection of pressure ulcers following traumatic spinal cord injury*. Doctoral Dissertation, University of Pittsburgh.

Kynes, P. (1986). A new perspective on pressure sore prevention. *Journal of Enterostomal Therapy, 13*(2), 42.

Levy, A., Kopplin, K., & Gefen, A. (2013). Simulation of skin and subcutaneous tissue loading in the buttocks while regaining weight bearing after a pushup in wheelchair users. *Journal of Mechanical Behavior of Biomedical Materials, 28*, 436–447.

Levy, A., Kopplin, K., & Gefen, A. (2014). An air-cell-based cushion for pressure ulcer protection remarkably reduces tissue stresses in the seated buttocks with respect to foams: Finite element studies. *Journal of Tissue Viability, 23*(1), 13–23.

Lindan, O. (1961). Etiology of decubitus ulcers: An experimental study. *Archives of Physical Medicine and Rehabilitation, 42*, 774–783.

Linder-Ganz, E., & Gefen, A. (2009). Stress analyses coupled with damage laws to determine biomechanical risk factors for deep tissue injury during sitting. *Journal of Biomechanical Engineering, 131*(1), 011003.

Linder-Ganz, E., Shabshin, N., Itzchak, Y., et al. (2008). Strains and stresses in sub-dermal tissues of the buttocks are greater in paraplegics than in healthy during sitting. *Journal of Biomechanics, 41*, 567–580.

Liu, L. Q., Moody, J., Traynor, M., et al. (2014). A systematic review of electrical stimulation for pressure ulcer prevention and treatment in people with spinal cord injuries. *Journal of Spinal Cord Medicine, 37*(6), 703–718.

Makhsous, M., Priebe, M., Bankard, J., et al. (2007). Measuring tissue perfusion during pressure relief maneuvers: Insights into preventing pressure ulcers. *The Journal of Spinal Cord Medicine, 30*(5), 497.

Manzano, F., Navarro, M. J., Roldán, D., et al. (2010). Pressure ulcer incidence and risk factors in ventilated intensive care patients. *Journal of Critical Care, 25*(3), 469–476.

Mathewson, C., Adkins, V., Lenyoun, M., et al. (1999). Using telemedicine in the treatment of pressure ulcers. *Ostomy/Wound Management, 45*(11), 58–62.

Mawson, A. R., Biundo Jr, J. J., Neville, P., et al. (1988). Risk factors for early occurring pressure ulcers following spinal cord injury. *American Journal of Physical Medicine and Rehabilitation, 67*(3), 123–127.

Mawson, A., Siddiqui, F., & Biundo, J. (1993). Enhancing host resistance to pressure ulcers: A new approach to prevention. *Preventive Medicine, 22*(3), 433–450.

McKinley, W. O., Jackson, A. B., Cardenas, D. D., et al. (1999). Long-term medical complications after traumatic spinal cord injury: A regional model systems analysis. *Archives of Physical Medicine and Rehabilitation, 80*(11), 1402–1410.

McKinley, W., Tewksbury, M., & Godbout, C. (2002). Comparison of medical complications following nontraumatic and traumatic spinal cord injury. *The Journal of Spinal Cord Medicine, 25*(2), 88.

Mortenson, W., & Miller, W. (2007). A review of scales for assessing the risk of developing a pressure ulcer in individuals with SCI. *Spinal Cord, 46*(3), 168–175.

National Spinal Cord Injury Statistical Center. (2011). Spinal Cord Injury Facts and Figures at a Glance. Retrieved July 18, 2013, from http://www.ncbi.nlm.nih.gov/pmc/articles/PMC3237291/pdf/scm-34-620.pdf

Norton, D. (1980). [Norton scale for decubitus prevention]. *Krankenpflege (Frankf), 34*(1), 16.

Noridian—Medicare Pricing, Data Analysis and Coding (PDAC). (2014). Application and Checklist for PDAC HCPCS Coding Verification Request: Wheelchair Cushions. Website https://www.dmepdac.com/review/apps_check.html. Accessed August 18, 2014.

NSCISC. (2006). *Annual Report for the Model Spinal Cord Injury Care Systems*. Birmingham, AL.

NSCISC. (2011). *Annual Report for the Model Spinal Cord Injury Care Systems*. Birmingham, AL.

Nussbaum, E. L., Biemann, I., Mustard, B. (1994). Comparison of ultrasound/ultraviolet C and laser for treatment of pressure ulcers in patients with spinal cord injury. *Physical Therapy, 74*(9), 812–825.

Nussbaum, E. L., Flett, H., Hitzig, S. L., et al. (2013). Ultraviolet C irradiation in the management of pressure ulcers in people with spinal cord injury: A randomized placebo-controlled trial. *Archives of Physical Medicine & Rehabilitation, 94*(4), 650–659.

Pagliacci, M. C., Celani, M. G., Zampolini, M., et al. (2003). An Italian survey of traumatic spinal cord injury. The Gruppo Italiano studio epidemiologico Mielolesioni study. *Archives of Physical Medicine and Rehabilitation, 84*(9), 1266–1275.

Patterson, R., Cranmer, H. H., Fisher, S. V., et al. (1993). The impaired response of spinal cord injured individuals to repeated surface pressure loads. *Archives of Physical Medicine and Rehabilitation, 74*(9), 947–953.

Peerless, J. R., Davies, A., Klein, D., et al. (1999). Skin complications in the intensive care unit. *Clinics in Chest Medicine, 20*(2), 453–467.

Portnoy, S., Vuillerme, N., Payan, Y., et al. (2011). Clinically oriented real-time monitoring of the individual's risk for deep tissue injury. *Medical and Biological Engineering and Computing, 49*(4), 473–483.

Rappl, L. M. (2008). Physiological changes in tissues denervated by spinal cord injury tissues and possible effects on wound healing. *International Wound Journal, 5*(3), 435–444.

Rappl, L. M. (2011). Effect of platelet rich plasma gel in a physiologically relevant platelet concentration on wounds in persons with spinal cord injury. *International Wound Journal, 8*(2), 187–195.

Reddy, M., Gill, S. S., & Rochon, P. A. (2006). Preventing pressure ulcers: A systematic review. *JAMA: The Journal of the American Medical Association, 296*(8), 974–984.

Regan, M., Teasell, R. W., Keast, D., et al. (2012). Pressure ulcers following spinal cord injury. In J. J. Eng, R. Teasell, W. C. Miller, et al. (Eds.), *Spinal Cord Injury Rehabilitation Evidence*. Vancouver.

Richardson, R. R., & Meyer, P. R. (1981). Prevalence and incidence of pressure sores in acute spinal cord injuries. *Spinal Cord, 19*(4), 235–247.

Rittweger, J., Gerrits, K., Altenburg, T., et al. (2006). Bone adaptation to altered loading after spinal cord injury: A study of bone and muscle strength. *Journal of Musculoskeletal and Neuronal Interactions, 6*, 269–276.

Rodriguez, G., & Claus-Walker, J. (1988). Biochemical changes in skin composition in spinal cord injury: A possible contribution to decubitus ulcers. *Spinal Cord, 26*(5), 302–309.

Rodriguez, G., & Markowski, J. (1995). Changes in skin morphology and its relationship to pressure ulcer incidence in spinal cord injury [ACRM abstract]. *Archives of Physical Medicine and Rehabilitation, 76*(6), 593.

Saladin, L. K., & Krause, J. S. (2009). Pressure ulcer prevalence and barriers to treatment after spinal cord injury: Comparisons of four groups based on race-ethnicity. *NeuroRehabilitation, 24*(1), 57–66. doi: 10.3233/NRE-2009-0454.

Salzberg, C. A., Byrne, D. W., Cayten, C. G., et al. (1996). A new pressure ulcer risk assessment scale for individuals with spinal cord injury. *American Journal of Physical Medicine and Rehabilitation, 75*(2), 96–104.

Salzberg, C., Byrne, D. W., Cayten, G. C., et al. (1998). Predicting and preventing pressure ulcers in adults with paralysis. *Advances in Skin and Wound Care, 11*(5), 237–246.

Scevola, S., Nicoletti, G., Brenta, F., et al. (2010). Allogenic platelet gel in the treatment of pressure sores: A pilot study. *International Wound Journal, 7*(3), 184–190.

Smith, B. M., Guihan, M., LaVela, S. L., et al. (2008). Factors predicting pressure ulcers in veterans with spinal cord injuries. *American Journal of Physical Medicine and Rehabilitation, 87*(9), 750–757. doi: 10.1097/PHM.0b013e3181837a50.

Sonenblum, S. E., & Sprigle, S. H. (2011). The impact of tilting on blood flow and localized tissue loading. *Journal of Tissue Viability, 20*(1), 3–13.

Sprigle, S. H., & Sonenblum, S. E. (2011). Assessing evidence supporting redistribution of pressure for pressure ulcer prevention: A review. *Journal of Rehabilitation Research & Development, 48*(3), 203–213.

Stefanovska, A., Vodovnik, L., Benko, H., et al. (1993). Treatment of chronic wounds by means of electric and electromagnetic fields. *Medical and Biological Engineering and Computing, 31*(3), 213–220.

Stover, S. L., DeLisa, J. A., & Whiteneck, G. G. (1995). *Spinal cord injury: clinical outcomes from the model systems*. Gaithersburg, MD: Aspen Publishers.

Teasell, R. W., Arnold, J. M. O., Krassioukov, A., et al. (2000). Cardiovascular consequences of loss of supraspinal control of the sympathetic nervous system after spinal cord injury. *Archives of Physical Medicine and Rehabilitation, 81*, 506–516.

Thakral, G., LaFontaine, J., Najafi, B., et al. (2013). Electrical stimulation to accelerate wound healing. *Diabetic Foot and Ankle, 4*.

Thijssen, D. H. J., Maiorana, A. J., O'Driscoll, G., et al. (2010). Impact of inactivity and exercise on the vasculature in humans. *European Journal of Applied Physiology, 108*, 845–875.

Thomason, S. S., Luther, S. L., Powell-Cope, G. M., et al. (2014). Validity and reliability of a pressure ulcer monitoring tool for persons with spinal cord impairment. *J Spinal Cord Med, 37*(3), 317–327.

University of Alabama Birmingham, School of Medicine, Department of Physical Medicine and Rehabilitation website, (2014). Pressure Ulcers and Skin Care. www.uab.edu/medicine/sci/daily-living/managing-personal-health/secondary-medical-conditions/pressure-ulcers-a-skin. Accessed August 14, 2014.

Vaishampayan, A., Clark, F., Carlson, M., et al. (2011). Preventing pressure ulcers in people with spinal cord injury: Targeting risky life circumstances through community-based interventions. *Advances in Skin and Wound Care, 24*(6), 275–284; quiz 285–276.

Vaziri, N. D., Eltorai, I., Gonzales, E., et al. (1992). Pressure ulcer, fibronectin, and related proteins in spinal cord injured patients. *Archives of Physical Medicine and Rehabilitation, 73*, 803–806.

Watts, D., Abrahams, E., MacMillan, C., et al. (1998). Insult after injury: Pressure ulcers in trauma patients. *Orthopaedic Nursing, 17*, 84–91.

Wilczweski, P., Grimm, D., Gianakis, A., et al. (2012). Risk factors associated with pressure ulcer development in critically ill traumatic spinal cord injury patients. *Journal of Trauma Nursing, 19*(1), 5–10. doi: 10.1097/JTN.0b013e31823a4528.

QUESTIONS

1. The wound care nurse is teaching a patient with a spinal cord injury (SCI) how to accomplish a "clean transfer." What intervention is recommended for this procedure?

A. Using a sliding board
B. Using extra attendants for the transfer if needed
C. Learning how to unweight bony prominences
D. Choosing a softer mattress and chair pad

2. The wound care nurse is teaching pressure ulcer prevention to a patient with a spinal cord injury (SCI). What teaching point reflects a recommended intervention for patients with SCI to restore normal blood flow and oxygen levels?

A. Sleep in the prone position if possible.
B. Off-weight by leaning backward with the elbows on a flat surface.
C. Tilt the seat-and-back unit to <65 degrees for 1 minute.
D. Perform wheelchair push-ups for 60 seconds every 30 minutes.

3. The wound care nurse recommends skin checks for a paraplegic being transferred to a rehabilitation facility. What sign would indicate that a pressure ulcer is developing?

A. Blanchable erythema that is present 15 minutes following off-weighting.
B. Warmth persisting 30 minutes following off-weighting.
C. An area of the skin feels cool to the touch compared to the rest of the skin.
D. A reddened area does not return to normal color when off-weighting 1 hour.

4. What assessment technique must the SCI individual (or caregiver) use to ensure a pressure ulcer is not developing unnoticed in the subdermal tissues?

A. Observation
B. Palpation
C. Auscultation
D. Percussion

5. The wound care nurse is teaching hygienic measures to protect the skin to a patient with a recently diagnosed spinal cord injury (SCI). What statement reflects a recommended guideline for this population?
   A. Bathe daily to remove irritating perspiration.
   B. Use pH-balanced no-rinse cleansers on the skin.
   C. Do not use baby wipes on the perineal area.
   D. Remove bowel or bladder incontinence with alcohol wipes.

6. For what two comorbidities does the risk of mortality increase for the person with a spinal cord injury (SCI) by 1.4- and 2-fold, respectively?
   A. Diabetes mellitus and congestive heart failure
   B. Diabetes mellitus and renal failure
   C. Pulmonary disease and bladder cancer
   D. Renal failure and hypertension

7. The wound care nurse is aware that 47% of all pressure ulcers occur over the ischial tuberosities and sacrum. What intervention would the nurse institute based on this statistic?
   A. Have the patient lie in a side-lying position to sleep.
   B. Tell the patient to stay out of the wheelchair as much as possible.
   C. Maintain the wheelchair and seat cushion in proper working order.
   D. Pad the bony prominences with foam overlays.

8. The wound care nurse is inspecting the wheelchair of a patient who just returned from a seating clinic. What is a recommended guideline for choosing a wheelchair seat?
   A. Shaped cushions are always contraindicated.
   B. A slightly reclined position should be maintained to improve function and prevent shearing forces.
   C. Thicker cushions should be used to facilitate dressing and transfers to other surfaces.
   D. The cushion should envelop the skeleton, spreading interface pressure across the whole seating surface.

9. The wound care nurse is investigating why modalities and treatments used in the management of wounds are less effective with spinal cord–injured patients. What is one reason that has surfaced?
   A. There is an increase in sympathetic innervation causing enhanced perfusion of the skin and soft tissues.
   B. $TcPO_2$ levels may be up to five times lower below the level of injury than above, decreasing oxygen to the wound.
   C. Collagen is not excreted as quickly through the urine of a person with SCI causing a buildup in the wound bed.
   D. SCI patients have a significantly higher concentration of fibronectin, which counteracts the function of collagen.

10. Based on the recommendations of the SCIRE (Spinal Cord Injury Rehabilitation Evidence) project, what priority intervention should the wound care nurse recommend for a patient with a spinal cord injury who develops pressure ulcers?
    A. Regular off-weighting exercises and sitting in safe cushion environment
    B. Extended periods of bed rest with limited sitting in safe cushion environment
    C. Negative pressure wound therapy (NPWT) with daily dressing changes
    D. Monitored healing using the PUSH tool and the BWAT

11. The wound care nurse is preparing a patient who has a spinal cord injury for tissue flap surgery to heal a pressure ulcer. What intervention is a recommended guideline for postsurgical care?
    A. Monitoring the site for ischemic changes
    B. Off-loading the site every 2 hours for 6 weeks
    C. Placing the patients on an alternating pressure overlay
    D. Initiating sitting 1 week after surgery

ANSWERS: 1.**B**, 2.**A**, 3.**D**, 4.**B**, 5.**B**, 6.**A**, 7.**C**, 8.**D**, 9.**B**, 10.**B**, 11.**A**

PART 2

Specific Wounds

CHAPTER 16

General Concepts Related to Skin and Soft Tissue Injury Caused by Mechanical Factors

Dorothy B. Doughty and Laurie L. McNichol

OBJECTIVES

1. Define the following terms: friction; shear; pressure.
2. Explain the pathology and clinical presentation of each of the following:
    - Friction injuries
    - Moisture associated skin damage
    - Pressure–shear injuries
3. Explain the concept of "top down" versus "bottom up" tissue damage
4. Explain the importance of accurate classification of pressure and nonpressure injuries
5. Identify the parameters most critical to accurate differential assessment of trunk wounds
6. Utilize patient history, wound location, and wound characteristics to determine probable wound etiology
7. Discuss current challenges in accurate wound classification

Topic Outline

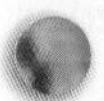

Introduction

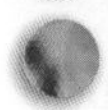

Overview of Mechanical Factors Causing Skin and Tissue Damage

Moisture-Associated Skin Damage
Friction
Shear
Pressure

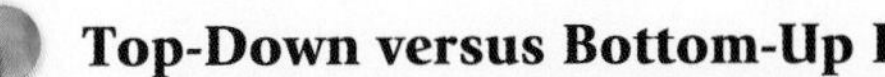

Top-Down versus Bottom-Up Injury

Importance Accurate Classification
Top-Down versus Bottom-Up Concept of Injury

Guidelines for Differential Assessment

Current Gaps

Conclusion

Introduction

The first half of this core curriculum focused on general concepts related to skin and soft tissue anatomy, the physiology of wound healing, guidelines for wound assessment, and the principles of wound management, to include both systemic factors and topical therapy; there were also chapters devoted to wound healing and wound management for specific patient populations. In the second half of the curriculum, the focus will be on specific types of wounds; this section will address wounds caused by mechanical factors, vascular and metabolic disease, infectious processes, dermatologic conditions, oncologic conditions, and trauma.

Mechanical factors contributing to skin and soft tissue breakdown include friction, shear, pressure, and moisture; management of these factors is essential for prevention of skin breakdown, which is a key nursing responsibility in all care settings. This chapter will provide an overview of these mechanical factors and the differences in breakdown that occurs from "top down" versus "bottom up." Guidelines for differential assessment are provided, and current gaps in our knowledge and research base are addressed.

CLINICAL PEARL

Mechanical factors contributing to skin and soft tissue breakdown include friction, shear, pressure, and moisture; management of these factors is essential for prevention of skin breakdown.

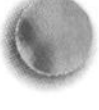

Overview of Mechanical Factors Causing Skin and Soft Tissue Damage

Incontinence-associated dermatitis, intertriginous dermatitis, other forms of moisture-associated skin damage, friction lesions, skin tears, and pressure ulcers are all examples of skin and soft tissue damage caused by mechanical factors. Effective management of these factors can significantly reduce the incidence of skin and soft tissue breakdown, and most wounds caused by mechanical factors are considered to be avoidable. Thus, the wound care nurse must educate her/his staff regarding the adverse effects of moisture, friction, shear, and pressure on tissue viability, and the specific strategies to be used to mitigate their effects.

Moisture-Associated Skin Damage

Normally hydrated skin is resistant to other types of mechanical damage, while overhydrated skin is associated with reduced tensile strength and increased vulnerability to breakdown caused by friction, shear, pressure, or exposure to pathogens, irritants, and enzymes. Recent consensus sessions and documents have introduced the concept of "moisture plus" in the etiology of skin and soft tissue breakdown (Gray et al., 2011, 2012). Overhydration (maceration) results in increased permeability of the cell wall, which renders the epithelium more vulnerable to invasion by pathogens, irritants, or enzymatic agents. In addition, overhydration increases the friction coefficient between the skin and the underlying linen or absorptive pads; this translates into increased "drag" (frictional forces and shear forces) when the patient is repositioned. Finally, multiple studies confirm the link between overhydration and pressure ulcer development, probably because macerated tissues are less able to provide normal pressure distribution (Doughty et al., 2012; Gray et al., 2011, 2012; Mahoney et al., 2013). As a result of increased understanding of the impact of moisture on skin health, there is now a focus on "skin microclimate control"; this will be addressed further in the chapter on support surfaces.

CLINICAL PEARL

Overhydrated skin is more vulnerable to invasion by pathogens, irritants, or enzymatic agents, is at greater risk for friction and shear damage, and is also at greater risk for pressure ulcer development.

The four most common types of moisture-associated skin damage are incontinence-associated dermatitis; intertriginous dermatitis; peristomal moisture-associated skin damage; and periwound moisture-associated skin damage (Gray et al., 2011). Each of these will be addressed in detail in Chapter 17, along with implications for management.

Friction

Friction (frictional force) is defined as "the resistance to a motion in a parallel direction relative to the common boundary of two surfaces, for example, when skin is dragged across a coarse surface, such as bed linens." Current evidence suggests that friction alone causes superficial skin loss that presents clinically as an abrasion or "rug burn." This type of skin damage should not be confused with or classified as a pressure ulcer; the most recent iteration of the Prevention and Treatment of Pressure Ulcers International Clinical Practice Guideline clearly states that friction is no longer considered an etiologic factor for pressure ulcers (Bryant, 2012; National Pressure Ulcer Advisory Panel/European Pressure Ulcer Advisory Panel/Pan Pacific Pressure Injury Alliance, 2014).

CLINICAL PEARL

Friction alone causes superficial skin damage that presents as an abrasion; friction alone is no longer considered an etiologic factor for pressure ulcers.

In contrast, friction combined with force can cause shear, which *is* an etiologic factor for pressure ulcer development. Frictional forces cause the skin to adhere to the bed or chair surface, while gravity pulls the deep tissues down toward the foot of the bed or chair; this causes the tissue layers to slide against one another, which causes distortion of the blood vessels that pass through the involved tissue layers. This distortion of the blood vessels causes ischemic damage that contributes to pressure ulcer development (Bryant, 2012; Pieper, 2012) (Figs. 16-1 and 16-2).

CLINICAL PEARL

Friction in combination with gravity causes shear, and shear is an etiologic factor for pressure ulcer development.

Shear

There are two components to shear: shear stress, defined as the force per unit area exerted parallel to the plane of interest, and shear strain, defined as the distortion or deformation of tissue as a result of shear stress (NPUAP/EPUAP/PPPIA, 2014). Shear strain can cause either superficial damage, as occurs with skin tears, or deep damage, as occurs with pressure ulcers (Bryant, 2012). Skin tears most commonly involve shearing of the epidermal layer from the dermal layer, as a result of patient handling or adhesive removal; this type of superficial shear force usually creates

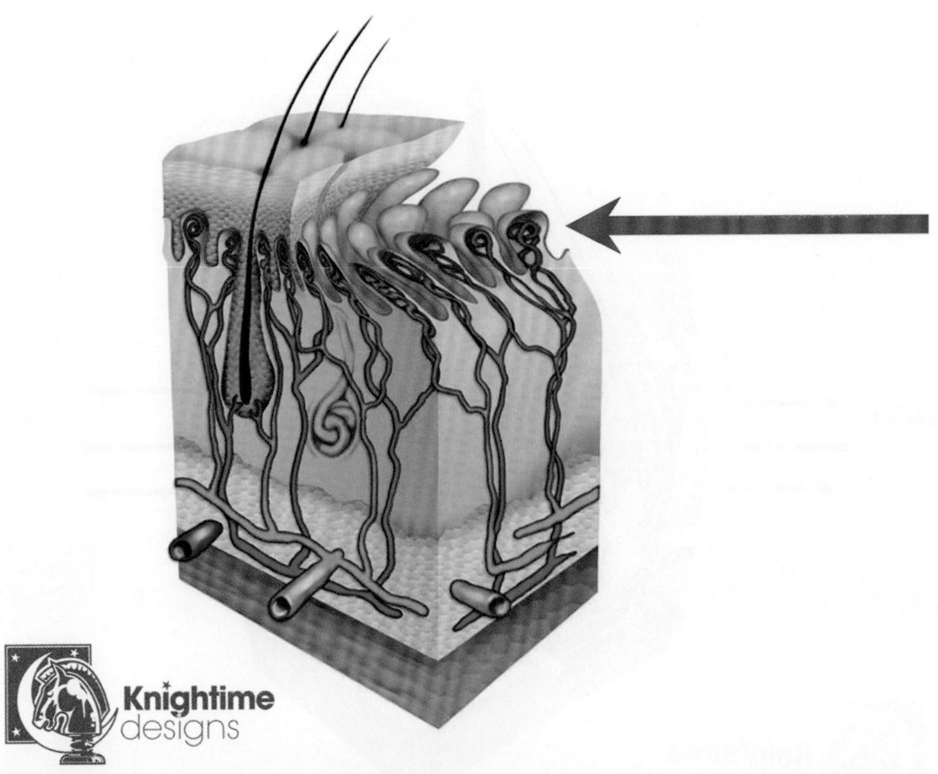

FIGURE 16-1. Shear is a force parallel to the surface of the skin. (Courtesy of Laura Edsberg, PhD.)

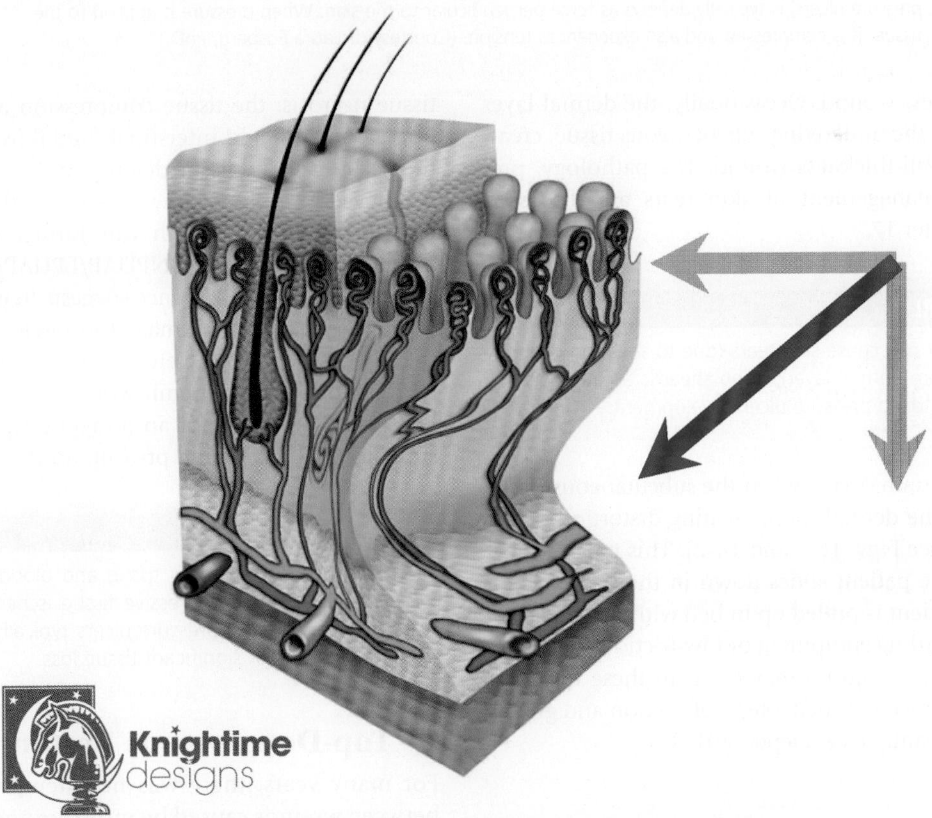

FIGURE 16-2. Tissue distortion as a result of shear force. The total force is the combination of both pressure and shear forces applied to the tissue. Depending on the magnitude of the components (pressure and shear), this force can significantly impact deep tissues. (Courtesy of Laura Edsberg, PhD.)

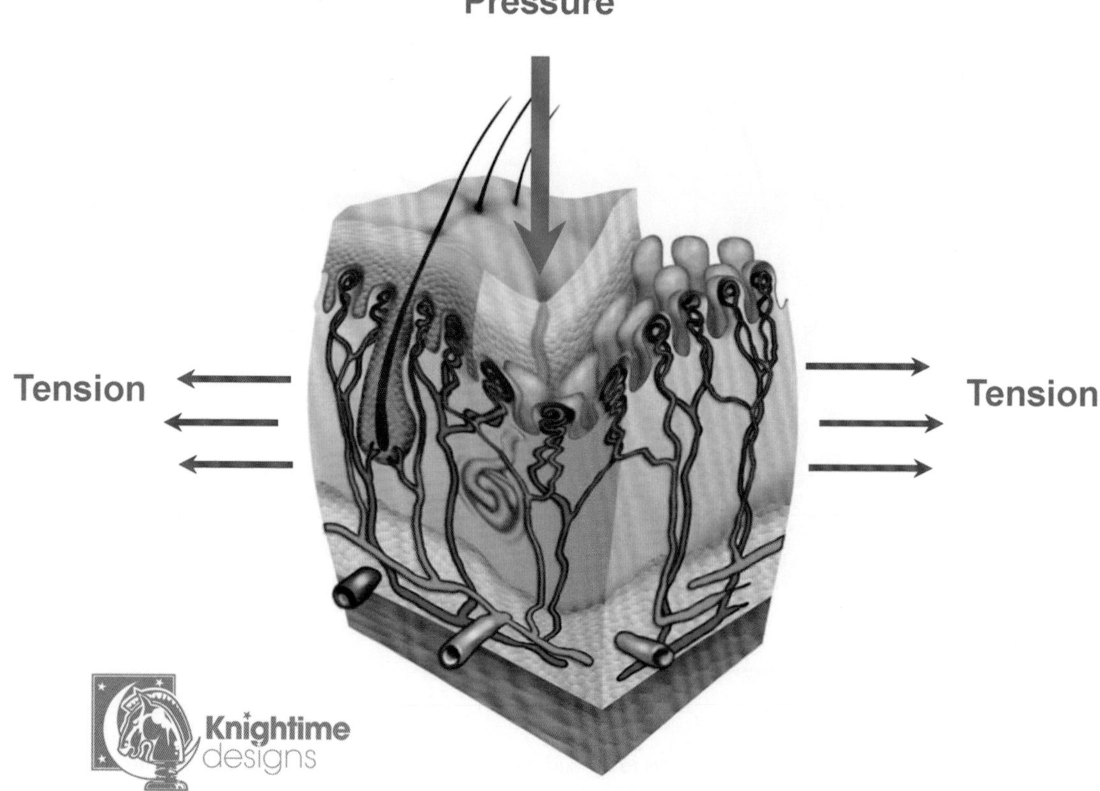

FIGURE 16-3. Pressure and tension: vertical compression of tissues leading to ischemia. Pressure (in pressure ulcers) is typically defined as force perpendicular to the skin. When pressure is applied to the tissue, it is compressed and also experiences tension. (Courtesy of Laura Edsberg, PhD.)

a partial-thickness wound. Occasionally, the dermal layer is sheared from the underlying subcutaneous tissue, creating a shallow full-thickness wound. The pathology, prevention, and management of skin tears are discussed further in Chapter 17.

CLINICAL PEARL

Superficial shear can cause skin tears (due to shearing of epidermal layer from dermal layer); deep shear is a causative or contributing factor to pressure ulcer development.

Deep shear strain occurs when the subcutaneous tissue shears against the dermal layer, creating distortion of the blood vessels (see Figs. 16-1 and 16-2). This type of shear occurs when the patient slides down in the bed or chair or when the patient is pulled up in bed without the use of safe patient handling equipment or low-friction coefficient linens. Deep tissue injuries may occur in these instances and are due to the combined effects of friction and gravity (i.e., shear) (Bryant, 2012; Pieper, 2012).

Pressure

Pressure is defined as "normal force per unit surface area." Sustained pressure causes tissue and blood vessel compression that results in progressive tissue ischemia and eventual tissue necrosis; the tissue compression also impairs lymphatic function and interstitial fluid flow, which increases the risk of cell and tissue death (Fig. 16-3). When pressure is relieved and blood flow is restored, there is the risk of reperfusion injury, which can further compromise the already damaged tissues (NPUAP/EPUAP/PPPIA, 2014). In addition, emerging evidence suggests that unrelieved pressure can cause direct damage to muscle cells unrelated to the ischemic damage (Gefen, 2012). Thus, pressure ulcers typically present as ischemic wounds with significant tissue loss (see Chapter 18 for an in-depth explanation of pressure ulcer pathology and presentation).

CLINICAL PEARL

Sustained pressure causes tissue and blood vessel compression that results in progressive tissue ischemia and eventual tissue necrosis; thus, pressure ulcers typically present as ischemic wounds with significant tissue loss.

Top-Down versus Bottom-Up Injury

For many years, there was no attempt to differentiate between wounds caused by moisture and/or friction versus those caused by pressure and/or shear; any wound located in the trunk area was typically labeled a "pressure ulcer."

Importance Accurate Classification

Over the past decade, there has been increasing recognition that most pressure ulcers are avoidable; as a result, third-party payers no longer provide reimbursement for agency-acquired pressure ulcers, and the incidence of agency-acquired pressure ulcers is a reportable quality-of-care indicator. Benchmarking of quality indicators is now standard, and such benchmarking data are available to the public. This means that agencies need to accurately assess and document any pressure ulcers present on admission and to accurately differentiate between pressure ulcers and other types of skin breakdown. Failure to accurately classify wounds based on etiology compromises the accuracy of benchmarking data and can potentially increase an agency's risk for fiscal penalties related to perceived poor quality of care. It is therefore critical for the wound care clinicians to accurately classify wounds and to educate and assist their staff to classify wounds correctly (Mahoney et al., 2013). However, this is difficult to achieve since clear guidelines for differential assessment are not yet available, and since some wounds are of mixed or unclear etiology.

Top-Down versus Bottom-Up Concept of Injury

One concept that can help to differentiate ischemic wounds (those caused by pressure and/or shear) from nonischemic wounds (those caused by moisture and/or friction) is the "top-down" versus "bottom-up" concept of injury. Current evidence indicates that most ischemic wounds develop from the "bottom up," because the muscle layer is much more vulnerable to ischemia than the epidermis, dermis, and subcutaneous tissue; this means that reduced perfusion will have the greatest effects at the muscle layer. In contrast, nonischemic wounds develop from the "top down" because overhydration and friction primarily affect the exposed surface of the skin (Sibbald et al., 2011). Thus, most pressure/shear wounds are full-thickness wounds that exhibit evidence of ischemic damage, while most nonpressure wounds present as superficial wounds with evidence of abrasive force (and possibly maceration) but no evidence of tissue ischemia. In teaching bedside clinicians to distinguish between pressure wounds and nonpressure wounds, it is sometimes instructive to have them ask: Is there evidence of ischemic damage or significant tissue loss? *or* Does this wound appear to have been caused by mechanical damage that removed the skin one layer at a time?

CLINICAL PEARL

Ischemic wounds develop from the "bottom up," because the muscle layer is more vulnerable to ischemia than the skin layers and subcutaneous tissue; in contrast, wounds caused by moisture and/or friction present as superficial wounds with evidence of abrasive force (and possibly maceration) but no evidence of ischemia.

Guidelines for Differential Assessment

As noted, accurate classification of wounds according to etiology is critical in today's health care environment, and this is frequently very challenging for the bedside clinician. While there is considerable evidence to support the "bottom-up" progression of pressure ulcers and the "top-down" progression of moisture and friction injuries, we currently lack any diagnostic tool or imaging technology that is readily available for use by bedside clinicians and that would clearly distinguish between superficial and deep tissue damage. The clinician is therefore challenged to determine probable etiology based on comprehensive wound assessment, patient history, and understanding of the mechanisms of injury involved in each type of wound.

The assessment parameters of greatest value to differential assessment of trunk wounds include (1) location; (2) wound depth (partial vs. full thickness) and characteristics (indicators of ischemia vs. indicators of maceration and/or friction); and (3) patient history (**Table 16-1**). The mechanism of injury for pressure ulcers is ischemia caused by soft tissue and blood vessel compression; thus, pressure ulcers are most likely to occur over bony prominences or under medical devices (where pressure and vessel compression is greatest). In terms of wound characteristics, pressure ulcers are typically full-thickness (because damage usually begins at the muscle–bone interface), they typically demonstrate evidence of necrosis (significant tissue loss, purple discoloration, or blood-filled blisters), and they usually are well-defined lesions with distinct borders. Patient history reveals prolonged immobility, exposure to shear force, or use of a medical device associated with ulcer development (Pieper, 2012). Occasionally, pressure ulcers occur over fleshy prominences in patients who have been immobile for a prolonged period of time or who have experienced a combination of unrelieved pressure and hypotension; however, the clinician will observe indicators of ischemic damage such as well-defined areas of purplish discoloration. In contrast, friction injuries are typically located over fleshy prominences exposed to repetitive "rubbing" force as the patient moves around in the bed or chair. The wounds are usually superficial with no evidence of ischemic damage; the edges may be well defined or irregular (Figs. 16-4, 16-5, and 16-6). Patient history reveals that the patient is restless or that the patient frequently slides down in the bed or chair and may reveal that the patient is malnourished, on steroids, or diaphoretic; however, the patient does not experience prolonged immobility (Mahoney et al., 2013). Moisture-associated skin damage occurs either between body folds (in a patient with diaphoresis) or in the perineal area, inner thighs, and buttocks (in a patient with incontinence). The lesions are typically superficial (partial thickness), and the edges

TABLE 16-1 Differential Assessment Friction Wounds, MASD, and Pressure Ulcers

Wound Type	Location	Depth	Characteristics	Patient History
Friction (Top Down)	Fleshy surfaces exposed to repetitive rubbing	Usually partial thickness (superficial)	Wound bed usually pink/red with no evidence necrosis Edges may be well defined or irregular	Restlessness Frequent sliding in bed or chair Patient may be malnourished, diaphoretic, or on steroids
Moisture-Associated Skin Damage (Top Down)	ITD: between body folds in a patient who is diaphoretic and/or obese IAD: perineal area, inner thighs, buttocks	Usually partial thickness (superficial)	ITD: linear breaks in skin at base of fold *or* superficial "kissing lesions" IAD: edges frequently indistinct; associated fungal rash common Both: Wound bed usually pink/red with no evidence necrosis	ITD: trapped moisture beneath body folds due to diaphoresis or obesity IAD: prolonged or recurrent exposure to urine and/or stool
Pressure/Shear (Bottom Up)	Over bony prominences Under medical devices Atypical: over fleshy prominences exposed to prolonged pressure (e.g., in a patient who was "found down")	Usually full thickness (Stage III, Stage IV, unstageable, or sDTI)	Well-defined lesions with distinct borders Tunneling and undermining common, especially when shear involved Tissue necrosis usually evident (i.e., purple discoloration, blood filled blister, slough or eschar, significant tissue loss)	Prolonged immobility Exposure to shear (sliding) force Use of medical device in area of damage May have periods of hypotension and/or vasopressor administration

are frequently indistinct and irregular. The surrounding skin is macerated, and the patient history includes either diaphoresis or incontinence (Mahoney et al., 2013) (See Figs. 17-1 and 17-3).

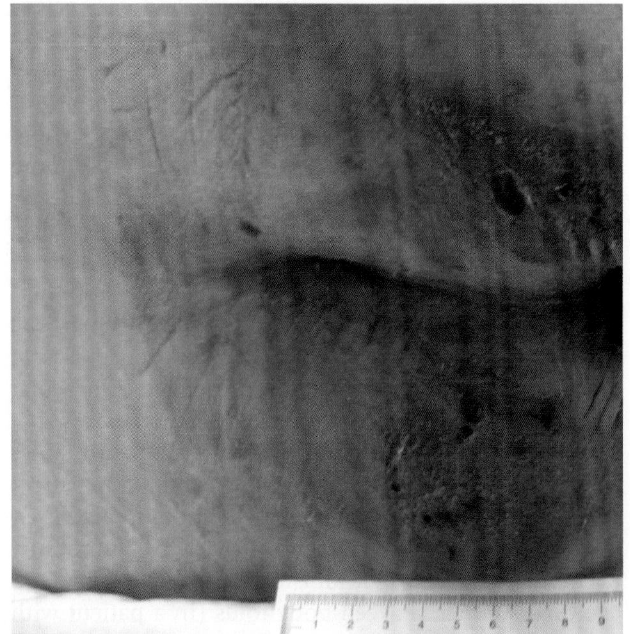

FIGURE 16-4. Friction damage characterized by hyperkeratosis, ridging, lichenification, scaling, blanching erythema, shallow full-thickness ulcers, and tissue deformation. (Courtesy of Chris Berke.)

CLINICAL PEARL

The parameters of greatest value to differential assessment of trunk wounds include (1) location; (2) wound depth (partial vs. full thickness) and characteristics (indicators of ischemia vs. indicators of maceration and/or friction); and (3) patient history.

In some cases, wounds are of mixed etiology; in this case, they may exhibit features of both top-down and bottom-up injury, that is, superficial skin loss with evidence of underlying ischemic damage. Patient history will reveal exposure to more than one mechanical stressor, for example, pressure and moisture.

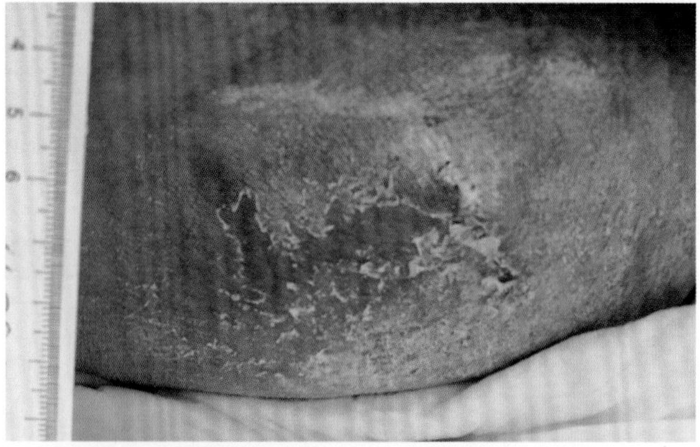

FIGURE 16-5. Mild friction damage characterized by hyperkeratosis, scaling, blanching erythema. (Courtesy of Chris Berke.)

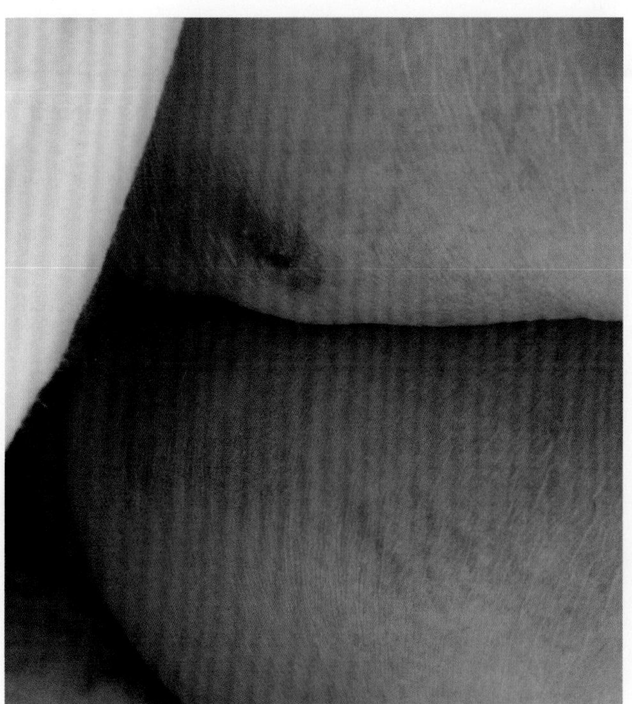

FIGURE 16-6. Friction damage characterized by lichenification, ulcer formation, and scaling. (Courtesy of Chris Berke.)

Current Gaps

There are two major "gaps" in the science and research underlying accurate determination of wound etiology. The first gap is our incomplete understanding of the specific mechanisms of damage leading to both superficial and deep injury; while there is general consensus that the majority of pressure ulcers are ischemic injuries that begin at the interface between deep tissue and bone, definitive "proof" does not yet exist. There is a growing body of evidence to support the impact of skin microclimate (humidity and temperature) on the development of both superficial and deep breakdown; however, more evidence is needed to determine the specific interplay between skin moisture and friction and between skin moisture and pressure/shear. Even more critically, we currently lack the diagnostic tools to determine whether a specific wound is limited to the superficial skin and tissue layers or extends to the deeper tissue layers. There is some evidence that ultrasound can help to determine the level of tissue damage and can provide early and accurate determination of superficial versus deep damage; however, these devices are not yet available for bedside clinical use. Thus, at present, clinicians must base wound classification on the parameters discussed in this chapter (location, characteristics, and patient history) and must "stay tuned" to advances in wound diagnostics.

CLINICAL PEARL

There is a growing body of evidence to support the impact of skin microclimate on both superficial and deep breakdown; hot wet skin is vulnerable skin!

Conclusion

Mechanical factors (moisture, friction, shear, and pressure) are common causative and contributing factors to skin breakdown, and accurate determination of the specific etiologic factors impacts on accurate wound management and on benchmarking and reimbursement. However, accurate classification is not always easy, because many patients are at risk for multiple types of wounds, and we currently lack accurate diagnostic tools for determining depth of injury. The concept of "top-down" versus "bottom-up" injury can be helpful to accurate classification, because it reminds the clinician to ask the following question when assessing a particular wound: does this wound appear to involve ischemic damage ("bottom-up" damage), or does it appear to be caused by mechanical abrasive forces that remove the skin one layer at a time ("top-down" damage)? The factors most critical to accurate differential assessment of wound etiology include wound location, wound characteristics, and patient history.

REFERENCES

Bryant, R. (2012). Types of skin damage and differential diagnosis. In R. Bryant & D. Nix (Eds.), *Acute and chronic wounds: current management concepts* (4th ed.). St. Louis, MO: Elsevier Mosby.

Doughty, D., Junkin, J., Kurz, P., et al. (2012). Incontinence associated dermatitis: Consensus statements, evidence-based guidelines for prevention and treatment, and current challenges. *Journal of Wound, Ostomy, and Continence Nursing, 39*(3), 303–315.

Gefen, A. (2012). Some basic science aspects of the etiology of deep tissue injury. Podium Presentation WOCN Society Annual Conference, Charlotte, NC.

Gray, M., Black, J., Baharestani, M., et al. (2011). Moisture associated skin damage: Overview and pathophysiology. *Journal of Wound, Ostomy, and Continence Nursing, 38*(4), 359–370.

Gray, M., Beeckman, D., Bliss, D. Z., et al. (2012). Incontinence associated dermatitis: A comprehensive review and update. *Journal of Wound, Ostomy, and Continence Nursing, 39*(1), 61–74.

Mahoney, M., Rozenboom, B., & Doughty, D. (2013). Challenges in classification of gluteal cleft and buttock wounds: Consensus session reports. *Journal of Wound, Ostomy, and Continence Nursing, 40*(3), 239–245.

National Pressure Ulcer Advisory Panel, European Pressure Ulcer Advisory Panel, Pan Pacific Pressure Injury Alliance. (2014). In Emily Haesler (Ed.), *Prevention and treatment of pressure ulcers: clinical practice guideline*. Osborne Park, Western Australia: Cambridge Media.

Pieper, B. (2012). Pressure ulcers: Impact, etiology, and classification. In R. Bryant & D. Nix (Eds.), *Acute and chronic wounds: current management concepts* (4th ed.). St. Louis, MO: Elsevier Mosby.

Sibbald, G., Krasner, D., & Woo K. (2011). Pressure ulcer staging revisited: superficial skin changes and deep pressure ulcer framework. *Advances in Skin and Wound Care, 24*(12), 571–580.

QUESTIONS

1. The wound care nurse is assessing a patient whose wounds were caused by mechanical factors. Which of the following is an example of this type of injury?
A. A pressure ulcer caused by sliding down in a wheelchair
B. A venous leg ulcer
C. Eczema
D. Malignant wound

2. What is the best descriptor of tissue damage caused by deep shear strain?
A. Superficial skin loss caused by separation of epidermal and dermal layers (abrasion)
B. Tissue ischemia caused by sustained pressure
C. Edema caused by impaired lymphatic function resulting from unrelieved pressure
D. Vessel angulation resulting from the combined effects of friction and gravity

3. Which type of wound develops from the "bottom up?"
A. Friction wounds
B. Ischemic wounds
C. Wounds associated with incontinence
D. Wounds caused by intertriginous dermatitis

4. What is the initial effect of sustained pressure on a body part?
A. Tissue necrosis
B. Tissue loss
C. Tissue and blood vessel compression
D. Tissue remodeling

5. What is the driving force for the prevention of agency-acquired pressure ulcers?
A. Patient satisfaction
B. Quality-of-care indicators
C. Infection control
D. Minimizing staff workload

6. Which statement accurately describes a guideline wound care nurses can use when differentiating ischemic wounds from nonischemic wounds?
A. Current evidence indicates that most ischemic wounds develop from the "bottom up."
B. Most pressure/shear wounds are partial-thickness wounds that exhibit evidence of ischemic damage.
C. Most nonpressure wounds present as superficial wounds with evidence of abrasive force and tissue ischemia.
D. Diagnostic tools and imaging technology are readily available for use by bedside clinicians to distinguish between superficial and deep tissue damage.

7. Which assessment parameter is of greatest value to differential assessment of trunk wounds?
A. Indicators of ischemia versus indicators of maceration or friction
B. Wound size
C. Type of eschar involved
D. Indicators of infected versus noninfected wounds

8. Which condition might the wound care nurse observe as an indicator of ischemic damage?
A. Maceration of surrounding tissue
B. Excessive granulation tissue
C. Edema
D. Purplish discoloration

9. A wound care nurse documents a wound as being of "mixed etiology." What do these data describe?
A. Patient history reveals exposure to only one mechanical stressor.
B. The wound is limited to the superficial skin and tissue layers.
C. Features of both top-down and bottom-up injury are manifested.
D. Comorbidities affect the development of the wound.

10. What type of skin is most vulnerable to pressure ulcers?
A. Dry, fragile skin
B. Hot, wet skin
C. Hyperkeratotic skin
D. Skin manifesting a rash

ANSWERS: 1.**A**, 2.**D**, 3.**B**, 4.**C**, 5.**B**, 6.**A**, 7.**A**, 8.**D**, 9.**C**, 10.**B**

CHAPTER 17

"Top-Down" Injuries

Prevention and Management of Moisture-Associated Skin Damage (MASD), Medical Adhesive–Related Skin Injury (MARSI), and Skin Tears

Debra M. Thayer, Barbara Rozenboom, and Sharon Baranoski

OBJECTIVES

1. **Explain the pathology and clinical presentation of each of the following:**
   - Incontinence-associated dermatitis (IAD)
   - Intertriginous dermatitis (ITD)
   - Peristomal moisture-associated skin damage (PMASD)
   - Periwound moisture-associated skin damage (PWMASD)
   - Medical adhesive–related skin injury (MARSI)
   - Skin tears (Type 1, Type 2, Type 3)
2. **Describe strategies for prevention and management of each of the following:**
   - Incontinence-associated dermatitis (IAD)
   - Intertriginous dermatitis (ITD)
   - Peristomal moisture-associated skin damage (PMASD)
   - Periwound moisture-associated skin damage (PWMASD)
   - Medical adhesive–related skin injury (MARSI)
   - Skin tears (Type 1, Type 2, Type 3)

Topic Outline

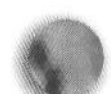

Introduction

The term "top down" has become increasingly popular to describe superficial cutaneous injuries. This perspective helps the wound nurse to distinguish damage that *begins* at the skin's surface from that beginning within soft tissue or at the soft tissue–bone interface. In contrast to "bottom-up" injuries that are often the result of ischemia, top-down injuries are initiated by mechanical forces, moisture, and/or the effects of inflammation. In this chapter, we will explore three common types of top-down injuries: moisture-associated skin damage (MASD), medical adhesive–related skin injury (MARSI), and skin tears.

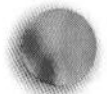

Moisture-Associated Skin Damage

MASD is defined as inflammation and erosion of the skin caused by prolonged exposure to various sources of moisture, including urine or stool, perspiration, wound exudate, and mucus or saliva (Gray et al., 2011). The four most common forms of MASD have been identified as: incontinence-associated dermatitis (IAD), intertriginous dermatitis (ITD), periwound moisture-associated skin damage, and peristomal moisture-associated skin damage. Wound nurses are frequently consulted to identify and mitigate the source of moisture and recommend interventions to treat the skin damage, prevent further skin damage, and promote healing.

A variety of terms have been used to describe MASD including irritant dermatitis, diaper rash, perineal dermatitis, moisture lesions, skin erosion, and perineal maceration. The skin changes associated with prolonged exposure to moisture have been traditionally linked to incontinence, but it is now realized that prolonged exposure to moisture from any source can cause skin damage (Voegeli, 2012).

As discussed in Chapter 1, healthy skin serves to prevent the entry of harmful pathogens and also prevents excess fluid loss from the body. Excessive moisture from any source can cause overhydration, which increases the skin's permeability and compromises its barrier function (Voegeli, 2012). Existing evidence and clinical experience suggest that moisture alone causes overhydration but is insufficient to cause significant inflammation or skin loss; this level of skin damage is attributable to overhydration complicated by one of the following: chemical irritants within the moisture source; mechanical factors such as friction; and/or invasion of pathogenic microorganisms. For example, when the skin is exposed to liquid stool for a period of time, the enzymes and irritants in the stool can cause inflammation and skin damage. Similarly, persistent urinary and/or fecal incontinence can create an environment favorable to overgrowth of yeast, and candidiasis is commonly seen in patients with IAD. Finally, the combination of overhydrated skin and minor friction can cause skin loss (Gray et al., 2011).

CLINICAL PEARL

Moisture alone causes maceration—acute inflammation and skin loss are usually due to a combination of maceration and some other source of injury (chemical irritant, friction, or pathogenic invasion).

Overhydration of the stratum corneum compromises the brick-and-mortar configuration of the epidermal layer and permits penetration by irritants, which results in inflammation. The overhydrated skin is also more prone to damage from the forces of friction and shearing, because overhydrated skin has less tensile strength and tends to "drag" against the underlying surface. Finally, the overhydrated stratum corneum allows common pathogens such as *Candida* and *Staphylococcus* to enter, leading to a secondary infection (Voegeli, 2012).

Other factors that affect the protective barrier of the skin include age, obesity, and the environment. As people age, the skin becomes thinner and dryer, and the barrier function is compromised. Obesity causes humans to store heat longer, and evaporative loss is diminished in a warm humid environment. Obese individuals produce more sweat, and this exposes the skin to increased moisture, especially in skin folds. Environmentally, the relative humidity affects transepidermal water loss (Gray et al., 2011); when humidity is reduced, transepidermal water loss (TEWL) is increased.

The National Pressure Ulcer Advisory Panel (NPUAP) defines friction as "the resistance to motion in a parallel direction relative to the common boundary of two surfaces" (NPUAP, 2001). Skin injury by friction initially appears as erythema and progresses to an abrasion. Friction primarily affects superficial layers and thus does not result in tissue necrosis, while shearing forces mainly affect deeper tissue layers (Bryant, 2012). Friction occurs when caregivers use vigorous rubbing during cleansing of the perineal area or when the skin rubs against incontinence garments or bed or chair surfaces. Overhydrated skin is more vulnerable to skin damage from friction than dry skin; caregivers should be instructed to use gentle cleansing techniques and soft cloths, and turn sheets and lift devices should be used to reduce friction during repositioning or transfer. Superficial skin loss due to a combination of friction and moisture is considered a "top-down" injury (Mahoney et al., 2011).

Incontinence-Associated Dermatitis

IAD is the most common form of MASD. A 2007 consensus statement defined IAD as inflammation of the skin that occurs when urine or stool comes in contact with perianal or perigenital skin (Gray et al., 2007). Gray and colleagues subsequently updated the definition to "an irritant dermatitis that develops from chronic exposure to urine or liquid stool" (Gray et al., 2007). Skin exposed to urine and stool, especially liquid stool, is at risk for IAD. The term dermatitis denotes inflammation and erythema with or without erosion or denudation; IAD specifically identifies the source of the irritant (urine or fecal incontinence) and acknowledges that the area of the skin affected commonly extends beyond the perineum (Bryant, 2012).

Prevalence

Urinary incontinence is the involuntary loss of urine, bowel incontinence is the unintentional loss of liquid or solid stool, and double incontinence is the involuntary loss of both urine and stool (Langemo et al., 2011). In a study of almost 60,000 long-term care residents, the reported prevalence of incontinence was 59.8%; 7.7% had only urinary incontinence, 12.4% had only fecal incontinence, and 39.7% had both urinary and fecal incontinence (Bliss et al., 2006). This is significant since patients with fecal or double incontinence are particularly high risk for IAD.

Pathology

Urine consists of 90% water mixed with solutes; as the urea in urine breaks down, ammonia is produced, and ammonia is highly alkaline. The overexposure of skin to urine changes the skin pH from acid to alkaline, thus compromising the protective acidic mantle. The longer the duration of exposure to urine, the greater the risk of developing IAD. Stool consists of undigested substances, water, and lipids. Skin exposed to liquid stool is at particularly high risk for IAD (Gray et al., 2007), because the alkaline pH of moisture-damaged skin activates enzymes in liquid stool that cause proteolytic damage and possible skin loss (Anderson et al., 1994). The pH properties of solid stool are more neutral and have fewer active enzymes; thus, solid stool is less damaging to the skin.

Additional risk factors for developing IAD include comorbidities, age, nutritional status, core body temperature, cleansing methods, inadequate oxygenation, poor skin condition at baseline, pain, and decreased mobility (Langemo et al., 2011).

Clinical Presentation

IAD due to urinary incontinence may involve the perineum and the area between the vulva or scrotum and the anus. IAD due to fecal incontinence may involve the anus, buttocks, and coccyx and can extend to the perigenital areas, groin folds, and posterior and medial thigh regions. Typical manifestations of IAD include moist, bright red skin, inflammation, denudement, erosion, and the formation of vesicles (Fig. 17-1). In people with darker skin tones, there will be more subtle redness or discoloration of the surrounding skin (Wound Ostomy Continence Nursing Society, 2011). IAD appears in a diffuse distribution with irregular edges. IAD is typically manifest as superficial damage, though there are anecdotal reports of progression to shallow full-thickness lesions. If exudate is present, it is clear, serous, and weepy. Sensations of burning, mild-to-severe pain, and itching are reported with IAD (Langemo et al., 2011).

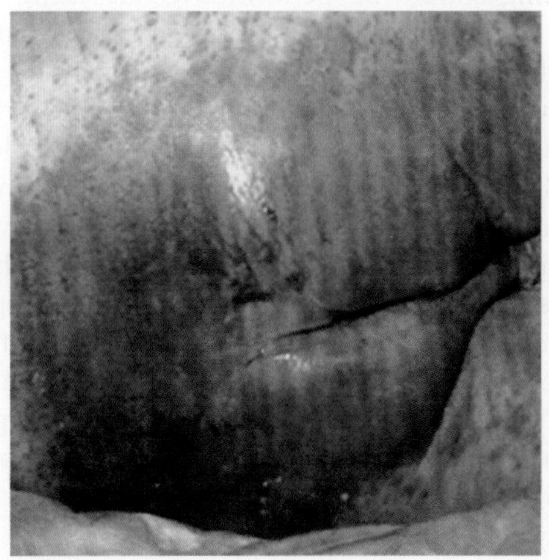
A

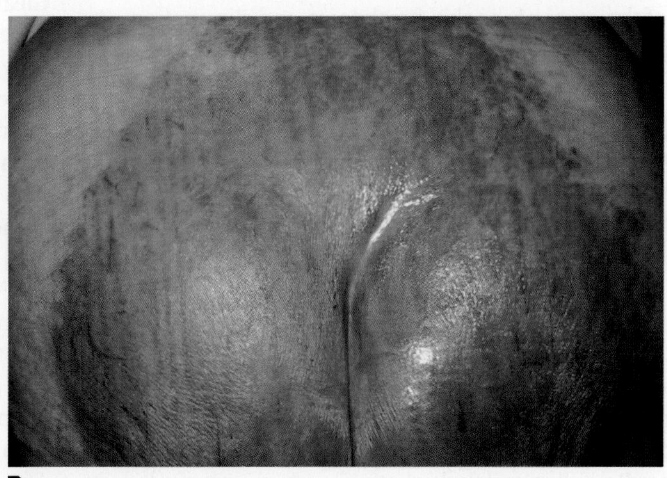
B

FIGURE 17-1. **A,B:** Incontinence-associated dermatitis (IAD). Note diffuse erythema, patchy areas of denudation, and coexisting candidiasis. (Courtesy of KDS Consulting.)

CLINICAL PEARL

IAD is manifest by erythema with or without vesicles and skin loss (or candidiasis) in areas exposed to stool and urine.

Prevention

Prevention of IAD should focus on identifying the population who are at risk of developing IAD. Identifying the cause of incontinence will assist in determining appropriate treatment interventions to help modify or eliminate the cause, such as toileting or appropriate use of containment products. In 2009, Beeckman et al. (2009) introduced a structured skin care protocol that was demonstrated to reduce the incidence of IAD. Prevention and treatment should consist of an individualized plan of care that includes the following:

1. Gentle cleansing—the skin should be cleansed with a no-rinse skin cleanser as an alternative to soap and water. No-rinse cleansers contain surfactants to loosen and remove irritants (Beeckman et al., 2011).
2. Moisturizing—moisturizers are intended to improve the appearance of skin and/or repair the skin barrier. Some also promote normal retention of water within the skin and reduce transepidermal water loss (Beeckman et al., 2011).
3. Protection—skin protectants, also referred to as moisture barriers, provide a coating that protects the skin from overhydration, chemical irritants, and pathogens in stool and urine (Doughty et al., 2012).

The addition of antifungal products, topical steroidal products, and topical antibiotics should be used only to treat specific issues and not used prophylactically. Interventions such as the use of containment devices to avoid skin exposure to urine and stool are indicated in specific situations (Gray et al., 2012).

When developing a plan of care for prevention or treatment of any form of MASD, it should begin with identification of the cause of the skin breakdown and elimination of the irritant.

CLINICAL PEARL

The three critical elements of any structured skin care protocol include gentle cleansing; moisturizing to replace skin lipids; and moisture barrier to limit contact between skin and urine and stool.

The ideal approach to prevention of IAD is prevention of incontinence. Bowel and bladder programs should be implemented in an attempt to decrease incontinence episodes. Providing toilet alternatives such as commodes and urinals can aid in minimizing incontinence (Wound Ostomy Continence Nursing Society, 2011). Toileting programs such as timed or prompted toileting should be implemented for patients who have communication and mobility limitations but who respond positively to toileting assistance.

Containment devices such as condom or Foley catheters and fecal containment systems can be utilized when appropriate to collect urine and liquid stool. These devices can be implemented to restore or maintain skin integrity by reducing or eliminating skin exposure to urine or stool (Beeckman et al., 2011). Indwelling Foley catheters may be indicated for patients with stage III or IV pressure ulcers but should not be used for management of incontinence or for prevention of IAD. Internal and external fecal containment devices can be used to contain liquid stool and protect the perianal skin (Wound Ostomy Continence Nursing Society, 2011). A skin protectant/moisture barrier should be used in conjunction with fecal management systems to protect the skin from small amounts of leakage around the tube (Junkin & Selekof, 2007).

Disposable incontinence garments and products with superabsorbent polymers can be used to absorb urine and feces and wick moisture away from the skin. Absorbent briefs should be used for patients who are being transported for diagnostic testing or treatment and may be needed in the home setting to contain incontinence and promote dignity (Gray, 2004). However, in the inpatient setting, absorptive products should be left open under the patient in order to avoid the occlusive environment that develops when the absorptive product is closed around the patient; an occlusive environment increases skin temperature and humidity and therefore is a significant risk factor for IAD. In patients managed with absorptive products, it is essential to check the product frequently and change promptly when soiled. In addition to increasing the risk of skin damage, the weight and bulk of a full pad or brief may make ambulation difficult and may increase fall risk. Absorptive pads for beds and chairs should be used and checked frequently to ensure the pad is dry (Zulkowski, 2012).

Cleansing should be performed gently using a pH-balanced liquid cleanser with nonionic surfactants for healthy skin. The use of soap is discouraged due to the alkaline nature typical of most soaps and the risk of resulting skin irritation (Fiers & Thayer, 2000). A soft cloth or disposable wipe should be used to minimize friction and trauma and to avoid disrupting the skin's protective barrier function (Gray et al., 2012). Cleansing should be performed as soon as possible after the incontinence episode occurs. Meticulous care should be taken to avoid further mechanical trauma to the skin when moist skin folds and buttocks are separated for cleansing. The intergluteal cleft is particularly prone to skin tears during the process of cleansing and turning a patient with overhydrated skin (Mahoney et al., 2013).

After cleansing, the skin should be moisturized with an emollient product to preserve the skin's protective barrier function; emollients are used to smooth skin and in some cases penetrate the stratum corneum to replace lost skin lipids and to fill the gaps between the epidermal cells. Many no-rinse combination products (such as disposable perineal cleansing wipes) and skin cleansers contain emollients (Gray et al., 2012); these products simplify perineal skin care by combining cleansing and moisturizing into one step. The wound nurse should be aware that some products classified as "moisturizers" contain humectants (e.g., urea or alpha-hydroxy acids). These products work by attracting water to the skin and are intended for use on very dry skin; they would obviously *not* be appropriate for the patient with overhydrated skin at risk for IAD. In contrast, occlusive skin-conditioning products moisturize by creating an oily film on the skin that prevents water loss; these products would be appropriate for the patient at risk for IAD. The wound nurse should also be aware that some ingredients found in skin care products (such as fragrance) may lead to the development of contact dermatitis; it is important to select products with limited fragrance and dyes and to monitor all patients for evidence of adverse reactions (Beeckman et al., 2011).

CLINICAL PEARL

Products classified as "moisturizers" include humectants and emollients; humectants attract water and are inappropriate for IAD prevention, while emollients smooth and protect the skin and are appropriate for IAD prevention.

The third step is to apply a skin protectant, which creates a barrier to penetration of the skin by water and irritants from urine and stool. Skin protectants can be formulated as barrier creams, ointments, or films. Barrier creams consist of a lipid/water emulsion base; some contain a metal oxide such as zinc. Ointments are formulations that typically have a petrolatum base and are anhydrous, meaning they do not contain water. A study by Hoggarth and colleagues tested water-in-oil–, oil-in-water–, and zinc-based products on their ability to protect against irritants, maintain skin hydration, and provide a barrier to maceration. Petroleum products are water-in-oil–based formulations; they provide effective protection of the skin from maceration. Oil-in-water products such as dimethicone provide greater hydration for the skin. Zinc-based products provide more effective protection against irritants than petroleum or dimethicone products. The study concluded that petrolatum-based products demonstrated protection against irritants and maceration and provided some skin hydration. Dimethicone products varied in their ability to provide protection against irritants but provided good skin hydration. Zinc-based products protected against irritants but had poor skin hydration properties and did not effectively prevent maceration (Hoggarth et al., 2005).

CLINICAL PEARL

Effective moisture barriers include liquid acrylate barrier films as well as moisture barrier ointments containing petrolatum, dimethicone, and zinc oxide.

In addition to assuring availability of appropriate products for preventive care, the wound nurse should be cognizant of the fact that simplified protocols with fewer steps have been demonstrated to result in improved staff adherence. For example, combination products such as the 3-in-1 washcloths that cleanse, moisturize, and protect, have been shown to be effective in reducing the incidence of IAD when staff is educated on proper usage (Beeckman et al., 2011; Gray et al., 2012). Another simplifying approach is the use of liquid acrylates as a moisture barrier product. These agents provide a semipermeable protective polymer barrier to the skin; they require fewer applications than creams or ointments (typically 3×/week as opposed to multiple times daily) because they are resistant to removal by repetitive cleansing (Langemo et al., 2011). Another potential advantage is the fact that they are clear, so it is easy for staff to monitor skin status.

Treatment

Once the cause of the IAD is identified and eliminated, treatment should focus on protecting the skin from further exposure to irritants, establishing a healing environment, and eradicating any cutaneous infections (Beeckman et al., 2011). The goal of treatment is to improve skin integrity and to minimize and/or eliminate redness, pain, and candidiasis. Evidence supports the use of a structured skin care program that includes cleansing, moisturizing, and protecting the skin and the use of quality products that wick moisture away from the skin (Gray et al., 2012). Management of denuded skin requires use of products that adhere to moist skin and commonly involves a zinc oxide–based agent and an absorbent such as karaya or carboxymethylcellulose. These products are often referred to as "pastes." Another approach involves application of pectin powder to the denuded skin, followed either by a moisture barrier ointment or paste or by a liquid acrylate barrier film.

Antifungal products may be added to treat secondary candidiasis infections, which manifest as an erythematous maculopapular rash with distinct satellite lesions at the periphery (Fig. 17-2). Two approaches involve use of a moisture barrier ointment containing an antifungal (e.g., azole products) or use of an antifungal powder (e.g., azole or nystatin) followed by a moisture barrier ointment or a clear acrylate. Topical steroid creams may be used with caution to help reduce inflammation of the skin (Black et al., 2011).

Application of topical antibiotics or antimicrobials may be used if a secondary bacterial infection is suspected; the optimal dosage and duration of therapy are individualized.

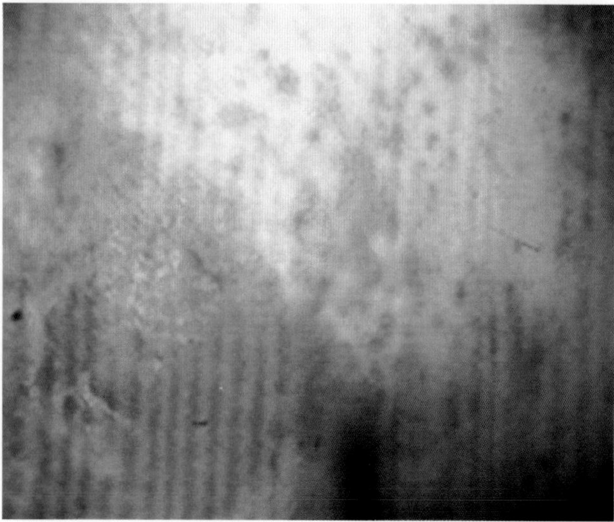

FIGURE 17-2. Candidiasis.

These additional treatments should be used on an as-needed basis. A treatment plan using these products should be reassessed after 2 weeks of use and discontinued when symptoms of secondary infection and inflammation are resolved (Gray et al., 2011; Voegeli, 2012).

IAD versus Pressure Ulcer: Differential Assessment

Mechanical damage traumatically abrades and disrupts the superficial layers of the skin from the "top down." Pressure and shearing forces cause vessel compression and ischemic damage; injury occurs from the "bottom up." IAD is a type of top-down injury. Skin that is macerated or inflamed is at increased risk for both friction damage and shear damage. These patients may develop complex lesions that are a combination of "top-down" injury (superficial damage caused by moisture and friction), and "bottom-up" damage (deep damage caused by pressure and shear) (Mahoney et al., 2013). Current studies indicate that muscle tissue is the layer most vulnerable to diminished blood flow; thus pressure and shear typically create damage that "begins at the bottom" (muscle–bone interface) and progresses to the surface (Sibbald et al., 2011).

Emerging evidence has helped delineate the difference between IAD and pressure ulcers, and there is increasing recognition that superficial skin breakdown is usually "top down" and caused by moisture and/or friction rather than pressure (Sibbald et al., 2011). However, accurate wound classification remains a challenge for clinicians. In 2010, a 14-member panel was convened to explore current thinking about pressure ulcer staging and causation with the intent to improve clinical care and patient outcomes. The Shifting of the Original Paradigm Expert Panel (S.O.P.E) proposed a conceptual framework to differentiate superficial lesions caused by moisture and friction from deep tissue damage that is usually caused by pressure and shear (Sibbald et al., 2011). In addition, the NPUAP has redefined stage II pressure ulcers to exclude lesions caused by moisture or friction (NPUAP, 2005). However, there is persistent confusion regarding wound classification, and many superficial wounds caused by friction and moisture are still incorrectly identified as pressure. Adding to the confusion is the factor that patients who are at risk for pressure ulcers are also frequently at risk for IAD and ITD (Doughty, 2012) (See Table 16-1 on page 278).

Intertriginous Dermatitis

ITD, also referred to as intertrigo, is an inflammatory skin condition that affects opposing skin surfaces. This condition can develop in any area of the body where two skin surfaces are in contact.

Pathology

Intertrigo is thought to be caused by a combination of two factors: overhydration of the skin due to trapped moisture and friction between the opposing skin folds (i.e., skin rubbing against skin). The overhydrated stratum corneum "drags" rather than glides over opposing skin surfaces, which leads to increased friction and the risk of skin damage. Intertrigo can coexist with IAD (Gray, 2004). ITD can also present as a linear skin tear at the base of the skin fold; the tear may occur when the overhydrated skin is "stretched" during routine assessment and hygienic care requiring separation of the skin folds. Contributing factors to ITD include the following: reduced perfusion (common in adipose tissue); diabetes; and concomitant administration of steroids and broad-spectrum antibiotics. Obese individuals are at high risk due to increased perspiration and the challenges of personal hygiene resulting from restricted dexterity and limited ability to reach the necessary areas to cleanse (Voegeli, 2013). Obese individuals also have deep folds with constant skin to skin contact; these folds may be difficult to separate for effective cleansing and drying.

Clinical Presentation

ITD is most commonly seen in the axillae, intergluteal cleft, and inguinal region; under the breasts; and in the abdominal folds. Obese individuals often develop ITD under an abdominal or pubic pannus (Voegeli, 2012). Intertrigo can also occur in the neck folds of infants with a short neck, where moisture from drooling is trapped in the deep creases of the neck (Janniger et al., 2005).

The earliest indicator of ITD is mild erythema; if left untreated, the condition can progress to severe inflammation with mirrored areas of skin erosion or linear fissure formation (Fig. 17-3). ITD lesions are typically partial thickness, though there are anecdotal reports of progression to full-thickness lesions when treatment is delayed or ineffective. The patient may report pain, itching, burning, and odor. Complications of ITD include secondary infections such as candidiasis, pseudomonas, staph, strep, and antibiotic-resistant infections; these organisms thrive in the moist, warm environment created by trapped moisture

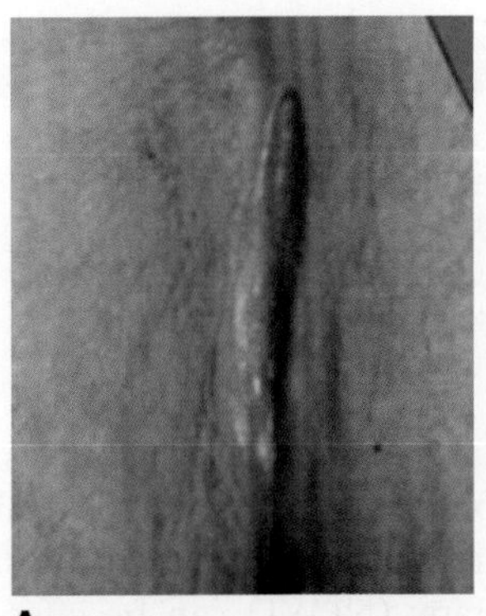
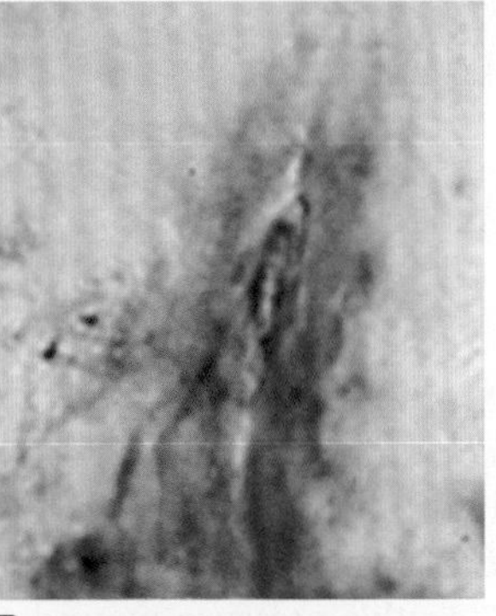

A B

FIGURE 17-3. **A,B:** Intertriginous dermatitis (ITD): linear lesions located at base of skin folds in areas of maceration.

and skin loss (Voegeli, 2012). If ITD is not well managed, the person is at greater risk for severe infections such as cellulitis and panniculitis (Gray, 2004).

CLINICAL PEARL

ITD is caused by trapped perspiration in a body fold (which causes maceration), and friction or slight mechanical stretch (which causes superficial breakdown or a linear "fissure" at the base of the fold).

Prevention

There is limited information about ITD, and no formal risk assessment tool is currently available. Prevention of ITD should be focused on measures to keep skin folds clean and dry and on measures to reduce friction. Skin folds should be cleansed gently with a soft cloth and a pH-balanced spray cleanser or premoistened no-rinse cloth. The skin fold should be patted dry or dried with a handheld dryer on a cool setting. The patient should be encouraged to wear lightweight and loose-fitting clothing in order to wick moisture away from the skin and should be taught to avoid the use of plain gauze pads, paper towels, or coffee filters between the skin folds, since these can actually trap the moisture and increase the risk for maceration of the skin. In the patient care setting, effective strategies include positioning to include air flow to the area and placement of wicking sheets or absorptive padding between the skin folds.

Treatment

Treatment of ITD begins with a thorough and complete examination of all skin folds. Air circulation to the deep skin folds should be improved by positioning to expose the affected area. A commercial textile product is available that effectively wicks moisture away from the body fold; the sheet is placed between the two folds of skin and should extend from the base of the fold to several inches beyond the fold (to allow for wicking and evaporation). These products are impregnated with an antimicrobial agent, which is intended to reduce the risk of cutaneous infections such as candidiasis. In addition, placement of the low-friction textile sheet provides separation of the body folds and significantly reduces the risk of friction damage. Alternatives to commercial products include use of absorptive products such as foam dressings, peripads, or abdominal dressing pads. In the home care setting, athletic socks are sometimes used to provide absorption of moisture and separation of body folds. If there are indicators of candidiasis, a light dusting of antifungal powder should be applied to the area; patients and clinicians should be cautioned to avoid excessive use of any powder, since "caking" is a common result, and this increases the risk of friction damage (Gray, 2004).

CLINICAL PEARL

Effective prevention and management of ITD include measures to wick or absorb the trapped moisture and separation of the fold to prevent friction damage.

Effective management of open lesions requires application of a dressing that absorbs moisture, maintains a moist wound surface, and maintains separation of the fold to prevent additional damage, for example, thin adhesive foam dressings. Moisture barrier ointments are also sometimes used but should be preservative and fragrance free and combined with use of a soft folded gauze sponge to maintain separation of the folds.

Periwound Moisture-Associated Skin Damage

The literature defines periwound skin as the area within 4 cm of a wound edge, and this is the area at greatest risk for skin damage caused by exposure to wound exudate. However, cases of more extensive periwound MASD have been noted when there is caustic drainage from a wound or fistula.

Pathology

The etiology and pathophysiology of periwound MASD are not well understood but are probably due to a combination of overhydration (maceration), inflammation, and friction. The production of exudate is normal during the inflammatory phase of wound healing due to osmotic and hydrostatic forces that cause fluid to leak from the blood vessels; the exposed stratum corneum responds by absorbing the exudate (Gray, 2004; Gray et al., 2011). As a result, the underlying epidermal layers become overhydrated and macerated; this renders the periwound skin more vulnerable to friction damage and to penetration by pathogens and irritants. Macerated skin is more prone to epidermal stripping with removal of adhesive dressings; the resultant loss of the epidermal layer causes denudement, which further increases exposure of the periwound tissue to moisture (Colwell et al., 2011).

Current evidence indicates a greater risk of periwound MASD with chronic wounds as opposed to acute wounds, and this seems to be due in large part to differences in the type of exudate produced by chronic wounds. All wound exudate contains cellular debris and enzymes, which are potentially damaging to the skin. However, the enzymes in acute wounds tend to be inactive, and there are lower levels of cellular debris. In contrast, the exudate produced by chronic wounds contains higher levels of active proteolytic enzymes such as matrix metalloproteinases (MMPs); in addition, chronic wounds are more likely to become infected, which further increases the volume of enzymatic exudate (Colwell et al., 2011; Cutting & White, 2002).

CLINICAL PEARL

Periwound MASD is more likely to occur with chronic wounds because the exudate produced by chronic wounds contains high levels of inflammatory agents.

Clinical Presentation

Clinical indicators of periwound MASD include erythema, maceration, and skin loss. Macerated skin typically appears wet, "water-logged," and somewhat wrinkled. It is important to realize that the presentation may be different in patients with darker skin tones; erythema may be masked, and maceration may present as gray-white, wrinkled skin (Voegeli, 2013) (Fig. 17-4).

Prevention

The goal in the prevention of periwound MASD is to maintain a moist wound bed while keeping the periwound skin dry (Colwell et al., 2011). Strategies to prevent periwound MASD include the selection of dressings that provide effective exudate control, appropriate frequency of dressing change to prevent overhydration and leakage of exudate onto the periwound skin, and protection of the periwound skin with moisture barrier products. Staff and caregivers should be educated to change saturated or leaking dressings rather than reinforcing them. Wet dressings will trap moisture against intact skin and lead to the development of periwound MASD.

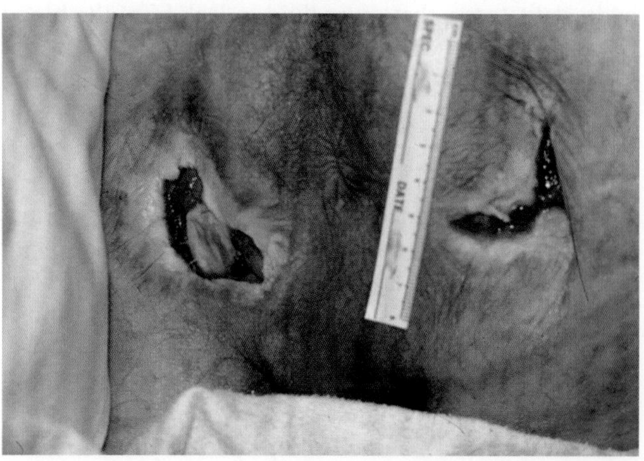

FIGURE 17-4. Periwound MASD.

CLINICAL PEARL

Prevention and management of periwound MASD include selection of dressings (and dressing change frequency) to effectively manage wound exudate and routine use of moisture barrier products to the periwound skin.

Management

Dressings designed to absorb moisture such as alginates, hydrofibers, foams, hydrocolloids, and antimicrobial dressings should be considered for treatment options. Negative-pressure wound therapy (NPWT) can be effective in removing edema and wound exudate, thus reducing the risk of periwound moisture; however, clinical experience demonstrates that inappropriate application of NPWT can paradoxically promote MASD. Windowed dressings with adhesive hydrocolloid or solid skin barriers can be used to contain wound effluent and protect the periwound skin from exposure to exudate. Pouching systems should be considered for wounds with >200 mL of exudate/day (Colwell et al., 2011). Many of these systems have detachable windows that provide access to the wound for assessment and care while containing the drainage and providing protection of the periwound skin (Hess, 2005).

Gray and Weir reviewed evidence on the prevention and management of periwound maceration and found a reduced risk of maceration with application of a liquid acrylate barrier film or a petrolatum- or zinc-based skin protectant (Gray & Weir, 2007). Protective barrier pastes and ointments can be effective in preventing exposure of periwound skin to exudate, but they often interfere with the adherence of the dressing and affect absorption of drainage into the dressing; thus, they are more appropriate for wounds managed with nonadhesive dressings. Pastes can also be difficult to remove. Liquid acrylate barrier films can be used for any wound requiring periwound protection. A study by Cameron and associates compared a zinc-based product and a no-sting barrier film for prevention of periwound maceration and irritation associated with venous leg ulcers. Both products proved effective; however, no-sting barrier films were found to be easier to apply and were transparent. The zinc-based product was messy to apply and difficult to remove, which increases nursing time for wound care (Cameron et al., 2005).

Peristomal Moisture-Associated Skin Damage

Peristomal MASD is inflammation and erosion of the skin related to moisture that begins at the stoma/skin junction and extends to include all skin under the pouching system, which is typically a 4-inch (10-cm) radius (Colwell et al., 2011).

Pathology

Peristomal MASD can occur when there is prolonged or recurrent exposure of the peristomal skin to the effluent from any type of stoma including urine and bowel ostomies, tracheostomies, and gastrostomies. The most common cause of peristomal skin damage is prolonged exposure to stool or urine. Peristomal skin damage can also be caused by prolonged exposure to perspiration, outside water sources (bathing, swimming), or wound drainage.

Several studies have been done on the prevalence and incidence of peristomal skin damage. One study reported that the majority of peristomal complications occur within the first 2 weeks following discharge (Persson et al., 2010). In a study by Bass and colleagues, the incidence of peristomal skin complications was 45% among patients who received preoperative education and marking of the stoma site compared to 77% among those who did not receive education and stoma siting (Bass et al., 1997). Patient education is often limited in the postoperative phase as a result of short acute care stays and limited options for ostomy education once the patient is discharged home (Colwell et al., 2011).

When the skin barrier of the ostomy appliance is dislodged or leaks, it allows effluent from the stoma to have contact with the skin around the stoma. The greatest risk occurs when the skin is exposed to highly enzymatic liquid stool, such as the effluent from an ileostomy. Enzymes from the small intestine cause erosion of the skin when the effluent is in contact for even a short period of time, and bacteria in the stool may lead to a secondary infection (Colwell et al., 2011). Fecal stomas with liquid output, such as ileostomies, are associated with a higher degree of skin breakdown complications (Ratliff, 2010). Thicker or formed stool contains less moisture and fewer enzymes and is less likely to lead to skin damage. Urine does not contain enzymes so is less damaging to the skin than liquid stool; however, prolonged exposure of the peristomal skin to urine can cause maceration, compromise of the epidermal barrier, and other complications.

There are factors other than the effluent that can contribute to peristomal MASD. For example, perspiration can become trapped under the skin barrier and interfere with an effective seal. The skin under the barrier can become macerated, with increased transepidermal water loss (Omura et al., 2010). Prolonged exposure to outside water sources may also contribute to the development of peristomal MASD. Pouching systems may require more frequent changes when the water-resistant adhesive on the ostomy appliance becomes impaired. Frequent appliance changes may cause mechanical stripping of the epidermal layer of skin. Finally, inflammatory skin ulcerations that develop around the stoma and cause drainage can lead to impaired peristomal skin integrity due to exposure to wound exudate. The skin becomes overhydrated, which interferes with maintenance of an effective seal between the barrier and the skin (Colwell et al., 2011).

Clinical Presentation

Assessment should begin with determining the source of the moisture. Assessment of peristomal MASD should include the integrity of the skin, the location of the affected area, and the distribution of the skin damage. Peristomal MASD is usually manifest by areas of maceration and erythema; superficial skin loss is common. The ostomy appliance should be assessed to help determine the cause and location of the leakage. The patient's technique for pouch removal and application should be assessed as well.

Prevention

Prevention of peristomal MASD begins with education on proper peristomal skin care and application of the skin barrier. The goal in preventing peristomal skin complications is to establish an appropriate pouching system that provides a reasonable wear time and maintains a seal that protects the peristomal skin.

Treatment

Treatment of peristomal MASD should initially focus on eliminating the cause of the moisture, that is, modifying the pouching system to eliminate exposure of the skin to urine or stool (or other sources of moisture). The peristomal skin damage should be treated with topical products that will promote adherence of the barrier seal. Ostomy appliances may require more frequent changes until the skin damage has healed.

CLINICAL PEARL

Correction of peristomal MASD requires correction of the underlying problem (such as a pouching system problem) as well as treatment of the damaged skin with topical products that promote ostomy pouch adherence.

Treatment may also include dietary modifications or pharmacologic interventions to thicken the stool output, wound care for the peristomal ulcerations, and treatment of secondary infections (Colwell et al., 2011). Prevention and management of peristomal MASD are discussed further in the Ostomy component of the core curriculum.

CASE STUDIES

CASE STUDY FOR MASD

Mr. Jones is an 80-year-old male who was admitted to home health care services following a recent hospitalization for pneumonia. Mr. Jones lives at home with his wife who is his primary caregiver.

Mr. Jones' medical history includes Parkinson's disease and hypertension. He has occasional fecal incontinence with episodes of loose stool. He wears an incontinence garment.

In addition to his prehospitalization medication regimen, he was prescribed an oral antibiotic for 7 days.

Mr. Jones had been ambulatory in his home prior to this illness but now requires assistance to stand and transfer from his bed to the chair or commode. He sits in a recliner chair when up.

His appetite is poor, but he has adequate fluid intake. He drinks one can of liquid nutritional supplement daily. He has had a five-pound weight loss since his recent illness.

Mrs. Jones provides daily hygiene and incontinence care. Personal care is often difficult for her to provide due to his weakness and limited mobility.

The home health nurse visits Mr. Jones twice a week. Upon assessment, the nurse observed that the scrotum was erythemic. The skin was moist and shiny, and Mr. Jones reported this area was sore. It was noted that the buttocks and intergluteal area were also reddened and moist, with scattered superficial lesions present.

The home health care nurse requested a consultation from the Wound Ostomy Continence (WOC) nurse to determine the etiology of the skin breakdown and develop a plan to manage incontinence and skin care.

QUESTION 1

What are the key factors contributing to skin breakdown?

ANSWER/RATIONALE

The key factors contributing to Mr. Jones skin breakdown include the following:

a. The skin is exposed to moisture and irritants from liquid stool. Stool may contain enzymes as well as other irritants that are damaging to the skin. Alteration in normal skin pH (change from acidic to alkaline) is also common. The presence of microbes can trigger a secondary infection.

b. Decreased mobility makes toileting difficult and incontinence care a challenge for his caregiver.

c. Friction from aggressive cleansing, moist or soiled incontinence garments, and transferring from a sitting to standing position contributes to skin breakdown. Moist skin is more prone to damage.

QUESTION 2

What are the clinical characteristics that will help the WOC Nurse determine that this is IAD vs. a pressure ulcer?

ANSWER/RATIONALE

The characteristics most critical to differential assessment include location, depth and distribution of the damage, and patient history. Mr. Jones' breakdown involved areas exposed to urine and stool, the lesions were superficial and scattered, and his history includes multiple episodes of fecal incontinence; all of these findings are consistent with IAD. Pressure ulcers are generally distinct open lesions that are located over and localized to a bony prominence.

QUESTION 3

What interventions must be included in the WOC Nurse's management plan?

ANSWER/RATIONALE

- Gentle cleansing with pH-balanced no-rinse cleanser and soft cloth (or 3-in-1 disposable cleansing wipe)
- Use of zinc oxide or zinc oxide/petrolatum combination ointment *or*
- Application of pectin powder followed with liquid acrylate barrier film

Use of the 3-in 1 disposable wipe would facilitate cleansing, but a pH-balanced no-rinse cleanser and disposable soft cloth would also be appropriate. Because he already has skin breakdown, he requires higher-level protection—a product that contains either zinc oxide or a layer of pectin powder covered with a liquid acrylate barrier film.

Additional measures would include the following:

- Use of a polymer-based absorptive product that wicks liquid away from the skin
- Bedside commode to facilitate toileting; scheduled toileting if indicated
- Gentle rectal exam to rule out impaction
- Consider physical therapy consult to provide strengthening exercises
- Nutritional assessment and modifications as indicated

Medical Adhesive–Related Skin Injury

Adhesive products are commonplace in institutional health care settings and allow clinicians to secure dressings, devices and equipment for both diagnostic procedures and treatment. In addition to tapes, adhesive wound dressings, ostomy pouches, condom catheters, catheter securement devices, electrodes, and surgical drapes are frequently used. Skin damage can accompany adhesive use and represents another example of "top-down" injury.

Because barrier function is critically dependent on the integrity of the stratum corneum, adhesive skin damage is an important clinical concern and one that is preventable. In 2012, a panel of 23 clinical experts from various disciplines and specialties were brought together to consider the topic and advance a best practice framework for this underappreciated problem. Following a literature review, a group of practice concepts were developed. A Delphi process was used to yield 25 consensus statements addressing the assessment, prevention, and treatment of adhesive-related skin damage (McNichol et al., 2013).

Definition

From that work, the term MARSI was developed to describe and define the clinical problem. The definition is as follows: A MARSI is an occurrence in which erythema and/or other manifestation of cutaneous abnormality (including, but not limited to, vesicle, bulla, erosion, or tear) persists 30 minutes or more after removal of the adhesive (McNichol et al., 2013).

Prevalence and Incidence

Despite the universal and frequent use of adhesive dressings and tapes in clinical settings, few papers addressing prevalence and incidence of adhesive injury have been published. In a study of 155 long-term care residents 65 years and older, Konya and colleagues (2010) reported a cumulative incidence rate of 15.5%. Maene (2013) reported on a European survey, in which an incidence of 7.1% was reported, with skin stripping being the most common type of injury. A pediatric survey done by Noonan et al. (2006) showed a prevalence rate of 8% for epidermal stripping; in a previous pediatric study, McLane and colleagues (2004) found a 17% prevalence. The majority of data have come from studies in operative orthopedic populations; in these studies, the reported incidence is 13% to 35% (Cosker et al. 2005; Jester et al., 2000; Koval et al., 2003; McNichol et al., 2013; Polatsch et al., 2004; Sellæg et al., 2012).

Risk Factors

Numerous and diverse intrinsic and extrinsic risk factors have been advanced (McNichol et al., 2013), but a risk assessment tool has yet to be developed (**Table 17-1**, Risk Factors for MARSI). Age has long been considered a significant risk factor, with individuals at each end of the lifespan being at greatest risk. The very old are at risk due to changes in the dermal–epidermal junction that compromise the attachment of the epidermis to the dermis; the reduced cohesion significantly increases the risk of adhesive-related injury. Interestingly, recent research using skin models suggests that age-related changes including the extent of *skin wrinkling* are risk factors for the development of superficial skin lesions (Sopher & Gefen, 2011). In preterm infants, maturation of skin structures has not yet occurred; as a result, the barrier function of the stratum corneum is absent or diminished, and there is very poor cohesion of the skin layers. In addition, the skin is much thinner in these infants. All of these factors place them at increased risk for adhesive-related damage.

TABLE 17-1 Intrinsic and Extrinsic Factors Increasing Risk of Skin Tears

Intrinsic Risk Factors

- Age: the very young and the very old are at increased risk; extremes of age impact not only how individuals heal but also their susceptibility to developing a wound
- Skin changes: dermal and subcutaneous tissue loss, epidermal thinning, reduced levels of skin lipids/skin moisture content, reduced elasticity and tensile strength of skin
- Dehydration, poor nutrition, cognitive impairment, altered mobility, and decreased sensation
- Neonates: decreased epidermal-to-dermal cohesion, deficient stratum corneum, impaired thermoregulation

Extrinsic Risk Factors

- Increased risk of mechanical trauma during ADLs
- Use of soap (reduces the skin's natural lubrication)
- Dry skin more susceptible to friction and shearing
- Inability to reposition independently
- Sharp corners/edges that are not padded to protect

(Please refer to Chapters 12 and 13 for additional details on age-related skin characteristics.)

Patients in intervention-intense environments such as Critical Care, the Operating Room and Post Anesthesia Care Unit, or the Emergency Department are exposed to numerous adhesive products that may require repeated application and removal over the course of therapy. Individuals with central venous catheters and peripherally inserted central catheters (PICCs) require frequent dressing changes and therefore comprise another at-risk population (Thayer, 2012). Patients with dermatologic diseases that disrupt epidermal barrier function are also at increased risk for adhesive injury. Patients who have degenerative, atrophic skin changes from long-term corticosteroid administration have very fragile skin and are another population at high risk for MARSI.

Oncology patients receiving cytotoxic therapy represent another high-risk group. All chemotherapeutic agents target rapidly dividing cells, including skin cells, which compromises skin health. Patients receiving *targeted therapies* present a special challenge to adhesive use. These drugs are designed to block epidermal growth factor receptors and commonly create severe acneiform skin reactions. Radiation therapy is also associated with high incidence of adverse skin changes (radiodermatitis); early changes are due to inflammation and loss of epidermal cells, and late changes are due to chronic ischemia and fibrosis. (Please refer to Chapter 29 for additional information on effects of cancer treatments.)

CLINICAL PEARL

MARSI is common, typically painful, and almost always preventable.

In addition, distortion of the skin caused by edema, distention, or movement of the skin under an adhesive can increase the risk of skin injury.

Mechanisms of Injury

Several types of common MARSI have been identified (Bryant, 1988; Bryant, 2012; McNichol et al, 2013). The wound nurse needs to understand the different mechanisms of injury and the key assessment findings for each type of damage, in order to provide appropriate preventive care and assessment.

Irritant Contact Dermatitis

The term *Irritant Contact Dermatitis* (ICD) describes cutaneous inflammation that is triggered by exposure to an irritant. The response is immune mediated but *nonallergic* and comprises a group of complex reactions that are not completely understood. Reaction threshold and severity are influenced by the offending irritant and vary from person to person. Reactions to products commonly used in clinical settings generally develop over hours to days. Erythema and edema are initial assessment findings (Fig. 17-5).

Vesicles may be present in addition to erythema and edema. Repeated exposure may result in a *cumulative irritant contact dermatitis,* which may persist for an extended period even if the offending substance has been discontinued (Widmer et al., 1994). The time required for resolution of adhesive-induced dermatitis in clinical settings has not been documented; however, data from healthy volunteers have demonstrated return of normal barrier function, as evidenced by normal TEWL, within 6 to 12 days after injury (Hoffman & Maibach, 1976).

Allergic Contact Dermatitis

Allergic contact dermatitis (ACD) is a well-defined immune-mediated inflammatory response. The initial phase, "sensitization," occurs when tiny protein molecules called haptens penetrate the stratum corneum. The Langerhans cells normally present in the epidermis for immune surveillance bind to the invading allergen (i.e., the *antigen*), and then transport the bound antigen to the lymph nodes for presentation to T lymphocytes. If the T-cell possesses a receptor that is complementary for the antigen, the T-cell becomes *sensitized* to that antigen. The sensitized T cells then proliferate, returning to the skin and circulating through the bloodstream. As a result, areas of skin distant to the site of exposure can become populated with sensitized T cells. During the *elicitation* phase, sensitized T lymphocytes accumulate at the site of exposure. When repeat exposure to the offending substance occurs, proinflammatory mediators (cytokines and lymphokines) are produced by both antigen-specific *and* nonspecific T cells. Some cytokines (e.g., tumor necrosis factor-beta [TNF-β]) exert significant, destructive effects on cells including epidermal lysis. Other inflammation-promoting chemicals such as histamine are released by mast cells and basophils during ACD (Rietschel & Fowler, 2008).

In the nursing literature, allergy has generally been described as consisting of two distinct phases with elicitation occurring as a result of subsequent exposure. It is now recognized that these phases can occur *simultaneously* in some patients upon initial exposure to the antigen. Allergy does require antigen-specific susceptibility. However, sensitization is more easily induced in individuals whose barrier integrity is already compromised; thus, the presence of ICD may increase risk for an allergic response in a susceptible individual.

In both ICD and ACD, there is erythema of variable severity, which manifests as shades of pink to red. Primary lesions such as macules, papules, and vesicles are often present in the form of a diffuse rash. Wheals may also be noted (Fig. 17-6). It is important to recognize that distinguishing ACD from ICD on clinical assessment alone is difficult and sometimes impossible (Belsito, 2000; Marzulli & Maibach, 2008). Patch testing can provide definitive confirmation of allergy.

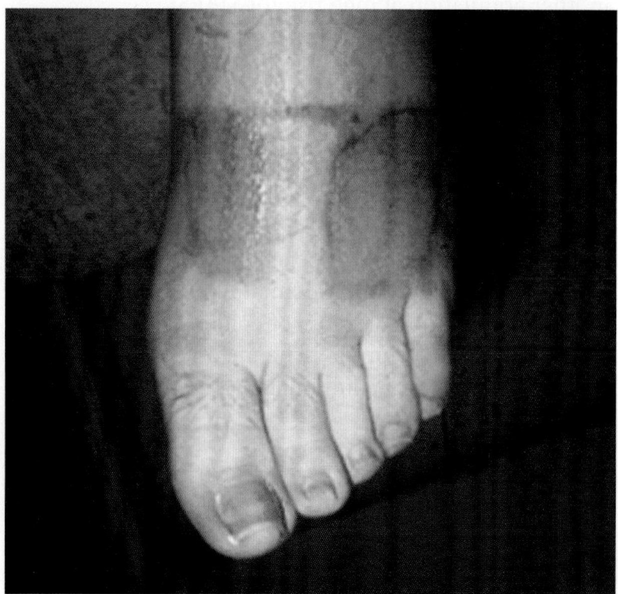

FIGURE 17-5. Irritant contact dermatitis.

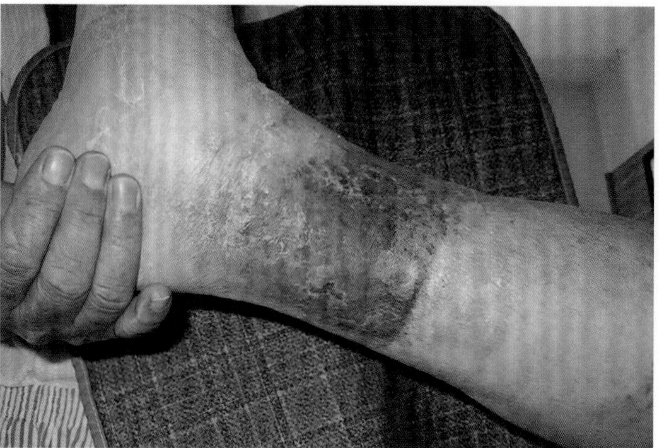

FIGURE 17-6. Allergic contact dermatitis (patient with sensitivity to hydrocolloid adhesive). (From Berke, C. T. (2015). Pathology and clinical presentation of friction injuries: Case series and literature review. *Journal of Wound Ostomy and Continence Nursing*, *42*(1), 47–61.)

Shelanski et al. (1996) observed that "every topically applied product has the potential to cause an adverse reaction in some individual…" This perspective speaks to the diversity of individual immune response and skin sensitivity and provides a meaningful perspective for wound nurses who routinely apply a wide variety of topical products including adhesives to the skin. Other potential etiologies of dermatitis should be considered if similar lesions are noted beyond or distant from the adhesive footprint. A referral to Dermatology may be indicated in these situations.

It is common for bedside nurses to presume an allergic reaction when erythema is observed after adhesive removal. This erroneous conclusion has resulted in many patients reporting they are allergic to adhesives. *Transient erythema* (also known as transient hyperemia) is commonly observed in light-skinned individuals when adhesives are removed. This represents a short-term inflammatory response triggered by corneocyte disruption (Pinkus, 1952) and typically resolves within several minutes. The inclusion of a time factor within the MARSI definition (McNichol et al., 2013) has provided clarity in differentiating this transient color change from actual injury.

At the time of this writing, data on incidence of contact dermatitis (either ICD or ACD) related to *adhesive product use* in populations of concern to the wound nurse are limited. Anecdotally, wound nurses report ACD to be much less common than ICD. In a study of ostomy patients, ACD occurred in only 0.7% (Lyon et al., 2000). Within the extensive literature on occupational dermatitis, 80% of skin damage is reported to be irritant versus allergic (NIOSH, 2010). Based on available data and expert opinion, an adverse skin response that persists for >30 minutes is *more likely* to be the result of a contact irritation or mechanical damage than true allergy.

Maceration

Maceration is another type of MARSI. (McNichol et al., 2013). The mechanism of damage involves overhydration of the skin under tape and has already been described in the section on MASD. Excessive hydration causes the epidermal cells (corneocytes) to swell with loss of the normal tight intercellular junctions (Zhai & Maibach, 2001); overhydration reduces tensile strength and increases the risk of skin disruption with adhesive removal. Overhydration presents clinically as wrinkling of the skin surface and a change in skin color (to white or gray or a tone lighter than the surrounding skin) (Fig. 17-7).

Maceration is promoted by the use of occlusive or minimally breathable adhesive products or by adhesive products being left in place for extended periods of time. It is also influenced by the skin's microclimate. Increases in skin surface moisture can contribute to maceration, even when breathable adhesive products are used.

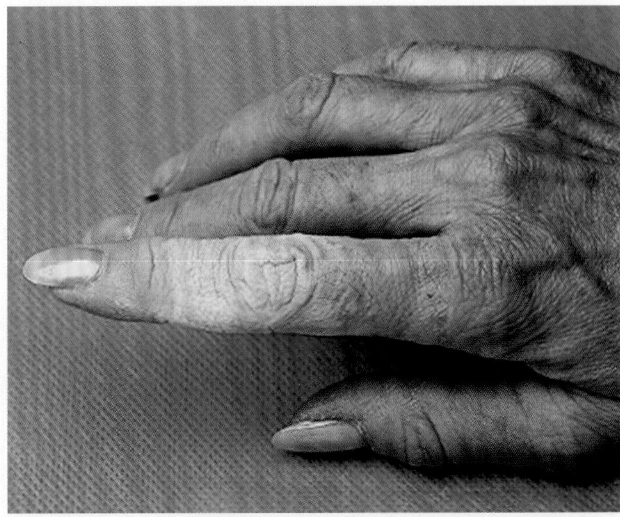

FIGURE 17-7. Maceration.

CLINICAL PEARL

Common types of MARSI include contact dermatitis, maceration, mechanical trauma (skin stripping), tension blisters, and folliculitis.

Mechanical Trauma

In the clinical setting, adhesives are often required over extended periods and removed repeatedly. Only a handful of published studies have examined the impact of this practice on skin integrity. The effects of postoperative dressings in total joint arthroplasty patients constitute the majority of these investigations, most of which focused on skin condition following a *single* adhesive application/removal or limited numbers of dressing changes (Cosker et al., 2005; Jester et al., 2000; Polatsch et al., 2004; Sellaeg et al., 2012). Published data are also limited within the ostomy population despite extensive and long-term adhesive use.

All adhesive products used in clinical practice can be expected to detach layers of cells to some degree (Alikahn & Maibach, 2009; Cutting, 2008; Dykes et al., 2001; Zhai et al., 2007), which can result in significant disruption of the epidermis. TEWL is a sensitive indicator of stratum corneum integrity and barrier function, with TEWL levels rising as the skin's barrier function diminishes. TEWL can be measured with specialized instruments and has been used in tape studies to show that TEWL increases in direct proportion to the extent of stratum corneum damage (Hoffman & Maibach, 1976; Shah et al., 2005).

The term "skin stripping" is used to describe delamination of epidermal layers or complete detachment of the epidermis from the dermis (Bryant, 1988; McNichol et al., 2013). Any degree of stripping triggers cell division in the stratum germinativum (basal layer of the epidermis) in an effort to repair the disrupted barrier. No obvious injury will be seen with removal of just a few cell layers *if* the

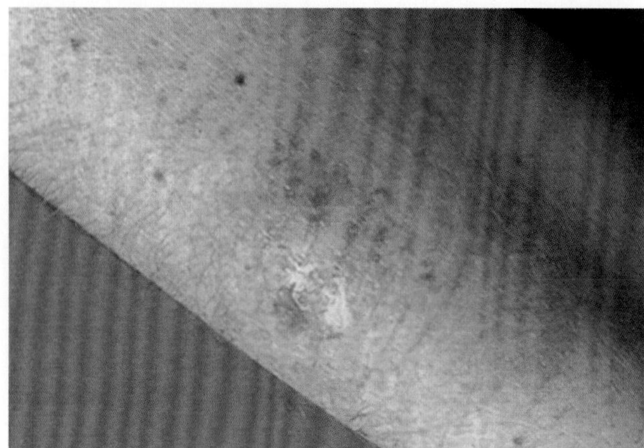

FIGURE 17-8. Skin Stripping.

patient can mount a healing response and *if* the recovery time (i.e., time between adhesive removal episodes) is sufficient for cell regeneration. A moist "glistening" surface is observed when sufficient layers are removed to expose the lower portion of the epidermis (Lund and Tucker, 2003); inflammation is obvious and the barrier is clearly compromised (Fig. 17-8).

Complete epidermal loss creates a partial-thickness wound. The underlying moist dermis is visible, and significant discomfort can be expected as nerve endings are exposed (Fig. 17-9).

The term "skin tear" is often used to describe the traumatic partial-thickness skin loss that results from adhesives. Skin tears are discussed later in this chapter.

Several factors are implicated in the development of skin stripping. Skin-related factors include overall health of the skin and the cohesive competence between the epidermal layers, or between the epidermis and dermis (in other words, the degree to which the cell layers are attached). Adhesive-related factors include *type of adhesive* (Dykes, 2007; Waring et al., 2011), *amount of tack to skin,* (i.e., "strength" of the adhesive (Tokumura et al., 2005), and the *peel force, angle, and speed* of adhesive product removal (Jackson, 1988; Klode et al., 2010; Lund & Tucker, 2003). The use of aggressive adhesives can delaminate the epidermis, especially when the epidermis is immature or fragile and poorly anchored. Occlusive adhesives cause excessive hydration and increase the risk of cell disruption (Tokomura et al., 1999). Indiscriminate use of adhesion promoters (i.e., "tackifiers"), as well as rapid and careless adhesive removal also disrupts epidermal cohesion and can create stripping injuries.

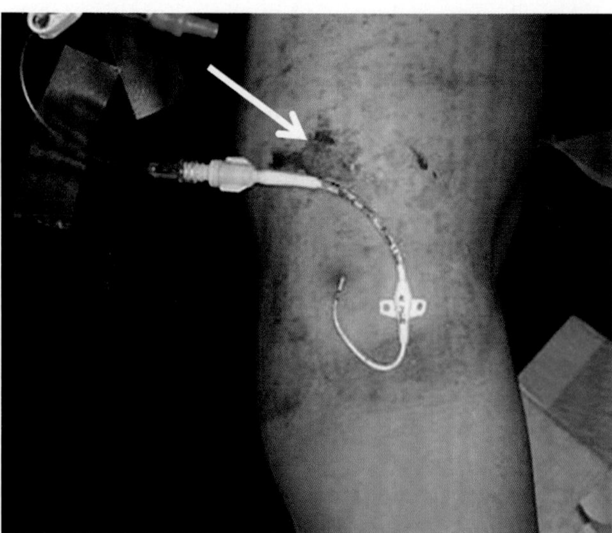

FIGURE 17-9. Skin stripping involving PICC line.

Barrier recovery after experimental stripping has been shown to require 2 weeks or more (Baker & Kligman, 1967).

Tension Blisters

The term *tension blisters* describes another variation of mechanical injury (McNichol, et al., 2013) (Fig. 17-10). When a shearing force is applied to skin and the skin to adhesive attachment is greater than that of skin to skin, the epidermis lifts from the dermis (Polatsch et al., 2004). Development of edema and the accompanying distortion of skin are believed to be a key factor contributing to tension underlying the adhesive. Tension blisters have also been shown to form when adhesive dressings or tapes are stretched or "strapped" during application (Fig. 17-11). When the tape is released following application under tension, the adhesive backing resumes its normal configuration and the resulting tension pulls the epidermis off the dermis, causing a blister to form. The blisters are typically "unroofed" when the adhesive is removed, resulting in a superficial partial-thickness

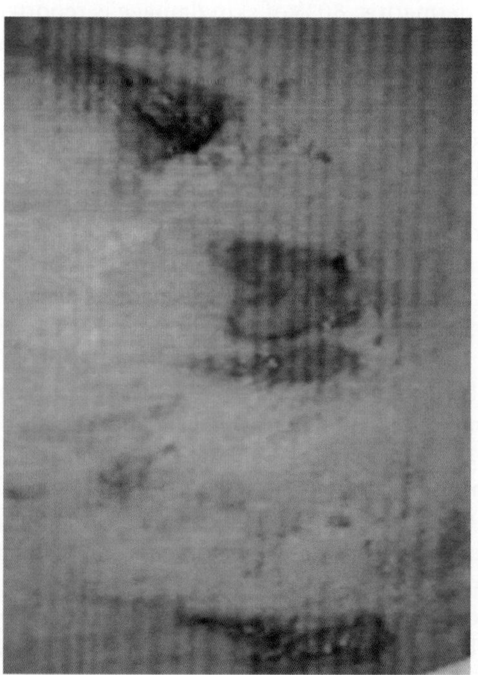

FIGURE 17-10. Tension blister. (From Berke, C. T. (2015). Pathology and clinical presentation of friction injuries: Case series and literature review. *Journal of Wound Ostomy and Continence Nursing*, *42*(1), 47–61.)

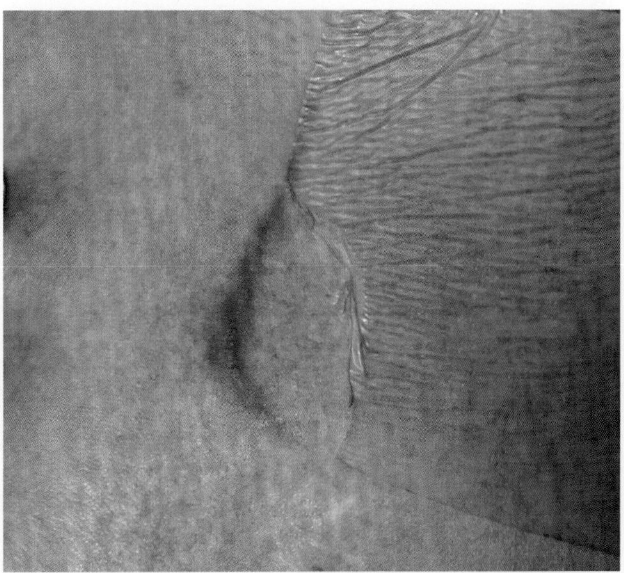

FIGURE 17-11. Tension blister at periphery of dressing.

wound that is open and extremely painful. Tension blisters have primarily been reported in the orthopedic population (Cosker et al., 2005; Jester et al., 2000; Koval et al., 2003; Polatsch et al., 2004; Sellæg et al., 2012) but have also been associated with intravenous securement dressings (Thayer, 2012). Critical adhesive-related factors contributing to tension blisters include lack of conformability and elasticity, and lack of breathability (Sivamani et al., 2003).

Erythema *without blister formation* can develop at the periphery of adhesive dressings and tapes. This results from frictional forces generated by skin movement under nonconformable adhesives (Tokumura et al., 2005). Frictional forces are increased when skin is moist or wet with an accompanying increase in the likelihood of skin injury (Sivamani et al., 2003). In a patient with significant diaphoresis, moisture *and* friction are probable factors contributing to skin injury under an adhesive product. This underscores the need for proper skin preparation prior to adhesive application.

Folliculitis

Folliculitis is a dermatologic condition also included in the MARSI framework (McNichol et al., 2013). It is characterized by inflammation of hair follicles, but is not exclusively associated with adhesive use. Causes include physical or chemical irritation or infection; staphylococcal species are the most common offending organisms for infectious folliculitis (Habif, 2010). Assessment findings include erythema that is localized to the follicles (Fig. 17-12).

Pustules are noted in the presence of infection. The distinct localized lesions of folliculitis should be differentiated from *Candidiasis,* a yeast-like fungus that manifests as an area of diffuse erythema with pinpoint maculopustular or maculopapular lesions at the *periphery* of the affected area.

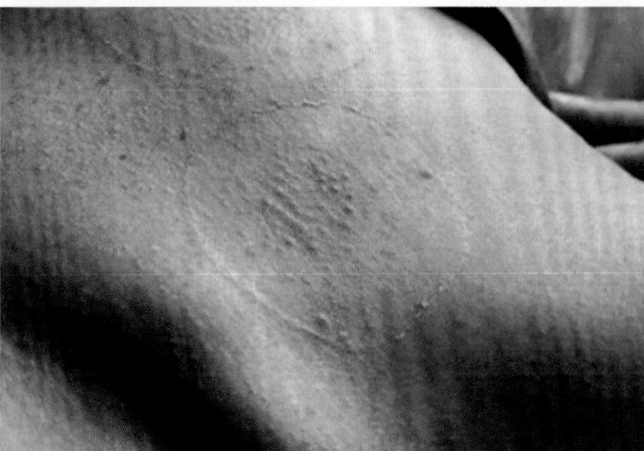

FIGURE 17-12. Folliculitis. (From McNichol, L., Lund, C., Rosen, T., et al. (2013). Medical adhesives and patient safety: State of the science. *Journal of Wound Ostomy and Continence Nursing, 40*(4), 365–380; quiz E1–E2.)

Prevention of MARSI

Five key interventions form the essential clinical approach to MARSI prevention (see Box 17-1).

Step 1: Assessment

A thorough assessment should be conducted to (1) identify risk factors associated with MARSI development (see Table 17-1) and (2) inspect the skin. Two areas of risk warrant special attention. A focused patient history should be obtained in order to uncover known or potential *allergies and sensitivities* (McNichol et al., 2013). Patch testing may be beneficial for patients: (1) undergoing chemotherapy or a surgical procedure requiring extended aftercare; (2) with complex skin problems; or (3) with a history of multiple allergies. This allows the clinician to evaluate the adhesive products that are commonly used as a part of a treatment regime in regard to patient tolerance and reactivity.

Assessment should also be focused on identifying patients at risk for *mechanical injury* (McNichol et al., 2013). As noted previously, patients in any age group with significant edema (e.g., anasarca in the critically ill) or distention are at high risk for stripping or tension blister formation.

Step 2: Selection of Correct Adhesive Product Based on Clinical Requirements and Patient Characteristics

Adhesives will adhere most effectively to a *clean, dry, flat, immobile* surface. Skin presents a challenging substrate due to its unique and dynamic characteristics. The epidermal

BOX 17-1. Prevention of MARSI

1. Assess the patient.
2. Select the correct adhesive product based on clinical requirements and patient characteristics.
3. Prepare the skin.
4. Apply the adhesive product correctly.
5. Remove the adhesive product correctly.

surface is "contaminated" by the presence of dead corneocytes and surface oil. The skin's microclimate—a combination of skin surface temperature and moisture—varies with body temperature and environmental humidity and can produce moist or extremely wet skin. Skin is highly contoured and extremely mobile, which creates an uneven surface for adhesion. Elasticity allows accommodation of mobile surfaces (e.g., over joints) but presents a major challenge to adhesives. Not surprisingly, adhesive products are better tolerated and less likely to fail in areas that are static.

Medical adhesive technology must overcome or accommodate these characteristics in order to provide effective clinical products. Understanding the fundamentals of this technology enables the wound nurse to optimize product selection for successful securement and avoidance of skin injury.

How Adhesives Work

The majority of adhesive products consist of at least two components: the adhesive *coating* that attaches to the skin and the material or *backing* to which the adhesive is applied (Fig. 17-13). The *combination* of these components determines the characteristics of the product. Some tapes may incorporate additional layers, for example, a release coating that allows easier release or unwinding from a roll.

CLINICAL PEARL

One key measure for MARSI prevention is selection of the best adhesive product based on clinical requirements and patient characteristics. In selecting an adhesive, the nurse must consider both the adhesive coating and the adhesive backing.

While there is evidence of adhesive use in ancient times, the first modern tapes for medical care incorporated natural rubber and appeared in the late 1800s. The Second World War created a shortage of rubber and spurred development of synthetic polymers. What we recognize as modern medical adhesives were introduced in the 1960s. These newer *acrylates* offered good tack, material stability and greater adaptability than rubber adhesives (Lucast, 2000). Today, the majority of medical products incorporate acrylate or silicone polymers, with natural rubber still used for some tapes. Other categories of adhesives include hydrocolloids (ostomy barriers and hydrocolloid dressings), hydrogels (incorporated into some electrodes), and zinc oxide–containing formulations (used in tapes).

Acrylate adhesives are considered pressure-sensitive adhesives (PSAs). PSAs behave like liquids and "flow" into the skin's irregular contours due to viscoelastic properties. When using a PSA product, the clinician should apply with firm but gentle pressure to promote adhesion of the adhesive product to the skin. PSAs should ideally demonstrate a "strong holding force," that is, remain attached for the desired time period, while also allowing atraumatic removal with no adhesive residue on the skin (Lund & Tucker, 2003).

CLINICAL PEARL

Acrylate adhesives (such as paper tape products) are PSAs; they should be applied with firm but gentle pressure, and the adhesive bond continues to increase over time; they may not be a good choice for situations in which only short-term adhesion is needed.

The adhesion of acrylate PSAs builds over time. This characteristic underscores the importance of understanding adhesive product characteristics and matching those features to the desired clinical wear time. The risk of skin trauma is increased when adhesives are removed during peak adhesion.

Adhesives characterized as *aggressive* typically have thick adhesive coatings. While they may utilize acrylates, these high adhesion materials more commonly incorporate natural or synthetic rubber–based agents.

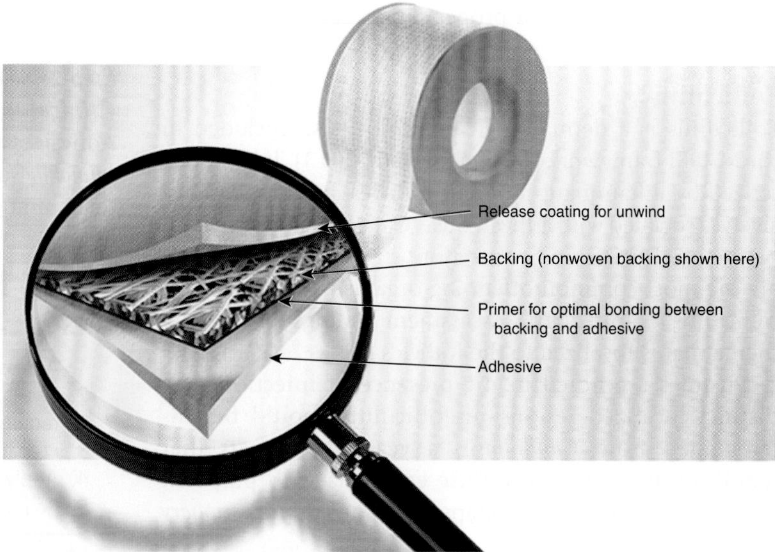

FIGURE 17-13. Common component layers of medical tape. (From Berke, C. T. (2015). Pathology and clinical presentation of friction injuries: Case series and literature review. *Journal of Wound Ostomy and Continence Nursing*, *42*(1), 47–61.)

Common backings used for adhesive tapes and dressings include: paper and paper blends, plastic, paper/plastic blends, fabric (cotton or woven polyesters), foam, and polyurethane film.

The breathability of an adhesive product can greatly impact the skin's normal TEWL. Occlusive products create a barrier on the skin surface and will cause overhydration. Overhydration causes the cells to swell, with an accompanying decrease in the cohesive strength between cells. As a result, removal of the adhesive product is more likely to create a stripping injury (Tokomura et al., 1999).

As noted previously, the combination of the adhesive and backing will determine breathability, gentleness, potential for sensitization, strength, conformability, ability to stretch, ability to be torn, and optimal clinical uses.

The introduction of an acrylate adhesive coating onto a *porous* paper backing in the 1960s has been described as the "single most important technical innovation in decreasing tape dermatitis" (Hoffman & Maibach, 1976). In addition to being breathable, this tape was the first minimally sensitizing and residue-free tape available for clinical use.

Matching Adhesive Product to Clinical Situation (Table 17-2)

Clinical considerations that influence adhesive product selection include intended clinical purpose, type of device to be secured, location on the body, intended duration of securement, and skin condition (McNichol et al., 2013; Lund & Tucker, 2003). Product properties such as tack, gentleness, breathability, stretch, conformability, and ability to tear should also be considered.

While maintenance of skin integrity is an important consideration, it must be balanced against the need for reliable securement of critical devices such as endotracheal tubes and vascular access devices. Dislodgment or detachment of life-sustaining or supporting devices due to adhesive failure is unacceptable. In these situations, securement is the priority, and products with higher adhesion are indicated. As a result, traditional cloth tapes coated with zinc oxide–containing adhesives or synthetic rubber or woven polyester ("silk") coated with acrylate adhesives are commonly used. Because of the challenges associated with use of these adhesive products, nonadhesive securement devices for endotracheal tubes have been adopted by some clinicians. When adhesive securement is desired or the only option available, critical tubes and devices should be anchored using a strong but conformable and breathable adhesive product.

CLINICAL PEARL

Securement of critical devices such as endotracheal tubes or vascular access devices should be done with high adhesion products such as cloth tapes or woven polyester ("silk") tapes with more aggressive adhesive coatings.

Higher adhesion has been correlated with increased risk of skin injury and pain (Bryant, 2012; Dykes et al., 2001). Silicone adhesives provide an effective solution for securement on fragile skin or where frequent adhesive product changes are required. In contrast to acrylate adhesives, silicone adhesives attach to skin with lower surface tension, and adhesion does not build over time. In addition, silicone adhesives detach fewer cells during removal (Cutting, 2006; Grove et al., 2013). Silicone adhesive tapes are best suited for securement of dressings and lightweight tubing. Generally, they do not provide sufficient adhesion for securing critical or heavy devices. Evidence of effectiveness should be provided if a manufacturer is making such a recommendation.

TABLE 17-2 Guidelines for Tape Selection

Clinical Need	Adhesion Level	Backing/Adhesive	Examples
Securing critical or heavy devices and tubes (dry or moist skin)	High to very high	Polyester ("silk")/acrylate; cloth/acrylate; cloth/latex rubber	"Silk" tape; Cloth adhesive tape; "Athletic tape"
Securing dressings; reinforcing dressings	Moderate	Cloth–paper combo/acrylate; cloth/acrylate; variable backings/silicone	Soft cloth tape; Paper tape; Paper–plastic blend tape
Securement of medium-light size/weight tubes/devices	Moderate	Cloth–paper combo/acrylate; cloth/acrylate; variable backings /silicone	Soft cloth tape; Paper tape; Paper–plastic blend tape
Noncritical securement on sensitive, compromised or at-risk skin; situations where removal anticipated to be traumatic (e.g., Pediatric population, cognitive impairment)	Lower	Variable backings /silicone	Silicone tape
Securement where movement/edema/distention is anticipated	Moderate	Cloth/acrylate	Soft cloth tape
Noncritical securement where skin is moist/damp	Moderate	Paper/acrylate; paper–plastic blend/acrylate	Paper tape

Medical tapes that are intended for a range of dressing securement or splinting needs are referred to as multipurpose and typically feature a gentle acrylate adhesive on a backing such as polyester ("silk") or soft cloth fabric. Some silicone tapes may also be suitable for multipurpose use.

CLINICAL PEARL

Silicone adhesive products are gentle adhesives in which the adhesion does not build over time; they are appropriate for application of dressings to fragile skin but not for securement of essential devices.

Achieving adhesion over contoured areas or within folds requires soft, conformable backings with adequate tack to skin. A backing that stretches is necessary over areas of the body that move or where edema or distention is anticipated. However, even if a stretchable adhesive product has been appropriately selected and applied, the product should be *removed and replaced* if underlying tension is noted. Silicone adhesives are the exception to this rule as they allow repositioning. At the time of this writing, a silicone tape with a stretchable backing is not available (Fig. 17-13).

An adhesive tape with lower adhesion properties and breathability is appropriate in clinical situations where frequent dressing changes are desired or necessary and the dressing is not large or bulky.

As noted earlier, adhesives perform optimally on dry surfaces. Some PSAs are formulated to adhere to moist surfaces but will not adhere optimally when skin is wet. This property reinforces the need to create as dry a surface as possible prior to adhesive application.

Step 3: Skin Preparation

Skin preparation is essential for successful adhesive product use. Attention to this step can prevent adhesive failures that create patient discomfort, increase the work of care, and waste supplies.

Excessive hair adversely impacts adhesion as well as markedly increasing discomfort during removal. In addition, hair is a reservoir for microbes. The effect of shaving has not been studied in the ostomy or chronic wound population; however, in a surgical population, shaving has been shown to increase infection risk (Tanner et al., 2006) and is associated with folliculitis (Habif, 2010). Therefore, at this time, recommendations include removal of excessive or coarse hair with scissors or surgical clippers and avoidance of shaving. For the infusion therapy population where sterile technique is required, Infusion Nursing Society guidelines recommend hair removal using sterile scissors or a clipper with disposable head (Infusion Nursing Society, 2006).

Next, skin should be cleansed and dried. The optimal product for skin preparation has not been identified, but principles of cleansing directed at maintaining normal skin pH and minimizing barrier disruption should be followed (Schmid & Kortig, 1995). Gentle, no-rinse pH-balanced cleansers or pH-balanced soaps are desirable based on their ability to remove dead skin cells, excessive oil, and adhesive or dressing residue. Cleansing formulations containing barrier or moisturizing ingredients (e.g., dimethicone) can potentially interfere with adhesion. Manufacturers' guidance should be consulted to determine if a specific no-rinse cleanser is suitable for use under adhesive products. Most bar soaps are alkaline and should be avoided. After cleansing, the skin should be gently dried.

The wound nurse may be consulted on MARSI prevention in patients receiving infusion therapy. In this population, considerations for skin preparation are different from those of ostomy or wound care patients. Antiseptic preparations must be allowed to completely dry prior to application of an adhesive securement dressing or device. The risk of ICD or MASD is increased when a wet solution is trapped under an adhesive product.

As previously noted, adhesive removal detaches cell layers of the stratum corneum. For many years, wound nurses have used barrier films effectively to minimize this effect and to help prevent stripping injuries associated with adhesive use. The effectiveness of this practice is supported by several small studies and by expert opinion (Bryant, 2012; Campbell et al., 2000; Korber et al., 2007; McNichol et al., 2013; Rolstad et al., 1994; Samann, 1999; Sanders et al., 2007).

CLINICAL PEARL

Effective skin preparation is a critical element in MARSI prevention and includes the following: removal of excess hair; gentle cleansing with no-rinse cleanser; thorough drying; and protection with liquid barrier film that is allowed to dry prior to tape application.

Barrier films consist of either a copolymer or terpolymer dissolved in a liquid solvent. When applied to the skin, the solvent evaporates and the polymer dries on the skin as a transparent coating that provides a protective interface between the epidermis and the adhesive. When the adhesive product is removed, the film is lifted from the skin rather than skin cells. Formulations of barrier films differ, and this should be considered when selecting a product for skin protection. Traditional formulations, while inexpensive, utilize alcohol as a solvent. Alcohol is a potent irritant that is unsuitable for use on compromised skin; alcohol can also elicit a sting or pain response on *intact* skin in some individuals (Rietschel & Fowler, 2008). Modern barrier film formulations utilize alcohol-free, nonstinging solvents that can be applied to damaged or sensitive skin.

Polymers also differ. The polymer providing the barrier film should create a waterproof, transparent coating that allows TEWL. Once on the skin, many barrier films tend to be "brittle" and ultimately fail over time by forming microcracks. This behavior compromises barrier function and ultimately results in failure of the coating. The incorporation of an additional polymer called a "plasticizer" is advantageous in that it softens the film, which allows it to flex with skin movement. This characteristic helps to maintain an intact coating over the desired area of protection.

The polymer in the barrier film should also be compatible with chlorhexidine gluconate (CHG) antiseptic preps when used for infusion therapy site protection. CHG is a positively charged (cationic) molecule. Use of nonionic formulations avoids the possibility of a chemical interaction that could diminish the prep's effectiveness (Senior, 1973).

The barrier film should be applied to any skin that will contact the adhesive product. As with antiseptics, barrier films should be allowed to dry completely prior to adhesive application. Most barrier films are removed when the adhesive product is lifted from the skin and require reapplication prior to placement of a new adhesive tape, dressing, or device.

The appropriateness of barrier films under electrodes and grounding pads should be verified with the device manufacturer prior to film application, because the presence of a film may increase skin impedance and reduce effectiveness of the device.

Adhesion promoters such as compound tincture of benzoin (CPT) or mastic are commonly referred to as *tackifiers*. It is important to distinguish these products from barrier films as their chemistry and indications differ. Adhesion promoters enhance or promote adhesion between the skin and adhesive product. Use should be based on specific patient need, and routine or indiscriminate use of these compounds should be avoided to prevent MARSI (McNichol et al., 2013). This is especially important in patients with fragile skin. Sensitization to both compounds has been reported in the literature (Rietschel & Fowler, 2008).

Step 4: Correct Application of Adhesive Product

Adhesive products should be applied without tension or stretch of the adhesive product to avoid deformation of the underlying skin and to prevent tension blisters or irritation at the product's periphery. Selection of an *appropriately sized* adhesive product reduces the tendency to stretch a dressing to fit the desired coverage area. Stretching an adhesive does not improve or increase tack. As noted previously, virtually all adhesives used in clinical practice today are *pressure* sensitive. Gentle but firm pressure upon application activates the viscoelastic polymers so that they behave like a liquid and flow into the sulci cutis (i.e., contours) of the epidermis; this assures optimal surface area contact.

Even with proper application, edema or distention of the underlying tissue can develop, resulting in deformation or compression of the skin. Acrylate adhesive products must be replaced when this occurs, whereas most silicone adhesive products can be repositioned.

Step 5: Correct Removal of Adhesive Product

Technique for removal is critical for maintenance of skin integrity, with attention directed to the *peel angle* and support of the *peel line*.

Peel force is associated with skin injury and is governed by the angle at which the adhesive is removed from the skin (Lund & Tucker, 2003). Removal at a 90-degree angle (i.e., perpendicular) to the skin surface generates significantly greater forces than narrow-angle or horizontal removal where the adhesive remains close to the skin surface (Breternitz et al., 2007; Jackson, 1988). The *peel line* describes the point where the adhesive separates from the skin. The skin that is immediately adjacent to the peel line should be supported as it is exposed to prevent pulling and distortion (Fig. 17-14).

Finally, the adhesive product should be slowly and deliberately removed. This "low and slow" approach of deliberate horizontal removal requires patience; thus, it is critical to emphasize the importance to all caregivers (Lavelle, 2004).

CLINICAL PEARL

Inappropriate removal technique is a common contributor to MARSI; the adhesive should be removed at a low (horizontal) angle, and the skin adjacent to the peel line should be supported to prevent pulling.

An alternative "stretch and release" technique may be used to remove nonbordered transparent film dressings. The edge of the film is gently pulled, allowing the film to lift from the skin (Fig. 17-15).

Placement of a small piece of tape at the edge or corner of the adhesive product can facilitate removal. A portion

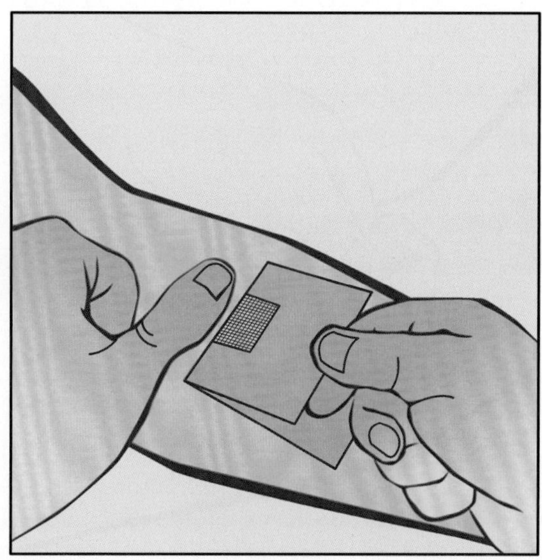

FIGURE 17-14. "Push/pull" approach to adhesive removal.

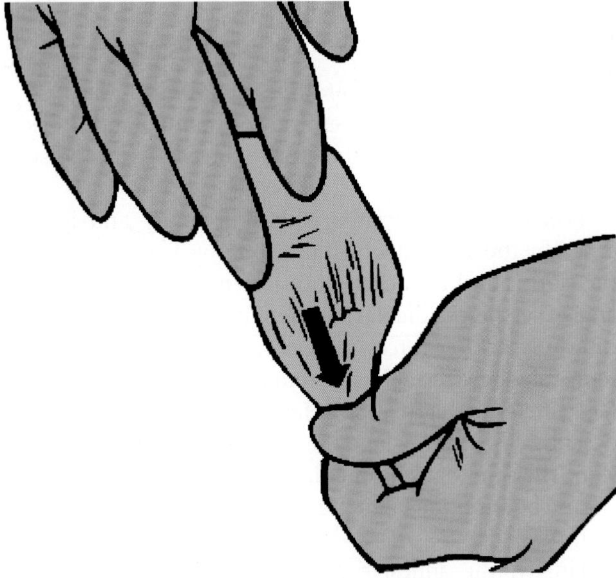

FIGURE 17-15. "Stretch and release" technique for tape removal.

of this "tape tab" is gently pressed onto the underlying adhesive product. The free edge of the tab serves as a handle to help lift the adhesive product and begin removal, thus avoiding the need to scratch or pick at the skin (Fig. 17-16).

Use of adhesive removers should be considered (McNichol et al., 2013), especially when removing aggressive adhesives or adhesive residue from skin. Ethanol, isobutene, naphtha, mineral spirits, and silicone are common ingredients in adhesive removal products. Other removers contain a chemical called D-limonene which is a citrus-derived oil. While this agent is "naturally occurring," it can remove skin lipids, disrupt the skin barrier, and serve as an irritant (Tornier et al., 2008). No studies have been conducted to show the benefit of one formulation over another. All adhesive removers should be completely removed from the skin prior to application of a new adhesive product. It is advisable to consult the manufacturer's recommendations for product removal as formulations may contain both water-soluble and water-*insoluble* ingredients such as silicone and isobutene. Products containing an ingredient called hexamethyldisiloxane (HMDS) will remove silicone. Isobutene can be removed with mineral oil; prior to adhesive reapplication, the skin should be washed with a surfactant-containing cleanser or gentle soap to remove any residual oil.

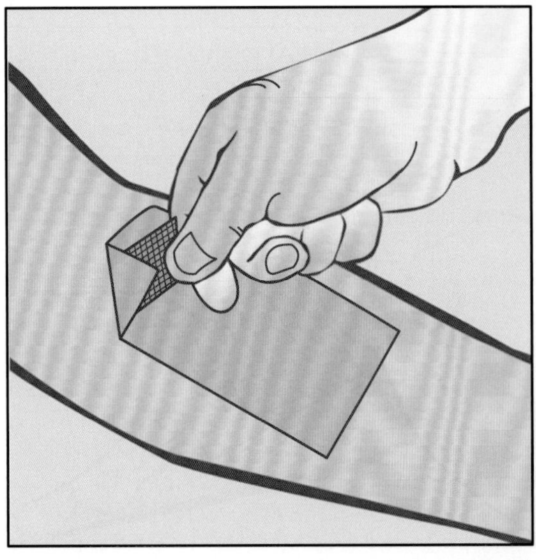

FIGURE 17-16. "Tape tab" technique for tape removal.

Creating a MARSI-Free Environment

Adhesive Alternatives

Alternatives to adhesives should be considered for dressing securement when skin is extremely fragile or silicone adhesives are not available. Options for nonadhesive dressing securement are listed in Table 17-3.

Both open-weave wrap gauze and elastic bandages (e.g., ACE wraps) are commonly used as adhesive alternatives

TABLE 17-3 Adhesive Alternatives for Dressing Securement

Device Description	Examples
Tubular elastic net dressing	Curad Tubular Elastic Retention Netting, Curad Hold Tite Tubular Stretch Bandage (Medline Industries Inc.); Medi-PakPerformance Tubular Elastic Net Dressing Retainer (McKesson Corp.); Surgilast Tubular Elastic Dressing Retainer (DermaSciences, Inc.); Stretch Net Tubular Elastic Bandage (DeRoyal Industries Inc.); Spandage (MEDI-TECH International Corporation)
Elastic tubular bandage	Tubigrip Elasticated Tubular Bandage, Tubifast Dressing Retention Bandage (Molnlycke Health Care); Medigrip Elasticated Tubular Bandage (Medline Industries Inc.)
Self adherent elastic bandages	3M Coban Self-Adherent Wrap (3M Health Care); CoFlex Self-Adherent Wrap (Andover Healthcare Inc.); Medi-Grip Self-Adherent Compression Bandage, Co-Lastic LF, Co-Wrap (Hartmann USA)
Conforming bandages (gauze)	Kling Conforming Bandage (Johnson & Johnson); Curity Stretch Bandage (Covidien); Conform Stretch Bandages (Kendall-Covidien); Duflex Synthetic Conforming Bandage (Derma Sciences Inc.)
Abdominal dressing holders	Medfix Montgomery Straps (Medline Industries Inc.) Montgomery Straps Adhesive Retention Dressing (DeRoyal Industries Inc.)

but are not ideal choices as both have the potential for slippage. In addition, there is variability in the subbandage pressures provided by elastic bandages or "Ace Wraps" related to wrapping technique (Mosti, 2014).

CLINICAL PEARL

Adhesive alternatives are an excellent approach for securing products to very fragile skin (e.g., wrap gauze, elastic net dressings, and commercial securement devices).

Nonadhesive stabilizing devices are available for endotracheal tubes and indwelling urinary catheters. There are also specifically designed feeding tubes with stabilizing bumpers or discs that avoid the need for adhesive securement. Routine use of these products should be encouraged as they typically provide both better securement for these devices and protection against MARSI.

Staff Education and Problem Surveillance

Because adhesive use is common and MARSI is a preventable complication, education on adhesive injury and preventive strategies should be built into orientation and ongoing training (McNichol et al., 2013). All disciplines that apply or remove adhesive products should be educated on securement protocols and prevention techniques.

Written protocols and procedures should be developed to guide technique for and frequency of adhesive product change. Change frequency should be based on the criticality and duration of desired securement and product capabilities rather than habit or convenience. Adding MARSI surveillance to pressure ulcer Prevalence and Incidence surveys can quantify the scope of the problem and target prevention efforts where needed.

Optimizing Adhesive Product Utilization

Acute care facilities commonly stock a wide variety of medical tapes. Unfortunately, all too often the characteristics and indicated uses are not well understood and products are inappropriately used, thus increasing the potential for MARSI (McNichol et al., 2013). A process of *standardization* can be extremely beneficial in reducing the number of adhesive products and clarifying appropriate use of each. The wound nurse should work with key clinical stakeholders and Materials Management to assure that tapes and other adhesive products are matched to the needs of the organization, aligned to protocols, and available where clinically needed. In addition to clinical benefits, this deliberate, collaborative approach can result in reduced waste, improved inventory control, and reduced supply costs (3M, 2014).

Management of MARSI

Adhesive-related skin injury should be managed according to the type of damage. When a contact dermatitis develops, the offending product should be discontinued. In situations where more than one product was used on the skin, (e.g., an antiseptic, a barrier film and an adhesive product), products should be removed and reintroduced systematically. For ACD confirmed by patch testing or when ACD is strongly suspected, the offending topical product should be discontinued. Both irritant and ACD are commonly treated with a limited course of low- to mid-potency topical corticosteroids (McNichol et al., 2013). A Dermatology referral should be considered for failure to respond to this first-line therapy.

Partial-thickness injuries associated with skin stripping and tension blisters should be managed using principles of wound bed preparation (Bryant, 2012; McNichol et al., 2013).

Maceration can be improved by discontinuing adhesive product use and allowing the affected skin to dry. In the event that adhesive securement cannot be discontinued, a more breathable adhesive product should be used.

Antibiotics (topical and/or oral) are used to treat folliculitis complicated by infection (McNichol et al., 2013; Habif, 2010). Other nursing considerations include (1) modification of hair removal technique (eliminate shaving, or modify shaving technique to leave hair longer) (Habif, 2010); (2) skin preparation to assure a clean surface; and (3) selection of a more breathable adhesive product.

The wound nurse may be consulted for MARSI at infusion catheter sites. The need for antiseptic site preparation, site visibility, and strict aseptic technique presents requirements and challenges not ordinarily present in wound and skin care. At the time of this writing, best practice guidelines for management of skin damage at central venous access device sites are being developed by a working group from the World Congress of Vascular Access (WoCoVA).

 Skin Tears

A skin tear is a wound caused by shear, friction, and/or blunt force resulting in separation of skin layers. A skin tear can be partial thickness (separation of the epidermis from the dermis) or full thickness (separation of both the epidermis and dermis from underlying structures) (Leblanc et al., 2011). Despite preliminary studies that suggest skin tears may be more prevalent than pressure ulcers, there remains a paucity of literature to guide prevention, assessment, and treatment of skin tears. Payne and Martin in the early 1990s established a classification system; however, it failed to gain universal acceptance. An international survey by LeBlanc, Baranoski, and Regan in 2011 indicated that health care professionals would like a simplified classification system.

Background

In an effort to increase awareness of this largely unheeded health care issue, a consensus panel of 13 internationally recognized key opinion leaders convened to establish consensus statements on the prevention, prediction, assessment, and treatment of skin tears. The initial ***International Skin Tear Advisory Panel (ISTAP)*** meeting was held in 2011 and resulted in the development and publication of 12 key consensus statements and a broader definition for skin tears that were supported by representatives from 18 different countries (LeBlanc et al., 2011).

This meeting provided the ground work for continued development of education tools to support the consensus statements.

In addition, the ISTAP group developed the ISTAP Skin Tear Classification System, (LeBlanc et al., 2013, 2014). The classification system was developed by consensus, with 100% agreement from the ISTAP group. Test–retest and intrarater reliability was established using the Fleiss k test (Fleiss, 1971). Interrater reliability was tested using the Cohen k test. This test was interpreted as satisfactory or not satisfactory, with the point of discrimination being 0.70 (Cohen, 1968). The external validity of the system was then tested on a sample of 327 individuals. The sample consisted of nurses with the credentials of registered nurse, registered practical nurse/licensed vocational nurse/licensed practical nurse/ certified nursing assistant, and nonnurses from Canada, the United States, Brazil, the United Kingdom, and China. There were only 24 nonnursing subjects in the sample; therefore, they were excluded from further analysis. The data indicated a moderate level of agreement on classification of Skin Tears by type (Fleiss k = 0.545). Interrater reliability based on wound care expertise was established using the Fleiss k statistic. The level of agreement was substantial (Fleiss k = 0.653, Cohen 1968). A moderate level of agreement was demonstrated (Fleiss k = 0.555).

A recent study in Denmark (Skiveren et al., 2014) replicated the ISTAP study (Leblanc et al., 2013). They conducted a two-phase study; Phase 1 included the translation of the classification system into Danish, and Phase 2 sought to replicate the ISTAP study. They reported a moderate level of agreement (Fleiss k = 0.464) in 270 registered nursing staff (non–wound care specialist). These results closely mirrored those found by LeBlanc et al. (2013) and added further support for the validation of the ISTAP skin tear classification system. These results support the integration of this classification system into practice.

Definition and Overview

For the purpose of this discussion, a skin tear is a tear or laceration of the skin caused by shear or friction or by minor blunt force trauma. Skin tears result in a separation of the epidermis from the dermis or of the epidermis and dermis from the underlying connective tissue, with creation of a flap or pedicle of skin. The skin flap may or may not be viable. Skin tears can produce either a partial- or a full-thickness injury. Skin tears are often jagged or irregular in nature and usually occur in high-risk areas, such as the extremities. These wounds may be dry with little or no drainage or may produce moderate amounts of drainage, depending on the location and extent of injury.

ISTAP Classification System

The ISTAP created a new simplified taxonomy for skin tears to better support management and documentation of this frequently ignored wound. The classification system is adapted from previous work done by Payne and Martin (1990, 1993) and Carville (2007). The scheme involves three categories of skin tears:

Type 1

No skin loss—linear or flap tear that *can be* repositioned to cover the wound bed.

Type 2

Partial flap loss—partial flap loss that *cannot* be repositioned to cover the wound bed.

Type 3

Total flap loss—total flap loss exposing the entire wound bed (Fig. 17-17).

CLINICAL PEARL

The ISTAP skin tear classification system is easy to use and provides guidance in management. Type 1 tears have no skin loss; Type 2 tears involve partial flap loss; and Type 3 tears involve full flap loss.

Etiology and Risk Factors

Populations at the highest risk for skin tears include those at extremes of age and the critically or chronically ill. These individuals typically have multiple comorbidities and are at higher risk for development of secondary wound infections (Carville et al., 2007; Payne & Martin, 1993; LeBlanc et al., 2008).

The most common cause of skin tears in the elderly population is from traumatic injury (Leblanc et al., 2011) due to wheelchair injuries, bumping into objects, transfers, falls, and inappropriate removal of dressings. In the neonatal and pediatric population, skin tears are listed as one of the more common wound injuries seen, along with mechanical device injury and occiput pressure ulcers (Irving et al., 2006; Baharestani, 2007). A key component to the prevention of skin tears in this population is to recognize fragile, thin, vulnerable skin and to modify care accordingly (Table 17-4).

According to the ISTAP Consensus report (LeBlanc et al., 2011), intrinsic risk factors, such as age, pertain to an individual's inherent biologic or genetic makeup. Extremes in age impact not only how individuals heal but also their susceptibility to developing a wound (Ovington, 2003). With increasing age, individuals

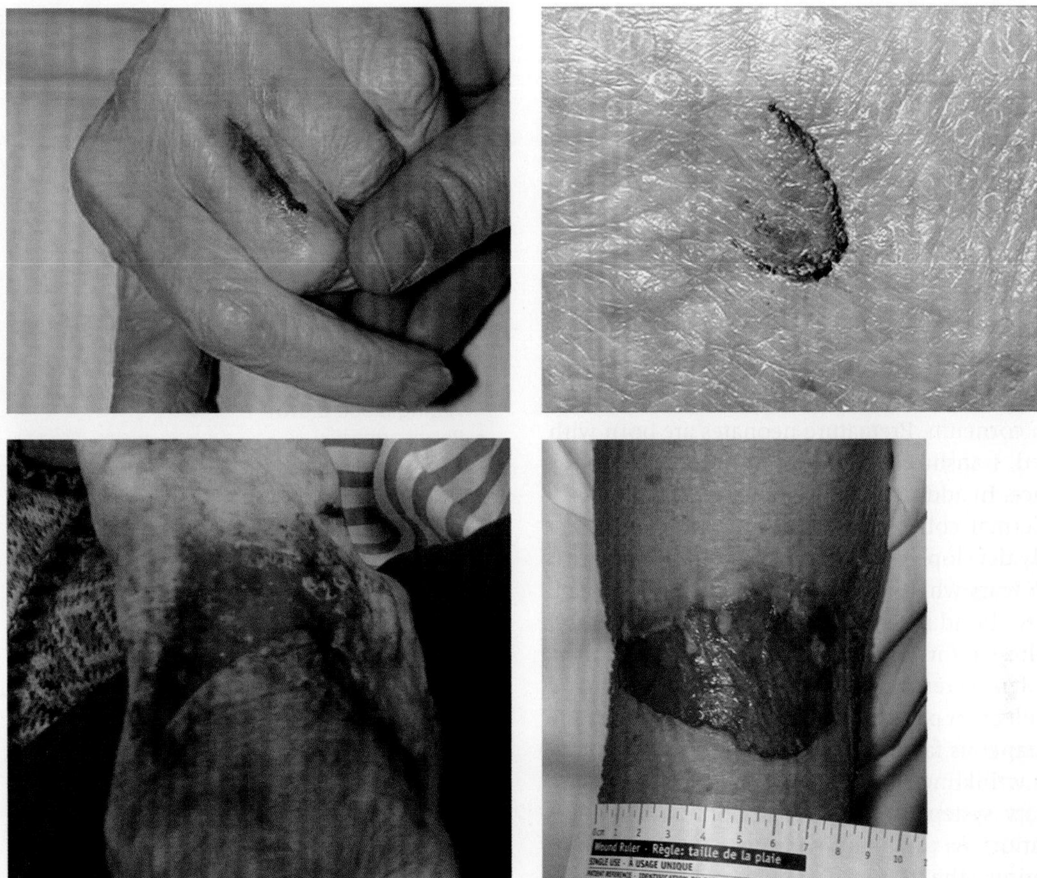

FIGURE 17-17. ISTAP skin tear classification system.

TABLE 17-4 Strategies for Prevention of Skin Tears

- Determine and remove potential causes for trauma. Ensure a safe environment with adequate lighting.
- Remove objects which can be a source of blunt trauma, declutter area, remove scatter rugs and excessive furniture.
- Hydrate skin with moisturizer at least twice a day, especially after bathing, with the skin still damp, not wet.
- Utilize soapless, no-rinse, and pH-balanced skin cleansers, tepid water, and gentle technique for bathing.
- Use appropriate lifting, turning aids, slide sheet, when moving patients; never drag the patient across bed.
- Encourage the patient to wear long sleeves, long trousers or knee high socks; provide shin guards for those who experience repeat skin tears; provide gloves for those in wheelchairs to protect the hands.
- Pad edges of furniture and equipment.
- Finger and toe nails should be kept cut short and filed to remove rough edges to prevent self-inflicted skin tears. (Good idea for health care workers to keep nail short as well).
- Avoid adhesive products on frail skin. If dressings or tapes are required, use paper tapes or soft nonadherent dressings to avoid skin stripping or tearing the skin with the removal of adhesives.
- Label dressings showing removal pulling away from the skin flap.
- Educate staff on the importance of "gentle care."

experience dermal and subcutaneous tissue loss, epidermal thinning, and reduced production of skin lipids, all of which contribute to the thin dry skin commonly seen in the elderly. This thin dry skin is much less resistant to minor stretch and trauma and much more likely to tear. In addition, the loss of subcutaneous tissue reduces protection against shear force and increases skin vulnerability to minor trauma, especially over the face, dorsum of the hands, and shins. In addition, there is progressive loss of the normal cohesion between the skin and soft tissue layers, due to flattening of the rete ridges; this results in diminished "anchoring" of the epidermis to the dermis, which is a significant risk factor for skin tears. Senile purpura is another common finding due to changes in the skin vasculature that cause the vessels to become thinner and more fragile; interestingly, skin tears frequently occur at sites of senile purpura. Finally, the skin's elasticity and tensile strength decrease as a result of sun damage and changes in fibroblast activity; reduced elasticity means the skin is less able to stretch and more likely to tear. The risk of skin tears is further increased by dehydration, poor nutrition, cognitive impairment, altered mobility, and decreased sensation (Baranoski & Ayello, 2014). These factors are common in the elderly in all care settings and combine to increase the skin's vulnerability to trauma.

CLINICAL PEARL

Common risk factors for skin tears include extremes of age (premature infants and the elderly), those who are chronically or critically ill, dependence on others for daily care, and purpuric lesions.

Neonates have underdeveloped skin, and children have only 60% of adult epidermal thickness (Baharestani, 2007; Baharestani & Pope, 2007; Coha et al., 2012). Neonates and infants are also susceptible to skin tears. The premature neonate at 24 weeks' gestation has minimal stratum corneum. Premature neonates are born with red, wrinkled, translucent skin that is almost gelatinous in appearance. In addition, neonates have decreased epidermal-to-dermal cohesion, because the rete ridges are incompletely developed; this places these infants at great risk for skin tears when adhesive products are removed. If the adhesive bond between the tape and skin is greater than the cohesive force between the epidermis and dermis, the epidermis remains attached to the tape and tape removal results in a painful skin tear.

As subcutaneous fat deposits begin to form (weeks 26 to 29), skin wrinkling starts to decrease. Maturity of the integumentary system is complete at approximately 33 weeks' gestation. As the infant continues to develop (40 weeks' gestation), the stratum corneum begins to increase in thickness. Additional characteristics of this fragile population that render them vulnerable include a thin and deficient stratum corneum; reduced subcutaneous tissue, and impaired thermoregulation; body surface/weight ratio nearly five times greater than an adult; and immaturities in the immune system as well as hepatic and renal function. The combination of these factors places this population at increased risk for epidermal stripping, secondary infection, increased TEWL and heat loss, and toxicity from percutaneous absorption (Baharestani, 2007; Noonan et al., 2006).

Extrinsic factors also play an important role in the development of skin tears. Individuals who require assistance for bathing, dressing, toileting, and transferring are at increased risk for mechanical trauma. All individuals who are critically ill, at the end of life, or who suffer from multiple intrinsic and extrinsic risk factors, regardless of age are at higher risk for skin tear development (see Box 17-2).

Often the cause of a skin tear is not known. When the cause is known, skin tears are frequently linked to blunt trauma from accidentally bumping into objects, wheelchair injuries, transfers, or falls (Bank & Nix, 2006; Leblanc et al., 2008). In the 2011 survey conducted by LeBlanc and colleagues, the most common causes of skin tears included blunt trauma, falls, activities of daily living, patient transfers, dressing- and treatment-related tears, and equipment injury (Fig. 17-18).

BOX 17-2. Risk Factors for Skin Tears

- Very young and very old (>75 years of age)
- Gender (female)
- Race (Caucasian)
- Immobility (chair or bed bound)
- Inadequate nutritional intake
- Long-term corticosteroid use
- History of previous skin tears
- Altered sensory status
- Cognitive impairment
- Stiffness and spasticity
- Neuropathy
- Having blood drawn
- Polypharmacy
- Presence of ecchymosis
- Dependence for activities of daily living
- Using assistive devices
- Applying and removing stockings
- Removing tape
- Vascular problems
- Cardiac problems
- Pulmonary problems
- Visual impairment
- Transfers and falls
- Prosthetic devices
- LE skin tears
- Continence/incontinence
- Skin cleansers
- Improper use of skin sealants

Risk Assessment

Just as pressure ulcer risk assessment may reduce the prevalence of pressure ulcers, identifying those individuals at high risk for skin tears and instituting prevention strategies may reduce the risk of skin tears (Krasner 2010; Stephen-Haynes et al., 2011).

While validated risk assessment tools are available to predict pressure ulcers and are well utilized, the same is not true for skin tears. Several tools have been proposed in the literature, but none have been validated and none are in common use. A comprehensive assessment of risk factors for skin tears is recommended for all individuals within the context of their environment but is difficult given the absence of a validated risk assessment tool. The ISTAP Skin Tear Risk Assessment pathway (Fig. 17-19) was developed to identify patients who are potentially at risk; this tool focuses on three main categories of identified risk factors (General Health, Mobility and Skin). At-risk individuals and all those involved in their care should be educated regarding critical preventive measures (Baharestani, 2007; Reddy et al., 2006; Reddy, 2008).

General Health

Chronic disease, critical illness, and extremes of age are associated with changes in the skin and soft tissues that increase the risk of skin tears (LeBlanc et al., 2011). Altered sensory function (including neuropathy) and diminished

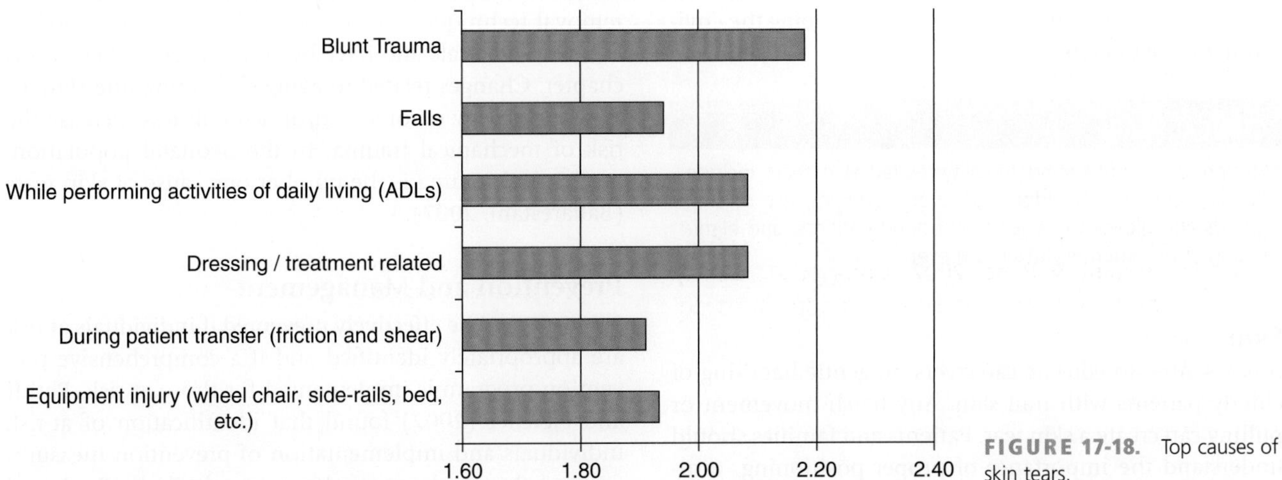

FIGURE 17-18. Top causes of skin tears.

visual and auditory acuity contribute to increased fall risk (Reddy, 2008; Reddy et al., 2006), and a history of falls has been strongly linked in the literature to an increased risk of skin tears (Bank & Nix, 2006; LeBlanc et al., 2011; LeBlanc et al., 2008; Ratliff & Fletcher, 2007).

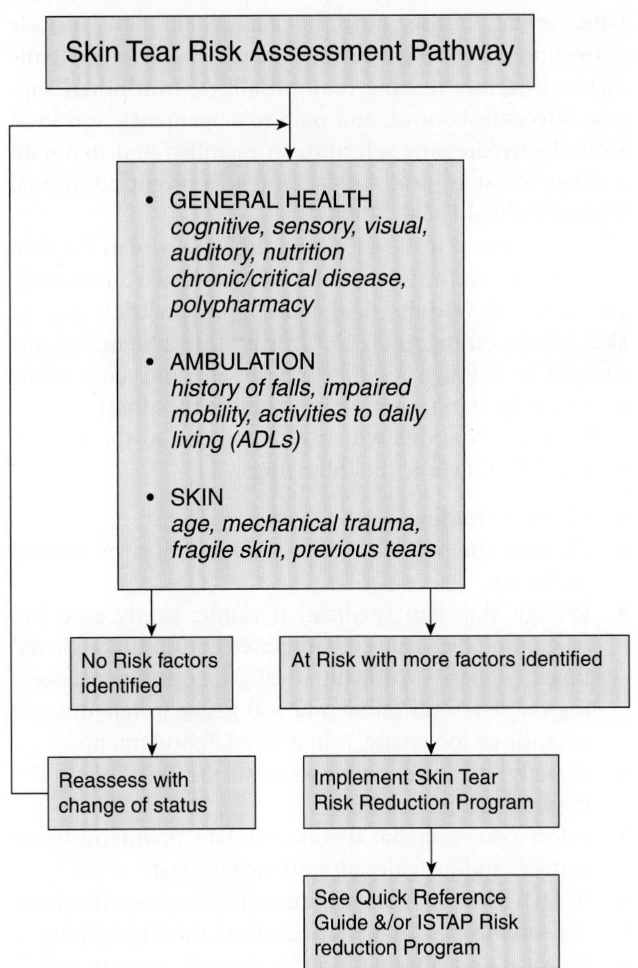

FIGURE 17-19. Skin tear risk assessment pathway.

Polypharmacy (i.e., the use of multiple medications that might predispose patients to drug interactions/reactions or confusion) is common among the elderly; corticosteroids and chemotherapeutic agents are a particular risk factor because they interfere with epidermal regeneration and collagen synthesis (Leblanc et al., 2008; Reddy, 2008).

Polypharmacy has also been found to be an independent risk factor for falls (Hajjar et al., 2007; Pervin, 2008; Smith, 2004). Pervin's (2008) research concluded that individuals receiving four or more medications or any medication associated with cognitive impairment, reduced mobility, hypotension, dizziness, or drowsiness increases risk of falls and resultant skin tears.

Malnutrition and dehydration are associated with thin dry skin that is higher risk for skin tears; adequate nutrition and hydration help maintain tissue viability (Dorner et al., 2009), and nutritionists can be valuable in providing accurate nutritional assessment and interventions.

Ambulation/Mobility

In the elderly population skin tears are often environmentally related (Baranoski & Ayello, 2014; LeBlanc & Baranoski, 2009). In 1990, Payne and Martin conducted a 3-month descriptive study in 10 long-term care facilities to describe skin tears, identify risk factors, and determine the rate of healing of skin tears. In this study, the predominant risk factors included impaired activity and mobility as well as sensory and cognitive impairment. McGough-Csarny and Kopac (1998) conducted a similar study in a veteran's affairs nursing home and found the major risk factors to be dependency for activities of daily living, sensory loss, limited mobility, use of assistive devices, and impaired cognition.

Specific mobility-related issues include blunt trauma to shins, hands, and arms secondary to hitting objects when seated in a wheelchair or when using canes and walkers, and inadvertent skin tears associated with use of transfer devices or other movement aids (LeBlanc et al., 2008).

Strategies for preventing *mobility-related* skin tears include padding areas of concern (corners, edges), using shin guards and gloves if in a wheel chair, and keeping the environment free of clutter.

CLINICAL PEARL

Strategies for preventing mobility-related skin tears include padding corners and edges in the environment, use of shin guards and gloves for wheelchair-bound patients, and eliminating environmental clutter to prevent falls.

Skin

It is essential to educate caregivers on gentle handling of elderly patients with frail skin. Any harsh movement or pulling can create a skin tear. Patients and families should understand the importance of proper positioning, turning, lifting, and transferring. Lift sheets should be used to move patients up in bed, and padding should be added to hard objects, including side rails, wheelchair arm and leg supports, and other equipment. Protective arm sleeves or wraps and trousers/pants or shin guards should be routinely used to protect the extremities (Baranoski & Ayello, 2014; Benbow, 2009; LeBlanc & Baranoski, 2009). In addition, patients and caregivers should keep their fingernails short to prevent mechanical trauma, should use no-rinse, pH-balanced cleansers for bathing, should use gentle technique and caution in assisting the patient to dress, and should moisturize the skin with creams rather than lotions (LeBlanc et al., 2011; LeBlanc et al., 2008; Stephen-Haynes et al., 2011). A study by Carville et al. (2014) found that twice-daily application of a moisturizer to the extremities of residents in an aged (long-term care) facility in Australia reduced the incidence of skin tears almost 50%.

CLINICAL PEARL

Measures for prevention of skin tears related to handling during daily care include protective arm sleeves, short nails for patient and caregivers, routine use of moisturizers, gentle approach when assisting with bathing and mobility, and appropriate tape removal technique.

Falls are a major risk factor for skin tears in the elderly; an average nursing home with 100 beds reports 100 to 200 falls annually (Bank & Nix, 2006; Ratliff & Fletcher, 2007). Implementation of a best practice fall prevention program has proven to be successful in reducing falls (and thus skin tears) in elderly long-term care patients. It should be noted that successful implementation of best practice guidelines requires adequate planning, resources, organization and administrative support, and appropriate facilitation (Brillhart, 2005; McCarthy et al., 2009).

Another source of mechanical trauma leading to skin tears is removal of adhesive tapes and dressings (Carville et al., 2007; LeBlanc et al., 2011; LeBlanc et al., 2008); adhesive alternatives, gentle adhesives, and appropriate removal techniques are critical to skin tear prevention in at-risk individuals and have been discussed earlier in this chapter. Changes related to aging skin, immature skin, or skin affected by chronic and/or acute illness increase the risk of mechanical trauma. In the neonatal population, mechanical trauma is the number one cause of skin tears (Baharestani, 2007).

Prevention and Management

Skin tears can be effectively prevented if individuals at risk are appropriately identified and if a comprehensive prevention program is implemented for those at risk. Ratliff and Fletcher (2007) found that identification of at-risk individuals and implementation of prevention measures reduced the incidence of skin tears; similarly, Bank and Nix (2006) conducted a study demonstrating the ability of a prevention program to reduce the incidence of skin tears.

Skin tears represent a specific type of wound; however, the same principles used to manage other wounds should be employed when treating skin tears. When developing any wound care treatment plan, regardless of the wound type, several factors must be addressed; these include correction of etiologic factors, management of systemic factors affecting healing (comorbidities, nutritional support, glycemic control, and pain management), and local wound care/dressing selection to establish and maintain a clean moist wound surface and to prevent additional trauma (Sibbald et al., 2004).

The first step in developing a treatment plan for skin tears is to assess the wound. Key assessment factors include presence and viability of the skin flap (pedicle), type of skin tear according to ISTAP Classification system, volume of exudate, any signs of infection present, and status of the surrounding skin (maceration, fragility, bleeding).

Recommendations will vary according to the type of skin tear, but include the following:

- Control bleeding.
- Cleanse the wound with normal saline or wound surfactant.
- Realign skin flap (pedicle) if viable; gently ease flap back into place using a dampened cotton tip or gloved finger; if flap is difficult to align, consider moistening the flap with saline and soft gauze to rehydrate; if necrotic or too crusty, it may need debridement.
- Classify, measure, and document the skin tear in the medical record.
- Select a dressing that absorbs exudate, maintains moist surface, and provides atraumatic removal.
- At each dressing change, gently lift and remove the dressing, working the dressing away from the attached flap.
- Monitor and observe for any changes, signs or symptoms of infection, and/or poor healing.

- Consider administration of tetanus immunoglobulin if source of skin tear is unknown, especially if full thickness or contaminated (Carden, 2004).

CLINICAL PEARL

Effective management of skin tears includes gentle cleansing, realignment of any viable flap, and application of a dressing that absorbs drainage, maintains a moist wound surface, and provides for atraumatic removal.

Based on available evidence (which is limited), the recommended dressing options for skin tears include nonadherent dressings such as nonadhesive foam secured with wrap or roller gauze, nonadherent contact layers secured with wrap or roller gauze, impregnated mesh, lipidocolloid mesh, silicone mesh, hydrogel, calcium alginate, hydrofiber, and clear acrylic dressings and those dressings with gentle adhesive properties. Dressings with aggressive adhesives and limited absorptive capacity can be problematic and should be avoided, for example, closure strips, hydrocolloids, and transparent adhesive dressings. The ISTAP committee has just begun its study of appropriate dressings for the care and management of skin tears. More research is needed in this area of practice.

CLINICAL PEARL

Consider drawing an arrow on the dressing to show best direction for removal so as to protect the flap from disruption. Avoid dressings with aggressive adhesion, such as hydrocolloid dressings.

The overall goal of care should be to treat the cause if known; use an appropriate moist wound therapy dressing that will manage exudate and promote a healing environment, assess for infection, and control any discomfort or pain at wound site. In addition, it is critical to assure that an appropriate prevention plan is in place to reduce further incidence and trauma to the area involved.

Conclusion

Moisture-Associated Skin Damage, Medical Adhesive–Related Skin Injury, and Skin Tears comprise three common types of skin damage commonly encountered in clinical practice. While superficial, these "top-down" injuries are by no means trivial. With all of these problems, the epidermis is disrupted, and the body's most fundamental protective barrier against invasion of microbes and irritants is compromised or destroyed. The wound nurse has a responsibility not only for providing expert care for skin injury but also for creating a culture where risk is recognized and best practice interventions are focused on prevention.

CASE STUDIES

CASE STUDY FOR SKIN TEAR MANAGEMENT

Mr. JP was a 75-year-old with a history of cardiac, pulmonary, and renal comorbidities. His skin was easily insulted due to the nature of his illnesses and longstanding medication regimen of Coumadin.

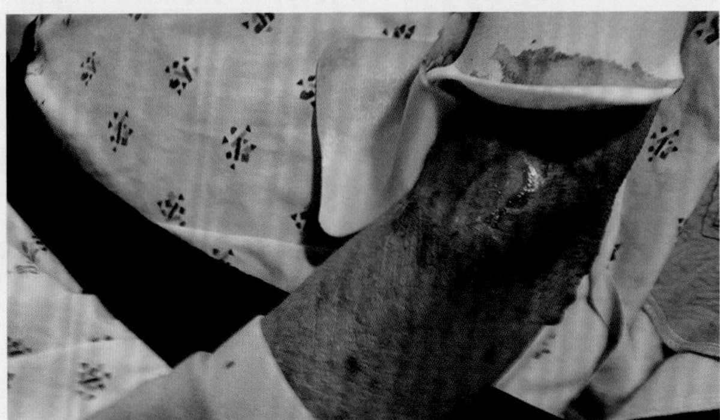

Day 1

The skin tear seen on his left arm is from the staff pulling him onto a stretcher to go to x-ray. He asked the staff to get more help but was told none were available. As JP was pulled to the stretcher, his skin was torn in the area where the health care worker was holding his arm. Wound care was notified.

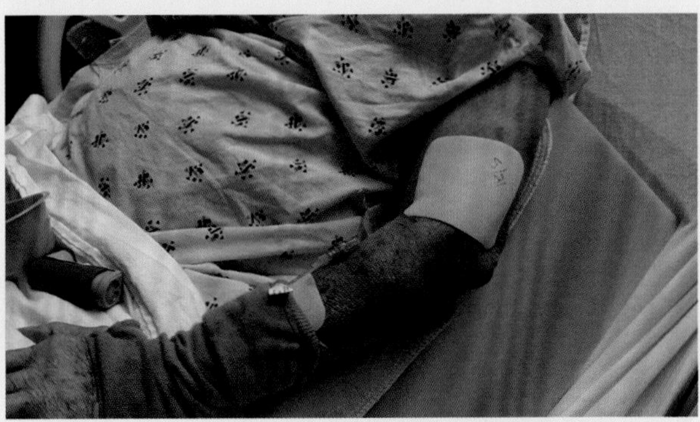

Nonadherent dressing.

Mr. JP's left arm was cleansed with saline, the bleeding was stopped, and the wound was assessed by the CWOCN as being a Type 3 skin tear. No flap or pedicle was present. Orders were received for a nonadherent dressing to be applied and changed every 3 to 4 days.

On Day 2, the wound care nurse stopped in to see how the patient was doing and found the dressings saturated and in need of being changed. She changed the dressings while educating the nurse taking care of Mr. JP. It was also decided to use a protective sleeve to reduce the risk of further injury to the area and help to secure the dressing. The CWOCN followed up 1 week later and found the skin tear much improved and healing.

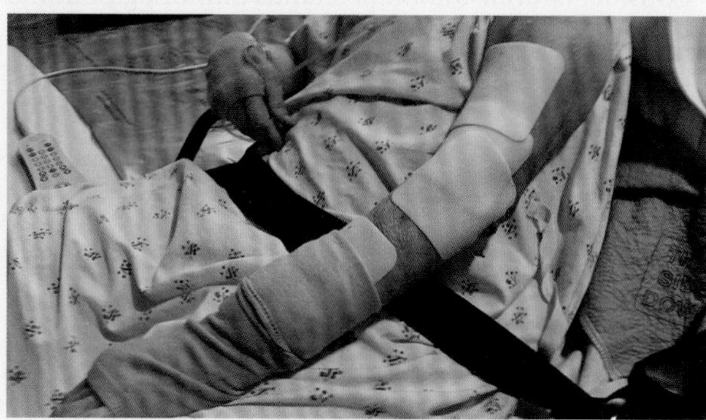

Protective sleeve.

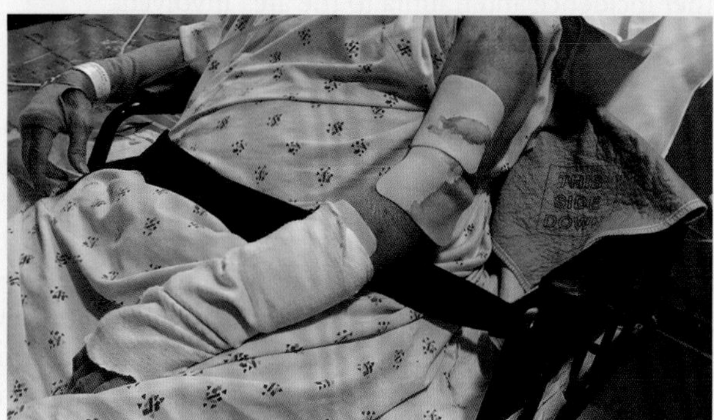

Day 2.

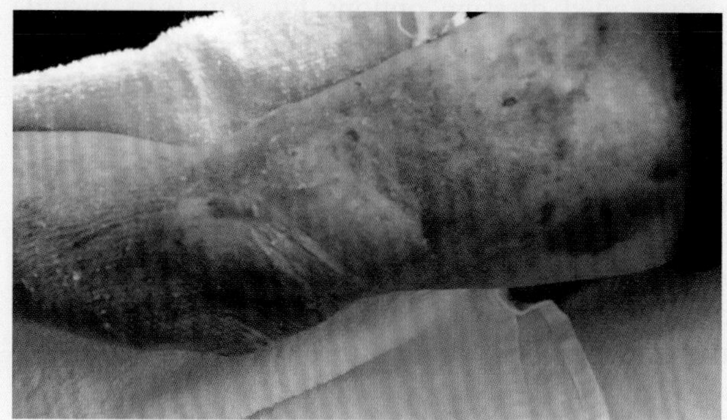

One week later.

REFERENCES

Alikahn, A., & Maibach, H. I. (2009). Biology of the stratum corneum: Tape stripping and protein quantification. In M. A. Firage, H. I. Maibach & K. W. Miller (Eds.), *Textbook of aging skin* (pp. 401–408). New York, NY: Springer-Verlag.

Anderson, P. H., Bucher, A. P., Saeed, I., et al. (1994). Faecal enzymes: In vivo human skin irritation. *Contact Dermatitis, 30*, 152–158.

Baharestani, M. (2007). An overview of neonatal and pediatric wound care knowledge and considerations. *Ostomy Wound Management, 53*(6), 34–55.

Baharestani, M., & Pope, E. (2007). Chronic wounds in neonates and children. In D. Krasner, G. T., Rodeheaver & G. T. Sibbald (Eds.), *Chronic wound care: A clinical source book for healthcare professionals* (pp. 679–693). Malvern, PA: HMP Communications.

Baker, H., & Kligman, A. M. (1967). Measurement of transepidermal water loss by electrical hygrometry. *Archives of Dermatology, 96*, 441–452.

Bank, D., & Nix, D. (2006). Preventing skin tears in a nursing and rehabilitation center: An interdisciplinary effort. *Ostomy Wound Management, 52*(9), 38–46.

Baranoski, S., & Ayello, E. A. A. (2014). Skin an essential organ. In S. Baranoski & E. A. A. Ayello (Eds.), *Wound care essentials: Practice principles* (pp. 60–85). Philadelphia, PA: Lippincott Williams & Wilkins.

Bass, E., Del Pino, A., Tan, A., et al. (1997). Does preoperative stoma marking and education by the enterostomal therapist affect outcome? *Diseases of the Colon and Rectum, 40*, 440–442.

Beeckman, D., Schoonhoven, L., Verhaeghe, S., et al. (2009). Prevention and treatment of incontinence-associated dermatitis: Literature review. *Journal of Advanced Nursing, 65*(6), 1141–1154.

Beeckman, D., Woodward, S., & Gray, M. (2011). Incontinence-associated dermatitis: Step-by-step prevention and treatment. *British Journal of Community Nursing, 16*(8), 382–389.

Belsito, D. V. (2000). The diagnostic evaluation, treatment and prevention of allergic contact dermatitis in the new millennium. *Journal of Allergy and Clinical Immunology, 105*(3), 409–420.

Benbow, M. (2009). Skin tears. *Journal of Community Nursing, 23*(1), 14–18.

Black, J., Gray, M., Bliss, D., et al. (2011). MASD Part 2: Incontinence-associated dermatitis and intertriginous dermatitis. *Journal of Wound, Ostomy, and Continence Nursing, 38*(4), 359–370.

Bliss, D., Savik, K., Harms, S., et al. (2006). Prevalence and correlates of perineal dermatitis in nursing home residents. *Nursing Research, 55*, 243–251.

Breternitz, M. Flach, M. Präßler, J., et al. (2007). Acute barrier disruption by adhesive tapes is influenced by pressure, time and anatomical location: Integrity and cohesion assessed by sequential tape stripping: A randomized controlled study. *British Journal of Dermatology, 156*, 231–240.

Brillhart, B. (2005). Pressure sore and skin tear prevention and treatment during a 10-month program. *Rehabilitation Nursing, 30*(3), 85–91.

Bryant, R. A. (1988). Saving the skin from tape injuries. *American Journal of Nursing, 88*(2), 189–191.

Bryant, R. A. (2012). Types of skin damage and differential diagnosis. In R. A. Bryant & D. P. Nix (Eds.), *Acute and chronic wounds: Current management concepts* (pp. 83–107). St Louis, MO: Mosby Elsevier.

Cameron, J., Hoffman, D., Wilson, J., et al. (2005). Comparison of two peri-wound skin protectants in venous leg ulcers: A randomized controlled trial. *Journal of Wound Care, 14*, 233–236.

Campbell, K., Woodbury, M. G., Whittle, H., et al. (2000). A clinical evaluation of 3M Cavilon No Sting Barrier Film. *Ostomy Wound Management, 46*(1), 24–30.

Carden, D. L. (2004). Tetanus. In J. E. Tindtinalli, G. Kelen, & J. S. Stapczynski (Eds.), *Emergency medicine: A comprehensive study guide* (pp. 34–37). Irving, TX: American College of Emergency Physicians.

Carville, K., Lewin, G., Newall, N., et al. (2007). STAR: A consensus for skin tear classification. *Primary Intention, 15*(1), 8–28.

Carville, K., Osseiran-Moisson, R., Newall, N., et al. (2014). The effectiveness of a twice-daily skin moisturizing regimen for reducing the incidence of skin tears. *International Wound Journal, 11*(4), 446–453.

Coha, T., Wysocki, A. B., Bryant, R. A., et al. (2012). Skin care needs of the pediatric and neonatal patient. In R. A. Bryant & D. P. Nix (Eds.), *Acute and chronic wounds: Current management concepts* (pp. 489). St Louis, MO: Mosby Elsevier.

Cohen, J. (1968). Weighted kappa: Nominal scale agreement with provision for scaled disagreement or partial credit. *Psychological Bulletin, 70*, 213–220.

Colwell, J., Ratliff, C., Goldberg, M., et al. (2011). MASD part 3: Peristomal moisture-associated skin dermatitis and periwound moisture-associated dermatitis. *Journal of Wound, Ostomy, and Continence Nursing, 38*(5), 541–553.

Cosker, T., Elsayed, S., Gupta, S., et al. (2005). Choice of dressing has a major impact on blistering and healing outcomes in orthopedic patients. *Journal of Wound Care, 14*(1), 27–29.

Cutting, K. F. (2006). Silicone and skin adhesives. *Journal of Community Nursing, 20*(11), 36–37.

Cutting, K. F. (2008). Impact of adhesive surgical tape and wound dressing on the skin with reference to skin stripping. *Journal of Wound Care, 17*(4), 157–162.

Cutting, K., & White, R. (2002). Avoidance and management of periwound maceration of the skin. *Journal of Professional Nursing, 18*, 33, 35–36.

Dorner, B. D., Posthauer, M. E., & Thomas, D. (2009). Role of nutrition in pressure ulcer healing clinical practice guideline. In National Pressure Ulcer Advisory Panel and European Pressure Ulcer Advisory Panel. *Prevention and treatment of pressure ulcers: Clinical practice guideline*. Washington, DC: National Pressure Ulcer Advisory Panel.

Doughty, D. (2012). Differential assessment of trunk wounds: Pressure ulceration versus incontinence-associated dermatitis versus intertriginous dermatitis. *Ostomy Wound Management, 58*(4), 20–22.

Doughty, D., Junkin, J., Kurz, P., et al. (2012). Incontinence-associated dermatitis: consensus statements, evidence-based guidelines for prevention and treatment, and current challenges. *Journal of Wound Ostomy Continence Nursing, 39*(3), 303–317.

Dykes, P. (2007). The effect of adhesive dressing edges on cutaneous irritancy and skin barrier function. *Journal of Wound Care, 16*(3), 97–100.

Dykes, P. J., Heggie, R., & Hill, S. A. (2001). Effects of adhesive dressings on the stratum corneum of the skin. *Journal of Wound Care, 10*(2), 7–9.

European Pressure Ulcer Advisory Panel (EPUAP) and National Pressure Ulcer Advisory Panel (NPUAP). (2009). *Pressure Ulcer Prevention and Treatment: Clinical Practice Guideline*. Washington, DC: NPUAP.

Fiers, S., & Thayer, D. (2000). Management of intractable incontinence. In D. Doughty (Ed.), *Urinary and fecal incontinence: Nursing management* (pp. 183–207). St Louis, MO: Mosby.

Fleiss J. L. (1971). Measuring nominal scale agreement among many raters. *Psychological Bulletin, 76*, 378–382.

Gray, M. (2004). Preventing and managing perineal dermatitis: A shared goal for wound and continence care. *Journal of Wound Ostomy & Continence Nursing, 31*(suppl 1), S2–S9.

Gray, M., & Weir, D. (2007). Prevention and treatment of moisture-associated skin damage (maceration) in the periwound skin. *Journal of Wound Ostomy & Continence Nursing, 34*, 153–157.

Gray, M., Bliss, D., Doughty, D., et al. (2007). Incontinence-associated dermatitis: A consensus. *Journal Wound Ostomy & Continence Nursing, 34*, 45–54.

Gray, M., Black, J., Baharestani, M., et al. (2011). Moisture-associated skin damage: Overview and pathophysiology. *Journal Wound Ostomy & Continence Nursing, 38*(3), 233–241.

Gray, M., Beeckman, D., Bliss, D., et al. (2012). Incontinence-associated dermatitis: A comprehensive review and update. *Journal of Wound Ostomy & Continence Nursing, 39*(1), 61–74.

Grove, G. L., Zerveck, C., Houser, T., et al. (2013). A randomized and controlled comparison of gentleness of 2 medical adhesive tapes in healthy human subjects. *Journal Wound Ostomy & Continence Nursing, 40*(1), 51–59.

Habif, T. S. (2010). *Clinical dermatology: A color guide to diagnosis and therapy*. New York, NY: Mosby Elsevier.

Hajjar, E. R., Cafiero, A. C., & Hanlon, J. T. (2007). Polypharmacy in elderly patients. *The American Journal of Geriatric Pharmacotherapy, 5*(4), 345–351.

Hess, C. (2005). *Preparing and managing the skin and the wound bed. Wound care* (pp. 94–117). Philadelphia, PA: Lippincott Williams & Wilkins.

Hoffman, H., & Maibach, H. (1976). Transepidermal water loss in adhesive tape induced dermatitis. *Contact Dermatitis, 2*, 171–177.

Hoggarth, A., Waring, M., Alexander, J., et al. (2005). A controlled, three part, trial to investigate the barrier function and skin hydration properties of six skin protectants. *Ostomy Wound Management, 51*(12), 30–42.

Infusion Nursing Society. (2006). Infusion nursing standards of practice. *Journal of Infusion Nursing, 29*(1 suppl), S1–S92.

Irving, V., Bethell, E., & Burtin, F. (2006). Neonatal wound care: Minimizing trauma and pain. *Wounds UK, 2*(1), 33–41.

Jackson, A. P. (1988). The peeling of pressure-sensitive adhesives at different angles. *Journal of Materials Science Letters, 7*, 1368–1370.

Janniger, C., Schwartz, R., Szepietowski, J., et al. (2005). Intertrigo and common secondary skin infections. *American Family Physician, 72*(5), 833–838.

Jester, R., Russell, L., Fell, S., et al. (2000). A one hospital study of the effect of wound dressings and other related factors on skin blistering following total hip and knee arthoplasty. *Journal of Orthopaedic Nursing, 4*, 71–77.

Junkin, J., & Selekof, J. (2007). Prevalence of incontinence and associated skin injury in the acute care inpatient. *Journal Wound Ostomy & Continence Nursing, 34*, 260–269.

Klode, J., Schöttler, L., Stoffels, I., et al. (2010). Investigation of adhesion of modern wound dressings: A comparative analysis of 56 different wound dressings. *Journal of European Academy of Dermatology and Venereology, 25*, 933–939.

Konya, C., Sanada, H., Sugama, J., et al. (2010). Skin injuries caused by medical adhesive tape in older people and associated factors. *Journal of Clinical Nursing, 19*, 1236–1242.

Korber, A., Holze, K., Grabbe, S., et al. (2007). Protection of wound edges with 3M cavilon no sting barrier film during vacuum-assisted closure therapy: Results of a clinical investigation in patients with chronic leg ulcers. *Zeitshrift for Wundheilung, 12*(1), 6–11.

Koval, K.J., Egol, K. A., Polatsch, D. B., et al. (2003).Tape blisters following hip surgery: A prospective, randomized study of two types of tape. *Journal of Bone and Joint Surgery (American), 85-A*(10), 1884–1887.

Krasner, D. (2010, April). Skin tears: Understanding the problem leads to prevention, and proper care. *Long Term Living Magazine*, 30–32.

Langemo, D., Hanson, D., Hunter, S., et al. (2011). Incontinence and incontinence-associated dermatitis. *Advances in Skin & Wound Care, 24*(3), 126–140.

Lavelle, B. (2004). Reducing the risk of skin trauma related to medical adhesives. *Managing Infection Control, 182*, 1289–1294.

LeBlanc, K., & Baranoski, S. (2009). Prevention and management of skin tears. *Advances in Skin & Wound Care, 22*(7), 325–334.

LeBlanc, K., Christensen, D., Orstead, H., et al. (2008). Best practice recommendations for the prevention and treatment of skin tears. *Wound Care Canada, 6*(8), 14–32.

LeBlanc, K., Baranoski, S., & Regan, M. (2011). International 2010 Skin Tear Survey (unpublished data).

LeBlanc, K., & Baranoski, S.; Skin Tear Consensus Panel Members. (2011). Skin tears: State of the science: Consensus statements for the prevention, prediction, assessment, and treatment of skin tears. *Advances in Skin & Wound Care, 24*(9S), 2–15.

LeBlanc, K., Baranoski, S., Christensen, D., et al. (2013). International Skin Tear Advisory Panel: A tool kit to aid in the prevention, assessment, and treatment of skin tears using a simplified classification system. *Advances in Skin & Wound Care, 26(10)*, 459–476.

LeBlanc, K., Baranoski, S., Holloway, S., et al. (2014). A descriptive cross-sectional study to explore current practices in the assessment, prevention, and treatment of skin tears. *International Wound Journal 11*(4), 424–430.

Lucast, D. (2000, October). Skin tight: Adhesive considerations for developing stick-to-skin products. *Adhesives Age*, 36–39.

Lund, C. H., & Tucker, J. A. (2003). Adhesion and newborn skin. In S. Hoath, & H. I. Maibach (Eds.), *Neonatal skin: Structure and function* (pp. 299–324). New York, NY: Marcel Dekker, Inc.

Lyon, C. C., Smith, A. J., Griffiths, C. E. M., et al. (2000). The spectrum of skin disorders in abdominal stoma patients. *British Journal of Dermatology, 143*, 1248–1260.

Maene, B. (2013). Hidden cost of medical tape-induced injuries. *Wounds UK, 9*, 46–50.

Mahoney, M., Rozenboom, B., Smith, H., et al. (2011). Issues related to accurate classification of buttock wounds. *Journal Wound Ostomy & Continence Nursing, 38*(6), 635–642.

Mahoney, M., Rozenboom, B., & Doughty, D. (2013). Challenges in classification of gluteal cleft and buttock wounds. *Journal Wound Ostomy & Continence Nursing, 40*(3), 239–245.

Marzulli, F. N., & Maibach, H. I. (2008). Allergic contact dermatitis. In H. Zhai, K.-P Wilhelm, & H. I. Maibach (Eds.), *Marzulli and Maibach's dermatotoxicology* (pp. 155–157). Boca Raton, FL: CRC Press.

McCarthy, R., Adedokum, C., & Moody F. (2009). Preventing falls in the long term care facilities. Retrieved July 29, 2014, from http://rnjournal.com/journal-of-nursing/preventing-falls-in-the-elderly-long-term-care-facilities .

McGough-Csarny, J., & Kopac, C. A. (1998). Skin tears in institutionalized elderly: An epidemiological study. *Ostomy/Wound Management, 44*, 14S–25S.

McLane, K., Bookout, K., McCord, S., et al. (2004). The 2003 national pediatric pressure ulcer and skin breakdown prevalence survey: Multisite study. *Journal of Wound Ostomy & Continence Nursing, 31*(4), 168–178.

McNichol, L., Lund, C., Rosen, T., et al. (2013). Medical adhesives and patient safety: State of the science: Consensus statements for the assessment, prevention, and treatment of adhesive-related skin injuries. *Journal Wound Ostomy & Continence Nursing, 40*(4), 365–380.

Mosti, G. (2014). Compression in leg ulcer treatment: Inelastic compression. *Phlebology, 29*, 146–151.

National Institute for Occupational Safety and Health. (2010). *Skin exposure and effects*. Retrieved August 26, 2010, from http://www.cdc.gov/niosh/topics/skin/.

National Pressure Ulcer Advisory Panel. (2001). National pressure ulcer advisory panel support surface standards initiative. http:www.npuap.org/NPUAP_S31_TD.pdf.

Noonan, C., Quigley, S. & Curley, M. A. Q. (2006). Skin integrity in hospitalized infants and children a prevalence survey. *Journal of Pediatric Nursing, 21*(6), 445–453.

Omura, Y., Yamabe, M., & Anazawa, S. (2010). Peristomal skin disorders in patients with intestinal and urinary ostomies: Influence of adhesive forces of various hydrocolloid wafer skin barriers. *Journal of Wound Ostomy & Continence Nursing, 37*, 289–298.

Ovington L. (2003). Bacterial toxins and wound healing. *Ostomy Wound Management, 49*(7A), 8–12.

Payne, R. L., & Martin, M. C. (1990). The Epidemiology and management of skin tears in older adults. *Ostomy Wound Management, 26*(1), 26–37.

Payne, R. L., & Martin, M. C. (1993). Defining and classifying skin tears: Need for a common language. *Ostomy Wound Management, 39*(5), 16–26.

Persson, E., Berndtsson, I., Carlsson, E., et al. (2010). Stoma-related complications and stoma size a two year follow up. *Colorectal Diseases, 12*, 971–976.

Pervin, L. (2008). *Polypharmacy and aging: Is there cause for concern? Gerontology Update: AJN Network.* Retrieved July 19, 2014, form www.rehabnurse.org/pdf/GeriatricsPolypharmacy.pdf

Pinkus, H. (1952). Examination of the epidermis by the strip method. II. Biometric data on regeneration of the human epidermis. *Journal of Investigative Dermatology, 19*, 431–446.

Polatsch, D. B., Baskies, M. A., Hommen, J. P., et al. (2004). Tape blisters that develop after hip fracture surgery: A retrospective series and a review of the literature. *American Journal of Orthopedics (Belle Mead, N.J.), 33*(9), 452–456.

Ratliff, C. (2010). Early peristomal skin complications reported by WOC nurses. *Journal Wound Ostomy & Continence Nursing, 37*(5), 505–510.

Ratliff, C. R., & Fletcher, K. R. (2007). Skin Tears: A review of the evidence to support prevention and treatment. *Ostomy Wound Management, 53*(3), 32–42.

Reddy, M. (2008). Skin and wound care: Important considerations in the older adult. *Advances Skin Wound Care, 21*(9), 424–436.

Reddy, M., Gill S. S., & Rochon, P. A. (2006). Prevention of pressure ulcers: A systematic review. *JAMA, 296*(8), 974–984.

Rietschel, R., & Fowler, J. F. (2008). *Fisher's contact dermatitis*. Hamilton, ON: B.C. Decker.

Rolstad, B., Borchert, K., Magnan, S., et al. (1994). A comparison of an alcohol-based and a siloxane-based peri-wound skin protectant. *Journal of Wound Care, 3*(8), 367–368.

Samann, S. (1999). Skin care for intensive care patients. *KrankenPflege Journal, 37*, 328–330.

Sanders, C., Young, A., McAndrews, H. F., et al. (2007). A prospective randomized trial on the effect of a soluble adhesive on the ease of dressing removal following hypospadias repair. *Journal of Pediatric Urology, 3*(3), 209–213.

Schmid, M. H., & Kortig, H. C. (1995). The concept of the acid mantle of the skin: Its relevance for the choice of skin cleansers. *Dermatology, 191*, 276–280.

Sellæg, M. S., Romild, U., & Kuhry, E. (2012). Prevention of tape blisters after hip replacement surgery: A randomized clinical trial. *International Journal of Orthopaedic and Trauma Nursing, 16*(1), 39–46.

Senior, N. (1973). Some observations on the formulation and properties of Chlorhexidine. *Journal Society of Cosmetic Chemists, 24*, 259–278.

Shah, J. H., Zhai, H., & Maibach, H. I. (2005). Comparative evaporimetry in man. *Skin Research and Technology, 11*, 205–208.

Shelanski, M. V., Phillips, S. B., & Potts, C. E. (1996). Evaluation of cutaneous reactivity to recently marketed dermatologic products. *International Journal of Dermatology, 35*(2), 137–140.

Sibbald, R. G., Orstead, H. L, Coutts, P., et al. (2004). Best practice recommendations for preparing the wound bed: Update. *Wound Care Canada, 4*(1), 15–29.

Sibbald, G., Krasner, D., & Woo, K. (2011). Pressure ulcer staging revisited: Superficial skin changes and deep pressure ulcer framework. *Advances in Skin & Wound Care 24*(12), 571–580.

Sivamani, R. K., Goodman, J., Gitis, N. V., et al. (2003). Friction coefficient of skin in real-time. *Skin Research and Technology, 9*(3), 235–239.

Skiveren, J., Bermark, S., LeBlanc, K., et al. (2014). *Danish translation and validation of the International Skin Tear Advisory Panel's Skin Tear Classification System.* Poster presentation, Canadian Association of Wound Care Annual Conference, Toronto, Canada.

Smith, M. (2004). Medication & the risk of falls in the older person. On behalf of WAM falls in elderly steering group produced by *B.Pharm MRPharmS*. Retrieved July 12, 2014, from www.rehab-nurse.org/pdf/GeriatricsPolypharmacy.pdf

Sopher, R., & Gefen, A. (2011). Effects of skin wrinkles, age and wetness on mechanical loads in the stratum corneum as related to skin lesions. *Medical and Biological Engineering and Computing, 49*(1), 97–105.

Stephen-Haynes, J., Callaghan, R., Bethell, E., et al. (2011). The assessment and management of skin tears in care homes. *British Journal of Nursing, 20*(11), S12–S22.

Tanner J., Woodings, D., & Moncaster K. (2006). Perioperative hair removal to reduce surgical site infection. *Cochrane Database Systematic Reviews*, (3), CD004122.

Thayer, D. (2012). Skin damage associated with intravenous therapy: Common problems and strategies for prevention. *Journal of Infusion Nursing, 36*(6), 390–401.

Tokomura, F., Ohyama, K., Fujisawa, H., et al. (1999). Time-dependent changes in dermal peeling force of adhesive tape. *Skin Research and Technology, 5*, 33–36.

Tokumura, F. et al. (2005). Skin irritation due to repetitive application of adhesive tape: The influence of adhesive strength and seasonal variability. *Skin Research and Technology, 11*, 102–106.

Tornier, C., Rosdy, M. & Maibach, H. I. (2008). *In vitro* skin irritation testing on SkinEthic™-Reconstituted Human Epidermis: Reproducibility for fifty chemicals tested with two protocols. In H. Zhai, K.-P. Wilhelm, & H. I. Maibach (Eds.), *Marzulli and Maibach's dermatotoxicology* (pp. 927–944). Boca Raton, FL: CRC Press.

Voegeli, D. (2012). Moisture-associated skin damage: Aetiology, prevention and treatment. *British Journal of Nursing, 21*(9), 517–521.

Voegeli, D. (2013). Moisture-Associated Skin Damage: An overview for community nurses. *British Journal of Community Nursing, 18*(1), 6, 8, 10–12.

Waring, M., Bielfeldt, S., Matzold, K., et al. (2011). An evaluation of the skin stripping of wound dressing adhesives. *Journal of Wound Care, 20*(9), 412–422.

Widmer, J., Elsner, P., & Burg, G. (1994). Skin irritant reactivity following experimental cumulative irritant contact dermatitis. *Contact Dermatitis, 199*(30), 33–39.

Wound Ostomy Continence Nursing Society. (2011). Incontinence Associated Dermatitis (IAD): Best Practice for Clinicians. Mt. Laurel, NJ: WOCN.

Zhai, H., & Maibach, H. I. (2001). Skin occlusion and irritant and allergic contact dermatitis: An overview. *Contact Dermatitis, 44*, 201–206.

Zhai, H., Dika, E., Goldovsky, M., et al. (2007). Tape-stripping method in man: Comparison of evaporimetric methods. *Skin Research and Technology, 13*, 207–210.

Zulkowski, K., (2012). Diagnosing and treating moisture-associated skin damage. *Advances in Skin & Wound Care, 25*(5), 231–236.

3M. (2014). Supply Standardization: The clinical and economic benefits of reducing waste in the supply chain. St Paul, MN: 3M.

QUESTIONS

1. A wound care nurse is assessing the wound of a patient and documents the wound as a "top-down" wound. This term refers to:
   A. A wound that begins within soft tissue and works its way downward
   B. A wound that begins at the skin's surface
   C. A wound that is caused by ischemia
   D. A wound that begins at the soft tissue–bone interface

2. A wound care nurse is performing skin assessments on patients in a long-term care facility. What type of skin injury might occur when caregivers use vigorous rubbing when cleansing the perineal area?
   A. Friction
   B. Shearing force
   C. Maceration
   D. Ulceration

3. The wound care nurse is preparing a teaching plan for prevention and treatment of incontinence-associated dermatitis (IAD) in long-term care facilities. What teaching point should the nurse include?
   A. Cleanse the skin vigorously using a soft cloth.
   B. Avoid using moisturizers on skin that is exposed to urine or stool.
   C. Use soap and water to cleanse the perineal area instead of no rinse cleansers.
   D. Use moisture barriers to protect the skin from moisture and chemical irritants.

4. A wound care nurse is preparing a treatment plan for a patient with MASD and denuded skin. Which intervention is recommended for this patient?
   A. Using an ointment containing glycerin and petroleum jelly on denuded skin
   B. Leaving the area open to air
   C. Using a zinc oxide–based agent on the denuded skin
   D. Applying liquid acrylate followed by pectin powder to the denuded skin

5. A wound care nurse is caring for a patient with periwound moisture-associated skin damage (MASD). Which intervention would be appropriate for this patient?
   A. Maintain a moist wound bed while keeping periwound skin dry.
   B. Reinforce saturated dressings rather than changing them.
   C. Use a pouching system for wounds with <200 mL of exudate.
   D. Use zinc-based products as opposed to no-sting barrier film on wound.

6. Which adhesive product would be the best choice to secure an endotracheal tube?
   A. Silicone adhesive tape
   B. Multipurpose tape with a gentle acrylate adhesive
   C. Traditional cloth tape coated with zinc oxide–containing adhesives
   D. Stretchable adhesive product

7. The wound care nurse documents a type 2 skin tear in a patient being treated for a pressure ulcer wound. What skin characteristics denote this category of skin tear?
   A. No skin loss; flap tear that can be repositioned to cover the wound bed
   B. Partial flap loss that cannot be repositioned to cover the wound bed
   C. Partial flap loss that can be repositioned to cover the wound bed
   D. Total flap loss exposing entire wound bed

8. Which anatomical skin difference related to aging predisposes the elderly to skin tears?
   A. Thickening of the epidermis
   B. Increased production of skin lipids
   C. Loss of subcutaneous tissue
   D. Increased "anchoring" of the epidermis to the dermis

9. The wound care nurse is managing an elderly patient who has a skin tear. Which of the following is a recommended guideline?
   A. Do not remove the skin flap even if it is necrotic.
   B. Cleanse the wound with hydrogen peroxide.
   C. Administer antibiotics prophylactically.
   D. Select a dressing that absorbs exudate.

10. What type of dressing is recommended for type 2 and type 3 skin tears?
   A. Nonadhesive foam dressings secured with wrap gauze
   B. Hydrocolloid dressings
   C. Transparent adhesive dressings
   D. Dressings should not be used for skin tears

ANSWERS: 1.**B**, 2.**A**, 3.**D**, 4.**C**, 5.**A**, 6.**C**, 7.**B**, 8.**C**, 9.**D**, 10.**A**

CHAPTER 18

Bottom-Up (Pressure Shear) Injuries

Joyce K. Stechmiller, Linda J. Cowan, and C. W. J. Oomens

OBJECTIVES

1. Explain the role of each of the following in pressure ulcer development:
   - Prolonged or intense pressure
   - Shear force
   - Compromised tissue tolerance
2. Discuss current theories of pressure ulcer pathogenesis, to include each of the following:
   - Vessel compression and tissue ischemia
   - Lymphatic vessel compression and edema
   - Reperfusion injury
   - Direct damage to cytoskeleton of muscle cell
3. Develop an evidence-based agency-wide program for pressure ulcer prevention that includes risk assessment and prompt initiation of prevention measures for any patient found to be at risk.
4. Correctly stage/categorize a pressure ulcer using the currently accepted classification system.
5. Identify limitations of the current classification system and implications for practice.
6. Describe the etiology and pathology of sDTI lesions, and address implications for documentation and management.

Topic Outline

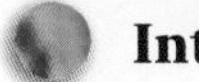

Introduction

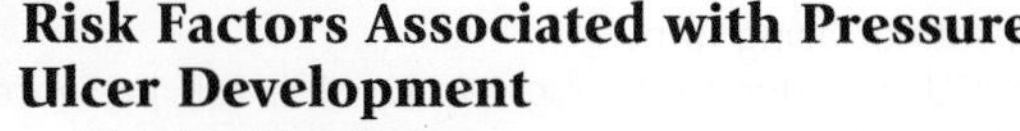

Risk Factors Associated with Pressure Ulcer Development

- Major Risk Factors
- Risk Assessment Tools
  - Braden Scale
  - Data Regarding Use of Risk Assessment Tools
  - Current Recommendations

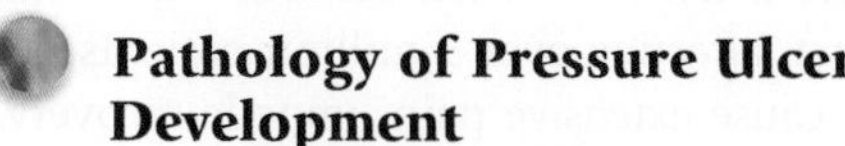

Pathology of Pressure Ulcer Development

- Top-Down versus Bottom-Up Tissue Damage
- Pressure Intensity and Pressure Duration
- Pathology of Pressure/Shear Damage
  - Vessel Compression Resulting in Tissue Ischemia
  - Lymph Vessel Occlusion and Edema Formation
  - Reperfusion Injury
  - Direct Damage to Cytoskeleton of Muscle Cell
- Pathology of Heel Ulcers/sDTIs

Staging of Pressure Ulcers

- Stage I versus sDTI
- sDTI versus Stage II Ulcer
- Challenges in Staging

sDTI (suspected Deep Tissue Injury)

- sDTI in Critical Care Patients
- sDTI in Long-Term Care Patients
- Risk Factors for sDTI
- sDTI Outcomes
- Early Detection and Assessment of sDTI

Management of sDTI

Perioperative Pressure Ulcers

Medical Device–Related Pressure Ulcers

Avoidable versus Unavoidable Pressure Ulcers

- Unavoidable Pressure Ulcer

Conclusion

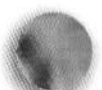

Introduction

This chapter provides an overview of pressure ulcers, to include risk factors, pathology, clinical presentation, and pressure ulcer staging, with a focus on the characteristics of bottom-up injury versus superficial skin breakdown. We will also provide an in-depth discussion of the epidemiology, risk factors, etiology, pathology, clinical presentation, and prevention of suspected deep tissue injury (sDTI). A discussion of avoidable versus unavoidable pressure ulcers is included, based on results of the NPUAP consensus conference held in February, 2014. Finally, the chapter introduces current recommendations for the assessment, staging, and prevention of medical device–related pressure ulcers (to include mucosal pressure ulcers).

Pressure ulcers (PUs) are a significant health care burden in the United States, accounting for over $10 billion in annual health care costs (NPUAP/EPUAP/PPPIA, 2014; Sen et al., 2009; Smith et al., 2013). In addition to the fiscal impact, pressure ulcers have a tremendous emotional and medical impact, affecting over 3 million patients per year. Indeed, PUs cause extensive pain, impede recovery, prolong hospitalization, and substantially increase the risk of sepsis and overall patient mortality (Sullivan, 2013).

CLINICAL PEARL

Pressure ulcers are a very costly and usually preventable complication associated with extensive pain, prolonged hospitalization, and significant increase in risk for sepsis and death.

Pressure ulcers have been defined by the National Pressure Ulcer Advisory Panel (NPUAP), in conjunction with the European Pressure Ulcer Advisory Panel (EPUAP), as follows: localized injury to the skin and/or underlying tissue, usually over a bony prominence, as a result of pressure, or pressure in combination with shear (NPUAP/EPUAP/PPPIA, 2014). The NPUAP revised the definition of a pressure ulcer and the stages of pressure ulcers in 2007, including the original four stages and adding two additional stages, sDTI and unstageable pressure ulcers. This work was the culmination of over 5 years of work that began with the identification of sDTI in 2001. Factors prompting the revision in definitions and the staging system included increasing awareness that the severity of injury at the time of initial presentation of a pressure ulcer had worsened; this was the stimulus for the addition of the new stage labeled "suspected deep tissue injury" (sDTI). These sDTI lesions are thought to occur as a result of bony compression and distortion of the deep tissues; this distortion produces severe ischemia and a highly painful compression injury that is difficult to treat (Coleman et al., 2014). In response to the increasing incidence of sDTI injuries and the lack of evidence regarding pathology, prevention, and management, the NPUAP has now established hospital-acquired (HA) sDTI as a national research priority (NPUAP/EPUAP/PPPIA, 2014). The critical need for research in this area was underscored by discussion at an NPUAP consensus conference in February 2013; the goal was to establish consensus regarding risk factors and measures for prevention of sDTI, but the group failed to reach consensus due to the lack of research and the complexities surrounding this condition (Coleman et al., 2014).

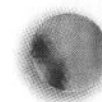

Risk Factors Associated with Pressure Ulcer Development

The purpose of risk assessment for the development of pressure ulcers is to provide early detection of at-risk individuals, followed by prompt implementation of prevention strategies (Stechmiller et al., 2008). Potential risk factors associated with PU development have been documented since at least the 1500s, when Fabricius Hildanus described his theories on the role of "internal supernatural" and "external natural" factors in the diminished tissue perfusion resulting in pressure ulcer or "bedsore" development. Mechanical pressure and incontinence were identified as key factors associated with PUs by French surgeon de la Motte in 1722 (Defloor, 1999). By 1996, the medical literature had described at least 200 risk factors associated with PU development (Byrne & Salzberg, 1996). Lyder reduced the list of significant PU risk factors in early 2000 to 100 (Lyder, 2003), and guidelines published by the Wound, Ostomy, and Continence Nurses Society in 2010 (WOCN, 2010), also identified more than 100 risk factors. The most significant of these risk factors are listed in Box 18-1.

BOX 18-1. Common Risk Factors for Pressure Ulcer Development

- General medical conditions, such as diabetes, stroke, multiple sclerosis, cognitive impairment, cardiopulmonary disease, cancer, hemodynamic instability, peripheral vascular disease, malnutrition, and dehydration
- Smoking
- History of a previous pressure ulcer (since scar tissue is weaker than the skin it replaced and will break down more rapidly than intact skin)
- Increased facility length of stay
- Prolonged surgical procedures (i.e., >3 hours)
- Significant weight loss
- Prolonged time on a stretcher, such as in the emergency room
- Medications, such as sedatives and analgesics
- Refusal of care, such as when a patient refuses to be turned or moved despite education
- Edema
- Obesity
- Patient not being turned
- An ICU stay, due to the high acuity of illness, presence of multiple comorbid conditions, and:
  - Mechanical ventilation
  - Vasopressors and hemodynamic instability
  - Multiple surgeries
  - Increased length of stay
  - Inability to report discomfort

CLINICAL PEARL

The purpose of risk assessment is to provide early detection of the at-risk individual, followed by prompt implementation of aggressive preventive measures.

Major Risk Factors

Advanced age is a significant risk factor; individuals >65 years of age are at high risk and those over age 75 are at even greater risk. Patients with a fractured hip are another high-risk group, especially for heel pressure ulcers. Individuals who have sustained spinal cord injuries are also at high risk; factors increasing risk in this group include spasticity, higher and more complete lesions resulting in greater sensorimotor impairment, younger age at time of injury, difficulty in managing preventive care, and reduced access to equipment and care (see Chapter 15 for an in-depth discussion of pressure ulcer prevention and management in the spinal cord–injured population.) Any individual with significant mobility impairment is at risk, specifically those who are wheelchair bound or bedbound and those for whom turning and repositioning requires significant or taxing effort (such as those who are morbidly obese). Excess exposure to moisture, due to either diaphoresis or incontinence, is another known risk factor for pressure ulcer development.

CLINICAL PEARL

Major risk factors include advanced age, fractured hip, spinal cord injury, significant mobility impairment, and exposure to excessive moisture.

Fogerty and colleagues (2008) identified risk factors associated with PU development in a large acute care sample, using the National Inpatient Sample (NIS) database. There were 94,758 incident pressure ulcers documented among a final discharge sample of 6,610,787 persons; discharge ICD-9 diagnosis codes were used as variables in multivariate logistic regression analysis to identify the top 45 diagnoses among persons with pressure ulcers. Odds ratios (estimate of relative risk) were reported for the most significant risk factors. Analysis was also conducted after stratifying the sample by age, race, and gender. In this study, age over 75 years was the strongest risk factor, with an odds ratio (OR) of 12.63. Age 59 to 75 years was a strong risk factor (OR 5.99, no confidence interval reported), as was African American race (OR 5.71, 95% CI, 5.35 to 6.10). Fogerty and colleagues also reported a statistically significant interaction between race and age; that is, aging was associated with greater increase in risk of pressure ulcer development among African Americans than among Caucasians, indicating noteworthy racial disparities. Other significant findings from this study include the differentiation between major risk factors that are nonmodifiable (age, paralysis, race) and those that are potentially modifiable (infection, nutritional deficiencies) (Fogerty et al., 2008).

Risk Assessment Tools

Risk assessment tools have been developed to assist the clinician to identify individuals at risk for pressure ulcer development.

Braden Scale

The most popular, widely used risk assessment tool in use today is the Braden Scale for Predicting Pressure Sore Risk (Bergstrom et al., 1987). The Braden Scale was first published in 1987 and has therefore been in use over 20 years in various settings. It includes six main risk factors for PU development (sensory status, mobility, activity, exposure to moisture, nutritional status, exposure to friction and shear), with a potential total score ranging from 6 to 23. Lower scores on the Braden Scale indicate greater risk for pressure ulcer development. Very high risk = 9 or below; high risk = 10 to 12; moderate risk = 13 to 14; and mild risk = 15 to 18. There is literature by Braden to suggest that if a person has other major risk factors present (e.g., advanced age, fever, or hemodynamic instability), his or her score should be advanced to the next highest level of risk, yet observational studies suggest this is not routinely done by nurses. On the contrary, research suggests that nurses frequently underestimate the level of pressure ulcer risk (Ayello & Braden, 2002; Bergstrom et al., 1987, 1996; Braden & Bergstrom, 1994; Stotts & Gunningberg, 2007).

CLINICAL PEARL

Braden recommends that, for persons with major risk factors not addressed by the Braden Scale (e.g., advanced age, fever, or hemodynamic instability), the risk score should be modified to reflect the next highest level of risk; however, studies suggest that this is not routinely done.

The theoretical framework for the Braden Scale is based on a physiological model depicting factors that contribute to the development of pressure ulcers. It includes factors affecting intensity and duration of pressure (decreased mobility, decreased activity, and decreased sensory perception) and other extrinsic factors (increased moisture, increased friction, and increased shear forces), as well as intrinsic factors (e.g., nutrition) that affect tissue tolerance (Reddy et al., 2006). Defloor (1999) criticized the inclusion of "tissue tolerance" in the conceptual model stating, "Tissue tolerance cannot cause pressure sores" (p. 207). The exposure to pressure and/or shear force was viewed by Defloor as the primary etiologic factor, and he considered tissue tolerance to be an intermediate variable and not a causal factor. Defloor (1999) also commented that the Braden and Bergstrom conceptual model (and Braden Scale) did not include factors identified in other studies as being strongly associated with pressure ulcer development such as specific diseases, dehydration, protein deficiency, body build, and position.

CLINICAL PEARL

The Braden Scale is based on a conceptual framework that includes duration and intensity of pressure, other extrinsic factors (moisture, friction, and shear), and intrinsic factors affecting tissue tolerance (e.g., nutritional status).

Cowan and colleagues (2012) conducted a retrospective study of 213 hospitalized veterans (100 with PU and 113 without PU) to test the Fogerty findings, with a secondary goal of identifying factors that could be used to enhance the Braden Scale. In this study, the Braden total score (with an "at-risk" cutoff score of 18) demonstrated a sensitivity of 65% and a specificity of 70%. The positive predictive value (PPV) of the total Braden score was 65.7% and the negative predictive value (NPV) was 69.3%. The prognostic separation index (PSI) was 0.35 (measure of overall predictive value calculated by PPV + NPV − 1) and the Youden Index was 0.35 (a measure of overall diagnostic value calculated by sensitivity + specificity − 1). The area under the ROC curve for this model was 0.70. In this study, a four–medical factor model that included pneumonia, poor nutrition, surgery, and candidiasis was found to be more predictive than the Braden 6-factor scale. The four–medical factor model demonstrated a sensitivity of 83% and specificity of 72% (PPV 0.72/NPV 0.83). The PSI for this model was 0.55, the Youden Index was 0.55, and the area under the ROC curve was 0.82. Interestingly, when only two subscores of the Braden tool were used (friction and activity), the two-factor scale was more predictive than the Braden total 6-factor model with a sensitivity of 80% and specificity of 65% (PPV 67% and NPV 79%). The PSI for the two-factor model was 0.46, the Youden Index was 0.46, and the area under the ROC curve was 0.75. This was a small study of a possibly unique patient population; however, it seems clear that risk factors may vary from population to population and that more study is needed in the area of risk assessment tools.

In an "Up to Date" literature review, Berlowitz (2014) states that the most important risk factors associated with pressure ulcer development include immobility, malnutrition, reduced perfusion, and sensory loss; this review is available at http://www.uptodate.com/contents/epidemiology-pathogenesis-and-risk-assessment-of-pressure-ulcers?source=see_link&anchor=H76126129#H76126129.

CLINICAL PEARL

In an "Up to Date" review, Berlowitz identified immobility, malnutrition, reduced perfusion, and sensory loss as major risk factors for pressure ulcer development.

Data Regarding Use of Risk Assessment Tools

It is important to emphasize that further research is needed to address risk of pressure ulcer development. In reviewing the current literature, there are significant limitations affecting most pressure ulcer predictive studies including small sample sizes, convenience sampling, potential bias due to underreporting of pressure ulcers or classification of other skin injuries (skin tears, incontinence-associated dermatitis) as pressure ulcers, and lack of scientific rigor of some studies (Bolton, 2007; Schoonhoven et al., 2006; VanGilder et al., 2008).

Berlowitz (2014) points out, "Identifying at-risk patients is central to preventing pressure ulcers. However, the effectiveness of formal risk assessment instruments compared with less standardized methods has not been clearly established." Furthermore, Schoonhoven and colleagues (2002) have criticized pressure ulcer risk assessment tools by stating, "Neither risk factors nor the weights attributed to them have been identified using adequate statistical techniques" (p. 65). To add to these criticisms, Papanikolaou et al. (2007) recommended that "differential weighting scoring techniques, advanced statistical methods, and large data sets be used to develop data driven and more robust PU risk assessment scales." (p. 285).

Of interest is a study performed by Pancorbo-Hildago and colleagues (2006). They conducted a systematic review of 33 studies involving three risk assessment tools: the Braden Scale, the Norton Scale, and the Waterlow Scale. They found no reduction in pressure ulcer incidence that could be attributed to use of a risk assessment tool, though they did note that the use of validated tools was associated with increased intensity and effectiveness of prevention interventions. In the studies they reviewed, the Braden Scale was associated with the best validity scores and the best sensitivity/specificity balance (57.1%/67.5%, respectively); they concluded that the Braden score is a good pressure ulcer risk predictor (odds ratio = 4.08, CI 95% = 2.56 to 6.48). The Norton Scale was found to have reasonable sensitivity (46.8%), specificity (61.8%), and risk prediction (OR = 2.16, CI 95% = 1.03 to 4.54). The Waterlow Scale was associated with high sensitivity (82.4%), but low specificity (27.4%), and was a good predictor of risk (OR = 2.05, CI 95% = 1.11 to 3.76). Nurses' clinical judgment was considered in only three studies; in these studies, clinical judgment was associated with moderately good sensitivity (50.6%) and specificity (60.1%) but was not found to be a good pressure ulcer risk predictor (OR = 1.69, CI 95% = 0.76 to 3.75). The investigators concluded there was no evidence that the use of risk assessment tools decreased pressure ulcer incidence, but also acknowledged that both the Braden and Norton scales provided more accurate results than nurses' clinical judgment in terms of identifying patients at risk.

More detailed information on PU risk assessment has been completed by the Agency for Healthcare Research and Quality (AHRQ), who published a Comparative Effectiveness Summary Report on Pressure Ulcer Risk Assessment and Prevention in May 2013 (Chou et al.,

2013). The report examined 120 studies and concluded that commonly used risk assessment tools (including the Braden, Norton, and Waterlow scales) can help to identify patients at risk for pressure ulcer development but are relatively weak predictors; they found no significant difference among the tools in terms of diagnostic accuracy.

Current Recommendations

In summary, there is strong evidence that, in regard to PU risk assessment tools, something is better than nothing! However, it is clear that further research is warranted to develop accurate risk identification tools and integrate these into evidence-based practice and to develop effective preventive interventions based on the individual's specific risk factors (Seongsook et al., 2004). In the current age of computer technology and decision-support programming that can be embedded into patient assessment documentation and order forms, it is conceivable that the future may provide more robust risk identification and prevention methods, whereby triggers in the documentation software are activated by entry of patient-specific data and result in an individualized pressure ulcer prevention plan. In addition, clinicians should work to assure that, regardless of the specific risk assessment tool being used, the professionals using it are proficient in its use and knowledgeable regarding potential risk factors within their patient population *not* accounted for by the assessment tool they are using.

CLINICAL PEARL

In regard to pressure ulcer risk assessment tools, something is better than nothing! However, further study is needed to develop accurate risk identification tools and to develop individualized prevention programs.

Pathology of Pressure Ulcer Development

Top-Down versus Bottom-Up Tissue Damage

Current theory suggests that skin and soft tissue damage can begin at the surface and progress inward, or begin at the muscle and progress outward, depending on the etiologic factors (Agam & Gefen, 2008; Bouten et al., 2003). Top-down (superficial) damage is caused primarily by superficial shear or friction and presents as a Stage I PU (nonblanchable redness); these lesions can almost always be treated effectively before they become Stage III to IV full-thickness PUs. Bottom-up (deep) damage is caused by sustained compression of the tissue, which originates at the muscle–bone interface. Sustained compression of the tissue can cause rapid development of extensive deep tissue necrosis, without initial visible changes at the skin surface; the first surface indicators may be a blood-filled blister with bruising that eventually progresses to Stage III to IV ulceration. This sustained compression form of damage is considered especially harmful because the subcutaneous, fascia, and muscle layers may suffer substantial necrosis, but there are only minor signs of tissue breakdown at the skin surface. The skin surface indicators do usually permit differentiation between an sDTI and a Category/Stage I pressure ulcer. A Stage I PU presents as intact skin with superficial inflammatory changes (nonblanchable redness) that resolves easily with pressure offloading; Stage I lesions rarely deteriorate to a Stage III to IV ulcer so long as they are managed properly. In contrast, sDTI lesions present with deep purple discoloration and can rapidly evolve to full-thickness tissue loss.

CLINICAL PEARL

Bottom-up damage is caused by intense or sustained compression of the tissue and begins at the muscle–bone interface.

Pressure Intensity and Pressure Duration

Research on pressure ulcers has focused on determining the minimal degree of loading that will consistently lead to tissue damage. These studies all show an inverse relationship between the magnitude and duration of loading, indicating that higher loads (pressure levels) require less time to cause deep tissue breakdown. However, to date, no specific level of pressure intensity has been identified as the "cut point" beyond which ischemic damage is inevitable. Evidence to date indicates that pressure-related damage may occur within a short period of time (minutes to hours), and the specific time frame and pressure intensity required to produce irreversible damage most likely vary from person to person depending on their clinical condition (e.g., age, hemodynamic status, and comorbid conditions). The data *do* clearly indicate that pressure ulcer prevention must include strategies to reduce both the magnitude of loading (intensity of pressure), and the duration of loading, specifically pressure redistribution surfaces and routine repositioning. These two strategies are the primary components of all recommended pressure ulcer prevention protocols.

CLINICAL PEARL

Evidence to date indicates that pressure-related damage may occur within minutes to hours, and the time frame and pressure intensity required to produce irreversible damage most likely vary from person to person depending on their clinical condition. No specific level of pressure intensity has been identified beyond which tissue damage is inevitable.

Pathology of Pressure/Shear Damage

The literature on pressure ulcer etiology and pathology identifies four major factors hypothesized to cause this type of "bottom to top" form of tissue damage:

1. Occlusion of blood vessels resulting in tissue ischemia (Bader et al., 1986; Daniel et al., 1981; Dinsdale, 1973, 1974; Edsberg et al., 2000)

2. Occlusion of lymph vessels resulting in impaired removal of waste products and increased risk of edema (Krouskop, 1983; Krouskop et al., 1978)
3. Ischemia/reperfusion damage resulting from an accumulation of oxygen free radicals during the ischemic period (Ikebe et al., 2001; Peirce et al., 2000; Reid et al., 2004; Unal et al., 2001)
4. Direct deformation damage of the cytoskeleton of muscle cells in situations involving high-pressure loads (Bouten et al., 2003; Loerakker et al., 2011; Stekelenburg et al., 2007, 2008)

Each of these factors will be addressed in more detail.

Vessel Compression Resulting in Tissue Ischemia

Even at relatively low pressures, there can be some reduction in perfusion related to vessel compression; smaller or damaged blood vessels may be totally occluded. As the tissue load (pressure) rises, the degree of interference to perfusion becomes greater and can lead to significant reduction in blood flow to the tissues; at very high loads, even larger vessels can be completely occluded. The reduced blood flow causes tissue ischemia, meaning that the delivery of oxygen and nutrients to the cells is compromised; the removal of metabolic waste products from the cells is also impaired. This does not cause immediate damage to the tissues, because the cells can and will shift from aerobic to anaerobic metabolism. Anaerobic metabolism is less effective and generates more waste products (lactate); nonetheless, anaerobic metabolism can meet the energy needs of the cells for a significant period of time. However, over time, metabolic waste products accumulate in the intercellular space and reduce the pH levels, which will eventually damage the cells. In animal experiments, cell damage becomes evident after a period of 2 to 3 hours.

Lymph Vessel Occlusion and Edema Formation

Lymphatic vessels play an important role in removal of waste products from the interstitial space and in control of the amount of free water in the interstitial space. Although we do not know the exact point at which pressure and shear forces begin to occlude the blood vessels and lymphatics, it is very likely that in many clinical situations, both the vascular and lymphatic transport systems are compromised, which causes worsening of the ischemia. Failure of the lymphatic system leads to increased accumulation of cellular waste and to accumulation of fluid in the interstitial space (edema).

Reperfusion Injury

It is well known from cardiovascular research that rapid reperfusion after a period of ischemia (e.g., an infarct) can add to the damage caused by the ischemic episode. This is due to two major factors. (1) The period of reduced blood flow can result in formation of small clots that obstruct small vessels once blood flow is reestablished. (2) Ischemia results in the accumulation of oxygen free radicals; when oxygen becomes available, it triggers chemical reactions that are damaging to the cells and tissue. A slower rate of reperfusion may reduce these negative effects; however, at present, we have no mechanisms for controlling the rate of reperfusion. In addition, the exact role that reperfusion injury plays in pressure ulcer development remains unknown. Although several studies have been published on this subject, it is very difficult to separate reperfusion damage from damage due to other causes.

CLINICAL PEARL

The pathology of pressure ulcer development is thought to involve the following four factors: vascular compression (reduced perfusion) and tissue ischemia, lymph vessel compression and edema, reperfusion injury, and direct damage to the cytoskeleton of the muscle cell.

Direct Damage to Cytoskeleton of Muscle Cell

Muscle deformation may cause direct damage to the cytoskeleton of the cell. Studies using cultured cells and tissue-engineered muscle constructs indicate that even moderate levels of deformation can compromise the cytoskeleton of the muscle cell. Extensive studies in which deformation was combined with different degrees of ischemia indicate that "deformation damage" occurs more rapidly than ischemic damage. The causes are not yet clear but may include membrane failure, rupture of the cytoskeleton, or activation of a biochemical pathway triggered by the deformation (Bouten et al., 2003; Breuls et al., 2002, 2003a, 2003b; Gawlitta et al., 2007a, 2007b). Animal studies have confirmed the phenomenon of "deformation damage" and have shown that the amount of damage is correlated to the degree of deformation. These in vivo studies also confirmed that deformation damage can occur quickly, with cellular damage becoming evident within minutes; however, the in vivo studies found that damage only occurred at high levels of strain and deformation. This is an important finding, because the level of strain associated with muscle cell damage is most likely to occur near the bony prominence of a person sitting or lying on a hard surface. This level of strain/deformation can also be caused by folds in the clothing or sheets or from stiff objects in pockets (Ceelen et al., 2008; Chow & Odell, 1978; Loerakker et al., 2011; Stekelenburg et al., 2007, 2008).

Clinically, it is very hard to totally protect the soft tissue from the ischemic effects of tissue loading; thus, it is imperative to routinely change the areas exposed to mechanical loading by repositioning the patient. Fortunately, it is usually possible to prevent "deformation damage" through the use of proper support surfaces and by increasing awareness of the problem among patients and caregivers.

CLINICAL PEARL

Pressure ulcer prevention must include strategies to reduce both the magnitude of loading (intensity of pressure) and the duration of loading, specifically pressure redistribution surfaces and routine repositioning. These two strategies are the primary components of all recommended pressure ulcer prevention protocols.

Pathology of Heel Ulcers/sDTIs

As noted, the heel is the most common site for development of sDTI (and the second most common site of all pressure ulcers). The heel bears the major portion of body weight in the standing position and is critical for walking because it transfers ground forces to the body by absorbing shear and pressure. During prolonged bedrest, the ability of the heel to compensate for positional changes is altered, especially in the presence of serious comorbidities, which may hamper protective biomechanical and kinesiologic mechanisms. The heel is at greater risk for development of pressure ulcer development because of the thin layer of overlying soft tissue and the small curvature of the bony prominence; these factors contribute to a greater degree of tissue and vessel compression and to high pressures (mechanical loading) exerted by the bony prominence against the overlying soft tissue. In addition, the heel may be exposed to shear forces if the bedbound individual uses the heel to "push off" during attempts to move up in bed. Because of the small surface area and high tissue-interface pressure, the heel is one of the most difficult anatomical areas to protect using pressure redistribution surfaces; current guidelines require use of pillows or other devices that elevate the heel off of the bed or chair and thus effectively off-load the pressure (Salcido et al., 2010).

CLINICAL PEARL

The heel is very difficult to protect using pressure redistribution surfaces; current guidelines require use of pillows or other devices that elevate the heel off of the bed or chair.

Staging of Pressure Ulcers

Pressure ulcers are commonly "staged" (or "graded") based on depth of tissue injury. In the United States, the staging system promulgated by the NPUAP is the accepted system for use (**Table 18-1**; **Figs. 18-1** to **18-7** for current staging system). Accurate staging of pressure ulcers is complex. Staging is dependent on accurate identification of the viable structures within the wound bed, which requires the clinician to be knowledgeable regarding the tissue layers and structures.

CLINICAL PEARL

Accuracy in staging is dependent on correct identification of the viable structures within the wound bed and requires the clinician to be knowledgeable regarding tissue layers and structures.

Stage I versus sDTI

Accurate differentiation between Stage I and sDTI lesions can be challenging, since both involve discoloration (or palpatory changes) of intact skin; accurate differential assessment is supported by knowledge of patient history and any episodes of prolonged immobility. Gefen and colleagues (2013) suggest use of the term PRIDAS (pressure-related intact discolored area of skin) as an umbrella term encompassing both Stage I ulcers (nonblanchable erythema) and sDTI. They recommend that the clinician consider the patient's risk factors (to include comorbidities) and their history of exposure to high level or prolonged pressure and that, when in doubt, they err on the side of deep tissue injury and immediately implement aggressive preventative measures. This is particularly important when assessing individuals with very dark skin, because it can be very hard to accurately distinguish between Stage I and sDTI lesions in these individuals. In assessing for sDTI lesions, it is important to include careful assessment of the skin within the natal cleft, as these lesions are often missed. Farid and colleagues (2012) point out that apparently superficial injury (Stage I) can progress to a more serious wound (sDTI) in very ill patients, which underscores the importance of aggressive preventive care for all at risk patients as well as those with apparently limited damage.

sDTI versus Stage II Ulcer

Confusion has also existed regarding the differential diagnosis of an sDTI versus a Stage II pressure ulcer. An sDTI should not be confused with a Stage II ulcer, which presents as a partial-thickness wound or a clear fluid-filled or open superficial blister that heals predictably; in Stage II ulcers, the damage is limited to the skin layers themselves and does not extend past the dermis into the subcutaneous tissue. In contrast, an sDTI is defined by EPUAP & NPUAP (2009) as the following: "Purple or maroon localized area of discolored intact skin or blood-filled blister due to damage of underlying soft tissue from pressure and/or shear. The area may be preceded by tissue that is painful, firm, mushy, boggy, warmer or cooler as compared to adjacent tissue." Evolution of sDTI may include a thin blister over a dark wound bed, followed by development of a thin layer of eschar; evolution is sometimes rapid, exposing additional layers of tissue even with optimal treatment (EPUAP & NPUAP, 2009).

CLINICAL PEARL

An sDTI should not be confused with a Stage II ulcer, which presents as a partial-thickness wound that heals predictably.

Challenges in Staging

One major problem with pressure ulcer classification and staging is the reliance on visual inspection to determine depth of injury and tissue layers involved. As noted, at present, clinicians are taught to use skin color as an indicator of inflammatory or ischemic changes; erythema is an indicator of hyperemia (Stage I ulcer), while deep purple or purple-black hues represent infarction and necrosis (Salcido et al., 2011). However, visual inspection is fraught with error. Researchers for Bruin Biometrics (White Paper, 2013) identified a number of problems with reliance on visual skin inspection for determining the presence or absence of pressure-related tissue damage. Two of their major criticisms include the following: (1) Skin assessments are subjective and unreliable; several studies have

TABLE 18-1 Pressure Ulcer Staging System (NPUAP)

Category/Stage I: Nonblanchable erythema
A Stage I pressure ulcer is characterized as intact skin with nonblanchable redness of a localized area usually over a bony prominence. Darkly pigmented skin may not have visible blanching; its color may differ from the surrounding area. The area may be painful, firm, soft, warmer, or cooler as compared to adjacent tissue. Category I may be difficult to detect in individuals with dark skin tones. It may indicate "at-risk" persons for the development of more severe injury including sDTI (NPUAP/EPUAP/PPPIA, 2014) (see Fig. 18-1).
Category/Stage II: Partial thickness
A Stage II pressure ulcer is characterized as partial-thickness loss of dermis presenting as a shallow open ulcer with a red-pink wound bed, without slough. A Stage II PU may also present as an intact or open/ruptured serum-filled or serosanguineous filled blister. A stage II PU presents as a shiny or dry shallow ulcer without slough or bruising*. This category should not be used to describe skin tears, tape burns, incontinence-associated dermatitis, maceration, or excoriation. Bruising is likely to indicate deep tissue injury (NPUAP/EPUAP/PPPIA, 2014) (see Fig. 18-2).
Category/Stage III: Full-thickness skin loss
A Stage III pressure ulcer is a full-thickness tissue loss lesion. Subcutaneous fat may be visible but bone, tendon, and muscle are *not* exposed. Slough may be present but does not obscure the depth of tissue loss. A Stage III PU *may* include undermining and tunneling. The depth of a Category/Stage III pressure ulcer varies by anatomical location. The bridge of the nose, ear, occiput, and malleolus do not have (adipose) subcutaneous tissue, and Category/Stage III ulcers can be shallow. In contrast, areas of significant adiposity can develop extremely deep Category/Stage III pressure ulcers. Bone/tendon is not visible or directly palpable with a Stage III PU (NPUAP/EPUAP/PPPIA, 2014) (see Fig. 18-3).
Category/Stage IV: Full-thickness tissue loss
A Stage IV PU is characterized as full-thickness tissue loss with exposed bone, tendon, or muscle. Slough or eschar may be present. Often, a Stage IV PU includes undermining and tunneling. The depth of a Category/Stage IV pressure ulcer varies by anatomical location. The bridge of the nose, ear, occiput, and malleolus do not have (adipose) subcutaneous tissue, and these ulcers can be shallow. Category/Stage IV ulcers can extend into muscle and/or supporting structures (e.g., fascia, tendon or joint capsule) making osteomyelitis or osteitis likely to occur. Exposed bone/muscle is visible or directly palpable with a stage IV PU (NPUAP/EPUAP/PPPIA, 2014) (see Fig. 18-4).
Additional categories/stages for the United States
Unstageable/unclassified: Full-thickness skin or tissue loss—depth unknown
This category/stage of PU is characterized as full-thickness tissue loss in which actual depth of the ulcer is completely obscured by slough (yellow, tan, gray, green, or brown) and/or eschar (tan, brown, or black) in the wound bed. Until enough slough and/or eschar are removed to expose the base of the wound, the true depth cannot be determined; but it will be either a Category/Stage III or IV. Stable (dry, adherent, intact without erythema or fluctuance) eschar on the heels serves as "the body's natural (biological) cover" and should not be removed (NPUAP/EPUAP/PPPIA, 2014) (see Fig. 18-5).
Suspected deep tissue injury—depth unknown
Definition of suspected deep tissue injury
Suspected deep tissue injuries usually develop over a bony prominence due to sustained mechanical loading (unrelieved pressure) and/or repeated shear forces to the involved tissues. This results in ischemic injury to the subcutaneous tissue and/or muscle due to deformation of the deep tissues and associated blood vessels. These lesions can deteriorate rapidly into a full-thickness "bottom-up" ulcer if pressure and shear are not relieved in a timely manner. The literature indicates that (1) DTI involves skeletal muscle tissue injury and is likely to initiate in muscle tissue, (2) compressive mechanical loading (such as compressive stress, deformation, or strain) is the most important cause of DTI, and (3) DTI cannot develop without such mechanical loading (Agam & Gefen, 2008). Clinically, these injuries may initially present as a deep purple or maroon "bruised" area or as a blood blister under intact skin, followed by rapid progression to an open full-thickness wound; this sequence of events is explained by the fact that the injury to the deep tissues occurs prior to the visual manifestation on the surface of the skin (Agam & Gefen, 2008) (see Figs. 18-6 and 18-7).

been done that suggest poor interrater reliability of skin assessments conducted by different clinicians. (2) Visual inspection is often inaccurate, since it is impossible to detect tissue damage at the initial point of injury (near the bone) by visual inspection of the intact skin; the color changes associated with deep tissue damage do not usually occur until hours or days later. In addition, visual skin inspection is often difficult (due to issues with patient positioning and lighting), and 24 hour a day visual monitoring of every inch of a patient's skin is not realistic. Thus, one challenge in early detection of pressure-related tissue damage is the current absence of inexpensive and accurate diagnostic tools that can be used by the bedside clinician to identify any areas of impending ulceration.

CLINICAL PEARL

One major problem with pressure ulcer classification and staging is the reliance on visual inspection to determine depth of injury and tissue layers involved—visual assessment is fraught with error.

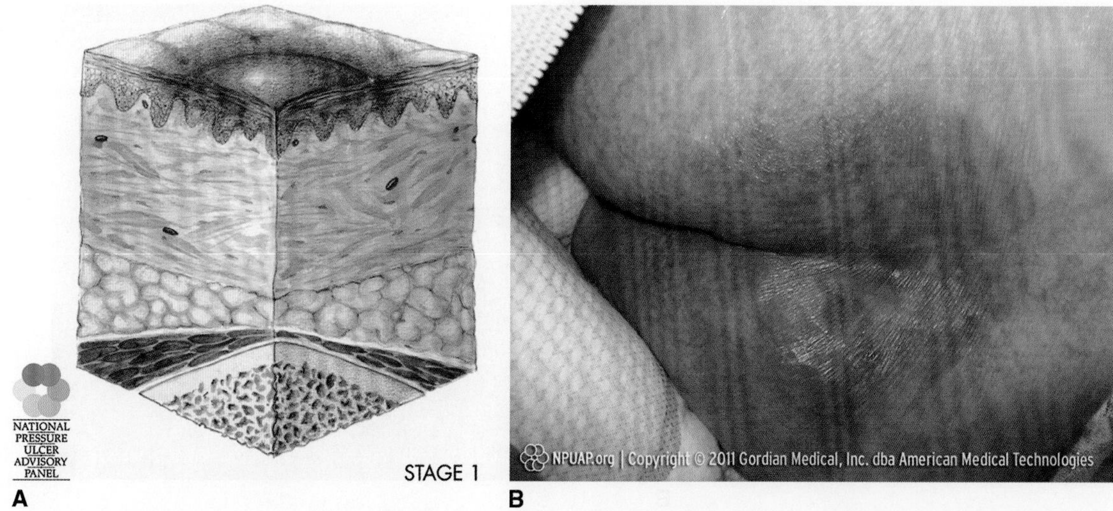

FIGURE 18-1. **A, B.** Stage I pressure ulcer. (Used with permission of the National Pressure Ulcer Advisory Panel, 2015. Copyright © NPUAP.)

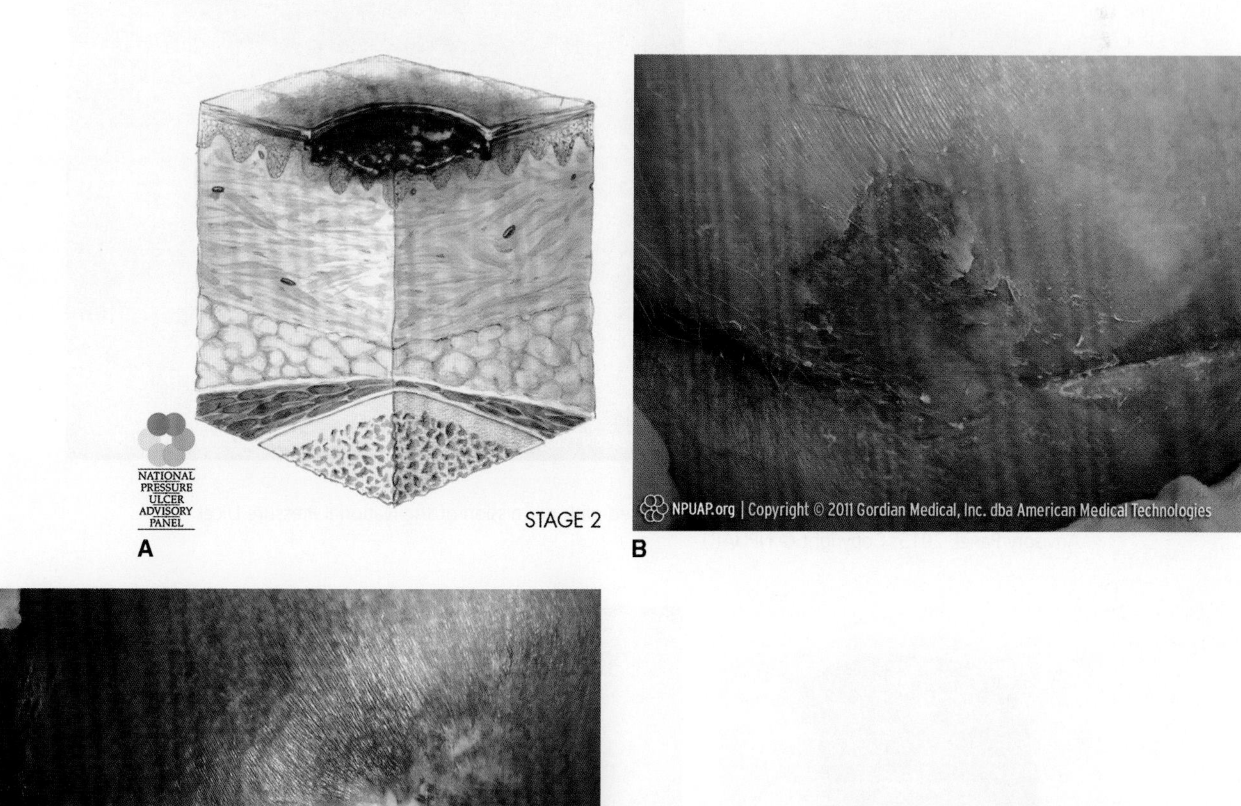

FIGURE 18-2. **A–C.** Stage II pressure ulcer. (Used with permission of the National Pressure Ulcer Advisory Panel, 2015. Copyright © NPUAP.)

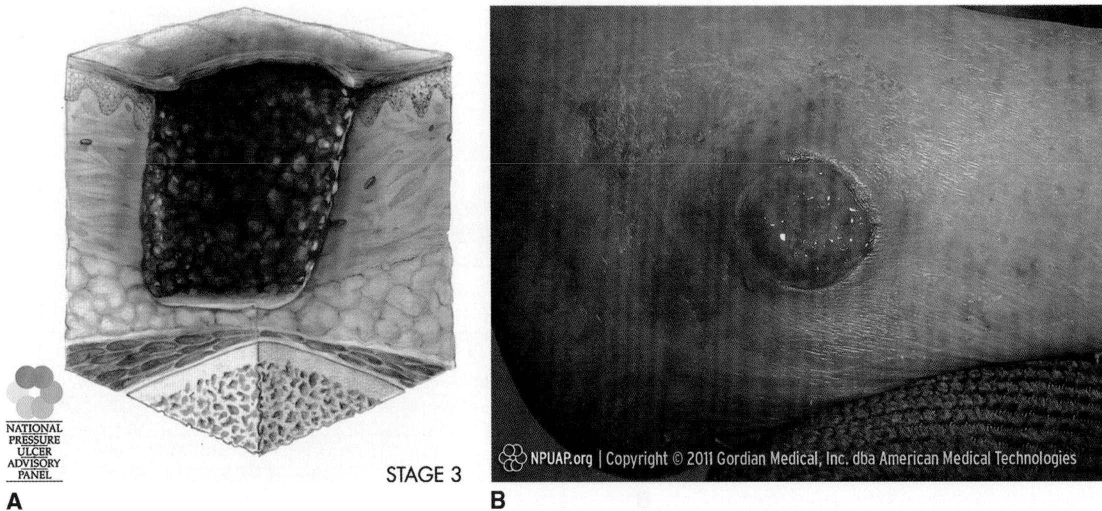

FIGURE 18-3. **A, B.** Stage III pressure ulcer. (Used with permission of the National Pressure Ulcer Advisory Panel, 2015. Copyright © NPUAP.)

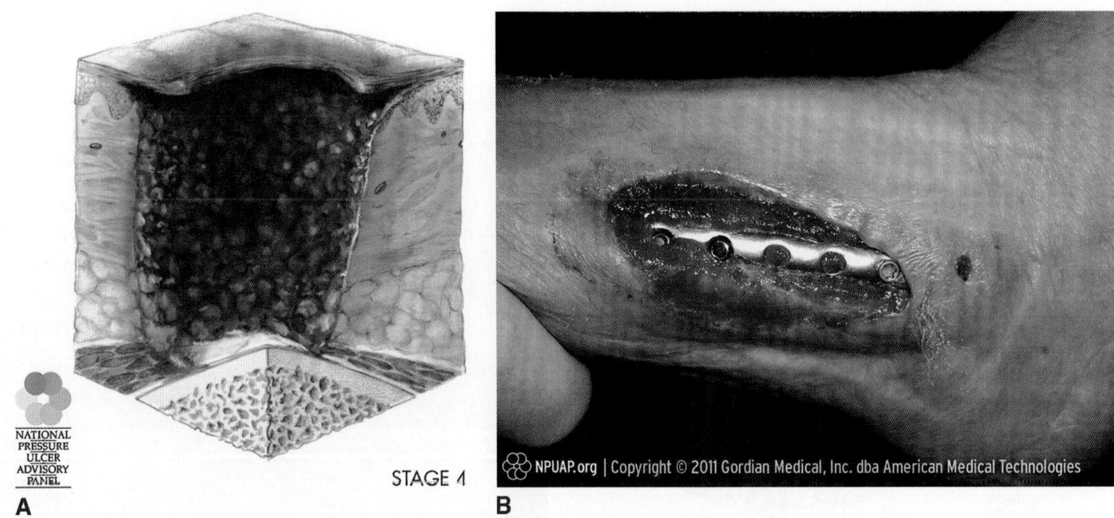

FIGURE 18-4. **A, B.** Stage IV pressure ulcer. (Used with permission of the National Pressure Ulcer Advisory Panel, 2015. Copyright © NPUAP.)

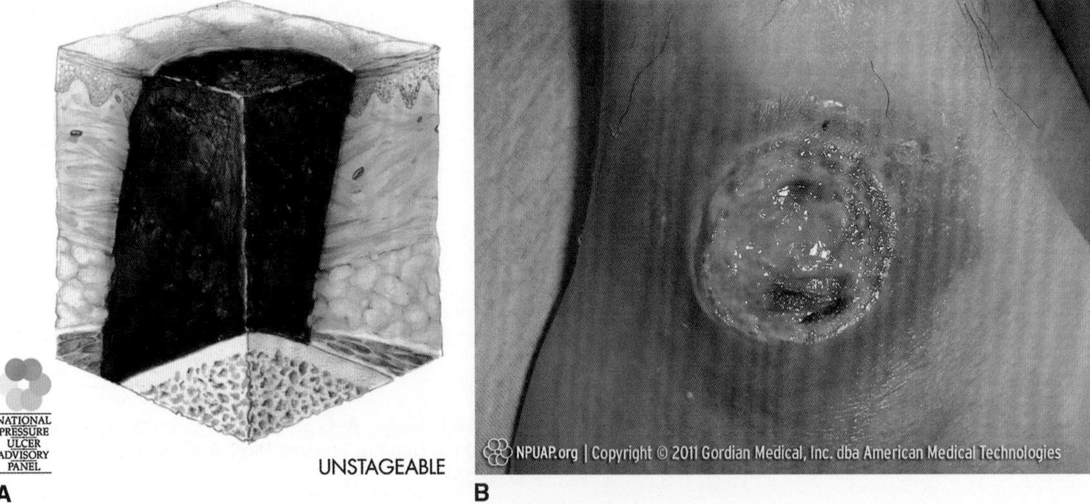

FIGURE 18-5. **A, B.** Unstageable pressure ulcer. (Used with permission of the National Pressure Ulcer Advisory Panel, 2015. Copyright © NPUAP.)

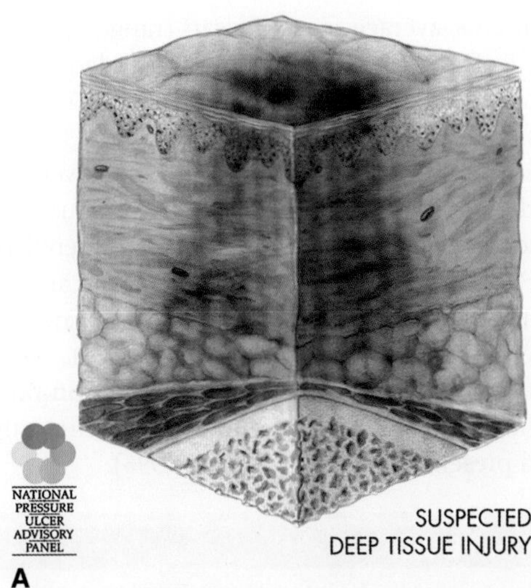

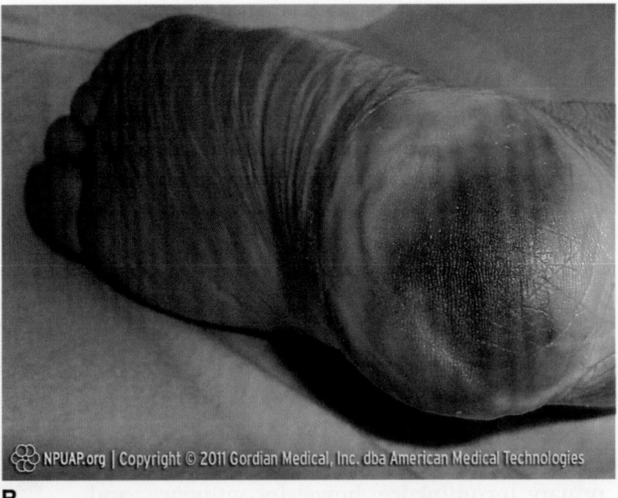

FIGURE 18-6. **A, B.** Suspected deep tissue injury (sDTI). (Used with permission of the National Pressure Ulcer Advisory Panel, 2015. Copyright © NPUAP.)

Lyder (2007) suggests that technology may soon provide answers to the challenge of early and accurate detection of pressure-induced tissue damage; studies suggest that ultrasound can be used to identify subepidermal moisture (SEM) and that SEM is a marker for inflammatory changes. In addition, Bates-Jensen and colleagues (2007, 2008, 2009) demonstrated measurable local tissue edema associated with inflammation in epidermal and dermal tissues up to 10 days before any visible skin changes or discoloration were present, suggesting that objective measures of epidermal and dermal edema could also be used in early detection of pressure damage.

Clearly, further research is needed to develop new technology, techniques, and diagnostic tools that permit early detection of pressure- and shear-related skin and soft tissue damage. In addition, we need to identify successful and cost-effective strategies for preventing, reducing, and reversing these changes *before* irreversible deep tissue injury occurs. Early intervention (off-loading and elimination of shear force) may help to limit the damage; thus, ongoing assessment and prompt identification of sDTI are essential.

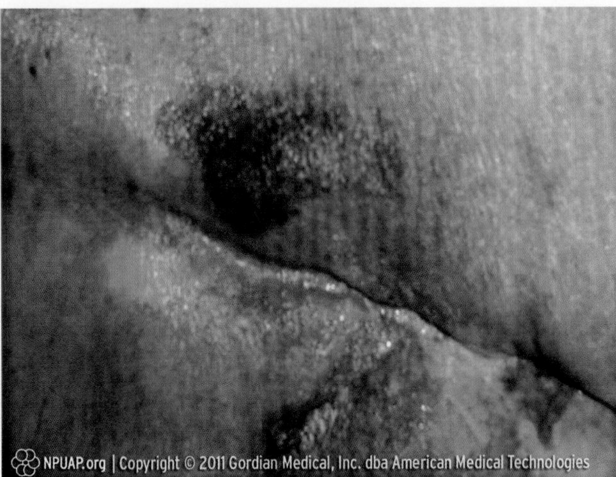

FIGURE 18-7. Discoloration characteristic of sDTI. (Used with permission of the National Pressure Ulcer Advisory Panel, 2015. Copyright © NPUAP.)

sDTI (suspected Deep Tissue Injury)

Health care providers are becoming more knowledgeable regarding the signs and symptoms of sDTI and are therefore becoming more vigilant; as a result, reported sDTI rates have increased three-fold since 2009. sDTI lesions now comprise 9% of all observed ulcers, making sDTI more prevalent than all Stage III and IV ulcers combined (VanGilder et al., 2010). The heel is the most common site of sDTI development, accounting for 41% of all sDTIs, followed by those involving the sacrum (19%) and buttocks (13%) (Salcido et al., 2011).

sDTI in Critical Care Patients

One population of patients at high risk for the development of sDTI pressure ulcers are those in the critical care unit; in a recently reported study by Gefen et al. (2013), 84.2% of sDTIs occurred in critical care patients. Critically ill patients are typically much less mobile, due to analgesics, conscious sedation, ventilator assistance, and the multiple lines and wires attached to their bodies. The use of vasopressors and anticoagulants is also common in this population, and these drugs have been associated with increased risk of sDTIs and pressure ulcers (Fleck, 2007). Honaker and colleagues (2014) found that the most common precipitating factor for the development of sDTI was patient transfers; other variables that appeared to contribute to the development of sDTIs were the use of anticoagulants and the presence of anemia. One hypothesis for the increased development of sDTI during transfers is the increased risk of shear injury during bed and surface transfer. Although some pressure ulcers may be unavoidable due to severe circulatory compromise and other comorbidities, most ulcers and sDTIs are preventable (Gefen et al., 2013). Even for patients who develop Stage I or sDTI lesions, early identification and intervention have the potential to prevent deterioration and to minimize tissue damage.

sDTI in Long-Term Care Patients

Residents of long-term care facilities are also at high risk for development of sDTI, as well as other pressure ulcers. A recent study by Ahn and colleagues (2014) utilized a retrospective analysis of the MDS 3.0 national database to provide a detailed summary of the relationship between sDTI and resident characteristics. In this study, nine resident characteristics were associated with sDTI in multivariate logistic regression analysis: increased age, impairment in activities of daily living, malnutrition, use of anticoagulant, urinary incontinence, bowel incontinence, and overweight/obesity were associated with increased risk of sDTI development (Elsner & Gefen, 2008), while female sex and Caucasian race were associated with reduced risk. Interestingly, cognitive status and dementia had no impact on risk for sDTI in this study.

Risk Factors for sDTI

Studies indicate that patients on bed rest following hip surgery are at particularly high risk for sDTI of the heels (Black, 2006). Advanced age may be another risk factor; a 2009 survey of hospitalized patients revealed that the mean age of patients with sDTI was 71.9, which is older than the mean age of patients with Stage III/IV pressure ulcers (Alderden et al., 2011). Obesity is another potential risk factor; in the 2009 survey, the mean body mass index (BMI) for acutely ill patients with sDTI was 27.9 kg/m2, which indicates overweight status. The use of safe patient handling equipment for moving patients with obese body habitus is recommended to reduce shear. Overall, sDTI incidence increased to ten percent in 2009 and continues to increase rapidly (Ahn et al., 2014), especially in acute and critical care settings (Alderden et al., 2011; Sullivan, 2013). One potential contributing factor to the increasing incidence of sDTI is the fact that the Braden Scale, which is commonly used to assess pressure ulcer risk, does not include some of the factors thought to contribute to sDTI (e.g., obesity, multiple comorbidities, anticoagulation, anemia, sepsis, and respiratory failure) (Cowan et al., 2012; Gefen et al., 2013; Liu et al., 2012).

A study by Sullivan (2013) provides additional insight into risk factors, presentation, and outcomes of sDTI. This single-site, 2-year, retrospective, IRB-approved study was designed to increase understanding of the evolution and outcomes of sDTI. Inclusion criteria were hospitalized patients, 18 years or older, with an sDTI confirmed by a wound care nurse. Patient charts and wound, ostomy, and continence nurse (WOC nurse) notes were examined and patient demographics and DTI variables were abstracted. All patients received standardized, comprehensive care for pressure ulcer prevention and treatment. Seventy-seven (77) patients, average age 67.5 years (range 32 to 91 years), with 128 sDTIs were identified and included in the study. The majority were men (52, 67.5%) and non-Hispanic Caucasian (68, 88.3%). Twenty-three (23, 31%) were overweight. The most common comorbidities were coronary artery disease (38, 50%) and diabetes mellitus (33, 43%), and the vast majority (67, 88.1%) had altered mobility (67, 88.1%), spent time in the intensive care unit (64, 84.2%), and were incontinent (64, 84.2%). The most common areas involved were the sacrum (51, 39.8%) and the heel/Achilles region (37, 28.9%). Maroon-purple discoloration of intact skin was the most commonly documented presentation (115 ulcers, 89.9%).

CLINICAL PEARL

The sacrum and heel areas account for almost 70% of sDTI lesions.

sDTI Outcomes

Average length of follow-up was 6 days (range 1 day to 14 weeks). At the final assessment, 85 sDTIs (66.4%) completely resolved or were progressing toward resolution, 31 remained unchanged and were still documented as purple-maroon discoloration or a blood-filled blister, and 12 (9.3%) had deteriorated to full-thickness tissue loss (Sullivan, 2013). These observations offer important and encouraging insights into the evolution of sDTIs, since the majority of these lesions had resolved or were improving. Additional research is needed to more clearly define the demographics, risk factors, prevention, and treatment of sDTI in acute and critical care settings.

CLINICAL PEARL

In a recent study, 66% of sDTI lesions either resolved or improved with appropriate management.

Early Detection and Assessment of sDTI

Clinically, these injuries may initially present as a deep purple or maroon "bruised" area or as a blood blister under intact skin, followed by rapid progression to an open full-thickness wound; this sequence of events is explained by the fact that the injury to the deep tissues occurs prior to the visual manifestation on the surface of the skin (Agam & Gefen, 2008). This is of major concern since identification of the sDTI is the critical first step in providing appropriate management. In addition, the lag time between development of the deep tissue damage and visible evidence of the damage creates legal and regulatory issues, since at present, the only way to determine underlying deep tissue damage is by recognition of visual or palpatory changes. This means that a patient admitted with deep tissue injury but no visual or palpatory manifestations of that injury will be assessed on admission as having intact skin; when the injury becomes manifest by color changes or palpatory changes some days later, the lesion will be incorrectly classified as a hospital-acquired pressure ulcer (HAPU) (Farid et al., 2012). This underscores the need for diagnostic measurements that can detect underlying tissue damage prior to visual changes.

CLINICAL PEARL

There is a need for diagnostic measurements that can detect underlying tissue damage prior to color and tissue changes that are visible and palpable at the skin surface.

Ultrasound technology has proven to be a highly sensitive diagnostic tool in detecting early DTI associated with an isolated shear or pressure injury and in determining the severity of muscle injury and destruction (Higashino et al., 2012; Honaker & Forston, 2011; Honaker et al., 2013). Aliano and colleagues (2014) also used ultrasonography to evaluate depth of tissue damage; their study was designed to test the hypothesis that clinically superficial PUs (Stage I and Stage II) are actually associated with greater depths of injury than predicted. In their study, subjects with sacral PUs on admission were staged according to the NPUAP classification system. Patients who were classified as having a Stage I or Stage II ulcer or sDTI were assessed with high-frequency (12-MHZ) ultrasonography (US) to identify any evidence of injury to the deep tissue. All twenty patients, regardless of PU stage, were found to have evidence of deep tissue injury upon ultrasonographic examination. In patients with clinical findings consistent with sDTI, ultrasound reliably confirmed the presence of deep tissue injury. The findings from this small study suggest that even PUs that appear to be superficial may have a component of deeper tissue damage (Aliano et al., 2014); more study is needed to confirm these findings and to determine whether there are any differences in the degree of tissue damage as assessed by ultrasonography. It is hoped that, as our understanding of DTI and pressure ulcer pathology continue to evolve, better tools will be developed that provide for better and earlier detection.

The Honaker Suspected Deep Tissue Injury Severity Scale (HSDTISS) is a new assessment scale that helps to classify the sDTI in terms of severity. The aims of the instrument are to (a) accurately evaluate the severity of the sDTI, (b) determine progression of SDTI, and (c) demonstrate utility of the instrument in the clinical setting. The HSDTISS includes three parameters: total surface area, skin integrity, and wound color/tissue assessment. The total surface area is scored on a scale of 1 to 8, the skin integrity item is scored on a scale from 1 to 3, and the wound color/tissue assessment item is scored on a scale of 1 to 7. Cumulative scores for the HSDTISS range from 3 to 18. Content validity and interrater reliability testing have been completed with positive psychometric outcomes. Findings to date suggest that the HSDTISS accurately classifies wound severity among patients with SDTI. However, further rigorous testing is needed to confirm these preliminary findings.

Management of sDTI

Management of sDTI lesions is essentially the same as management of any pressure-related injury and is focused primarily on reducing pressure and shear forces to the area. Specific measures include routine turning and repositioning with particular attention to effective off-loading of the sDTI area. Therapeutic bed and chair surfaces should be utilized and should be selected based on documented ability to provide effective pressure redistribution and to reduce shear. In selecting a therapeutic device for the bed or chair, the clinician must also consider cost, the patient's specific clinical needs, type of care setting, whether or not the patient can be turned effectively off of the involved area, caregiver support, and the need for heel elevation (Allen et al., 2012; Mao et al., 2010). For example, the patient with an sDTI who is also diaphoretic would need a surface that provides microclimate control in addition to pressure redistribution and shear reduction. The obese patient with a sacral sDTI will need a surface that provides very high-level pressure redistribution, since it is unlikely that the care team will be able to keep the patient totally off of the sacral area. For more information on support surfaces, refer to Chapter 20.

CLINICAL PEARL

Management of sDTI lesions is essentially the same as management of any pressure-related injury and is focused primarily on reducing pressure and shear forces to the area (through use of therapeutic support surfaces and routine repositioning).

Special attention to pain assessment and management is of utmost importance for all patients with pressure-related injuries, and Ahn and colleagues (2014) have determined that sDTI is associated with moderate pain.

There is a paucity of research related to potential strategies for reversing the damage associated with sDTI; therefore, at present, the focus is on prevention of additional damage, as previously addressed. There is currently no evidence that topical therapy has any impact on the damage that has already occurred; thus, dressings are usually not indicated, and the skin is typically left untreated unless there is clear demarcation of necrosis, breakdown to a visible ulcer, or a specific issue that can be addressed with topical agents. Once there is clear demarcation of necrotic tissue, it is appropriate to proceed with debridement, if the goal is healing. Similarly, once the DTI has progressed to an open ulcer, the basic principles of wound bed preparation and moist wound healing should be followed. Finally, wicking agents and moisture barrier products should be used for the patient who is diaphoretic or incontinent, in order to prevent further skin damage (Mao et al., 2010). Systemic measures such as glycemic control, interventions to improve perfusion, and nutritional support should be provided for all patients.

CLINICAL PEARL

There is currently no evidence that topical therapy has any impact on the damage that has already occurred; thus, dressings are usually not indicated, and the skin is typically left untreated unless there is clear demarcation of necrosis, breakdown to a visible ulcer, or a specific issue that can be addressed with topical agents.

The major limitation in current pressure ulcer and sDTI management is our inability to accurately determine the extent of injury and our incomplete understanding of the specific pathological mechanisms. Fortunately, research is ongoing in regard to the pathology, assessment, and management of these wounds. For example, computer modeling is being used to assess the effects of sitting and lying on mechanical loads (pressure) applied to tissues. Animal and computer modeling studies are also being used to characterize the changes in muscle tissue associated with development of DTI and full-thickness pressure ulcers. Finally, investigators are evaluating practical and effective methods for early detection of DTI and for early intervention to minimize or prevent skin breakdown and tissue loss (Honaker & Forston, 2011; Honaker et al., 2013).

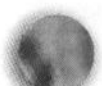

Perioperative Pressure Ulcers

The incidence of pressure ulcers in surgical patients during the perioperative period has been reported to range from 4% to 45%; this is an area where additional study is desperately needed. The patient who undergoes a long complicated orthopedic, cardiac, or abdominal surgery and is not repositioned for several hours during the intraoperative period is potentially at risk for development of pressure ulcers (Price et al., 2005). There are limited data regarding risk factors that are specific to the perioperative patient; however, at a minimum, patients with any of the following risk factors should be considered at high risk for pressure ulcer development in the operating/procedure room:

- Procedures lasting >3 hours
- Cardiac, vascular, trauma, transplant, and bariatric procedures
- BMI of <19 or >40
- Bedbound, chairbound, or unable to reposition
- Impaired sensation
- History of pressure ulcers/existing skin breakdown
- Hospital-specific risk factors (patients determined to be higher risk based on hospital data).

Prevention of perioperative pressure ulcers requires meticulous attention to padding of bony prominences, use of table pads that provide effective immersion and envelopment (e.g., high-specification foam), and consistent heel elevation (see Chapter 20 for further discussion of therapeutic surfaces). It can also be helpful to maintain the individual on an effective pressure redistribution surface pre- and postoperatively and to avoid postoperative positioning in the position the patient was in during the operative procedure (NPUAP/EPUAP/PPPIA, 2014).

CLINICAL PEARL

Prevention of perioperative pressure ulcers requires meticulous padding of bony prominences, use of a surface that provides effective envelopment and immersion, and heel elevation.

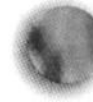

Medical Device–Related Pressure Ulcers

Acutely ill patients require a variety of medical devices (e.g., casts, traction boots, compression hose, pulmonary devices [oxygen masks and tubing, BIPAP and CPAP devices, and tracheostomy tubes], vascular access devices, and enteral feeding devices); these devices can restrict movement and increase the risk for pressure ulcers, and they can also cause localized tissue compression that can result in skin and tissue breakdown. MDrPUs are therefore receiving increased attention in terms of pathology, prevention, and management. Current guidelines for prevention of medical device–related pressure ulcers include the following key interventions:

1. Secure the device in a way that minimizes pressure against the underlying tissue; for example, tape tubes such as nasogastric tubes in a way to avoid tension/pressure against the nasal tissue.
2. Utilize foam (or comparable) dressings underneath or around rigid devices such as cervical collars, oxygen tubing, tracheostomy tubes, or gastrostomy tubes.
3. Whenever possible, remove or reposition the device at least daily, and inspect the underlying and surrounding tissue for any evidence of impending ulceration. If the device cannot be removed or repositioned, the skin around the device should be inspected.

CLINICAL PEARL

Prevention of medical device–related pressure ulcers requires tension-free taping, padding of rigid devices, and routine replacement and repositioning of the device when possible.

It is recognized that in selected situations, essential tubing and devices cannot be retaped (e.g., ECMO), and in these situations, MDrPUs may be unavoidable; however, in *most* situations, simple preventive measures can effectively prevent these wounds.

In describing/documenting MDrPUs, the nurse should be aware of two differences in staging: (1) ulcers involving mucosal tissue should not be staged as the staging system is based on the anatomy of the skin and soft tissues;

and (2) if the ulcer involves an anatomic site that lacks the standard tissue layers (epidermis, dermis, subcutaneous tissue, muscle, bone), staging must be modified accordingly; for example, a full-thickness ulcer over the bridge of the nose would be classified as Stage IV since there is no adipose tissue (NPUAP/EPUAP/PPPIA, 2014).

The wound nurse should also be aware that MDrPUs are reportable to state and federal agencies, as are those caused by pressure over bony prominences.

Avoidable versus Unavoidable Pressure Ulcers

During the NPUAP consensus conference on avoidable versus unavoidable pressure ulcers held in 2014, consensus was established for the following statements:

- Most PUs are avoidable.
- Not all PUs are avoidable.
- There are situations that render PU development unavoidable, including hemodynamic instability that is worsened with physical movement, and inability to maintain nutrition and hydration status and the presence of an advanced directive prohibiting artificial nutrition/hydration.
- Pressure redistribution surfaces cannot replace turning and repositioning.
- If enough pressure was removed from the external body, the skin cannot always survive.

CLINICAL PEARL

Pressure ulcers can be considered unavoidable only when all appropriate preventive care was provided, and the ulcer occurred anyway—it is always a retrospective determination.

Consensus was not obtained on the practicality or standard of turning patients every 2 hours or on concerns surrounding the use of medical devices vis-à-vis their potential to cause skin damage. Research is needed to examine these issues, refine preventive practices in challenging situations, and identify the limits of prevention (NPUAP/EPUAP/PPPIA, 2014).

Panelists reviewed the only existing definition of avoidable and unavoidable pressure ulcers and revised the definitions as follows: *Avoidable pressure ulcer:* An avoidable pressure ulcer can develop when the provider did *not* do one or more of the following:

- Evaluate the individual's clinical condition and pressure ulcer risk factors;
- Define and implement interventions consistent with individual needs, individual goals, and recognized standards of practice;
- Monitor and evaluate the impact of the interventions; or
- Revise the interventions as appropriate.

Unavoidable Pressure Ulcer

An unavoidable pressure ulcer can develop even though the provider evaluated the individual's clinical condition and pressure ulcer risk factors; defined and implemented interventions consistent with individual needs, goals, and recognized standards of practice; monitored and evaluated the impact of the interventions; and revised the approaches as appropriate. The panelists unanimously voted that not all pressure ulcers are avoidable because there are patient situations where pressure cannot be relieved and perfusion cannot be improved. However, the determination regarding avoidability is made after the fact, when the processes of care can be evaluated. It cannot be predetermined that an unavoidable ulcer will develop.

The purposes of the conference were realized in that consensus was reached regarding the following clinical issues:

1. There are some individuals in whom pressure ulcer development is unavoidable.
   a. Conditions were identified that may lead to unavoidable pressure ulcers (e.g., hemodynamic instability and impaired perfusion); however, these conditions do not make pressure ulcers inevitable. The duty to provide preventive care remains.
   b. There are situations and conditions that limit preventive interventions.
2. Skin failure at end of life is not the same as pressure ulcers (NPUAP/EPUAP/PPPIA, 2014).

For each of the content areas explored at this conference, current evidence suggests that prevention, early identification, and intervention have the potential to prevent deterioration and minimize tissue destruction in all settings. Goal # 1 is prevention, and most ulcers are considered preventable through simple measures such as heel elevation, routine repositioning, and use of therapeutic surfaces that provide high-level pressure redistribution as well as shear reduction. However, Curry and colleagues (2012) reported sDTIs in critically ill patients that occurred despite turning and positioning; these apparently unavoidable lesions occurred several days following a febrile state, hemodynamic instability, or respiratory acidosis. Unavoidable ulcers and sDTIs may also occur at the end of life, with skin failure, and following cardiac/respiratory arrest (Sibbald et al., 2010).

Conclusion

Pressure ulcers are a life-threatening problem among vulnerable individuals, including those who are bedbound or chairbound and those who are critically ill. The pathology of pressure ulcer development is thought to include vessel occlusion and ischemia, lymphatic vessel compression and edema, reperfusion injury, and possibly direct damage to the cytoskeleton of the muscle cell.

The major etiologic factors for pressure ulcer development are prolonged or high-intensity pressure and shear force, and individuals with multiple comorbid conditions adversely affecting tissue tolerance are at greater risk. Pressure ulcer severity ranges from preulcerative conditions (such as Stage I lesions) to full-thickness tissue loss (Stage III and IV ulcers). Pressure ulcers of particular interest at present include sDTI, which are rapidly developing lesions typically associated with very high-intensity or prolonged pressure, perioperative pressure ulcers, and medical device–related pressure ulcers. Pressure ulcer prevention requires prompt identification of the at-risk individual followed by prompt initiation of an aggressive prevention protocol.

CASE STUDIES

CASE STUDY

Mr. M. is a 68-year-old male with type II diabetes who was admitted to the hospital following a fall at home. He was cleaning out his gutters and fell off a 6′ ladder onto the ground below. He could move all extremities, but he is a large man and was unable to right himself following the accident. He stayed on his back on the ground for approximately 6 hours until his grandson came to his home to check on him after school.

Mr. M. was transported by EMS to the emergency department of the local feeder hospital where his blood glucose was regulated and radiographic studies were performed overnight. It was determined that he had sustained a fracture to the left femur. He was held in the emergency department on a stretcher and was transported to the larger community hospital the following morning.

The admitting nurse on the orthopedic unit noted a 6 cm × 8 cm purple-red discoloration at the apex of the gluteal cleft, or coccyx. It presented as symmetrical in appearance and did not blanch.

The staff nurse who noted the abnormality in the skin indicated in the electronic record that it was an area of ecchymosis from trauma sustained during the fall. Mr. M. went for orthopedic surgery (an open reduction and internal fixation, or ORIF) within an hour after being admitted. The surgery lasted just under 3 hours; MR. M. recovered for about an hour in the postanesthesia care unit and returned to the orthopedic unit.

Within 72 hours following admission, the area surrounding Mr. M's coccyx was indurated and the top layer of skin was peeling away from the discolored area. The tissue revealed beneath was dark purple with a black center. A WOC nurse was consulted for suggestions for topical care. Simultaneously, it was determined that Mr. M. could be better turned off the affected area in a bariatric bed with a low air loss feature and one was obtained. A soft, silicone foam dressing was placed over the affected area with instructions for the nursing staff to peel it back twice daily to inspect the ulcer and record their findings. The dressing was to be changed twice weekly and PRN for loosening of dressing edges or strike-through of any drainage onto the exterior of the dressing.

Mr. M. began to complain of pain in this area and the dark center evolved into a dry eschar. On day 5 following admission, wound care was changed to an enzymatic debriding agent topped with a saline-dampened gauze dressing and covered with dry dressing. Mr. M. was discharged to home with a home health care nurse and home physical therapy.

On day 9, Mr. M.'s home health nurse called the orthopedic surgeon to report that the sDTI ulcer had "opened" and revealed itself to be a Stage IV pressure ulcer. The measurements were 6 cm × 8 cm × 2.5 cm. The surgeon referred Mr. M. to the outpatient wound care center where he underwent serial debridements, pulsatile lavage sessions, and continued topical wound care using moisture retentive dressings. He required assistance and oversight for topical wound care by the home health nursing staff for 12 weeks at which time the Stage IV pressure ulcer was determined to have closed. On the advice of his physical therapist, Mr. M. limits the time he spends reclining in his recliner chair, uses a pressure redistribution chair cushion, and contracts with a local gutter-cleaning service.

DISCUSSION POINTS

1. No documentation exists for the turning and repositioning of Mr. M. in the emergency department of the feeder hospital, although we have to assume he was moved for the radiographic procedures. There is no notation of an alteration in his integumentary system. We know that the focus of his stay there was to regulate his blood glucose level and to determine the extent of his LE injury. Might a comprehensive skin assessment have revealed a tissue abnormality at that point of care?
2. Mr. M. was transported via EMS twice following his fall, once from his home to the feeder hospital and a second time from the feeder hospital to the community hospital for his surgery.
3. Upon admission to the orthopedic unit at the community hospital, the red-purple area of discoloration

that did not blanch is not captured as an area of sDTI, nor was it captured as a pressure ulcer that was present on admission (POA). Do you think this is a common error? Do you think that having two members of the nursing staff perform admission assessments might have resulted in different documentation?

4. It is known that patients who undergo operative procedures lasting >3 hours have an increased incidence of pressure ulceration. Do you think that this particular operative procedure contributed to the tissue injury and subsequent ulceration sustained by Mr. M?
5. What role would having a sleep surface of the appropriate size play in the adequate turning and repositioning of this patient off of an area that is known to be compromised?
6. It has been noted by the NPUAP that areas of sDTI *evolve* and occasionally *resolve*. There is no specific time frame agreed upon for evolution, but some suggest that it is between 3 and 10 days, even with appropriate interventions. Does Mr. M.'s presentation and evolution occur during this time frame?
7. Mr. M. is considering litigation pertaining to his "bedsore" as a result of talking to neighbors, parishioners, and some of his care providers. Do you think that there is enough information provided to substantiate a claim that any care providers were negligent?

REFERENCES

Agam, L., & Gefen, A. (2008). Toward real-time detection of deep tissue injury risk in wheelchair users using Hertz contact theory. *Journal of Rehabilitation Research and Development, 45*(4), 537–550.

Ahn, B., Rice, R., Horgas, A., & Stechmiller, J. (2014). Factors associated with suspected deep tissue injury in nursing homes: Analysis of national MDS 3.0 dataset. *Proceedings of the 26th annual Wound Healing Society and Symposium of Advanced Wound Care*, Orlando, FL.

Alderden, J., Whitney, J. D., Taylor, S. M., et al. (2011). Risk profile characteristics associated with outcomes of hospital-acquired pressure ulcers: A retrospective review. *Critical Care Nurse, 31*(4), 30–43. doi: 10.4037/ccn2011806.

Aliano, K., Low, C., Stavrides, S., et al. (2014). The correlation between ultrasound findings and clinical assessment of pressure-related ulcers: Is the extent of injury greater than what is predicted? *Surgical Technology International, 24*, 112–116.

Allen, L., McGarrah, B., Barrett, D., et al. (2012). Air-fluidized therapy in patients with suspected deep tissue injury: A case series. *Journal of Wound, Ostomy, & Continence Nursing, 39*(5), 555–561.

Ayello, E., & Braden, B. (2002). How and why to do pressure ulcer risk assessment. *Advanced Wound Care, 15*(3), 125–131.

Bader, D. L., Barnhill, R. L., & Ryan, T. J. (1986). Effect of externally applied skin surface forces on tissue vasculature. *Archives of Physical Medicine and Rehabilitation, 67*(11), 807–811.

Bates-Jensen, B. M., McCreath, H., & Pongquan, V. (2007). Testing threshold values for sub-epidermal moisture: Identifying stage I pressure ulcers in nursing home residents. *L'Escarre [French], 36*(4), 9–15.

Bates- Jensen, B. M., McCreath, H., Pongquan, V., et al. (2008). Subepidermal moisture differentiates erythema and stage I pressure ulcers in nursing home residents. *Wound Repair and Regeneration, 16*, 189–197.

Bates-Jensen, B., McCreath, H. E., & Pongquan, V. (2009). Subepidermal moisture is associated with early pressure ulcer damage in nursing home residents with dark skin tones. *Journal of Wound, Ostomy, & Continence Nursing, 36*(3), 277–284.

Bergstrom, N., Braden, B., Laguzza, A., & Holman, V. (1987). The Braden scale for predicting pressure sore risk. *Nursing Research, 36*, 205–210.

Bergstrom, N., Braden, B., Kemp, M., et al. (1996). Multi-site study of incidence of pressure ulcers and the relationship between risk level, demographic characteristics, diagnosis, and prescription of preventive intervention. *Journal of American Geriatric Society, 44*(1), 22–30.

Berlowitz, D. (2014). http://www.uptodate.com/contents/prevention-of-pressure-ulcers

Black, J. (2006). Saving the skin during kinetic bed therapy. *Nursing, 36*(10), 17. No abstract available.

Bolton, L. (2007). Which pressure ulcer risk assessment scales are valid for use in the clinical setting? *Journal of Wound Ostomy & Continence Nursing, 34*(4), 368–381.

Bouten, C. V. C., Oomens, C. W. J., Baaijens, F. P. T., et al. (2003). The aetiology of pressure sores: Skin deep or muscle bound? *Archives of Physical Medicine and Rehabilitation, 84*(4), 616–619,

Braden, B., & Bergstrom, N. (1994). Predictive validity of the Braden Scale for pressure sore risk in a nursing home population. *Research in Nursing and Health, 17*, 459–470.

Breuls, R. G., Sengers, B. G., Oomens, C. W., et al. (2002). Predicting local cell deformations in engineered tissue constructs: A multilevel finite element approach. *Journal of Biomechanical Engineering, 124*(2), 198–207.

Breuls, R. G., Bouten, C. V., Oomens, C. W., et al. (2003a). Compression induced cell damage in engineered muscle tissue: An in vitro model to study pressure ulcer aetiology. *Annals of Biomedical Engineering, 31*(11), 1357–1364.

Breuls, R. G., Bouten, C. V., Oomens, C. W., et al. (2003b). A theoretical analysis of damage evolution in skeletal muscle tissue with reference to pressure ulcer development. *Journal of Biomechanical Engineering, 125*(6), 902–909.

Bruin Biometrics (2013). *White Paper: Can Pressure Ulcers be Prevented?* http://www.bruinbiometrics.com/images/White_Papers/WP_CanPressureUlcersBePrevented_20131011_VF.pdf

Byrne, D. W., & Salzberg, C. A. (1996). Major risk factors for pressure ulcers in the spinal cord disabled: A literature review. *Spinal Cord, 34*(5), 255–263.

Ceelen, K. K., Stekelenburg, A., Loerakker, S., et al. (2008). Compression-induced damage and internal tissue strains are related. *Journal of Biomechanics, 41*(16), 3399–3404.

Chou, R., Dana, T., Bougatsos, C., et al. (2013). *Prevention: Comparative effectiveness*. Comparative Effectiveness Review No. 87. (Prepared by Oregon Evidence-based Practice Center under Contract No 290–2007-10057I) AHRQ Publication No. 12(13) -EHC148-EF. Rockville, MD: Agency for Healthcare Research and Quality. www.effectivehealthcare.ahrq.gov/reports/final.cfm

Chow, W. W., & Odell, E. I. (1978). Deformations and stresses in soft body tissues of a sitting person. *Journal of Biomechanical Engineering, 100*, 79–87.

Coleman, S., Nixon, J., Keen, J., et al. (2014). A new pressure ulcer conceptual framework. *Journal of Advanced Nursing, 70*(10), 2222–2234. doi: 10.1111/jan.12405.

Cowan, L. J., Stechmiller, J. K., & Rowe, M. (2012). Enhancing Braden pressure ulcer risk assessment in acutely ill adult veterans. *Wound Repair and Regeneration, 20*(2), 137–148. doi: 10.1111/j.1524-475X.2011.00761.x.

Curry, K., Kutash, M., Chambers, T., et al. (2012). A prospective, descriptive study of characteristics associated with skin failure in critically ill adults. *Ostomy Wound Management, 58*(5), 36–38, 40–43. Erratum in: *Ostomy Wound Management,* 58(6), 6.

Daniel, R. K., Priest, D. L., & Wheatley, D. C. (1981). Etiologic factors in pressure sores: An experimental model. *Archives of Physical Medicine and Rehabilitation, 62*(10), 492–498.

Defloor, T. (1999). The risk of pressure sores: A conceptual scheme. *Journal of Clinical Nursing, 8,* 206–216. doi: 10.1046/j.1365-2702.1999.00254.x.

Dinsdale, S. M. (1973). Decubitus ulcers in swine: Light and electron microscopy study of pathogenesis. *Archives of Physical Medicine and Rehabilitation, 54*(2), 51–56.

Dinsdale, S. M. (1974). Decubitus ulcers: Role of pressure and friction in causation. *Archives of Physical Medicine and Rehabilitation, 55*(4), 147–152.

Edsberg, L. E., Cutway, R., Anain, S., et al. (2000). Microstructural and mechanical characterization of human tissue at and adjacent to pressure ulcers. *Journal of Rehabilitation Research and Development, 37*(4), 463–471.

Elsner, J. J., & Gefen, A. (2008). Is obesity a risk factor for deep tissue injury in patients with spinal cord injury? *Journal of Biomechanics, 41*(16), 3322–3331. doi: 10.1016/j.jbiomech.2008.09.036. Epub 2008 Nov 20.

EPUAP & NPUAP. (2009). *Prevention and Treatment of Pressure Ulcers: Clinical Practice Guidelines*. Washington, DC: NPUAP.

Farid, K. J., Winkelman, C., Rizkala, A., et al. (2012). Using temperature of pressure-related intact discolored areas of skin to detect deep tissue injury: An observational, retrospective, correlational study. *Ostomy Wound Management, 58*(8), 20–31.

Fleck, C. A. (2007). Review. *Advances in Skin & Wound Care, 20*(7), 413–415.

Fogerty, M., Abumrad, N., Nanney, L., et al. (2008). Risk factors for pressure ulcers in acute care hospitals. *Wound Repair and Regeneration, 16,* 11–18.

Gawlitta, D., Li, W., Oomens, C. W., et al. (2007a). The relative contributions of compression and hypoxia to development of muscle tissue damage: An in vitro study. *Annals of Biomedical Engineering, 35*(2), 273–284.

Gawlitta, D., Oomens, C. W., Bader, D. L., et al. (2007b). Temporal differences in the influence of ischemic factors and deformation on the metabolism of engineered skeletal muscle. *Journal of Applied Physiology, 103*(2), 464–473.

Gefen, A., Farid, K., & Shaywitz, I. (2013). A review of deep tissue injury development, detection, and prevention: Shear savvy. *Ostomy Wound Management, 59*(2), 26–35.

Higashino, T., Nakagami, G., Kadono, T., et al. (2012). Combination of thermographic and ultrasonographic assessments for early detection of deep tissue injury. *International Wound Journal,* 1742–1748.

Honaker, J., & Forston, M. (2011). Adjunctive use of noncontact low-frequency ultrasound for treatment of suspected deep tissue injury: A case series. *Journal of Wound, Ostomy, & Continence Nursing, 38*(4), 394–403. doi: 10.1097/WON.0b013e31821e87eb.

Honaker, J. S., Forston, M. R., Davis, E. A., et al. (2013). Effects of noncontact low-frequency ultrasound on healing of suspected deep tissue injury: A retrospective analysis. *International Wound Journal, 10*(1), 65–72. doi: 10.1111/j.1742-481X.2012.00944.x.

Honaker, J., Brockopp, D., & Moe, K. (2014). Suspected deep tissue injury profile: A pilot study. *Advances in Skin & Wound Care, 27*(3), 133–140; quiz 141–142.

Ikebe, K., Kato, T., Yamaga, M., et al. (2001). Increased ischemia-reperfusion blood flow impairs the skeletal muscle contractile function. *Journal of Surgical Research, 99*(1), 1–6.

Krouskop, T. A. (1983). A synthesis of the factors that contribute to pressure sore formation. *Medical Hypotheses, 11*(2), 255–267.

Krouskop, T. A., Reddy, N. P., Spencer, W. A., et al. (1978). Mechanisms of decubitus ulcer formation—An hypothesis. *Medical Hypotheses, 4*(1), 37–39.

Liu, P., He, W., & Chen HL. (2012). Diabetes mellitus as a risk factor for surgery-related pressure ulcers: A meta-analysis (Review). *Journal of Wound Ostomy & Continence Nursing, 39*(5), 495–499. doi: 10.1097/WON.0b013e318265222a.

Loerakker, S., Manders, E., Strijkers, G. J., et al. (2011). The effects of deformation, ischemia, and reperfusion on the development of muscle damage during prolonged loading. *Journal of Applied Physiology, 111*(4), 1168–1177.

Lyder C. l. (2003). Pressure ulcer prevention and management. *Journal of American Medical Association, 289*(2), 223.

Lyder, C. (2007). The use of technology for improved pressure ulcer prevention. *Ostomy Wound Management, 53*(4), 14–16.

Mao, C., Rivet, A., Sidora, T., et al. (2010). Update on pressure ulcer management and deep tissue injury. *Annals of Pharmacotherapy, 44,* 325–332.

National Pressure Ulcer Advisory Panel, European Pressure Ulcer Advisory Panel and the Pan Pacific Pressure Ulcer Injury Alliance (NPUAP/EPUAP/PPPIA). (2014). Prevention and treatment of pressure ulcers: Clinical practice guideline. In E. Haesler (Ed.), Perth, Australia: Cambridge Media.

Pancorbo-Hidalgo P. L., Garcia-Fernandez F. P., Lopez-Medina I. M., et al. (2006). Risk assessment scales for pressure ulcer prevention: A systematic review. *Journal of Advanced Nursing, 54*(1), 94–110.

Papanikolaou, P., Lyne, P., & Anthony, D. (2007). Risk assessment scales for pressure ulcers: A methodological review. *International Journal of Nursing Studies, 44*(2), 285–296.

Peirce, S. M., Skalak, T. C., & Rodeheaver, G. T. (2000). Ischemia-reperfusion injury in chronic pressure ulcer formation: A skin model in the rat. *Wound Repair and Regeneration, 8*(1), 68–76.

Price, M., Whitney, J., & King, C. (2005). Development of a risk assessment tool for intraoperative pressure ulcers. *Journal of Wound Ostomy & Continence Nursing, 19–30.*

Reddy, M., Gill, S., & Rochon, P. (2006). Preventing pressure ulcers: A systematic review. *Journal of American Medical Association, 296*(8), 974–984.

Reid, R. R., Sull, A. C., Mogford, J. E., et al. (2004). A novel murine model of cyclical cutaneous ischemia-reperfusion injury. *Journal of Surgical Research, 116*(1), 172–180.

Salcido, R., Lee, A., & Ahn, C. (2011). Heel pressure ulcers: Purple heel and deep tissue injury. *Advances in Skin & Wound Care, 24*(8), 374–380.

Schoonhoven, L., Haalboom, J. R., Bousema, M. T., et al. (2002). Prospective cohort study of routine use of risk assessment scales for prediction of pressure ulcers. *British Medical Journal, 325,* 797–802.

Schoonhoven, L., Grobbee, D., & Donders, A., et al. (2006). Prediction of pressure ulcer development in hospitalized patients: A tool for risk assessment. *Quality & Safety in Health Care, 15*(1), 65–70.

Sen, C. K., Gordillo, G. M., Roy, S., et al. (2009). Human skin wounds: A major and snowballing threat to public health and the economy. *Wound Repair and Regeneration, 17*(6), 763–771.

Seongsook, J., Ihnsook, J., & Younghee, L. (2004). Validity of pressure ulcer risk assessment scales: Cubbin and Jackson, Braden, and Douglas scale. *International Journal of Nursing Studies, 41,* 199–204.

Sibbald, R. G., Krasner, D. L., & Lutz, J. (2010). SCALE: Skin changes at life's end: Final consensus statement: October 1, 2009. *Advances in Skin & Wound Care, 23*(5), 225–236; quiz 237–238. doi: 10.1097/01.ASW.0000363537.75328.36.

Smith, M. E., Totten, A., Hickam, D. H., et al. (2013). Pressure ulcer treatment strategies: A systematic comparative effectiveness review. *Annals of Internal Medicine, 159*(1), 39–50. doi: 10.7326/0003-4819-159-1-201307020-00007.

Stechmiller, J., Cowan, L, Whitney, J., et al. (2008). Guidelines for the prevention of pressure ulcers. *Wound Repair and Regeneration, 16*, 151–168.

Stekelenburg, A., Strijkers, G. J., Parusel, H., et al. (2007). Role of ischemia and deformation in the onset of compression-induced deep tissue injury: MRI-based studies in a rat model. *Journal of Applied Physiology, 102*(5), 2002–2011.

Stekelenburg, A., Gawlitta, D., Bader, D. L., et al. (2008). Deep tissue injury: How deep is our understanding? *Archives of Physical Medicine and Rehabilitation, 89*(7), 1410–1413.

Stotts, N., & Gunningberg, L. (2007). How to try this: Predicting pressure ulcer risk. *American Journal of Nursing, 107*(11), 40–48.

Sullivan, R. (2013). A two-year retrospective review of suspected deep tissue injury evolution in adult acute care patients. *Ostomy Wound Management, 59*(9), 30–39.

Unal, S., Ozmen, S., Demlr, Y., et al. (2001). The effect of gradually increased blood flow on ischemia-reperfusion injury. *Annals of Plastic Surgery, 47*(4), 412–416.

VanGilder, C., MacFarlane, G., & Meyer, S. (2008). Results of nine international pressure ulcer prevalence surveys: 1989 to 2005. *Ostomy Wound Management, 54*(2), 40–54.

VanGilder, C., MacFarlane, G. D., Harrison, P., et al. (2010). The demographics of suspected deep tissue injury in the United States: An analysis of the International Pressure Ulcer Prevalence and Suspected deep tissue injury. *Advances in Skin & Wound Care, 23*(6), 254–261. doi: 10.1097/01.ASW.0000363550.82058.7f.

QUESTIONS

1. What is the greatest risk factor for the development of pressure ulcers?
   A. Diabetes mellitus that is long-standing (>10 years)
   B. Age >75
   C. Exposure to excessive moisture
   D. African American ethnicity

2. Which of the following is NOT considered an etiologic factor for pressure ulcers?
   A. Shear force
   B. Prolonged pressure
   C. Friction
   D. Medical device–related injury

3. Which statement accurately describes one of the four major factors hypothesized to cause pressure/shear damage?
   A. Excessive perfusion of blood vessels resulting in tissue ischemia
   B. Increased risk of dehydration due to occlusion of lymph vessels
   C. Edema resulting from accumulation of oxygen free radicals
   D. Direct deformation damage of muscle cells during high-pressure loads

4. Which area of the body is the most difficult to protect using pressure redistribution surfaces?
   A. Sacrum
   B. Heel
   C. Ischial spine
   D. Skull

5. The wound care nurse is responsible for staging pressure ulcers for hospitalized patients. Which statement accurately describes a guideline for staging?
   A. sDTI lesions should always be considered as Stage I pressure ulcers.
   B. sDTI presents as a partial-thickness wound that heals predictably.
   C. Visual inspection alone is prone to error in pressure ulcer staging.
   D. Tissue damage should be inspected at the initial point of injury for staging.

6. The wound care nurse is assessing the development of a potential sDTI on a patient in the critical care unit. How do these pressure ulcers present initially?
   A. Deep purple or maroon "bruised area"
   B. Open full-thickness wound
   C. Open wound caked with black eschar
   D. Reddened patch of skin

7. Which statement describes the primary focus of management of sDTI lesions?
   A. Surgical debridement
   B. Topical therapy
   C. Use of appropriate dressings
   D. Reducing pressure and shear forces

8. Which surgical patient would the wound care nurse consider high risk for the development of pressure ulcers?
   A. A patient whose surgery lasted >2 hours
   B. A patient having a cesarean birth
   C. A patient with a BMI <19
   D. A patient with a BMI >30

9. The wound care nurse is planning care for a patient with a tracheostomy tube. What intervention would the nurse institute to prevent a medical device–related pressure ulcer?

A. Avoid using tape to secure the device.
B. Pad the device with a foam dressing.
C. Remove or reposition the device every day.
D. Use antiseptic cleansers on the skin surrounding the device.

10. Which patient would the nurse classify as high risk for developing an unavoidable pressure ulcer while hospitalized?

A. A patient who is at end of life and has severely impaired perfusion
B. A patient with long-standing diabetes mellitus and peripheral neuropathy
C. A patient with a spinal injury
D. A patient with a cardiac condition

ANSWERS: 1.**B**, 2.**C**, 3.**D**, 4.**B**, 5.**C**, 6.**A**, 7.**D**, 8.**C**, 9.**B**, 10.**A**

CHAPTER 19

Pressure Ulcer Prevention

Specific Measures and Agency-Wide Strategies

JoAnn Maklebust and Morris A. Magnan

OBJECTIVES

1. Utilize evidence-based risk assessment tool to accurately identify patients at risk for pressure ulcer development and to develop an individualized prevention plan.
2. Select/recommend appropriate redistribution devices for bed, chair, and heels.
3. Design a system to monitor prevalence of agency-acquired pressure ulcers in a clinical agency.
4. Develop an evidence-based agency-wide program for pressure ulcer prevention that includes risk assessment on admission and at appropriate intervals thereafter and prompt initiation of prevention measures for any patient found to be at risk.
5. Discuss strategies that can be used to promote an agency-wide culture of pressure ulcer prevention.

Topic Outline

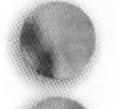

Introduction

Monitoring Pressure Ulcer Prevalence and Incidence

Calculation of Prevalence and Incidence Rates

Strategies to Promote Accuracy in Prevalence and Incidence Data Collection

Benchmarking

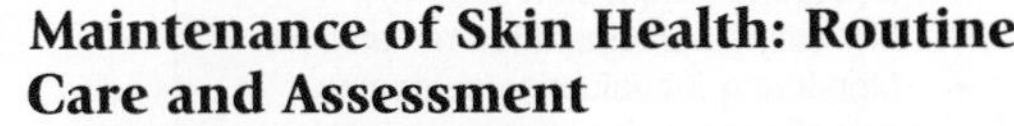

Maintenance of Skin Health: Routine Care and Assessment

Routine Skin Care

Skin Assessment

Pressure Ulcer Risk Assessment

Timing, Frequency, and General Principles

Risk Assessment Tools

The Braden Scale

Common Errors in Use of Braden Scale

Measures to Improve Accuracy in Risk Assessment

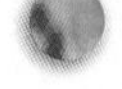

Assessment and Management of Risk Factors

Limitations in Mobility

Magnitude of Pressure versus Duration of Pressure

Preventive Measures for Limited Mobility

Support Surfaces

Protecting the Heels from Pressure Ulceration

Foam Positioning Wedges

Exposure to Friction and Shear

Friction

Shear

Prevention Strategies

Moisture

Nutrition

Program Management

Program Management at the Organizational Level

Program Management at the Departmental and Interdepartmental Level

Program Management at the Unit Level

Program Management Related to the Use of Medical Devices

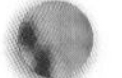

Conclusion

Introduction

The body of knowledge that informs our understanding of pressure ulcer prevention has grown immensely over the last four decades. Still, knowledge related to pressure ulcer prevention, no matter how vast, is of little value to humanity if it is not used to protect *individuals* from harm. It is the individual who is at the center of care, and it is the individual who needs to be protected from harm. In the arena of pressure ulcer prevention, the best defense against pressure ulcers is a well-developed, evidence-based prevention plan that is tailored to the individual's specific needs, conscientiously implemented, and revised as needed based on the patient's response to care.

CLINICAL PEARL

Knowledge related to pressure ulcer prevention, no matter how vast, is of little value unless it is used to protect individuals from harm.

Developing an individualized plan of care requires effort, and implementing the plan of care requires leadership and team work. A pressure ulcer prevention plan should be based on knowledge and assessment data related to the following: clinical condition (current health state and comorbidities), current skin condition, overall pressure ulcer risk status and specific risk factors, and resource availability (human and environmental) (Fig. 19-1 and Table 19-1). Knowledge pertaining to the patient's clinical presentation, skin condition, and specific risk factors provides information needed to determine what *should* be done to prevent the development of pressure ulcers. Knowledge pertaining to the availability of resources helps to determine what *can* be done. *What will be done* depends largely upon the knowledge base, motivation, commitment, and involvement of the entire health care team (i.e., patient, family, physician, nurse, physical therapist, pharmacist, dietitian, and nursing assistants). The goal of this chapter is to provide current information regarding pressure ulcer prevention and strategies for ensuring that preventive care is routinely incorporated into patient care.

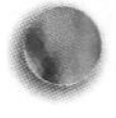

Monitoring Pressure Ulcer Prevalence and Incidence

The first step in building a successful pressure ulcer prevention program is to establish an effective monitoring system that provides periodic and ongoing assessment of pressure ulcer prevalence and incidence across the entire health care system. The wound care nurse should also monitor the degree to which best practices for pressure ulcer prevention are being used throughout the facility. In order to understand the severity of the pressure ulcer problem and the degree to which preventive care is being incorporated, information must be collected and analyzed on a routine basis, by nursing and by those responsible for quality care and performance improvement. This information includes

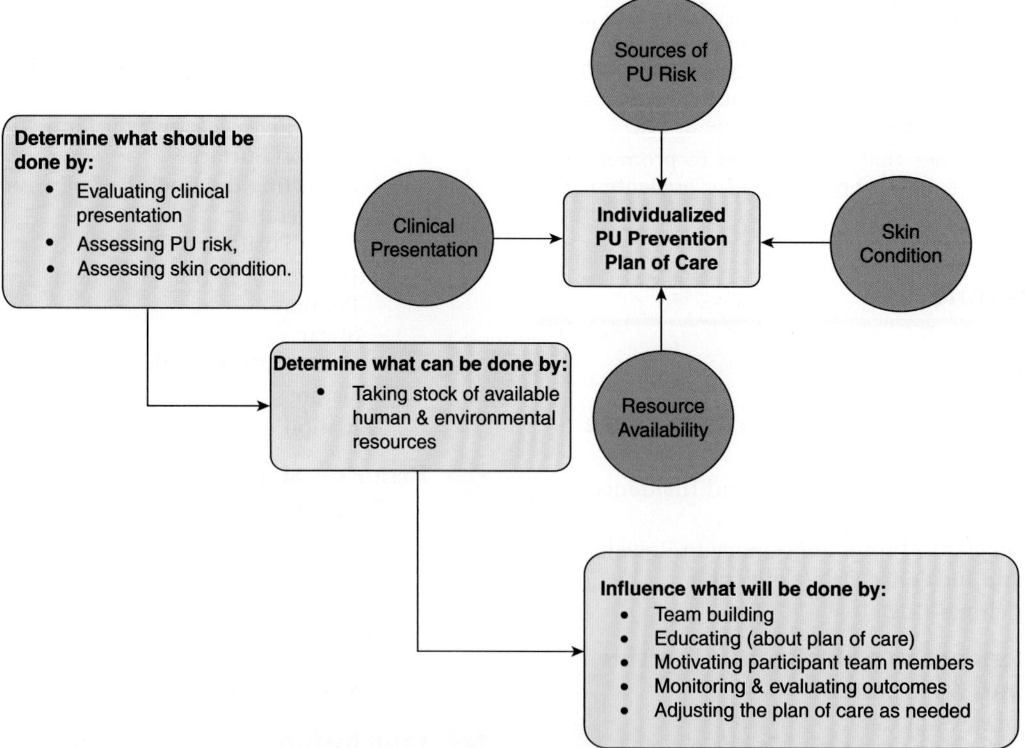

FIGURE 19-1. Model for individualized pressure ulcer prevention. (Used with permission of the National Pressure Ulcer Advisory Panel, 2015. Copyright NPUAP.)

TABLE 19-1 Example of Individualized Pressure Ulcer Prevention Plan

Risk Factors	Data	Intervention	Supportive Rationale from NPUAP/EPUAP/PPPIA Guidelines (2014) and the Literature
Limitations in mobility/activity	**PU Risk assessment data:** Braden mobility score = 1 Braden activity score 1 **Clinical presentation data:** BMI = 45; poor tolerance of lateral positioning, heart rate increase from 120 up to >200 with repositioning **Skin condition data:** Blanchable erythema right heel	Place the patient on a bariatric bed with alternating pressure low air loss mattress. Start progressive bed mobility by alternating between supine position and right lateral 15-degree tilt (monitor tolerance by assessing vital signs 10 minutes after lateral positioning). Reposition slowly to optimize adaptation to position change Use a foam wedge (with special textile covering) to help maintain position. Reposition every 2 hours; post a turning clock at the head of the bed and adjust frequency of repositioning based upon tolerance Apply protective boots to both the feet. Remove protective boots daily for heel inspection.	Select a support surface that meets the individual's needs. Consider the individual's need for pressure redistribution based on the following factors: level of immobility and inactivity, need for microclimate control and shear reduction, size and weight of the patient (NPUAP/EPUAP/PPPIA, p. 28) Use an active support surface (overlay or mattress) for individuals at higher risk of pressure ulcer development when frequent manual reposition is not possible (NPUAP/EPUAP/PPPIA, p. 29). Consider the need for additional features such as ability to control moisture and temperature when selecting a support surface (NPUAP/EPUAP/PPPIA, p. 18). Consider selecting a support surface with enhanced pressure redistribution, shear reduction, and microclimate control for bariatric individuals (NPUAP/EPUAP/PPPIA, p. 53). Consider the condition of the individual and the pressure redistribution support surface in use when deciding if repositioning should be implemented as a prevention strategy (NPUAP/EPUAP/PPPIA, p. 23). Consider slow, gradual turns allowing sufficient time for stabilization of hemodynamic and oxygenation status (NPUAP/EPUAP/PPPIA, p. 55). Establish pressure relief schedules that prescribe the frequency and duration of weight shifts (NPUAP/EPUAP/PPPIA, p. 23). Ensure that the heels are free of the surface of the bed. Use heel suspension devices that elevate and off-load the pressure completely (NPUAP/EPUAP/PPPIA, p. 27). Remove the heel suspension device periodically to assess skin integrity (NPUAP/EPUAP/PPPIA, p. 27).
Skin exposure to moisture	**PU risk assessment data:** Braden moisture score = 1 **Clinical presentation:** Sweating profusely, frequent liquid diarrhea stools contaminated with *C. difficile* **Skin condition data:** Perianal skin and skin on the buttocks intact but fire-engine red with blanchable erythema Skin under the breast and pannus intact, moist, and red	Change sheets as needed to minimize moisture contact with the skin Insert FDA-approved internal bowel management system to divert stool away from the skin Apply moisture barrier cream to the buttocks and perianal area tid and prn. Use prepackaged, pH-adjusted wipes for cleaning as needed. Place wicking textile or surgical pads under the breasts and pannus to interrupt skin-to-skin contact and wick moisture away	Develop and implement an individualized continence management program (NPUAP/EPUAP/PPPIA, p. 17). Protect the skin from exposure to excessive moisture with a barrier product in order to reduce the risk of pressure damage. Differentiate intertriginous dermatitis from category I/stage I and II pressure ulcers (NPUAP/EPUAP/PPPIA, p. 53).

(Continued)

TABLE 19-1 Example of Individualized Pressure Ulcer Prevention Plan (*Continued*)

Risk Factors	Data	Intervention	Supportive Rationale from NPUAP/EPUAP/PPPIA Guidelines (2014) and the Literature
Skin exposure to friction and shear	**PU risk assessment data:** Braden friction/shear score = 1 **Clinical presentation data:** BMI = 45; requires maximum assistance for positioning (3 to 4 care givers) **Skin condition data:** Elbows red and chafed.	Use special textile sheets only. Use a lift sheet (special textile) to lift patient up toward the head of the bed. Use a lift team of 3 to 4 nursing personnel to move patient up in bed. Contact materials management regarding bariatric lift system. Apply transparent protective dressing to both elbows.	Avoid subjecting the skin to pressure and shear forces (p. 23). Consider using silk-like fabrics rather than cotton or cotton-blend fabrics to reduce shear and friction (NPUAP/EPUAP/PPPIA, p 19). Provide safe, respectful care and avoid injuries to both the individual and health professionals (NPUAP/EPUAP/PPPIA, p. 53). Consider applying a polyurethane foam dressing to bony prominences for the prevention of pressure ulcers in anatomical areas frequently subjected to friction and shear. When selecting a prophylactic dressing consider: ability of the dressing to manage microclimate, ease of application and removal; ability to regularly asses the skin; anatomical location where the dressing will be applied;… (NPUAP/EPUAP/PPPIA, p. 18).
Nutrition	**PU risk assessment data:** Braden nutrition score = 1 **Clinical presentation data:** NPO since admission 4 days ago, increased metabolic demands from fever and agitation, fresh surgical wound	**Consult dietitian for nutritional screening.**	Screen nutrition status for each individual at risk of or with a pressure ulcer with each significant change of clinical condition (NPUAP/EPUAP/PPPIA, p. 20)

the number and percentage of patients with pressure ulcers and whether these ulcers occurred before or after admission to the facility. Determining the number and percentage of patients with pressure ulcers provides information about the size of the pressure ulcer problem in various inpatient care departments. Determining the number and percentage of ulcers that developed prior to and/or following admission provides critical information regarding the effectiveness of the current pressure ulcer prevention program. This information can be used to build a pressure ulcer best practice program for the health care facility. The same pressure ulcer data set needs to be collected periodically (usually quarterly) to determine whether the best practice program is working well or needs some improvement. In addition, many agencies find it helpful to track agency-acquired pressure ulcers on an ongoing basis and to carefully analyze the preventive care provided those patients to determine any correctable gaps (root cause analysis). Root cause analysis (RCA) is a very important study method to help determine the exact cause of a serious problem (Box 19-1). It usually requires a team of individuals who were involved in the problem to review the steps taken that may have inadvertently caused the problem. The goal is not to place blame but to determine if any steps in the care process can be changed in order to avoid having the same problem recur. As changes in the process are made, they must be made clear to all who use the process.

CLINICAL PEARL

The first step in establishing an effective pressure ulcer prevention program is to set up a program for monitoring pressure ulcer incidence on an ongoing basis.

Calculation of Prevalence and Incidence Rates

Accurate interpretation and utilization of data regarding pressure ulcer rates requires a basic understanding of how these rates are determined and factors affecting accuracy.

Traditionally research studies and quality improvement efforts that center on pressure ulcers have relied on calculations of incidence and prevalence rates. Both incidence and prevalence rates are measures of disease frequency. They each provide a perspective on the scope of the pressure ulcer problem in a given setting and at a given time. At its most basic level prevalence is the proportion of all persons who have a pressure ulcer in a specific setting at a specific point in time [point prevalence], or period of time [period prevalence]. In contrast, incidence

BOX 19-1. Sample Root Cause Analysis Form

Root Cause Analysis
Unit:____________
Site of Ulcer:____________
Date Ulcer First Identified:____________
Ulcer Stage When First Identified:____________
Risk Assessment Done on Admission? Yes (score)________
No________
Risk Assessment Done At Least Daily Following Admission?
Yes, Consistently________ Sometimes________
No________
Risk Assessment Scores Consistent with Pt Status as Documented in Record?
Yes________ No (explain)____________________
If pt found to be at risk:
Prevention Protocol Initiated Immediately? Yes____ No____
Not Clear____

Trunk Wound:
- Pt on appropriate support surface? Yes____ No____

Date patient placed on current surface:____________
- T & P q2 to 3hrs and documented? Yes____ No____ Partial____
- Skin status documented at least daily? Yes ____ No____ Partial____
- Nutritional consult? Yes ____ No____ Not indicated (no evidence nutritional compromise) ____

Ulcer Under Medical Device:
- Type of medical device:____________
- Duration of use prior to ulcer development:____________
- Protective measures utilized? Yes____ No____ Yes, but inconsistently or only after breakdown noted:____________

Heel Ulcer:
- Heel elevation consistently maintained? Yes ____ No____ Partial____
- Support stockings/SCDs removed at least bid & skin status doc? Yes____ No____ N/A____

Contributing Factors:
- Hemodynamic instability (describe severity, duration, and time frame in relation to ulcer development): ____________
- Patient/family nonadherence to prevention program despite education (specify areas of program in which pt not in compliance, education provided, frequency and duration of non compliance, time frame in relation to ulcer development):
- Has pt been off unit for >4 consecutive hours within past 3 days?

Yes (specify)________ No________
- Other:____________

Conclusion:
____All appropriate preventive measures implemented; ulcer not avoidable
____Gaps in preventive measures
Specify:____________
____Ulcer most likely began when pt off unit
Recommendations:

is the proportion of persons at risk who develop new pressure ulcers during a specific period of time [cumulative incidence], or who develop new ulcers relative to the number of ulcer free days [incidence density]. While prevalence and incidence rates are a standard tool for use in epidemiology research and quality improvement, they do have limitations. For example, prevalence of pressure ulcers provides information about the number of persons with the problem, but does not tell the clinician whether or not the ulcers developed following admission. To address some of these limitations, efforts to describe pressure ulcer rates are increasingly using a "hybrid" approach that incorporates elements of both prevalence and incidence studies in order to calculate what is known as the "facility-acquired" prevalence rate (e.g., Hospital Acquired Pressure Ulcer rate, or HAPU rate) (Berlowitz, 2012, p. 19).[1]

Formulas used to calculate prevalence and incidence rates are shown in **Table 19-2**. Berlowitz (2012) provided excellent, detailed information about the interpretation of prevalence, incidence, and facility-acquired rates, but the most critical data for the clinician developing and monitoring a pressure ulcer prevention program are the incidence or "facility-acquired" rates. In most agencies, studies are conducted quarterly, and this is a requirement for all Magnet facilities; typically, the data required are "point prevalence" data. In addition, some agencies have implemented an ongoing tracking system that allows them to do root cause analysis for any new ulcer that is pressure related. With this system, the staff immediately reports any lesion thought to be pressure related to the wound care team; a member of the wound care team then assesses the patient to determine whether or not the lesion is pressure related. If the lesion *is* determined to be pressure related, all preventive care is reviewed to determine whether there were any areas in which preventive care could be improved (root cause analysis). With this approach, the data used for monitoring also provide the specific information needed to improve the prevention program. For example, if root cause analysis reveals heel ulcers associated with failure to provide consistent heel elevation, a very targeted improvement program can be initiated. In contrast, if root cause analysis reveals that all preventive care *is* being consistently implemented and that ulcers are occurring only in critically ill patients on vasopressors, no corrective action is needed.

CLINICAL PEARL

Root cause analysis involves critical assessment of the care provided to patients with agency-acquired pressure ulcers to identify any gaps in care, with the intent of improving care processes.

[1]Reprinted with permission from Berlowitz, D. (2012). Prevalence, incidence and facility-acquired rates. In B. Pieper (Ed.), *Pressure ulcers: Prevalence, incidence, and implications for the future* (pp. 19–24). Washington, DC: National Pressure Ulcer Advisory Panel. Used with permission of the National Pressure Ulcer Advisory Panel 2014.

TABLE 19-2 Formulas Used to Calculate Prevalence and Incidence

Formula Name	Calculation
Pressure Ulcer Point Prevalence	$\frac{\text{Number of persons with a pressure ulcer} \times 100}{\text{Number of persons in population at a particular point in time}}$
Pressure Ulcer Period Prevalence	$\frac{\text{Number of persons with a pressure ulcer} \times 100}{\text{Number of persons in population at a particular time period}}$
Pressure Ulcer Cumulative Incidence	$\frac{\text{Number of persons developing new pressure ulcers} \times 100}{\text{Total number of persons in population at beginning of time period}}$
Pressure Ulcer Incidence Density	$\frac{\text{Number of persons developing new pressure ulcers} \times 100}{\text{Total patient days free of ulcers}}$
Facility Acquired Rate	$\frac{[(\text{\# of persons with a pressure ulcer}) - (\text{\# of people with same ulcer on admission})] \times 100}{(\text{\# of person in a population at a particular point}) - (\text{\# of people with same ulcer on admission})}$

Adapted from Berlowitz, D. (2012). Prevalence, incidence and facility-acquired rates. In B. Pieper (Ed.), *Pressure ulcers: Prevalence, incidence, and implications for the future* (pp. 19–24). Washington, DC: National Pressure Ulcer Advisory Panel. Used with permission of the National Pressure Ulcer Advisory Panel (2014).

Strategies to Promote Accuracy in Prevalence and Incidence Data Collection

In order for the data provided by prevalence and incidence studies to be of value, the studies must be done correctly and consistently. Directions for conducting a house-wide pressure ulcer audit can be accessed from the National Data Base for Nursing Quality Indicators (Press Ganey's NDNQI, 2014) Module III. It is advisable for everyone on the NDNQI audit team to read the entire module and to complete the competency exercises included in the module. In addition, the wound care team must continually reinforce key points and must take measures to ensure accuracy. Strategies to promote accuracy of prevalence and incidence data obtained during quarterly studies include the following: (1) ongoing education to all survey team members regarding wound classification and pressure ulcer staging, (2) wound team member availability during surveys to assist with classification or staging of challenging wounds, and (3) spot audits conducted by wound team members to verify the accuracy of wound classification and wound staging.

CLINICAL PEARL

Strategies to improve accuracy in prevalence and incidence studies include education of all survey team members, wound nurse support, and spot audits.

Benchmarking

The data obtained from facility-wide surveys should be compared to data from similar facilities as one indicator of the effectiveness of the prevention program; this "benchmarking" data is also used by independent quality monitoring programs as one indicator of the quality of nursing care.

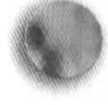

Maintenance of Skin Health: Routine Care and Assessment

Key components of any skin protection program include appropriate routine skin care to maintain skin health and routine skin assessment to detect any impending or actual alteration in skin status. As explained in Chapter 1, the skin plays a critical role in protecting the body from excess water loss and from infection, in addition to contributing to temperature regulation and vitamin D production (Dealy, 2009). In neonates and in the elderly, the skin is thinner and less resilient; this is also true of the skin in malnourished individuals and those on long-term steroids. Thus, these individuals require even more meticulous skin care and assessment.

Routine Skin Care

Maintaining the skin in a healthy state and early detection of injury to the skin are nursing responsibilities that should not be taken lightly. Regular cleansing can help keep the skin healthy but can be damaging if harsh, alkaline soaps are used. Often warm water is all that is needed to cleanse the skin adequately (Maklebust & Sieggreen, 2001). Moisturizing agents applied immediately after bathing while the skin is still damp but not wet will help to keep the skin supple. With respect to cleansing equipment, the washbasin has been the standard piece of equipment used by nurses for many years. However, research has shown that washbasins are a source of bacteria and may be linked to the transmission of hospital-acquired infections (HAIs) (Johnson et al., 2009; Marchaim et al., 2012). The human and economic costs of HAIs are high: approximately two million patients suffer from HAIs with hospital admission rates averaging 5% to 10%, and cost of HAIs in the United States is estimated at $20 billion each year (Palmore, 2010). For these reasons, using prepackaged, premoistened, rinse-free, disposable cleansing cloths are gaining greater acceptance as an alternative to use of conventional bath basins and washcloths.

CLINICAL PEARL

Use of commercially available disposable cleansing wipes helps to maintain skin health and also reduces the risk of infection associated with use of bath basins.

Skin Assessment

Regular assessment and examination of the skin is a critical component of pressure ulcer prevention. Assessment of the skin should include identification of factors that may decrease the resilience of the skin such as age-related thinning of the skin, malnutrition and dehydration, exposure to moisture, excessive dryness, and the individual's overall health status (Dealy, 2009). Specifically, the EPUAP/NPUAP (2009) recommends the following in regard to skin assessment: (1) ensuring a complete skin assessment as part of the pressure ulcer risk assessment, (2) educating professionals about how to do a comprehensive skin assessment, and (3) regular inspection of the skin for signs of redness.

For patients at risk for pressure ulcers, the skin should be inspected daily with special attention to the skin over bony prominences (e.g., sacrum and coccyx, ischial tuberosities, greater trochanters, and heels) (NPUAP/EPUAP/PPPIA, 2014) and the skin in contact with medical devices (e.g., the area where a nasal cannula is looped over the ear). In addition, the nursing team should be alert to components of medical supplies and equipment that are frequently found in the patient's bed as "bed trash" (e.g., needle covers, rolls of tape, ink pens and covers, disposable instruments). Skin inspection should also involve a careful inspection of the bed to ensure that these unwanted components are removed and do not act as an additional source of pressure on the skin.

CLINICAL PEARL

Daily skin inspection is a critical element of care for individuals at risk for pressure ulcers. Stockings, heel protectors, and anything obstructing the skin must be removed for skin inspection.

With respect to inspection of the heels, heel protectors/boots, dressings, stockings, and anything that obstructs direct visual inspection of the skin must be removed to adequately assess the condition of the skin and underlying tissues. Inspection of the lateral and medial malleoli should be conducted during inspection of the heels. A body diagram (Fig. 19-2) can be used to accurately document the location of any abnormal findings such as bruises, abrasions, and areas of nonblanchable erythema. It is particularly important to "name" pressure-related injuries based on the underlying prominence and to avoid vague anatomical terms (e.g., trochanter as opposed to the "hip," medial malleolus as opposed to the "ankle").

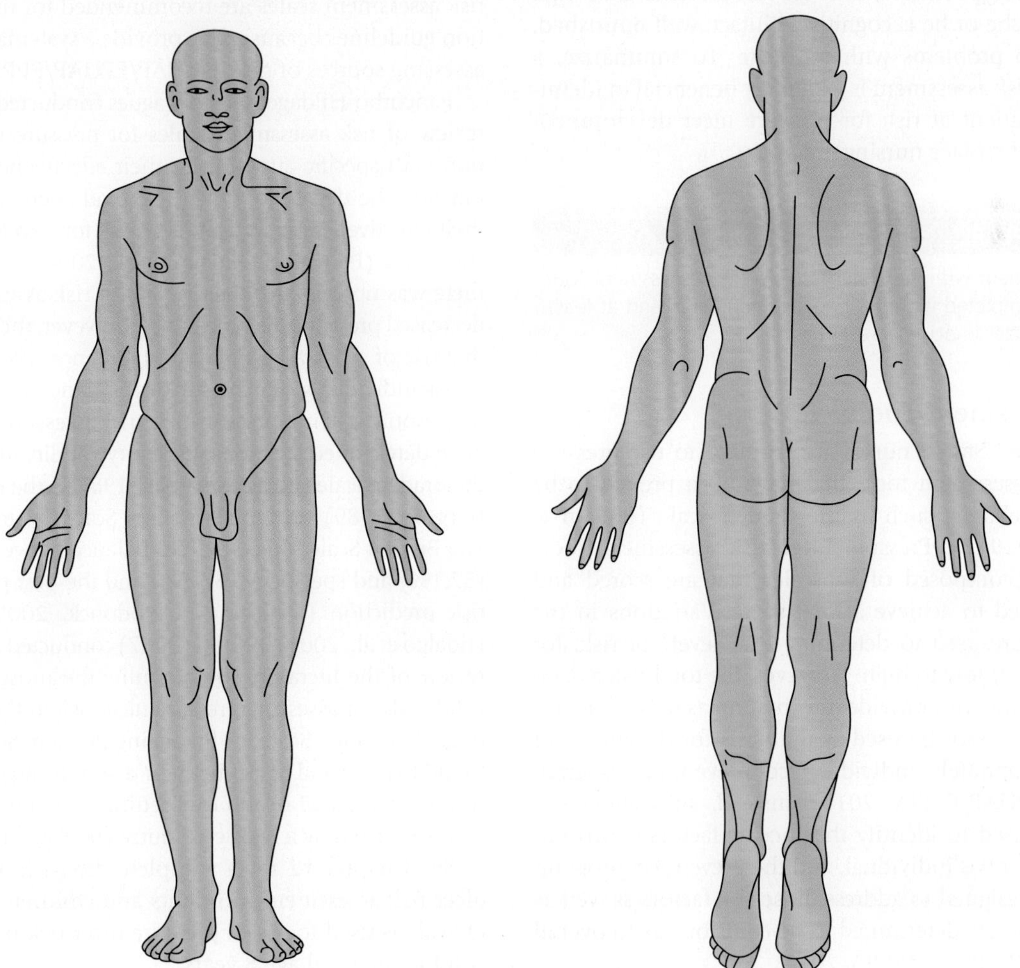

FIGURE 19-2. Body diagram for recording skin injuries.

Pressure Ulcer Risk Assessment

Pressure ulcer (PU) prevention begins upon admission with a structured assessment of the individual's risk for developing a pressure ulcer. There is no agreed upon best approach to assessing risk. However, there is some consensus that using a "structured" approach will yield better determinations about level of risk and sources of risk because it facilitates consideration of all relevant risk factors (NPUAP/EPUAP/PPPIA, 2014).

Timing, Frequency, and General Principles

Risk for pressure ulcer development should be determined within 8 hours of admission and at regular intervals thereafter (NPUAP/EPUAP/PPPIA, 2014). Typically, the frequency of reassessment of risk is every 24 hours for acute care patients deemed to be at risk. However, more frequent reassessments may be needed based upon the patient's clinical presentation and/or institutional policy. At minimum, determinations about risk and sources of risk should be based upon data obtained from completion of a valid and reliable pressure ulcer risk assessment tool. Additional data obtained from a comprehensive clinical assessment (including skin assessment) further informs decisions about risk status; for example, an elderly individual who is critically ill, hypotensive, and on vasopressors is at high risk even if she or he is cognitively intact, well nourished, and has no problems with moisture. To summarize, a structured risk assessment is extremely beneficial in identifying the patient at risk for pressure ulcer development but does not replace nursing judgment.

CLINICAL PEARL

Risk assessment with an evidence-based risk assessment tool must be completed within 8 hours of admission and at least daily thereafter in acute care settings.

Risk Assessment Tools

In the United States, nurses are required to use pressure ulcer risk assessment tools that have been proven to be valid and reliable, such as the Braden Scale (Braden & Bergstrom, 1987). Pressure ulcer risk assessment tools are usually composed of subscales that are scored and then summed to achieve a total score. Variations in the total score are used to determine the "level" of risk, for example, from low to high. However, the total risk assessment score does not provide information as to specific risk factors and cannot be used as the basis for development of an appropriately individualized prevention program (NPUAP/EPUAP/PPPIA, 2014). Instead, subscale scores should be used to identify the specific factors contributing to risk for *this* individual, and the prevention program should be designed to address those risk factors as well as any other factors determined to be contributors to overall risk (NPUAP/EPUAP/PPPIA, 2014).

CLINICAL PEARL

Prevention protocols should not be based only on the total risk assessment score; subscale scores should be used to identify specific risk factors for the individual patient.

Pressure ulcer risk assessment was haphazard prior to the introduction of risk assessment scales and usually consisted of a nurse caregiver's clinical judgment. Edwards (1994) reported on the rationale for use of risk assessment calculators in pressure ulcer prevention and on the reliability and validity of published scales. There are multiple intrinsic and extrinsic factors that have been associated with increased risk for pressure ulcers; risk assessment tools were developed in an attempt to incorporate these multiple factors into a simple assessment tool that would accurately identify patients at greatest risk, thus permitting appropriate allocation of prevention equipment and prevention interventions. At least 40 pressure ulcer risk assessment scales have been developed by researchers and clinicians from the United States and Europe (Nixon et al., 2005). These scales are used to identify the level of pressure ulcer risk along a severity continuum of low, medium, or high risk. The relationship between pressure ulcer risk assessment scores and pressure ulcer incidence is not firmly established. Still, risk assessment scales are recommended for use in prevention guidelines because they provide a systematic means of assessing sources of risk (NPUAP/EPUAP/PPPIA, 2014).

Pancorbo-Hildago and colleagues conducted a systematic review of risk assessment scales for pressure ulcer prevention with specific attention to their effectiveness in clinical practice, the degree to which they had been validated, and their effectiveness as indicators of risk for developing a pressure ulcer (Pancorbo-Hildago et al., 2006). In this review, there was no evidence that the use of risk assessment scales decreased pressure ulcer incidence; however, there *is* evidence that use of a risk assessment tool enhances identification of at-risk individuals, which provides guidance in use of preventive resources. Three pressure ulcer risk assessment scales have been determined to have satisfactory validity and reliability: the Braden Scale (Bergstrom et al., 1987a), the Norton Score (Norton, 1989), and the Waterlow Scale (Waterlow, 1985). The Braden Scale offers the best balance between sensitivity (57.1%) and specificity (67.5%) and the best pressure ulcer risk prediction (Defloor & Grypdonck, 2005; Pancorbo-Hidalgo et al., 2006). Bolton (2007) conducted an integrated review of the literature to determine the most reliable and valid scale for assessing pressure ulcer risk in the clinical setting. The Braden Scale for Predicting Pressure Sore Risk© was found to be a valid instrument for determining pressure ulcer risk in a variety of health care settings when the assessment was conducted by a registered nurse (Bolton, 2007).

See Chapter 12 for a complete discussion of pressure ulcer risk assessment in infants and children. The Braden Q Scale is used to assess pressure ulcer risk in infants and children up until age 8 years.

The Braden Scale

The Braden Scale for Predicting Pressure Sore Risk© was introduced into the literature in 1987 by Braden and Bergstrom (Braden & Bergstrom, 1987; Bergstrom et al., 1987a; Bergstrom et al., 1987b) and was based on a conceptual model of the etiologic factors contributing to pressure ulcer development. Their schema (Fig. 19-3) included two main etiologic factors: pressure against the tissue and the tissue's ability to tolerate pressure. Together, these two etiologic factors were theorized to determine a person's likelihood for developing pressure ulcers. Individual risk factors either increased the likelihood of prolonged pressure or reflected reduced tissue tolerance to pressure.

The Braden Scale (Fig. 19-4) directs nurses to assess and score six specific risk factors that contribute to pressure ulcer risk: sensory–perceptual level, exposure of the skin to moisture, activity level, mobility level, nutritional intake, and exposure to friction and shear. Each of these subscales is rated from 1 to 4 except the friction–shear subscale, which is rated from 1 to 3. Each rating is accompanied by a brief description of the criteria for assigning the rating. When the six subscales are summed, the total Braden Scale score ranges from 6 to 23.

Braden Scale scores reflect five levels of pressure ulcer risk: generally not at risk (19 to 23), mild risk (15 to 18), moderate risk (13 to 14), high risk (10 to 12), and very high risk (≤9) (Bergstrom & Braden, 2002; Braden & Maklebust, 2005). The Braden Scale score is an inverse measurement of risk; that is, a lower Braden Scale score indicates higher risk for developing pressure ulcers. A cut-off score of 18 or below is considered predictive of pressure ulceration in all care settings and all ethnic groups (Braden & Bergstrom, 1994; Bergstrom & Braden, 2002; Braden & Maklebust, 2005; Lyder et al., 1999).

Since its inception in 1987, the Braden Scale has undergone extensive reliability and validity testing. Validity refers to the ability of an instrument to accurately reflect or represent what it is intended to measure (Polit & Beck, 2011). The ability of the Braden Scale to accurately predict pressure ulceration has been studied extensively across settings including intensive care (Bergstrom et al., 1995), acute care (Bergstrom et al., 1987b), multisite, acute tertiary care, Veterans Administration Medical Center (VAMC) (Bergstrom et al., 1998), skilled rehabilitation (Braden & Bergstrom, 1987, 1994), home care (Bergquist & Frantz, 2001), and nursing home settings (Bergstrom

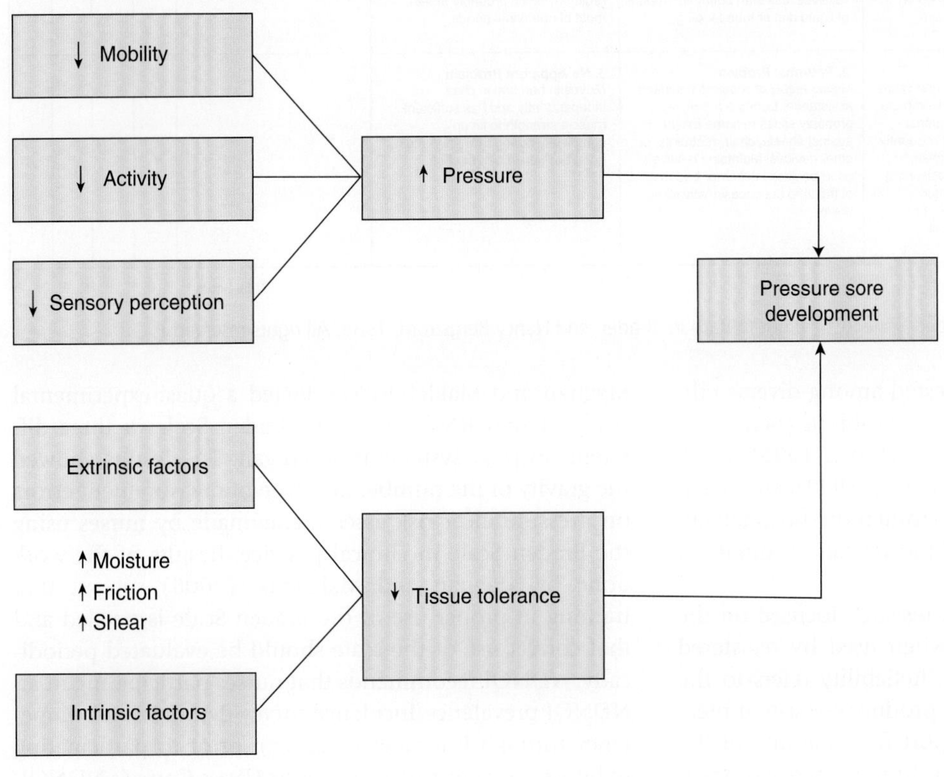

FIGURE 19-3. Braden Scale schema. (Reprinted from Braden, B. (1987). A conceptual schema for the study of the etiology of pressure sores. *Rehabilitation Nursing*, *12*(1), 9, with permission of the Association of Rehabilitation Nurses. Copyright © 1987 by the Association of Rehabilitation Nurses.)

BRADEN SCALE FOR PREDICTING PRESSURE SORE RISK

Patient's Name ____________ Evaluator's Name ____________ Date of Assessment

SENSORY PERCEPTION Ability to respond meaning-fully to pressure-related discomfort	**1. Completely Limited** Unresponsive (does not moan, flinch, or grasp) to painful stimuli, due to diminished level of consciousness or sedation, OR limited ability to feel pain over most of body.	**2. Very Limited** Responds only to painful stimuli. Cannot communicate discomfort except by moaning or restlessness, OR has a sensory impairment which limits the ability to feel pain or discomfort over ½ of body.	**3. Slightly Limited** Responds to verbal com-mands but cannot always communicate discomfort or the need to be turned, OR has some sensory impairment which limits ability to feel pain or discomfort in one or two extremities.	**4. No Impairment** Responds to verbal commands. Has no sensory deficit which would limit ability to feel or voice pain or discomfort.				
MOISTURE Degree to which skin is exposed to moisture	**1. Constantly Moist** Skin is kept moist almost constantly by perspiration, urine, etc. Dampness is detected every time patient is moved or turned.	**2. Very Moist** Skin is often but not always moist. Linen must be changed at least once a shift.	**3. Occasionally Moist** Skin is occasionally moist, requiring an extra linen change approximately once a day.	**4. Rarely Moist** Skin is usually dry; linen only requires changing at routine intervals.				
ACTIVITY Degree of physical activity	**1. Bedfast** Confined to bed.	**2. Chairfast** Ability to walk severely limited or non-existent. Cannot bear own weight and/or must be assisted into chair or wheelchair.	**3. Walks Occasionally** Walks occasionally during day, but for very short distances, with or without assistance. Spends majority of each shift in bed or chair.	**4. Walks Frequently** Walks outside room at least twice a day and inside room at least once every 2 hours during waking hours.				
MOBILITY Ability to change and control body position	**1. Completely Immobile** Does not make even slight changes in body or extremity position without assistance.	**2. Very Limited** Makes occasional slight changes in body or extremity position but unable to make frequent or significant changes independently.	**3. Slightly Limited** Makes frequent though slight changes in body or extremity position independently.	**4. No Limitations** Makes major and frequent changes in position without changes.				
NUTRITION Usual food intake pattern	**1. Very Poor** Never eats a complete meal. Rarely eats more than 1/3 of any food offered. Eats two servings or less of protein (meat or dairy products) per day. Takes fluids poorly. Does not take a liquid dietary supplement, OR is NPO and/or maintained on clear liquids or IVfor more than 5 days.	**2. Probably Inadequate** Rarely eats a complete meal and generally eats only about ½ of any food offered. Protein intake includes only three servings of meat or dairy products per day. Occasionally will take a dietary supplement OR receives less than optimum amount of liquid diet or tube feeding.	**3. Adequate** Eats over half of most meals. Eats a total of four servings of protein (meat, dairy products) each day. Occasionally will refuses a meal, but will usually take a supplement when offered, OR is on a tube feeding or TPN regimen, which probably meets most of nutritional needs.	**4. Excellent** Eats most of every meal. Never refuses a meal. Usually eats a total of four or more servings of meat and dairy products. Occasionally eats between meals. Does not require supplementation.				
FRICTION & SHEAR	**1. Problem** Requires moderate to maximum assistance in moving. Complete lifting without sliding against sheets is impossible. Frequently slides down in bed or chair, requiring frequent repositioning with maximum assistance. Spasticity, contractures, or agitation leads to almost constant friction.	**2. Potential Problem** Moves feebly or requires minimum assistance. During a move, skin probably slides to some extent against sheets, chair, restraints, or other devices. Maintains relatively good position in chair or bed most of the time but occasionally slides down.	**3. No Apparent Problem** Moves in bed and in chair independently and has sufficient muscle strength to lift up completely during move. Maintains good position in bed or chair.					
				Total Score				

FIGURE 19-4. Braden Scale. (Copyright © Barbara Braden and Nancy Bergstrom, 1988. All rights reserved.)

et al., 1987a). It has also been tested among diverse ethnic groups, including Black and White subjects (Bergstrom & Braden, 2002), ethnic minorities (Lyder, 1996), Black and Latino/Hispanic elders (Lyder et al., 1999), and Asian patients, including those in rehabilitation hospitals in China (Pang & Wong, 1998) and acute care hospitals in China (Kwong et al., 2005).

Until recently, there was little research focused on the reliability of the Braden Scale when used by registered nurses (RNs) in clinical settings. Reliability refers to the capacity of a measuring device to produce consistent measures (Polit & Beck, 2011). Support for reliability of the Braden Scale as a screening tool in clinical practice is based on five studies, most of which involved nurses participating in research studies in nursing home settings (Bergstrom et al., 1987a; Bergstrom et al., 1987b; Halfens et al., 2000).

Common Errors in Use of Braden Scale

Empirical support for the reliability of the Braden Scale when used by RNs in acute care settings is sparse. In 2008, Magnan and Maklebust conducted a quasi-experimental study of staff RNs' use of the Braden Scale in three different hospital systems in Michigan. The results showed the gravity of the number and type of measurement errors on pressure ulcer risk assessments made by nurses using the Braden Scale in clinical practice. Results of the work done by Magnan and Maklebust (2008) suggest that training in proper use of the Braden Scale is needed and that correct use of the scale should be evaluated periodically. NDNQI recommends that nurses participating in an NDNQI prevalence/incidence survey demonstrate competency through interrater agreement prior to participating in housewide pressure ulcer audits (Press Ganey's NDNQI, 2014, Module III).

Clinical nurse specialists, wound nurse specialists, and other wound team members report seeing staff nurses make repeated errors and misapplications of the Braden Scale in daily clinical practice. Perhaps the most egregious misapplication occurs when nurses arbitrarily assign a Braden Scale total score of "19" or juggle subscale scores to achieve a total score of "19" to avoid having to design and implement a pressure ulcer prevention plan. Other errors and misapplications include copying the score obtained by a previous provider, using the same score every day, choosing a subscale score without comparing the clinical data to the defined subscale criteria, choosing a numerical rating from the subscale without reading the criteria, and choosing poor nutrition when the patient is only NPO overnight for a procedure.

CLINICAL PEARL

Common errors in risk assessment include copying results obtained by a previous provider, underestimation of risk, and choosing a subscale score without comparing clinical data to the defined criteria.

Measures to Improve Accuracy in Risk Assessment

Strategies that can be used to improve accuracy in risk assessment include ongoing education for nurses using interactive teaching strategies (such as the NDNQI module) and emphasizing the caveat "when in doubt, score low" to assure that at-risk patients are identified and protected. It is also helpful to conduct periodic spot audits of Braden Scale score accuracy by comparing Braden subscale scores with an expert validator. Some clinicians incorporate Braden Scale risk assessment and prevention planning into annual skills days by creating a patient scenario and having the nurses complete a risk assessment and select prevention measures for the "scenario patient." Data obtained from audits and skills fairs can be used to enhance ongoing staff education related to pressure ulcer prevention.

CLINICAL PEARL

One strategy for improving accuracy in risk assessment is to follow the caveat "when in doubt, score low"; another is to teach risk assessment using interactive strategies.

Assessment and Management of Risk Factors

Limitations in Mobility

Mobility is considered limited whenever there is a reduction in an individual's frequency of movement or ability to move (e.g., ability to independently reposition oneself in a bed or chair). Limitations in mobility are distinguished from restrictions in activity such as when a patient is bedfast or chairfast (NPUAP/EPUAP/PPPIA, 2014). Limited and/or impaired mobility is an especially worrisome risk factor for pressure ulcer development because of the increased potential for exposure of tissues to prolonged and/or intense pressure. Moreover, the prevalence of more severe ulcers (stage III and stage IV) is greater among those who are completely immobile (Lahmann & Kottner, 2011).

Magnitude of Pressure versus Duration of Pressure

Research has shown that the damaging effects of pressure are related to both the magnitude of the pressure and the duration of the pressure. As early as 1959, Kosiak, using an animal (anesthetized dogs) model, demonstrated that pressure ulcers occurred when tissues were exposed to high-pressure loads for short periods of time and when tissues were exposed to low-pressure loads for longer periods of time (Kosiak, 1959). From Kosiak's work, it can be shown that plotting the amount of time tissue is exposed to pressure against the amount of pressure applied to the tissue (the time-at-pressure curve) takes the form of an inverse parabola. Reswick and Rogers (1976) studied time–pressure relationships in human subjects with spinal cord injury and found the same time–pressure relationship in humans that Kosiak observed in dogs. The now famous Reswick-Rogers curve is shown in Figure 19-5.

Insights into the time–pressure relationships revealed by the work of Kosiak (1959) and Reswick and Rogers (1976) make it clear that off-loading pressure and limiting the amount of time tissues are exposed to pressure are critical components of pressure ulcer prevention. Persons with normal sensation and no limitations in mobility can independently off-load pressures as often as is needed to prevent tissue damage. For example, after sitting in one position without moving, the unimpaired person will sense discomfort in the buttocks and independently change position to off-load or redistribute pressure, even in his or her sleep. Persons with limited mobility may sense discomfort, but they need assistance because they may not or cannot off-load pressure independently.

CLINICAL PEARL

Reducing the intensity of pressure (through use of support surfaces) and reducing the duration of pressure (through repositioning) are critical strategies in pressure ulcer prevention.

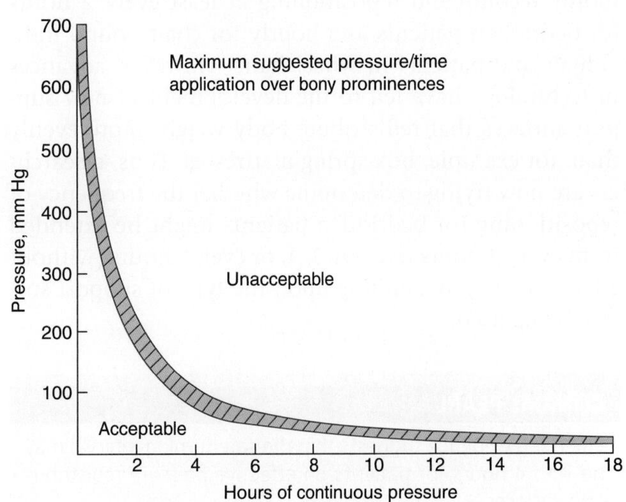

FIGURE 19-5. Reswick-Rogers curve.

Preventive Measures for Limited Mobility

Pressure ulcer prevention for persons with limited mobility must focus on proactively limiting the magnitude of pressure (load) over bony prominences and limiting the duration (length of time) the tissue is exposed to pressure.

Support Surfaces

Limiting the magnitude of pressure on vulnerable areas is managed by proper selection and use of support surfaces to redistribute pressure (Sprigle, 2000). Limiting the duration of exposure to pressure is managed by repositioning and weight shifting (Sprigle, 2000). Even small shifts in body weight can be helpful.

Routine Repositioning

Repositioning (e.g., turning) patients is a well-recognized and long-standing nursing intervention and is a consistent element of evidence-based pressure ulcer prevention guidelines in the United States, Europe, and Australia (NPUAP/EPUAP/PPPIA, 2014). Repositioning is commonly understood as manually moving the patient into another position to relieve pressure off a particular part of the body or to redistribute the pressure on a body part. In a recent meta-analysis, Gillespie et al. (2014) noted that the evidence to support the use of repositioning to prevent pressure ulcers is low in both volume and quality; however, this does not mean that repositioning is ineffective or unnecessary (Gillespie et al., 2014). To the contrary, a pressure ulcer prevention program that does not include a repositioning schedule would be deemed deficient based on current best practice prevention guidelines (NPUAP/EPUAP/PPPIA, 2014).

As noted earlier, pressure intensity and the amount of time body tissues are exposed to pressure work together to cause pressure ulcers. Therefore, the twofold aim of repositioning should be to (1) reduce or relieve pressure at the interface between bony prominences and the support surface and (2) limit the amount of time the tissues are exposed to pressure. Best practice guidelines commonly recommend repositioning at least every 2 hours for bedridden patients and hourly for chair-bound individuals and patients in wheelchairs. However, advances in technology have led to the development of new support surfaces that redistribute body weight more evenly than, for example, box-spring mattresses. Thus, researchers are now trying to determine whether the frequency of repositioning for bedridden patients might be extended from every 2 hours to every 3, 4, or even 6 hours (without adverse effect), depending upon the type of support surface being used.

CLINICAL PEARL

Emerging evidence suggests that the safe turning interval may be 3 to 4 hours for patients on effective pressure redistribution surfaces.

In a well-designed randomized clinical trial (RCT) involving nursing home patients ($N = 942$) in the United States and Canada, Bergstrom and colleagues (2013) compared the effects of repositioning at 2-, 3-, and 4-hour intervals on the incidence of pressure ulcers. In this study, all nursing homes were using high-density foam mattresses, and patients were admitted to the study if they were aged 65 years or older and at moderate (Braden score = 13 to 14) or high (Braden score = 10 to 12) risk for developing pressure ulcers. Findings showed an overall low incidence (2% of participants) of superficial pressure ulcers, stage I or stage II, and no statistically significant difference in the incidence of pressure ulcers observed by risk category or turning schedule. Thus, when elderly nursing home patients are bedded on high-density foam mattresses turning at 3- and 4-hour intervals seems to be as effective in preventing pressure ulcers as turning every 2 hours. However, one needs to consider that the study protocol called for consistent and careful documentation every time the patient was repositioned. This documentation included position, brief checks for incontinence, skin condition, and skin care provided. The authors of the study have speculated that the level of documentation required may have been an effective reminder for the caregivers that added a dimension of safety and thereby contributed to the low incidence of pressure ulcers observed. In a similar study involving nursing home patients ($N = 235$) bedded on a viscoelastic foam (7 cm) mattress, patients in the experimental group were repositioned at varying intervals (2 hours lateral then 4 hours supine then 2 hours lateral), whereas patients in the control group were repositioned at equal intervals (4 hours lateral then 4 hours supine then 4 hours lateral) (Vanderwee et al., 2007). Patients in both the experimental and control group developed pressure ulcers, but between the two groups, there was no statistically significant difference in the incidence, severity, or time to development of pressure ulcers (Vanderwee et al., 2007). In another well-designed study of nursing home patients, Defloor and colleagues (2004) reported a low incidence (3%) of grade II and higher pressure ulcers among patients bedded on viscoelastic foam mattresses and turned every 4 hours, as compared to incidence ranging from 14.3% to 24.1% among patients on a standard hospital mattress who were turned every 2, 3, and 6 hours. Collectively, the results of these studies raise questions about the value of more frequent turning (e.g., every 2 hours) and suggest that repositioning at 4-hour intervals is an effective preventative intervention when nursing home patients are bedded on a pressure-reducing foam mattress. Such findings are likely to hold true for patients in other care settings as well who are managed on effective pressure redistribution surfaces.

While research can help to define general parameters for turning and repositioning intervals, all preventive care must be tailored to the specific needs of individuals and their unique responses to the care provided. Blanchable, reactive hyperemia is an expected response when tissue is exposed to pressure loads that compromise arteriolar flow to the tissues

(Maklebust & Sieggreen, 1993); however, this "normal" reactive hyperemia should resolve within 20 to 30 minutes of off-loading pressure with no residual effects. Evidence of nonblanchable erythema that persists following off-loading is by definition equivalent to a stage I pressure ulcer (Maklebust & Sieggreen, 1993; NPUAP, 2007a) and an indication that the intervals between repositioning need to be shortened. Turning clocks placed in the patient's room at the head of the bed are helpful reminders for repositioning (Maklebust & Sieggreen, 1993; Magnan & Maklebust, 2009) and may be of particular benefit whenever a patient's repositioning interval varies from the agency's standard-of-care (i.e., "routine") repositioning intervals.

CLINICAL PEARL

Normal reactive hyperemia should resolve within 30 minutes of off-loading; if it persists, either the support surface or the repositioning schedule should be modified to provide higher-level tissue protection.

Repositioning for Hemodynamically Unstable Patients

Repositioning of critically ill and hemodynamically unstable patients is another special area of concern. Critical care nurses have sometimes reported unstable vital signs and low levels of respiratory and energy reserves as reasons for not repositioning patients (Winkleman & Peereboom, 2010). In addition, decisions made about repositioning critically ill patients often are based on the nurse's perception of what might happen if the patient is repositioned rather than on an actual test of the patient's tolerance to repositioning (Brindle et al., 2013). Experts recommend that most critically ill patients, even those receiving vasoactive medications, should undergo repositioning trials to evaluate their tolerance to repositioning (Brindle et al., 2013; Dammeyer et al., 2013; Vollman, 2012). Repositioning hemodynamically unstable patients does frequently result in changes in SVO_2, BP, and heart rate; however, research has shown that these changes are usually transient and most patients return to baseline within 5 minutes of completing the turn (Winslow et al., 1995). Experts therefore suggest that critically ill patients should be monitored for time to recovery to baseline hemodynamic parameters and that timely recovery is a better indicator of tolerance to repositioning than the changes seen immediately after repositioning. Thus, the patient's ability to tolerate a position change should not be assessed until 5 to 10 minutes after repositioning (Vollman, 2012).

CLINICAL PEARL

Current evidence suggests that repositioning is important for hemodynamically unstable patients, that slow small shifts may be tolerated even when major repositioning is not tolerated, and that recovery to baseline within 10 minutes should be used as the measure of tolerance to repositioning.

Repositioning should begin shortly after admission to the ICU and certainly within 8 hours of admission. Vollman (2012) has noted that orthostatic tolerance to repositioning deteriorates quickly with immobility and failure to reposition. Thus, the longer the patient is left immobile in a supine position, the more apt he or she is to develop what has been referred to as "gravitational disequilibrium." Gravitational disequilibrium inhibits the patient's ability to adapt to position changes. This situation can be aggravated by turning the patient too rapidly. Turning the critically ill patient slowly and in small increments gives the body time to adjust to the position change.

Critically ill patients seem to tolerate the right lateral tilt position better than the left lateral position (Vollman, 2012). While the reasons for this difference have not been fully elucidated, experts currently recommend beginning with a supine to right lateral tilt and incorporating the left lateral position as repositioning tolerance improves (Vollman, 2012). Using pillows and wedges to achieve small incremental lateral position changes of 15 degrees may be needed before moving the patient to the 30-degree lateral position. Repositioning from the 30-degree lateral position to the supine position may require a similar cautious approach, with a gradual reduction in the lateral angle, 15 degrees at a time.

There is no consensus regarding absolute contraindications to repositioning the critically ill patient. It has been suggested that the presence of life-threatening arrhythmias, active fluid resuscitation to maintain systemic blood pressure, and active hemorrhage may render the patient too unstable to tolerate turning; unstable spinal fractures and fractures of the pelvis are also considered contraindications to turning (Brindle et al., 2013). For all other patients, the decision regarding repositioning should be made on a case-by-case basis and with due consideration given to the patient's demonstrated hemodynamic response to repositioning. For patients who fail repositioning trials due to hemodynamic instability, the use of a lateral rotation bed should be considered; however, this surface should not be considered an alternative to repositioning because the trunk is minimally affected by the lateral rotation. Thus, repositioning should be implemented as soon as possible.

There are occasions when critically ill patients must be placed in a prone position for an extended period of time (e.g., 6 to 10 hours). Indications for prone positioning include poor oxygenation, mobilization of secretions, and pressure relief (Gattinoni et al., 2001; Vollman, 2004). These patients should be assessed for evidence of facial ulcers as well as ulcers in other areas of the body (e.g., breast region, knees, toes, penis, clavicles, anterior iliac crests, symphysis pubis) that are usually considered "low risk" or "no risk" for pressure ulcer development (NPUAP/EPUAP/PPPIA, 2014).

Side-Lying Tilt

To avoid pressure on the trochanters, patients at risk for pressure ulcers should not be placed in a 90-degree lateral position (NPUAP/EPUAP/PPPIA, 2014). Instead, the 30-degree

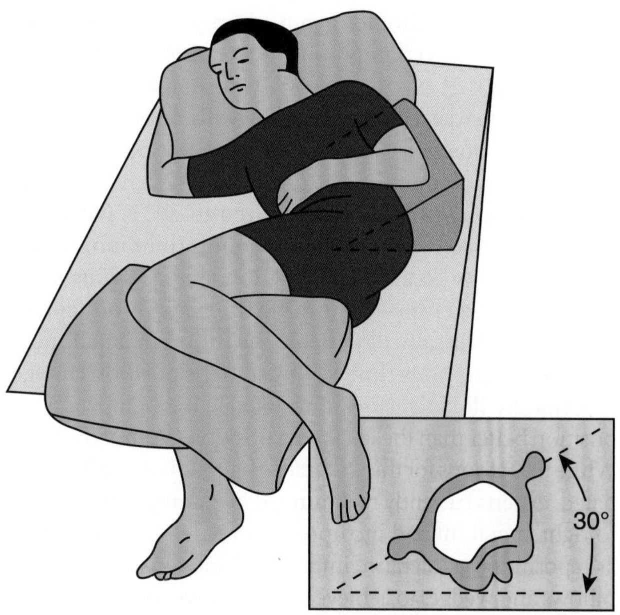

FIGURE 19-6. 30-degree tilt for side-lying position.

lateral tilt position is recommended for lateral positioning (Fig. 19-6). When using the 30-degree lateral tilt position, it is prudent to ensure the correct position has been achieved by observing the angle of the hips in relation to the long axis of the bed and by performing a hand check. To perform a hand check, slip your hand, palm up, under the patient's hip and push upward to validate that the patient is resting on the fleshy part of the buttocks and not on the trochanter (Fig. 19-7). Pillows and wedges can be used to help maintain the desired position. Whenever patients are positioned laterally, pillows or folded bath blankets should be used to separate opposing bony prominences such as the knees and ankles so they do not put pressure on each other.

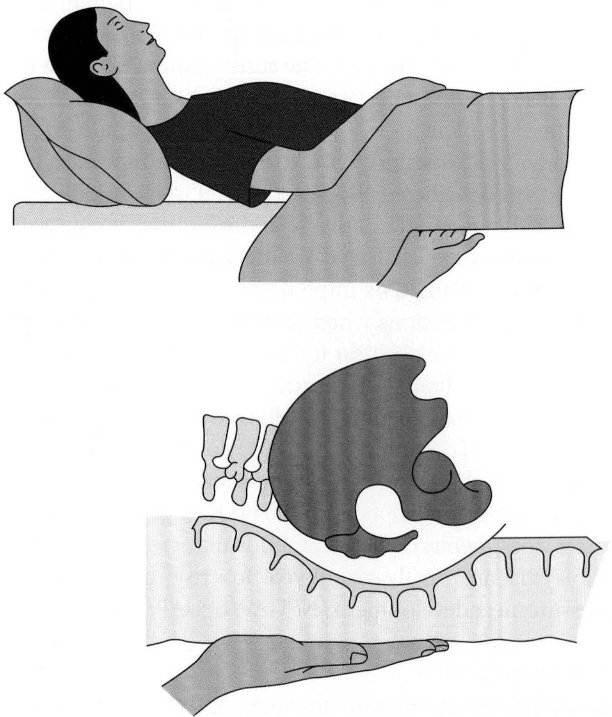

FIGURE 19-7. Hand check between mattress and overlay to assess for "bottoming out."

CLINICAL PEARL

A 30-degree lateral tilt is recommended for the side-lying position; this position protects both the trochanter and the sacrococcygeal area.

Support Surfaces

Support surfaces play a vital role in both the prevention and the treatment of pressure ulcers (Thompson et al., 2009). The National Pressure Ulcer Advisory Panel (NPUAP) defines *support surface* as "a specialized device for pressure redistribution designed for management of tissue loads, microclimate, and/or other therapeutic functions (i.e., any mattresses, integrated bed system, mattress replacement, overlay or seat cushion, or seat cushion overlay)" (NPUAP, 2007b, p. 1). This lengthy definition draws immediate attention to one critical feature of support surfaces, that is, the "redistribution…of tissue loads." Support surfaces redistribute tissue loads by immersion and envelopment. Immersion is a measure of how deeply one sinks into the support surface (Sprigle & Sonenblum, 2011). Envelopment is the capability of a support surface to deform around and evenly encompass the contours of the body, thus evenly distributing pressure across the entire contact surface (Sprigle & Sonenblum, 2011).

A great number of support surfaces are available for use, and they can generally be classified as reactive (constant low pressure) or dynamic (alternating pressure) (McInnes et al., 2011; Thompson et al., 2008). Reactive systems increase the contact area between the loaded point of the body and the surface the individual is lying on or sitting on. Dynamic (alternating) surfaces contain air-filled cells that inflate and deflate in a cyclical fashion, thereby changing the points of tissue loading on a frequent basis (Moore et al., 2014). When used appropriately, support surfaces can help prevent pressure ulcers by cushioning vulnerable parts of the body and by redistributing body weight across the lying or seating surface, thus minimizing interface pressures between the bony prominences and the lying or seating surface. However, the use of a support surface alone will not prevent pressure ulceration. Instead, treatment with a support surface must be accompanied by other preventive measures including repositioning, moisture management, nutritional support, and protection from friction and shear (Thompson et al., 2008).

The NPUAP (2007b), through its Support Surface Standards Initiative (S3I), has defined the components, features, and categories of support surfaces. These definitions can be found online and in Chapter 20. The S3I was founded in 2001 to fill the need for performance and reporting standards related to support surfaces. Still, there is a pressing need to develop standards for reporting support surface performance data in a way that would make it easier for health care professionals to compare the performance of different support surfaces and to make informed choices about which support surface should be used for which type of patient (Hermans et al., 2014).

Choosing a support surface to prevent pressure ulcers should not be based solely on the patient's level of risk for pressure ulcer development (EPUAP & NPUAP, 2009). Instead, additional factors such as the patient's clinical presentation, age, size, level of mobility within the bed, patient comfort, the need for microclimate control, maintenance, and costs should be considered (Moore et al., 2014; EPUAP & NPUAP, 2009; Thompson et al., 2009). However, for patients who are at high risk and cannot be repositioned manually, a dynamic support surface that can change the load distribution should be considered (see Chapter 20).

CLINICAL PEARL

A dynamic support surface (alternating pressure device) should be considered for patients who cannot be repositioned.

A number of studies have been conducted to compare the effectiveness of different support surfaces to standard bed mattresses as well as studies that compare the relative effectiveness of different support surfaces to each other. Typically, the outcome of interest in these studies is the incidence of pressure ulcers. In a recent meta-analysis of support surface studies, McInnes and colleagues (2011) analyzed the results of published and unpublished randomized controlled trials (RCTs) and quasi-randomized studies from any patient group or setting that measured pressure ulcer incidence as the outcome. According to these authors, "the clearest conclusion that can be drawn is that standard hospital mattresses have been consistently outperformed by a range of foam-based, low-pressure mattresses and overlays, and also by higher-specification pressure-relieving beds and mattresses in the prevention of pressure ulcers" (McInnes et al., 2011, p. 17).

Although evidence shows that pressure redistribution support surfaces (PRSSs) outperform standard hospital mattresses in reducing the incidence of pressure ulcers (McInnes et al., 2011), wound care nurses may still need to advocate for the use of PRSSs. Baumgarten and colleagues (2010) studied the use of PRSSs among elderly hip fracture patients, a high-risk group. These investigators found that PRSS use was only 57% in the acute care setting, the odds of PRSS use in the rehabilitation setting were less than half those in the acute care setting, and the odds of PRSS use in the nursing home setting were less than one quarter those in the acute care setting. Moreover, despite the fact that guidelines recommend that prevention efforts be based on each patient's pressure ulcer risk status (Ratliff, 2005), neither Braden score nor any other pressure ulcer risk factors were significantly associated with PRSS use (Baumgarten et al., 2010). Results of this study suggest that vigilance is needed to ensure that the quality of care delivered is consistent with available evidence and adheres to recommended guidelines for pressure ulcer prevention.

Seating surfaces and cushions constitute a special class of support surfaces. Unlike mattresses and mattress overlays, which may be static or dynamic, seating surfaces are primarily static and made out of foam, gel, air, or some combination. Seating surfaces play an important role in preventing sitting-induced pressure ulcers especially for individuals who are wheelchair bound. Choosing a seating surface for long-term use by wheelchair-bound individuals (e.g., those with spinal cord injury) is a complex task that must address patient comfort, pressure relief, moisture accumulation, and heat accumulation and loss as well as the postural stability of the patient (Brienza & Geyer, 2000). A seating specialist who has received comprehensive training in the clinical evaluation of patients, the biomechanics of sitting, and cushion fabrication techniques should be consulted. See Chapter 15 for further discussion regarding options and considerations for selection of wheelchair cushions.

For individuals who require only short-term use of a wheelchair and cushion, the clinician can use a hand-check to determine if the chair cushion has enough depth to offer pressure redistribution. With the hand flat and the palm facing upward the clinician's hand is inserted between the chair surface and the chair cushion to see if the ischial tuberosities can be felt through the chair cushion. About 1 inch of air or other cushioning material should be felt between the lowest portion of the body and the chair surface—in other words, the patient's body should not be sitting on the clinician's hand but instead should be "floating" on about 1 inch of air or foam or gel.

For persons who require long-term use of wheelchairs, it is best if the seating surface and the wheelchair are ordered at the same time, and selection should be done by a specialist who can use real-time pressure mapping to guide decision making about seating cushion selection (Bain & Ferguson-Pell, 2002).

Nursing home (NH) patients are particularly vulnerable to sitting-induced pressure ulcers because they often spend long hours of the day seated or confined to a wheelchair. The risk for sitting-induced pressure ulcers among NH patients increases considerably if they are mobility impaired and unable to reposition themselves independently (Shaw & Taylor, 1991). Characteristics of the patient, the wheelchair, and the support surface work together to influence the development of sitting-induced pressure ulcers. A number of studies have shown that the use of pressure-redistributing wheelchair cushions designed to maintain tissue integrity reduce the incidence and/or the severity of sitting-induced pressure ulcers among NH patients (Bardsley, 1993; Brienza et al., 2001; Conine et al., 1994; Geyer et al., 2001; Lim et al., 1988). However, much of the research that examines the effect of wheelchair seat cushions on pressure ulcer prevention has failed to control for the wheelchair effect. In contrast, Brienza and colleagues (2010) conducted a well-designed RCT examining the effect of wheelchair seat cushions on the incidence of ischial tuberosity (IT) pressure ulcers among NH patients and did control for the wheelchair effect. Specifically, these investigators provided subjects in both the control group and the research arms of the study with properly fitted wheelchairs. All patients in the study were at risk for developing pressure ulcers (Braden Scale total score of 18 or less), aged 65 years or older, free of IT pressure ulcers at the start of the study, and able to withstand wheelchair sitting times of 6 hours or longer. Subjects were randomly assigned to a skin protection cushion group (SPC; experimental arm) or a segmented foam cushion group (SFC; control group). The SPC group received an air, viscous fluid and foam, or gel and foam cushion based upon individualized assessment (by a seating specialist) of patient's need, preference, and comfort. Results of the study showed that the incidence of IT pressure ulcers was statistically significantly less in the SPC group who were seated on cushions deemed to be more suitable to their needs than in the SFC group who received foam cushions only.

Some research has shown that bedridden obese patients are at greater risk for developing pressure ulcers (Swanson et al., 2011). However, it is important to note that obese individuals are not necessarily more vulnerable to sitting-induced pressure ulcers. Obese individuals typically have more fat and muscle padding, which provides a larger seating surface over which the weight of the upper body can be distributed. In comparison, emaciated individuals with flaccid gluteal tissues *are* at greater risk for sitting-induced pressure ulcers (Sprigle, 2000). The combination of decreased padding and poor muscle tone contributes to poor weight distribution over the seating surface. As a result, tissues over the ischial tuberosities are at greater risk for pressure ulceration. Positioning the seated individual to distribute weight evenly across the seating surface is critical for preventing sitting-induced pressure ulcers. Even when a pressure-reducing cushion is used, care should be taken to ensure that (1) the depth of the chair seat (back to front) is sufficient to provide support from the buttocks to the back of the knees, (2) the floor-to-seat height (from floor-to-seating surface) is sufficient to maintain the thighs in a position parallel to the floor (with hip flexion at 90 degrees), and (3) the pelvis is not rotated posteriorly or obliquely (Maklebust & Sieggreen, 2001) (Fig. 19-8).

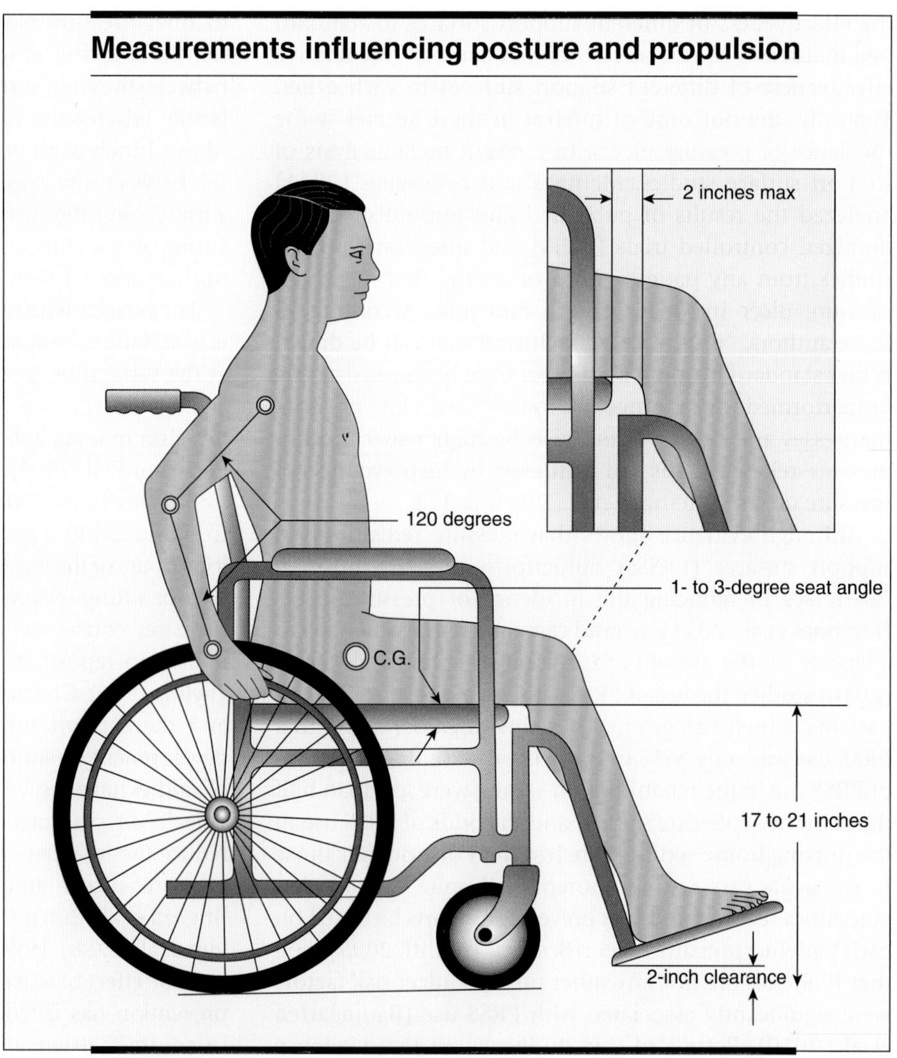

FIGURE 19-8. Proper position for wheelchair seating.

Protecting the Heels from Pressure Ulceration

Tymec et al. (1997) compared two pressure-relieving devices to protect the heels from pressure ulceration. They compared heel pressure ulcer rates among individuals managed with hospital bed pillows under the lower leg to float the heels off the mattress and those managed with a commercial boot (heel elevation device). Fifty-two patients participated in this study and were randomized to one of the two groups. Heel interface pressure measurements were taken with patients in supine and right lateral positions. In this study, logistic regression demonstrated a statistically significant difference in interface pressures on the left and right (left > right), and the generalized estimating equation (GEE) method revealed that the commercial foot elevation boot was four times less likely to suspend the right heel off the bed than the hospital pillow. There was no statistically significant difference in the number of pressure ulcers between groups, but the patients wearing the commercial boot with a heel elevator developed pressure ulcers earlier (10 days vs. 13 days). This study reminds clinicians that they cannot simply rely on use of a commercial device but must ensure that the device does effectively elevate the heel off the bed. Heels have a very small surface area and a very heavy bony structure resulting in high compressive force. Heels are the second most common site for pressure ulcer development, with the sacral area being the most common site; in addition, heel ulcers are frequently refractory to healing. Thus, heel protection must be a high-priority component of care for all at-risk patients.

CLINICAL PEARL

Heels are the second most common site for pressure ulcer development; thus, heel protection must be a high priority.

Foam Positioning Wedges

Many years ago, the 30-degree lateral tilt body position was introduced as being more desirable for pressure ulcer prevention than the 90-degree side-lying position; in response, the nurses at Harper Hospital in the Detroit Medical Center began cutting foam mattresses into 30-degree wedges to effectively support patients in the recommended position. Based on observed effectiveness (and when no longer allowed to cut their own wedges), they worked with a company to make these wedges commercially available, and they are now widely used across the country. These wedges can also be modified to serve as effective heel elevation devices. Specifically, the device is placed horizontally across the foot of the bed, and two divots are removed to accommodate the legs. These wedges are not easily kicked away by restless patients, and they seem to suspend the heels more effectively than most other positioning devices.

Exposure to Friction and Shear

While it is well known that "pressure" causes pressure ulcers, in theory (Bergstrom et al., 1987a; 1987b), friction and shear increase the risk for pressure ulcers by adversely affecting tissue tolerance (Antokal et al., 2012). While friction alone causes superficial damage only, friction combined with gravity creates shear force that can disrupt or compress blood vessels, resulting in significant ischemic damage (see Chapters 16 and 18). Thus, a comprehensive pressure ulcer prevention program must address and manage friction and shear. Sansom and Flynn (2007) have noted that "a successful ulcer prevention program will address contributing factors such as pressure, shear forces, friction, and moisture."

Friction

Friction occurs when skin rubs against an external surface. Many patient care situations can cause friction. For example, friction occurs when a patent is pulled or dragged up in bed rather than lifted. Friction may also occur when a brace or other orthotic device rubs against the skin. The independent or improper use of an overhead bed trapeze can result in a friction injury as well, especially if only the upper torso is lifted off the bed and the buttocks and heels are left to drag across the surface of the bed. There is significant potential for causing a friction injury during the placement and removal of bedpans, especially if care is not taken to ensure that the surface of the bedpan is not dragged across the skin during placement or removal. Agitated patients and those who are resistant to care may be unduly exposed to friction as a result of repetitive and resistive movement. Abrasive fabrics used in washcloths and vigorous rubbing during cleansing care are another source of friction.

Some body locations and body types are more vulnerable to the mechanical forces of friction. The heels and elbows are particularly vulnerable to friction (Hansen et al., 2010). Friction to the heels and elbows is especially problematic for patients who use their elbows and heels to wiggle themselves up toward the head of the bed. Wearing long sleeves on the arms and socks on the feet can help to minimize the frictional forces on these areas, as can protective dressings such as transparent adhesive dressings. Obesity may increase the risk of friction damage; research suggests that low scores on the friction and shear subscale (of the Braden Scale) are more highly associated with pressure ulcer development among obese patients ($BMI \geq 30$) than among patients with a $BMI < 30$ (Swanson et al., 2011). However, this does not mean that friction is not a problem for thin patients. Laboratory research suggests that among very thin patients with protruding bony prominences, the magnitude of the mechanical forces of friction can be quite severe and damaging, especially over the protruding bony prominences (Ohura, 2013). One strategy for protecting the sacrococcygeal area against friction damage is application of adhesive foam dressings (Brindle, 2013).

CLINICAL PEARL

One strategy for protecting the sacrococcygeal area against friction is use of gentle adhesive foam dressings.

Shear

Shear is defined as the "force per unit area exerted parallel to the plane of interest" (Maklebust, 1987; NPUAP, 2007a, p. 2). Shear is further defined as a mechanical force that acts on an area of the skin in a direction parallel to the body's surface. Shear is affected by the amount of pressure exerted, the coefficient of friction between the materials contacting each other, and the extent to which the body makes contact with the support surface (Bergstrom et al., 1994). In the body, tissue consists of several layers or planes including the skin, adipose tissue, fascia, muscle, periosteum, tendon, and bone; shearing forces cause one layer of tissue to move in relation to one or more of the other layers (Ohura, 2013), thus distorting the tissues involved (Nakagami et al., 2006). A common example of a shearing force is the movement of the axial skeleton in the body sack; for example, when a patient is sitting in a less than fully upright position, the skin and surface tissues adhere to the surface of the bed while the axial skeleton and attached muscle slides downward inside the body sack. It is the adipose tissue and perfusing vessels that are most often involved in this type of shear damage. Another example of shearing occurs when the patient is sitting (e.g., on the side of the bed or in a chair) and is dragged toward the front edge of the seating surface. In this situation, the surface tissues of the buttocks remain somewhat stationary while the deeper tissues slide forward. Shear injuries may also occur when the patient is repositioned by being dragged up toward the head of the bed instead of being lifted completely off the bed surface. Similarly, using slide boards to transfer from bed to gurney or bed to chair can cause shearing injuries in the deep body tissue—especially if the patient "sticks" to the sliding surface. For this reason, patients are advised not to use a slide board against their bare skin. If the patient is not wearing long pants, a sheet or blanket or pillow case can be used to cover the slide board before use to mitigate the tendency of the skin to adhere to the sliding surface (Maklebust, 1987). A shear injury will not be immediately visible at the skin surface because the damage occurs in deeper tissue planes.

CLINICAL PEARL

Patients are at risk for shear damage when they slide down in bed or when they use sliding boards against the bare skin for transfers.

It is difficult to separate friction and shear for clinical research purposes. The Braden Scale (Braden, 1987), which is used widely to assess the risk for pressure ulceration, combines the assessment of friction and shear into one subscale. However, a number of studies have demonstrated a significant relationship between low scores on the "friction and shear" subscale and pressure ulcer development; thus, management of friction and shear is an important component of a pressure ulcer prevention program (Lahmann et al., 2010; Lahmann & Kottner, 2011; Lahmann et al., 2011).

Prevention Strategies

Strategies used to minimize the adverse effects of friction should be directed at lowering the coefficient of friction, which is the "amount of friction existing between two surfaces." One very important strategy is to keep the skin dry; wet skin is known to have a much higher friction coefficient (Gerhardt et al., 2008; Zhong et al., 2006). Thus, an effective moisture management program can help minimize the friction problem. Dry lubricants such as cornstarch can be used on bedpans to lower the coefficient of friction. Protective covers for the elbows and heels will lower the friction coefficient; however, these "protectors" frequently slide out of position and have no impact on protection against pressure. Therefore, use of protective dressings such as transparent adhesive dressings, gentle adhesive foam dressings, and solid glycerin gel dressings may be of greater benefit. As noted, there is increasing data to support the use of gentle adhesive foam dressings over the sacrococcygeal area as one component of a comprehensive prevention program.

CLINICAL PEARL

Measures to keep the skin cool and dry (microclimate control) reduce the risk for friction and shear injury.

Low Friction Textiles

Patient care textiles, such as bed linens and patient gowns, have recently received increased recognition as a significant contributor to skin health or skin damage; specifically, linens can compromise the skin by increasing the friction coefficient and abrasive force and/or trapping heat and moisture against the skin, thus adversely affecting the skin's microclimate (Zhong et al., 2006; Zhong et al., 2008). Tissue tolerance to friction and shear is reduced when moisture accumulates at the skin surface, which is common among febrile and diaphoretic patients (Pan & Sun, 2011; Zhong et al., 2006). Textiles that have the ability to wick moisture away from the skin and linens that reduce frictional forces can contribute to pressure ulcer prevention and overall skin health.

Special textiles that reduce friction and optimize moisture transport are now available, and there is increasing evidence of their beneficial effects. These "special" textiles differ from conventional bedding textiles (e.g., cotton and cotton blends) both in fiber type and fabric construction. The moisture channels in these textiles facilitate moisture transport from the skin to the environment rather than allowing it to be trapped in the fabric or between the fabric and the skin, and the reduced friction coefficient reduces the risk of friction and shear injury.

Clinical research demonstrating the effectiveness of these special textiles in pressure ulcer prevention is limited but growing. In a study involving 46 male nursing home residents, Twersky and colleagues (2012) reported significantly fewer pressure ulcers among residents bedded on silk-like fabric sheets constructed from nylon and polyester yarns and using high absorbency briefs compared to residents bedded on conventional cotton–polyester sheets (approximately 50% cotton and 50% polyester) and "usual care adult incontinence brief." In addition, the number of new non–stage I ulcers was significantly lower in the intervention group. Smith et al. (2013) used a retrospective research design to examine pressure ulcer incidence in an acute care setting before and after introducing hospital-wide use of synthetic silk-like fabric bed linens and patient gowns. Conventional cotton–blend linens were used in the "before" segment of the study. In total, the data from 1,427 patients were examined. These researchers reported that the number of patients with hospital-acquired pressure ulcers in the group that used the silk-like fabric textiles was statistically significantly less (for all pressure ulcers, for stage I only, and for stage II and higher only) than the number of patients with pressure ulcers in the group using conventional cotton–blend linens. Results of these studies provide an early indication that using special textiles for bedding and gowns may help prevent pressure ulcers. While further research is needed, especially among special needs groups (e.g., neonates, infants, paraplegic patients, obese patients), current evidence-based guidelines list use of therapeutic linens at "B" level of evidence (NPUAP/EPUAP/PPPIA, 2014).

CLINICAL PEARL

There is increasing evidence that low-friction linens (bedding and gowns) can help to prevent pressure ulcers.

Lifting and Positioning

Strategies used to minimize the adverse effects of shearing forces should be directed at minimizing the contralateral movement between tissue planes. Proper lifting, positioning, and repositioning techniques are perhaps the best defense against injury from shearing forces. The use of lift sheets and having sufficient help to actually lift (not drag) patients when moving them to the head of the bed is critical. When positioning in a semi-Fowler's position, elevating the head of the bed to 30 degrees or less will minimize the risk for shearing that comes from sliding down in bed. In addition, measures to reduce the friction coefficient between the skin and the bed or chair surface will also reduce shear force, since friction is essential to shear; thus, strategies to keep the skin cool and dry, use of therapeutic linens, support surfaces with low-friction low-shear covers, and use of protective dressings can help to reduce both superficial friction damage and deep shear damage.

Moisture

Moisture alone will not cause skin damage (Gray et al., 2011); however, as explained in Chapter 17, overhydrated skin is much more vulnerable to friction and shear damage and is also less able to distribute weight normally. Moisture contributes to pressure ulcer development by decreasing tissue tolerance (Braden & Bergstrom, 1987) and by increasing susceptibility to friction and to pressure and shear (EPUAP & NPUAP, 2009). Thus, a comprehensive pressure ulcer prevention program should include measures to protect the skin from excessive exposure to moisture from wound exudate, perspiration, and urinary and fecal incontinence.

Exposure to moisture from urine and stool can lead to hyperhydration of the skin and alter the skin pH, both of which compromise tissue tolerance (Gray et al., 2011). Tissue tolerance may be further compromised by exposure to fecal contents including fecal enzymes and intestinal flora (Gray et al., 2011). Strategies for moisture management must include strategies for managing both internally produced moisture (perspiration) and external sources of moisture (urine, stool, and wound exudate). As noted earlier in this chapter and in Chapter 17, internally produced moisture is best managed by use of wicking products or absorbing products that keep the skin dry. In contrast, protection against external moisture sources usually involves application of products that repel moisture and help to keep the skin dry, in addition to use of containment devices or absorptive products for urine, stool, and wound exudate (Sibbald et al., 2009). Moisture barrier products include liquid barrier films in spray form and moisture barrier ointments (e.g., dimethicone, petrolatum, zinc oxide). Zinc oxide is very commonly used for protection against high-volume liquid stool or for management of denuded skin; while it provides effective protection, caregivers must be taught appropriate use and should be cautioned not to aggressively remove all of the ointment with each incontinent episode (Penzer, 2009). Instead, the soiled layers should be gently removed and new ointment applied following each incontinent episode; cleansing down to the skin (for assessment) should be limited to daily or every other day and must be done gently using a soft cloth and perineal cleanser or mineral oil (Beeckman et al., 2011).

See Chapter 17 for an in-depth discussion of prevention and management of MASD. Other strategies for protecting the skin against stool and urine include diverting devices such as urinary catheters and fecal incontinence systems. The risk of catheter-associated urinary tract infections makes the use of internal urinary catheters a less than desirable strategy for moisture management. Instead, alternatives such as frequent toileting, barrier creams, incontinence briefs, and absorbent underpads that wick moisture away from the skin are preferred. For male patients, condom catheters can be an effective way of diverting urine away from the skin, but care must be taken to apply them properly.

External fecal incontinence collectors (e.g., pouches) can be used to keep feces from coming in contact with the skin. However, these devices are difficult to apply and usually require two caregivers to place the device properly (Scardillo & Aronovitch, 1999). Also, because an adhesive is used to secure the collection device to the skin, removal of the device can damage fragile perianal skin. Tubes inserted into the rectum offer another alternative for diverting frequent, liquid diarrheal stools, such as those caused by *Clostridium difficile*. Tube systems may be makeshift or manufactured. Makeshift devices include the use of tubes designed for other purposes such as urinary catheters, mushroom catheters, and nasal trumpets inserted into the rectum and connected to a drainage collection system (e.g., a urinary drainage bag). While the literature suggests that these makeshift devices perform effectively in diverting stool away from the skin (Blair et al., 1992; Grogan & Kramer, 2002), there are no data as to safety, and these devices are therefore considered to be *contraindicated*. Manufactured fecal incontinence systems are superior to makeshift systems because they are designed specifically for the purpose of internal placement to divert feces and have undergone extensive testing for both performance and safety.

Irritation and erosion of the rectal mucosa with subsequent bleeding is a safety risk whenever any device is inserted into the rectum. Manufactured fecal incontinence systems are designed to provide low-pressure contact with the rectal mucosa and to minimize mucosal irritation. Still, reports of patient harm from pressure necrosis as well as harm from traumatic removal of these systems can be found in the literature (Sparks et al., 2010). Therefore, care should be taken to minimize the risk of traumatic removal of fecal management systems, either by the patient (e.g., by grabbing or hooking with the foot) or by caregivers, during routine care and repositioning. Any evidence of trauma, such as bloody drainage or complaints of discomfort, mandates removal. In addition, these devices must be removed after 29 days of continuous use based on FDA regulations.

Minimizing the amount of time skin comes in contact with moisture is one of the essential components of any moisture management program. The longer the skin is exposed to incontinence moisture and the contaminants in the moisture, the greater the risk of skin damage. Therefore, skin care and pressure ulcer prevention for the individual who requires use of absorptive products must include frequent checks of briefs and absorbent underpads and prompt changes for soiling. It is difficult to make solid recommendations regarding the timing and frequency of checks for incontinence. The time from moisture exposure to skin damage cannot be predicted accurately but may be very short, especially if the pH of the moisture is alkaline and/or proteolytic enzymes are present and active; thus, absorptive products should be composed of super absorbent polymers that wick moisture away from the skin, and the "check and change" program must be used in conjunction with the use of moisture barrier products. In addition, clinical judgment must be used in making decisions about how often the patient should be checked for exposure to moisture; this information should be communicated in handoff reports. The importance of prompt cleaning after incontinence cannot be overstated. Many studies have demonstrated a relationship between incontinence and pressure ulcers. As early as 1994, in a secondary analysis of pressure ulcer audits from 2,189 acute care patients, Maklebust and Magnan reported that the odds of pressure ulceration among patients with fecal incontinence was 22 times greater than the odds of pressure ulceration among patients without fecal incontinence. Moreover, an analysis of the interactive effects of fecal incontinence and immobility showed that the odds for pressure ulceration among those with immobility and fecal incontinence were 37.5 times greater than the odds of pressure ulceration among patients who were continent and mobile (Maklebust & Magnan, 1994). These findings make it clear that patients who are both incontinent and immobile are at great risk for tissue damage and in desperate need of the most conscientious, hypervigilant nursing care possible.

CLINICAL PEARL

In some studies, the risk of pressure ulceration was 22 times greater among individuals with fecal incontinence than among individuals without fecal incontinence.

As noted, underpads and absorbent incontinence briefs should be chosen based on their ability to wick moisture away from the patient's skin; it is much more important to keep the interface between the patient and the underpad or brief dry than to keep the bed dry. In general, absorptive products should be left open under the patient to avoid the occlusive environment and hot wet skin that results from closure of the brief around the patient.

Selection of products for perineal cleansing is another area where recent evidence contradicts conventional wisdom. For example, the common sense use of soap and water to cleanse the skin does not make as much sense as it might seem. Soaps often have an alkaline pH that is not compatible with the normal acid mantle of the skin (Lambers et al., 2006). Alkaline products can dry the skin and alter the surface pH, making it more vulnerable to infection. Therefore, pH-adjusted no-rinse cleansers and soft disposable cloths are now recommended for perineal cleansing; impregnated cleansing wipes that also contain moisturizers and moisture barriers simplify the incontinence care regimen.

Nutrition

Nutritional status is widely recognized as an important determinant of overall health, and malnutrition is recognized as a risk factor for impaired healing, because adequate protein intake is essential for collagen synthesis. Incorporation of nutritional status into the Braden Scale was initially based on Dr. Braden's study of nutritional status among the elderly residents of an RWJ Teaching Nursing Home project. She observed that the healthiest residents fed themselves and ate more protein, and based on this observation, she conducted an in-depth study of the relationship between dietary intake and pressure ulcer development. While the scientific evidence regarding the relationship between nutritional status and pressure ulcer prevention and management remains sparse, general consensus supports nutritional management as an important aspect of a comprehensive care plan for pressure ulcer prevention and treatment (Pinchofsky-Devin & Kaminski, 1986; Thomas, 2007; Thomas et al., 1996). It is essential to address nutrition in every patient with a pressure ulcer, because adequate calories, protein, fluids, vitamins, and minerals are required for healing; these nutrients are also required for health and tissue maintenance.

CLINICAL PEARL

General consensus supports nutritional management as an important aspect of a comprehensive care plan for pressure ulcer prevention and treatment.

In a large cohort study of 1,534 residents in 95 nursing facilities, pressure ulcer development was positively correlated with advancing age, frailty, severity of illness, pressure ulcer history, and significant weight loss and difficulty eating (Bergstrom et al., 2005; Horn et al., 2004). Nutrition-related risk factors for pressure ulcers include compromised nutritional status with unintended weight loss, impaired ability to eat independently, low BMI, and reduced food intake (Center for Medicare & Medicaid Services State Operations manual: Guidance for surveyors of long-term care facilities, 2008).

Reddy et al. (2006) conducted a systematic review of pressure ulcer prevention studies and found five RCTs on nutrition and pressure ulcers; however, only one of them (Bourdel-Marchasson et al., 2000) supported use of nutritional supplementation to reduce the risk for pressure ulcers. The purpose of this multicenter trial was to assess the effect of nutritional supplementation on dietary intake and pressure ulcer development in critically ill older patients. The study involved 19 wards stratified according to specialty and recruitment for critically ill older patients; 9 wards were randomly selected for nutritional intervention (nutritional intervention group). The intervention consisted of daily administration of two oral supplements, each of which contained 200 kcal, for 15 days. Pressure ulcer incidence was prospectively recorded for stages I (erythema), II (superficial broken skin), and III (subcutaneous ulcer) for 15 days. There were 672 subjects older than 65 years; 295 were in the nutritional intervention group versus 377 in the control group. At baseline, the patients in both groups were similar for age, gender, and C-reactive protein. During the trial, energy and protein intake were higher in the nutritional intervention group (day 2: 1,081 ± 595 kcal vs. 957 ± 530 kcal, $P = 0.006$; 45.9 ± 27.8 g protein vs. 38.3 ± 23.8 g protein in the control group, $P < 0.001$). At 15 days, the cumulative incidence of pressure ulcers was 40.6% in the nutritional intervention group versus 47.2% in the control group. The proportion of stage I ulcers relative to the total number of cases was 90%. In conclusion, according to the data collected, it was possible to increase the dietary intake of critically ill elderly subjects by systematic use of oral supplements. This intervention was associated with a decreased incidence of pressure ulcer development.

Ek and colleagues (1991) hypothesized that nutritional supplementation might prevent pressure ulcers from developing and help improve healing of existing pressure ulcers. All newly admitted residents who were to stay more than 15 days were randomized into treatment and control groups. Nutritional state was evaluated weekly with serum protein analyses, anthropometry, the delayed hypersensitivity skin test, and the Norton Score. The treatment group residents were given extra nutritional support. Significantly more residents with protein energy malnutrition (PEM) had or developed pressure ulcers. Regression analyses indicated **albumin, mobility, activity, and food intake were predictors** for pressure ulcer development. Patients who received nutritional supplements developed fewer pressure ulcers.

In summary, while data regarding the specific impact of nutritional status on pressure ulcer risk are limited, clinical consensus supports nutritional assessment and nutritional intervention as essential for overall health and an important component of pressure ulcer prevention.

To make sure that nutrition is not overlooked during patients' hospitalization, a nutritionist should be a member of the pressure ulcer prevention team; in addition, the nursing staff should be taught the correct meaning of each Braden scale rating criteria (e.g., "usual eating pattern" means at least 1 week, not 1 or 2 days, and not just NPO for a procedure), and a house-wide Braden subscale trigger should be established for a nutrition consult (e.g., a nutrition subscale score <3 initiates a nutrition consult). It is also helpful to offer malnourished individuals their favorite foods after making sure that these foods are allowed. For a more in-depth review of nutrition and nutritional needs of individuals with protein energy malnutrition (PEM), please see Chapter 6.

CASE STUDIES

CASE STUDY

At the beginning of this chapter, the assertion was made that "the best defense against pressure ulcers is a well-developed, evidence-based prevention plan that is tailored to the individual's specific needs, conscientiously implemented, and revised as needed based on the patient's response." In addition, the authors stated that "the pressure ulcer prevention plan should be based on knowledge and assessment data related to the following: clinical condition (current health state and comorbidities), current skin condition, overall pressure ulcer risk status and specific risk factors, and resource availability (human and environmental) (see Fig. 19-1)." Up to this point, detailed information has been provided about specific risk factors and strategies used to minimize the risk of pressure ulcer development. In this section, a case study exemplar is used to demonstrate how data from the assessment of the patient's clinical condition, skin condition, and pressure ulcer risk status are brought together to develop an individualized evidence-based pressure ulcer prevention plan of care.

Clinical Presentation

Mrs. S. is a 55-year-old Caucasian female patient admitted to the ICU 4 days ago after a below the knee amputation of a gangrenous left lower extremity. She is 5′6″ and weighed 278 pounds before amputation with a BMI = 45. She has a history of insulin-dependent diabetes, peripheral vascular disease, hypertension, and hypothyroidism. She was initially detained in the ICU due to failure to wean from the ventilator. However, within 24 hours of admission to ICU she spiked a fever of 104°F and started defecating frequent liquid diarrhea stools. Laboratory studies confirmed the presence of *C. difficile* in the stool specimens. The fluid loss from the diarrhea has been massive. Saturated linens are being changed at least three to six times each shift. She is receiving aggressive fluid replacement therapy but her blood pressure remains low at 90/40 with a heart rate of 120. She is delirious, agitated with frequent thrashing of the arms and right leg, unable to follow simple commands, sweats profusely, does not reposition self, and resists nursing efforts directed at perineal cleansing and repositioning. Her bed is maintained flat because blood pressure drops below 80 mm Hg with any attempt at elevating the bed. The patient's weight and restlessness make it difficult to reposition her without assistance from three to four caregivers. Turning laterally increases agitation and heart rate from baseline of 120 to over 200 bpm. She is NPO since before surgery, has NG tube in place, and a Foley catheter, which was placed in the operating room.

Skin Condition

Skin over the sacrum is intact, warm to touch, with blanchable erythema. Skin over ischial tuberosities and greater trochanters is warm to touch, without redness or evidence of edema, and tissue consistency is comparable to the consistency of surrounding tissues. Skin on the right heel shows blanchable erythema. No redness on lateral or medial malleolus. Elbows are red and chafed looking, but skin is intact. Skin under the breasts and pannus is intact, moist, and red but without evidence of fungal infection. Perianal skin and skin of the buttocks remains intact but is fire-engine red and blanches to pressure. Stump incision line of the left leg is well approximated, with no redness and no drainage. Skin on surfaces of the stump is normal in color without redness and warm to touch with capillary refill <3 seconds. No evidence of edema on torso or extremities. No evidence of circumoral or lip irritation from endotracheal tube.

Pressure Ulcer Risk Assessment

The patient's Braden Scale total score is 7, which places her at a "very high" level of risk for pressure ulceration. Braden Scale subscale scores are as follows:

Sensory perception = 2
Moisture = 1
Activity = 1
Mobility = 1
Nutrition = 1
Friction/shear = 1

Resource Availability

Specialty beds and support surfaces can be ordered with wound care nurse approval. Internal bowel management systems are stocked in limited supply by wound nurse practitioner, and ICU nurses have received special training in the use of these systems. Specialty textiles are available for use but only when authorized by the wound nurse.

Nurse:patient ratio is 1:2 in ICU with two to four nurse assistants available on each shift.

The hospital has a pressure ulcer prevention and treatment team that rounds daily during the week on all ICU patients, all patients at high risk for pressure ulcers, and patients who currently have pressure ulcers. The team includes a medical intensivist, the wound nurse practitioner who sees all patients, and the clinical manager and the pressure ulcer prevention champion (usually a staff nurse) who see the patients on their respective units. Hospital administration, nurses, and nursing assistive personnel value pressure ulcer prevention and take great pride in consistently maintaining their rate of hospital-acquired pressure ulcers well below national benchmarks.

Program Management

Creating a pressure ulcer prevention program is a complex process that involves many areas of institutional operations. Developing an effective pressure ulcer prevention program takes a great deal of coordinated effort by many people with specialized knowledge and skill. Every heath care organization needs to develop an integrated program at the institutional level, the unit level, and across departments (e.g., transportation, radiology, OR, ER, PACU, etc.) and disciplines. The Agency for Health Care Research and Quality (AHRQ, 2012) has published a toolkit to guide hospitals in the development of high-quality pressure ulcer prevention programs. This comprehensive toolkit is available online at: www.ahrq.gov/professionals/systems/long-term-care/resources/pressure-ulcers/pressureulcertoolkit/putool4.html

CLINICAL PEARL

The Agency for Health Care Research and Quality has published a toolkit to guide hospitals in the development of high-quality pressure ulcer prevention programs.

Many of the principles and components addressed in the AHRQ toolkit can be adapted for use in other settings.

Program implementation is never flawless. Still, it is possible to learn from others' experiences and missed steps. Wound care nurses are well positioned to establish comprehensive programs that minimize "program gaps." Jankowski and Nadzam (2011) conducted a study involving four hospitals and identified the following as commonly occurring "gaps": (1) use of an abbreviated version of the Braden Scale scoring form that provides only the risk factor title but does not include the rating criteria for the levels of risk, (2) failure to include Braden Scale risk score information during routine RN "handoff" reports, (3) lack of teamwork between RNs and nursing assistants, (4) PU prevention supplies not always readily available, and (5) physicians unaware of PU prevention program. Wound care nurses are well equipped to address each of these issues.

Pressure ulcer prevention programs should be grounded in evidence. Evidence-based guidelines for pressure ulcer prevention are now available (e.g., NPUAP/EPUAP/PPPIA, 2014; WOCN, 2010). Both research and expert opinion suggest that when prevention guidelines are implemented, the prevalence of pressure ulcers decreases (Cuddign et al., 2001; Lahmann et al., 2010). However, wound nurses must exercise caution when selecting prevention guidelines upon which to base their agency's program. First, one must consider that advances in knowledge about pressure ulcer prevention are occurring rapidly. Therefore, it is important to make certain that the guideline being implemented is the most recent version and that it has been developed, reviewed, or revised within the last 5 years (Coopey et al., 2006). Secondly, wound care nurses need to be astute in determining which agency-wide prevention measures must be implemented immediately and which measures can be implemented at a later point. These determinations need to be based upon a critical evaluation of the organization's readiness for change, existing threats to patient safety, and the availability of human and environmental resources. It may not be feasible to initiate a whole new prevention program all at once. Careful planning and attention to feedback will provide guidance in terms of program success and readiness for the next phase of implementation; important indicators include the amount of pushback against the program, the amount of enthusiasm for the program, the increasing or decreasing incidence of hospital-acquired pressure ulcers, the number of nurses and assistants who want to sit on the prevention team, and the number of people who contribute good suggestions.

CLINICAL PEARL

When prevention guidelines are implemented, the incidence of pressure ulcers decreases.

Program Management at the Organizational Level

At the organizational level, the prevention program should include a planning and oversight committee that is strongly committed to developing and implementing an effective prevention program. The focus at this level should be on having the right level of expertise and authority at the planning table and ensuring that the planning and oversight committee has direct access to and the support of upper-level management (AHRQ, 2012). At a minimum, the members of the planning and oversight committee should have sufficient knowledge and authority to ensure: (1) resource adequacy and availability, (2) an appropriate level of program monitoring and evaluation, (3) implementation of continuous quality improvement initiatives, (4) establishment of policies and procedures as well as standards of care and standards of practice, and (5) completion of a root cause analysis (RCA) whenever a hospital-acquired pressure ulcer is identified. A root cause analysis is a process used to identify the causes of an undesirable event. (See Box 19-1 for a simple root cause analysis form.)

Program Management at the Departmental and Interdepartmental Level

Departmental and interdepartmental programs are needed to ensure that patients at risk for pressure ulcers are not exposed to preventable pressure and mechanical forces while under the temporary care of another department (e.g., ER, OR, PACU, radiology, transportation). Each department should have its own set of policies related to pressure ulcer prevention. For example, ER polices may include statements related to (1) identification of patients who require pressure ulcer risk assessment at time of admission to the ER department, (2) acceptable time frame for placement on a stretcher, (3) frequency of repositioning for immobile and critically ill patients, and (4) documentation of skin condition at time of admission. Documentation of skin status on admission is especially important for patients admitted from nursing homes, and patients who were "found down," that is, patients who fell and were on the floor for an unknown period of time. In addition, each department should have ready access to supplies and equipment needed for pressure ulcer prevention in their setting; for example, mattress overlays for stretchers, absorbent underpads, and pillows for heel elevation would be routinely needed in the emergency department.

CLINICAL PEARL

An effective agency-wide program for pressure ulcer prevention must include all departments and all levels of personnel.

Interdepartmental collaboration and education about best practices related to pressure ulcer prevention are essential if an agency-wide culture of prevention is to be established. For example, prevention is supported by an agency-wide standard that includes communication regarding pressure ulcer risk and prevention at each "handoff": for example, from nursing to transportation to interventional radiology and back again. Specifically, all transport gurneys should be equipped with pressure redistribution mattresses, and patient transporters need to be taught to routinely "float heels" for at-risk patients. Personnel who work in radiology need to be educated regarding the potential for ischemic damage related to prolonged placement in one position on the radiology table and should also be taught that repetitive exposure to high-intensity pressure can cause cumulative damage that is not immediately obvious. Radiology staff should be taught to reposition patients when possible and to assist the patient to make small shifts in body weight when a full-body rotation is not feasible. Patients may wait for a long time (often in the hallway) before a transporter returns them to their room; if there is a delay in transport, the patient should be repositioned if at all possible. Simple strategies can be used to improve communication with staff in other departments regarding a patient's level of risk for pressure ulcer development. For example, pink wrist bands may be used to readily identify at-risk patients who are in transit from one area of the hospital to another or left to lay unattended in hallways while waiting for tests. The pink wrist band would serve as a visual cue that the patient is at risk and *in need of repositioning*.

Program Management at the Unit Level

Unit-level prevention programs are needed to ensure that quality of care delivered at the point of service on a day-to-day basis is evidence-based, in keeping with established standards, and achieves desired outcomes. Pressure ulcer prevention rounds are an ideal approach for exchanging information about patients and for team building. It is important to understand that teams are different than small groups. Teams come together for a specific, goal-directed purpose, and team members have specific roles, perform specific tasks, and interact, communicate, and coordinate to achieve a common goal or outcome (Sargent et al., 2008). As noted above, contact among team members should not be haphazard. Instead, a deliberate effort is needed to ensure that team members come together to clarify and talk about their shared goal (pressure ulcer prevention) and their specific, individual responsibilities related to goal attainment.

The precise division of labor and responsibilities of team members may vary across institutions. What is important is that team member responsibilities are communicated and understood. During pressure ulcer prevention rounds, team members should be able to provide information about activities that fall within their scope of responsibility and provide additional information about barriers and facilitators that impact their ability to achieve goal-specific tasks. Including PCAs and nursing assistants in patient care rounds is critical. These providers are well positioned to provide high-quality preventative care and to observe, document, and report conditions that increase the risk for pressure ulcer development and report when prescribed interventions are not effective (e.g., amount of food left on tray suggests insufficient caloric intake).

Effective pressure ulcer teams gather members together on a regular basis to review the status of the prevention program on their unit. Each unit should have assigned team members who rotate on and off the team so that each nursing staff member has a chance to serve on the committee. Each member of the pressure ulcer management team should have assigned duties for the unit, and each member should know exactly what their duties entail. Essential team members include the wound care nurse, the unit manager, staff nurses (one from each shift), nursing assistants, off-shift supervision, and a representative from performance improvement and risk management. Each member reports on needed supplies, needed education, ideas for improving the prevention program, and initiatives to identify and correct any gaps in the unit's program. During routine meetings, each member of the PU prevention team should report on her or his areas of responsibility and other team members should respond with suggestions or recommendations. Responsibilities for recording meeting minutes are typically rotated among team members. The PU prevention team minutes should be shared with all the unit nursing staff at their regular practice council meetings so that everyone can benefit from any changes in the program.

It is unfortunate, but nurses and nursing assistants sometimes have difficulty working together as a team. Nurses accuse nursing assistants of not wanting to do their assignments and nursing assistants accuse nurses of assigning them the undesirable tasks such as incontinence care. The nursing assistants sometimes state that nurses think they are better than the assistants and that they assign all the "dirty work" to the assistants. In turn, nurses sometimes "blame" nursing assistants for failing to provide critical care such as turning and ambulating; this causes further disagreement between nurses and nursing assistants. In one large nursing study involving several hospitals, Kalisch et al. (2009, 2011) found that the nursing activities most often "missed" are assisting patients to ambulate and providing mouth care, tasks that are commonly delegated to nursing assistants. Ideally, all team members work together to respond to patients' care needs, and nurses and nursing assistants recognize that each team member has an important role in pressure ulcer prevention. For example, nursing assistants can play a critical role in both prevention and early detection of skin breakdown, because they are the front line care providers and the team members who provide direct patient care and who can therefore monitor skin for early changes. Factors contributing to friction among team members include communications issues and lack of clarity when tasks are delegated. Sometimes, the nurse who delegates the assignment does not make the assignment clear and the nursing assistant does not understand her or his responsibility for the delegated task. This communication gap often becomes a source of friction because the two parties may not understand delegation. The RN may not know how to delegate tasks, and the nursing assistant may not know how to receive delegated tasks. Both parties can become frustrated over miscommunication, which is the main source of team problems. Each person on a team must learn to show respect for other team members. It may be useful to set some ground rules for team member communication. This may seem simplistic to some, but good communication rules may save a lot of misunderstanding in the long run.

Program Management Related to the Use of Medical Devices

Effective pressure ulcer prevention programs must include standards of care related to the use of medical devices. Most pressure ulcers occur over bony prominences, but medical device–related (MDR) pressure ulcers are becoming more common (Black et al., 2010). Critically ill patients and neonates are particularly vulnerable to MDR pressure ulcers. Wound care nurses need to be acutely aware of the medical devices used in their institution, the correct application of these devices, expected points of contact with skin, areas of skin that need additional protection from pressure (e.g., edematous or fragile tissue under a medical device), and acceptable ways of cushioning contact with MDRs to redistribute pressure. MDRs commonly associated with ulceration include devices such as nasal cannulas, cervical collars, external braces, support stockings (especially the infrapopliteal area), endotracheal tubes, and digital and aural (ear lobe) pulse oximetry devices. The NPUAP (2013) has recommended specific "best practice" interventions to prevent MDR pressure ulcers and has posted photographic examples of MDR pressure ulcers observed among critical care, pediatric, and long-term care patients. These best practice recommendations include interventions such as (1) ensuring that the size of the device used is appropriate for the patient, (2) using cushioning dressings under the device (e.g., gauze or adhesive foam), (3) inspecting the skin under the device daily (or more often as indicated), (4) observing for edema under devices since it can make the tissues more vulnerable to breakdown, and (5) removing or repositioning the device daily. In addition, staff education related to correct use of MDRs and prevention of MDR pressure ulcers is critical.

CLINICAL PEARL

Medical device–related pressure ulcers are becoming more common; prevention includes padding, retaping and repositioning when possible, and daily inspection.

Conclusion

The stated goal for this chapter was "to provide current information regarding pressure ulcer prevention and strategies for ensuring that preventive care is routinely incorporated into patient care." To achieve this goal, the authors started by making the assertion that "the best defense against pressure ulcers is a well-developed, evidence-based prevention plan that is tailored to the individual's specific needs." Then, a conceptual model (see Fig. 19-1) was used to depict four domains that must be assessed to gather data needed to develop an individualized plan of care. A brief discussion of the concepts of incidence and prevalence followed to help wound nurses distinguish between these concepts and recognize that "facility-acquired" incidence is the best indicator of the effectiveness of a pressure ulcer prevention program. Detailed information about risk factors and specific strategies used to mitigate risk was provided. Then, a case study was included to demonstrate application of this knowledge to the development of an individualized prevention plan of care. Finally, some points related to program management were presented to help the reader understand and appreciate that the full scope of an effective pressure ulcer program extends across departments and disciplines.

While it is true that the knowledge base that informs our understanding of pressure prevention is growing at an accelerated pace, it is also true that pressure ulcers persist at an alarming rate. Deep ulcers are painful and costly and can even cause death; however, they are preventable if the individual is promptly identified as being "at risk" and if an individualized prevention program is immediately implemented. Preventing the occurrence of these costly and potentially life-threatening lesions is of intense national concern (Joint Commission, 2007; U.S. Department of Health and Human Services. Healthy People 2010, November 2000). Wound nurses, by virtue of their education and scope of practice, are well positioned to help us overcome this national health crisis, patient by patient and agency by agency.

REFERENCES

AHRQ. (2012). Preventing pressure ulcers in hospitals: A toolkit for improving quality of care. Retrieved October 15, 2014, from www.ahrq.gov/professionals/systems/long-term-care/resources/pressure-ulcers/pressureulcertoolkit/putool4.html

Antokal, S., Brienza, D., Bryan, N., et al. (2012). Friction induced skin injuries: Are they pressure ulcers? A National Pressure Ulcer Advisory Panel White Paper. Retrieved September 15, 2014, from http://www.npuap.org/wp-content/uploads/2012/01/NPUAP-Friction-White-Paper.pdf

Bain, D. S., & Ferguson-Pell, M., (2002). Remote monitoring of sitting behavior of people with spinal cord injury. *Journal of Rehabilitation Research and Development, 39*(4), 513–520.

Bardsley G. (1993). Wheelchairs and seating. *Current Opinion in Orthopedics, 4*(6), 110–116.

Baumgarten, M., Margolis, D., Orwig, D., et al. (2010). Use of pressure-redistributing support surfaces among elderly hip fracture patients across the continuum of care: Adherence to pressure ulcer prevention guidelines. *The Gerentologist, 50*(2), 253–262.

Beeckman, D., Woodward, S., & Gray, M. (2011). Incontinence-associated dermatitis: Step-by-step prevention and treatment. *British Journal of Community Nursing, 16*(8), 382–389.

Bergquist, S., & Frantz, R. (2001). Braden scale: Validity in community-based older adults receiving home health care. *Applied Nursing Research, 14*(1), 36–43.

Bergstrom, N., Bennett, M. A., Carlson C. E., et al. (1994). *Treatment of pressure ulcers: Clinical practice guideline, No. 15. AHCPR Publication No. 95-0652.* Rockville, MD: Agency for Health Care Policy and Research.

Bergstrom, N., & Braden, B. J. (2002). Predictive validity of the Braden scale among Black and White subjects. *Nursing Research, 51*(6), 398–403.

Bergstrom, N., Braden, B., Boynton, P., et al. (1995). Using a research-based assessment scale in clinical practice. *Nursing Clinics of North America, 30*(3), 539–551.

Bergstrom, N., Braden, B., Kemp, M., et al. (1998). Predicting pressure ulcer risk. A multi-site study of the predictive validity of the Braden scale. *Nursing Research, 47*(5), 261–269.

Bergstrom, N., Braden, B. J., Laguzza, A., et al. (1987a). The Braden scale for predicting pressure sore risk. *Nursing Research, 36,* 205–210.

Bergstrom, N., Demuth, P. J., & Braden, B. J. (1987b). A clinical trial of the Braden scale for predicting pressure sore risk. *Nursing Clinics of North America, 22*(2), 417–428.

Bergstrom, N., Horn, S. D., Smout, R. J. et al. (2005). The National Pressure Ulcer Long-term Care Study: Outcomes of pressure ulcer treatments in long-term care. *Journal of the American Geriatrics Society, 53*(10), 1721–1729.

Bergstrom, N., Horn, S. S., Rapp, M. P., et al. (2013). Turning for Ulder Reduction: A multisite randomized clinical trial in nursing homes. *Journal of the American Geriatrics Society, 61*(1), 1705–1713.

Berlowitz, D. (2012). Prevalence, incidence and facility-acquired rates. In B. Pieper (Ed.), *Pressure ulcers: Prevalence, incidence, and implications for the future* (pp. 19–24). Washington, DC: National Pressure Ulcer Advisory Panel.

Black, J. M., Cuddigan, J. E., Walko, M. A., et al. (2010). Medical device related pressure ulcers in hospitalized patients. *International Wound Journal, 7*(5), 358–365.

Blair, G. J., Djonlic, K., Fraser, G. C., et al. (1992). The bowel management tube: An effective means for controlling fecal incontinence. *Journal of Pediatric Surgery, 27,* 1269–1272.

Bolton, L. (2007). Which pressure ulcer risk assessment scales are valid for use in the clinical setting? *Journal of Wound, Ostomy, and Continence Nursing, 34*(4), 368–381.

Bourdel-Marchasson, I., Barateau, M., Rondeau, V., et al. (2000). A multi-center trial of the effects of oral nutritional supplementation in critically ill older inpatients. *Nutrition, 16*(1), 1–5.

Braden, B., & Bergstrom, N. (1987). A conceptual schema for the study of the etiology of pressure sores. *Rehabilitation Nursing, 12*(1), 8–12.

Braden, B., & Bergstrom, N. (1994). Predictive validity of the Braden scale for pressure sore risk in a nursing home population. *Research in Nursing and Health, 17*(6), 459–470.

Braden, B., & Maklebust, J. (2005). Preventing pressure ulcers with the Braden scale: An update on this easy-to-use tool that assesses a patient's risk. *American Journal of Nursing, 105*(6), 70–72.

Brienza, D. M., & Geyer, M. I. (2000). Understanding support surface technologies. *Advances in Skin and Wound Care, 13*(5), 237–244.

Brienza, D., Kelsey, S., Karg, P., et al. (2010). A randomized clinical trial on preventing pressure ulcers with wheelchair seat cushions. *Journal of the American Geriatrics Society, 58*(12), 2308–2314.

Brindle, C. T. (2013). Ten top questions and answers on the use of dressings for pressure ulcer prevention. *Wounds International, 4*(4), 16–21.

Brindle, C. T., Malhotra, R., O'Rourke, S., et al. (2013). Turning and repositioning the critically ill patient with hemodynamic instability: A literature review and consensus recommendations. *Journal of Wound, Ostomy, and Continence Nursing, 40*(3), 254–267.

Center for Medicare & Medicaid Services State Operations manual: Guidance for Surveyors of Long Term Care Facilities. (2008). Appendix PP. Revision 26. Retrieved September 1, from http://www.cms.hhs.gov/GuidanceforLawsAndRegulations/12_NHs.asp

Conine, T. A., Hershler, C., Daechsel, D., et al. (1994). Pressure ulcer prophylaxis in elderly patients using polyurethane foam or Jay wheelchair cushions. *International Journal of Rehabilitation Research, 17*(2), 123–137.

Coopey, M., Nix, M. P., & Clancy, C. M. (2006). Translating research into evidence-based nursing practice and evaluating effectiveness. *Journal of Nursing Care Quality, 21*(5), 195–202.

Cuddign J., Ayello E., & Sussman, C. (Eds.). 2001. *Pressure ulcers in America.* Reston, VA: NPUAP.

Dammeyer, J., Dickson, S., Packard, D., et al. (2013). Building a protocol to guide mobility in the ICU. *Critical Care Nursing Quarterly, 36*(1), 37–49.

Dealy, C. (2009). Skin care and pressure ulcers. *Advances in Skin and Wound Care, 22*(9), 421.

DeFloor, T., De Bacquer, D., & Grypdonck, M. H. F. (2004). The effect of various combinations of turning and pressure reducing devices on the incidence of pressure ulcers. *International Journal of Nursing Studies, 42*(1), 37–46.

Defloor, T., & Grypdonck, M. F. H. (2005). Pressure ulcers: Validation of two risk assessment scales. *Journal of Clinical Nursing, 14,* 373–382.

Edwards, M. (1994). The rationale for the use of risk calculators in pressure sore prevention, and the evidence of the reliability and validity of published scales. *Journal of Advanced Nursing, 20,* 288–296. doi:10.1046/j.1365-2648.1994.20020288.x.

Ek, A. C., Unosson, M., Larsson, J., et al. (1991). The development and healing of pressure sores related to the nutritional state. *Clinical Nutrition, 10*(5), 245–250.

European Pressure Ulcer Advisor Panel & National Pressure Ulcer Advisory Panel (EPUAP/NPUAP). (2009). *International guideline prevention and treatment of pressure ulcers: Quick reference guide.* Washington, DC: National Pressure Ulcer Advisory Panel.

Gattinoni, L., Tognoni, G., Pesenti, A. et al. (2001). Effect of prone positioning on the survival of patients with acute respiratory failure. *New England Journal of Medicine, 345*(8), 568–573.

Gillespie, B. M., Chaboyer, W. P., McInnes, E., et al. (2014). Repositioning for pressure ulcer prevention in adults (review). *The Cochrane Library,* Issue 4.

Gerhardt, L. C., Strassle, V., Lenz, A., et al. (2008). Influence of epidermal hydration on the friction of human skin against textiles. *Journal of the Royal Society Interface, 5,* 1317–1328.

Geyer, M. J., Brienza, D. M., Karg, P., et al. (2001). A randomized control trial to evaluate pressure-reducing seat cushions for elderly wheelchair users. *Advances in Skin and Wound Care, 14*(3), 120–132.

Grogan, T. A., & Kramer, D. J. (2002). The rectal trumpet: Use of a nasopharyngeal airway to contain fecal incontinence critically ill patients. *Journal of Wound, Ostomy, and Continence Nursing, 29,* 193–202.

Gray, M., Black, J. M., Baharestani, M. M., et al. (2011). Moisture-associated skin damage. *Journal of Wound, Ostomy, and Continence Nursing, 38*(3), 1–7.

Halfens, R. J. G., Van Achterberg, T., & Bal, R. H. (2000). Validity and reliability of the Braden scale and the influence of risk factors: A multi-centre prospective study. *International Journal of Nursing Studies, 37*(19), 313–319.

Horn, S. D., Bender, S. A., Ferguson, M. et al. (2004). The National Pressure Ulcer Long-Term Care Study: Pressure ulcer development in long-term care residents. *Journal of the American Geriatrics Society, 52*(3), 359–367.

Hansen, D., Langemo, D. K., Anderson, J., et al. (2010). Friction and shear considerations I pressure ulcer development. *Advances in Skin and Wound Care, 23*(1), 21–24.

Hermans, M. H. E., Weyl, C., & Roger, S. I. (2014). Performance parameters of support surfaces: Setting measuring and presentation standards. *Wounds, 26*(1), 28–36.

Jankowski, I. M., & Nadzam, D. M. (2011). Identifying gaps, barriers, and solutions in implementing pressure ulcer prevention programs. *The Joint Commission Journal on Quality and Patient Safety, 37*(6), 253–264.

Johnson, D., Lineweaver, L., & Maze, L. (2009), Patients' bath basins as potential sources of infection. A multicenter sampling study. *American Journal of Critical Care, 118*(1), 31–38.

Joint Commission. (2007). Preventing pressure ulcers: The goal is zero. *Joint Commission Journal on Quality and Patient Safety, 33*(10), 605–610.

Kalisch, B. J., Landstrom, G., & Williams, R. A. (2009). Missed nursing care: Errors of omission. *Nursing Outlook, 57*(1), 3–9.

Kalisch, B. J., Tschannen, D., & Friese, C. R. (2011). Hospital variation in missed nursing care. *American Journal of Medical Quality, 28*(4), 291–292.

Kosiak, M. (1959). Etiology and pathology of ischemic ulcers. *Archives of Physical Medicine and Rehabilitation, 40*, 62–69.

Kwong, E., Pang, S., Wong, T., et al. (2005). Predicting pressure ulcer risk with the modified Braden, Braden, and Norton scales in acute care hospitals in Mainland China. *Applied Nursing Research, 18*(2), 122–128.

Lahmann N. A., Halfens, R. J. G., & Dassen, T. (2010). The impact of prevention structures and processes on pressure ulcer prevalence in nursing homes and acute-care hospitals. *Journal of Evaluation in Clinical Practice, 16*(1), 50–56.

Lahmann, N. A., & Kottner, J. (2011). Relation between pressure, friction and pressure ulcer categories: A secondary data analysis of hospital patients using CHAID methods. *International Journal of Nursing Studies, 48*(12), 1487–1494.

Lahmann, N. A., Tannen, A., Dassen, T., et al. (2011). Friction and shear highly associated with pressure ulcers of residents in long-term care—Classification tree analysis (CHAID) of Braden items. *Journal of Evaluation in Clinical Practice, 17*, 168–173.

Lambers, H., Piessens, S., Bloem, A., et al. (2006). Natural skin surface pH is on average below 5, which is beneficial for its resident flora. *International Journal of Cosmetic Science, 28*(5), 359–370.

Lim, R., Sirett, R., Conine, T. A., et al. (1988). Clinical trial of foam cushions in the prevention of decubitus ulcers in elderly patients. *Journal of Rehabilitation Research and Development, 25*(2), 19–26.

Lyder, C. H. (1996). Examining the inclusion of ethnic minorities in pressure ulcer prediction studies. *Journal of Wound Ostomy Continence Nursing, 23*(5), 257–260.

Lyder, C. H., Yu, C., Emerling, J., et al. (1999). The Braden Scale for pressure ulcer risk: Evaluating the predictive validity in Blacks and Hispanic elderly patients. *Applied Nursing Research, 12*(2), 60–68.

Magnan, M. A., & Maklebust, J. (2008). The effect of web-based Braden Scale training on the reliability and precision of Braden scale pressure ulcer risk assessments. *Journal of Wound, Ostomy, and Continence Nursing, 35*(2), 199–208.

Magnan, M. A., & Maklebust, J. (2009). The nursing process and pressure ulcer prevention: Making the connection. *Advances in Skin & Wound Care, 22*(2), 83–92.

Maklebust, J., & Magnan, M. A. (1994). Risk factors associated with having a pressure ulcer: A secondary data analysis. *Advances in Skin and Wound Care, 7*(6), 27–28, 30–34.

Maklebust J. (1987). Pressure ulcers: Etiology and prevention, *Nursing Clinics of North America, 22*(2), 359–377.

Maklebust, J., & Sieggreen, M. (1993). *Pressure ulcers: Guidelines for prevention and management* (3rd ed.). Springhouse, PA: Springhouse Corporation.

Maklebust, J., & Sieggreen, M. (2001). *Pressure ulcers: Guidelines for prevention and management* (3rd ed.). Springhouse, PA: Springhouse Corporation.

Marchaim, D., Taylor, A. R., Hayakawa, K., et al. (2012). Hospital bath basins are frequently contaminated with multi-drug resistant human pathogens. *American Journal of Infection Control, 40*(6), 562–564.

McInnes, E., Jammeli-Blasi, A., Bell-Syer, S. E. M., et al. (2011). Support surfaces for pressure ulcer prevention. *Cochrane Collaboration*, Issue 4. Published by John Wiley & Sons Ltd., pp. 1–17.

Moore, Z., Haynes, J. S., & Callaghan, R. (2014). Prevention and management of pressure ulcers: Support surfaces. *British Journal of Nursing, 33*(6), S636.

Nakagami, G., Sanada, H. Konya, C., et al. (2006). Comparison of two pressure ulcer preventive dressings for reducing shear force on the heel. *Journal of Wound, Ostomy, and Continence Nursing, 33*(3), 267–272.

National Pressure Ulcer Advisory Panel. (2007a). Pressure ulcer stages and categories. Retrieved September 1, 2014, from www.npuap.org/resources/educational-and-clinical-resouces/npuap-pressure-ulcer-stagescategories

National Pressure Ulcer Advisory Panel Support Surface Standards Initiative. (2007b). Terms and definitions related to support surfaces. Retrieved September 15, 2014, from http://www.npuap.org/resources/educational-andclinical-resources/support-surface-standards

National Pressure Ulcer Advisory Panel (NPUAP) and European Pressure Ulcer Advisory Panel (EPUAP). (2009). *Prevention and Treatment of Pressure Ulcers*. Washington, DC: NPUAP.

National Pressure Ulcer Advisory Panel, European Pressure Ulcer Advisory Panel and the Pan Pacific Pressure Ulcer Injury Alliance (NPUAP/EPUAP/PPPIA). (2014). *Pressure ulcer prevention: Pressure, shear, friction, and microclimate in context. A consensus document.* London, UK: Wounds International. Emily Haesler (Ed.). Perth, Australia: Cambridge Media.

NDNQI. (2014). NNQDI Module III: Pressure ulcer survey team training. Retrieved October 15, 2014, from https://members.nursingquality.orgNDNQPressureUlcerTraining/Module3/PressureUlcerTeamTraining_2aspx

Nixon, J., Thorpe, H., Barrow, H., et al. (2005). Reliability of pressure ulcer classification and diagnosis. *Journal of Advanced Nursing, 50*, 613–623. doi:10.1111/j.1365-2648.2005.03439.x.

Norton, D. (1989). Calculating the risk: Reflections on the Norton Scale. *Decubitus, 2*(3), 24–31.

Ohura, T. (2013). External force and its clinical influence—The relationships between fundamental biomechanics and clinical findings. *World Council of Enterostimal Therapists Journal, 33*(2), 14–20.

Palmore, T. N. (2010). Enhancing patient safety by reducing healthcare associated infections: The role of discovery and dissemination. *Infection Control Hospital Epidemiology, 31*(2), 118–123.

Pan, N., & Sun, G. (2011). *Functional textiles for improved performance, protection and health.* Cambridge, UK: Woodhead Publishing Ltd.

Pancorbo-Hidalgo, P. L., Garcia-Fernandez, F. P., Lopez-Medina, I. M., et al. (2006). Risk assessment scales for pressure ulcer prevention: A systematic review. *Journal of Advanced Nursing, 54*(1), 94–110.

Pang, S. M., & Wong, T. K. (1998). Predicting pressure sore risk with the Norton, Braden, and Waterlow Scales in a Hong Kong Rehabilitation Hospital. *Nursing Research, 47*(3), 147–153.

Penzer, R. (2009). Best practice when applying topical barrier creams. *Wound Essentials, 4*, 75–77.

Pinchofsky-Devin, G. D., & Kaminski, M. V. (1986). Correlation of pressure sores and nutritional status. *Journal of the American Geriatrics Society, 34*, 435–440.

Polit, D. R., & Beck, C. T. (2011). *Nursing research: Principles and methods* (9th ed.). Philadelphia, PA: Lippincott Williams & Wilkins.

Ratliff, C. R. (2005). WOCN's evidence-based pressure ulcer guideline. *Advances in Skin and Wound Care, 18*(4), 204–208.

Reddy, M., Gill, S. S., & Rochan, P. A. (2006). Preventing pressure ulcers: A systematic review. *JAMA, 296*(8), 974–984.

Reswick, J., & Rogers, J. (1976). Experiences at Rancho Los Amigos Hospital with devices and techniques to prevent pressure sores. In R. M. Kenedi, J. M. Cowden, & J. T. Scales (Eds.) *Bedsore biomechanics* (pp. 301–310). Baltimore, MD: University Park Press.

Sansom W, Flynn K (2007) Risk assessment and anatomical foam heel dressings in emergency department to contribute to reduced development of pressure ulcers. *Australian Journal of Wound Management, 15*(3), 114–117.

Sargent, J., Loney, E., & Murphy, G. (2008). Effective interprofessional teams: "Contact is Not Enough" to build a team. *Journal of Continuing Education in the Health Professions, 28*(4), 228–234.

Scardillo, J., & Aronovitch, S. A. (1999). Successfully managing incontinence-related irritant dermatitis over the lifespan. *Ostomy/Wound Management, 45*, 36–44.

Shaw, G., & Taylor, S. J. (1991). A survey of wheelchair seating problems of the institutionalized elderly. *Assistive Technologies, 3*(1), 5–10.

Sibbald, R. G., Norton, L., & Woo, K. Y. (2009). Optimized skin care can prevent pressure ulcers. *Advances in Skin and Wound Care, 22*(9), 392.

Smith, A., McNichol, L. L., Amos, M. A., et al. (2013). A retrospective, nonrandomized, before-and-after study of the effect of linens constructed of synthetic silk-like fabric on pressure ulcer incidence. *Ostomy/Wound Management, 59*(4), 28–34.

Sparks, D., Chase, K., Heaton, B., et al. (2010). Rectal trauma and associated hemorrhage with the use of the ConvaTec Flexi-Seal Fecal Management System: Report of 3 Cases. *Diseases of the Colon and Rectum, 53*(3), 346–349.

Sprigle, S. (2000). Effects of forces and the selection of support surfaces. *Topics in Geriatric Rehabilitation, 16*(2), 47–62.

Sprigle, S., & Sonenblum, S. (2011). Assessing evidence supporting redistribution of pressure for pressure ulcer prevention: A review. *Journal of Rehabilitation Research and Development, 48*(3), 203–213.

Swanson, M. S., Rose, M. A., Baker, G. et al. (2011). Braden subscales and their relationship to the prevalence of pressure ulcers in hospitalized obese patients. *Bariatric Nursing and Surgical Patient Care, 6*(1), 21–23.

Thomas, D. R. (2007). Loss of skeletal muscle mass in aging: Examining the relationship of starvation, sarcopenia and cachexia. *Clinical Nutrition, 26*(4), 389–399.

Thomas, D. R., Goode, P. S., Tarquine, P. H., et al. (1996). Hospital acquired pressure ulcers and the risk of death. *Journal of the American Geriatrics Society, 44*(12), s1435–s1440.

Thompson, P., Anderson, J., Langemo, D., et al. (2008). Support surfaces: Definitions and utilization for patient care. *Advances in Skin and Wound Care, 21*(6), 264–266.

Thompson, P., Anderson, J., Langemo, D., et al. (October, 2009). Support surfaces: Reducing pressure ulcer risk. *Nursing Management, 40*(11), 49–51.

Twersky, J., Montgomery, T., Sloane, R., et al. (2012). A randomized, controlled study to assess the effect of silk-like textiles and high-absorbency adult incontinence briefs on pressure ulcer prevention. *Ostomy/Wound Management, 58*(12), 18–24.

Tymec, A. C., Pieper, B., & Vollman, K. (1997). A comparison of two pressure-relieving devices on the prevention of heel pressure ulcers. *Advances in Wound Care, 10*(1), 39–44.

US Department of Health and Human Services. (2010). *Healthy People 2010*. Hyattsville, MD: National Center for Health Statistics.

Vanderwee, K., Grydonck, M. H., De Bacquer, D., et al. (2007). Effectiveness of turning with unequal time intervals on the incidence of pressure ulcer lesions. *Journal of Advanced Nursing, 57*(1), 59–68.

Vollman, K. M. (2004). Prone positioning for the patient who has acute respiratory distress syndrome: The art and science. *Critical Care Nursing Clinics of North America, 16*(3), 319–336.

Vollman, K. M. (2012). Hemodynamic instability: Is it really a barrier to turning critically ill patients? *Critical Care Nursing Quarterly, 32*(1), 70–75.

Waterlow, J. (1985). A pressure sore risk assessment card. *Nursing Times, 81*, 49–55.

Winkleman, C., & Peereboom, K. (2010). Staff perceived barriers and facilitators. *Critical Care Nurse, 30*(2), S13–S16.

Winslow, E. H., Lane, L. D., & Woods, R. J. (1995). Dangling, a review of relevant physiology: Research and practice. *Heart and Lung, 24*(4), 263–272.

WOCN Society. (2010). *Guideline for management of pressure ulcers: WOCN clinical practice guidelines series # 2*. Glenview, IL: WOCN.

Zhong, W., Xing, M. M. Q., Pan, N., et al. (2006). Textiles and human skin, microclimate, cutaneous reactions: An overview. *Cutaneous and Ocular Toxicology, 25*(1), 23–39.

Zhong, W., Ahmad, A., Xing, M. M., et al. (2008). Impact of textiles on formation and prevention of skin lesions and bedsores. *Cutaneous and Ocular Toxicology, 24*(1), 21–28.

QUESTIONS

1. A wound care nurse is using root cause analysis (RCA) to determine the cause of a patient's necrotic pressure ulcer. What is the primary goal of this study method?

A. Prevent fiscal penalties related to poor quality of care
B. Place blame on the individuals responsible for the problem
C. Identify potential areas for improvement in prevention protocols
D. Change agency protocols for pressure ulcer prevention

2. The wound care nurse in a long-term care facility is calculating the cumulative incidence of pressure ulcers in the current residents. What does this ratio represent?

A. The number of persons at risk who develop new pressure ulcers during a specific period of time
B. The number of persons at risk who develop new ulcers relative to the number of ulcer-free days
C. The proportion of all persons who have a pressure ulcer in a specific setting at a specific point in time
D. The proportion of all persons who have a pressure ulcer in a specific setting at a specific period of time

3. The wound care nurse is calculating the pressure ulcer point prevalence for a nursing home population. The data obtained are as follows: On a particular date, 15 persons have a pressure ulcer out of 120 residents. The pressure ulcer point prevalence is:
   A. 1.00 = 10%
   B. 1.25 = 12.5%
   C. 1.50 = 15%
   D. 2.00 = 20%

4. The wound care nurse is benchmarking the data on pressure ulcer incidence obtained in a critical care unit. What is the goal of this process?
   A. To determine the severity of the pressure ulcers discovered
   B. To obtain reimbursement from third-party payers and reduce litigation risk
   C. To determine pressure ulcer treatment protocols
   D. To determine effectiveness of the prevention program by comparing outcomes to those of other (similar) agencies/settings

5. The wound care nurse uses risk assessment tools to determine which patients in an acute care setting are at risk for pressure ulcers. What is the primary purpose of these tools?
   A. To use as a basis to design an agency-wide pressure ulcer prevention program
   B. To obtain information as to specific risk factors throughout the agency
   C. To identify other factors contributing to overall risk
   D. To identify patients at risk and their particular risk factors

6. The wound nurse assessing a patient for pressure ulcers places the patient as an 11 on the Braden Scale. What risk level does this number represent?
   A. Mild risk
   B. Moderate risk
   C. High risk
   D. Very high risk

7. What measures can wound care nurses take to improve accuracy in risk assessment?
   A. When in doubt, score high on the Braden Scale.
   B. Refrain from using data obtained from audits and skills fairs.
   C. Use the NDNQI module as a teaching strategy.
   D. Assign a Braden Scale total score of 19 to save time with patient care.

8. A wound care nurse off-loading a patient every 2 hours notes that normal reactive hyperemia does not resolve within 30 minutes of off-loading. What is the significance of this finding?
   A. A stage I pressure ulcer is developing.
   B. This is a normal finding unrelated to pressure ulcer development.
   C. The nurse should discontinue off-loading and concentrate on the surface.
   D. The patient has developed a stage II pressure ulcer.

9. The wound care nurse is repositioning patients in a critical care unit. Which statement accurately describes a therapeutic effect of this intervention?
   A. Critically ill patients seem to tolerate the right lateral position better than the left lateral position.
   B. Wedges should be used to achieve small incremental lateral position changes of 30 degrees before moving the patient to the 45-degree lateral position.
   C. The presence of life-threatening arrhythmias or active hemorrhage in a patient requires more frequent positioning.
   D. The use of a lateral rotation bed should be considered as an alternative to repositioning.

10. The wound care nurse uses proven strategies to protect patients from pressure ulcer development. What is one recommended technique?
    A. Use a commercial foot elevation boot rather than a bed pillow to suspend the heel off the bed and prevent pressure ulcers.
    B. Use a sliding board against bare skin when transferring a patient from bed to gurney or bed to chair.
    C. Protect the sacrococcygeal area against friction damage by applying adhesive foam dressings.
    D. Take measures to keep the skin warm and moist to reduce the risk for friction and shear injury.

11. Which of the following describes an effective strategy for minimizing the adverse effects of shearing forces?
    A. Maintain the head of the bed elevation at 45 degrees unless medically contraindicated
    B. Use foam redistribution surfaces whenever possible.
    C. Use two to three layers of underpads to keep the perineal skin dry and to prevent contamination of the support surface
    D. Elevate the head of the bed to 30 degrees or less when positioning in a semi-Fowler's position.

ANSWERS: 1.C, 2.A, 3.**B**, 4.**D**, 5.**D**, 6.**C**, 7.**C**, 8.**A**, 9.**A**, 10.**C**, 11.**D**

CHAPTER 20

Therapeutic Surfaces for Bed and Chair

Dianne Mackey and Carolyn Watts

OBJECTIVES

1. Explain the role of each of the following in pressure ulcer development: prolonged or intense pressure, shear force, moisture, and tissue tolerance.
2. Explain how therapeutic bed and chair surfaces contribute to prevention and management of pressure ulcers.
3. Select/recommend appropriate pressure redistribution devices for bed, chair, and heels.
4. Design a decision-making algorithm for appropriate use of off-loading devices and therapeutic support surfaces.

Topic Outline

Introduction

As discussed in the chapter on pressure ulcer pathology and presentation, key etiologic factors for pressure ulcer injuries include prolonged or high-intensity pressure, friction and shear, and hot wet skin, and each of these factors can be at least partially controlled by an appropriate surface for the bed and chair. Appropriate selection and use of these surfaces are the focus of this chapter. A support surface is a specialized mattress or mattress overlay, chair cushion, or stretcher/operating room pad designed for the management of tissue loads, microclimate, and/or other therapeutic functions (National Pressure Ulcer Advisory Panel [NPUAP], 2007). Knowledge of the components of a support surface along with the product's performance is key in selecting a product that reduces pressure, shear, friction, and moisture between the patient's skin and the support surface. Support surfaces are available in a variety of sizes and shapes and include mattresses, mattress overlays, operating room (OR) surfaces, examination and procedure table surfaces, and pads for emergency and transport stretchers or gurneys. For the purposes of this chapter, the term support surface refers to both horizontal surfaces (overlay, mattress, or integrated bed system) and seat cushions, unless otherwise stated.

Clinicians are expected to make care recommendations based on current research, and we do have evidence that pressure redistribution devices can help reduce the incidence of pressure ulcers by up to 60% (Cullum et al., 2004; Whitney et al., 2006). However, research related to support surface utilization is very limited, and at present, there is no evidence that one particular type or brand of support surface is better than another (NPUAP & EPUAP, 2014; Whitney et al., 2006; WOCN Society, 2010). Thus, at present, clinicians must base product selection on a clear understanding of the therapeutic features of various products as compared to the patient's needs. This chapter addresses (1) risk factors and support surfaces; (2) components, categories, and features of support surfaces; (3) selection/evaluation of a support surface based on an individual patient's needs; and (4) the development/evaluation of a facility- or agency-wide support surface decision tree or algorithm. General guidelines for care of the patient requiring a support surface are provided in Box 20-1.

CLINICAL PEARL

Studies indicate that pressure redistribution devices can reduce the incidence of pressure ulcers by up to 60%; however, there is currently no evidence that one type or brand of support surface is better than another.

Risk Factors Addressed by Support Surfaces

Prevention of pressure ulcers is accomplished primarily by effective management of tissue loads and shear forces. Support surfaces are an integral component of a pressure ulcer prevention and treatment program because they can enhance perfusion of at-risk or injured soft tissue. It is important to remember that support surfaces are only one component of a comprehensive pressure ulcer prevention and treatment program; they should *not* be considered a stand-alone intervention. Recent research suggests that pressure is not the only contributing factor to tissue breakdown and therefore not the only factor to be addressed by a therapeutic support surface; other causative factors include shear, friction, moisture, and heat. However, in most situations, pressure redistribution is the most important feature of a support surface. Research has clearly shown that the damaging effects of pressure are related to both its

BOX 20-1. General Recommendations for Support Surfaces

- Support surfaces are not a stand-alone intervention for the prevention and treatment of pressure ulcers but are to be used in conjunction with proper nutritional support, moisture management, pressure redistribution when in bed and chair, turning and repositioning, risk identification, and patient and caregiver education.
- Support surfaces do not eliminate the need for turning and repositioning.
- Consider concurrent use of a pressure redistribution seating surface or cushion of an appropriate type along with use of any support surface.
- When choosing a support surface, consider contraindications for use of specific support surfaces as specified by the manufacturer.
- In order to achieve the full benefits of a support surface, the support surface must be functioning properly and used correctly according to the manufacturer instructions.
- When choosing a support surface, consider current patient characteristics and risk factors, including weight and weight distribution; fall and entrapment risk; risk for developing new pressure ulcers; number, severity, and location of existing pressure ulcers; as well as previous support surface usage and patient preference.
- The person who exceeds the weight limit or whose body dimensions exceed his or her current support surface should be moved to an appropriate bariatric support surface.
- For persons who are candidates for progressive mobility, consider a support surface that facilitates getting out of bed.
- Persons who meet facility protocol for a low bed frame and who have a pressure ulcer, or are at risk for developing a pressure ulcer, should also receive an appropriate support surface.
- Persons who have medical contraindications for turning should be considered for an appropriate support surface and repositioning with frequent small shifts.
- For persons experiencing intractable pain, consider providing an appropriate alternative to the current support surface.
- Persons with a new myocutaneous flap on the posterior or lateral trunk or pelvis should be provided with an appropriate support surface per facility protocol.
- Minimize the number and type of layers between the patient and the support surface.
- Support surfaces must be compatible with the care setting while meeting the individual needs of the patient.
- Consider fall/entrapment risk when choosing between a mattress and an overlay.
- A support surface that dissipates moisture (low air loss) may be indicated when moisture/incontinence cannot be managed by other means.
- At present, guidelines for prevention of heel ulcers require elevation of the heel off the bed; support surfaces cannot provide sufficient envelopment to protect the soft tissue of the heel (even very high level support surfaces).

Source: WOCN Support Surface Consensus Conference Statements (2014).

magnitude and duration; simply stated, tissues can withstand higher loads for shorter periods of time (Brienza & Geyer, 2005) and lower loads for longer periods of time. A surface that effectively redistributes pressure across the entire contact surface effectively reduces the *magnitude* of the pressure and extends the time that the patient can safely remain in one position.

CLINICAL PEARL

Support surfaces are only one element of a comprehensive pressure ulcer prevention program; they should *not* be considered a stand-alone intervention.

The clinician must remember that the risk of skin and soft tissue breakdown is affected not only by the extrinsic factors already addressed (pressure, shear, friction, moisture, and heat) but also by intrinsic risk factors such as advanced age, low blood pressure, smoking, elevated body temperature, poor protein intake, anemia, generalized edema, and hemodynamic instability. This again underscores the fact that a support surface is only one element of a comprehensive management plan and does not replace attention to perfusion, nutritional support, and management of comorbidities.

Tissue Loading and Interface Pressure

Tissue interface pressure is defined as the force per unit area that acts perpendicularly between the patient's skin and the support surface (Cullum et al., 2004). As noted, the intensity (magnitude) and duration of pressure exerted against the skin and soft tissue is a critical factor in risk for skin breakdown, and therapeutic support surfaces "work" primarily by reducing the intensity of interface pressure. Thus, a critical question to be addressed in relation to any surface is the degree to which it reduces pressure, and interface pressure measurements have been used for years to compare various products in terms of their pressure redistribution ability. This noninvasive test involves placement of a mat equipped with a single pressure sensor or multiple pressure sensors between the patient's skin and the underlying support surface. This "tissue interface pressure" measurement provides an approximation of the pressure exerted over a specific bony prominence and the surrounding area (Le et al., 1984; Miller et al., 2013; Reger et al., 1988). For years, research efforts have focused on establishment of a critical "cutoff" for interface pressure (i.e., the pressure reading beyond which pressure ulcers are likely to develop); however, to date, it has not been possible to establish a specific reading that represents the physiologic "limit" for the majority of patients. Thus, the value of tissue interface pressure measurements is primarily in comparison of one product to another (assuming the availability of valid interface pressure measurements for the various devices).

CLINICAL PEARL

In most situations, pressure redistribution is the most important feature of the support surface; effective pressure redistribution reduces the intensity of the pressure and extends the time the patient can safely remain in one position.

Physical Concepts

Physical concepts are performance-related terms used to guide discussions and evaluations of the performance of various support surfaces (Christian & Lachenbruch, 2007).

Life Expectancy

The term "life expectancy" refers to the period of time during which a product is expected to effectively fulfill its purpose.

Fatigue

Life expectancy may be impacted by *fatigue*, that is, reduced performance capacity due to intended or unintended use and/or prolonged exposure to chemical, thermal, or physical forces (NPUAP, 2007). Life expectancy and fatigue will impact the ability of the support surface to redistribute pressure, control friction and shear, and manage the microclimate (temperature and humidity). Staff who have the opportunity to observe support surfaces during linen or room changes should be alert to indicators that the surface is no longer performing as expected: reduced height or thickness; discoloration; altered integrity of the cover, seams, zipper/zipper cover flap, or backing; degradation of internal components; or presence of odor. If any of these are observed, the surface should be referred to engineering/maintenance for evaluation, whether or not it has exceeded its stated product life span. Staff members to be involved in monitoring include nursing staff, certified nursing assistants (CNAs), housekeeping, and engineering and maintenance personnel (E. Call, *personal communication*, 2014).

CLINICAL PEARL

All staff should be alert to evidence of product *fatigue* (e.g., reduced height or thickness, discoloration, odor, visible damage) and should have the product evaluated by engineering/maintenance, *even if it is still under warranty and has not exceeded its stated lifespan.*

Pressure Redistribution (Immersion and Envelopment)

Support surfaces are designed to prevent pressure ulcers and promote pressure ulcer healing through effective pressure redistribution and reduction in pressure intensity/magnitude. By conforming to the contours of the body, support surfaces redistribute pressure over a larger surface area rather than having pressure concentrated in a more circumscribed location (e.g., directly over the bony prominence); the end result is reduced interface pressure. The therapeutic function of pressure redistribution is accomplished through immersion and envelopment.

Immersion

The term immersion refers to the depth to which the body is allowed to penetrate or "sink into" the surface; as the body sinks into the surface, the pressure is spread out over the entire contact area rather than being concentrated directly over the bony prominence (NPUAP, 2007). Immersion is dependent on factors such as the stiffness and thickness of the support surface and the flexibility of the cover.

Envelopment

The term envelopment refers to the ability of the support surface to conform evenly to irregularities (e.g., clothing, bedding, bony prominences) without causing a substantial increase in pressure; by creating a very close "match" between the support surface and the body surface, envelopment maximizes pressure redistribution (Brienza & Geyer, 2005; Christian & Lachenbruch, 2007; NPUAP, 2007).

CLINICAL PEARL

Most support surfaces provide pressure redistribution through *immersion* and *envelopment* (i.e., allowing the patient to sink into the product and evenly conforming to his or her bodily contours).

Bottoming Out

In contrast to the therapeutic functions of immersion and envelopment, *"bottoming out"* is the term used to denote excessive penetration of the surface; if the surface provides inadequate support for the patient's weight, the body may sink so deeply into the surface that the patient's bony prominences are actually resting against the underlying bed frame. Whitney et al. (2006) defined bottoming out as <1 inch of material between the support surface and the skin surface; to evaluate for bottoming out, the clinician should place her or his hand palm up beneath the support surface in the area underlying the patient's bony prominence. Factors that contribute to bottoming out include (1) patient weight that exceeds support surface's weight limits, according to the manufacturer; (2) disproportion between weight and size, such as with bilateral lower extremity amputation; (3) persistent head-of-bed elevation exceeding 30 degrees; and (4) inadequate support surface settings, such as over or under inflation. An essential clinical caveat in effective use of *all* support surfaces is to limit the layers (sheets, briefs, and underpads) between the patient and the support surface.

CLINICAL PEARL

"Bottoming out" means the overlay or mattress is providing insufficient support and the patient's bony prominences are resting on the underlying bed frame; this mandates a change in support surface.

Friction and Shear Reduction

Friction and shear are physical forces that increase the risk of pressure ulcer formation, with shear being of tremendous significance. *Shear stress* refers to the deformation that occurs when the tissue is exposed to lateral strain (Christian & Lachenbruch, 2007); specifically, the patient is at risk for shear damage when exposed to the dual forces of friction and gravity. This occurs when the patient slides down in bed; typically, frictional forces hold the skin stationary while gravitational forces cause the deep tissue layers (muscle and bone) to slide down. This causes shear and deformation of the subcutaneous tissue and blood vessels, which is a major contributor to ischemic injury. Support surfaces with low-friction covers (e.g., Gore-Tex type covers) reduce frictional forces and thereby reduce tissue deformation when the patient slides down in bed. An alternative approach is to reduce sliding, but this is very difficult to accomplish in situations requiring head-of-bed elevation. However, a support surface cannot provide total protection against shear and does not eliminate the need for additional interventions to minimize friction and shear.

CLINICAL PEARL

Surfaces with low-friction covers reduce tissue deformation and underlying tissue damage when the patient slides down in bed.

Microclimate (Temperature and Moisture) Control

Microclimate control is a therapeutic function provided by some support surfaces; this feature may be of particular benefit to patients who are diaphoretic. Excessively moist skin is a well-known risk factor for pressure ulcer development, as is abnormally warm skin. Control of temperature at the interface surface (patient–bed boundary) helps to maintain normal skin temperature, which in turn inhibits sweating and reduces skin moisture (Mackey, 2005). An ideal support surface would therefore be designed to help maintain normal skin hydration and temperature (Brienza & Geyer, 2005). This can be accomplished through porous covers that reduce moisture by promoting air transfer between the skin and surface, with resultant dissipation of moisture and body heat. Another approach is to provide constant airflow against the skin by pumping air through microperforations in the support surface cover.

CLINICAL PEARL

Microclimate control can be provided by providing airflow against the skin or by increasing the transfer of air between the skin and the support surface.

Components of a Support Surface

Perhaps the most important component of a support surface is the medium used to provide pressure redistribution. Mediums include air, fluid, or solid and can be used alone or in combination. The ability to encapsulate the medium is another component of the support surface and is called a cell or bladder (NPUAP, 2007). Cells can be configured in a longitudinal or latitudinal pattern and can be individual or interconnected.

Foam

Foam is available in chair cushions, overlays, mattresses for beds, and pads for transport gurneys, stretchers, and OR and procedure tables. Most foam overlays and cushions are indicated for single-patient use, whereas mattresses are intended for multiple-patient use. All foam products are designed for a specific weight limit and life span. Foam can be the sole medium or may be included in hybrid products that include gel, air, or other fluid materials that enhance envelopment in key areas. Benefits associated with foam support surfaces include their relatively low cost, light weight, and minimal maintenance. Disadvantages include a limited life span due to fatigue caused by flexion and compression over time. There is also a high risk for moisture penetration and resulting potential for infection. Additional disadvantages include the cost of disposal and negative environmental impact.

Foam can be closed cell or open cell. *Closed-cell* foam is a nonpermeable formulation with a barrier between the cells that prevents gases or liquids from passing through the foam (NPUAP, 2007); closed-cell foam products have the potential to increase skin temperature by preventing dissipation of body heat (Nicholson et al., 1999). *Open-cell* foam is a higher-specification foam that has been shown to be more effective in preventing pressure ulcers than closed-cell foam. Examples of higher-specification foams are elastic and viscoelastic. There is no evidence that one type of high-specification foam is better than another (McInnes et al., 2011, NPUAP & EPUAP, 2014).

Elastic Foam

Elastic foam is high-specification foam made of a porous polymer material that conforms in proportion to the applied weight; air enters and exits the open-cell foam rapidly due to its greater density (NPUAP, 2007). The surface continues to conform until the resistance to compression exceeds the weight being applied (Christian & Lachenbruch, 2007). The combination of density and hardness determines compressibility and conformability, which determines the ability of the support surface to mechanically redistribute loading force. Density refers to the weight of the foam and is reported as either pounds per cubic foot or kilograms per cubic meter. Greater density provides more durability.

Indentation force deflection (IFD), known previously as indentation load deflection (ILD), is a measure of firmness or resistance to compression. In the United States, IFD is reported as the force in pounds required to compress a specific area of foam by 25%. Surfaces can be made with a combination of foams strategically placed to optimize pressure redistribution in targeted locations (Polyurethane Foam Association [PFA], 2010). For example, a mattress or cushion may be constructed with a lower-density and more compressible foam located close to the surface to enhance conformability and a higher-density and less compressible foam located more deeply in the mattress to prevent compression or bottoming out. See Figure 20-1 for an example of a foam pressure redistribution device.

A foam overlay is a single-use form of support surface placed on the top of a mattress. If used for pressure redistribution, an overlay should have a base height of at least 3 inches measured from the base (or bottom) to the lower level of convolution, sufficient density to ensure durability (1.3 to 1.6 lb/ft^3), and an IFD of 30 (Whittemore, 1998).

Viscoelastic (Memory) Foam

A viscoelastic foam is another high-specification open-cell foam made of a porous polymer material that conforms in proportion to the applied weight. Air enters and exits the foam cells slowly, which means the material responds more slowly than elastic foam. Viscoelastic foams are a subset of urethane polymer foams that exhibit a slow recovery (memory) property; these products generally have high density and low IFD, meaning they provide both conformability and support. Because of its fluid nature and low resistance, viscoelastic foam is rapidly displaced and conforms readily to the shape of any object placed on the surface. Viscoelastic foam is available in many grades and qualities; each has properties that affect pressure redistribution and microclimate performance in unique ways. Some viscoelastic foams are engineered to change hardness within a specific temperature range. These materials tend to get softer as the material warms to body temperature, resulting in conformability similar to that provided by a gel. Viscoelastic support surfaces are often used in the OR (Association of periOperative Registered Nurses [AORN], 2008) and have been shown to effectively decrease the

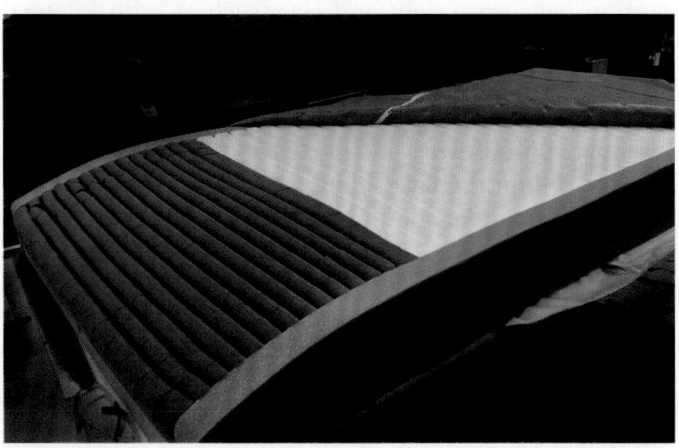

FIGURE 20-1. Foam pressure redistribution device.

incidence of pressure ulcers in high-risk elderly patients with fractures of the neck and femur (Cullum et al., 2001). In one study of 838 patients at risk for pressure ulcers, patients turned every 4 hours on a viscoelastic foam surface had lower incidence of pressure ulcer development than patients on a standard mattress who were turned every 2 hours (Defloor et al., 2005). (See Fig. 20-2 for an example of viscoelastic foam.)

CLINICAL PEARL

There are many variations in foam products; foam devices with proven effectiveness in pressure ulcer prevention or management include elastic foam and viscoelastic foam.

Gel

Gel contains a network of solid aggregates, colloidal dispersions, or polymers that may exhibit elastic properties (NPUAP, 2007). Some gel products are called *viscoelastic gel* because they respond similarly to viscoelastic foam. Gel support surfaces are intended for multiple-patient use. Because of the consistency of the medium, gels have been found to be especially effective in preventing shear. Other advantages include ease of cleaning and the fact that it is nonpowered and therefore requires no electricity. Disadvantages of gel support surfaces are that they tend to be heavy and are difficult to repair. In addition, the nonporous nature of the gel and lack of airflow can result in increased skin moisture; although the gel is cool upon initial contact, skin temperature may rise after hours of constant contact. Gel must be carefully monitored for migration, and the material must be manually moved back to the areas under bony prominences if this has occurred (Brienza & Geyer, 2005).

Fluids (Viscous Fluid, Water, Air)

Fluids are considered substances whose molecules flow freely past one another. Fluids have no fixed shape, so they take on the shape of the load with less resistance than a gel or solid, providing a high degree of immersion. Fluid mediums include viscous fluid, water, and air. Moisture control characteristics are dependent on the ability of the medium to conduct heat and the composition of the product's cover.

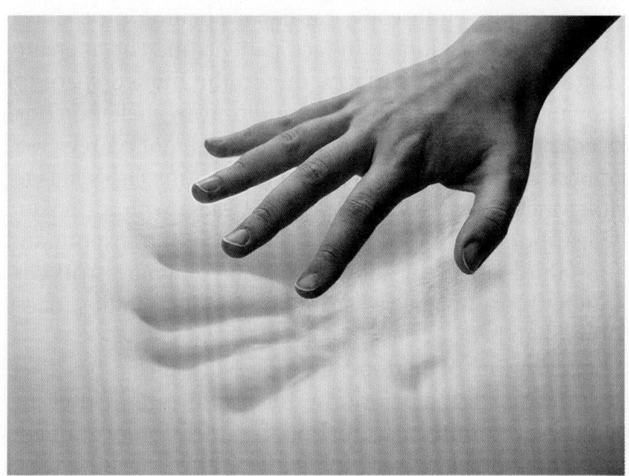

FIGURE 20-2. Viscoelastic foam device. (Courtesy Tempur-Pedic.)

Viscous Fluid

Viscous fluid is composed of materials such as silicon elastomer, silicon, or polyvinyl (Brienza & Geyer, 2005). At first glance, viscous fluid can be mistaken for gel. Although many of the advantages and disadvantages are similar to those of gels, viscous fluid is free flowing and has a similar pressure redistribution response as air or water. Compared to air and water, viscous fluid is thicker, with a relatively higher resistance to flow (NPUAP, 2007).

Water

Water is a moderate-density fluid with moderate resistance to flow (NPUAP, 2007). Studies have demonstrated that water-filled support surfaces provide lower interface pressure than a standard mattress (Cullum et al., 2001). Although popular for use in the home, water mattresses are undesirable in the hospital or long-term care setting due to multiple management concerns including the need for a heater to control temperature; potential for leakage; difficulty associated with repositioning, transfers, and performance of cardiopulmonary resuscitation (CPR); and the time and labor required to drain and move the bed.

Air

Air is a low-density fluid with minimal resistance to flow (NPUAP, 2007) and is a frequently used medium for support surfaces. Air may be the sole redistribution medium, or it may be combined with other mediums (NPUAP, 2007). Support surfaces that incorporate air are available as chair cushions, overlays, mattresses, and bed systems. Most air support surfaces are easy to clean and can be reused. Air products have the potential to leak if damaged and require either periodic reinflation (nonpowered device) or a pump to maintain continuous inflation (powered device). Air mattresses and overlays have the advantage of being lightweight and easy to clean.

Categories and Features

Categories of pressure redistribution support surfaces include overlays, mattresses, and integrated bed systems. Pressure redistribution products may be purchased in the form of a mattress, mattress overlay, chair cushion, transport pad, procedure pad, emergency room pad, or perioperative surface. All of these surfaces may be powered or nonpowered, active or reactive. A feature is a therapeutic (functional) component of a support surface that can be used alone or in combination with other features and includes low air loss, air fluidization, lateral rotation, and alternating pressure (AP). Pressure redistribution surfaces can be either single- or multizoned surfaces; a zone is a segment with a single pressure redistribution capability. Therefore, a multizoned surface has different segments with different pressure redistribution capabilities (NPUAP, 2007).

Overlays

The mattress overlay is a support surface that is placed on the top of an existing mattress (Christian & Lachenbruch, 2007; NPUAP, 2007). Gel, water, and some air-filled overlays are intended for multiple-patient use and have the advantage of requiring much less storage space than mattresses and bed systems. Other overlays, such as foam and some air products, are for single-patient use and present environmental concerns relative to disposal of the product. Overlays are thinner than mattress replacements, so there is the risk for bottoming out, especially if the patient is heavy. Because they are applied over an existing mattress, mattress overlays increase the height of the sleep surface and may complicate patient transfers, alter the fit of linens, or increase the risk for patient entrapment and falls (U.S. Food and Drug Administration [U.S. FDA], 2006).

CLINICAL PEARL

Overlays should be used with caution, as they increase the risk for entrapment and falls and may permit the patient to "bottom out."

Mattresses

A mattress is composed of any medium or combination of mediums and is placed on an existing compatible frame. Mattresses reduce some of the high-profile-related disadvantages experienced with overlays and generally present less risk for bottoming out. When therapeutic support surfaces were first introduced, the available options were essentially limited to rental beds (integrated support surfaces) or overlays that were rented or purchased. As the market evolved, manufacturers began to produce nonpowered mattresses that incorporated the features of pressure redistribution along with the "usual" features of hospital mattresses (e.g., durability, multiple-patient use following cleaning, etc.). These surfaces were initially known as "replacement mattresses" because agencies began to "replace" their standard mattresses with the therapeutic mattresses; for most agencies, this change resulted in improved skin and wound outcomes as well as reduced expenditures related to rental surfaces (Cullum et al., 2004; Gray et al., 2001). In addition, replacement mattresses eliminated "wait time" for delivery of bed systems and the need for staff to transfer the patient once they were identified as being "at risk" for pressure ulcer development. Today, most companies (in the United States) no longer make mattresses that do not redistribute pressure, so their standard mattress *is* a support surface, and therapeutic surfaces have become the "standard of care" for inpatient facilities. Mattresses may provide a variety of therapeutic functions in addition to pressure redistribution, depending on the support medium and cover; selected products also provide shear and friction reduction and management of the microclimate between the patient's skin and the support surface.

CLINICAL PEARL

Today, almost all hospital mattresses (in the United States) combine pressure redistribution features with durability and multiple-patient use; therefore, pressure redistribution has become the "standard of care" for inpatient facilities.

Integrated Bed Systems

An integrated bed system is a bed frame and support surface combined into a single unit. It may be either a rented or purchased unit, but its components do not function separately (Christian & Lachenbruch, 2007; NPUAP, 2007); therefore, it is used in place of an existing bed. When recommending an integrated bed system, the clinician must evaluate the features of both the frame and the support surface. Frames come in different heights, widths, and lengths and support a specified amount of weight. Some frames have the ability to adjust or fold for storage or for transport through narrow doors and elevators. Most frames today are electric, but alternatives are available. When selecting a frame, the population to be served and the setting in which it will be used should be considered. For example, frames with built-in bed exit alarms may be needed for patients who are confused and at risk for falls. This same patient population also needs a pressure-redistributing support surface since many are either at risk or have an existing pressure ulcer. Frames with built-in bed scales may be needed for units where daily weights are a necessity and, for many frames, scales are a standard feature. The primary advantages and disadvantages of integrated bed systems relate to whether they are purchased or rented.

Procedure, Transport, Emergency Room, and OR Mattresses

It stands to reason that patients who require a support surface in bed would benefit from a support surface during transport on gurneys, while in the emergency department awaiting admission, and during special procedures (for example, endoscopy, cardiac evaluation/procedures, or surgical procedures). In fact, patients may be at greater risk while on these surfaces, due to the limited space for moving and repositioning in addition to their potential need for sedation or anesthesia. Although not yet reviewed in peer-reviewed publications, manufacturers now are creating mattresses (sometimes called *pads*) with a pressure redistribution option for emergency room, transport, and procedure tables. In addition, some companies will custom fit their pressure redistribution products to fit surfaces other than beds.

Prevention of perioperative pressure ulcers has been identified as a major priority for health care institutions across the country. International guidelines recommend that individuals at risk for perioperative pressure ulcer development be placed on mattresses that provide higher level pressure redistribution than standard OR mattresses (AORN, 2008; NPUAP & EPUAP, 2014). (A standard OR mattress is defined as a 2-inch foam surface covered with a vinyl or nylon fabric.) (AORN, 2008). Recent literature takes this recommendation a step further; authors note that there are a number of uncontrolled variables in the surgical environment that could alter a patient's risk during the procedure (e.g., reaction to anesthesia, unexpected prolongation of the surgical procedure, unanticipated hypotensive episodes). As a result, authors concur that all surgical patients should be considered at risk and placed on a mattress with higher level pressure distribution properties (Walton-Geer, 2009).

CLINICAL PEARL

It stands to reason that patients who need pressure redistribution when in bed also need pressure redistribution during transport and during procedures; therefore, it is critical to assure appropriate mattresses for gurneys, emergency department beds, and OR tables.

A number of support surface options are now available for the OR, including air, gel, and high-specification foam mattresses. The best OR surface for preventing pressure ulcers has not been determined. McInnes et al. (2011) concluded that pressure redistribution overlays reduced the incidence of postoperative pressure ulcers, but this finding may not apply to *all* pressure-redistributing overlays; a study by Schultz et al. (1999) found evidence that certain overlays were actually associated with harmful postoperative skin changes. Therefore, selection of an OR support surface requires careful analysis of a number of factors to ensure that the product provides effective pressure redistribution while also demonstrating compatibility with the facility's surgical positioning procedures, safety protocols, transfer equipment, and budget.

Of note, pads and blankets (such as warming and cooling blankets) placed between the patient and the OR mattress will interfere with the pressure redistribution properties of the mattress. As a result, AORN (2008) specifically recommends use of a higher-grade pressure redistribution mattress when a cooling blanket is placed between the patient and the OR mattress.

Chair Cushions

Individuals who remain seated for prolonged periods of time are predisposed to pressure ulcer development, particularly in the ischial area. Wounds that develop from sitting are located on the ischia during upright sitting and on the sacrum when slouching, sliding, or reclining. Pressure redistribution chair cushions should be used with seated individuals who are at risk for pressure ulcers and have reduced mobility (NPUAP & EPUAP, 2014). General guidelines for chair cushion selection include matching the chair cushion to the individual patient, with attention to body size and configuration, postural effects, mobility, and lifestyle needs. A critical aspect in product selection is to assure that the cushion and cover provide for heat dissipation and air exchange at the skin–cushion interface (NPUAP & EPUAP, 2014). Selecting a cushion of appropriate size and depth is also essential; in the seated position, the weight of the body is supported by a relatively small surface area, which increases the risk for bottoming out. Cushions are available in both regular and bariatric size, and the appropriate size should be chosen based on the patient's weight and width. Individuals who are wheelchair dependent should be evaluated by a seating specialist (if available) to assure the optimal selection of chair cushion (Fig. 20-3).

Chair cushions are available in a variety of support mediums, including foam, air, and gel. Some cushions also provide AP therapy; however, this therapy must be used with caution. Specifically, construction and operation of the cushion must be evaluated, and the benefits of off-loading must be weighed against the risk for instability and shear (NPUAP & EPUAP, 2014). The data regarding effectiveness of AP cushions are limited; their use has been studied in young spinal cord–injured patients (Makhsous et al., 2009) and in older hospitalized patients (Clark, 1998). There were mixed outcomes, leading Saha et al. (2013) to state that the strength of evidence is insufficient to draw generalizable conclusions.

Once implemented, chair cushions must be inspected regularly for wear and tear. Improper inflation, overcompression, or displaced gel can compromise pressure redistribution and lead to bottoming out. Appropriate training and maintenance must occur on a regular basis to ensure that the device is functioning properly and effectively meets the patient's needs.

In general, patients with existing ischial or sacral ulcers should strictly avoid long-term seating until the ulcer has completely healed. Individuals with existing pressure ulcers should be referred to a seating specialist for evaluation if seating is unavoidable.

CLINICAL PEARL

Pressure redistribution chair cushions must be used for all at-risk patients when up in the chair; they are available in a variety of sizes and support mediums. Ring cushions (doughnut devices) should *never* be used for pressure ulcer prevention or management.

Ring cushion (doughnut) devices increase venous congestion and edema and should not be used for pressure ulcer prevention and management (NPUAP & EPUAP, 2009; Whitney et al. 2006; WOCN Society, 2003, 2010).

Active (Alternating Pressure)

An *active* support surface is a powered mattress or overlay that changes its load distribution properties with or without an applied load (NPUAP, 2007). An active support surface moves even if no one is in the bed

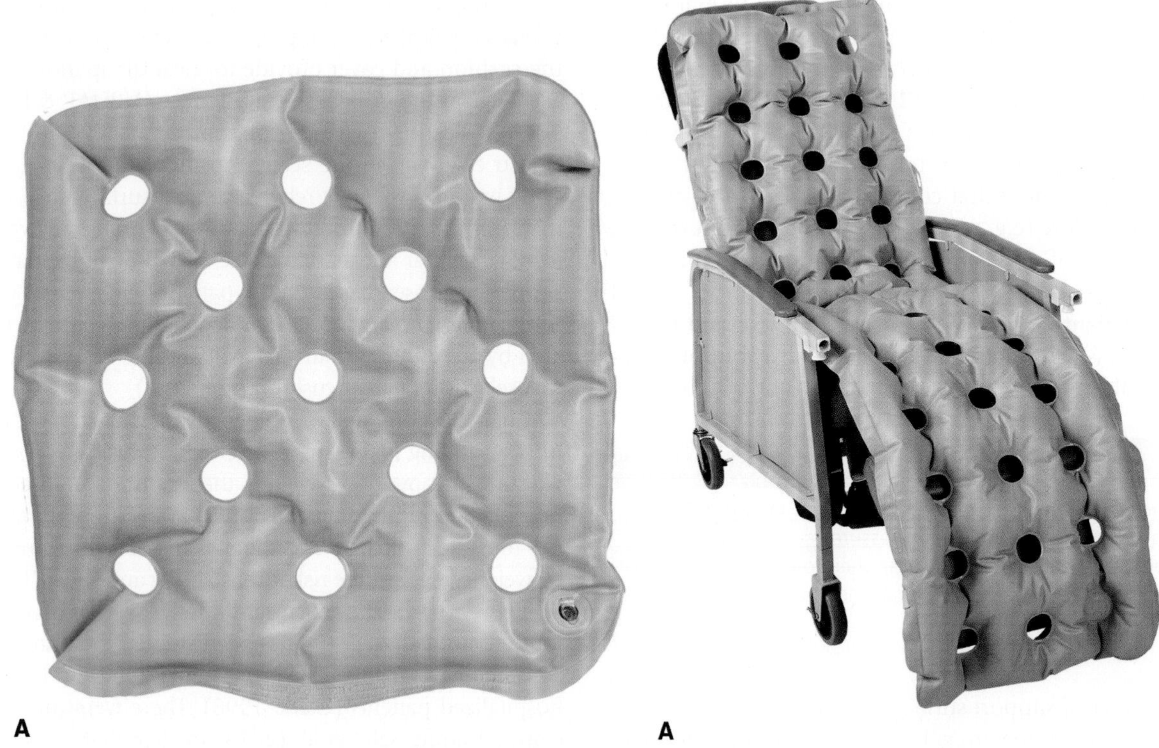

FIGURE 20-3. **A.** A simple chair cushion. **B.** A full geri-chair cushion. (Courtesy EHOB, Inc.)

(Christian & Lachenbruch, 2007). High-risk patients should be placed on an active mattresses or overlay when frequent repositioning is not possible (NPUAP & EPUAP, 2009). As of 2010, the only active support surfaces on the market are those that include the feature of alternating pressure therapy.

Alternating pressure is a feature found in both overlays and mattresses. These products are comprised of air cells that can be cyclically inflated and deflated, and they periodically change the areas of the body under pressure by inflating and deflating the cells of alternating zones. (They do not work through the principles of immersion and envelopment.) The individual cell that composes the alternating pressure mattress and/or overlay must be 10 cm or greater in depth to effectively redistribute pressure (NPUAP & EPUAP, 2009). *Pulsating pressure* refers to shorter-duration inflation and higher-frequency cycling; there is less direct evidence supporting use of these products (Gunther & Clark, 2000). Alternating pressure and pulsating pressure can be found in combination with foam and low-air-loss products.

International pressure ulcer guidelines recommend use of an active support surface (mattress or overlay) for patients at higher risk for pressure ulcer development where frequent manual repositioning is not possible. However, this recommendation was derived indirectly from two studies, one of which was recognized as a poor-quality study. Thus, further study is needed before definitive recommendations can be made.

Iglesias et al. (2006) noted that pressure ulcers occurred almost 11 days sooner on an alternating pressure overlay when compared to an alternating pressure mattress. However, in another study (cited by International Pressure Ulcer Guidelines), there was no significant difference in outcomes among patients managed with alternating pressure mattresses and those managed with overlays. This is the basis for the guidelines statement that alternating pressure mattresses and overlays have similar efficacy in terms of pressure ulcer prevention (Nixon et al., 2006; NPUAP & EPUAP, 2009) (Fig. 20-4).

Reactive

A *reactive* support surface moves or changes its load distribution properties only in response to an applied load, such as the patient's body (Christian & Lachenbruch, 2007). Unlike active support surfaces that must be powered, reactive support surfaces can be either powered or nonpowered; the advantages of nonpowered surfaces are the lack of dependency on electricity or battery and the absence of noise associated with a motor. Examples of reactive support surfaces include mattresses and overlays filled with foam, air, or a combination of foam–air. Reactive surfaces are available as chair cushions, overlays, mattresses, and pads for stretchers, OR tables, and procedure tables. Nonpowered air-filled support surfaces range from low-end prevention products that encapsulate air into a single bladder or cell to therapeutic products containing hundreds of individual interconnected cells. All reactive support surfaces are appropriate for pressure ulcer prevention in the patient who is frequently repositioned.

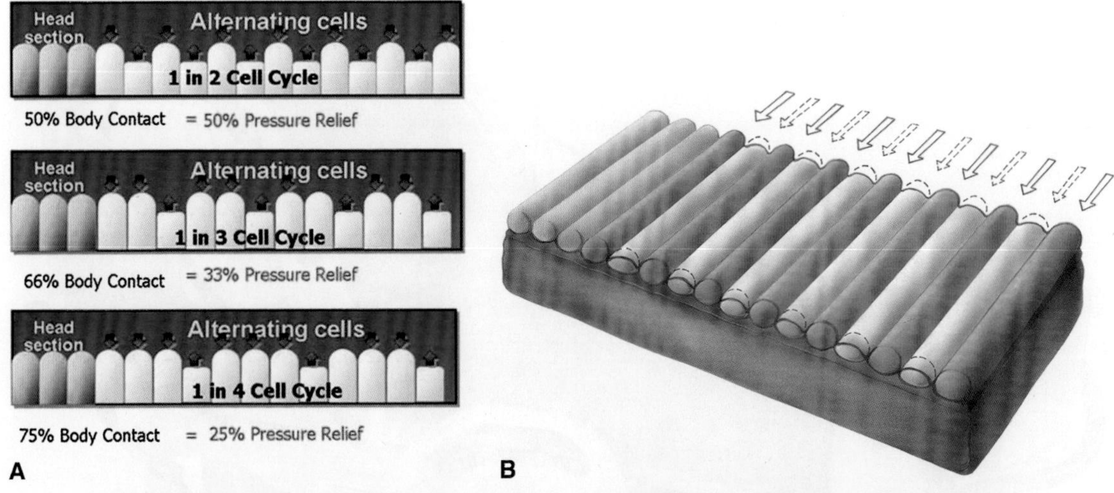

FIGURE 20-4. Alternating pressure device. **A.** Diagram depicting options for alternating pressure devices (2 versus 3 versus 4 cell models). **B.** Example of 2-cell model. (Courtesy Joerns, Inc.)

Some are also appropriate for patients with existing pressure ulcers. With few exceptions, reactive support surfaces are appropriate for use in long-term care facilities, hospitals, and home settings.

CLINICAL PEARL

Active surfaces are powered devices that change their load-bearing properties even if no weight is applied (alternating pressure devices); *r*eactive surfaces may be powered or nonpowered devices and change their load-bearing properties only in response to applied weight (such as the patient's body).

Low Air Loss

One commonly misunderstood feature related to support surfaces is low air loss. The NPUAP (2007) defines low air loss as a feature that provides a flow of air to assist in managing the heat and humidity (microclimate) of the skin. Low air loss surfaces are comprised of a series of connected pillows. A pump provides slow continuous airflow allowing for even distribution into the porous mattress and continuous airflow across the skin. The amount of pressure in each pillow is controlled and can be calibrated according to height and weight distribution to meet the individual needs of the patient. As the patient settles down into the mattress, weight is distributed more evenly for pressure redistribution. There may be an additional component placed at the base of the product, such as foam or air pillows, when "bottoming out" is problematic. Low air loss can be found alone or in combination with alternating pressure, lateral rotation, and air-fluidized technology, and can be incorporated into overlays, mattresses, bed systems, and even a chair cushion.

CLINICAL PEARL

Products with a low-air-loss feature assist with microclimate control either by providing low-volume airflow to the skin or by pulling heat and water vapor away from the skin for elimination out the sides or end of the mattress.

The construction of a low-air-loss surface that addresses the microclimate of the skin can be achieved in two ways; with airflow under the cover or with an air-permeable cover. Most familiar to clinicians is the air-permeable cover, which allows for the slow, evenly distributed release of air *through* the cover and directly to the skin. Low-air-loss surfaces with airflow *under* the cover addresses skin microclimate by receiving heat, gas, and water molecules through a moisture vapor-permeable cover (conducted downward from the skin), into the air stream inside the mattress, which eventually exits along the sides or ends of the mattress.

The smooth covers for low-air-loss surfaces are generally made of nylon or polytetrafluoroethylene fabric and have a low coefficient of friction. The covers are waterproof, impermeable to bacteria, and easy to clean. In order to obtain the full benefits of low air loss, linen should be minimized and special underpads with a high level of moisture vapor permeability (rather than plastic back pads) should be used.

Low-air-loss support surfaces have been reported as an effective treatment surface and may improve healing rates of pressure ulcers (Saha et al., 2013). Because of the two aforementioned constructions (air-permeable cover versus airflow under the cover), low air loss helps to reduce moisture and may help to prevent skin damage such as incontinence-associated dermatitis or maceration (Cullum et al., 2004; WOCN Society, 2010). However, there is some potential for wound desiccation, which can be prevented by using a hydrating rather than absorptive dressing (if necessary).

Low-air-loss surfaces come with important safety features, such as controls that instantly inflate the cushions, thus facilitating patient positioning. Fowler boost controls help prevent bottoming out by adding more air under the buttocks when the patient's head is elevated. Controls that instantly flatten the air cushions are activated prior to administration of CPR so that effective chest compressions are possible.

Due to the lack of stability compared to a firmer mattress, low air loss is contraindicated for patients with an

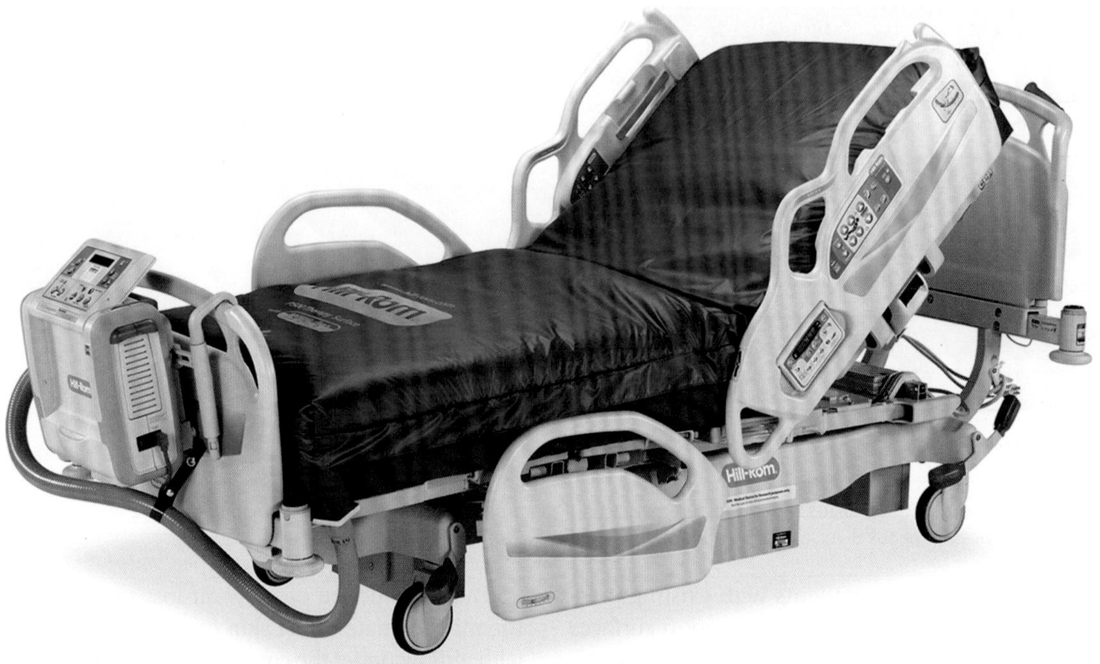

FIGURE 20-5. Surface with low-air-loss feature. (Courtesy Hill-Rom, Inc.)

unstable spine. Some patients lose their ability to effectively self-position on a low-air-loss surface, again due to the lack of firmness in the surface. Additional disadvantages of low-air-loss surfaces include increased risk of bed entrapment, especially if the device is not properly adjusted. It is imperative that clinicians and involved staff are familiar with the manufacturer's recommended instructions for use. Once the proper weight setting is established, it is prudent to record the setting to assure consistency of product use. Low-air-loss surfaces can be costly and require electricity and special underpads that cost more than the standard underpad.* See Figure 20-5 for example of bed with LAL feature.

Air Fluidized

The feature of air fluidization can only be found in an integrated bed system and was initially developed to treat patients with burns. Also known as high air loss, the surface contains silicone-coated beads that become incorporated into both air and fluid support; when air is pumped through the beads, the beads behave like a liquid. The person "floats" on a sheet, with one third of the body above the surface and the rest of the body immersed in the warm, dry, fluidized beads. Body fluids flow freely through the sheet and cover, but contamination is prevented through continuous pressurization (Holzapfel, 1993). When the air-fluidized bed is turned off, it quickly becomes firm enough for repositioning or CPR.

*Reprinted with permission from Nix, D. P., & Mackey, D. (2010). Support surfaces. In R. Bryant & D. Nix (Eds.). Acute and chronic wounds: Current management concepts (4th ed., pp. 162–163). New York, NY: Elsevier Health Sciences. Reprinted by permission of Elsevier.

Air-fluidized beds are most commonly used for patients with burns, myocutaneous skin flaps, and multiple stage III or IV pressure ulcers. Using a subset of retrospectively collected National Pressure Ulcer Long-Term Care Study data, Ochs et al. (2005) compared pressure ulcer outcomes of 664 residents placed on several types of support surfaces, including air-fluidized, low-air-loss, powered, and nonpowered overlays and hospital mattresses. Results indicated that residents placed on air-fluidized support surfaces had larger and deeper pressure ulcers and higher illness severity scores than did residents placed on the other support surfaces. However, residents who used air-fluidized surfaces had better healing rates, fewer emergency visits, and fewer hospital admissions. Saha et al. (2013) reviewed five studies conducted in the 1980s and 1990s and found that AF beds produced better healing in terms of reduction in ulcer size compared to several non-AF surfaces. These findings, although significant, warrant more research on variables such as initial wound size, use of dressing, debridement, nutritional status, and presence of infection and incontinence.

In the institutional environment, these products are not ideally suited to facility ownership because of the complexity and the high costs of maintenance. An air-fluidized bed system is one of the most expensive support surfaces. Air-fluidized products have a warming feature for the pressurized air, which can be comforting or harmful depending on the overall condition of the patient. Hydration issues may be more pronounced than that experienced with low-air-loss surfaces. Because air-fluidized beds are heavy, they may not be safe for use in

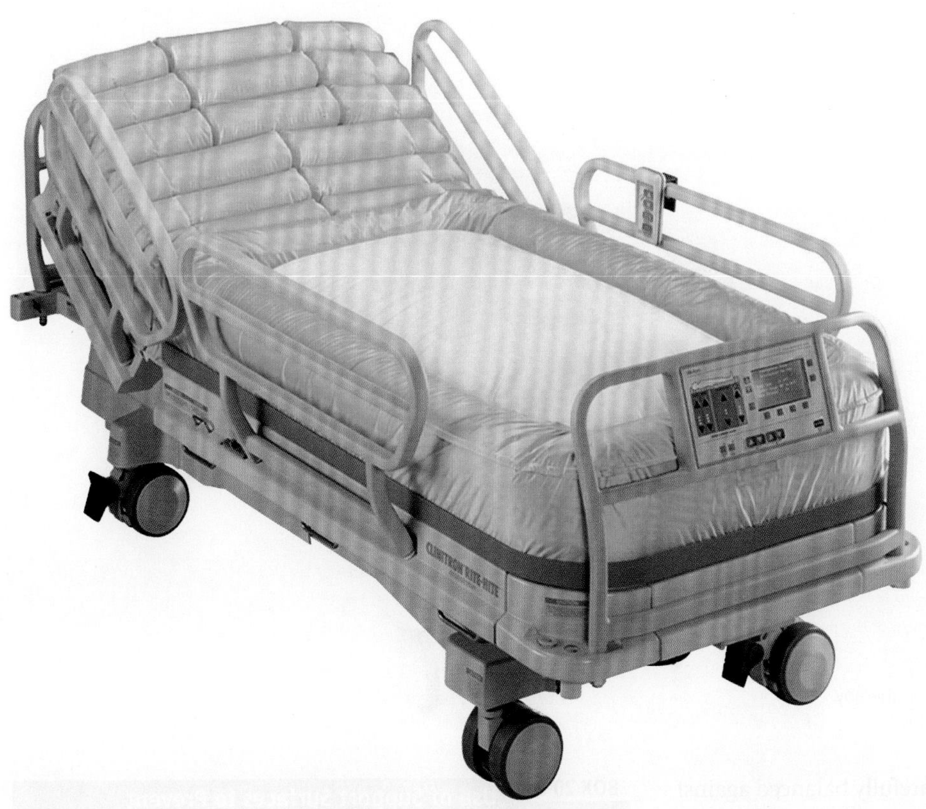

FIGURE 20-6. Bed with air-fluidized feature in lower section (low air loss in upper section). (Courtesy Hill-Rom, Inc.)

older homes. Traditional air-fluidized beds are not recommended for the patient with pulmonary disease or an unstable spine. However, air-fluidized therapy in the lower half of the bed has been combined with low air loss in the upper portion of the surface to create an adjustable bed for the patient who needs to be more upright. This bed is similar in size to a hospital bed, the head of the bed is readily adjustable, and the bed is lighter than a total air-fluidized system.† See Figure 20-6 for example of air-fluidized bed.

CLINICAL PEARL

Air-fluidized beds are one of the most expensive support surfaces and should be used only for patients who require very high level therapy, such as those with multiple full-thickness wounds or those S/P myocutaneous flap procedures.

Continuous Lateral Rotation

Continuous lateral rotation is a feature that has been used for the past 30 years for the prevention and treatment of selected cardiopulmonary conditions. Continuous lateral rotation therapy involves rotation of the patient in a regular pattern around a longitudinal (i.e., head-to-foot) axis; rotation is limited to 40 degrees *or less* to each side over a prescribed length of time ranging from minutes to hours. In contrast, kinetic therapy is defined as the side-to-side rotation of 40 degrees *or more* to each side. As noted, these surfaces are primarily used to facilitate pulmonary hygiene in the patient with acute respiratory conditions, and it is difficult to draw firm conclusions regarding their effectiveness in pressure ulcer prevention. We do know that use of adult specialty beds in the rotation mode is ineffective for small children because their small bodies are confined to one section or pillow of the surface (McCord et al., 2004).

Lateral rotation has been incorporated into some low-air-loss and air/foam mattresses, overlays, and integrated bed systems. One descriptive study of 30 patients on a foam mattress replacement with continuous lateral rotation therapy reported 0% incidence of new pressure ulcers and improvement in existing trunk and pelvis wounds (Anderson & Rappl, 2004); however, further data regarding the effects of continuous lateral rotation therapy on pressure ulcer prevention are needed.

It is important to emphasize that continuous lateral rotation therapy does not eliminate the need for routine manual repositioning. In addition, the staff needs to incorporate measures to protect the patient against shear, including aligning and securing the patient with bolster pads provided by the manufacturer, and frequent skin inspection for any indications of shear damage. Optimally, if the staff discovers a new shear injury, the patient should be positioned off the involved area and placed on an alternative support surface if clinically feasible. However, if the patient is still in respiratory distress, the pulmonary benefits of continuous

†Reprinted with permission from Nix, D. P., & Mackey, D. (2010). Support surfaces. In R. Bryant & D. Nix (Eds.). *Acute and chronic wounds: Current management concepts* (4th ed., pp. 162–163). New York, NY: Elsevier Health Sciences. Reprinted by permission of Elsevier.

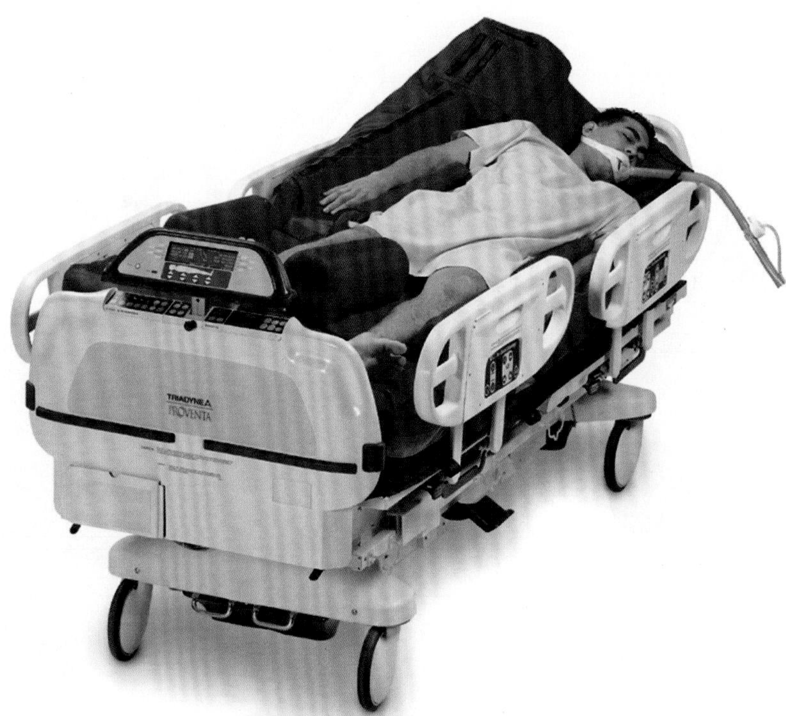

FIGURE 20-7. Continuous lateral rotation therapy. (TriaDyne images courtesy of ArjoHuntleigh Inc.)

lateral rotation therapy should be carefully balanced against the potential for additional skin damage, with the decision based on the patient's overall condition and need for therapy (NPUAP & EPUAP, 2009). See Figure 20-7 for example of continuous lateral rotation surface.

CLINICAL PEARL

Continuous lateral rotation devices are designed for pulmonary care and do not replace manual repositioning for pressure ulcer prevention.

 Matching the Product to the Patient

Despite the paucity of evidence to indicate that any one support surface is better than another, knowledge of the therapeutic features of various surfaces assists the clinician to develop decision-making guidelines that permit staff to appropriately match products to patients. Manufacturers now provide a full range of support surfaces with various therapeutic features; it is therefore possible to create setting-specific formularies with options that address the needs of patients typically managed in that setting. Boxes 20-2 and 20-3 provide the clinician with consensus driven and evidence-based statements regarding the use of support surfaces to prevent and treat pressure ulcers.

Individual Patient Needs

Individuals with pressure ulcers or those at risk for pressure ulcers should be placed on a support surface rather than on a standard hospital mattress (Cullum

BOX 20-2. Use of Support Surfaces to Prevent Pressure Ulcers

- Patients with mobility subscale scores of 2 or 1 who are at risk for the development of pressure ulcers should be placed on a reactive/CLP (continuous low pressure) support surface or an active support surface with an alternating pressure (AP) feature.
- Postoperative use of high-specification foam mattresses is more effective in reducing the incidence of pressure ulcers in persons at risk than standard hospital foam mattresses.
- There is no evidence of the superiority of any one high-specification foam mattress over an alternative high-specification foam mattress.
- Sheepskin overlays (Australian Medical grade) are effective in reducing the incidence of pressure ulcers compared to standard care.
- There is insufficient evidence to determine comparative effectiveness of various reactive/CLP support surfaces.
- Active support surfaces with an AP feature are more effective than standard hospital mattresses in the prevention of pressure ulcers.
- Active overlays and mattresses with AP features demonstrate similar efficacy in reducing pressure ulcer incidence.
- Mattresses with a multistage AP feature are more effective than overlays with an AP feature in preventing full-thickness pressure ulcers.
- Mattresses with a single-stage AP feature and overlays with an AP feature are equally effective for prevention of partial-thickness pressure ulcers.
- There is no difference between reactive/CLP support surfaces and active support surfaces with an AP feature with regard to efficacy in pressure ulcer prevention.
- Postoperative use of a support surface reduces the incidence of surgery-related pressure ulcers.

Source: WOCN Support Surface Consensus Conference Statements (2014).

BOX 20-3. Use of Support Surfaces in the Treatment of Pressure Ulcers

- There is insufficient evidence to suggest that there are differences among the efficacies of reactive/CLP devices, AP devices, LAL therapy, profiling beds, or Australian Medical grade sheepskin for the treatment of existing pressure ulcers.
- Current evidence suggests that there is no difference between reactive/CLP support surfaces and active support surfaces with an AP feature for pressure ulcer treatment.
- Persons with Braden Mobility subscale scores of 4 or 3, existing pressure ulcers on the trunk or pelvis, and 2 available turning surfaces should be placed on a reactive/CLP (air, foam, gel, or viscous fluid) support surface.
- Persons with Braden Mobility subscale scores of 2 or 1 and Braden Moisture subscale scores of 4 or 3 should be placed on a reactive/CLP support surface or an active support surface with an AP feature.
- Persons with Braden Mobility subscale scores of 2 or 1, existing pressure ulcers on the trunk or pelvis, and 2 available turning surfaces should be placed on a reactive/CLP support surface or an active support surface with an AP feature.
- Persons with Braden Mobility subscale scores of 2 or 1 and Braden Moisture subscale score of 1 with moisture that cannot be managed by other means, along with existing pressure ulcers on the trunk or pelvis, should be placed on a reactive/CLP support surface with an LAL or AF feature.
- Persons with multiple stage II, or large (of sufficient size to compromise a turning surface) or multiple stage III or stage IV pressure ulcers on the trunk or pelvis involving more than 1 available turning surface, should be placed on a reactive support surface with an LAL or AF feature.
- Persons who have ulcers (stages II to IV) on 2 or more turning surfaces, or have 1 or no available turning surfaces, should be placed on an active support surface with an AP feature or a reactive support surface with an LAL or AF feature.
- In cases of suspected deep tissue injury (sDTI) located on the trunk or pelvis, intervention should include strategies that facilitate tissue temperature reduction between the patient and the support surface (e.g., implementation of a turning regimen and use of a support surface that facilitates temperature reduction, e.g., gel surface or an AP, LAL, or AF feature).
- Persons with pressure ulcers on the head or upper or lower extremities should be off-loaded and may not require a change in the current support surface.
- If while on a reactive/CLP support surface with an LAL or AF feature, a person's condition improves such that the person no longer has a pressure ulcer or no longer is at high risk for the development of a pressure ulcer, the person should be placed on a reactive/CLP support surface or an active support surface with an AP feature.

Source: WOCN Support Surface Consensus Conference Statements (2014).

et al., 2004; NPUAP & EPUAP, 2014; Whitney et al., 2006; WOCN Society, 2010). As described throughout this chapter, each support surface has disadvantages and contraindications. Therefore, support surfaces should be selected based on assessment of the *patient* and his or her needs and not *solely* on the patient's wound (NPUAP & EPUAP, 2009). Optimal decision making regarding support surfaces is based on a comprehensive assessment that includes condition and location of wounds (if applicable); need for head-of-bed elevation; need for microclimate control; activity and positioning limitations; risk for falls and entrapment; physical appearance and size, including height and weight; and patient reports of comfort or discomfort when lying or sitting on the support surface.

CLINICAL PEARL

Selection of the best surface for an individual patient must be based on comprehensive assessment of the patient that includes risk status, number and location of any wounds, need for microclimate control, positioning needs and limitations, and weight and size.

Clinical Considerations

All patients with existing ulcers should be placed on a surface that provides an effective level of pressure redistribution (e.g., high-density foam, low-air-loss, alternating pressure, viscous fluid, or air-fluidized surface). A support surface that dissipates moisture (low air loss) may be indicated for the diaphoretic patient or the patient with copious wound drainage or incontinence not contained by dressings and absorptive products (Cullum et al., 2004; Whitney et al., 2006; WOCN Society, 2003). In addition, patients who require head-of-bed elevation may benefit from a surface that provides shear reduction. As discussed in the Chair Cushion section of this chapter, patients with sitting surface pressure ulcers require a support surface for the chair as well as the bed.

CLINICAL PEARL

All patients with existing pressure ulcers on positioning surfaces should be placed on a surface with effective pressure redistribution properties; if the patient requires head-of-bed elevation, a low shear cover is recommended, and a low-air-loss feature is recommended for patients who are diaphoretic.

Activity and Positioning

If frequent repositioning is not possible, an active support surface is recommended (NPUAP & EPUAP, 2009). When prolonged head-of-bed elevation is required, there is increased risk for bottoming out, and the clinician should consider changing from an overlay to a mattress. The patient who self-repositions, gets in and out of the bed, or is attempting to increase mobility and independence should be placed on a surface that facilitates rather than impairs activity and mobility.

CLINICAL PEARL

Active support surfaces (alternating pressure devices) are recommended for individuals who cannot be routinely and effectively repositioned.

Risk for Falls or Entrapment

A surface that increases the patient's overall height in bed (overall distance from the underlying bed frame) or creates more distance between the mattress and side rails increases the risk for entrapment and falls. In general, a pressure redistribution surface that also minimizes height and gaps should be selected for patients at risk for falls (U.S. FDA, 2006); some facilities are now adding fall risk assessment scores to support surface selection criteria to ensure that this is factored into the selection process. If the patient becomes at risk for falls or entrapment on a selected support surface, additional monitoring will be necessary or an alternative support surface should be selected (Nix & Mackey, 2012). Some facilities now utilize bed frames that go down close to the floor (low beds); combining a low bed with a pressure redistribution mattress addresses both safety concerns and the need for pressure ulcer prevention.

Size and Weight

Bed frame and mattress specifications for weight capacity must be considered. Low-air-loss products designed for adults do not provide options to accommodate the height and weight of small children (WOCN Society, 2010). Children and infants can sink into and between cushions, leading to risk for entrapment and falls (McLane et al., 2004).

The obese patient presents many challenges in terms of skin integrity, including increased risk for pressure ulcer development and for moisture-associated skin damage. Thus, appropriate support surface selection and frequent skin assessment are critical elements of care (Davidson & Callery, 2001). Admission assessment and initial support surface selection should include the potential need for a bariatric frame and support surface; in addition, a trapeze should be in place to reduce shear over the sacrum during repositioning. Bariatric support surfaces are available in foam, air, gel, and water with or without microclimate and moisture control features. Many adult hospital bed frames currently available have weight limits up to 500 lb. However, older frames may not be designed to support more than 350 lb; in addition, the width of older frames frequently precludes effective repositioning by obese patients. In addition to weight, the clinician must consider the patient's build and width when choosing a surface; shorter patients and those with truncal obesity may fall within the weight restrictions of the bed, but their width may prevent safe repositioning, and it may be difficult to prevent prolonged contact between the soft tissues and the side rails or other rigid components of the bed. Bariatric patients should be educated regarding the importance of repositioning and should be encouraged to make small position changes at regular intervals and to keep the head of the bed below 30 degrees. Care of the bariatric patient is further discussed in Chapter 14.

Patient Response

Once a product is selected, its effectiveness for that patient must be reevaluated at regular intervals to ensure that expected outcomes are being achieved. Expected outcomes may include prevention of pressure ulcers, patient comfort, or moisture control. Wound healing may or may not be an expected outcome, depending on the overall goals of care; if wound healing is an expected outcome, the support surface must be used in conjunction with a comprehensive pressure ulcer management plan (Nix & Mackey, 2012).

If expected outcomes are not being met, the surface must be reevaluated and an alternative surface should be considered, using the same decision-making guidelines as were used for selection of the original surface. Discontinuing or changing a support surface may be warranted when there are changes in a patient's overall condition. For example, the patient who once was hemodynamically unstable but is now improving may require a different support surface to facilitate independence with activity and mobility, including turning and repositioning himself or herself. Similarly, the patient on an overlay whose respiratory condition deteriorates and who now requires head-of-bed elevation may require transfer to a mattress in order to prevent bottoming out. Another example is the patient who develops delirium and is at increased risk for falling; in this case, the patient may need a low bed and a pressure redistribution mattress (Nix & Mackey, 2012).

Care Setting–Specific Formulary

The development and implementation of a standardized formulary describing the support surfaces that are available in a specific care setting is critical for minimizing staff confusion, managing costs, and improving access to appropriate and safe products (Whittemore, 1998). Considerations for compatibility with care setting include reimbursement, rental versus purchase, product maintenance, safety, and facility response. Once these considerations are analyzed, a formulary can be created with a range of products intended to meet the needs of the patient population. Innovative and creative decision-making tools are essential in educating staff regarding guidelines for support surface selection. See Figure 20-8 for sample decision tree/algorithm for support surface selection.

CLINICAL PEARL

A setting-specific formulary should be developed, and staff should be provided with a decision tree or algorithm to guide appropriate surface selection.

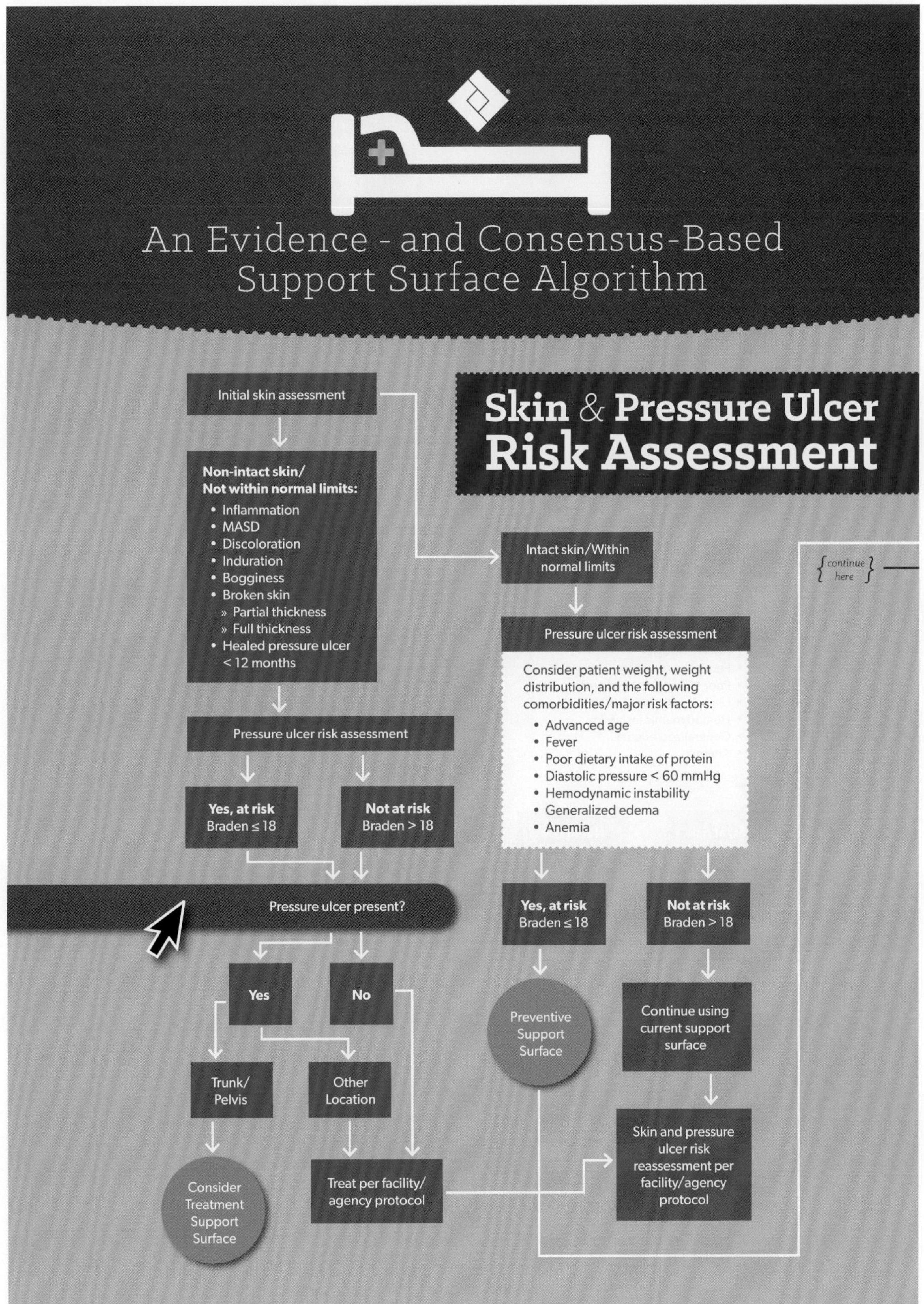

FIGURE 20-8. Decision tree/algorithm for support surface selection. (Copyright WOCN.)

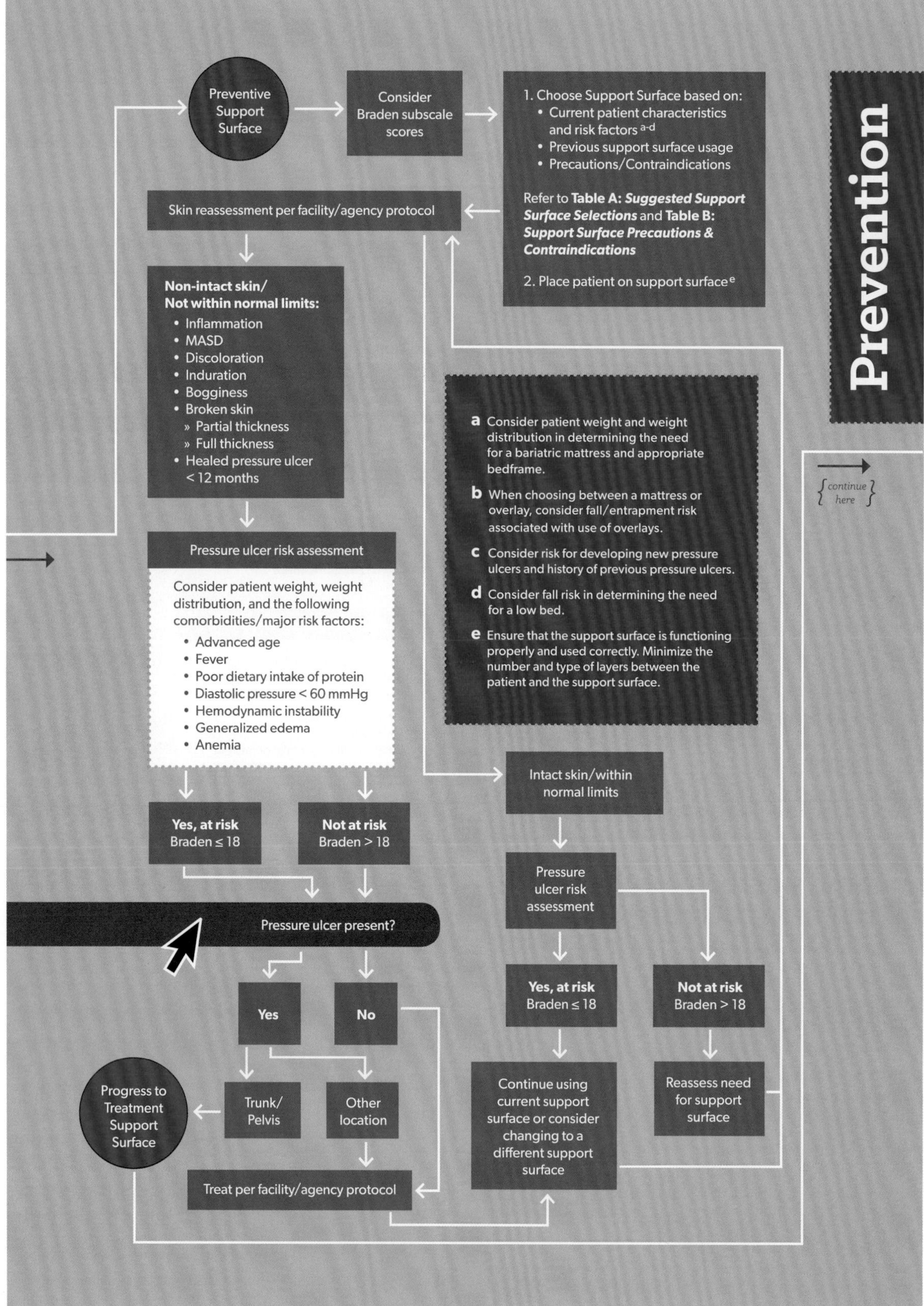

FIGURE 20-8. *(Continued)*

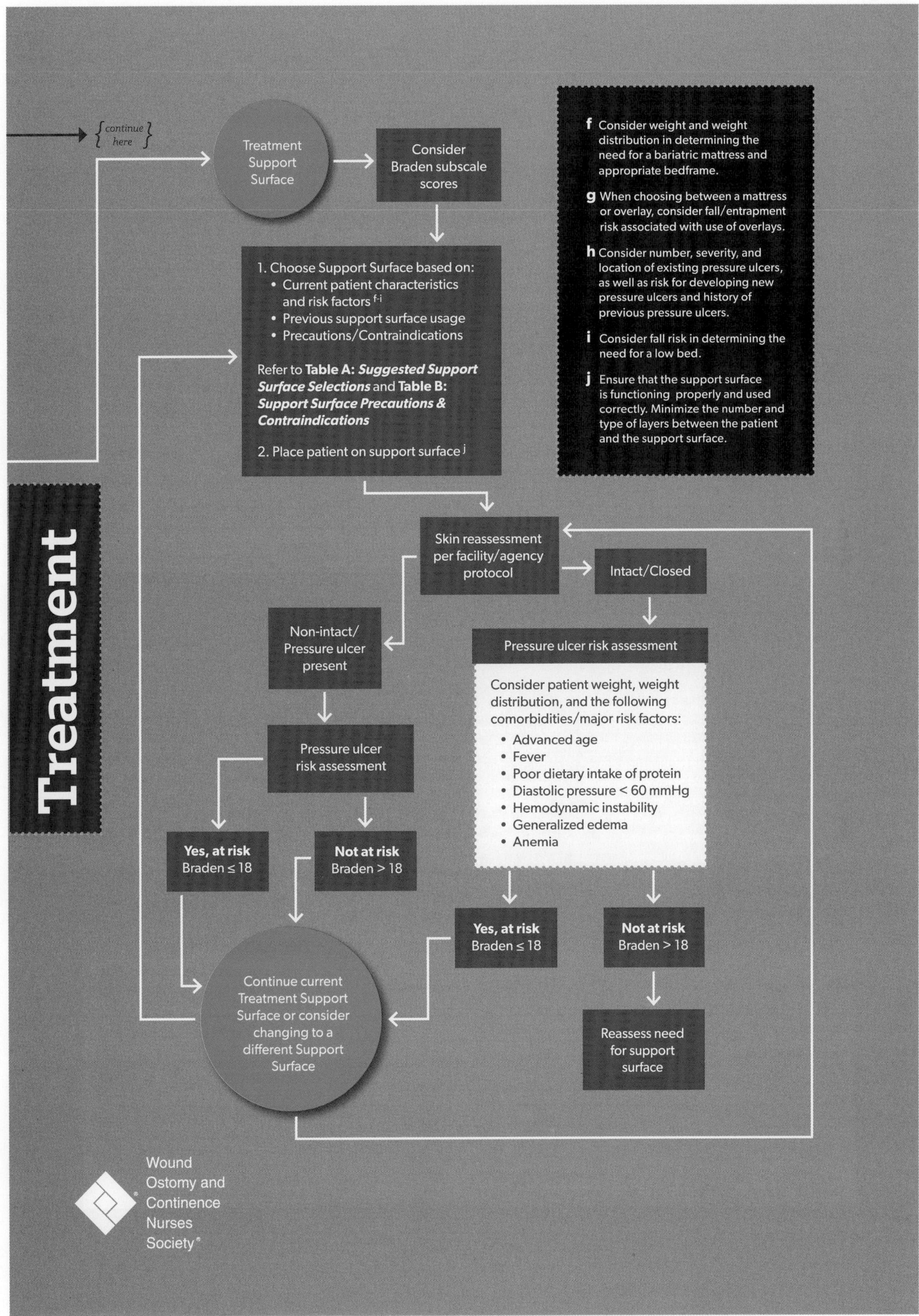

FIGURE 20-8. *(Continued)*

TABLE A:

Suggested Support Surface Overlay or Mattress Selections for Pressure Ulcer Prevention & Treatment Based on Braden Mobility & Moisture Subscores

a Braden B, Bergstrom N. http://bradenscale.com/images/bradenscale.pdf. Copyright 1988. Accessed August 8, 2014.

b In this table, Reactive/CLP refers to all types of Support Surfaces in this category with the exception of AMG sheep skin overlays, which are noted separately.

c AMG sheepskin is available for purchase through online suppliers.

Note: Persons with multiple Stage II, or large (of sufficient size to compromise a turning surface) or multiple Stage III or Stage IV pressure ulcers on the trunk or pelvis involving more than one available turning surface should be placed on a support surface with a low air loss or an air fluidized feature.

	BRADEN MOBILITY SUBSCALE SCORES[a]	
BRADEN MOISTURE SUBSCALE SCORES	**4 or 3** No limitation or slightly limited	**2 or 1** Very limited or completely immobile
4 or 3 Rarely or occasionally moist	• Reactive/CLP[b] (air, foam, gel, fiber, or viscous fluid, or combinations) • AMG sheepskin overlay (Prevention only)[c]	• Reactive/CLP • Active with AP feature
2 Very moist	• Reactive/CLP • Reactive/CLP with LAL feature	• Reactive/CLP with LAL feature
1 Constantly moist	• Reactive/CLP • Reactive/CLP with LAL feature	• Reactive/CLP with LAL feature • Reactive/CLP with AF feature (Treatment only)

AF = air fluidized; AMG = Australian Medical grade; AP = alternating pressure; CLP = constant low pressure; LAL = low air loss.

TABLE B:

Select Support Surface Precautions & Contraindications[a]

a Refer to manufacturer specifications, including product lifespan. Staff who have ongoing exposure to support surfaces during bedding or room changes should practice a continual awareness and opportunity-based observation of support surface lifespan indicators, including reduced height or thickness; discoloration; altered integrity of cover, seams, zipper/ zipper cover flap, or backing; degradation of internal components, or presence of odor. If any of these are observed, it is recommended that the surface be referred to engineering/ maintenance for testing or evaluation for continued use, irrespective of stated product lifespan.

b High risk for moisture penetration with potential for infection.

SUPPORT SURFACE	PRECAUTIONS	CONTRAINDICATIONS
High-specification foam	• Braden moisture subscale score of 2 or 1[b]	• Weight limitations for surface–may require another product in this category with higher weight limit
Reactive/CLP	• NA	• Unstable cervical, thoracic or lumbar spine • Cervical or skeletal traction • Weight limitations for surface– may require another product in this category with higher weight limit
Active with AP feature	• NA	
Reactive/CLP with LAL feature	• Combative/restless/agitated state	
Reactive/CLP with AF feature	• Combative/restless/agitated state • Need for aggressive pulmonary toilet • Need for frequent head elevation • Need for mobilization • Claustrophobia	• Unstable cervical, thoracic or lumbar spine • Cervical or skeletal traction • Weight limitations for surface– may require another product in this category with higher weight limit • Trendelenburg positioning

AF = air fluidized; AP = alternating pressure; CLP = constant low pressure; LAL = low air loss.

FIGURE 20-8. *(Continued)*

Support Surface Initiative (S3I)

There is a tremendous need for well-designed clinical studies that evaluate the effectiveness of various support surfaces. NPUAP's Support Surface Initiative (S3I) has focused efforts on the clear definition, objective testing, and comparable reporting of therapeutic features such as immersion, envelopment, and microclimate management. Next steps include introducing these standardized tests into the clinical setting and connecting the test results to clinical efficacy. Under the best of circumstances, outcomes such as pressure ulcer incidence, patient comfort, and cost should be included in the design and conduct of clinical trials. In addition, sample sizes should be appropriate to allow for the most relevant and meaningful type of statistical analysis. Many studies done to date involve small sample sizes, which increases the risk of false-positive results (i.e., the conclusion that a product makes a significant difference when it does not).

It is essential for nurses and other health care providers involved in tissue integrity management to maintain up-to-date knowledge regarding pressure redistribution along with the other therapeutic features provided by support surfaces. The astute wound specialist must be familiar with the performance characteristics of existing support surfaces in order to match individual patient needs to the appropriate support surface, with consideration as to care setting.

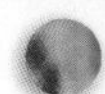

Conclusion

Support surfaces are a critical element of a comprehensive pressure ulcer prevention program, but they do not represent a stand-alone intervention and do not eliminate the need for routine repositioning. The primary therapeutic feature for all support surfaces is pressure redistribution; selected surfaces also provide shear reduction and microclimate control. Effective use of support surfaces requires a thorough understanding of the various features and products available, coupled with a comprehensive patient assessment. Development of an agency-specific formulary and decision-making algorithms guides the staff in making appropriate decisions regarding support surfaces.

REFERENCES

Anderson, C., & Rappl, L. (2004). Lateral rotation mattresses for wound healing. *Ostomy/Wound Management, 50*(4), 50–62.

Association of periOperative Registered Nurses (AORN). (2008). AORN standards of perioperative professional practice. In *Perioperative standards and recommended practices*. Denver, CO: AORN.

Brienza, D. M., & Geyer, M. J. (2005). Using support surfaces to manage tissue integrity. *Advances in Skin & Wound Care, 18*(3), 151–157.

Christian, W., & Lachenbruch, C. (2007). Standardizing the language of support surfaces. *Remington Report, 15*(3), 11–14.

Clark, D. I. (1998, November). A randomised controlled trial comparing the healing of pressure sores upon two pressure-redistributing seat cushions. *Proceedings of the 7th European Conferences on Advances in Wound Management*, 122–125.

Cullum, N., Nelson, E. A., Flemming, K., et al. (2001). Systematic reviews of wound care management: (5) beds; (6) compression; (7) laser therapy, therapeutic ultrasound, electrotherapy and electromagnetic therapy, *Health Technology Assessment, 5*(9), 1–221.

Cullum, N., McInnes, E., Bell-Syer, S. E., et al. (2004). Support surfaces for pressure ulcer prevention. *Cochrane Database of Systematic Reviews*, (3), CD001735.

Davidson, J., & Callery, C. (2001). Care of the obesity surgery patient requiring immediate-level care or intensive care. *Obesity Surgery, 11*, 93–97.

Defloor, T., De Bacquer, D., & Grypdonck, M. H. (2005). The effect of various combinations of turning and pressure reducing devices on the incidence of pressure ulcers. *International Journal of Nursing Studies, 42*(1), 37–46.

Gray, D., Cooper, P. J., & Stringfellow, S. (2001). Evaluating pressure-reducing foam mattresses and electric bed frames. *British Journal of Nursing, 10*(Suppl 22), s23.

Gunther, R. A., & Clark, M. (2000). The effect of dynamic pressure-redistributing bed support surface upon systemic lymph flow and composition. *Journal of Tissue Viability, 10*(3), 10–15.

Holzapfel, S. K. (1993). Support surfaces and their use in the prevention and treatment of pressure ulcers. *Journal of ET Nursing, 20*(6), 251.

Iglesias, C., Nixon, J., Cranny, G., et al. (2006). Pressure relieving support surfaces (PRESSURE) trial: Cost effectiveness analysis. *British Medical Journal, 332*(7555), 1416.

Le, K. M., Madsen, B. L., Barth, P. W., et al. (1984). An in-depth look at pressure sores using monolithic silicon pressure sensors. *Plastic and Reconstructive Surgery, 74*(6), 745.

Mackey, D. (2005). Support surfaces: Beds, mattresses, overlays-oh my! *The Nursing Clinics of North America, 40*(2), 251–265.

Makhsous, M., Lin, F., Knaus, E., et al. (2009). Promote pressure ulcer healing in individuals with spinal cord injury using an individualized cyclic pressure-relief protocol. *Advances in Skin & Wound Care, 22*(11), 514–521.

McCord, S., McElvain, V., Sachdeva, R., et al. (2004). Risk factors associated with pressure ulcers in the pediatric intensive care unit. *Journal of Wound, Ostomy, and Continence Nursing, 31*(4), 179–183.

McInnes, E., Jammali-Blasi, A., Bell-Syer, S. E., et al. (2011). Support surfaces for pressure ulcer prevention. *Cochrane Database of Systematic Reviews*, (4), CD001735.

McLane, K. M., Bookout, K., McCord, S., et al. (2004). The 2003 national pediatric pressure ulcer and skin breakdown prevalence survey: A multisite study. *Journal of Wound, Ostomy, and Continence Nursing, 31*(4), 168–178.

Miller, S., Parker, M., Blasiole, N., et al. (2013). A prospective, in vivo evaluation of two pressure-redistribution surfaces in healthy volunteers using pressure mapping as a quality control instrument. *Ostomy/Wound Management, 59*(2), 44–48.

National Pressure Ulcer Advisory Panel (NPUAP). (2007). NPUAP support surface standards initiative: Terms and definitions related to support surfaces. Retrieved May 11, 2009, from http://www.npuap.org/NPUAP_S3I_TD.pdf

National Pressure Ulcer Advisory Panel (NPUAP) and European Pressure Ulcer Advisory Panel (EPUAP). (2009). *Prevention and treatment of pressure ulcers*. Washington, DC: NPUAP.

National Pressure Ulcer Advisory Panel (NPUAP), European Pressure Ulcer Advisory Panel (EPUAP), Pan Pacific Pressure Ulcer Injury Alliance (PPPIA). (2014). *Prevention and Treatment of Pressure Ulcers: Clinical Practice Guideline*. Washington, DC: NPUAP.

Nicholson, G. P., Scales, J. T., Clark, R. P., et al. (1999). A method for determining the heat transfer and water vapour permeability of patient support systems. *Medical Engineering & Physics, 21*(10), 701.

Nix, D., & Mackey, D. (2012). Support surfaces. In R. Bryant & D. Nix (Eds.), *Acute and chronic wounds; Current management concepts* (4th ed., pp. 154–167). St. Louis, MO: Mosby Elsevier.

Nixon, J., Iglesias, C., Nelson, E. A., et al. (2006). Randomised, controlled trial of alternating pressure mattresses compared with alternating pressure overlays for the prevention of pressure ulcers: PRESSURE (pressure relieving support surfaces) trial. *British Medical Journal, 332*(7555), 1413.

Ochs, R. F., Horn, S. D., van Rijswijk, L., et al. (2005). Comparison of air-fluidized therapy with other support surfaces used to treat pressure ulcers in nursing home residents. *Ostomy/Wound Management, 51*(2), 38.

Polyurethane Foam Association (PFA). (2010). Joint industry foam standards and guidelines. Indentation force deflection (IFD) standards and guidelines. Retrieved October 5, 2010, from http://www.pfa.org/jifsg/jifsgs4.html

Reger, S. I., McGovern, T. F., Chung, K.-C., et al. (1988). Correlation of transducer systems for monitoring tissue interface pressures. *Journal of Clinical Engineering, 13*(5), 365–371.

Saha, S., Smith, M. E. B., Totten, A., et al. (2013). *Pressure ulcer treatment strategies: Comparative effectiveness*. Comparative Effectiveness Review No. 90. (Prepared by the Oregon Evidence-based Practice Center under Contract No. 290-2007-10057-I.) AHRQ Publication No. 13-EHC003-EF. Rockville, MD: Agency for Healthcare Research and Quality.

Schultz, A., Bien, M., Dumond, K., et al. (1999). Etiology and incidence of pressure ulcers in surgical patients. *AORN Journal, 70*(3), 434, 437–440, 443–449.

U.S. Food and Drug Administration (U.S. FDA), Center for Devices and Radiological Health. (2006). *Hospital bed system dimensional and assessment guidance to reduce entrapment*. Retrieved May 11, 2009, from http://www.fda.gov/MedicalDevices/DeviceRegulationandGuidance/GuidanceDocuments/ucm072662.htm

Walton-Geer, P. (2009). Prevention of pressure ulcers in the surgical patient. *AORN Journal, 89*(3), 538–552.

Whitney, J., Phillips, L., Aslam, R., et al. (2006). Guidelines for the treatment of pressure ulcers. *Wound Repair and Regeneration, 14*(6), 663–679.

Whittemore, R. (1998). Pressure-reduction support surfaces: A review of the literature. *Journal of Wound, Ostomy, and Continence Nursing, 25*, 6.

WOCN Society. (2003). *Guideline for management of pressure ulcers, WOCN Clinical Practice Guideline Series #2*. Glenview, IL: WOCN.

WOCN Society. (2010). *Guideline for management of pressure ulcers, WOCN Clinical Practice Guideline Series #2*. Glenview, IL: WOCN.

QUESTIONS

1. The wound nurse is recommending a support surface for a patient at risk for pressure ulcer development. What guideline would the nurse follow?

A. Support surfaces should be used as a stand-alone intervention for the prevention and treatment of pressure ulcers.
B. Correctly using support surfaces eliminates the need for turning and repositioning.
C. Australian Medical-grade sheepskins overlays are effective in reducing the incidence of pressure ulcers compared to standard care.
D. Active support surfaces with an AP feature are not more effective in preventing pressure ulcers than standard hospital mattresses.

2. For which patient would the wound nurse recommend placement on a reactive support surface with an LAL or AF feature?

A. A patient with multiple stage II pressure ulcers
B. A patient with Braden Mobility score of 2
C. A patient at risk for pressure ulcers with a mobility subscale score of 1
D. A patient who exceeds the weight limit of his or her current support system

3. A postsurgical patient who is on a reactive/CLP support surface with an LAL feature improves to the point that the patient is no longer at high risk for developing a pressure ulcer. What would be an appropriate recommendation for this patient?

A. Discontinue the use of support surfaces.
B. Place a sheepskin overlay between the patient and the hospital bed.
C. Move the patient to an appropriate bariatric support surface.
D. Place the patient on an active support surface with an AP feature.

4. Which general practice point for using support surfaces follows recommended guidelines for prevention and management of patients with pressure ulcers?

A. Choose a support surface based on availability within the facility and cost of product.
B. Make sure that the patient can assume a variety of positions on the surface without "bottoming out."
C. Use an overlay over a mattress if the patient has a considerable risk for fall or entrapment.
D. Choose a regular mattress over a support surface when patient incontinence cannot be managed by other means.

5. In most cases what is the most important therapeutic feature of a support surface to prevent or treat pressure ulcers?

A. Pressure redistribution
B. Cooling effect
C. Moisture barrier
D. Friction reduction

6. A wound nurse recommends a support surface for a patient who is at risk for pressure ulcers. The nurse explains to the patient that the mechanism works by:

A. Increasing tissue load
B. Reducing fatigue
C. Decreasing interface pressure
D. Increasing air pressure

7. The wound nurse is assessing the "envelopment" feature of a support surface being used for a patient who has a sacral pressure ulcer. What factor would the nurse check?
   A. Depth to which the body is allowed to penetrate the surface
   B. Reduced performance capacity due to use
   C. Ability of the support surface to conform evenly to irregularities
   D. Degree to which the surface reduces pressure

8. A wound nurse is investigating the use of a foam overlay for a patient with chronic wounds. Which statement correctly describes a characteristic of a type of foam product?
   A. *Closed-cell* foam is a higher-specification foam that has been shown to be more effective in preventing pressure ulcers than open-cell foam.
   B. *A viscoelastic* foam allows air to enter and exit the foam cells slowly, which means the material responds more quickly than elastic foam.
   C. Gel support surfaces are intended for single-patient use and have been found to be effective in preventing shear.
   D. Indentation force deflection (IFD), known previously as indentation load deflection (ILD), is a measure of firmness or resistance to compression.

9. The wound nurse recommends an active (alternating pressure) surface for a patient with an ischial pressure ulcer. What is the advantage of this type of surface?
   A. It does not need power to operate it.
   B. It is effective for high-risk patients when frequent positioning is not available.
   C. It does not make noise when it is operating.
   D. It facilitates pulmonary hygiene in the patient with acute respiratory condition.

10. The wound nurse is deciding on a support surface for a patient who requires head-of-bed elevation for tube feedings. What additional benefit might influence the choice?
   A. Provision of shear reduction
   B. Dissipation of moisture
   C. Facilitation of activity
   D. Minimization of the height of the bed and gaps

ANSWERS: 1.**C**, 2.**A**, 3.**D**, 4.**B**, 5.**A**, 6.**C**, 7.**C**, 8.**D**, 9.**B**, 10.**A**

CHAPTER 21

Venous Insufficiency, Venous Ulcers, and Lymphedema

Jan Johnson, Stephanie S. Yates, and Joanna J. Burgess

OBJECTIVES

1. Compare and contrast arterial, venous, neuropathic, and mixed ulcers in terms of risk factors, pathology, clinical presentation, and management guidelines.
2. Describe critical parameters to be included in assessment of the individual with a lower extremity ulcer.
3. Use assessment data to determine causative and contributing factors for a lower extremity ulcer and to develop individualized management plans that are evidence based.
4. Identify indications, contraindications, options, and guidelines for implementation of the following:
   - Therapeutic level static compression therapy
   - Modified static compression therapy
   - Dynamic compression therapy
   - Complex decongestive physiotherapy
5. Demonstrate correct technique for application of compression wraps.
6. Describe clinical characteristics and management options for venous dermatitis.
7. Describe indications for referral to vascular surgeon, lymphedema specialist, or dermatologist.
8. Describe the etiology and pathology of lymphedema, to include differentiation between primary and secondary lymphedema.
9. Describe the various stages of lymphedema, to include clinical characteristics and implications for management.
10. Identify indications that a lower extremity ulcer is "atypical" and requires additional diagnostic workup and/or medical–surgical intervention.

Topic Outline

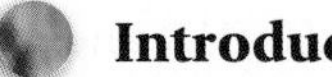

Introduction

Prevalence and Incidence of Venous Insufficiency and Venous Ulcers

Pathology of Venous Insufficiency and Venous Ulceration

- Normal Function
- Pathology of Venous Insufficiency
- Pathology of Venous Ulceration

Assessment and Diagnosis

- History
  - Conditions Leading to Valvular Dysfunction
  - Conditions Resulting in Calf Muscle Pump Dysfunction
  - Impediments to Healing
  - History of Healed and/or Current Ulceration
  - Triggers for Ulceration
- Symptoms
- Physical Examination
- CEAP Classification
- Wound Assessment
- Diagnostic Studies

Primary Prevention

Management of CVI

- Compression Therapy
  - Static Compression
  - Inelastic Compression
  - Dynamic Compression

Introduction

Lower extremity ulcers are a common type of chronic wound, especially among the elderly, and venous ulcers are the most common type of lower extremity wound. This chapter addresses the prevalence and incidence, pathology, diagnosis, clinical presentation, and management of venous insufficiency and venous ulcers. The prevalence, pathology, presentation, and management of lymphedema and lipedema are also addressed.

Prevalence and Incidence of Venous Insufficiency and Venous Ulcers

Lower extremity venous disorders (LEVDs), also known as chronic venous disorders (CVDs), cover a broad spectrum of morphologic and/or functional abnormalities of the venous system (Porter & Moneta, 1995). Severity ranges from mild conditions such as uncomplicated telangiectasias and spider veins to more complex conditions such as deep vein thrombosis (DVT) and venous ulcers (VU). Varicose veins are present in 10% to 30% of the general population with increasing prevalence associated with aging. In the Framingham Study, 1,720 men and 2,102 women were examined for varicose veins every 2 years over a 16-year span; during this time period, 23% of the men (396) and 30% of the women (629) developed varicose veins. On average, the 2-year incidence of varicose veins was 39.4 per 1,000 for men and 51.9 per 1,000 for women; interestingly, the highest incidence rates were among women 40 to 49 years of age (Brand et al., 1988). An estimated 7 million individuals worldwide have LEVD with 3 million progressing to ulceration (Bergen et al., 2006). Venous ulcers, also known as venous stasis ulcers, venous insufficiency ulcers, and venous leg ulcers, affect approximately 1% of the U.S. population with reports of 600,000 new venous ulcers each year (Wound, Ostomy, and Continence Nurses Society [WOCN], 2011). Venous ulcers account for 80% to 90% of all leg ulcers (O'Meara et al., 2008) and cost the U.S. health care system an estimated $1.9 to $3.5 billion per year (WOCN, 2011). Recurrence rates of 57% to 97% reflect the chronicity of this condition (Milic et al., 2009). Quality of life (QOL) issues are significant and include absence from work due to pain, frequent clinic visits, and treatment requirements (WOCN, 2011). In one study on the impact of leg ulcers (all types) on QOL, 81% of patients believed their mobility was adversely affected by the ulcer, 58% found caring for the ulcer burdensome, and 68% reported that the ulcer had a negative emotional impact (Phillips et al., 1994).

CLINICAL PEARL

Venous ulcers affect about 1% of the U.S. population and have a significant negative effect on QOL.

Pathology of Venous Insufficiency and Venous Ulceration

Normal Function

With normal venous function, blood is drained from the superficial vessels of the skin and subcutaneous fat by three major vascular pathways: the superficial veins

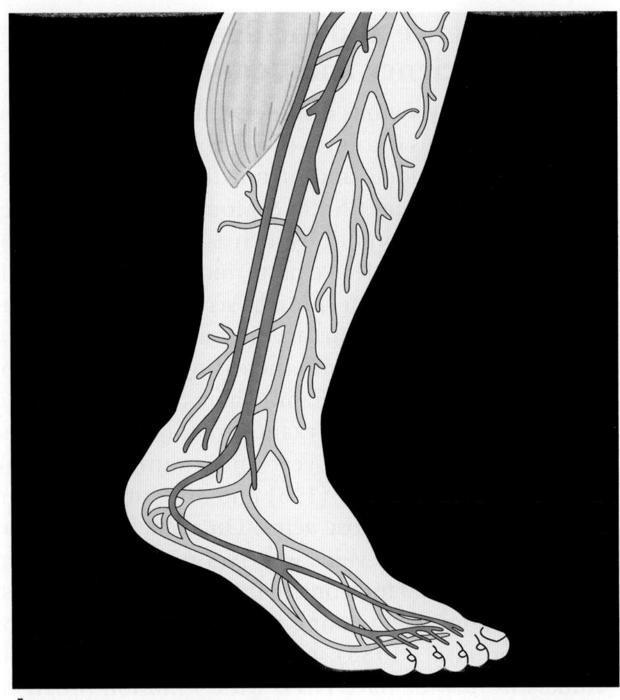

A

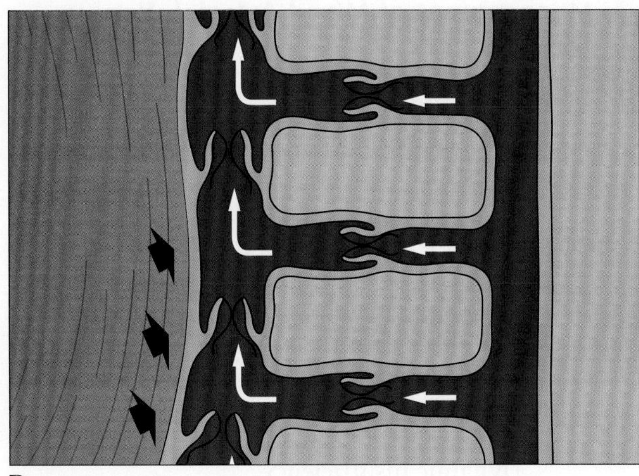

B

FIGURE 21-1. Normal venous system. **A.** Anatomy of venous system: superficial, perforator, and deep veins. **B.** One-way valves in perforator and deep veins for prevention of venous reflux.

(low-pressure system), the deep veins (high-pressure system), and the perforating veins (veins that transfer blood between the superficial and deep systems) (Fig. 21-1). The superficial veins are located above the deep muscular fascia and include the great saphenous and small saphenous veins. The deep veins lie within the muscle compartments (intramuscular) or between the muscles (intermuscular). The latter are more critical in the development of chronic venous insufficiency (CVI) because they are exposed to high subfascial pressures during calf muscle contraction. The intermuscular veins parallel the lower extremity arteries and include the anterior tibial, posterior tibial, peroneal, popliteal, and femoral veins. Perforator veins, also known as communicating veins, connect the two systems, passing through the deep fascia at the mid-thigh, knee, and ankle. There are more than 90 perforating veins in each leg; the perforators are equipped with unidirectional bicuspid valves that open to permit blood flow out of the legs toward the heart and then close to prevent the return of blood toward the feet. This series of valves is essential to normal venous function and unidirectional blood flow, particularly when the individual is in the upright position. The calf muscle pump and the valves normally work in concert to promote the return of blood, against gravity, to the heart (Eberhardt & Raffetto, 2014). When the calf muscle is relaxed, the valves open, allowing blood to fill the deep veins; filling increases the pressure in the deep venous system. Contraction of the calf muscle then empties the veins and reduces venous pressure.

CLINICAL PEARL

Normal function of the venous valves are essential to unidirectional blood flow and effective venous return; the one-way valves and calf muscle pump work together to promote the return of blood, against gravity, back to the heart.

Pathology of Venous Insufficiency

Pathology develops when there are abnormalities in any part of the system that result in impaired venous return and persistent high pressures within the deep venous system (venous hypertension), such as a DVT that causes obstructed venous return and valvular dysfunction (Fig. 21-2). Venous hypertension is the etiologic factor common to all people with LEVD (Bergan, 2007). Impaired venous return and venous hypertension eventually result in pathologic changes in the superficial venous system and the microvascular system (capillary bed). These changes include development of high pressures and possibly varicosities within the superficial system, which is usually a low-pressure system. In addition, the impaired venous return eventually results in capillary bed congestion and extravasation of intravascular molecules into the surrounding tissues.

CLINICAL PEARL

Venous hypertension occurs when the venous system does not empty effectively and is the primary etiologic factor for lower extremity venous disease; venous hypertension causes capillary bed congestion, and leakage of fluid and molecules into the surrounding tissues.

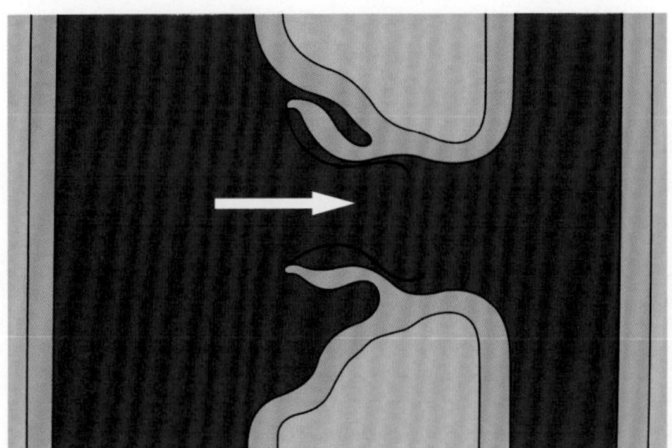
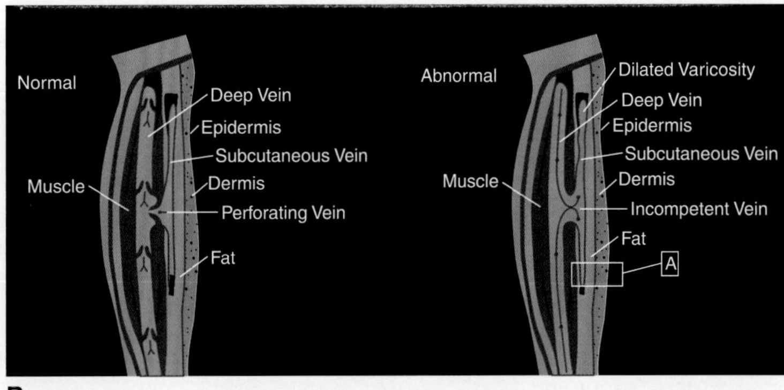

A B

FIGURE 21-2. **A, B.** Valvular dysfunction/venous reflux.

Pathology of Venous Ulceration

While the pathology of venous insufficiency is clear, the specific pathologic mechanisms resulting in venous ulceration and impaired healing are not well understood at present. Theories include damage to the endothelial lining of the vessels, platelet aggregation, activation of white blood cells, abnormal levels of inflammatory cytokines such as matrix metalloproteases (MMPs), inflammation, and fibrotic changes in the soft tissues, due in part to the extravasation of cells and plasma proteins into the tissues (Collins & Seraj, 2010; De Araujo et al., 2003; Nicolaides et al., 2008). While the specific pathology of venous ulceration remains unclear, the underlying cause is venous hypertension secondary to venous reflux and obstruction.

CLINICAL PEARL

The specific pathology of venous ulcers is not clear but is thought to be due to inflammatory and fibrotic changes in the soft tissues that render them very vulnerable to minor trauma.

 Assessment and Diagnosis

The diagnosis of lower extremity venous disease is primarily made based on patient history and clinical examination.

History

A thorough history should include inquiry into family history of venous disease as well as factors that result in valvular dysfunction, calf muscle pump dysfunction, impediments to healing, and impediments to treatment.

CLINICAL PEARL

The history for a patient with suspected venous disease should include any family history of venous problems and questions about any conditions resulting in valvular dysfunction, calf muscle pump dysfunction, and/or impediments to healing and treatment.

Conditions Leading to Valvular Dysfunction

The patient should be asked about pathologic conditions that compromise function of the one-way valves critical to normal venous function, which include the following:

- Conditions that increase resistance to venous return, such as obesity, multiple pregnancies, or pregnancies close together
- Conditions that directly damage the valves, such as DVT or phlebitis, and conditions associated with undiagnosed DVT (e.g., pulmonary embolism, leg trauma, head injury, or other trauma)
- Thrombophilic conditions such as protein S deficiency, protein C deficiency, or factor V Leiden mutations
- Inflammatory autoimmune diseases such as systemic lupus erythematosus (SLE) and antiphospholipid syndrome, which may involve venous inflammation that results in microthrombi

CLINICAL PEARL

Conditions that interfere with normal valvular function include obesity, DVT or phlebitis, thrombophilic conditions, and inflammatory autoimmune conditions.

Conditions Resulting in Calf Muscle Pump Dysfunction

The patient should also be queried regarding conditions that adversely affect function of the calf muscle pump, such as:

- Advanced age, which may lead to stiffening of the calf muscle tendon and reduced range of motion in the ankle
- Any alteration in gait that results in loss of the normal heel strike—toe-off mechanics that cause calf muscle contraction (e.g., a "shuffling" gait)

CLINICAL PEARL

Conditions that cause impaired calf muscle function include paralysis, gait alterations, advanced age, and sedentary lifestyle or reduced mobility.

- Sedentary lifestyle or reduced mobility, that is, occupations that require long periods of standing without walking, morbid obesity that limits mobility, or musculoskeletal disorders such as paralysis, arthritis, or prior surgery to the knee, ankle, or foot resulting in fixation of the joint.

Impediments to Healing

The wound nurse should also ask the patient about factors that would impact on his or her ability to heal (e.g., diabetes, tobacco use, nutritional status, and medications) and factors that would affect treatment (such as activity restrictions, impaired mobility, or heart failure) (WOCN, 2011).

History of Healed and/or Current Ulceration

The individual should also be asked about any prior ulcers and the current ulcer, to include location, description, duration, and treatment. The individual with a past history of ulceration should be carefully queried to determine his or her understanding of the pathology underlying the ulcer, the treatment resulting in healing, and the need for continued compression following healing. Specifically she or he should be asked about any prescription for compression hosiery, factors impacting on consistency of use, and the relationship between compression therapy use and ulcer recurrence.

Triggers for Ulceration

Seventy-four percent of venous ulcers begin with a specific "trigger." Therefore, the history should include queries related to known triggering events: cellulitis, penetrating injury/trauma, contact dermatitis, rapid onset of leg edema, burns, dry skin with itching/scratching, and insect bites (Shai & Halevy, 2005).

CLINICAL PEARL

Seventy-four percent of venous ulcers begin with a specific "trigger," such as cellulitis, trauma, contact dermatitis, rapidly developing edema, burns, dry skin resulting in scratching, and/or insect bites.

Symptoms

The initial presentation/clinical symptomatology related to venous disease varies widely; common symptoms include "heaviness" or aching of the legs, pain, swelling, dry skin, a feeling of tightness in the lower limb, skin irritation, and itching. Pain is typically reported as worsening with prolonged dependency and improving with elevation. Pain may be severe enough to limit ambulation.

CLINICAL PEARL

Pain associated with venous ulcers and venous disease is typically described as "aching" pain that is worsened by dependency and relieved by elevation.

TABLE 21-1 Common Physical Findings in Venous Disease

Telangiectasias	Small (<1 mm diameter) linear blood vessels visible under the skin, usually red or purple; commonly referred to as "spider veins"
Reticular veins	Slightly larger (1–3 mm diameter) veins that are visible under the skin, usually blue and slightly bulging in venous disease
Varicose veins	Superficial veins that are large, thickened, twisting, dilated, and often painful
Hemosiderosis	Reddish brown/black pigmentation, usually in the ankle area, resulting from extravasated red blood cells; as the cells break down, iron from the hemoglobin is released into the tissue causing the staining
Atrophie blanche	Smooth localized areas of ivory white atrophic skin with or without tiny dilated capillaries that appear as red dots throughout the area, often confused with scar tissue
Lipodermatosclerosis	Skin changes in the lower leg with induration, fibrosis, and hyperpigmentation resulting in "inverted champagne bottle" or "inverted bowling pin" appearance

Physical Examination

Physical assessment includes a thorough examination of the limb, to include skin status, perfusion status, edema, and any ulcerations that are present. Common physical signs include dilated veins (telangiectasias, reticular veins, varicose veins), edema, skin changes (hemosiderosis, atrophie blanche, and/or dermatitis), and/or ulceration (See **Table 21-1** for common physical findings and descriptions; see Fig. 21-3 for hemosiderosis). The presence of edema is a particularly significant finding and requires differential assessment to rule out causes other than venous insufficiency (WOCN, 2011) (**Table 21-2**). The edema is often long-standing and typically worsens when the leg

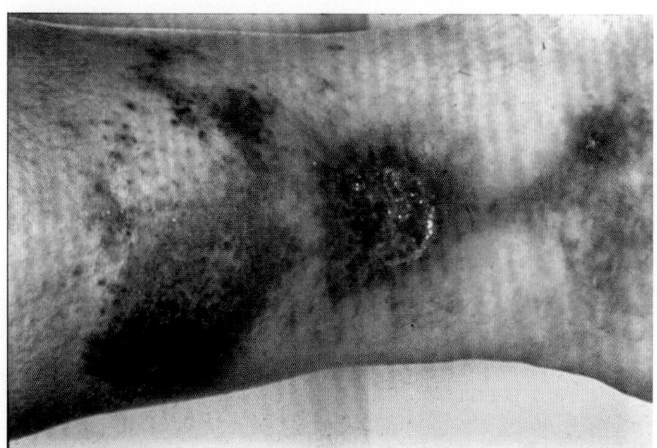

FIGURE 21-3. Hemosiderosis around venous ulcer.

TABLE 21-2 Differences between Edema, Lymphedema, and Lipedema

	Skin and Pigment Alterations	Edema Characteristics	Part Involved	Treatment
Venous insufficiency edema				
Elevated venous pressures related to venous valve incompetence and/or obstruction	Skin thickens, becomes fibrotic and woody. Dark pigmentation common. Ulceration common.	Insidious onset; heaviness and pain in the legs at the end of the day; increasing soft, pitting swelling; when chronic becomes hard and irregular with venous eczema common.	Lower legs and feet.	Skin care; compression therapy; possibly manual drainage (note limited evidence on the benefits of manual drainage for edema associated with venous insufficiency).
Lymphedema				
Damage and/or blockage of lymph flow, which causes accumulation of high-protein edema	Skin thickened, becomes firm and fibrotic; lymphangitis and cellulitis common. Ulceration not common.	May be congenital; may be sudden onset; otherwise may be gradual increase in edema over months or years; pitting if recent onset; indurated and hard if long-standing.	Any extremity or body part; may be one part, one entire side, or one, two, or all extremities.	Weight control; skin care; manual lymphatic drainage; localized procedures such as liposuction; exercise; compression.
Lipedema				
Increase in fat deposition of lower extremities ("painful fat syndrome")	Accumulation of loosely textured fat, most commonly limited to the lower extremities. Usually occurs in women, beginning in adolescence. Bruising is common and involved areas are tender to palpation.	Bilateral and symmetrical. No ulcerations.	Legs and buttocks; feet not involved.	Weight loss; reduction of size by surgery is done in some centers but not enough evidence to determine long-term effect.

Sources: Fife, C. E., & Carter, M. J. (2008). Lymphedema in the morbidly obese patient: Unique challenges in a unique population. *Ostomy Wound Management, 54*(1), 44–56; Molski, P., Ossowski, R., Hagner, W., et al. (2009). Patients with venous disease benefit from manual lymphatic drainage. *International Angiology, 28*(2), 151–155; Radhakrishnan, K., & Rockson, S. G. (2008). The clinical spectrum of lymphatic disease. *Annals of the New York Academy of Sciences, 1131*, 155–184; Schmeller, W., & Meier-Vollrath, I. (2006). Tumescent liposuction: A new and successful therapy for lipedema. *Journal of Cutaneous Medicine and Surgery, 10*(1), 7–10.

is in a dependent position for prolonged periods of time; edema that is venous in origin is normally reduced by elevation of the leg above the level of the heart. Venous dermatitis is another common finding and should be distinguished from cellulitis (WOCN, 2011). Scars from previous ulcers should be noted as well as "ankle flaring," which is a cluster of reticular and spider veins along the ankle.

Perfusion status must always be thoroughly assessed for any individual with a lower extremity wound; this includes assessment of pedal pulses, which are commonly palpable in patients with venous disease, and validation of perfusion status with measurement of the ankle–brachial index (ABI). ABI measurement is critical not only to rule out significant arterial disease but also to determine the level of compression therapy that can be safely used for treatment of the venous disease (see Chapter 22 for directions on ABI testing and interpretation).

CLINICAL PEARL

Common physical findings in the patient with a venous ulcer include edema, hemosiderosis, palpable pulses, warm feet, and possibly venous dermatitis.

Peripheral sensory neuropathy is often present in patients with LEVD; thus, physical assessment should include monofilament testing (see Chapter 23 for directions on monofilament testing and interpretation).

CEAP Classification

Venous disease is sometimes classified as to severity using the CEAP (Clinical–Etiology–Anatomy–Pathophysiology) system (Table 21-3) (Eklof et al., 2004). While additional testing is required for fully accurate classification using this system, many clinicians use the section on clinical manifestations when documenting the severity of disease. It should be noted that the term "chronic venous insufficiency" (CVI) is reserved for use with C4-C6 disease. Thus, varicose veins alone without skin changes do not indicate CVI.

Wound Assessment

Assessment of the wound should include location; dimensions; appearance of the wound bed; status of wound edges and periwound skin; volume, color, and odor of exudate; and bleeding. The classic location for these ulcers is superior to the medial malleolus; however, venous ulcers may occur anywhere on the lower leg including the posterior

TABLE 21-3 Revised CEAP Classifications: Summary

Clinical Classification	
C_0:	No visible or palpable signs of venous disease
C_1:	Telangiectasias or reticular veins
C_2:	Varicose veins
C_3:	Edema
C_{4a}:	Pigmentation or eczema
C_{4b}:	Lipodermatosclerosis or atrophie blanche
C_5:	Healed venous ulcer
C_6:	Active venous ulcer
S:	Symptomatic, including ache, pain, tightness, skin irritation, heaviness, and muscle cramps, and other complaints attributable to venous dysfunction
A:	Asymptomatic
Etiologic Classification	
Ec:	Congenital
Ep:	Primary
Es:	Secondary (postthrombotic)
En:	No venous cause identified
Anatomic Classification	
As:	Superficial veins
Ap:	Perforator veins
Ad:	Deep veins
An:	No venous location identified
Pathophysiologic Classification	
Basic CEAP	
Pr:	Reflux
Po:	Obstruction
Pr,o:	Reflux and obstruction
Pn:	No venous pathophysiology identifiable

Example:
A patient has painful swelling of the leg and varicose veins, lipodermatosclerosis, and active ulceration. Duplex scanning on May 17, 2004, showed axial reflux of the great saphenous vein above and below the knee, incompetent calf perforator veins, and axial reflux in the femoral and popliteal veins. There are no signs of postthrombotic obstruction.

Classification according to basic CEAP: C6,S, Ep,As,p,d, Pr. Reprinted with permission from Eklof, B., Rutherford, R. B., Bergan J. J., et al. (2004). Revision of the CEAP classification for chronic venous disorders: Consensus statement. *Journal of Vascular Surgery*, *40*(6), 1248–1252. doi: 10.1016/j.jvs.2004.09.027.

calf and dorsum of the foot. The wound bed is usually shallow, with a ruddy red color; a yellow film may also be present and may be adherent or loose (Fig. 21-4 for classic venous ulcer). There is seldom tunneling or undermining. The periwound skin is often macerated, and there may be crusting and scaling as well as hyperpigmentation (hemosiderosis). Exudate is usually moderate to heavy, and odor and bleeding may or may not be present (WOCN, 2011).

CLINICAL PEARL

Venous ulcers are typically shallow, exudative, ruddy in appearance (or covered with a yellow film), and located around the malleolus.

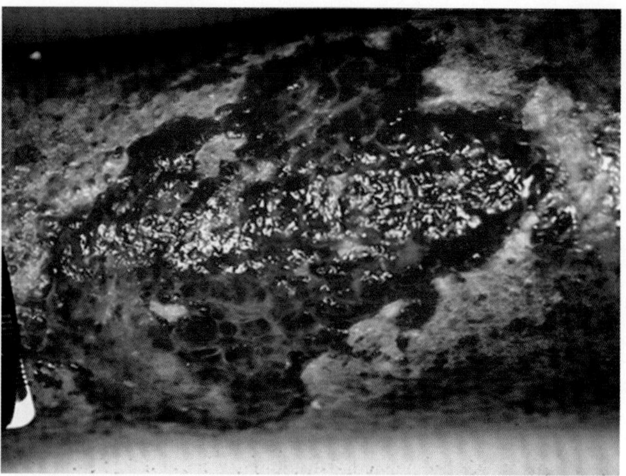

FIGURE 21-4. Classic venous ulcer with periwound maceration and dermatitis.

Diagnostic Studies

Vascular laboratory studies can assist in determining the extent and severity of venous disease. Decisions regarding which, if any, tests are needed should be made after considering whether the diagnosis of CVI is clear or questionable and whether the patient is a candidate for and interested in vascular intervention. Vascular studies are very helpful when the clinical presentation is unclear or atypical and for patients who fail to respond to conservative treatment. Venous duplex ultrasound is the most reliable and commonly used noninvasive test. It is used to identify the presence and direction of blood flow and to detect venous reflux or venous obstruction and the anatomic location of the obstruction; this information confirms the diagnosis of venous insufficiency and can be used to plan for vein ablation or other interventions. Other noninvasive tests sometimes used to assess the presence and severity of venous reflux include air plethysmography and photoplethysmography (PPG); however, these are not widely used given the availability and utility of venous duplex ultrasonography (Alguire & Mathes, 2014). PPG can be performed relatively quickly and provides a reading of the overall venous refill time. (Normal is approximately 20 seconds) Handheld versions of the PPG device have been shown to provide valid results and may be used in selected settings to provide earlier diagnosis of CVI (Kelechi & Bonham, 2008).

CLINICAL PEARL

Venous duplex ultrasound is the most reliable and commonly used noninvasive test for diagnosing venous disease; it detects venous reflux or obstruction and the anatomic location of the obstruction.

As previously noted, pulse palpation and ABI measurement are critical elements of the assessment; thus, a handheld Doppler is an essential diagnostic tool (Carmel, 2012). The handheld Doppler can also be used to verify pulses when edema makes palpation difficult.

Primary Prevention

Early identification of venous disease (CEAP levels C1-C3) allows for earlier treatment, which is directed toward reducing symptoms and preventing progression to ulceration. Patients with known risk factors (**Table 21-4**) or early signs of CVI should begin wearing compression garments (stockings/hosiery) immediately and should wear them consistently to prevent venous edema and ulceration.

In addition to compression, there are three additional categories of preventive strategies: weight management, exercise/physical activity, and treatment of varicosities. Obesity is a strong risk factor for CVI; thus, all efforts to attain and maintain a healthy weight should be considered including dietary alterations, counseling, drug therapy, and weight loss surgery. Because the calf muscle pump plays a critical role in normal function and in the pathophysiology of CVI, exercise programs aimed at improving function have proven helpful. Physical therapy may be needed to improve range of motion and/or gait followed by a more aggressive exercise program. Interventional treatment of varicosities, such as endovenous laser ablation, radiofrequency ablation, and other approaches to repair veins and valves, have proven to prevent the progression of venous disease and the development of ulcerations (Eberhardt & Raffetto, 2014).

CLINICAL PEARL

Preventive care for individuals at risk for venous ulceration includes compression, weight management, exercise/physical activity, and treatment of varicosities.

TABLE 21-4 Risk Factors for LEVD

Related to valvular dysfunction	Related to calf muscle pump dysfunction
• Family history of venous disease	• Sedentary lifestyle
• Pregnancy (multiple or close together)	• Prolonged standing
• Thrombophilia (protein S or protein C deficiency)	• Prolonged sitting
• Anticardiolipin antibody	• Surgery/trauma to the foot/ankle/leg
• Systemic inflammation	• Altered gait
• Venous thromboembolism (VTE)/phlebitis/pulmonary embolism	• Paralysis
• Obesity	• Restricted range of motion of the ankle
• Injectable drug use	• Advanced age

Adapted from Wound, Ostomy, and Continence Nurses Society (WOCN). (2011). *Guideline for management of wounds in patients with lower-extremity venous disease*. Mount Laurel, NJ: Author; Carmel, J. E. (2012). Venous ulcers. In R. A. Bryant & D. P. Nix (Eds.), *Acute & chronic wounds: Current management concepts* (4th ed., pp. 194–213). St. Louis, MO: Elsevier.

Management of CVI

Management of CVI, with or without ulceration, involves compression therapy, leg elevation, selected use of pharmaceuticals, and surgical intervention for selected patients.

CLINICAL PEARL

Management of CVI, with or without ulceration, involves compression therapy, leg elevation, selected use of pharmaceuticals, and surgical intervention for selected patients.

Compression Therapy

Compression and elevation have long been considered to be essential elements of any comprehensive venous ulcer management program (Vowden & Vowden, 2006); both help to reduce edema and improve venous return. Compression therapy "works" mechanically by partially compressing the distended superficial veins; this reduces the diameter of the vessels and makes previously incompetent valves competent, which restores the normal pattern of one-way blood flow. Compression also supports the calf muscle pump, which further promotes venous return and reduces venous hypertension; the normal ejection fraction of the calf muscle pump is approximately 65% (Black, 2014; Brem et al., 2004). Compression therapy also increases the level of pressure in the interstitial space, which reduces edema by preventing leakage of fluid out of the capillary bed and by promoting return of edema fluid to the lymphatic system and capillary bed. While the primary effects of compression therapy are reduction of venous hypertension and control of edema, recent studies suggest that there may be other ways in which compression therapy contributes to venous ulcer healing. For example, in a 2008 study, Beidler and colleagues (2008) concluded that compression therapy also reduces the proinflammatory environment (matrix metalloproteinases) characteristic of chronic venous ulcers.

Long-term compression therapy has been demonstrated in numerous randomized clinical trials to be beneficial in management of edema and venous ulcers and remains the gold standard of venous ulcer therapy, despite the fact that there are no internationally accepted performance standards (O'Meara et al., 2009). The most recent Cochrane review (O'Meara et al., 2012) summarized the current evidence regarding the various approaches to compression therapy as follows:

1. Compression increases healing rates when compared with no compression.
2. Multicomponent systems are more effective than single-component systems.
3. Multilayer systems with an elastic bandage component appear to be more effective than those mainly made up of inelastic components.
4. Two component bandages appear to perform as well as four-layer bandages (4LB).
5. 4LB systems heal ulcers faster than the short-stretch bandage (SSB).

The goals of compression therapy are to improve symptoms, reduce edema, and heal ulcers. Compression can be provided by wraps, garments, bandages, or devices and is available in both static devices and dynamic "pump" devices.

CLINICAL PEARL

Compression can be provided by wraps, garments, bandages, or devices and is available in both static and dynamic forms.

Static Compression

Static compression therapy involves application of constant gradient pressure to the lower extremity, with highest pressures exerted distally (at the ankle) and lowest pressures exerted proximally (usually at the knee). Therapeutic level compression is generally considered to be 30 to 40 mm Hg at the ankle. Examples of static therapy are compression bandages, leggings with Velcro straps, and compression hosiery. While compression bandages can be composed of both elastic and inelastic materials, hosiery by necessity is elastic (WOCN, 2011) (**Table 21-5**). Static compression is considered first-line therapy for most individuals with venous disease; however, static compression is contraindicated for individuals with uncompensated (symptomatic) heart failure and for individuals with advanced lower extremity arterial disease (LEAD), as evidenced by an ABI $\leq$ 0.5. For individuals with moderately severe LEAD (ABI $\geq$ 0.5 to $\leq$0.8), modified compression is recommended (i.e., 23 to 30 mm Hg compression at the ankle) (see Chapter 22 for detailed discussion of compression therapy for patients with mixed arterial and venous disease).

TABLE 21-5 Compression Stocking Classifications between United States and United Kingdom

US Class	Descriptor	Ankle Pressure
Class 1	Light support	20–30 mm Hg
Class 2	Medium support	30–40 mm Hg
Class 3	Strong support	40–50 mm Hg
Class 4	Very strong support	50–60 mm Hg
UK Class	**Descriptor**	**Ankle Pressure**
Class 1	Light support	14–17 mm Hg
Class 2	Medium support	18–24 mm Hg
Class 3	Strong support	25–35 mm Hg

Adapted from: O'Meara, S., Cullum, N. A., & Nelson, E. A. (2009). Compression for venous leg ulcers. *Cochrane Database of Systemic Reviews*, (1), CD000265; Partsch, H., Clark, M., Mosti, G., et al. (2008). Classification of compression bandages: Practical aspects. *Dermatologic Surgery*, *34*(5), 600–609.

CLINICAL PEARL

Therapeutic level static compression is contraindicated in patients with uncompensated heart failure and patients with coexisting arterial disease (ABI <0.8). For individuals with moderately severe arterial disease (ABI > 0.5 to <0.8), modified compression is indicated; for individuals with ABI < 0.5, compression is totally contraindicated.

Compression Stockings

Prescription hosiery (also known as compression stockings) are widely used for primary and secondary prevention of venous ulcers; they are not a good choice for early therapy when the limb is very edematous, because hosiery must be sized to fit the leg and is intended for repetitive use over time. Thus, compression wraps are typically used for initial therapy, and the patient is then "crossed over" to compression hosiery or an alternative product for maintenance therapy.

Compression stockings are designed to provide a pressure gradient across the length of the stocking, with the greatest pressure exerted at the ankle and the least pressure exerted at the proximal end of the stocking.. A new form of stocking with higher pressures over the calf has been described in European studies but at this time is not considered standard therapy (Armstrong & Meyr, 2014). It is generally accepted that an external pressure of 35 to 40 mm Hg at the ankle is necessary to prevent leakage from capillaries affected by venous disease; however, the optimal level of pressure needed to overcome the underlying venous hypertension has not been determined.

Hosiery are available in a variety of lengths: knee-high, thigh-high, chaps (unilateral waist high), standard pantyhose, and maternity pantyhose. Knee-high stockings are sufficient for most patients and are generally well tolerated; however, thigh-high stockings are often prescribed following venous surgery. It is important to instruct the patient to pull the thigh-high stockings up on the thigh so they do not wrinkle at the knee, which causes binding, stricturing, and discomfort.

Stockings are also available in five pressure gradients (<20, 20 to 30, 30 to 40, 40 to 50, and >50 mm Hg). To be effective, compression stockings need to exert a minimum of 20 to 30 mm Hg pressure at the ankle. It is important to realize that the "antiembolism" stockings usually used in the hospital exert only 8 to 10 mm Hg at the ankle and are ineffective for treatment of venous insufficiency. Patients should be provided with a prescription that specifies length of stocking and level of compression and must be correctly fitted. In some clinics, the patient is measured for the stockings by the wound care nurse, who also instructs the patient in application. In other clinics, the patient is provided with a prescription and referred to a pharmacy or supply center with a qualified fitter. The critical issues in assuring effective therapy include stockings that provide therapeutic level compression, stockings that are correctly fitted, and collaboration with the patient to assure appropriate application and consistent use.

A common problem reported by patients wearing compression hosiery is difficulty with application; this is an even greater problem for obese individuals, those who cannot bend over, and those with limited hand strength and dexterity. Fortunately, there are a number of hosiery options and application devices that make it easier to don the stockings. For example, patients with foot deformities typically find it easier and more comfortable to use open toe stockings. There are zippered stockings and layered stockings that may be beneficial for patients who lack the mobility and hand strength to don regular compression stockings; in addition, there are stocking butlers and silken footies and liners that frequently make application easier. All patients should be advised to apply the stockings in the morning when edema is minimal; if there is a delay between getting out of bed and donning the stockings, the patient should be instructed to elevate the legs for 20 to 30 minutes prior to application. Patients should also be told that it is easier and safer to don the stockings while sitting in a chair with a firm back (rather than sitting on the edge of the bed). It is critical for the wound care nurse to become knowledgeable regarding the available stocking options and donning devices and to work with the patient to find a stocking and application technique that work effectively for that individual. For patients who are unable to effectively don the stockings, even with the various assistive devices, an inelastic reusable device such as CircAid might be appropriate. This device is secured with overlapping bands that provide inelastic compression and can easily be reapplied and readjusted when edema fluctuates. It also permits easy removal for bathing and wound care (Carmel, 2012). These devices must also be correctly fitted, and the patient must be instructed in their use.

CLINICAL PEARL

A common problem reported by patients is difficulty with application of compression stockings; fortunately, there are a number of options and devices that make it easier to don the stockings.

Care of hosiery is equally important since inappropriate laundering can reduce the level of compression and thereby compromise therapy. The following points should be included when teaching patients how to care for their stockings:

- Wash new stockings before wearing to reduce stiffness.
- Wash daily if possible; hand wash or machine wash on delicate cycle, and hang to dry.
- Moisturize the skin in the evening before going to bed as stockings absorb skin oils causing dryness.
- Purchase two pairs if possible and alternate wearing.
- Replace at least every 6 months or when stockings no longer have adequate compression.

Compression Bandages

Compression bandaging systems are commonly used in the initial treatment of venous insufficiency and venous ulceration; they are typically applied by a health care professional at 3- to 7-day intervals, with the specific interval determined by volume of exudate and level of edema. Compression wraps can be classified as elastic and/or inelastic and as single layer (one component) or multilayer (two to four components). An international expert consensus group (Partsch et al., 2008) recommended that classification of compression systems be based on components rather than layers, since multilayer wraps can have both elastic and inelastic components and since even single layer wraps overlap, actually creating two layers. The 2009 Cochrane Review on Compression for Venous Ulcers opted to follow these recommendations. Therefore, the terms multicomponent and single component should be used to describe compression bandages, rather than multilayer and single layer. The terms elastic and inelastic refer to the degree of "stretch" (extensibility) of the wrap. Sometimes clinicians use the terms elastic and long stretch (maximum extensibility >100%) interchangeably, to indicate wraps that exhibit high resting pressures and low working (walking) pressures. Inelastic and short stretch (maximum extensibility of <100%) are also used interchangeably to denote products that exhibit high working (walking) pressures and low resting pressures (WOCN, 2011).

CLINICAL PEARL

Compression wraps/bandaging systems are usually the best choice for initial treatment and until edema has been eliminated; data indicate that elastic systems provide better results than inelastic and that systems with at least two components (layers) provide better results than single-component systems.

Inelastic Compression

An inelastic system has no "give"; it exerts high "working" pressures (i.e., when the person is ambulating and the calf muscle is contracting) but is unable to tighten to provide continued support when the leg is at rest. In addition, inelastic systems cannot adapt to any changes in leg volume, such as increased edema with dependency or reduced edema resulting from leg elevation or due to the compression wrap itself. Inelastic systems are typically changed every 3 to 7 days and, as with all compression wrap systems, should be applied by trained personnel. The most commonly used inelastic compression system is the Unna's boot, an inexpensive and readily available compression product named after its inventor, German dermatologist Dr. Paul Unna (1850–1929). Today's zinc paste wraps come in different widths (common size is 4 inches width and 10 feet length) and can be impregnated with several different products including zinc paste, glycerin, gelatin, and calamine lotion. The goal in applying the zinc paste layer is to achieve a smooth conformable "boot" that supports the calf muscle pump; flat "pleats" are usually needed to assure a smooth fit over the foot and ankle. In most settings, the zinc paste layer is covered by a cohesive self-adherent bandage, which provides some additional compression. Advantages of this inelastic bandage system include its ability to provide high working pressure during walking, its relatively low cost and ready availability, the fact that it is a relatively thin wrap that usually permits the patient to wear his or her shoes, and the beneficial effects of the impregnated gauze on venous dermatitis. In addition, because the wrap is inelastic, it may be better tolerated by patients who feel that elastic wraps are "too tight." However, the zinc paste wrap is no longer considered "optimal" for most patients due to the following disadvantages: inability to adapt to any change in leg volume, inability to provide sustained compression (loss of subbandage pressure over time), potential allergic reactions to selected components (e.g., wraps containing calamine), high skill level needed for accurate application, and the need for frequent changes/reapplication when there is significant exudate.

CLINICAL PEARL

Limitations of inelastic systems (such as Unna's boot) are the inability to adjust to changes in leg volume and the inability to provide sustained compression over time.

Elastic Wraps

The category of elastic compression wraps includes two-component, three-component, and four-component wraps (often provided in a kit). These wraps are disposable and can be applied to provide either therapeutic or a modified level of compression; because they are elastic, they are able to provide both walking and resting support, which means that they are effective whether the patient is resting or active. Absorption of exudate is another key advantage of the multicomponent wrap. Skill is required to apply the wraps correctly so that they provide therapeutic level pressure.

CLINICAL PEARL

Elastic wraps (such as two layer/component, three layer/component, and four layer/component) provide both walking and resting support, which means that they are effective whether the individual is walking or resting.

If a protocol requires frequent dressing changes, a single-component wrap may be useful. However, the bandage tends to stretch with ambulation, which means that frequent rewrapping may be required. This wrap is most effective for the patient with minimal edema and small ulcers.

The multicomponent wraps with three and four components usually contain the following: (1) base layer: absorbent padding or cast padding that pads and protects the bony prominences and can be layered to assure a diameter of at least 18 cm at the ankle; (2) cotton crepe layer that smooths the padding layer and provides better conformability for the active compression layers (layers three and four); (3) elastic conformable bandage that provides 18 to 25 cm of compression when applied as directed (50% stretch, 50% overlap, and with figure 8 technique); and (4) cohesive self-adherent bandage that brings total compressive force to 40 mm Hg when applied at 50% stretch and 50% overlap with spiral technique. Two-component wraps include a base layer that provides padding and protection and that is typically applied in a spiral fashion from the base of the toes to 1″ below the knee, with the heel left out; the second layer is the active compression layer and is typically made of a modified cohesive material that provides therapeutic level compression when applied at full stretch (with the heel included). The advantage of the two-component wrap is the fact that it is lower profile and typically allows the patient to wear her or his own shoes.

The advantages of multicomponent wraps include the following: sustained compression and edema control for up to 1 week (so long as the patient does not require more frequent dressing changes), absorption of moderate-to-large volumes of exudate, and the ability to modify the level of compression by modifying the layers and amount of padding used. Disadvantages include the fact that they cannot be reused and the fact that they are bulky, which means the patient cannot wear her or his own shoes; in addition, patients sometimes complain that they feel "hot and tight." Accurate application of the compression wrap is essential to therapeutic outcomes; clinicians should utilize the following general guidelines and should follow the manufacturer's guidelines for the specific wrap.

1. Clean the leg with warm water, avoiding the use of soap. Dry well.
2. Moisturize the periwound skin with a fragrance-free ointment such as petrolatum.
3. Position the ankle in a neutral position at a right angle.
4. Pad depressions with cotton cast padding or similar material to equalize pressure.
5. Wrap each layer starting at the base of the toes; wrap to the patellar notch just distal to the knee.
6. Include the heel in the wrap unless instructed otherwise by manufacturer of wrap.

Dynamic Compression

Dynamic (intermittent) compression therapy or intermittent pneumatic compression (IPC) does not involve bandaging and may benefit patients who cannot tolerate static compression. It is especially useful for immobile patients or those needing higher pressures than can be obtained with stockings or wraps. Studies have indicated that IPC facilitates healing when compared with no compression, but there are no studies to support improvement in healing rates when paired with compression wraps or when used instead of compression wraps (WOCN, 2011). There is some evidence that IPC enhances fibrinolysis in addition to generating external pressure (Tarnay et al., 1980). However, IPC is contraindicated in patients with uncompensated (symptomatic) heart failure, acute cellulitis, and acute venous thrombosis.

CLINICAL PEARL

Dynamic compression therapy (intermittent pneumatic compression) is contraindicated for patients with uncompensated heart failure, acute cellulitis, and acute venous thrombosis.

The IPC device involves use of a pump and a single-chamber sleeve that is inflated intermittently, or a sleeve with multiple compartments that inflate sequentially, providing a "milking" action (from distal to proximal). Patients are usually instructed to use the pump one to two times daily, for 1 to 2 hours per treatment session. Benefits include mobilization of interstitial fluid back into the circulation and the ability to enhance venous return without impairing arterial blood flow, which provides safe therapy for the patient with venous disease complicated by moderately severe arterial disease (Bonham & Kelechi, 2008; Carmel, 2012). Disadvantages include the fact that the patient has to be immobile during therapy, potential difficulty with application and removal for the patient who lives alone, and the fact that Medicare and Medicaid reimbursement is limited to patients who have "failed" 6 months of conservative therapy (static compression).

Elevation

Leg elevation is a practical and simple way to improve venous return using gravitational forces. While few formal studies have proven its usefulness in preventing or treating CVI, most organizations include leg elevation in guidelines for care (Wipke-Tevis & Sae-Sia, 2004). The most common recommendation is to elevate the feet to at least the level of the heart for 30 minutes three to four times per day. Symptoms of mild venous disease may be relieved by this practice alone, but in more severe cases, this will likely be inadequate. Elevation below the level of the heart is ineffective (Alguire & Mathes, 2014). While helpful, many patients find this intervention difficult to consistently perform.

Pharmacologic Therapy

A variety of medications and supplements have been used to treat CVI with varying success and levels of evidence. The most commonly used agents in the United States include pentoxifylline and horse chestnut seed extract. Pentoxifylline (Trental) has been shown in a number of studies to be an effective addition to compression therapy, specifically through its beneficial effects on the microcirculation; mechanisms of action include its fibrinolytic properties, antiplatelet effects, and ability to reduce adhesion of leukocytes to the endothelium (Stellin & Waxman, 1989). Dosages of 400 mg three times per day have been shown to accelerate healing and are recommended for ulcers that are slow to heal. However, the potential benefits must be weighed against the cost and side effects, which are commonly GI related; pentoxifylline is primarily used in patients who fail to progress with standard therapy and not for routine care.

CLINICAL PEARL

Pentoxifylline is indicated for patients who fail to progress with standard therapy; it provides additive benefits when used in conjunction with compression therapy.

Multiple studies have shown horse chestnut seed extract (escin/aescin) to be beneficial in controlling pain and pruritus and in reducing edema and leg circumference in patients with CVI. It works by stimulating the release of prostaglandins (e.g., PGF2-alpha), which induce venoconstriction and reduce the permeability of vessel walls to low molecular proteins, water, and electrolytes (Pittler & Ernst, 2012). The suggested dose is 300 mg, containing 50 mg of the active ingredient aescin, taken twice daily for 12 weeks. It is available over the counter in the United States as an herbal supplement; therefore, purity and standardization of dose is not guaranteed. While it is generally considered safe, it may be toxic in high doses.

While not available in the United States, the phlebotropic drug known as micronized purified flavonoid fraction (MPFF) has been show to improve outcomes for patients with CVI including ulcerations and is used in Europe and other countries. MPFF used in combination with standard therapy has been shown to improve healing rates compared to standard therapy alone or to placebo. Its side effect profile is similar to placebo, and cost analysis studies have demonstrated a significant reduction in cost of healing. It has also been shown to improve QOL in patients with CVI. Hydroxyethylrutoside is another flavonoid compound that has been used extensively in Europe but is not available in the United States. It has been shown to be effective in reducing leg volume, edema, and symptoms of CVI (Alguire & Mathes, 2014).

Diuretics are sometimes used to treat edema from other conditions that aggravate venous disease, but they have no effect on venous edema or the underlying pathology of CVI. This is because the edema in CVI is caused by venous hypertension, which is a mechanical issue and unrelated to fluid overload. In addition, diuretic use can lead to hypovolemia and metabolic complications, particularly in the elderly; thus, diuretics should be used cautiously and only when indicated for systemic conditions causing edema (Alguire & Mathes, 2014).

There is limited or mixed evidence regarding the use of multiple other agents, including aspirin, granulocyte–macrophage colony-stimulating factor (GM-CSF), defibrotide, stanozolol, solcoseryl, iloprost, and topical growth factors.

Other pharmacologic agents are not readily available despite demonstrated efficacy, including sulodexide and hydroxyethylrutoside (AAWC, 2010; Carmel, 2012; WOCN, 2011).

Surgical Interventions

Evidence is mixed on the effectiveness of surgical/endovascular interventions to improve healing rates for current venous ulcers; however, surgical intervention has been shown to be quite effective in reducing venous hypertension and preventing recurrence. The subfascial endoscopic perforator surgery (SEPS) procedure has been shown to benefit most patients by reducing healing time and should be considered, especially to reduce recurrence. Procedures such as endovenous laser ablation, radiofrequency ablation, foam sclerotherapy, and valvuloplasty can also help to reduce venous hypertension and to prevent recurrence of ulcerations (**Table 21-6**) (Biemans et al., 2013; Vowden & Vowden, 2006). More recent studies have shown a positive effect on healing rates in addition to reduced recurrence rates using minimally invasive techniques (Alden et al., 2013).

CLINICAL PEARL

Surgical procedures to reduce venous hypertension have been shown to reduce the incidence of ulcer recurrence and to possibly improve healing rates.

Topical Therapy Guidelines

Dermatitis is common in patients with CVI; thus, management of these patients requires ongoing attention to prevention, early detection, and prompt intervention. Routine care should include gentle cleansing with a mild nonsoap cleanser that has no artificial colors or fragrances (e.g., Dove, Olay, Cetaphil, Neutrogena) to remove scales, crusts, and bacteria. Emollients such as petrolatum should be applied to the intact periwound skin while it is damp to prevent excessive drying of the skin surface. Emollients with known sensitizing agents, such as lanolin, should be avoided since patients with venous ulcers are at high risk for allergic contact dermatitis. In patients with very heavy wound exudate, it may be necessary to provide high-level protection of the periwound skin; zinc oxide preparations are commonly used in this situation. When the patient has venous dermatitis (also known as venous eczema), as evidenced by increased pruritis, erythema, and scaling, topical corticosteroids may be required. While scant data exist to inform the use of topical corticosteroids, use of a midpotency steroid, such as triamcinolone 0.1% in an ointment form, has been shown to be effective. Once started, the steroid should be continued for at least 2 weeks to clear the dermatitis before switching to a plain emollient. It should be used episodically thereafter for flares (Morton & Phillips, 2013; Nazarko, 2009) (Fig. 21-5 for illustration of venous dermatitis).

CLINICAL PEARL

Venous dermatitis is typically treated with a midpotency steroid ointment for 2 weeks.

Topical therapy for venous ulcers is based on characteristics of the wound. If nonviable tissue is present, debridement should be undertaken; the one exception would be a closed wound with dry eschar in a patient with significant arterial compromise. However, venous ulcers are typically well perfused, so any avascular tissue is usually limited and is more likely to represent a fibrinous exu-

TABLE 21-6 Common Surgical/Interventional Procedures for Management Venous Insufficiency

Procedure	Methods	Considerations
Surgical vein stripping (SVS)	Surgical procedure where the greater saphenous vein (GSV) is ligated at the groin and removed (stripped) to the knee	Surgical procedure requiring general anesthesia Seldom done now that minimally invasive techniques have been developed Used as the "gold standard" to which all subsequent procedures are compared
Endovenous laser ablation (EVLA)	Performed in endovascular suite; a laser fiber is used to produce heat that destroys the vascular endothelium along the GSV, closing the vein	Requires local anesthesia and light sedation Highly effective compared to SVS, verified with multiple studies Fewer complications than SVS with better long-term outcomes
Radiofrequency ablation (RFA)	Thermal energy is delivered using a catheter directly to the GSV walls resulting in closure of the vein	Requires local anesthesia and light sedation Effectiveness has been demonstrated
Ultrasound-guided foam sclerotherapy (USFS)	A sclerosing foam is injected under ultrasound guidance into the GSV—volume depends on length and diameter of vessel	Requires local anesthesia and light sedation Slightly less effective than EVLA and RFA but equal to SVS
Subfascial endoscopic perforator surgery (SEPS)	Surgical procedure done via a scope to close incompetent perforator veins	Used to address perforators when GSV closure was not adequate for symptom relief or ulcer healing

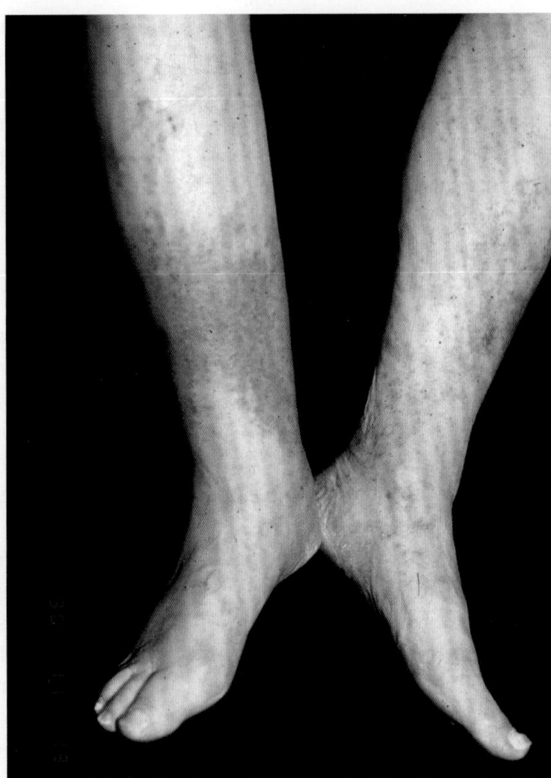

FIGURE 21-5. Venous dermatitis.

date or biofilm due to high bacterial loads. Options for debridement include use of a blunt curette to remove yellow tissue due to biofilm, autolytic debridement using moisture-retentive dressings, biodebridement with larval therapy, or sharp debridement (following application of a topical anesthetic such as EMLA [eutectic mixture of local anesthetics]). Enzymatic debriding agents have shown little effect.

Routine swab cultures of venous ulcers are not necessary; cultures should be performed only when there are clinical signs and symptoms of significant infection requiring systemic antibiotics. In this case, a culture is done to determine the specific organism and the antibiotics to which it is sensitive. Signs of infection that would warrant culture-based antibiotic therapy include the following:

- Local heat and tenderness
- Increasing erythema of the surrounding skin
- Lymphangitis (red streaks traversing up the limb)
- Rapid increase in the size of the ulcer
- Fever

Most venous ulcers are heavily colonized with both gram-positive and gram-negative bacteria. Topical antibiotics are of little use and, as noted, systemic antibiotics should be used only for signs and symptoms of invasive infection. Topical antimicrobials are frequently used though there is no firm evidence to support their use on a routine basis; commonly used agents include manuka honey, cadexomer iodine, various silver dressings, peroxide-based products, acetic acid, and sodium hypochlorite. Of these agents, manuka honey and cadexomer iodine have the strongest data. Anecdotally, any of these products can be used when the wound is not progressing and when there is no negative effect on healing or pain (O'Meara et al., 2013).

Most venous ulcers are relatively superficial with significant exudate. While no dressing has been proven to provide better healing rates than another, studies have shown several types of dressings to be effective, including alginates, hydrofiber dressings, foam dressings, and composite dressings. When selecting or recommending dressings, the clinician should focus on minimizing exposure to potential allergens, protecting the periwound skin from maceration and dermatitis, managing exudate, and controlling bioburden. Dressing characteristics should be matched to wound characteristics with changes in products as the wound improves or changes.

CLINICAL PEARL

Topical therapy for venous ulcers is determined by the characteristics of the wound; most ulcers are exudative so absorptive dressings are usually needed, and antimicrobial dressings (such as cadexomer iodine, silver, and manuka honey) may be used when indicated.

Skin grafting has been suggested for ulcers of >12-month duration or very large ulcers. Several biologic skin substitutes have been developed and have proven effective in promoting healing of recalcitrant wounds. These products are categorized by the layer of skin they are designed to replace, that is, epidermal, dermal, or bilayered substitutes. Epidermal substitutes are fragile and have not proven useful in venous ulcers. Dermal substitutes are composed of a bioabsorbable matrix; these "matrix" dressings may be acellular or may be populated with donor cells, such as fibroblasts. Acellular matrix dressings commonly used for venous ulcer treatment include Integra, Oasis, MatriStem PriMatrix, and Endoform. Dermagraft is a cell-populated dermal substitute but is not approved for use with venous ulcers. The bilayered skin substitute, Apligraf, has the strongest evidence and is reimbursed for venous ulcer treatment in the United States (Greaves et al., 2013). These skin substitutes are used in conjunction with compression and should be considered when healing is delayed. Other adjuncts to healing, including hyperbaric oxygen, electromagnetic therapy, electrical stimulation, low-level laser therapy (LLLT), negative pressure wound therapy, and therapeutic ultrasound, have not demonstrated a significant effect on healing of venous ulcers (AAWC, 2010; Alguire & Mathes, 2014; WOCN, 2011).

CLINICAL PEARL

The advanced therapy product with the strongest evidence base for use with refractory venous ulcers is a bilayered skin substitute such as Apligraf.

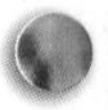

Secondary Prevention: Preventing Recurrence

Patients must understand that compression therapy will be a lifelong requirement. Once a venous ulcer has healed, a compression garment providing the appropriate amount of compression must be used daily. The prescription for elastic compression stockings must include both the length (calf vs. thigh vs. waist) and the amount of tension or compression. Based on clinical severity, patients with CEAP class C2 to C3 disease should use products that provide 20 to 30 mm Hg, those with CEAP class C4 to C6 should use products providing 30 to 40 mm Hg, and patients with recurrent ulcers should use products with 40 to 50 mm Hg. Knee length is most commonly used for increased patient compliance so long as symptom relief is adequate (Eberhardt & Raffetto, 2014). Consideration must be given to the patient's ability to don and doff the stockings independently or with available assistance. Many aids for donning and doffing stockings are available. Referral to occupational therapy may be needed to determine the best device for the patient. If the patient is unable to use stockings, other methods of compression are available such as tubular elastic bandages (e.g., Compressogrip by Knit-Rite Inc. or Tubigrip by Mölnlycke Health Care) or inelastic compression leggings with Velcro straps (e.g., CircAid by Medical Products, Inc. or FarrowWrap). The goal is always to provide the level of compression determined to be most appropriate for the patient's level of disease severity; however, consistent use of lower-level compression provides better outcomes than inconsistent use of higher-level compression. Thus, the wound nurse must collaborate with the patient and caregivers to develop a realistic plan for long-term management of CVI (Vowden & Vowden, 2006).

CLINICAL PEARL

Prevention of recurrent ulceration requires long-term adherence to compression therapy; while the goal is to provide the level of compression most appropriate for the individual's level of disease severity, consistent use of lower-level compression provides better outcomes than inconsistent use of higher-level compression.

Surgical/interventional correction of varicosities and valve dysfunction can also contribute positively to secondary prevention, as shown in the ESCHAR study (Barwell et al., 2004). In this study, surgical intervention did not provide significantly better ulcer healing rates but did help to reduce the rates of recurrence. However, more recent studies have shown a positive effect on healing rates in addition to reduced recurrence rates using minimally invasive techniques (Alden et al., 2013).

In addition, all of the measures previously discussed for management of CVI should be continued. These include lifelong exercise programs, weight control, and protection against injury. Patient education is paramount in assuring adherence to these lifelong practices. Education should include a practical explanation of venous disease and lifestyle factors that contribute to progression or recurrence, a practical plan for use of compression garments, information about the care and replacement of compression garments, and early symptoms of ulcer recurrence.

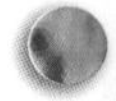

Management of Mixed Arterial–Venous Disease

Patients with concomitant arterial insufficiency require special adjustments to their treatment plan. Knowledge of the ABI as well as the systolic pressure at the ankle and/or toe is key to selecting an appropriate level of compression for treatment. For patients with an ABI > 0.5 to <0.8 and ankle pressures >0.70 who have edema and open ulcers, a trial of reduced compression (23 to 30 mm Hg) should be undertaken with close supervision. In a European study, Mosti et al. (2012) found that inelastic compression wraps, using a German self-adherent wrap, could be safely used with no interference to perfusion in patients with ABI > 0.5 to <0.8. Because the exact pressure applied with a wrap is difficult to determine, the wound care nurse must do all of the following to assure appropriate use of reduced level compression: (1) obtain ABI and note ankle pressure measurements, (2) apply the wrap using guidelines for reduced compression application from the manufacturer, and (3) educate the patient regarding signs of developing ischemia (numbness, pain, pallor, or cyanosis of toes) and proper response (removal of wrap and notification of wound care clinician). Some patients may tolerate light compression when legs are dependent but will experience pain with elevation to level of the heart; these patients should use a removable compression legging or reusable wrap and should be instructed to remove the wrap or legging at bedtime and reapply in the morning. These individuals may also be candidates for a compression pump. Patients with neuropathy should be cautioned to visually inspect the toes if a traditional compression wrap is used to prevent complications from compression (WOCN, 2014).

Compression is not recommended for individuals with an ABI <0.5, ankle pressure <70 mm Hg, or toe pressure <50 mm Hg; these individuals should be referred for a vascular workup and possible revascularization. Percutaneous interventions are favored as these patients are often poor surgical candidates. Following revascularization, use of compression should be reevaluated, including during the postprocedure period when edema may be increased due to a combination of lymphatic and inflammatory processes (Humphreys et al., 2007; WOCN, 2014).

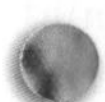

Lymphedema

Lymphedema is a chronic condition with no known cure and is generally recognized as an overlooked, underdiagnosed, and undertreated condition. Many patients with long-standing venous disease develop secondary lymphedema; thus, any patient with long-standing venous disease should be evaluated for coexisting lymphedema. All patients with lymphedema require treatment and ongoing care and maintenance for life. For cancer patients, specifically, it has been described as a significant survivorship issue with physical, functional, QOL, social, and economic consequences (Cormier et al., 2010). The diagnosis and treatment of lymphedema is based on a clear understanding of the lymphatic system. Increased attention to the lymphatic system translates into more accurate diagnoses, improved treatment, and enhanced education for patients with lymphedema.

CLINICAL PEARL

Many patients with long-standing venous disease develop secondary lymphedema; lymphedema is also common among individuals after cancer therapy. Unfortunately, lymphedema is frequently underdiagnosed and undertreated.

Anatomy and Physiology of Lymphatic System

The lymph system is the third component of the circulatory system (Ambroza & Geigle, 2010), and it plays a critical role in the transport of interstitial fluid and molecules back into the circulatory system. However, historically, the lymph system and lymphatic pathologies have received much less attention than pathologies associated with venous and arterial diseases.

The normal perfusion cycle involves movement of fluid and molecules out of the arterial capillary bed into the tissues, and most of the fluid and molecules are then returned to the capillary bed on the venous side. However, large molecules (such as plasma proteins) are unable to diffuse back into the venous capillary bed and are trapped in the interstitial space along with limited volumes of fluid. The return of these molecules and fluid to the circulatory system is dependent upon a normally functioning lymphatic system. Approximately 90% of the interstitial fluid is reabsorbed into the blood capillaries and the remaining 10% is handled by the lymphatic system.

CLINICAL PEARL

The lymphatic system plays a critical role in transport of fluid and molecules out of the tissues and back into the blood stream; the lymphatic system handles about 10% of the total interstitial fluid load.

Functions

The main functions of the lymph system are as follows:

- To collect and transport excess tissue fluid from the interstitium back to the veins in the blood system (Kunkel, 2010).
- To maintain normal plasma volumes by returning plasma proteins to the bloodstream. The lymphatic vessels absorb 2 to 4 L of protein-rich fluid retained in the interstitial tissue daily due to the venous system's inability to absorb all tissue fluids (Doughty & Holbrook, 2007).
- To prevent edema through its reserve capacity. During times of increased lymphatic load, the capacity for lymph transport is considerably greater than during times of normal lymphatic load (Doughty & Holbrook, 2007).
- To remove toxins from the tissue and protect the body against infection (Doughty & Holbrook, 2007).
- To produce antibodies to help fight disease states (Zuther & Norton, 2013) (see Lymph Nodes).

Overview of Lymphatic System

The lymphatic system is composed of lymphatic vessels and lymphatic tissue (Lawenda et al., 2009). Lymphatic vessels provide a one-way path for the movement of lymph back into the circulatory system (Kunkel, 2010). As shown in Figure 21-6, the lymphatic system is an open system as compared to the closed cardiovascular system; thus, some refer to the lymph system as a transport system rather than as a circulatory system. The lymphatic system also differs from the cardiovascular system in that there is no central pump and lymph transport is interrupted by lymph nodes (Zuther & Norton, 2013).

Lymph is a protein-rich fluid that also contains water, fatty acids, salts, white blood cells, cellular particles, microorganisms, and foreign debris (Lawenda et al., 2009). The lymph will appear as clear in color with the exception of the milky white chylous fluid (chyle) found in vessels

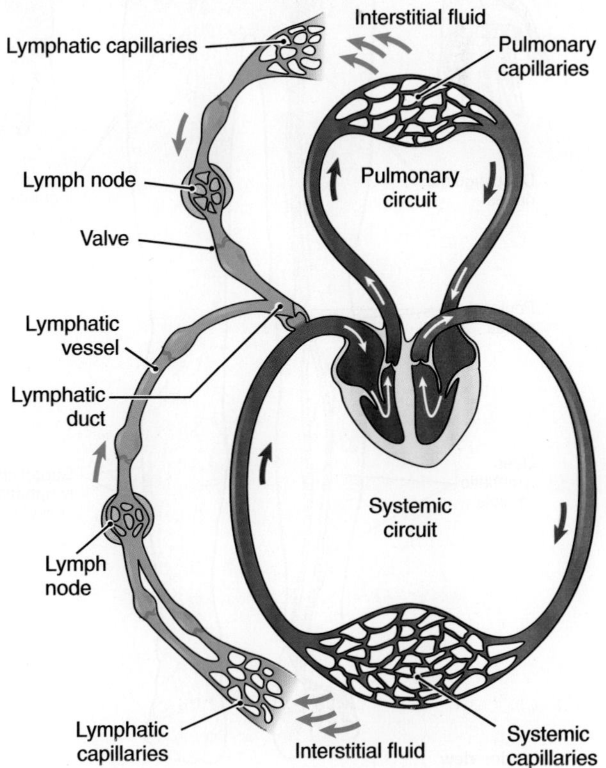

FIGURE 21-6. Lymphatic system.

draining the intestinal system, which contains digested fatty acids. The components of the lymph fluid are referred to as the lymphatic load (Zuther & Norton, 2013).

The lymphatic vessels run along similar paths as the arteries, veins, and capillaries and are composed of two distinguishable systems, a superficial system and a deep system (Quirion, 2010; Zuther & Norton, 2013). As depicted in Figure 21-7, the superficial vessels run close to the skin surface and drain the skin and subcutaneous tissues (Lawenda et al., 2009), while the deep vessels drain

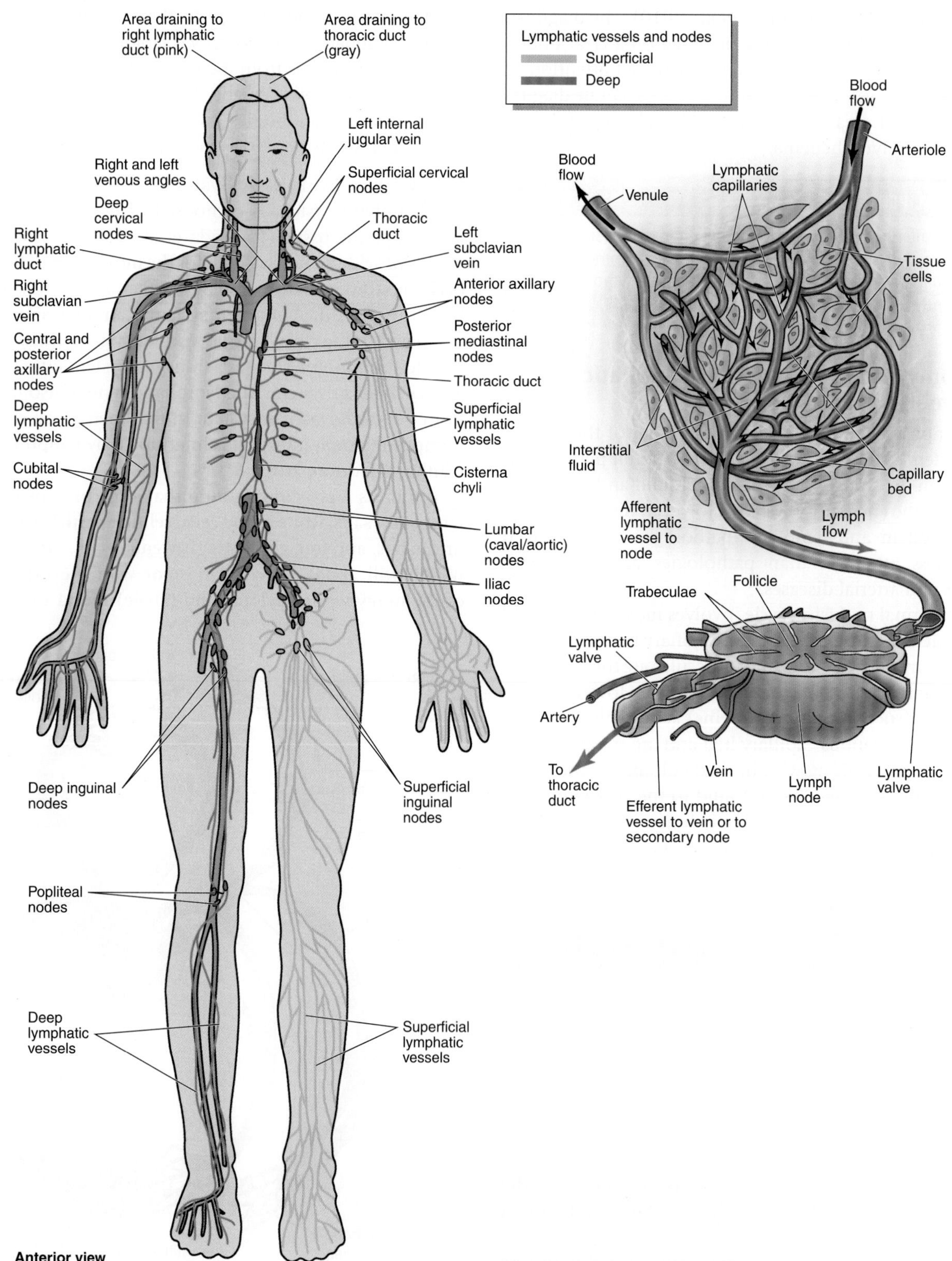

FIGURE 21-7. Lymphatic vessels (superficial and deep system).

the tissues deep to the fascia (Zuther & Norton, 2013). The two systems communicate through perforating vessels that pass through the fascia. In visceral regions, the deep lymphatic system drains organs and provides additional filtration and purification of lymph through the lymph nodes (Zuther & Norton, 2013).

Lymph Capillaries

The lymph capillaries (see Fig. 21-6) are the first component of the lymphatic system (Zuther & Norton, 2013); they are open-ended tubes that are in close proximity to the blood capillaries (Kunkel, 2010), and they form a complex dermal network that covers the entire surface of the body. They differ from blood capillaries in that they are larger and more permeable, which allows them to absorb fluids and molecules that are often too large to be reabsorbed into the venous system (Ambroza & Geigle, 2010; Lawenda et al., 2009). Lymph capillaries also have a unique structural support network called "anchoring filaments" that enable the vessels to stay open even when interstitial tissue pressures are elevated; the anchoring filaments act like swinging flaps to open the lymphatic lumen so that interstitial fluid can drain into the capillary (Lawenda et al., 2009). Lymph capillaries do not have valves, so the flow of lymph is controlled by pressure gradients through the process of filtration (Lawenda et al., 2009).

CLINICAL PEARL

The lymph capillaries are larger than blood capillaries, which allows them to absorb large molecules that cannot be reabsorbed by the venous system.

Precollector and Collector Vessels

Lymph flows from the capillaries through precollector vessels to collector vessels (see Fig. 21-6). The precollectors contain valves to control the direction of flow; they also have a layer of smooth muscle but do not display any detectable vasomotor activity (Kunkel, 2010). The collector vessels range in diameter from 0.1 to 0.6 mm and are responsible for transporting lymph to the lymph nodes and the lymphatic trunks (Zuther & Norton, 2013). These vessels are histologically similar to veins (though thinner), and they contain paired semilunar valves that assure unidirectional movement of the lymph, from distal to proximal (peripheral to central) (Kunkel, 2010). The interval between valves varies from 6 to 20 mm, and the segment of the collector located between two sets of valves is called a lymphangion. Lymphangions are innervated by the sympathetic nervous system and contract at a frequency of 10 to 12 contractions per minute at rest. This is known as lymphangiomotoricity or lymphangioactivity (Zuther & Norton, 2013). When a lymphangion contracts, the valve at the distal end of the lymphangion closes and the proximal valve opens to propel lymph proximally (Kunkel, 2010). Lymph collectors react to an increase in lymph formation by increasing contraction frequency. Other factors that increase contraction frequency include external stretch on the wall of the lymphangion (effect of manual lymph drainage [MLD]), temperature, activity of muscles and joints, diaphragmatic breathing, pulsation of adjacent arteries, and certain tissue hormones (Zuther & Norton, 2013).

Lymphatic Territories

As mentioned earlier, the superficial collectors drain lymph from the skin and subcutaneous tissue toward the lymph nodes; the superficial lymphatic system is subdivided into lymphatic territories. These territories consist of several collectors that all drain the same body area and to the same group of lymph nodes (regional lymph nodes). Watershed (Fig. 21-8) is the term used to describe linear, functional divisions of the superficial lymphatic system. Watersheds are characterized by a predictable pattern of lymph flow (Zuther & Norton, 2013). For example, the watershed territories of the right and left head and neck regions drain to the right and left cervical lymph nodes. The right and left upper quadrant watersheds include the upper extremities and upper trunk and drain into the right and left axillary nodes, respectively, while the right and left lower quadrant watersheds include the lower extremities and lower trunk and drain into the right and left inguinal nodes, respectively (Kunkel, 2010). Once lymph drains through a specific watershed territory, it then drains into the deeper lymphatic collectors, which run parallel to the larger blood vessels and organ vessels. An understanding of lymph territories and watersheds is very important in the treatment of lymphedema.

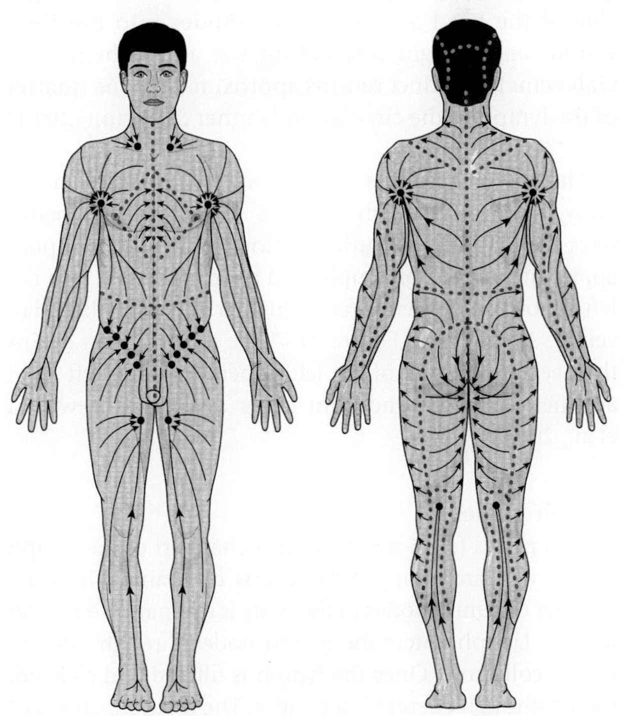

FIGURE 21-8. Lymphatic watershed.

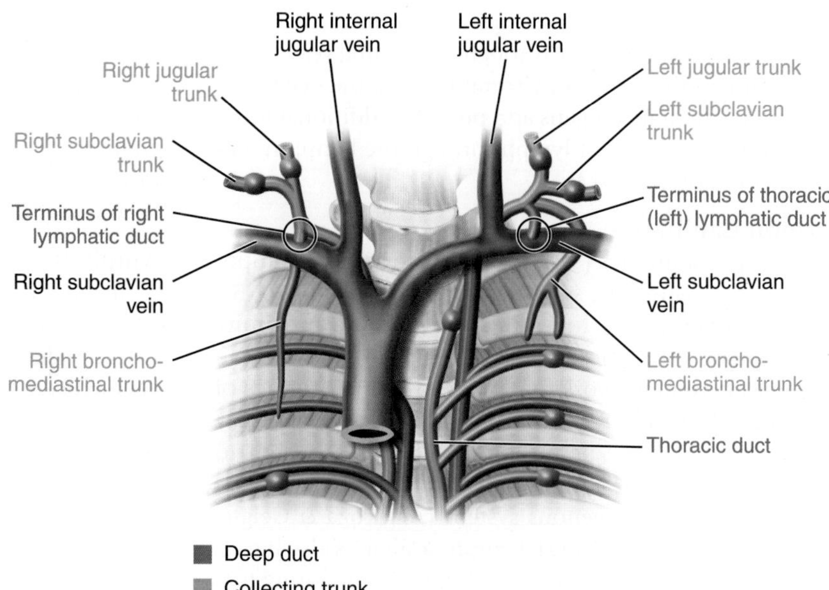

FIGURE 21-9. Right and Left venous angles.

Lymphatic Trunks and Ducts

Lymphatic trunks are the next larger classification of lymph vessels. Trunks are formed by the union of efferent lymph vessels (vessels that exit the lymph node) from individual lymph node groups (Kunkel, 2010). They are similar to lymph collectors in that they are equipped with valves, innervated by the sympathetic nervous system, and contractile (Lawenda et al., 2009). The trunks merge to form ducts. The right lymphatic duct (see Fig. 21-7) drains the superficial and deep lymphatics of the right upper limb, thorax, and right side of the head and neck and empties into the right venous angle (right internal jugular and right subclavian veins); this duct returns approximately one quarter of the lymph to the circulation (Zuther & Norton, 2013) (Fig. 21-9).

The thoracic duct is the largest lymph vessel in the body, varying in length from 36 to 45 cm, and perforates the diaphragm (Zuther & Norton, 2013). It empties approximately 3 L of lymph fluid per day directly into the left venous angle (left internal jugular and left subclavian veins). As shown in Figure 21-7, the thoracic duct drains the deep lymphatics of the left upper quadrant, left head and neck, and left and right lower quadrants (Lawenda et al., 2009).

Lymph Nodes

Lymph nodes (see Fig. 21-7) are a vital part of the lymph system and are arranged in groups or chains. The total number of lymph nodes in the body is estimated to be 600 to 700. Lymph enters the lymph nodes through afferent lymph collectors. Once the lymph is filtered and cleaned, it exits through efferent lymphatics. The main functions of the lymph nodes are as follows:

- To filter out harmful material in the lymph fluid (Zuther & Norton, 2013)
- To generate lymphocytes thus promoting immune function (Zuther & Norton, 2013)
- To thicken the lymph by reabsorbing water—much less lymph exits a lymph node than enters the node (Zuther & Norton, 2013)

Epidemiology

The most common cause of lymphedema worldwide is filariasis, a parasitic infection of the lymph vessels and lymph nodes found in certain developing countries (Avraham et al., 2010). The Centers for Disease Control and Prevention (CDC) considers filariasis to be a neglected tropical disease and the most frequent cause of permanent disability worldwide (CDC, 2014) (Fig. 21-10). However, in the Western world, lymphedema is almost always caused by significant trauma to the lymphatic system and is classified as secondary lymphedema. Specific causes of secondary lymphedema include cancer treatment that involves lymph node dissection and/or radiation therapy, severe burns or orthopedic trauma causing disruption of lymphatic vessels, CVI resulting in soft tissue fibrosis and disruption of lymphatic structures, and damage or obstruction of the lymphatics due to obesity, vascular reconstruction, severe infection, joint replacement surgery, or harvesting of veins for coronary artery bypass procedures (Doughty & Holbrook, 2007) (Fig. 21-11). Primary lymphedema is the second category of lymphedema and is far less prevalent. Primary lymphedema is due to developmental abnormalities of the lymphatic system and may be either congenital or hereditary (Zuther & Norton, 2013) (Fig. 21-12).

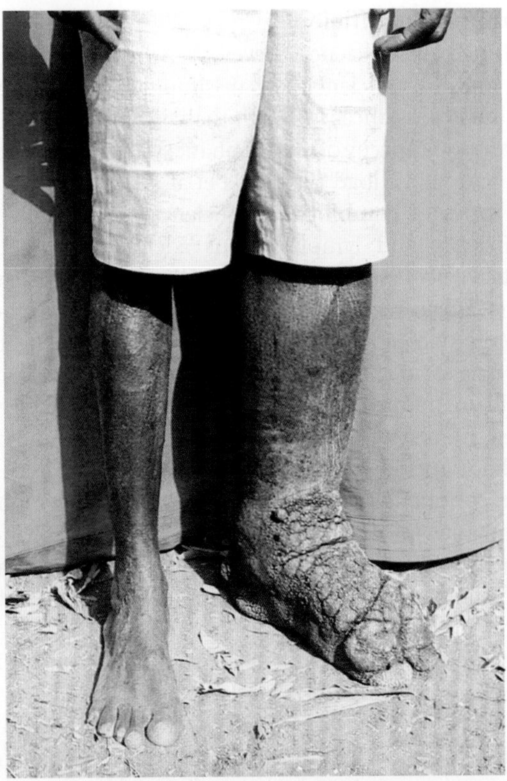

FIGURE 21-10. Lymphatic filariasis.

CLINICAL PEARL

In the Western world, lymphedema is almost always caused by significant trauma to the lymphatic system (cancer therapy, prolonged venous disease, severe trauma or burns, etc.) and is classified as secondary lymphedema.

No specific studies have been conducted on the global incidence of lymphedema (Maree, 2011). Although data on the prevalence of lymphedema are limited, it is estimated that over 3 million people in the United States suffer from lymphedema, with a significant proportion of cases caused by cancer and cancer treatment (McNeely et al., 2011). Estimates of the incidence of secondary lymphedema resulting from cancer vary greatly due to the absence of uniform criteria for measuring, defining, and reporting the condition. Most of the estimates that are available come from the breast cancer population, which has been the most studied and researched group (McNeely et al., 2011). In the breast cancer population, the incidence ranges from 10% to 60% (Quirion, 2010) and is influenced by patient factors (i.e., obesity), the extent of treatment (i.e., lymphadenectomy/radiation), and disease-related factors such as tumor size and location (Balci et al., 2012). Few estimates of lymphedema related to other cancers have been published.

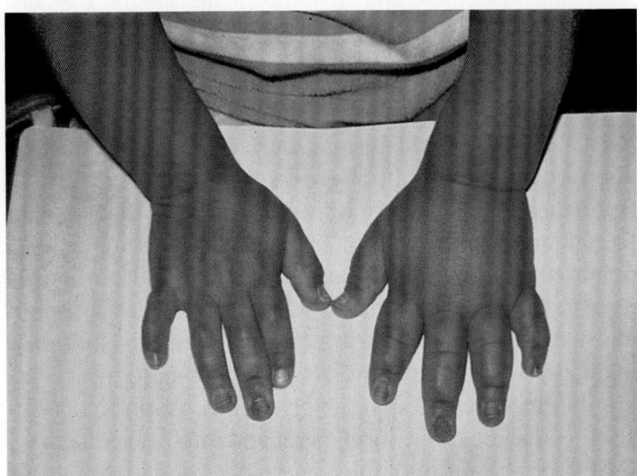

FIGURE 21-11. Secondary lymphedema in breast cancer patient.

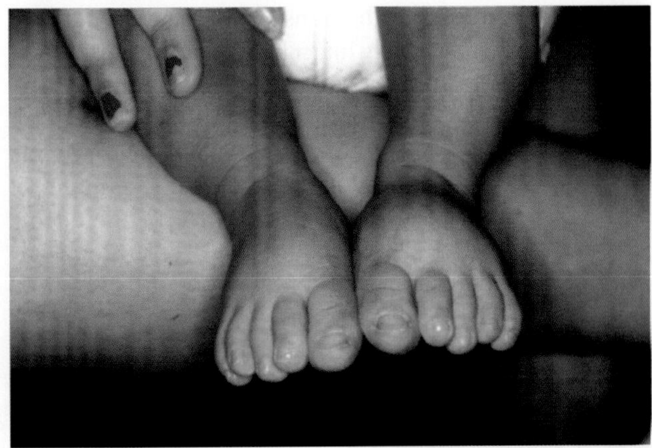

FIGURE 21-12. Congenital lymphedema in infant.

Classification of Edema

Chronic edema is a broad term encompassing a variety of conditions and etiologies. It is important to conduct a thorough assessment to identify the underlying cause for the edema and an appropriate treatment regimen (Cooper, 2013; Lay-Flurrie, 2011). The word edema means an abnormal accumulation of fluid in the interstitial tissue that is visible and palpable; it develops when the capillary filtration rate overwhelms the lymphatic drainage rate over a period of time (Hampton, 2010). Edema is not a disease but a symptom associated with a variety of conditions, including congestive heart failure, CVI, immobility, pregnancy, or even pressure from constrictive garments or clothing. Whatever the underlying cause of the edema, the result is the accumulation of fluid in the interstitial space due to either dynamic insufficiency or mechanical insufficiency of the lymphatic system (or a combination of both) (Zuther & Norton, 2013).

CLINICAL PEARL

Edema is not a disease but a symptom associated with a variety of conditions.

Dynamic Insufficiency

Dynamic insufficiency (high-volume insufficiency) is the most common type of problem and occurs whenever the lymphatic load exceeds the transport capacity of the anatomically and functionally intact lymphatic system (Zuther & Norton, 2013). It is also known as high-volume insufficiency. Increased filtration of fluid out of the blood capillaries results in excess interstitial fluid and edema characterized by high fluid and low protein. Examples of dynamic insufficiency–related edema include the edema caused by congestive heart failure, CVI, postthrombotic syndrome, and dependency. Kidney disease, starvation, severe anemia, and diseases of the liver also result in dynamic insufficiency due to low plasma protein levels (hypoproteinemia) that permit excess movement of fluid out of the vessels into the tissues (also known as third spacing). If dynamic edema persists for a long period of time, the chronic excess workload for the lymph vessels may result in damage to the vessel walls and the lymphatic valvular system (Zuther & Norton, 2013). To avoid secondary damage to the lymphatic system, edema caused by systemic disease should be treated medically. For example, edema due to venous insufficiency (localized edema) should be treated with elevation, compression, and exercise, while edema due to congestive heart failure (generalized edema) usually requires diuretic therapy in addition to treatment of the underlying heart condition (Zuther & Norton, 2013).

CLINICAL PEARL

Dynamic insufficiency edema refers to edema caused by abnormal loss of fluid from the bloodstream into the tissues; edema results because the fully functional lymphatic system is overwhelmed by the volume of fluid to be transported.

Mechanical Insufficiency

Mechanical insufficiency (low-volume insufficiency) occurs as a result of congenital or acquired damage to the lymphatic system that impairs its ability to provide normal transport of lymphatic fluid. Congenital malformation or absence of lymphatic tissue (primary lymphedema) is one cause of low-volume insufficiency; another is damage to the lymphatic system from functional or organic causes that lead to a reduction in the capacity for lymph transport (secondary lymphedema) (Lawenda et al., 2009). Mechanical insufficiency can result from surgery, radiation, trauma, infection, inflammation, and CVI (organic causes). Functional factors causing mechanical insufficiency include loss of lymphatic contractility due to certain toxins and drugs (Zuther & Norton, 2013). The appropriate treatment of choice for mechanical insufficiency is complete decongestive therapy (CDT).

CLINICAL PEARL

Mechanical insufficiency edema occurs when lymphatic system function is compromised, and it is therefore unable to provide normal levels of fluid transport. This is the type of edema that occurs in patients who have sustained damage to the lymphatic system.

Combined Insufficiency

Combined insufficiency develops when dynamic and mechanical insufficiencies occur simultaneously. This happens in circumstances in which there is both a reduction in the transport capacity of the lymphatic system and an increase in the lymphatic load (Lawenda et al., 2009). The two primary types of combined insufficiency are hemodynamic insufficiency and lymphovenous edema. Hemodynamic insufficiency causes edema because sustained cardiac insufficiency affects the right side of the heart as well as the left; when the right side of the heart does not empty effectively, there is resistance to venous return and increased volumes of fluid are trapped in the tissues. The persistent congestion of the venous system impairs lymphatic drainage and causes lymphatic overload. The end result is structural damage to the lymphatic vessels, dilation of the large lymphatics, and valvular insufficiency. MLD and compression therapy are strictly contraindicated in edema caused by cardiac insufficiency due to the risk of cardiac overload (Zuther & Norton, 2013). Lymphovenous edema is caused by venous disease (chronic venous insufficiency) that results in localized hemodynamic pathology (Lay-Flurrie, 2011). If venous insufficiency is not appropriately diagnosed and treated, the high volumes of fluid leaking into the interstitial space can cause dynamic lymphatic insufficiency and subsequent edema. With CVI, the dynamic insufficiency can be further complicated by mechanical insufficiency of the lymphatics; this is because the high levels of tissue proteins and chronic inflammation can cause fibrosis of the lymphangion walls and damage to the lymphatic vessels (Zuther & Norton, 2013). As CVI progresses, there are extensive fibrotic changes to the dermis caused by tissue reaction to the cells and proteins leaking into the soft tissues. These fibrotic changes can damage or obliterate lymphatic channels, leading to obstruction of lymph flow (Doughty & Holbrook, 2007). CDT can be an effective treatment for advanced stages of CVI (**Table 21-7**) resulting in lymphovenous edema.

CLINICAL PEARL

Accurate assessment and diagnosis of the specific type of edema is critical to appropriate and effective management.

Pathology

As stated, mechanical insufficiency lymphedema may be due to congenital malformations of the lymphatic system (primary lymphedema) or by injury to the lymphatic system (secondary lymphedema) (Kunkel, 2010). Lymphedema occurs when the lymphatic load exceeds the transport capacity of the impaired lymphatic system and results in an abnormal accumulation of protein-rich fluid in the interstitium. It manifests as swelling of the involved body part; most commonly the extremities are involved, but lymphedema can also involve the trunk, head, neck, and external genitalia.

It is important for clinicians to identify patients at risk for lymphedema (**Table 21-8**), to follow these patients

TABLE 21-7 Stages of Chronic Venous Insufficiency as It Relates to Lymphatic Function

Stage	Status of Lymphatic Vessels	Symptoms	Therapeutic Approach
0	Normal function; normal protein load	None	Compression therapy; elevation; exercise
1	Normal function; increased load	Mild edema	Compression therapy; elevation; exercise
2	High protein load; morphological changes	Moderate edema with pigmentation, varicosities, pain	CDT
3	Very high-protein load; morphological changes	Severe edema with hypoxia, tissue destruction, pain	CDT with needed wound care

CDT, combined decongestive therapy.

Adapted from Zuther, J., & Norton, S. (2013). *Lymphedema management: The comprehensive guide for practitioners* (3rd ed.). New York, NY: Thieme, with permission.

closely, and to educate patients regarding measures they should take to reduce their risk for lymphedema. Clinicians must inform patients at risk for secondary lymphedema that the risk is lifelong. The onset may occur at the time of the causative event or may be delayed for several decades (Lawenda et al., 2009).

Lymphedema is a progressive and chronic condition. The International Society of Lymphology (ISL) has identified four stages of lymphedema (**Table 21-9**). Stage 0 (latent stage) has recently been added to represent patients who are at risk for lymphedema but have no clinical signs of lymphedema. Stages I, II, and III lymphedema represent progressive changes in the severity of edema and skin and soft tissue changes (Armer et al., 2012).

CLINICAL PEARL

Nurses must educate individuals at risk for lymphedema about strategies for prevention and early intervention; early intervention is the key to effective therapy.

TABLE 21-8 Risk Factors for the Development of Secondary Lymphedema

Cancer surgery that involves excision of lymph nodes in the axilla and/or radiation therapy
Postsurgical complications from breast cancer surgery (seroma formation, axillary cording)
Postbreast cancer trauma in the extremity (injection, blood pressure)
Cancer surgery involving excision of inguinal nodes and or pelvic radiation therapy
Advanced cancer
Obesity
Recurrent soft tissue infections
Varicose vein stripping and vein harvesting
Chronic venous insufficiency, stages I and II
Thrombophlebitis and postthrombotic syndrome
Orthopedic injuries and traumas
Burn injuries
Immobility (paralysis)

Sources: Lymphoedema Framework. (2006). *Best practice for the management of lymphoedema. International consensus.* London, UK: MEP Ltd; Wigg, J., & Lee, N. (2014). Redefining essential care in lymphoedema. *British Journal of Community Nursing, 19*(Suppl. 4), S20–S27.

Diagnosis

To date, there are no universally accepted standards for diagnosing lymphedema (Zuther & Norton, 2013); in most cases, the diagnosis is made based on detailed patient history and clinical presentation. It is important to exclude other causes of edema before a confirmation of the diagnosis of lymphedema is made. In some instances, advanced diagnostics (ultrasound, lymphoscintigraphy, CT, and MRI) are indicated to confirm the diagnosis or to determine the diagnosis

TABLE 21-9 International Society of Lymphology—Stages of Lymphedema

Stage 0—Latency (subclinical lymphedema)

Edema is not evident despite impaired lymph transport
Extremity may feel heavy, full, tight, or achy
This stage may exist for months or years before edema is observable

Stage I—Early-onset edema

Edema is observable and measureable
Edema may pit with pressure
Edema resolves with elevation
Tissue feels soft (no fibrosis)
Clothing and jewelry may feel tight and produce constriction

Stage II (May be divided into early and late stage II)

There will be a combination of pitting and nonpitting edema (late stage II)
Edema does not resolve with elevation
Fibrosis present in the tissue (late stage II)
The patient may begin to experience decreased range of motion, difficulty fitting into clothing

Stage III

Significant skin changes present (generalized fibrosis and pitting response is absent)
Hypertrophy of the subcutaneous tissue
Papillomas and warty overgrowths may develop on the skin
Skin folds and lobules begin to develop
Disfigurement of the extremity
Ongoing infections of the tissue likely

Adapted from The International Society of Lymphology. (2013, March). Consensus document on diagnosis and treatment of peripheral lymphedema. *Lymphology*, (1), 1–11.

when the clinical picture is unclear (Lymphoedema Framework, 2006). Lymphoscintigraphy uses radiotracers to evaluate the anatomy and function of the lymphatic system (Muldoon, 2011).

Primary lymphedema is usually diagnosed by confirming lymphedema and excluding secondary lymphedema as the cause. Primary lymphedema may present clinically soon after birth (Milroy's disease), may develop at the onset of puberty (lymphedema praecox or Meige disease), or may not become apparent until many years into adulthood (lymphedema tarda); adult onset usually occurs between the ages of 35 and 45 (Korpan et al., 2011).

Lymphedema Assessment

Lymphedema assessment should be performed at the time of diagnosis and repeated periodically throughout treatment. Assessment is performed by a practitioner specifically trained in the treatment of lymphedema. The International Lymphedema Framework (ILF) recommends that the following be included in a comprehensive lymphedema assessment (Lymphoedema Framework, 2006).

Measurement of Limb Volume

The most widely used method for measuring limb volume is circumferential limb measurements, which are easily and cost-effectively obtained. The clinician should use a reproducible set of measurement points, with the circumference measured at each point (usually every 4 cm) and at fixed time intervals (Balci et al., 2012). Often a nonelastic tape measure is used with an attached tensioning device (Gulick) to ensure the same amount of tension at each measurement point and time (Muldoon, 2011). There are software programs that can be used to determine individual limb volume and excess limb volume based on the measurement data. Other measurement methods less frequently used are the water displacement method, perometry, and bioelectrical impedance spectroscopy. Perometry (Fig. 21-13) is an optoelectronic volumetry device consisting of arrays of optoelectronic sensors that measure limb volume (Balci et al., 2012). Bioelectrical impedance spectroscopy uses a single-frequency low-voltage electrical current passing through the water content of body tissue; this tool can detect alterations in extracellular fluid before clinical signs of edema are present (Muldoon, 2011).

Skin Assessment

The skin should be examined for dryness, color and pigmentation, temperature, scars, wounds, ulcers, skin folds, fragility, inflammation, pitting response, and fibrosis. A tonometer is a tool used to assess the resistance of tissue to compression and can aid in determining the extent of fibrosis (Muldoon, 2011). The clinician should also assess for Stemmer's sign; a positive Stemmer's sign is the inability to pinch or lift the skin fold at the base of the second toe (or middle finger). Finally, the skin should be assessed for excessive dryness, thickening, and hyperkeratosis and for the presence of cellulitis, open wounds, fungal infection, lymphorrhea (leakage of lymph onto the skin), and papillomatosis (raised projections on the skin due to dilation of lymphatic vessels and fibrosis) (Lymphedema Framework).

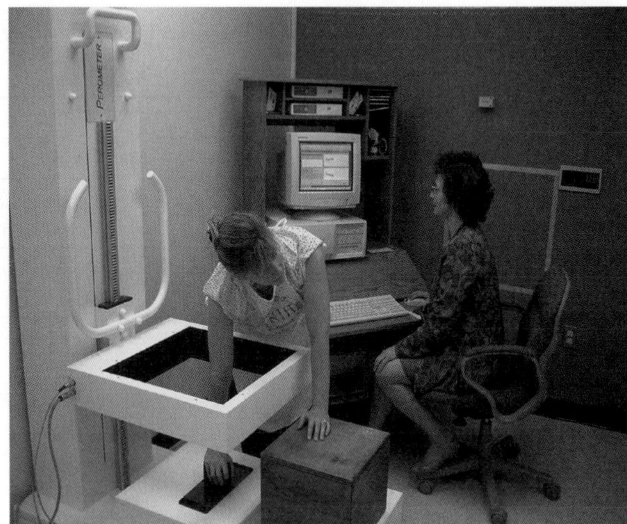

FIGURE 21-13. Perometry.

Vascular Assessment

It is important to rule out peripheral arterial occlusive disease as this is a contraindication for compression therapy or may indicate the need for a modified level of compression; a screening vascular assessment should include pulse palpation and ABI measurement (see Chapter 22 for in-depth discussion of ABI measurement and interpretation).

Pain Assessment

Pain may be caused by inflammation, infection, distention of the tissue, nerve entrapment, radiation fibrosis, cancer recurrence, or degenerative joint disease. It is important to note the cause, nature, frequency, site, and severity of pain; it is also important to determine whether the pain is related to the lymphedema or caused by other factors. Lymphedema is not associated with a "typical" pain pattern; some patients report no pain, while others report sensations such as aching, tingling, tightness, and weakness.

Psychosocial Assessment

Lymphedema can have a significant negative impact on an individual's QOL; thus, it is critical to evaluate the patient for depression, anxiety, ability to cope, and understanding of the disease process and treatment. It is also important to assess for the involvement of significant others and the patient's support system, health insurance issues and finances, living circumstances, and accommodations.

Mobility and Functional Assessment

Lymphedema can cause a marked reduction in mobility and functional status; the nurse should assess range of motion in the arms and legs, strength of the limbs, and ability to lift and move. The nurse should also query the patient regarding the ways in which lymphedema has affected activities of daily living.

Nutritional Assessment

The patient's weight and BMI should be determined, and the patient should be encouraged to maintain a healthy body weight. The clinician may need to refer the patient to a nutritionist to work on weight reduction in order to facilitate treatment. It is important to note that obesity contributes to the onset of lymphedema and often worsens the symptoms of existing lymphedema.

CLINICAL PEARL

Clinicians working with lymphedema patients should provide comprehensive periodic assessment to monitor response to treatment and to promptly detect any deterioration in status; limb volume and skin status are two particularly critical elements of assessment.

Management

Treatment depends on the stage of disease. For patients with stage 0 disease, the focus is on prevention (Lawenda et al., 2009).

Prevention

Prevention education should be provided to all at-risk patients (Table 21-10). Breast cancer–related lymphedema (BCRL) is the area of most intense research; thus, much of what we know regarding the incidence, prevention, and treatment of lymphedema is based on this population. The use of sentinel node biopsy represents a major advance in prevention of lymphedema. Until recently, curative procedures for solid tumors such as breast cancer involved removal of multiple lymph nodes. Current practice typically involves injection of dye into the tumor bed and removal of any lymph nodes that pick up the dye. If the sentinel node(s) is/are found to be negative for cancer, axillary node dissection can be avoided, thus reducing the risk for the development of lymphedema. Another approach to prevention of BCRL is the use of axillary reverse mapping (ARM). The concept of ARM is to map the lymphatics draining the arm with blue dye in order to create a roadmap for their preservation. However, there are limitations to this procedure, and preservation of lymphatics is not always possible (Balci et al., 2012).

Key preventive measures for all at-risk patients include the following:

- Obtaining baseline girth and volume measurements for affected and nonaffected limbs
- Educating the patient concerning arm or leg care guidelines (see **Table 21-10** and the National Lymphedema Network (NLN) position papers at Lymphnet.org)
- Implementing measures to reduce concurrent risk factors (e.g., obesity, venous disease)

TABLE 21-10 Risk Reduction Strategies for Patients at Risk for Lymphedema

Skin Care
Meticulous care of the skin and nails
Keep the skin clean and dry and well moisturized with low-pH lotions
Avoid trauma and injury to reduce infection risk (including injections and blood draws if possible)
Wear gloves when doing activities that may cause skin injury
Protect exposed skin with sunscreen and insect repellent
Activity and Lifestyle
Maintain an optimal body weight—obesity is a known risk factor for lymphedema
Eat a well-balanced diet
Avoid tight clothing including underwear, watches, and jewelry
Avoid blood pressures in the affected extremity
Avoid carrying a heavy bag or purse on the affected side
Undertake exercise and movement therapy
Avoid extreme temperatures—both heat and cold
Compression Garment
Wear prophylactic compression garments if prescribed
Consider wearing prophylactic compression garment during strenuous exercise and for travel by air to support the extremity at risk

Please note that prevention guidelines are anecdotal and based on clinical experience by experts in the field of lymphology. To see the full position paper, refer to The National Lymphedema Network Position Paper, May 2012, Summary of Lymphedema Risk Reduction Practices. Adapted from The National Lymphedema Network.

CLINICAL PEARL

Risk reduction strategies are a major component of patient education and lymphedema prevention. Organizations such as the NLN and American Cancer Society offer printable handouts that can be used as educational tools for patients.

Treatment Goals

Currently, lymphedema is considered a noncurable condition because damage to the lymphatics is usually irreversible, as is the absence of various components of the lymphatic system. However, it can be effectively managed with the goals of reducing and maintaining limb size, alleviating symptoms, preventing infection, improving limb function, and improving overall psychological well-being (Kunkel, 2010). Intervention should occur as soon as possible following diagnosis to prevent progressive tissue damage and advancement of the disorder. Treatment may be initiated at any stage of lymphedema; however, outcomes are less optimal when treatment is delayed until the later stages due to the significant fibrotic changes that occur in the tissue (Lawenda et al., 2009).

CLINICAL PEARL

Lymphedema is at present a noncurable condition; goals of therapy include reducing and maintaining limb size, preventing infection, improving limb function, alleviating symptoms, and improving overall well-being.

Complete Decongestive Therapy

This therapy is also known as comprehensive decongestive therapy, complex physical therapy, and complex decongestive physiotherapy and is the cornerstone of lymphedema treatment.

History of CDT

The technique of MLD, a component of combined decongestive therapy, was developed in 1932 by Emil Vodder, a PhD from Denmark. While working as a medical therapist on the French Riviera, he discovered that a very light form of massage therapy performed gently over the lymph nodes caused dramatic improvement among patients with colds and sinusitis. With the contributions of many scientists within the German Society of Lymphology (founded by Johannes Asdonk, 1976), the method has evolved into a comprehensive physical therapy approach to management that combines MLD with compression bandaging, skin care, and exercise (Williams, 2010).

Considerations Related to CDT

CDT is currently accepted as the international gold standard for the treatment of lymphedema and should be provided by a certified lymphedema health care practitioner (Uzkeser, 2012). The components of CDT are MLD, compression bandaging, compression garments, therapeutic exercises, meticulous skin care, and patient education. CDT consists of two phases. Phase one is the acute intensive (or reductive) phase. In phase one, patients are typically seen in an outpatient setting 3 to 5 days a week for 1 to 4 weeks or longer. Length and duration of treatment is determined by the clinician according to the severity and stage of lymphedema (Korpan et al., 2011). The goal of phase one treatment is to reduce the limb to the smallest possible size and to alleviate symptoms such as tightness, discomfort, and decreased range of motion (Fu et al., 2009). Phase II is the maintenance and home care component of the treatment. This phase is individualized based on the specific needs of the patient and focuses on maintaining limb reduction. Education includes continued skin care and infection prevention, exercises, self-massage, and use of garments and compression aids/devices (Balci et al., 2012; Quirion, 2010). It is important to note that there are absolute and relative contraindications to CDT, which reiterates the need for thorough assessment and diagnosis prior to initiation of therapy. Precautions must be taken with patients with hypertension because CDT can increase central venous blood volume (Lawenda et al., 2009). Other patients who require cautious use of CDT include those with compromised sensation, for example, individuals with paralysis or diabetic neuropathies. These patients may not detect pain, which means that improperly placed bandages or garments could result in injury. Such individuals must be followed closely and must be compliant with daily self-examination of the skin. CDT in patients with bronchial asthma could result in a bronchial asthma attack due to the effects of MLD on the parasympathetic nervous system (Lawenda et al., 2009). It should also be noted that lymphedema affecting the head, neck, trunk, or genitalia can be very challenging and requires a modified CDT approach. Absolute contraindications to CDT include patients with acute infections, symptomatic congestive heart failure, and DVT (Lawenda et al., 2009).

CLINICAL PEARL

CDT is currently accepted as the international gold standard for the treatment of lymphedema; the therapy includes MLD, compression bandaging, compression garments, therapeutic exercises, meticulous skin care, and patient education.

CDT Components: Manual Lymph Drainage

MLD is a gentle procedure that involves manual movement of the skin (a skin technique) using very light hand and finger movements. MLD works by promoting flow of lymph through the lymphatic structures located in the subcutaneous tissue. MLD should not be confused with massage therapies, which, in general, apply considerable pressure to treat conditions of muscle tissue, tendons, and ligaments. Massage therapy should not be used in the treatment of lymphedema as these techniques can increase vascular flow (which increases lymph formation) (Zuther & Norton, 2013).

MLD enhances the efficiency of the lymph system in several ways. It stretches the smooth muscle sheath of the superficial lymphatic vessels, which increases their pumping rate (lymphangiomotoricity) (Lawenda et al., 2009). MLD redirects lymph flow out of the compromised areas and into healthy functioning areas of the lymphatic system by opening and dilating the collateral vessels that cross lymphatic watersheds; in essence, it "bypasses" the ineffective or damaged lymphatics (Kunkel, 2010). The sequence in which MLD is performed on the body is very important and requires a full understanding of lymphatic watersheds and patterns of lymphatic drainage. It involves first stimulating the nonaffected areas of the body. Edema fluid is then massaged across the lymphatic watershed toward the functional lymphatic structures and regional lymph nodes.

The affected areas are treated last and always in the direction of proximal to distal. The benefits of MLD include a reduction in swelling that is produced by decongestion of the impaired lymphatic pathways, reduction in lymphatic load, enhanced development of collateral drainage routes, and stimulation of the functional and patent components of the system (Lymphoedema Framework, 2006). MLD also improves the quality of the tissue by reducing fibrosis.

CLINICAL PEARL

Manual lymphatic drainage uses very light and strategically directed touch to improve lymphatic flow; it should not be confused with massage, which uses high pressure touch and is totally contraindicated in the management of lymphedema.

Compression Therapy: Multilayer Compression Bandaging

The use of SSBs with low extensibility (inelastic bandages) is indicated for the treatment of lymphedema. SSBs are applied in multiple layers with more layers applied to the distal end of the extremity and less applied at the proximal end of the extremity (Fig. 21-14). This creates a gradient pressure to facilitate lymph flow. The bandages have a high working pressure and a low resting pressure. Muscle contraction facilitates lymph flow due to the antagonistic force between the muscle and the bandage (Uzkeser, 2012). Compression bandages are primarily used during the intensive phase (phase one) of treatment to achieve limb reduction. Once the clinician feels that the limb has reached maximum reduction in size, the patient is fitted for a compression garment.

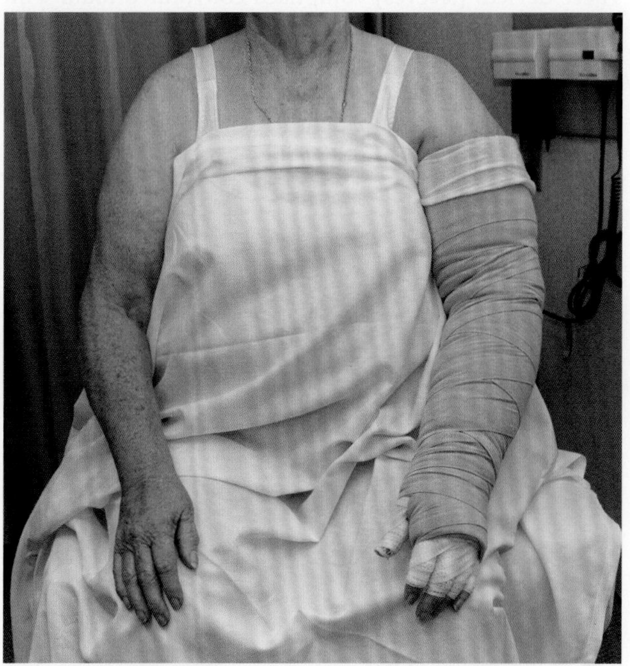

FIGURE 21-14. Short stretch multilayer bandages.

CLINICAL PEARL

Short-stretch layered bandages are used during the intensive phase of treatment to promote lymphatic flow and to reduce edema; once maximum edema reduction has been obtained, the patient should be fitted for a compression garment.

Compression Therapy: Compression Garments

Compression garments are used in phase II of therapy and are meant for long-term management of lymphedema. They assist in maintaining edema reduction by accelerating lymph flow. Garments are meant for daytime use as their effect is facilitated by muscle movement. Circular knit garments (ready to wear garments) have no seams, are made of thinner material, and for some patients are cosmetically more acceptable. Flat knit garments (custom-made garments) have seams and can be adapted to fit the special needs of some lymphedema patients. Garments come in a variety of pressure strengths (measured as mm Hg) and are determined by the clinician or by the garment fitter in collaboration with the patient and clinician. Compression garments (custom or readymade) can also be used to control lymphedema of the head and neck, breast, trunk, or genitalia.

CLINICAL PEARL

Compression garments are a critical element of long-term lymphedema management; they must be fitted by the clinician or a specially trained garment fitter.

Contraindications to compression garments are arterial insufficiency, extreme shape distortion of the limb, deep skin folds, extensive skin damage or ulcerations, acute cardiac failure, and severe peripheral neuropathy (Lymphoedema Framework, 2006). The wearing of compression garments is a lifelong commitment in order to reduce swelling and prevent further accumulation of lymphatic fluid in the tissues (Lay-Flurrie, 2011).

Therapeutic Exercises

Compression bandages are worn coupled with exercises during the intensive phase of treatment. Remedial exercises are geared toward increasing muscle strength, flexibility, and range of motion and improving lymphatic circulation (Cheifetz & Haley, 2010). Exercise protocols are established that are easy to learn and perform in order to promote compliance. Exercises are also encouraged for ongoing maintenance therapy and should be performed while the patient is wearing a compression garment.

Skin Care

Skin care focuses on optimizing skin health and treating any skin conditions. The skin should be cleaned using a low pH or neutral body wash or soap followed by the application of low pH or neutral lotion. Compression bandages are then applied. Patients are educated and encouraged to continue ongoing skin care throughout maintenance therapy (Quirion, 2010). It is important to note that most manufacturers do not provide the pH of their products. It will take diligence from the practitioner to seek out this information from the company whose products they are using and make changes as needed. Typically, body washes provide a lower pH than bar soaps and nonperfumed body lotions such as the Eucerin brand provide low pH options.

Patient Education

The patient's participation in a program of CDT is crucial if maximum results are to be achieved and maintained. It is recommended that prior to initiation of any intervention, the patient must have a thorough understanding of all components of treatment (Quirion, 2010). Patients must commit to the lifelong daily regimen of prescribed skin care, exercises, garments, and compression aids. Patient education focuses on proper skin care, the use and care of compression garments, ongoing remedial exercises, and, if needed, counseling on weight reduction with referral. Some patients require ongoing use of compression bandages or other compression aids to improve fibrosis and maintain edema reduction. Instruction in bandaging and use of these devices is then provided (see Assistive Devices for Lymphedema). Limitations that may affect compliance are physical difficulties in providing self-care, time constraints felt by the patient, and cost of products (bandages and garments) if not covered by insurance (Fu et al., 2009).

CLINICAL PEARL

Patients must commit to the lifelong daily regimen of prescribed skin care, exercises, garments, and compression aids. Patient education focuses on proper skin care, the use and care of compression garments, ongoing remedial exercises, and, if needed, counseling on weight reduction with referral.

Assistive Devices for Lymphedema

Due to an increase in awareness of the treatment for lymphedema over the past decade, many assistive devices are now available that can enhance treatment for someone going through CDT.

Advanced Pneumatic Therapy: Pneumatic Compression Devices

The gold standard of treatment for lymphedema as stated previously is CDT. However, pneumatic compression devices (PCDs) have been used for the medical management of swelling since the early 1950s. These devices initially were single-chambered pressure cuffs that applied uniform compression to the entire limb. Multichambered sequential devices were developed in the 1970s and evolved to provide a gradient sequential compression. These were often used at home by patients for management of edema; however, they used high pressures, and the compression was applied distal to proximal, while the sequence of MLD is proximal to distal. These differences led to concerns that these devices could potentially damage healthy functioning lymphatics (Scheiman, 2011). However, the most recently developed PCDs are believed to be safer than the older models; advanced PCDs (see Fig. 21-10) exert lower pressures and are meant to mimic the therapeutic techniques of MLD. Newer systems permit variation in the compression patterns to meet individualized needs and apply a light and variable pressure to the affected limb and to the trunk/chest wall as needed (Ridner et al., 2010) (Fig. 21-15). These advanced PCDs are being used both for accelerating the in-clinic treatment phase and for the home care phase. PCDs can be an adjunctive treatment for appropriate patients but cannot be considered as solo therapy for treatment of lymphedema (Ashforth, 2012). PCDs are contraindicated for patients with congestive heart failure, active infection, or deep venous thrombosis (Balci et al., 2012).

CLINICAL PEARL

PCDs can be appropriate adjunctive therapy for selected patients but cannot be considered solo therapy for treatment of lymphedema.

Compression Devices

For patients who are in need of ongoing lymphatic drainage during the maintenance (self-management) phase of lymphedema therapy, compressive devices (i.e., ReidSleeve, JoviPak, Solaris) have been developed that can be worn at home while sleeping or during the day if preferred by the patient. These devices are easy to don and can be a beneficial alternative to learning self-bandaging techniques. These devices (sleeves) comprised convoluted foam with an outer sleeve or straps that can be adjusted to provide the desired compression. Most companies offer both custom-made and standard options and work in collaboration with the therapist and patient to achieve the desired outcomes. Some therapists utilize these special devices during

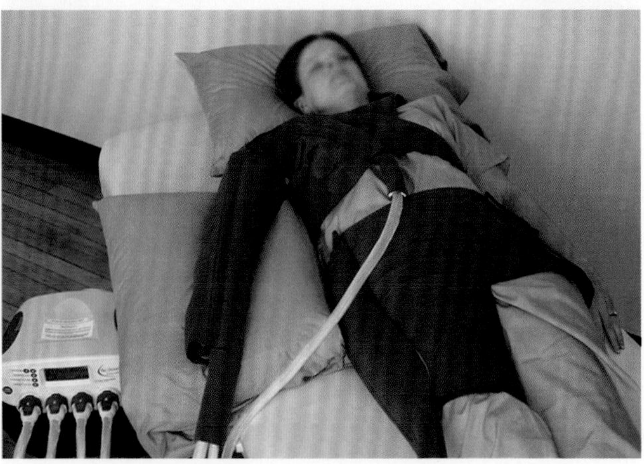

FIGURE 21-15. Pneumatic compression devices.

the intensive phase of therapy as they facilitate the breakdown and softening of fibrotic tissue.

Compressive Strapping Devices

Several companies have devised a wrapping system (e.g., FarrowWrap, CircAid) secured with Velcro straps that can be used as an alternative to short-stretch compression bandages and garments (Fig. 21-16). Indications for use include patients who are intolerant to bandaging or garments, have distorted limb shapes, have hand weakness or back problems, have skin sensitivities, or have compliance issues. These products are available in both standard and custom-made options (Hobday & Wigg, 2013).

Lymphatic Taping

Kinesio tape is a type of medical tape that is applied to the skin to facilitate lymphatic drainage. It has been shown to reduce lymphatic congestion and feelings of tightness and to improve function and movement. Additionally, it can improve the appearance of scar tissue (Hardy, 2012). Although medical taping concepts have only become popular over the last 10 years, lymph taping is now recognized as an effective adjunctive therapy in the management of lymphedema. Lymph taping works by increasing pressure differences within the lymph vessels, promoting opening of the lymphatic capillaries by lifting the skin, and providing a micro-massaging effect. However, it should be noted that taping cannot replace short-stretch bandaging and must be applied by someone who has been trained in the application technique. Lymphatic taping can be considered an alternative choice for patients with lymphedema in areas where compression is difficult or impossible to use (i.e., genital or facial edema) (Bosman, 2014).

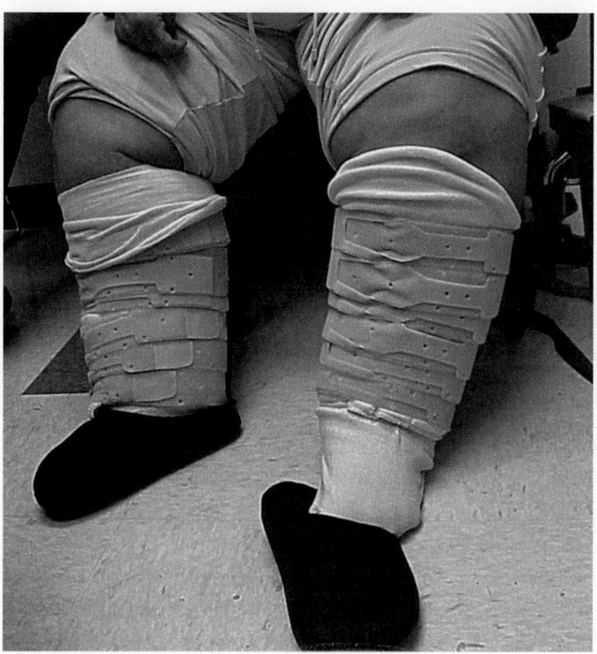

FIGURE 21-16. Velcro strapping system.

Low-Level Laser Therapy

LLLT was first introduced in 2006 and is sometimes used as an adjunct to combined decongestive therapy (Low Level Laser Therapy, 2011). Research has shown that LLLT can facilitate wound healing; improve lymphatic function; reduce inflammation, pain, and scar tissue; and enhance the effects of MLD (Wigg & Lee, 2014). LLLT treats the cells by delivering an infrared laser at a wavelength of 904 nm. This wavelength penetrates deeply into the tissue where it is absorbed by cells and converted into energy; the result is a photochemical reaction at the cellular level (Kozanoglu et al., 2009). To date, the RianCorp LTU-904 laser therapy unit has been cleared by the FDA for the treatment of postmastectomy lymphedema to reduce swelling (Low Level Laser Therapy, 2011). Therapists who have used the device also report softening of fibrosis, improvement of scars, and reduced pain. The device must be used by a trained professional as it requires correct positioning. LLLT should not be used for patients with infection, active cancer, or other medically prohibitive conditions.

CLINICAL PEARL

Patients should be provided with resources and referrals to facilitate self-care and management.

Surgical Techniques for Lymphedema

Surgical management of lymphedema is reserved for patients who are refractory to conservative measures and for most is palliative rather than curative (Avraham et al., 2010). Research support for surgical treatment of lymphedema remains limited (Williams, 2012).

Excisional Procedures (Reduction of Limb Volume Through Resection)

Excisional procedures (debulking procedures) are performed in a staged manner with repeated primary closure. Many complications can arise from excisional procedures including poor wound healing, extensive scarring, skin ulcerations, nerve damage, poor cosmetic outcomes, and increased edema from damage to residual normal functioning lymphatics (Avraham et al., 2010). This approach is rarely used now that MDs are more educated to the process of CDT. It may be reserved for patients who have failed CDT and who struggle with ongoing QOL issues such as the morbidly obese who often have large pendulous fibrotic lobules of edema.

Microsurgical Reconstruction

Microsurgical approaches are used to improve or restore lymphatic pathways or to bypass damaged lymphatics (Williams, 2012). These approaches are showing promising results and are considered to be the future trend in surgical management of lymphedema. Surgeons and researchers are working to develop improved techniques for directly reconnecting the lymphatics and restoring lymphatic flow. Derivative microsurgery focuses on redirecting lymph flow to the venous circulation at the level of obstruction through lymphatic–venous anastomoses. Reconstructive microsurgery repair focuses on restoring lymphatic flow by bypassing the site of obstruction either directly or with interposition of a vein or a lymphatic graft (Avraham et al., 2010). All researchers agree that additional study and research is indicated for further advancements in surgical procedures.

Tissue Transplantation
Another emerging therapy is surgical transplantation of lymph nodes and lymphatic vessels into areas where the lymphatics are missing or damaged. The technique is mainly used in upper limb swelling, and evidence for use is limited (Williams, 2012).

Liposuction
Liposuction is a technique that removes fat through a small metal cannula. Most professionals who treat and manage patients with lymphedema believe that great caution should be used with this approach. Surgeons need to have the appropriate skills and experience in treating lymphedema with liposuction. Liposuction may only be an option for selected patients and should be undertaken only in a multidisciplinary environment with appropriate follow-up and monitoring of results (Munnoch, 2012). Liposuction is usually only considered after more conservative methods have been tried (CDT) without response, and the patient has manifestations of late-stage lymphedema. The patient must maintain any reduction that is achieved with the lifetime use of compression garments.

Lipedema

Many medical practitioners are unfamiliar with the condition of lipedema, and it is often misdiagnosed as bilateral primary lymphedema or morbid obesity (Zuther & Norton, 2013). Lipedema (see Fig. 21-14) is a chronic condition of unknown etiology that results in the abnormal deposition of fat in the subcutaneous tissue (Hampton, 2010). It is sometimes known as painful fat syndrome. It manifests as swelling in the lower extremities but does not involve the feet (foot sparing) (Fig. 21-17). It can affect the upper extremities, but this is less likely, and it does not involve the hands. Lipedema almost exclusively affects women and is thought to possibly be related to a hormonal disorder. It often starts at times of hormonal changes such as puberty or pregnancy (Lymphoedema Framework, 2006). Lipedema complicated by weight gain can lead to the development of lymphedema (lipolymphedema). Characteristics of lipedema include the following:

- The swelling is bilateral and symmetrical.
- The feet and hands are spared of swelling.
- Stemmers sign is negative.
- The tissue is often painful and patients bruise easily.
- Hard nodules may be palpated in the tissue.

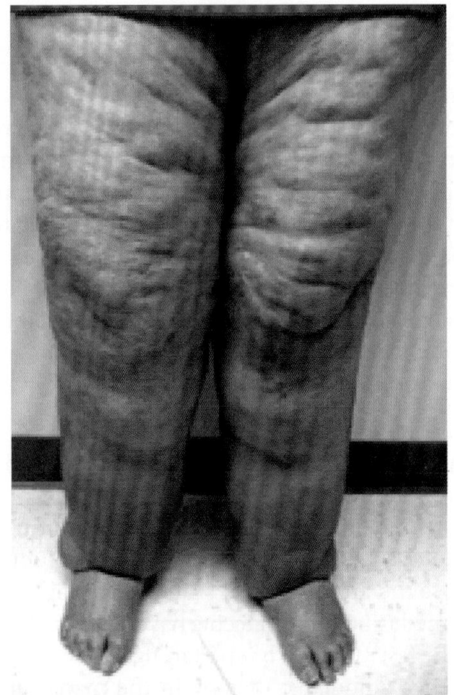

FIGURE 21-17. Lipedema.

- Tissue often does not pit when pressed.
- There is often a family history of lipedema.

CLINICAL PEARL

Lipedema is also known as "painful fat syndrome"; it involves abnormal deposition of fat in the lower (and sometimes upper) extremities with sparing of the feet (and hands, if upper extremities are involved). CDT and compression garments may provide some benefit.

Treatment for lipedema includes the following: nutritional guidance if the lipedema is associated with obesity, instruction and guidance in routine exercise therapy, medical management for any hormonal imbalance, CDT, and compression garments. It should be noted that the results obtained with CDT are typically slower and less dramatic than those obtained with lymphedema patients and that patients usually require custom-made compression garments. Liposuction is sometimes listed as a treatment option but must be used with extreme caution due to the risk of lymphatic damage.

Skin/Wound Care and Lymphedema

Patients with lymphedema are prone to skin problems which, if not treated, can quickly progress to the development of open wounds. Skin care should include patient education regarding proper daily skin care with low-pH soaps or soap substitutes followed by application of emollients. Skin folds should be kept clean and dry. Common skin conditions for those with lymphedema

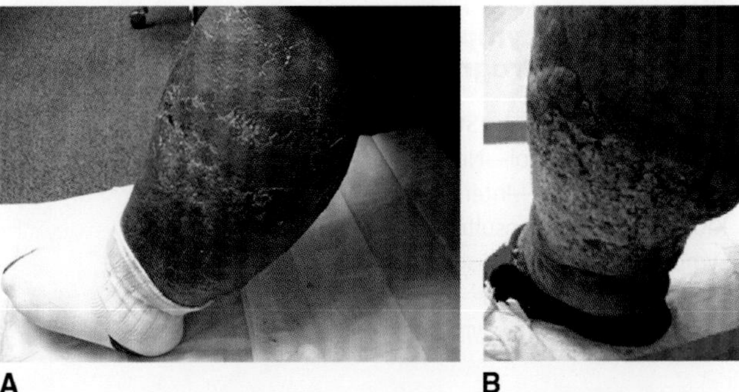

FIGURE 21-18. **A.** Hyperkeratosis. **B.** Stage III lymphedema with papillomatosis.

include hyperkeratosis (Fig. 21-18A), folliculitis, and fungal infections. Patients with lymphedema are also at risk for recurrent episodes of cellulitis. Good skin care is vital for the prevention of cellulitis, and prompt recognition and treatment of cellulitis is essential to prevent further soft tissue and lymphatic damage, which would predispose the patient to worsening disease and recurrent episodes.

CLINICAL PEARL

Patients with lymphedema are at risk for recurrent episodes of cellulitis, which can worsen the underlying condition; thus, meticulous preventive skin care and prompt response to any signs of infection are key elements of patient education.

Advanced skin conditions such as lymphangiectasia (fluid-filled projections from dilation of lymphatic vessels) and papillomatosis (raised projections on the skin due to dilation of lymphatic vessels and fibrosis, Fig. 21-18B) require management by a lymphedema practitioner in collaboration with an MD and dermatologist. In cases where lymph is leaking from the skin surface (lymphorrhea), the surrounding skin should be protected with a moisture barrier cream and/or a nonadherent absorbent dressing to avoid maceration of the skin (Lymphoedema Framework, 2006). Patients with lymphedema may develop skin tears and open wounds related to the poorly functioning lymphatic system or as a result of other comorbid conditions. Wounds can also result from trauma, allergies, or therapeutic procedures (e.g., surgery and radiation therapy). It is important to note that any wounds resulting from excessive accumulation of interstitial fluid (CVI and lymphedema, see Fig. 21-19) may be appropriately treated with combined decongestive therapy. Any associated open wounds, whether acute or chronic, superficial or deep, should be treated based on the principles of wound care discussed in this textbook. Advanced wound care products designed to manage large volumes of fluid should be used to control exudate and to facilitate debridement (if needed). As noted, vascular status must always be evaluated prior to initiation of any form of compression therapy (Zuther & Norton, 2013).

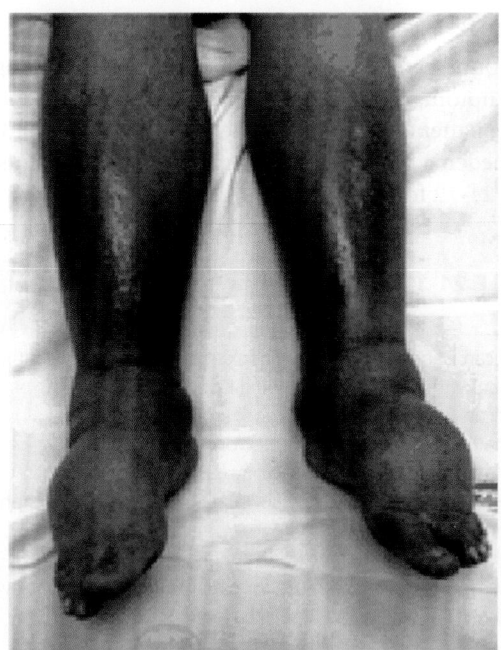

FIGURE 21-19. CVI and lymphedema.

CLINICAL PEARL

Wound management for the patient with lymphedema requires a dual focus: lymphedema management using the principles of complex decongestive therapy and wound care based on the principles of moist wound healing.

Referral for Lymphedema Services

The majority of lymphedema services are provided in the outpatient clinic setting through the physical therapy/occupational therapy department. In addition, more nurses are pursuing the study of lymphedema and incorporating it into advanced nursing wound care practice. Any wound care clinician needs to recognize the signs and symptoms of lymphedema and needs to be able to identify appropriate providers and initiate a referral. One option is to contact local physical therapy groups to determine groups that provide lymphedema services. The National Lymphedema Network (www.lymphnet.org) and the Lymphology Association of North America (LANA) (www.clt-lana.org) maintain a database of lymphedema practitioners across the country; the clinician can access this database by going to their Web sites. According to the NLN, a therapist should meet the following requirements: successful completion of 135 hours of CDT course work from a lymphedema training program with 1/3 theory hours and 2/3 lab hours and certification through the LANA (Quirion, 2010). Unfortunately, some patients may need to travel to find a qualified therapist.

Keynote

The wound care nurse may be the first person to recognize the symptoms of lymphedema in a patient and must be able to refer patients to a qualified therapist. See Table 21-11 for lymphedema resources for practitioners and patients and Table 21-12 for therapy training programs.

TABLE 21-11 Lymphedema Resources for Practitioners and Patients

American Cancer Society's free booklet, Lymphedema: What Every Woman with Breast Cancer Should Know.
American Lymphedema Framework Project (ALFP)
International Lymphedema Framework (ILF)
International Society of Lymphology (ISL)
Little Leakers—Web site for families with children with lymphatic malformations
Lymphology Association of North American (LANA)
Lymph Notes—online Web site for patients and professionals
Lymphatic Education and Research Network (LERN)
Lymphedema Resources, Inc.
Lymphoedema Support Network (LSN)— A British Lymphedema Society
Lymphedema Treatment Act (Legislative Organization)
Medicine Wheel and Lymphedema Impact on the Spirit
National Cancer Institute's PDQs for health care professionals
National Cancer Institute's PDQs for patients
National Lymphedema Network (NLN)
National Organization of Vascular Anomalies (NOVA)
Native American Cancer Research
North American Lymphedema Education Association (NALEA)
Oncology Nursing Society's Putting Evidence into Practice Lymphedema Resources

TABLE 21-12 Lymphedema Therapy Training Programs

Academy of Lymphatic Studies (ACOLS)—Florida
Boris-Lasinski School—New York
Dr. Vodder School—International
Klose Training & Consulting, LLC—Colorado
Lymphatic Care Specialists Training Programs—Virginia
Lymphedema Seminars—California
The Norton School of Lymphatic Therapy—New Jersey

Conclusion

The venous and lymphatic systems are intricately connected by the capillary system at the tissue level in order to transport venous blood and lymph fluid out of the tissue and back into the systemic circulation. This interconnectedness has long been overlooked or ignored. The systems function in a complementary fashion when both are functioning normally. When either of the systems is compromised by pathology (i.e., CVI or lymphedema), the interdependence creates an additional burden or load on the other system. Understanding this unique relationship is key to the management of patients with chronic venous disease and/or lymphedema. Early diagnosis and intervention is key in both conditions, and wound care nurses are in an optimal position to recognize the problems and provide guidance in treatment.

CASE STUDIES

CASE STUDY: LYMPHEDEMA

The patient is a 42-year-old male with a >10-year history of bilateral lower extremity lymphedema R>L. The edema began following a crush injury of the R thigh on a construction site where the patient worked. Patient's history also includes morbid obesity. He has had repeated episodes of cellulitis to the right thigh for which hospitalization was required. The patient presented with significant palpable fibrosis involving both lower extremities. Prior to the initiation of CDT, the patient was counseled on nutrition and lost 35 pounds. The patient was treated with CDT five times a week for 4 weeks. Compression therapy included the use of convoluted foam sleeves under SSBs used to soften fibrosis. Skin care included daily cleaning and application of Eucerin cream. Following therapy, the patient had redundant skin folds on the medial thighs, which were surgically excised. Complications after surgery included dehiscence of the suture line to the right thigh. This required an additional 2 weeks of treatment with MLD and SSBs until the suture line was healed. He was then fit into compression garments providing 40 to 50 mm Hg.

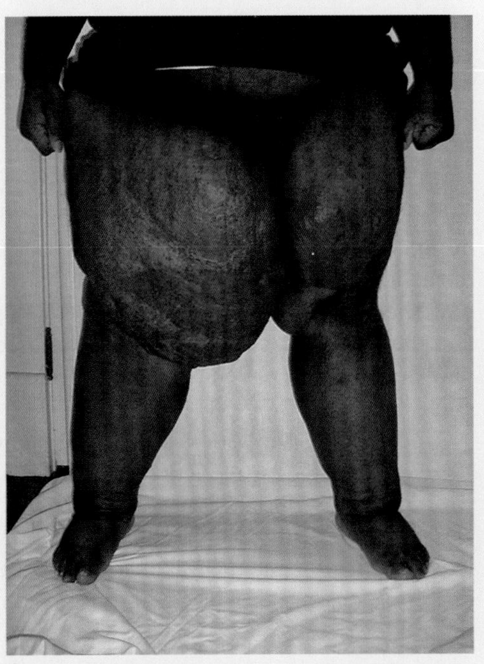

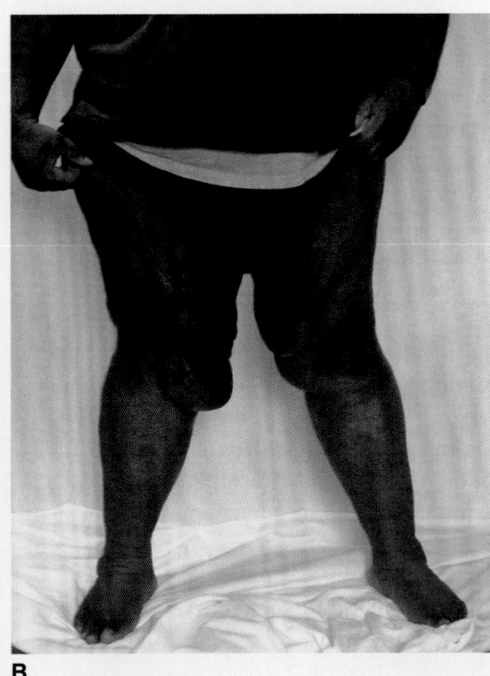

A. Stage III lymphedema. B. After treatment.

CASE STUDY: LYMPHEDEMA WITH VENOUS STASIS AND WOUND

The patient is a 68-year-old female with a 12-year history of venous stasis disease with lymphedema. She sustained a laceration to her right anterior lower leg after falling into a pipe that was protruding through a city street. The patient also has a history of type 2 diabetes. The wound was unhealed after 2 months of topical care, which included daily cleaning, application of Neosporin, and a protective cover dressing as prescribed by her MD. The patient presented with hemosiderin staining of the bilateral lower extremities (BLEs), palpable fibrotic edema from the ankles to knees, and soft edema from the knees to upper thighs. The wound to the right lower extremity (RLE) was dry and cracking with lymphorrhea. The patient was treated with 2 weeks of daily CDT to the BLEs. Skin care included daily cleaning and application of Eucerin cream. Xeroform gauze was placed daily over the wound site. The patient had a 35% reduction of the RLE and a 20% reduction of the LLE. The wound healed and skin condition improved with improved color and palpable softening of fibrosis.

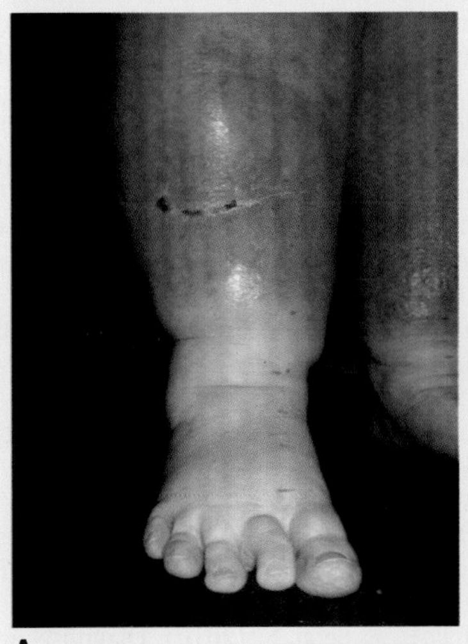

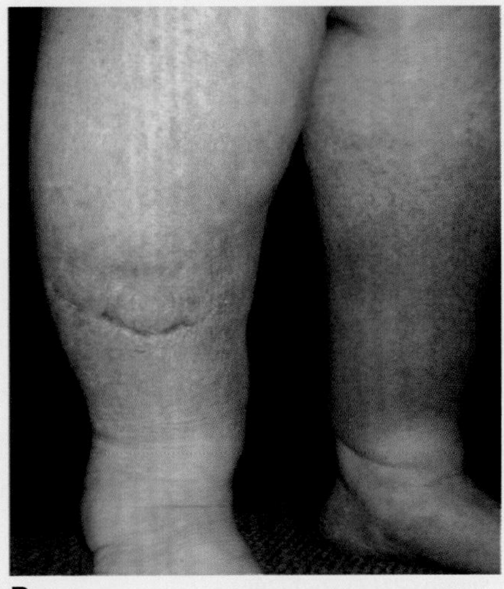

A. Venous stasis with lymphedema and wound. B. After treatment.

CASE STUDY: VENOUS

The patient, AJ, a 78-year-old retired female office worker, is referred to an outpatient wound clinic by her primary care provider for a nonhealing ankle ulcer of 3-month duration. Her complaints include a dull pain (5/10 on a 0/10 pain scale) that is relieved with leg elevation, swelling, tenderness, and intense itching in the ulcer area. She denies any previous ulcer history or trauma to the affected leg. She denies family history of leg ulcers but states her older sister did wear "jelly boots" on her lower leg before she died 20 years ago at age 70. The shallow, irregular ulcer on the medial aspect of the right ankle is 2 × 3 cm and has a ruddy red base with serous drainage. The skin is hyperpigmented in the gaiter area and varicose veins are noted. Pedal pulses are difficult to palpate due to edema, skin is warm to the touch, and the patient can feel a 5.07 monofilament when tested for neuropathy.

Medical history includes degenerative joint disease in the right knee, hypertension, and dyslipidemia.

She is currently taking multivitamins, naproxen, atenolol, and simvastatin.

ABI measurement revealed ABI 0.88 on the right and 0.90 on the left.

Compression therapy was initiated with a two-layer bandaging system; in addition, the patient was encouraged to elevate her legs above the level of the heart for 30 to 45 minutes twice daily and was instructed to perform "ankle pump exercises" every 2 hours during the day. The periwound skin was protected with petrolatum, and the wound was dressed with an antimicrobial alginate dressing. The patient was scheduled to return to the clinic in 5 days.

Upon return, the patient reported reduced pain, and there was a marked reduction in edema; in addition, the ulcer had reduced in size to 1.8 × 2.6 cm. Therapy was continued, and the ulcer healed within 8 weeks, at which point the patient was instructed in use of compression stockings providing 30 mm Hg compression at the ankle.

REFERENCES

Alden, P. B., Lips, E. M., Zimmerman, K. P., et al. (2013). Chronic venous ulcer: Minimally invasive treatment of superficial axial and perforator vein reflux speeds healing and reduces recurrence. *Annals of Vascular Surgery, 27*(1), 75–83.

Alguire, P. C., & Mathes, B. M. (2014). Medical management of lower extremity chronic venous disease. In T. W. Post (Ed.), *UpToDate*. Waltham, MA: UpToDate.

Ambroza, C., & Geigle, P. R. (2010). Aquatic exercise as a management tool for breast cancer-related lymphedema. *Topics in Geriatric Rehabilitation, 26*(2), 120–127.

Armer, J. M., Stewart, B. R., Wanchai, A., et al. (2012). Rehabilitation concepts among aging survivors living with and at risk for lymphedema. *Topics in Geriatric Rehabilitation, 28*(4), 260–268.

Armstrong, D. G., & Meyr, A. J. (2014). Compression therapy for the treatment of chronic venous insufficiency. In T. W. Post (Ed.), *UpToDate*. Waltham, MA: UpToDate.

Ashforth, K. (2012). Proper pressure. *Advance for Physical Therapy & Rehab Medicine, 23*(15), 19–21.

Association for the Advancement of Wound Care (AAWC). (2010). *Venous ulcer guideline*. Malvern, PA: Author.

Avraham, T., Daluvoy, S. V., Kueberuwa, E., et al. (2010). Anatomical and surgical concepts in lymphatic regeneration. *Breast Journal, 16*(6), 639–643.

Balci, F. L., DeGore, L., & Soran, A. (2012). Breast cancer-related lymphedema in elderly patients. *Topics in Geriatric Rehabilitation, 28*(4), 243–253.

Barwell, J. R., Davies, C. E., Deacon, J., et al. (2004). Comparison of surgery and compression with compression alone in chronic venous ulceration (ESCHAR study): Randomised controlled trial. *Lancet, 363*(9424), 1854–1859. doi: 10.1016/S0140-6736(04)16353-8.

Bergan, J. (2007). Molecular mechanisms in chronic venous insufficiency. *Annals of Vascular Surgery, 21*(3), 260–266.

Bergan, J. J., Schmid-Schönbein, G. W., Coleridge Smith, P. D., et al. (2006). Chronic venous disease. *New England Journal of Medicine, 355*(5), 488–498.

Beidler, S. K., Douillet, C. D., Berndt, D. F., et al. (2008). Multiplexed analysis of matrix metalloproteinases in leg ulcer tissue of patients with chronic venous insufficiency before and after compression therapy. *Wound Repair and Regeneration, 16*(5), 642–648.

Biemans, A. A., Kockaert, M., Akkersdijk, G. P., et al. (2013). Comparing endovenous laser ablation, foam sclerotherapy, and conventional surgery for great saphenous varicose veins. *Journal of Vascular Surgery, 58*(3), 727–734. doi: 10.1016/j.jvs.2012.12.074.

Black, C. M. (2014). Anatomy and physiology of the lower-extremity deep and superficial veins. *Techniques in Vascular and Interventional Radiology, 17*(2), 68–73. doi: http://dx.doi.org/10.1053/j.tvir.2014.02.002

Bonham, P., & Kelechi, T. (2008). Evaluation of lower extremity arterial circulation and implications for nursing practice. *Journal of Cardiovascular Nursing, 23*(2), 144–152.

Bosman, J. (2014). Lymphtaping for lymphoedema: An overview of the treatment and its uses. *British Journal of Community Nursing, 19*(Suppl. 4), S12–S18.

Brand, F. N., Dannenberg, A. L., Abbott, R. D., et al. (1988). The epidemiology of varicose veins: The Framingham study. *American Journal of Preventive Medicine, 4*(2), 96–101.

Brem, H., Kirsner, R. S., & Falanga, V. (2004). Protocol for the successful treatment of venous ulcers. *The American Journal of Surgery, 188*(1), 1–8.

Carmel, J. E. (2012). Venous ulcers. In R. A. Bryant & D. P. Nix (Eds.), *Acute & chronic wounds: Current management concepts* (4th ed., pp. 194–213). St. Louis, MO: Elsevier.

Centers for Disease Control and Prevention. (2014). Parasites-lymphatic filariasis. Retrieved from http://www.cdc.gov/parasites/lymphaticfilariasis/

Cheifetz, O., & Haley, L. (2010). Management of secondary lymphedema related to breast cancer. *Canadian Family Physician, 56*(12), 1277–1284.

Collins, L., & Seraj, S. (2010). Diagnosis and treatment of venous ulcers. *American Family Physician, 81*(8), 989–996.

Cooper, G. (2013). Compression therapy in oedema and lymphoedema. *British Journal of Cardiac Nursing, 8*(11), 547–551.

Cormier, J. N., Askew, R. L., Mungovan, K. S., et al. (2010). Lymphedema beyond breast cancer: A systematic review and meta-analysis of cancer-related secondary lymphedema. *Cancer, 116*(22), 5138–5149.

De Araujo, T., Valencia, I., Federman, D. G., et al. (2003). Managing the patient with venous ulcers. *Annals of Internal Medicine, 138*(4), 326–334.

Doughty, D., & Holbrook, R. (2007). Lower extremity ulcers of vascular etiology. In R. A. Bryant & D. P. Nix (Eds.), *Acute and chronic wounds* (3rd ed., pp. 298–303). St. Louis, MO: Elsevier.

Eberhardt, R. T., & Raffetto, J. D. (2014). Chronic venous insufficiency. *Circulation 130*(4), 333-346. doi: 10.1161/CIRCULATIONAHA.113.006898.

Eklof, B., Rutherford, R. B., Bergan, J. J., et al. (2004). Revision of the CEAP classification for chronic venous disorders: Consensus statement. *Journal of Vascular Surgery 40*(6), 1248-1252. doi: 10.1016/j.jvs.2004.09.027.

Fu, M. R., Ridner, S. H., & Armer, J. (2009). Post-breast cancer lymphedema: Part 2. *American Journal of Nursing, 109*(8), 34–42.

Greaves, N. S., Iqbal, S. A., Baguneid, M., et al. (2013). The role of skin substitutes in the management of chronic cutaneous wounds. *Wound Repair and Regeneration, 21*(2), 194–210. doi: 10.1111/wrr.12029.

Hampton, S. (2010). Chronic oedema and lymphoedema of the lower limb. *British Journal of Community Nursing, 15*(Suppl 6), S4–S12.

Hardy, D. (2012). Management of a patient with secondary lymphedema. *Cancer Nursing Practice, 11*(2), 21–26.

Hobday, A., & Wigg, J. (2013). FarrowWrap: Innovative and creative patient treatment for lymphoedema. *British Journal of Community Nursing, 18*(10), S24–S31.

Humphreys, M. L., Stewart, A. H., Gohel, M. S., et al. (2007). Management of mixed arterial and venous leg ulcers. *British Journal of Surgery, 94*(9), 1104–1107.

International Society of Lymphology. (2013). The diagnosis and treatment of peripheral lymphedema: 2013 consensus document. *Lymphology, 46*, 1–11.

Kelechi, T., & Bonham, P. (2008). Measuring venous insufficiency objectively in the clinical setting. *Journal of Vascular Nursing, 26*(3), 67–73.

Korpan, M. I., Crevenna, R., & Fialka-Moser, V. (2011). Lymphedema: A therapeutic approach in the treatment and rehabilitation of cancer patients. *American Journal of Physical Medicine & Rehabilitation, 90*(5), S69–S75.

Kozanoglu, E., Basaram, S., Paydas, S., et al. (2009). Efficacy of pneumatic compression and low-level laser therapy in the treatment of postmastectomy lymphedema: A randomized controlled trial. *Clinical Rehabilitation, 23*(2), 117–124.

Kunkel, K. R. (2010). Identification and impact of standard treatment protocols on the impairments and activity limitations related to lower extremity lymphedema (Doctoral dissertation). Open Access Dissertations. Paper 403. http://scholarlyrepository.miami.edu/oa_dissertations/403

Lawenda, B. D., Mondry, T. E., & Johnstone, P. A. (2009). Lymphedema: A primer on the identification and management of a chronic condition in oncologic treatment. *Cancer Journal for Clinicians, 59*(1), 8–24.

Lay-Flurrie, K. (2011). Use of compression hosiery in chronic oedema and lymphoedema. *British Journal of Nursing, 20*(7), 418–422.

Low Level Laser Therapy. (2011). Retrieved July 25, 2014, from http://www.lymphnotes.com/article.php/id/370/

Lymphoedema Framework. (2006). *Best practice for the management of lymphoedema. International consensus*. London, UK: MEP Ltd.

Maree, J. E. (2011). Yes, breast cancer related lymphoedema can be managed. *Health SA Gesondheid, 16*(1), 1–7. doi:10.4102/hsag.v16i1.578.

McNeely, M. L., Peddle, C. J., Yurick, J. L., et al. (2011). Conservative and dietary interventions for cancer-related lymphedema: A systematic review and meta-analysis. *Cancer, 117*(6), 1136–1148.

Milic, D. J., Zivic, S. S., Bogdanovic, D. C., et al. (2009). Risk factors related to the failure of venous leg ulcers to heal with compression treatment. *Journal of Vascular Surgery, 49*(5), 1242–1247.

Morton, L. M., & Phillips, T. J. (2013). Venous eczema and lipodermatosclerosis. *Seminars in Cutaneous Medicine and Surgery, 32*(3), 169–176.

Mosti, G., Iabichella, M. L., & Partsch, H. (2012). Compression therapy in mixed ulcers increases venous output and arterial perfusion. *Journal of Vascular Surgery, 55*(1), 122–128.

Muldoon, J. (2011). Assessment and monitoring of oedema. *Journal of Community Nursing, 25*(6), 26–28.

Munnoch, A. (2012). Liposuction for chronic lymphoedema–NICE251 (online article). Retrieved from http://www.lymphoedema.org/news/Story73.asp

Nazarko, L. (2009). Diagnosis and treatment of venous eczema. *British Journal of Community Nursing, 14*(5), 188–194.

Nicolaides, A. N., Allegra, C., Bergan, J., et al. (2008). Management of chronic venous disorders of the lower limbs: Guidelines according to scientific evidence. *International Angiology, 27*(1), 1–59.

O'Meara, S., Al-Kurdi, D., Ologun, Y., et al. (2013). Antibiotics and antiseptics for venous leg ulcers. *Cochrane Database of Systematic Reviews*, (1), CD003557.

O'Meara, S., Al-Kurdi, D., & Ovington, L. G. (2008). Antibiotics and antiseptics for venous leg ulcers. *Cochrane Database of Systematic Reviews, 23*(1), CD003557. doi: 10.1002/14651858.CD003557.pub2.

O'Meara, S., Cullum, N. A., & Nelson, E. A. (2009). Compression for venous leg ulcers. *Cochrane Database of Systematic Reviews*, (1), CD000265. doi: 10.1002/14651858.CD000265.pub2.

O'Meara, S., Cullum, N., Nelson, E. A., et al. (2012). Compression for venous leg ulcers. *Cochrane Database of Systematic Reviews, 11*, CD000265. doi: 10.1002/14651858.CD000265.pub3.

Partsch, H., Clark, M., Mosti, G., et al. (2008). Classification of compression bandages: Practical aspects. *Dermatologic Surgery, 34*(5), 600–609.

Phillips, T., Stanton, B., Provan, A., et al. (1994). A study of the impact of leg ulcers on quality of life: Financial, social, and psychologic implications. *Journal of the American Academy of Dermatology, 31*(1), 49–53.

Pittler, M., & Ernst, E. (2012). Horse chestnut seed extract for chronic venous insufficiency: Update. *Cochrane Database of Systematic Reviews*, CD003230; PMID: 16437450.

Porter, J. M., & Moneta, G. L. (1995). Reporting standards in venous disease: An update. *Journal of Vascular Surgery, 21*(4), 635–645. doi: 10.1016/S0741-5214(95)70195-8.

Quirion, E. (2010). Recognizing and treating upper extremity lymphedema in postmastectomy/lumpectomy patients: A guide for primary care providers. *Journal of the American Academy of Nurse Practitioners, 22*(9), 450–459.

Ridner, S. H., Murphy, B., Deng, J., et al. (2010). Advanced pneumatic therapy in self-care of chronic lymphedema of the trunk. *Lymphatic Research and Biology, 8*(4), 209–215.

Scheiman, N. (2011). To pump or not to pump: Is newer technology solving pumping issues in lymphedema? *Advance for Occupational Therapy Practitioners, 27*(4), 8–9.

Shai A., & Halevy S. (2005). Direct triggers for ulceration in patients with venous insufficiency. *International Journal of Dermatology, 44*(12), 1006–1009.

Stellin, G. P., & Waxman, K. (1989). Current and potential therapeutic effects of pentoxifylline. *Comprehensive Therapy, 15*(5), 11–13.

Tarnay, T. J., Rohr, P. R., Davidson, A. G., et al. (1980). Pneumatic calf compression, fibrinolysis, and the prevention of deep venous thrombosis. *Surgery, 88*(4), 489–496.

Uzkeser, H. (2012). Assessment of postmastectomy lymphedema and current treatment approaches. *European Journal of General Medicine, 9*(2), 130–134.

Vowden, K. R., & Vowden, P. (2006). Preventing venous ulcer recurrence: A review. *International Wound Journal, 3*(1), 11–21.

Wigg, J., & Lee, N. (2014). Redefining essential care in lymphoedema. *British Journal of Community Nursing, 19*(Suppl. 4), S20–S27.

Williams, A. (2010). Manual lymphatic drainage: Exploring the history and evidence base. *British Journal of Community Nursing, 15*(4), S18–S24.

Williams, A. (2012). Surgery for people with lymphedema. *Journal of Community Nursing, 26*(5), 27–29, 31–33.
Wipke-Tevis, D. D., & Sae-Sia, W. I. P. A. (2004). Caring for vascular leg ulcers. *Home HealthcareNurse, 22*(4), 237–247.
Wound, Ostomy, and Continence Nurses Society (WOCN). (2011). *Guideline for management of wounds in patients with lower-extremity venous disease.* Mount Laurel, NJ: Author.
Wound, Ostomy, and Continence Nurses Society (WOCN). (2014). *Guideline for management of wounds in patients with lower-extremity arterial disease.* Mount Laurel, NJ: Author.
Zuther, J., & Norton, S. (2013). *Lymphedema management: The comprehensive guide for practitioners* (3rd ed.). New York, NY: Thieme.

QUESTIONS

1. The wound care nurse is assessing the legs of a patient and documents: "2-mm veins visible under skin; veins are blue and slightly bulging." What condition do these data describe?
A. Telangiectasias
B. Reticular veins
C. Hemosiderosis
D. Lipodermatosclerosis

2. Which risk factor for LEVD is related to calf muscle pump dysfunction?
A. Altered gait
B. Pregnancy
C. Thrombophilia
D. Obesity

3. The wound care nurse is preparing a patient for radiofrequency ablation (RFA). Which statement accurately describes the method used to perform this procedure?
A. The greater saphenous vein (GSV) is ligated at the groin and removed (stripped) to the knee.
B. A laser fiber is used to produce heat that destroys the vascular endothelium along the GSV, closing the vein.
C. A sclerosing foam is injected under ultrasound guidance into the GSV—volume depends on length and diameter of the vessel.
D. Thermal energy is delivered using a catheter directly to the GSV walls resulting in closure of the vein.

4. The wound care nurse clinically classifies a patient's ulcers as C_2. What condition does this classification represent?
A. Telangiectasias
B. Varicose veins
C. Edema
D. Lipodermatosclerosis

5. Which of the following represent critical elements of therapy for all patients with chronic venous insufficiency?
A. Pharmacologic interventions such as pentoxifylline
B. Surgical intervention to eliminate venous reflux
C. Elevation of the leg to the level of the heart for at least 4 hours daily
D. Compression therapy to improve venous return

6. The wound care nurse is devising a management plan for a patient with stage 1 lymphedema and chronic venous insufficiency. What therapeutic approach would the nurse recommend?
A. Compression therapy, elevation, exercise
B. Combined decongestive therapy (CDT)
C. CDT with needed wound care
D. Surgical intervention

7. The wound care nurse documents stage II lymphedema on a patient chart. What characteristic distinguishes this condition from earlier stages?
A. Edema is observable and measurable.
B. Edema resolves with elevation.
C. Fibrosis is present in the tissue.
D. Ongoing infections of the tissue are likely.

8. The wound care nurse is teaching a patient who has had radical mastectomy how to lower her risk for lymphedema. Which strategy would the nurse recommend?
A. Keep the skin well moisturized with high-pH lotions.
B. Avoid carrying a heavy bag or purse on the affected side.
C. Avoid loose clothing and jewelry.
D. Avoid wearing compression garments during strenuous exercise.

9. Which condition is the pathological factor responsible for lower extremity venous disease?
   A. Damage to the endothelial lining of the vessels
   B. Platelet aggregation
   C. Venous hypertension
   D. Activation of white blood cells

10. Which of the following is the most reliable and commonly used noninvasive test for diagnosing venous disease?
    A. Venous duplex ultrasound
    B. Air plethysmography
    C. Photoplethysmography
    D. ABI measurements

11. The wound care nurse recommends therapeutic level static compression therapy for patients with venous insufficiency. For which patient is this therapy contraindicated?
    A. A patient with diabetes mellitus
    B. A patient with an ABI <0.8
    C. A patient who has varicose veins
    D. A patient with hypertension

12. The wound care nurse is teaching a patient with venous insufficiency how to care for prescribed compression stockings. What is a recommended guideline?
    A. Do not wash new stockings before wearing them.
    B. Wash stockings every other day.
    C. Moisturize the skin in the evening before going to bed.
    D. Replace the stockings annually.

13. Which general guideline for compression wrap use would the wound care nurse teach a new patient?
    A. Clean the leg well with soap and water prior to applying the wrap.
    B. Avoid using moisturizers on the periwound skin.
    C. Do not include the heel in the compression wrap.
    D. Position the ankle in a neutral position at a right angle.

14. Which pharmaceutical agent is indicated for patients who fail to progress with standard therapy and also provides additive benefits when used in conjunction with compression therapy?
    A. Pentoxifylline
    B. Horse chestnut seed extract
    C. Steroid ointment
    D. Diuretics

ANSWERS: 1.**B**, 2.**A**, 3.**D**, 4.**B**, 5.**D**, 6.**A**, 7.**C**, 8.**B**, 9.**C**, 10.**A**, 11.**B**, 12.**C**, 13.**D**, 14.**A**

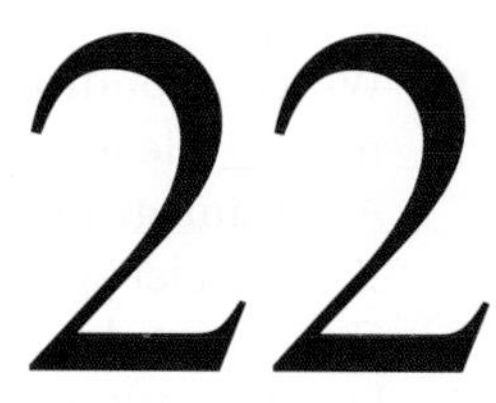

CHAPTER 22

Assessment and Management of Patients with Wounds due to Lower-Extremity Arterial Disease (LEAD)

Phyllis A. Bonham

OBJECTIVES

1. Compare and contrast arterial, venous, neuropathic, and mixed ulcers in terms of risk factors, pathology, clinical presentation, and management guidelines.
2. Describe critical parameters to be included in assessment of the individual with a lower extremity ulcer.
3. Demonstrate the procedure for ABI testing.
4. Interpret findings from
   - ABI testing
   - TBI testing
   - $TcPO_2$ testing
   - Sensory testing with Semmes-Weinstein monofilaments
5. Use assessment data to determine causative and contributing factors for a lower extremity ulcer and to develop individualized management plans that are evidence based.
6. Describe the impact of lifestyle modifications, pharmacologic options, surgical options, and hyperbaric oxygen therapy on improving lower extremity perfusion in the patient with an arterial ulcer.
7. Explain why debridement is contraindicated in a noninfected ischemic ulcer covered with dry eschar.
8. Describe indications for referral to vascular surgeon.

Topic Outline

Introduction

Lower-extremity arterial disease (LEAD) is also known as peripheral arterial occlusive disease (PAOD), peripheral vascular disease (PVD), peripheral arterial disease (PAD), and arterial insufficiency (Kravos & Bubnic-Sotosek, 2009). LEAD is not the most common cause of lower-extremity wounds, but its presence complicates the healing of lower-extremity wounds and can be limb threatening due to ischemia. Less common causes of ischemic lower extremity ulcers include sickle cell disease, embolism, clotting disorders, thromboangiitis obliterans (Buerger's disease), and vasospastic diseases such as Raynaud's disease (Bonham & Kelechi, 2008; Brevetti et al., 2010).

CLINICAL PEARL

LEAD is not the most common cause of lower extremity wounds, but its presence complicates the healing of wounds caused by other etiologic factors, and wounds caused by LEAD can be limb threatening.

A thorough assessment is essential to determine the correct etiology as a basis for an accurate diagnosis and appropriate management. All patients with leg wounds should be carefully examined to determine the presence or absence of LEAD, which is often asymptomatic (Aponte, 2011). Lower-extremity wounds present complex problems and require collaborative, multidisciplinary, and holistic care and management.

Prevalence, Incidence, and Significance of LEAD

In the United States, LEAD is estimated to affect 8 to 12 million adults (Aponte, 2011). The prevalence of LEAD, as defined by an ankle–brachial index (ABI) of 0.90 or less, is 19% to 32% in individuals 40 to 70 years of age (Aponte, 2011; Kravos & Bubnic-Sotosek, 2009). In individuals 80 years of age and older, the prevalence of LEAD is 40% (Bergiers et al., 2011). According to a review of population-based studies in the United States, the prevalence of LEAD is slightly higher in men than women (Hirsch et al., 2012). However, the severity of symptoms and impact of the disease on function and mobility are greater for women (Kumakura et al., 2011; McDermott et al., 2011a). Also, women have more complications associated with surgery and higher mortality than men (Vouyouka et al., 2010).

The incidence of LEAD has not been well documented. According to a French study, the 6-year incidence of LEAD was 5.1% in 3,805 individuals (30 to 65 years of age) with a normal fasting glucose at baseline, and 10.2% in individuals who progressed to diabetes over 6 years (Tapp et al., 2007). In another study of over 12,000 men in Australia, aged 65 years of age and older, the mean annual incidence of LEAD was 0.85% (Lakshmanan et al., 2010).

It has been reported that up to 80% of patients with LEAD are undiagnosed and untreated or undertreated, and many health care providers and patients lack awareness of the serious health-related consequences of LEAD (Bergiers et al., 2011). LEAD is a manifestation of systemic atherosclerosis and is associated with an increased risk of myocardial infarction (MI), stroke, and vascular death (Cimminiello et al., 2011). Individuals with LEAD have six times greater risk of death by cardiovascular disease and seven times higher risk of death from coronary artery disease than those without LEAD (Aponte, 2011).

CLINICAL PEARL

LEAD can be asymptomatic until late in the disease process, and it has been reported that up to 80% of patients with LEAD are undiagnosed and untreated or undertreated.

LEAD has socioeconomic implications for individuals and the overall health care system. There are high costs for treating LEAD due primarily to expenses for hospitalization and surgical care (e.g., bypass, angioplasty, amputation). Medicare hospitalization costs in the United States are estimated at $4.37 billion (Hirsch et al., 2008). Based on the total US census, overall costs for LEAD are projected to be $21 billion (Mahoney et al., 2010). LEAD also impacts the quality of life for patients due to caused by functional limitations leg-related symptoms (Regensteiner et al., 2008).

Pathophysiology/Etiology of LEAD and Ischemic Wounds

LEAD is a chronic and progressive disease due to atherosclerosis, which is a systemic condition (Aponte, 2011). Figure 22-1 illustrates common sites of atherosclerotic

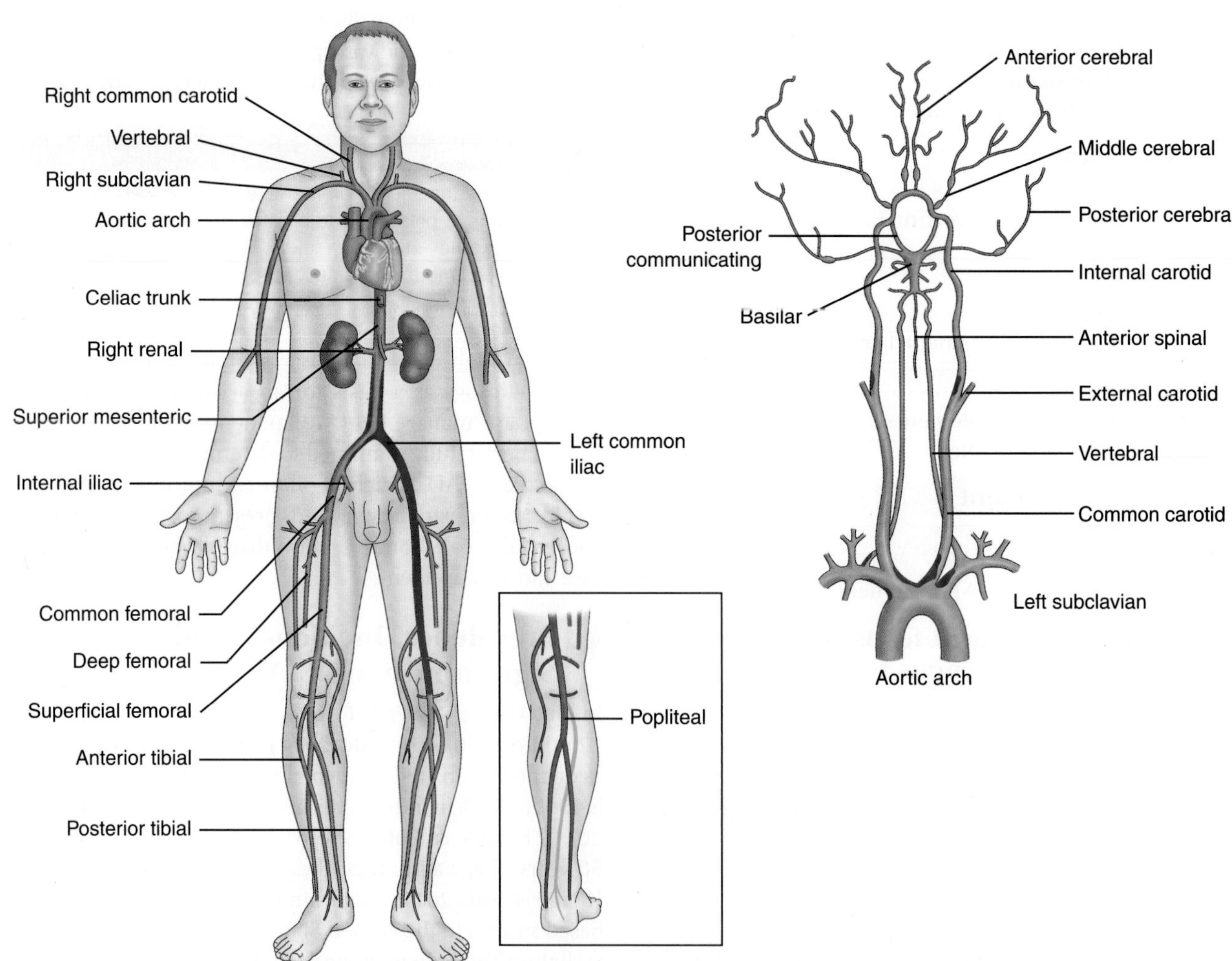

FIGURE 22-1. Example of common sites of atherosclerotic obstruction in major arteries in the body: cerebral, coronary, and lower extremities.

obstruction. Atherosclerosis is a dynamic disorder that involves both endothelial dysfunction and inflammation (Brevetti et al., 2010). In the lower-extremity arteries, atherosclerosis primarily affects the intimal layer, causing plaque formation and endothelial damage that results in stenosis; the injury to the vessel also triggers inflammation, which causes progressive fibrosis and hardening of the arterial walls (Berger et al., 2011; Bonham & Kelechi, 2008). Atherosclerosis and plaque formation can be characterized as developing in the following four stages (Bell, 2013):

- Initial lesion develops: Endothelial damage causes white blood cells to migrate into the area and become activated.
- Fatty streaks form: Fatty streaks, which are collections of lipid-filled macrophages, develop in the inner artery and trigger replacement of the smooth endothelial cells in the intimal layer with muscle cells from the medial layer.
- Atheroma develops: An atheroma, which contains large numbers of smooth muscle cells filled with lipids, forms from the fatty streaks.
- Advanced lesion develops: The atheromatous lesion, which contains endothelial cells, smooth muscle cells, and inflammatory cells, continues to develop and is characterized by a lipid core covered by a fibrous cap; disruption of the fibrous cap can result in thrombus formation and an acute occlusive arterial event.

As atherosclerosis progresses, the narrowed lumen and increased rigidity of the arterial walls prevent dilatation in response to tissue demands for increased blood and oxygen (Fig. 22-2); clinically this is manifest as progressive pain with activity, such as walking, that is relieved by rest (i.e., intermittent claudication). Advanced disease can severely impair tissue perfusion and can result in ischemic wounds.

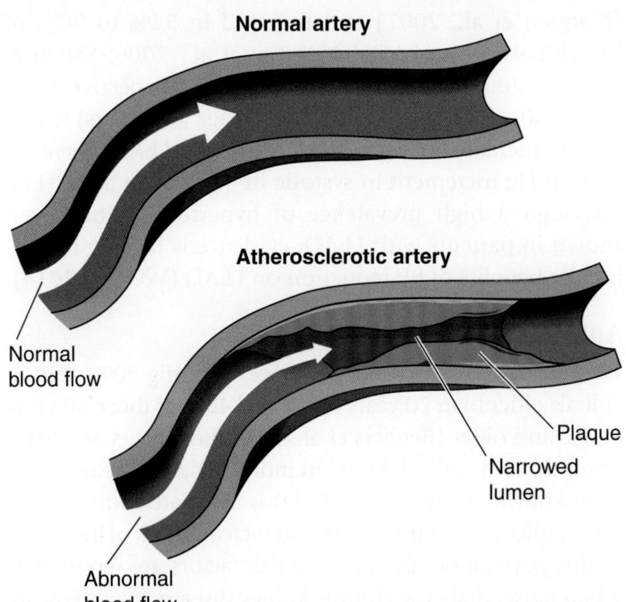

FIGURE 22-2. Example of impaired blood flow in an atherosclerotic artery. (Adapted from NHLBI Atherosclerosis homepage; http://www.nhlbi.nih.gov/health/health-topics/topics/atherosclerosis/)

Symptomatic and Asymptomatic LEAD

Symptomatic LEAD is defined as intermittent claudication or a prior vascular event (e.g., revascularization, amputation), regardless of the ABI (Diehm et al., 2009). However, patients with LEAD may not experience (or recognize) the classic symptoms of LEAD, such as intermittent claudication.

Asymptomatic LEAD is defined as a low resting ABI (<0.90), without a previous lower-extremity vascular event or intermittent claudication (Diehm et al., 2009). Asymptomatic LEAD has been found in 12% to 90% of individuals with the disease (Aronow et al., 2009; Diehm et al., 2009) and is associated with an increased risk of cardiovascular and cerebrovascular morbidity and mortality that is similar to symptomatic LEAD (Diehm et al., 2009; Monreal et al., 2008; Norgren et al., 2010).

CLINICAL PEARL

Individuals with LEAD may not experience (or recognize) the classic symptoms of LEAD, such as intermittent claudication. Both symptomatic and asymptomatic LEAD are associated with increased risk of cardiovascular and cerebrovascular morbidity and mortality.

Risk Factors

All patients with LEAD should undergo risk assessment to guide primary and secondary preventive interventions (Ali & Carman, 2012; Liapis et al., 2009). The risk factors for LEAD parallel those for systemic atherosclerotic conditions such as coronary and cerebrovascular disease (Ali & Carman, 2012; Bonham & Kelechi, 2008). The evidence suggests that many of the risk factors play a predisposing/contributing role as opposed to an independent causative role (Liapis et al., 2009; Norgren et al., 2007). Primary risk factors include smoking tobacco, diabetes mellitus, dyslipidemia, hypertension, and advanced age (Bell, 2013). Additional risk factors include chronic kidney disease, elevated homocysteine levels, family history of cardiovascular disease, ethnicity, inflammation, infection, hypercoagulable states, and vessel calcification (Bell, 2013; Liapis et al., 2009; WOCN, 2014). Some risk factors are modifiable (e.g., smoking, diabetes, abnormal lipids, hypertension), and others are nonmodifiable (e.g., age, family history, ethnicity); comprehensive management for the patient with LEAD includes attention to modifiable risk factors.

CLINICAL PEARL

Primary risk factors for LEAD parallel those for cerebrovascular and cardiovascular disease and include tobacco use, diabetes mellitus, dyslipidemia, hypertension, and advanced age.

Smoking Tobacco

Smoking tobacco is associated with a low ABI and is a strong predictor of LEAD (Cimminiello et al., 2011; Kravos & Bubnic-Sotosek, 2009; Sana et al., 2011). Starting smoking at/or before 16 years of age more than doubles the risk, regardless of the amount of exposure (Planas et al., 2002). Tobacco smoking is known to contribute to tissue hypoxia and has a negative influence on fibroblast activity, epithelialization, and the immune response (Ahn et al., 2008). In addition, smoking has been associated with a threefold increase in vascular graft failure (Willigendael et al., 2005).

The risk of LEAD is particularly high in women who smoke and is greater in premenopausal women with a strong relationship to the exposure defined by pack-years of smoking (Conen et al., 2011). Compared to individuals who never smoked, the risk of LEAD for current smokers is increased 10-fold in women and 4.3-fold in men, and for former smokers, the risk is increased 3-fold for women and 2.3-fold in men (Conen et al., 2011; Lee et al., 2011).

Exposure to secondhand smoke may also increase the risk of LEAD. While findings from the National Health and Nutrition Examination Survey 1999–2004 (NHANES) indicated there was no association between secondhand smoke exposure and LEAD (Agarwal, 2009), He and colleagues (2008) found the risk of LEAD was significantly higher in individuals exposed to secondhand smoke as compared to those who were not exposed.

Diabetes Mellitus (Diabetes)

Diabetes accelerates the natural course and distribution of atherosclerosis (Jalili, 2011), with a two- to fourfold increased risk for LEAD (Hirsch et al., 2006), and multiple studies have shown that diabetes is a strong predictor of LEAD (Kravos & Bubnic-Sotosek, 2009; Subramaniam et al., 2011; Tekin et al., 2011). Factors increasing the risk of LEAD in patients with diabetes include duration of disease, age, and possibly ethnicity (Escobar et al., 2011; Roy & Peng, 2008).

CLINICAL PEARL

Diabetes accelerates the natural course of atherosclerosis and is associated with a two- to fourfold increase in risk for LEAD.

The pathogenesis of diabetes-related atherosclerosis is complex and multifactorial. Hyperglycemia and insulin resistance play key roles in the development of atherosclerosis through mechanisms associated with overproduction of reactive oxygen species (ROS), which contributes to endothelial dysfunction and development of a proinflammatory and prothrombotic state contributing to atherosclerosis (Paneni et al., 2013). Chronic hyperglycemia is believed to be a primary factor in development of microvascular disease, but macrovascular disease is most likely caused by the combined effects of hyperglycemia, dyslipidemia, and hypertension (Jalili, 2011).

CLINICAL PEARL

Chronic hyperglycemia is thought to be a primary factor in development of microvascular disease; macrovascular disease is most likely caused by the combined effects of hyperglycemia, dyslipidemia, and hypertension.

Dyslipidemia

Abnormal lipid levels (i.e., elevated total cholesterol, low-density lipoprotein [LDL] cholesterol, and triglycerides and decreased high-density lipoprotein [HDL] cholesterol) play an important role in atherosclerosis and LEAD (WOCN, 2014). For example, there is a 10% increase in the risk of LEAD for each 10 mg per dL rise in total cholesterol (Hirsch et al., 2006). In contrast, Hussein and colleagues (2011) reported that LDL levels <70 mg/dL were associated with decreased progression and significantly less volume of atheroma ($p < 0.001$) in patients with and without LEAD. The American Heart Association (AHA, 2012) recommends the following for heart health: total cholesterol <200 mg/dL, HDL cholesterol equal to or greater than 60 mg/dL, LDL cholesterol <100 mg/dL (<70 mg/dL in individuals at very high risk), and triglyceride level <150 mg/dL.

CLINICAL PEARL

The AHA recommends the following lipid levels for heart health: total cholesterol <200 mg/dL; HDL cholesterol ≥60 mg/dL; LDL cholesterol ≤100 mg/dL, and triglyceride <150 mg/dL.

Hypertension

Hypertension (i.e., systolic blood pressure >140 mm Hg and/or diastolic blood pressure >90 mm Hg) has been associated with a two- to threefold increased risk for LEAD (Norgren et al., 2007) and is found in 52% to 90% of individuals with LEAD (Goessens et al., 2006; Selvin & Erlinger, 2004; Tekin et al., 2011). One prospective study of 39,260 women with LEAD (mean age ≥45 years) found a 43% increase in the adjusted risk for LEAD per each 10 mm Hg increment in systolic BP (Powell et al., 2011). Although a high prevalence of hypertension has been shown in patients with LEAD, evidence is lacking regarding the benefits of BP reduction on LEAD (WOCN, 2014).

Age

The risk of LEAD increases with age, affecting 30% of individuals older than 70 years of age and 40% of those 80 years of age and older (Bergiers et al., 2011; Bozkurt et al., 2011; Garofolo et al., 2007). LEAD in individuals <60 years of age (also known as premature LEAD) is associated with significant cardiovascular morbidity and increased risk of limb loss; in this population, the primary risk factors are reported as tobacco use, diabetes, chronic kidney disease, hypertension, elevated homocysteine levels, coronary artery disease, and elevated fibrinogen (Hirsch et al., 2006; Lane et al., 2006).

CLINICAL PEARL

LEAD affects 30% of individuals >70 years of age and 40% of those >80 years of age.

Chronic Kidney Disease

Chronic kidney disease affects approximately 13% of adults in the United States and is strongly associated with risk for LEAD, adverse cardiovascular events, and increased morbidity and mortality, particularly for individuals on dialysis (Ix et al., 2009; Tanaka et al., 2011). Coll and colleagues (2010) found that 84% of 409 patients with CKD or on dialysis had LEAD (ABI < 0.90), and 15.6% had an ABI > 1.41. Also, Ohtake and colleagues (2011) reported that 46 of 97 (47%) patients on dialysis had LEAD and 11 (11.3%) had critical limb ischemia (CLI). LEAD is also associated with higher mortality rates in patients with CKD; Otsubo and colleagues (2012) reviewed almost 9 years of data from 86 patients on hemodialysis (>60 years of age) and documented a survival rate of 29% in patients with LEAD versus 62% in those without LEAD.

Elevated Homocysteine Levels

Elevated homocysteine levels have been associated with increased risk for major cardiac events and for LEAD and are reported to be present in 30% to 40% of persons with LEAD (Cheng et al., 2009; Dunkelgrun et al., 2009; Hirsch et al., 2006; Veeranna et al., 2011; WOCN, 2014). It is believed that homocysteine, an amino acid produced by the body, is toxic to vascular endothelial cells (Dunkelgrun et al., 2009). However, treatment to lower homocysteine levels (with folic acid and vitamin B_{12}) remains controversial because lowering homocysteine levels has not reduced the incidence of atherosclerotic disease (Rooke et al., 2011).

Family History

A family history of cardiovascular disease is associated with an almost twofold increased risk for LEAD (Wassel et al., 2011). In a study of twins, individuals who had an identical twin with LEAD were at three times higher risk for LEAD than nonidentical twins (Wahlgren & Magnusson, 2011). Genetic factors accounted for 58% of the variance in risk among the twins and nonshared environmental factors accounted for 42%, suggesting that genetics play a key role in the development of LEAD.

Ethnicity

Studies have shown that Black individuals have a higher risk of LEAD compared to individuals who are White (Ix et al., 2008) or Hispanic (Allison et al., 2010b) and similar rates to South Asians (Bennett et al., 2010). However, a study of individuals with heart failure in Louisiana and Florida found that the prevalence of LEAD in White individuals was 26% compared to 14% for Black individuals and 13% for Hispanic individuals (Hebert et al., 2010); thus, the impact of ethnicity remains unclear.

Inflammation and Infection

Chronic inflammation and infection are believed to contribute to the development of atherosclerosis. However, the specific role of infectious and inflammatory agents remains uncertain (Berger et al., 2011; Watson & Alp, 2008).

Chlamydia pneumoniae

Chlamydia pneumoniae has been associated with LEAD in several older studies (Bloemenkamp et al., 2002; Freidank et al., 2002; Kaperonis et al., 2006; Krayenbuehl et al., 2005; Linares-Palomino et al., 2004; Signorelli et al., 2006, 2010; Ustunsoy et al., 2007; Wiesli et al., 2002). In a later study, Al-Bannawi and colleagues (2011) reported that proinflammatory chemokines played a key role in the development of atherosclerosis, and *C. pneumoniae* was a triggering agent. However, there are contradictory reports regarding the benefits of treatment (Jaff et al., 2009; Joensen et al., 2008; Vainas et al., 2005); thus, more research is needed to determine the specific role of *C. pneumoniae* and the implications for interventions.

CLINICAL PEARL

Chronic inflammation and infection are believed to contribute to the development of atherosclerotic disease although the specific role remains unclear.

Periodontal Disease

An association between periodontal disease and atherosclerotic vascular disease has been demonstrated in multiple observational studies, but a causal relationship or benefits of periodontal interventions have not been demonstrated (Hung et al., 2003; Lockhart et al., 2012; Lu et al., 2008; Soto-Barreras et al., 2013). Further research is needed to determine if a causal relationship exists between periodontal disease and LEAD and if treatment of periodontal disease is effective in preventing or diminishing the development or progression of atherosclerosis.

Biomarkers of Inflammation, Hypercoagulability and Vascular Calcification

Multiple investigators have found that individuals with LEAD have high levels of inflammatory proteins and thrombotic biomarkers. Elevated C-reactive protein, a marker of inflammation, has been found to be an independent risk factor for cardiovascular disease and LEAD, and levels >3.0 mg/L are associated with high risk for cardiovascular disease (Aboyans et al., 2006; Dhangana et al., 2011; Hogh et al., 2008; Khawaja et al., 2007; Schlager et al., 2009). In addition, studies have shown high levels of interleukins (IL-1, IL-6, IL-10, IL-13) in patients with LEAD and CLI (Chaparala et al., 2009; McDermott et al., 2005, 2008), and elevated levels of the proinflammatory enzyme myeloperoxidase have been associated with LEAD and increased risk of major cardiovascular events (Ali et al., 2009; Brevetti et al., 2008; Haslacher et al., 2012). All of these findings support the hypothesis that inflammation is a contributing factor to LEAD.

Hypercoagulability is also likely to play a role in LEAD, and recent studies demonstrate a positive association between markers of hypercoagulability and LEAD. For example, fibrinogen plays a key role in blood clot formation, platelet aggregation, inflammation, and blood viscosity (Khaleghi et al., 2009), and high levels of fibrinogen (>400 mg/dL) have been associated with an increased prevalence of LEAD (Dhangana et al., 2011; Khaleghi et al., 2009; Khawaja et al., 2007). High levels of D-dimer (formed by breakdown of the fibrin component of blood clots) are also associated with LEAD and increased mortality (Khaleghi et al., 2009; McDermott et al., 2008; Vidula et al., 2008).

Markers of vascular calcification (glycoproteins osteoprotegerin and fetuin-A) have also been associated with LEAD (Mogelvang et al., 2012; Szeberin et al., 2011). High concentrations of osteoprotegerin have been associated with increased risk of LEAD, coronary artery atherosclerosis, and hypertension (Mogelvang et al., 2012). Low levels of fetuin-A have been associated with the severity of arterial calcifications in patients with LEAD, which suggests that fetuin-A may play an important role in inhibiting arterial calcification (Szeberin et al., 2011).

Clinical Implications of Biomarkers

The specific clinical implications of biomarkers for screening and/or treatment of LEAD remain unclear, and routine measurement of these biomarkers is not currently recommended (Berger et al., 2011; Brevetti et al., 2010). Further studies are necessary to determine whether these novel biomarkers provide any additional prognostic information over the traditional measures of risks such as lipid levels.

 Assessment and Diagnosis

History

It is essential to identify the presence/absence of LEAD for any patient with a lower-extremity wound to guide treatment, evaluate the potential for healing, and determine the need for referrals for additional vascular testing, surgical interventions, or adjunctive therapies (WOCN, 2014). It is important to differentiate wounds due to LEAD from other etiologies, which require different management strategies. Risks, contributing factors, and coexisting problems that may complicate the care and management of the patient should be identified. Due to the systemic effects of atherosclerosis, a history of cardiovascular or cerebrovascular disease or surgeries should be determined (Subramaniam et al., 2011; Tekin et al., 2011).

Several diseases and conditions have been shown to coexist or be associated with LEAD.

In multiple studies, atherosclerosis and an increased prevalence of LEAD have been found in patients with rheumatoid arthritis (Stamatelopoulos et al., 2010), spinal cord injury (Bell et al., 2011), migraines (Jurno et al., 2010), atrial fibrillation (Masanauskiene & Naudziunas, 2011), human immunodeficiency virus (Palacios et al., 2008), and low testosterone (Tivesten et al., 2007). Patients with sickle cell disease have leg wounds that often are confused with wounds due to LEAD or venous disease. In sickle cell anemia, the abnormally shaped red blood cells (RBC) clump together and cause occlusion of the vessels, which can result in ischemia and chronic leg wounds, particularly in males (Madu et al., 2013). These ulcers are discussed further in Chapter 25.

Obesity (body mass index [BMI] > 30 kg/m^2) and metabolic syndrome (MetS) are also associated with LEAD. An observational study found that for each 5-unit increase in BMI (i.e., per 5 kg/m^2), there was a 30% greater prevalence of LEAD and adverse clinical events (Ix et al., 2011). Adults in the United States with MetS (i.e., altered glucose and insulin metabolism, abdominal obesity, abnormal lipid levels, hypertension) have been reported to have almost twice the risk of LEAD (Sumner et al., 2012), and the reported prevalence of MetS in patients with LEAD ranges from 24% to 60% (Cang et al., 2012; Maksimovic et al., 2009). Even more significantly, 97% of individuals with advanced claudication or CLI also have MetS (Qadan et al., 2008). Although the effects of obesity and MetS are documented, we currently lack data regarding the effects of weight/BMI reduction on LEAD.

CLINICAL PEARL

Obesity and metabolic syndrome are associated with increased risk for LEAD.

A history of alcohol use should also be determined. In one study, consumption of moderate to high levels of alcohol was associated with asymptomatic LEAD (Sana et al., 2011). However, two other studies found that moderate alcohol consumption (i.e., 1 to 13 drinks per week of beer, wine, or liquor) by patients with LEAD was associated with less decline in ABI, a lower risk of hospitalization for LEAD, and lower risk of mortality compared to abstainers (Garcia et al., 2011; Mukamal et al., 2008). Heavier drinking (i.e., >14 drinks per week) did not lower the risks.

LEAD has been associated with decreased walking endurance and performance (McDermott et al., 2010a), and limited exercise capacity in patients with LEAD has been associated with increased mortality (Gardner et al., 2008; Jain et al., 2012; Leeper et al., 2013). Therefore, the history should include a review of the patient's functional ability, limitations in ambulation and physical activity, and whether walking aids are required. Ischemia can negatively affect lower-extremity nerves, and studies have documented impaired muscle function due to reduced sural and peroneal nerve function (McDermott et al., 2004; McDermott et al., 2006); thus, the patient should be queried regarding signs and symptoms of neuropathy (e.g., decreased sensation, weakness of the ankles or feet, gait abnormalities, foot drop/foot drag). Additionally, it is important to obtain a history of all prescribed and over-the-counter medications. The review should include previous and current medication use (e.g., vasodilators, anticoagulants, antiplatelets, statins, analgesics, diuretics, herbal products).

CLINICAL PEARL

Ischemia can negatively affect nerve function; therefore, patients with LEAD should be screened for evidence of neuropathy.

Pain History

A detailed pain history is essential and should include the location, type, and characteristics of pain; exacerbating and alleviating factors; onset and duration; and use and effectiveness of analgesics. Also, it is important to determine if a painful wound is present.

The location of pain may indicate the location of stenosis or occlusion; pain typically occurs one joint below the site of the stenosis or occlusion (Doughty, 2012; Rumwell & McPharlin, 2009). Pain in the buttock indicates aortoiliac disease and suggests iliofemoral disease if the symptoms are unilateral. Pain in the thigh indicates distal external iliac/common femoral disease. Pain in the calf indicates femoral/popliteal disease, and pain localized to the foot indicates infrapopliteal disease.

Intermittent Claudication

The classic type of pain associated with LEAD is intermittent claudication, which occurs with approximately 50% occlusion of the vessel (Doughty, 2012). Intermittent claudication is defined as reproducible pain that is brought on by exercise such as walking. Claudication may be described as cramping, aching, fatigue, weakness, and/or pain in the buttock, thigh, or calf muscles (rarely the foot) that is relieved with approximately 10 minutes' rest (Doughty, 2012; Hirsch et al., 2006). However, it is estimated that only one third of patients with LEAD report intermittent claudication (Aponte, 2011; Hopf et al., 2008); it is important for health care providers to understand that persons with LEAD may not recognize and report the classic symptoms of claudication because they might limit their ambulation or activities to avoid leg pain or may have other comorbid conditions that limit their activities. Some individuals mistakenly believe their symptoms are due to aging. Also, the symptoms of claudication can be confused with pain due to other conditions such as arthritis, intervertebral disc disease, or spinal stenosis (Armstrong et al., 2010; Doughty, 2012; Lau et al., 2011). Finally, patients with impaired sensation due to neuropathy might not experience the classic claudication symptoms (Hopf et al., 2008).

CLINICAL PEARL

The type of pain most often associated with LEAD is intermittent claudication, which is defined as reproducible pain that is brought on by walking or similar activity and relieved by rest.

Positional and Rest Pain

As the severity of LEAD progresses, patients may experience positional or resting pain in the absence of walking or activity. Positional pain occurs when the legs are elevated and diminishes when the legs are placed in a dependent position (Doughty, 2012). Rest pain occurs in the absence of activity, most typically at night when the patient is supine or in bed, and the legs are not in a dependent position. Often, patients will dangle their leg(s) over the side of the bed or sit up in a chair in an effort to relieve ischemic pain; many patients report routinely sleeping in a recliner with their legs down. With very advanced LEAD, the pain can become continuous even with the legs in a dependent position. Ischemic rest pain is commonly localized in the distal part of the foot and toes (Rumwell & McPharlin, 2009) and is associated with >90% vessel occlusion (Doughty, 2012).

CLINICAL PEARL

Advanced LEAD is manifest by positional pain (pain with elevation) and eventually pain that persists even when the leg is dependent (rest pain); rest pain is associated with >90% vessel occlusion.

Differentiation Acute versus Critical Limb Ischemia

Assessment of the onset and duration of pain is necessary to differentiate acute from chronic limb ischemia. Acute limb ischemia is due to a sudden occlusion from a thrombus, embolism, or trauma (Rumwell & McPharlin, 2009). The hallmark signs of an acute limb-threatening occlusion are the sudden onset of the six "Ps": pulselessness, pain, pallor, paresthesia, paralysis, and polar/coldness (Rumwell & McPharlin, 2009; WOCN, 2014). Rumwell and McPharlin (2009) suggest including a seventh "P" for the purplish, cyanotic color seen in patients with acute occlusions. Findings should be compared to the contralateral limb. An immediate referral for a vascular surgical evaluation and intervention is indicated for patients with signs and symptoms of acute limb ischemia (Rumwell & McPharlin, 2009; WOCN, 2014).

CLINICAL PEARL

The hallmark signs of acute limb-threatening occlusion are sudden onset of the six "Ps": pulselessness, pain, pallor, paresthesia, paralysis, and polar (coldness).

CLI refers to patients with objectively proven arterial occlusive disease and chronic ischemic rest pain, wounds, or gangrene that, if untreated, would require a major amputation in 6 months (Hirsch et al., 2006; Norgren et al., 2007). CLI represents the end stage of LEAD and most often is due to multilevel, occlusive disease (Becker et al., 2011). It is estimated that CLI occurs in 1% to 3% of individuals with LEAD (Bunte & Shishehbor, 2013; Varu et al., 2010). The body's initial response to limb ischemia usually involves the development of collateral vessels through angiogenesis, with the goal of increasing blood flow to adequate levels. However, the patient with advanced LEAD lacks the blood flow and oxygen delivery required for support of neoangiogenesis, even with maximal dilation of the stenosed and damaged vessels (Varu et al., 2010). Chronic ischemia is associated with multiple changes in the microvasculature, endothelial dysfunction, and microthrombi formation, all of which impede oxygen exchange at the capillary level (Varu et al., 2010).

CLINICAL PEARL

CLI is defined as objectively proven LEAD (ABI < 0.4) and rest pain, wounds, or gangrene; CLI is associated with a high mortality rate.

It is important to validate the clinical diagnosis of CLI with objective data such as the following: ankle systolic pressure <50 mm Hg, ABI 0.40 or less, toe pressure (TP) <30 mm Hg (<50 mm Hg with diabetes), or transcutaneous oxygen ($TcPO_2$) <30 mm Hg (Hirsch et al., 2006; Hopf et al., 2008; Norgren et al., 2007). Half of the individuals with CLI require revascularization for limb salvage (Becker et al., 2011; Hirsch et al., 2006), and 30% of patients undergo a major amputation within 1 year following the diagnosis of CLI (Bunte & Shishehbor, 2013). CLI is associated with a high mortality rate: 20% or higher in the first year (Hirsch et al., 2006), and 70% in 5 years (Sultan et al., 2011). Due to the high morbidity and mortality, timely referral to a vascular surgical specialist is required for patients with signs and symptoms of CLI (WOCN, 2014).

Wound History

The history of a current or previous wound should include a description of the onset and precipitating factors, course (e.g., improvement/regression), duration, and prior treatment regimens and their effectiveness. Ischemia should be suspected in patients with lower-extremity wounds that do not heal despite proper management.

Laboratory Tests

A review of available laboratory tests can provide relevant information about risk factors for LEAD and the effectiveness of current interventions (e.g., cholesterol, triglycerides, homocysteine). While not specific to LEAD, other tests such as hemoglobin and hematocrit, prothrombin time, and international normalized ratio (INR) for patients on anticoagulants (e.g., warfarin) provide valuable information for patient management (WOCN, 2014). Although the values can be affected by numerous conditions, assessment of albumin or prealbumin may provide information about nutritional deficiencies that contribute to impaired wound healing. Routine monitoring of hemoglobin A1c (HbA_{1c}) and blood sugar levels is also indicated for individuals with LEAD and diabetes (Hopf et al., 2008). If nonhealing wounds are present and infection is suspected, a white blood cell count is warranted.

Psychosocial/Environmental Factors

It is important for health care providers to determine the psychological, sociological, and environmental factors that affect patients and their quality of life (e.g., self-care ability, availability of caretakers, length of illness, employment, recreational activity). An area that is often overlooked in patients with LEAD is depression, which can impact the patient's prognosis and quality of life. Smolderen and colleagues (2008) reported that 16% of 166 patients with LEAD had clinical depression that was associated with pain and impaired walking, and they suggested that health care workers make a greater effort to identify depression in patients with LEAD.

Lower-Extremity Assessment

A comprehensive examination of both lower extremities should be performed on any patient with or at risk for wounds due to LEAD to determine skin and tissue integrity, sensation, and peripheral circulatory status. It is necessary to examine both limbs because LEAD is often asymptomatic and may not be confined to one limb. A thorough assessment provides the foundational data required for correctly managing the patient and evaluating the effectiveness of therapeutic interventions (Bonham & Kelechi, 2008).

CLINICAL PEARL

The physical examination of a patient with LEAD must include both legs, since the disease process is often asymptomatic and may not be confined to one leg.

Status of Skin and Tissue

After removing the patient's shoes and any hosiery or compression devices, the nurse should carefully examine the lower limbs and feet (i.e., toes and skin between the toes, nails, and heels) for signs of ischemia, injury, or wounds; findings from each limb should then be compared. Footwear should also be assessed for fit. See **Table 22-1** for common clinical characteristics and skin changes in ischemic limbs.

Individuals with LEAD are at increased risk for developing pressure ulcers involving the heels or malleoli due to decreased perfusion; thus, individuals with limited mobility (e.g., bed/chair bound) should be assessed two to three times per day for evidence of early ischemic damage involving the heel or other bony prominences of the foot (Langemo et al., 2008). The heel is at particular risk due to the limited subcutaneous tissue and muscle and the limited blood supply to the skin (Bangova, 2013; Gefen, 2010). Meaume and Faucher (2007) reported that the

TABLE 22-1 Common Clinical Characteristics and Skin Changes in Ischemic Limbs

Clinical Characteristic	Common Skin and Limb Changes in Ischemia
Color	• Pallor on elevation of legs • Rubor (purplish red color) in dependent position
Temperature	• Skin feels cool to touch
Texture/turgor	• Shiny, taut, and dry skin • Thin, fragile skin • Atrophy of skin, subcutaneous tissue, and muscle
Capillary refill	• Delayed capillary refill (i.e., more than 3 s), which can be affected by environmental temperature
Venous refill	• Prolonged venous refill time (i.e., more than 20 s)
Nails	• Abnormal nails (thin and ridged)
Hair	• Minimal or absent hair
Sensation	• Paresthesia

Adapted with permission from Wound, Ostomy and Continence Nurses Society. (2014). *Guideline for management of wounds in patients with lower-extremity arterial disease. WOCN clinical practice guideline series1* (p. 46). Mt. Laurel, NJ: Author.

prevalence of LEAD did not differ between hospitalized patients with and without heel pressure ulcers (58% and 57%, respectively); however, pressure ulcer severity was greater among the individuals with LEAD. In a study of 84 patients in a nursing home with heel PrU, Clegg and colleagues (2009) reported that LEAD was present in 24 (39%). Because LEAD can be a significant contributing factor to heel PrU, vascular assessment (i.e., examination of pedal pulses and ABI) is indicated for individuals with PrU on the heel, foot, or lower limb (Ousey, 2009).

CLINICAL PEARL

Individuals with LEAD and limited mobility are at increased risk for pressure ulcers involving the heels and malleoli.

Sensory Status

The sensory status of both limbs should be assessed using simple noninvasive tests. Patients with LEAD may have neuropathy due to the impact of ischemia on peripheral nerve function; thus, patients should be screened for loss of protective sensation in the feet (Hopf et al., 2008; McDermott et al., 2006). Loss of protective sensation can be quickly determined by testing the feet with a 5.07/10 g Semmes-Weinstein monofilament, assessing vibratory sensation with a tuning fork (128 Hz), and testing ankle reflexes (WOCN, 2012, 2014). The inability to feel the pressure of the monofilament on one or more anatomic sites on the plantar and dorsal surface of the foot indicates a loss of protective sensation: At least four plantar sites should be tested to include the first, third, and fifth metatarsal head and distal great toe (WOCN, 2012). It is recommended to test the vibratory sensation over the base of the great toe at the first metatarsal bone; an abnormal response is when the patient loses the vibratory sensation while it is still felt by the examiner (WOCN, 2012). It is also helpful to check deep tendon reflexes on the ankle by stretching the Achilles tendon until the foot is in a neutral position and striking the tendon with a percussion hammer, which should result in plantar flexion of the foot. Total absence of the ankle reflex is an abnormal result indicating impaired motor nerve function (WOCN, 2012).

Pulses

The most common approach to assessment of perfusion status is pulse palpation, which includes palpation of the dorsalis pedis (DP) on the dorsum of each foot and the posterior tibial pulse on the medial aspect of the limb behind the ankle. See Figure 22-3 for location of pedal pulses. It is important to keep the room warm during pulse palpation to prevent vasoconstriction. It is recommended to assess and record the intensity of the pulse as: 0—absent, 1—diminished, 2—normal, and 3—bounding (Hirsch et al., 2006; WOCN, 2014). It is important to recognize that the presence of palpable pulses does not rule out arterial disease, because a palpable pulse does not provide an accurate indicator of vessel health and volume of blood flow. (In addition, clinicians may actually be feeling their own pulses rather than the pedal pulse of the patient.) Similarly, an absent pulse, alone, is not a sensitive indicator of LEAD because 4% to 12% of individuals have congenitally absent DP arteries (Collins et al., 2006; Criqui et al., 1985). The importance of conducting a comprehensive assessment and not relying simply on pulse palpation is underscored by the findings of Bozkurt and colleagues (2011), who evaluated 530 individuals with both pulse

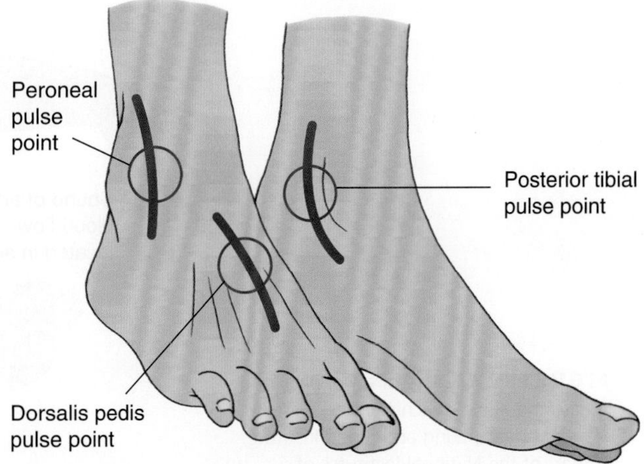

FIGURE 22-3. Location of pedal pulses: peroneal, dorsalis pedis, and posterior tibial. (Reprinted with permission from Weber, J., & Kelley, J. (2003). *Health assessment in nursing* (2nd ed.). Philadelphia, PA: Lippincott Williams & Wilkins.)

assessment and ABI. The investigators reported 6.5% were determined to have LEAD when absence of palpable pulses was the only diagnostic criterion, whereas the true prevalence was 20% as confirmed by ABI.

CLINICAL PEARL

Palpation of pedal pulses is an important component of the physical assessment; however, presence of palpable pulses does not rule out arterial disease, and the absence of a pedal pulse is not in and of itself a sensitive indicator of LEAD.

Femoral and popliteal arteries can be auscultated for bruits using the bell of a stethoscope; bruits are indicative of turbulent blood flow through stenotic vessels (Khan et al., 2006; Rumwell & McPharlin, 2009). However, bruits are low-frequency sounds and may not always be detected.

Noninvasive Assessment/Diagnostic Techniques

Because of the unreliability of pulse palpation and a history of claudication, additional tests using noninvasive techniques are needed to detect the presence and severity of LEAD. Several noninvasive, portable testing methods are available that can be used at the bedside to assess perfusion status including the ABI, TPs or toe–brachial index (TBI), and transcutaneous oxygen tension ($TcPO_2$).

Ankle Brachial Index (ABI)

One of the most commonly used noninvasive tests is the ABI, which provides an indirect assessment of arterial blood flow in the lower limbs by comparing the brachial systolic pressure to the systolic pressure at the ankle. ABI is recommended as a first-line, noninvasive test to establish a diagnosis in individuals at high risk or suspected of having LEAD such as individuals who have leg pain with walking, have nonhealing wounds, are 65 years of age or older, or are 50 years of age or older with a history of smoking or diabetes (Rooke et al., 2011).

CLINICAL PEARL

ABI is recommended as a first-line noninvasive test for individuals at risk for or suspected of having LEAD.

Measurement of ABI Using Continuous-Wave Doppler

The ABI should be tested bilaterally because LEAD may not develop or progress in the same manner in both limbs (Aboyans et al., 2012). An ABI is obtained by measuring the brachial systolic pressures in both arms and the DP and posterior tibial arteries (PT) in both ankles (Fig. 22-4). Doppler technique is the preferred method for measuring the arm and ankle pressures for the ABI (Aboyans et al., 2012; Kim et al., 2012; Nicolai et al., 2009; WOCN, 2014; Xu et al., 2010), because it is more accurate in measurement of low blood pressures than other methods using automated/oscillometric devices (Korna et al., 2009; Verbeck et al., 2012), stethoscope (Carmo et al., 2009), or pulse palpation (Aboyans et al., 2008; Akhtar et al., 2009).

Doppler ultrasound waveforms reflect the velocity of RBC passing through the vessel (Bonham & Kelechi, 2008).

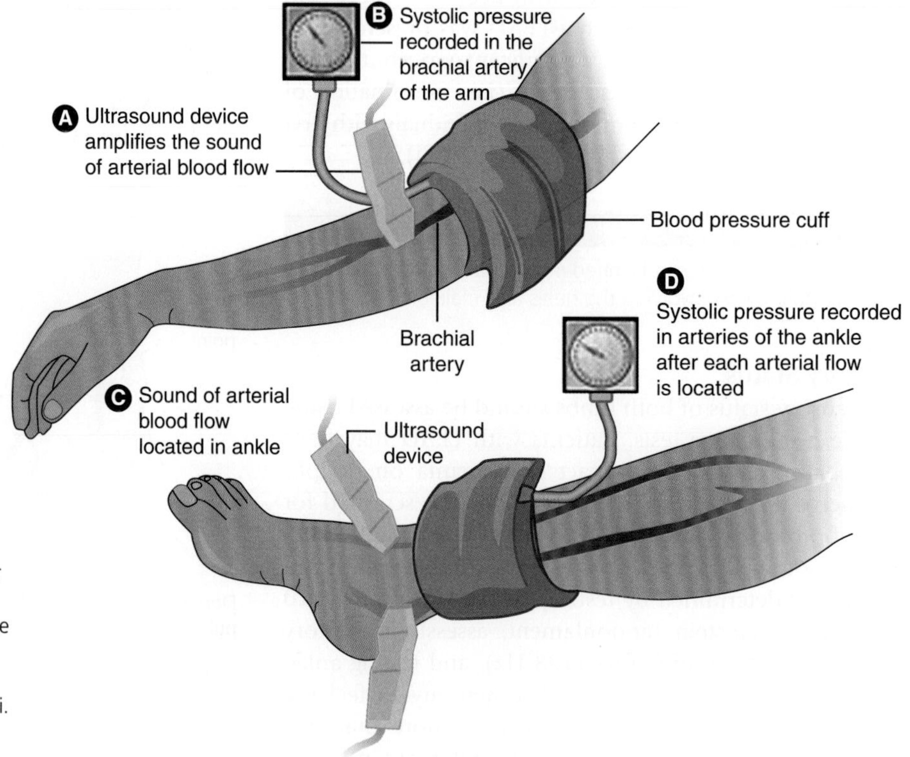

FIGURE 22-4. Use of a Doppler for measuring ankle–brachial index. (From National Heart, Lung and Blood Institute as part of the National Institutes of Health and the U.S. Department of Health and Human Services, www.nhlbi.nih.gov/health/dci/Diseases/pad/paddiagnsis.html)

Blood flow through a normal pedal vessel produces a triphasic waveform and a pressure comparable to brachial pressures, but if the pedal artery is stenosed or occluded, fewer RBCs pass through and the wave form is blunted (either biphasic or monophasic) depending on the severity of occlusion (Doughty, 2012; Rumwell & McPharlin, 2009). Pressures obtained from damaged vessels are typically lower than the brachial pressures. The exception is a vessel that is very rigid and therefore poorly compressible or noncompressible; these vessels generate pressures that are higher than the brachial pressures (Rumwell & McPharlin, 2009).

The Doppler-derived ABI is 94% sensitive and 99% specific, compared to arteriographically diagnosed disease (Dieter et al., 2003; Ouriel & Zarins, 1982; Yao et al., 1969), and studies have shown that ABIs measured with pocket Dopplers are interchangeable with ABIs measured in the vascular laboratory (Bonham et al., 2007; Nicolai et al., 2008). See **Table 22-2** for the recommended procedure for measuring and calculating the ABI with a continuous-wave Doppler.

TABLE 22-2 Procedure for Measuring and Calculating the ABI

Action	Procedure
Prepare equipment and supplies	1. Gather equipment and supplies for the ABI. • Portable continuous wave Doppler with 8- to 10-MHz probe (5 MHz if a large amount of edema is present at the ankle) • Aneroid sphygmomanometer and pressure cuff • Ultrasound transmission gel • Alcohol pads to clean the Doppler and gauze, tissue, or pads to remove the transmission gel from the patient's skin • Towels, sheets, or blankets to cover the trunk and extremities • Paper and pen for recording test results; calculator • Inspect the equipment and check the batteries if a battery-operated Doppler is used and replace equipment that is damaged or not calibrated 2. Pressure cuffs for arms and ankles should be long enough to fully encircle the limb. The width of the cuff's bladder should be 40% of the limb's circumference and the length sufficient to cover 80% of the limb's circumference. • Typically, 12-cm-wide cuffs are used for arms and 10 cm wide cuffs at the ankles. • Extralarge adult cuffs might be needed (14 cm).
Prepare patient and environment	1. Inquire about recent use of tobacco, caffeine, or alcohol; recent heavy activity; and presence of pain. Note: When possible, advise the patient to avoid stimulants or heavy exercise for an hour prior to the test. 2. Perform the ABI in a quiet, warm environment to prevent vasoconstriction of the arteries (21°C to 23°C ± 1°C). 3. The best ABI results are obtained when the patient is relaxed, comfortable, and has an empty bladder. 4. Explain the procedure to the patient. 5. Remove shoes, socks, and tight clothing to permit placement of the pressure cuff and access to the pulse sites by the Doppler probe. 6. Place the patient in a flat, supine position. Place one small pillow behind the patient's head for comfort. 7. Cover the trunk and extremities to prevent cooling. 8. Ensure the patient is comfortable and have the patient rest for a minimum of 10 min prior to the test to allow pressures to normalize. 9. After the rest period, measure the arm and ankle pressures.
Measure brachial pressures with Doppler	1. The arm should be relaxed, supported, and at heart level. 2. Prior to placement of the cuff, apply a protective barrier (e.g., plastic wrap) on the extremity if any wounds or alterations in skin integrity are present. 3. Place the pressure cuff with the bottom of the cuff approximately 2 to 3 cm above the cubital fossa on the arm. 4. The cuff should be wrapped without wrinkles and placed securely to prevent slipping and movement during the test. 5. Palpate the brachial pulse to determine the location to obtain an audible pulse. 6. Apply transmission gel over the pulse site. 7. Place the tip of the Doppler probe at a 45 degrees angle pointed toward the patient's head until an audible pulse signal is obtained. 8. Inflate the pressure cuff 20 to 30 mm Hg above the point where the pulse is no longer audible. 9. Deflate the pressure cuff at a rate of 2 to 3 mm Hg per second, noting the manometer reading at which the first pulse signal is heard and record that systolic value. 10. Cleanse/remove gel from the pulse site. 11. Repeat the procedure to measure the pressure on the other arm. 12. If a pressure needs to be repeated, wait 1 min before reinflating the cuff. 13. Use the higher of the brachial pressures from the right or left arm to calculate the ABI for both legs.

(Continued)

TABLE 22-2 Procedure for Measuring and Calculating the ABI (*Continued*)

Action	Procedure
Measure ankle pressures with Doppler	1. Prior to placing the cuff, apply a protective barrier (e.g., plastic wrap) on the extremity if there are any wounds or alterations in skin integrity. 2. Place the cuff on the patient's lower leg with the bottom of the cuff approximately 2 to 3 cm above the malleolus. 3. The cuff should be wrapped without wrinkles and placed securely to prevent slipping and movement during the test. 4. Measure both dorsalis pedis and posterior tibial pulses on each leg. 5. Locate the pulses by palpation or with the Doppler probe. 6. Apply transmission gel to the pulse site. 7. Place the tip of the Doppler probe at a 45° angle pointed toward the patient's knee until an audible pulse signal is obtained. 8. Inflate the pressure cuff 20 to 30 mm Hg above the point where the pulse is no longer audible. 9. Deflate the cuff slowly at a rate of 2 to 3 mm Hg per second noting the manometer reading at which the first pulse signal is heard and record that systolic value. 10. Cleanse/remove gel from the pulse site. 11. Repeat the procedure to measure pressures on the other ankle. 12. If a pressure needs to be repeated, wait 1 min before reinflating the cuff. 13. Use the higher of the ankle pressures of each leg to calculate the ABI for each leg.
Calculate the ABI	1. Divide the higher of the dorsalis pedis or posterior tibial systolic pressure for each ankle by the higher of the right or left brachial pressures to obtain the ABI for each leg. $$\text{ABI} = \frac{\text{Higher of either the dorsalis pedis or posterior tibial pressures}}{\text{Higher of the brachial pressures}}$$ 2. Interpret and compare the ABI values from each leg (see Table 22-3). 3. Refer the patient for further testing and evaluation if the ABI is < 0.90, >1.30, or unmeasurable due to noncompressible vessels and/or if the patient's clinical symptoms and ABI are inconsistent. 4. Document findings, follow-up plans, and referrals.

Adapted with permission from Wound, Ostomy and Continence Nurses Society. (2011). *Ankle brachial index: Quick reference guide for clinicians*. Mt. Laurel, NJ: Author.

CLINICAL PEARL

Doppler-derived ABI measurements have been shown to have 94% sensitivity and 99% specificity when compared to arteriographically diagnosed arterial disease.

The ABI is a ratio calculated by dividing the higher of the ankle pressures (DP or PT) for each leg by the higher of the brachial pressures from the right or left arm (Rumwell & McPharlin, 2009; WOCN, 2011a). When calculating ABI, the higher of the ankle pressures is preferred to minimize the overdiagnosis of LEAD in healthy individuals (Aboyans et al., 2012). Using the highest ankle pressure avoids overdiagnosis because both ankle arteries must have clinically significant disease for the ABI to be 0.90 or less, whereas only one of the ankle arteries must have significant disease if the lowest ankle pressure is used (Allison, et al., 2010a).

ABI Limitations

The ABI is an indirect test for large vessel arterial disease, and it cannot be used to determine the anatomic location of a stenotic/occlusive lesion (Rumwell & McPharlin, 2009). In addition, severe vessel calcification renders the ABI ineffective; it is common to obtain elevated (>1.30) readings when the vessels are rigid and calcified, and if the vessels are extremely rigid, it is impossible to compress the vessels enough to obtain a systolic pressure measurement. Conditions in which vessel calcification is common include diabetes, renal insufficiency, and rheumatoid arthritis (Brooks et al., 2001; del Rincon et al., 2005; O'Hare et al., 2004; Silvestro et al., 2006; Stein et al., 2006). There is also concern that in patients with some degree of calcification, the ABI may underestimate LEAD due to the possibility that mild to moderate calcification may affect the pressure measurement even though the artery can be compressed and the systolic blood pressure can be measured (Aerden et al., 2011). It is important to recognize high ABI levels because an ABI > 1.40 predicts cardiovascular risk, cardiac events, and mortality with similar strength to an ABI < 0.90 (Aboyans et al., 2012; Criqui et al., 2010; Fowkes et al., 2008; Resnick et al., 2004). A high ABI (>1.40) has also been found to be more strongly associated with stroke than low ABI (Criqui et al., 2010).

CLINICAL PEARL

There are concerns that ABI may underestimate LEAD in patients with some degree of vessel calcification, since this may affect the pressure measurement even though the artery can be compressed and a systolic pressure can be obtained.

We lack the data to identify a specific level of arterial calcification that correlates definitively with vessel rigidity, occlusion, stenosis, or ABI values. The distinction between an elevated ABI and noncompressible vessels (i.e., an unmeasurable ABI) has not been clearly differentiated in most studies, and it is unclear if the two findings have equivalent clinical significance. For example, if the pulse signal can be obliterated with inflation of the pressure cuff and the return of the pulse signal detected upon deflation of the cuff, the ABI may be high but is measurable. In contrast, if the pulse signal cannot be obliterated at high cuff pressures (>250 mm Hg) or detected with cuff deflation, the ABI is unmeasurable due to noncompressible arteries (Criqui et al., 2010).

It is important to realize that some individuals have claudication symptoms with activity but a normal ABI at rest; those individuals should be referred to a vascular laboratory for exercise testing (Aboyans et al., 2012; Rumwell & McPharlin, 2009). Ankle pressures and/or ABI should be obtained at baseline and repeated following exercise. Treadmill testing is the preferred method of exercise testing, but walking a predetermined distance or toe stands can be used if treadmill testing is not available (Hirsch et al., 2006; Rumwell & McPharlin, 2009). A drop in ankle pressure of more than 30 mm Hg or a decrease in ABI of more than 20% after exercise is considered significant for LEAD (Aboyans et al., 2012).

ABI Interpretation

If arterial blood flow is normal, the pressure in the ankle should be equal to/or only slightly higher than that in the arm with an ABI ratio of 1.00 or higher (Rumwell & McPharlin, 2009; WOCN, 2014). An ABI equal to or less than 0.90 indicates LEAD (Aboyans et al., 2012; Fowkes et al., 2006; Hirsch et al., 2006; Hopf et al., 2006; Norgren et al., 2007; Rooke et al., 2011; WOCN, 2014). When interpreting the ABI, clinical judgment is important, taking into consideration the overall findings from the comprehensive lower-extremity examination (Aboyans et al., 2012). See Table 22-3 for interpretation of the ABI.

TABLE 22-3 Interpretation of Ankle Brachial Index

ABI	Interpretation
Unable to obliterate the pulse signal at cuff pressure >250 mm Hg	Noncompressible arteries
>1.30	Elevated
≥1.00	Normal
≤0.90	LEAD
≤0.60 to 0.80	Borderline perfusion
≤0.50	Severe ischemia
≤0.40	CLI (limb threatened)

Reprinted with permission from Wound, Ostomy and Continence Nurses Society. (2014). *Guideline for management of wounds in patients with lower-extremity arterial disease. WOCN clinical practice guideline series1* (p. 60). Mt. Laurel, NJ: Author.

Frequency of ABI testing

Routine ABI measurement is recommended for patients with/or at high risk for LEAD or cardiovascular disease as part of the annual primary care exam to facilitate preventive care and timely referrals for further vascular testing or surgical evaluation (Aboyans et al., 2012; Hopf et al., 2008; WOCN, 2014). Patients with nonhealing lower-extremity wounds and LEAD should have the ABI rechecked every 3 months (WOCN, 2014). ABI can also be used to monitor patients for restenosis following revascularization, but it should not be used as a stand-alone measure of perfusion (Aboyans et al., 2012; Bundo et al., 2010).

Toe Pressures

Toe pressures and/or TBI are recommended for individuals with noncompressible ankle arteries or when the ABI is >1.30, inconclusive, or unmeasurable due to presence of a wound (Brooks et al., 2001; Carter & Tate, 1996; Hirsch et al., 2006); this is because digital (toe) arteries are usually less affected by calcification than ankle arteries (Sahli et al., 2004). According to several studies, a TBI < 0.64, as confirmed by angiography, indicates LEAD and is the most commonly cited cutoff value for LEAD (Carter, 1993; Carter & Lezack, 1971; Hoyer et al., 2013; Lezack & Carter, 1973; Makisalo et al., 1998). Studies have shown that a systolic toe pressure of <30 mm Hg (<50 mm Hg with diabetes) indicates CLI and is predictive of nonhealing wounds (Carter & Tate, 2001; de Graaff et al., 2003; Norgren et al., 2007; Wütschert & Bounameaux, 1998).

CLINICAL PEARL

Toe pressures or TBI measurements are recommended for individuals with noncompressible arteries or high ABI readings (i.e., >1.30), because toe arteries are less affected by calcification than ankle arteries.

Toe Pressure Technique

The toe pressure is measured on the digital artery of the first (great) toe or second toe using a small digital pressure cuff. A TBI is derived by dividing the toe pressure by the higher of the two brachial systolic pressures. Toe pressures and TBI are most commonly obtained in a vascular laboratory with a photoplethysmograph (PPG); a PPG detects pulsatile cutaneous blood flow from a transducer attached to the skin of the distal toe pad. Portable PPG devices are also available for use outside the vascular laboratory that have good sensitivity (79%) and high specificity (95%) for detection of LEAD (Bonham et al., 2010); PPGs with automatic cuff inflators may be more accurate than those that are manually controlled (Scanlon et al., 2012). Use of continuous-wave Dopplers to measure toe pressures is not recommended because the Doppler is unable to detect the flow of RBCs through constricted arteries when the toes are cold or there is vasospastic disease, and studies have shown that Doppler-derived toe pressures are not equivalent to those obtained in the vascular lab with a PPG (Bonham et al., 2007; Kroger et al., 2003). If clinicians do not have the equipment or skill to perform TP/TBI with specialized equipment such as PPG, patients should be referred to a vascular laboratory.

Transcutaneous Oxygen Tension

$TcPO_2$ measures oxygen levels in the periwound tissues and is indicated when a lower-extremity wound is not healing or if an accurate ABI or TBI cannot be obtained (Hopf et al., 2006; WOCN, 2014). A $TcPO_2$ of 40 mm Hg or above is considered normal, while levels <40 mm Hg are indicative of some degree of ischemia/hypoxia (Arsenault et al., 2012). $TcPO_2$ < 30 mm Hg is consistent with CLI and failure to heal (Norgren et al., 2007), while $TcPO_2$ > 30 mm Hg is 60% sensitive and 87% specific for prediction of healing (Yamada et al., 2008). Yamada and colleagues reported that 63% of 93 wounds on ischemic limbs healed when the $TcPO_2$ was >30 mm Hg, compared to only 14% if the $TcPO_2$ was <30 mm Hg.

CLINICAL PEARL

$TcPO_2$ levels <30 mm Hg is consistent with CLI and failure to heal, while $TcPO_2$ > 30 mm Hg is 60% sensitive and 87% specific for prediction of healing.

If the ABI, toe pressure/TBI, or $TcPO_2$ is inconclusive, inconsistent, or unmeasurable, patients should be referred for further vascular testing. Vascular laboratories can provide additional noninvasive studies that confirm or diagnose LEAD.

Segmental Pressures

Segmental pressures can be used to determine the anatomic location of stenosis or occlusion if surgery is planned (Hirsch et al., 2006; Lau et al., 2011). Consecutive and contralateral levels of pressures (i.e., high thigh, low thigh above knee, below knee, and ankle) are measured with pressure cuffs and a continuous-wave Doppler, and the measurements and limbs are compared. A decrease in pressure >20 to 30 mm Hg between two consecutive levels on the same leg indicates stenosis or occlusion, and a 20 to 30 mm Hg difference in pressure between the two legs at the same location indicates obstructive disease in the leg with the lower pressure (Lau et al., 2011; Rumwell & McPharlin, 2009). See Figure 22-5 for an example of segmental pressures, ABI, and wave forms.

Skin Perfusion Pressure

SPP is measured with a laser Doppler probe enclosed in a pressure cuff placed on the forefoot and can be used to assess blood flow in the microvasculature; it is helpful when calcification prevents accurate ABI measurement or when skin lesions or toe amputations prevent toe pressure measurements (Doughty, 2012; Okamoto et al., 2006). In a study of 36 patients on hemodialysis (42% with diabetes), an SPP of 50 mm Hg was 85% sensitive and 77% specific for detection of LEAD (Okamoto et al., 2006). Rumwell and McPharlin (2009) state that an SPP < 30 mm Hg predicts

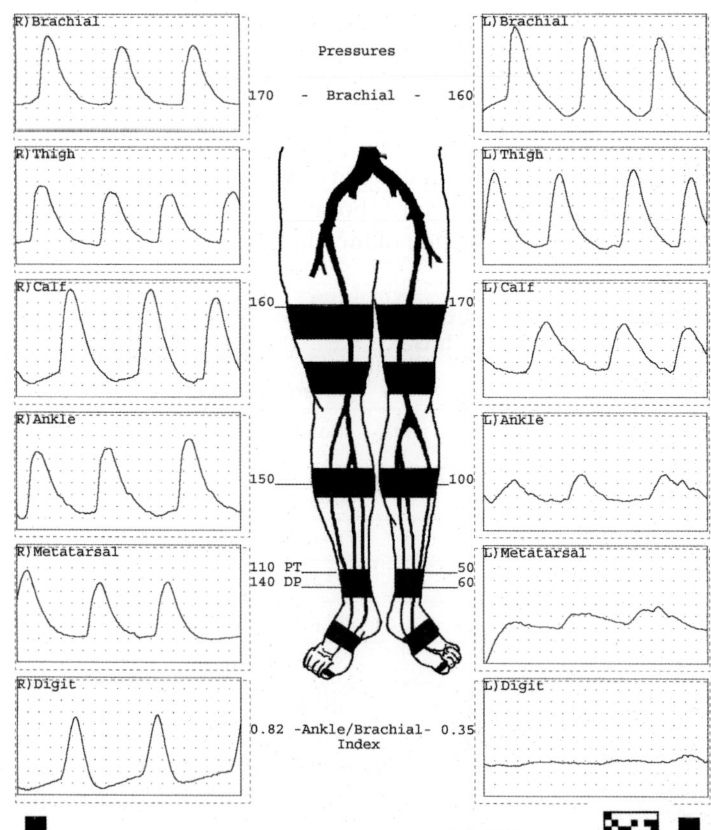

FIGURE 22-5. Segmental pressures including ankle–brachial index (ABI) and pulse volume recording (PVR). Right ABI is slightly reduced at 0.82 and left ABI of 0.35 indicates critical ischemia. PVR tracings on the left show diminution in amplitude t the calf and ankle, and the digit PVR tracing is flat suggesting severe small vessel disease in the left foot.

failure to heal, and Yamada and colleagues (2008) found that an SPP > 40 mm Hg plus a toe pressure >30 mm Hg predicted healing of wounds on ischemic limbs.

Pulse Volume Recordings

Pulse volume recordings (PVRs) provide qualitative and quantitative information about limb perfusion; plethysmography is used to measure changes in the volume of the lower limb throughout the cardiac cycle, which is a reflection of arterial inflow (Hirsch et al., 2006; Lau et al., 2011). PVRs are used to establish an initial diagnosis of LEAD for patients with noncompressible arteries or an elevated ABI (>1.30) and to monitor patients following lower-extremity revascularization (Rooke et al., 2011). In normal vessels, PVRs are triphasic; there is a clearly defined sharp upward stroke during peak systole followed by a prolonged downstroke during diastole and a dicrotic notch about half way through the downstroke, which represents reversed blood flow in early diastole (Rumwell & McPharlin, 2009). In the presence of LEAD, the dicrotic notch is diminished or absent and the amplitude of the waveform decreases. In mild LEAD, the waveforms are biphasic, and in advanced disease, they are monophasic (Doughty, 2012; Lau et al., 2011). See Figure 22-5 for examples of PVR wave forms.

Duplex Ultrasound Scanning

Duplex ultrasound (DUS) produces images of blood flow through vessels and is used to identify the precise anatomic location and severity of stenosis or occlusion when planning surgery and/or to monitor patency after surgery (Lau et al., 2011; Rooke et al., 2011). Studies have shown that DUS can accurately diagnose LEAD and detect femoral popliteal lesions (Eiberg et al., 2010; Khan et al., 2011). However, DUS has lower sensitivity than magnetic resonance angiography (MRA) and computed tomographic angiography (CTA), provides less accurate assessment of the aortoiliac vessels, and does not provide a detailed road map of the vascular system, particularly in the distal small vessels of the feet (Kayhan et al., 2012; Lau et al., 2011).

Magnetic Resonance Angiography

MRA is used to identify candidates for endovascular procedures or surgical revascularization and to plan treatment. Gadolinium-enhanced MRA provides highly accurate detection of stenosis and occlusion of the arteries in the lower extremity (Ouwendijk et al., 2008; Vahl et al., 2008). Because of the strong magnets in the machine, MRA cannot be used on patients with pacemakers, defibrillators, metallic stents, clips, or coils, and gadolinium should be avoided in individuals who have kidney failure or are on dialysis (Hirsch et al., 2006; Lau et al., 2011). Other limitations of MRA are that it does not reliably detect calcifications (Doughty, 2012) and can overestimate stenosis (Lau et al., 2011).

Computed Tomographic Angiography

CTA provides accurate identification of the anatomic location and degree of stenosis in arterial disease (Met et al., 2009). CTA uses specialized x-ray equipment and an intravenous injection of an iodine-containing contrast agent that makes the vessels opaque and creates cross-sectional images, which are processed to produce three-dimensional images of the vessels (Lau et al., 2011). CTA is less invasive than digital subtraction, is faster than MRA, and can be used for patients with pacemakers or other devices that prohibit use of MRA, but its accuracy is limited if extensive calcification is present (Hirsch et al., 2006; Lau et al., 2011). CTA should be avoided in patients with renal disease due to the use of an iodine-containing contrast agent (Hirsch et al., 2006).

Multidetector Computed Tomographic Angiography

Multidetector computed tomographic angiography (MDCTA) is a fast and accurate noninvasive test that detects stenotic and/or obstructed arteries and is more accurate than DUS in patients with mild LEAD (Kayhan et al., 2012). MDCTA uses a contrast agent delivered via a venous catheter and provides scanning of large areas of the body in a short period of time with high resolution to produce good delineation of arterial inflow and outflow. Limitations of MDCTA are the use of ionizing radiation and overestimation of stenosis if severe calcifications are present (Kayhan et al., 2012); however, a recent RCT found that reduced levels of radiation can be used for MDCTA without decreasing the quality or diagnostic accuracy of the test (Iezzi et al., 2012).

Invasive Diagnostic Studies

Invasive tests are associated with risks of bleeding, infection, and contrast nephropathy (Hirsch et al., 2006; WOCN, 2014) and are therefore reserved for patients who require surgery. Angiography is commonly utilized to map blood flow and determine the extent of disease. Contrast catheter angiography (CCA) provides definitive anatomic evaluation of LEAD (Hirsch et al., 2006; WOCN, 2014). A catheter is inserted through the skin into an artery and guided to the area of concern; contrast material is then injected through the catheter, and images are captured with x-rays. Unfortunately, CCA provides only limited visualization of the tibial–pedal vessels in patients with CLI.

Digital subtraction angiography (DSA) has been considered the gold standard for diagnosis of LEAD because it provides good visualization of the arterial system and can be used simultaneously with treatment (Kayhan et al., 2012). DSA is a technique in which the image prior to the injection of the contrast agent is electronically subtracted from the postcontrast image to provide the final image (Bonham & Kelechi, 2008). Because of potential limitations of DSA (i.e., invasiveness, need for hospitalization, high radiation doses, potential nephrotoxicity from iodine contrast agents), DSA is used primarily for planning surgical interventions or for patients in whom MRA or MDCTA are contraindicated or inconclusive (Doughty, 2012; Kayhan et al., 2012; Lau et al., 2011).

CLINICAL PEARL

DSA provides good visualization of the arterial system but is used primarily for planning surgical intervention because it is invasive and involves high radiation doses and potential nephrotoxicity from iodine contrast agents.

Wound Assessment

A thorough assessment of the wound along with consideration of the history, etiology, and other clinical findings is essential as a basis for planning care. Assessment of the wound includes location, shape and size (e.g., length, width, depth, tunneling, undermining), appearance of the wound base (e.g., presence or absence of necrosis, slough, granulation or epithelialization), wound edges (e.g., rolled, punched out, smooth, undermined), periwound skin and tissue (e.g., presence or absence of erythema, induration, increased warmth, local edema, sensitivity to palpation, fluctuant or boggy tissue), and exudate (e.g., color, amount, odor, consistency). In addition to the initial assessment, measurement and reassessment of wounds are needed on an ongoing basis. Also it is important to assess for complications such as infection, cellulitis, gangrene, or osteomyelitis. See Table 22-4 for common characteristics of lower-extremity ischemic wounds and Figure 22-6 for an example of leg wounds due to arterial insufficiency.

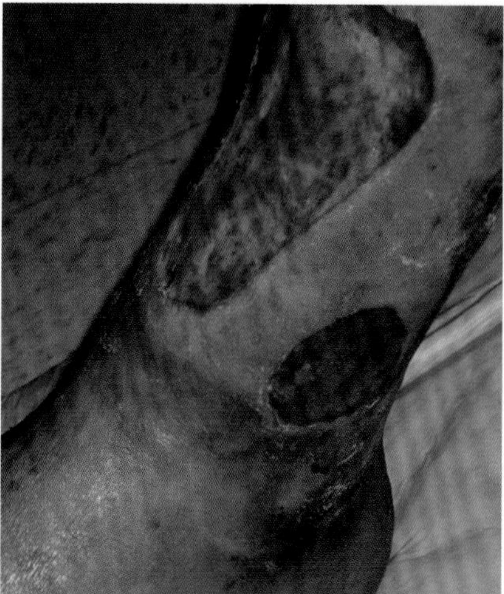

FIGURE 22-6. Example of leg wounds due to arterial insufficiency. (Reprinted with permission from Berg, D., & Worzala, K. (2006). *Atlas of Adult physical diagnosis*. Philadelphia, PA: Lippincott Williams & Wilkins.)

CLINICAL PEARL

"Classic" assessment findings for wounds caused by LEAD include the following: location either on distal foot and toes or nonhealing traumatic injury; ulcer bed commonly necrotic or pale with no granulation tissue; minimal exudate; and infection common but signs of infection frequently muted.

TABLE 22-4 Common Characteristics of Lower-Extremity, Ischemic Wounds

Assessment Parameter	Common Characteristics
Location	• If LEAD primary etiology: distal foot and toes; nonhealing traumatic wounds over lower leg or foot • If LEAD contributing factor: over areas exposed to pressure or repetitive trauma (heels, phalangeal heads, malleoli)
Pain	• Often painful; pain usually worsened by activity or elevation
Size and shape	• Often small • Shape and depth vary—can be deep • Tunnelling and undermining may be present
Wound edges	• Well defined, smooth edges; punched out appearance
Wound base	• Minimal or no granulation tissue • Often appears desiccated • Necrosis • Eschar • Wet or dry gangrene
Color	• Pale, nonviable; gray
Exudate	• Usually minimal
Periwound skin and tissue	• Edema is *not* typical of arterial wounds, and if present is generally due to other systemic condition such as chronic heart failure • Localized edema may indicate infection
Possible complications	• Infection/cellulitis: Erythema, induration, warmth, fluctuation, pain, or tenderness with palpation may be present. Often signs of infection are subtle with only a faint halo of erythema around the wound • Gangrene • Osteomyelitis

Adapted with permission from Wound, Ostomy and Continence Nurses Society. (2014). *Guideline for management of wounds in patients with lower-extremity arterial disease. WOCN clinical practice guideline series 1* (pp. 44–45). Mt. Laurel, NJ: Author.

TABLE 22-5 Indications for Referral: Complications and/or Findings from Vascular Tests

Complications	Findings from Vascular Tests
• Signs or symptoms of infection or cellulitis	• Absence of both dorsalis pedis and posterior tibial pulses
• Gangrene—Urgent referral	• Inconclusive vascular tests
• Suspected osteomyelitis (exposed bone)	• ABI 0.90 or less *plus* a nonhealing wound, intermittent claudication, and/or severe pain
• Atypical wounds	
• Nonhealing wounds: wounds that deteriorate, or fail to improve after 2 to 4 wk of appropriate therapy	• Toe pressure <30 mm Hg (<50 mm Hg with diabetes) • TBI < 0.64 • Ankle pressure <50 mm Hg • ABI 0.50 or less
• Intractable pain: rest pain or intermittent claudication that interferes with activities of daily living, work, or quality of life	• ABI 0.40 or less—urgent referral • ABI >1.30 or noncompressible vessels

Adapted with permission from Wound, Ostomy and Continence Nurses Society. (2014). *Guideline for management of wounds in patients with lower-extremity arterial disease. WOCN clinical practice guideline series 1* (p. 71). Mt. Laurel, NJ: Author.

Classification of LEAD

Based on clinical findings, LEAD can be categorized according to Fontaine's stages or Rutherford's grades (WOCN, 2014). Fontaine's stages are as follows: I—asymptomatic, IIa—mild claudication, IIb—moderate to severe claudication, III—ischemic rest pain, and IV—ulcerations or gangrene. Rutherford's grades are as follows: 0—asymptomatic, I—mild claudication, II—moderate claudication, III—severe claudication, IV—ischemic rest pain, V—minor tissue loss, and VI—ulceration or gangrene.

Indications for Referral

If a wound is atypical in appearance or location or does not respond to 2 to 4 weeks of appropriate therapy, a referral is warranted for further testing and/or a surgical evaluation and biopsy to determine other etiological factors. See Table 22-5 for a summary of complications or findings from vascular tests warranting a referral.

CLINICAL PEARL

If a wound is atypical in appearance or location or does not respond to therapy within 2 to 4 weeks, a referral is warranted for further testing and possibly biopsy.

Primary and Secondary Prevention

Primary prevention deals with delaying or preventing the onset of a disease, and secondary prevention is used after the disease has occurred to prevent further progression of the disease (Mohamad et al., 2013). The goals and interventions for primary and secondary prevention of LEAD are essentially the same.

A clinical priority for patients with LEAD is secondary prevention aimed at reducing the risks for adverse cardiovascular events, progression of atherosclerosis, and mortality. The success of secondary prevention relies on early detection of LEAD and interventions to prevent progression of the disease rather than waiting until patients develop severe ischemia (Mohamad et al., 2013).

CLINICAL PEARL

A high priority for management of the patient with LEAD is implementation of measures to reduce the risk for adverse cardiovascular events, progression of atherosclerosis, and mortality.

General Measures

Secondary preventive measures involve lifestyle modifications and therapies (e.g., exercise, dietary modifications, pharmacologic interventions) to address major risk factors and includes aggressive management of diabetes, dyslipidemia, and hypertension; weight control or reduction if needed; and tobacco cessation (Brassard, 2009). Diabetes is a significant contributor to the morbidity and mortality in patients with LEAD and glucose control is essential (Clair et al., 2012). The American Diabetes Association (ADA) recommends keeping HbA_{1c} at a target level of 7% or less for most individuals (ADA, 2013). In addition, a lipid profile should be assessed and dyslipidemia treated with an appropriate level of statin therapy to reduce cardiovascular events (Stone et al., 2013).

CLINICAL PEARL

The ADA recommends a target goal for HbA_{1c} as 7% or less for most individuals with diabetes.

Current national guidelines recommend maintaining blood pressure at 140/90 mm Hg or less for individuals with LEAD (Rooke et al., 2011), diabetes, and chronic kidney disease to reduce coronary and cerebrovascular morbidity and mortality (James et al., 2014). ACE inhibitors, beta-blockers, and thiazide diuretics can be utilized to manage hypertension and to reduce cardiovascular events for patients with LEAD (Lane & Lip, 2009; Norgren et al., 2007; WOCN, 2014). Antiplatelet therapy has been recommended to reduce the risk of MI, stroke, or vascular death in asymptomatic and symptomatic individuals with LEAD (Rooke et al., 2011). A more detailed discussion of medications used for LEAD is included under the section for primary management/interventions.

Tobacco Cessation

Tobacco cessation is of paramount importance for patients with LEAD. Several studies have reported that tobacco cessation is associated with a decreased risk of LEAD after 9 to 11 years, particularly in men (He et al., 2006; Jensen et al.,

2005; Lee et al., 2011). However, for women, studies have found that 10 to 20 or more years of cessation are required to significantly affect the risk of LEAD (Conen et al., 2011; Jensen et al., 2005). Also, smoking cessation after revascularization has been associated with improved vessel patency (Willigendael et al., 2005). The benefit of tobacco cessation on overall survival of patients with LEAD is less clear. Alvarez and colleagues (2013) found that, compared to nonquitters, smoking cessation was associated with a decrease in mortality in patients with coronary artery and cerebrovascular disease, but patients with LEAD had a slight, nonsignificant increase in mortality; this suggests that risk factors may not affect all arterial beds in the same manner, but more data are needed.

CLINICAL PEARL

Tobacco cessation is of paramount importance for the patient with LEAD; the wound nurse should educate the patient regarding the relationship between tobacco use and LEAD and should assist the patient to make and implement a plan for quitting (to include medications and nicotine replacement therapy [NRT] when indicated).

The effects of tobacco cessation on postoperative complications have also been explored. Based on a meta-analysis (not specific to LEAD), Mills and colleagues (2011) reported that preoperative tobacco cessation of at least 4 or more weeks resulted in a 41% reduction in postoperative wound healing and pulmonary complications. A later meta-analysis found that compared to nonsmokers, former and current smokers had more postoperative wound and healing complications such as necrosis, wound dehiscence, and surgical site infections (Sorensen, 2012). Therefore, tobacco cessation should be encouraged for surgical patients.

It is recommended that health care providers use brief interventions to encourage tobacco cessation such as the 5 As and 5 Rs (Fiore et al., 2008; WOCN, 2014). The 5 As include asking about current tobacco use every visit, advising to quit, assessing the extent of addiction and the readiness to quit, assisting in selecting and agreeing on a quit plan (e.g., behavioral counseling, NRT, pharmacotherapy), and arranging a follow-up plan. If patients are unwilling to quit tobacco, health care providers can help motivate the patient with a discussion of the 5 Rs: relevance of quitting to personal health, risks of continued tobacco use, rewards for quitting, roadblocks that interfere with quitting, and repetition of these factors with each encounter.

In an RCT of 124 outpatients with LEAD who were cigarette smokers, Hennrikus and colleagues (2010) found that a LEAD-specific, intensive intervention resulted in 21.3% abstinence at the 6-month follow-up compared to 6.8% abstinence in a minimal intervention group. The intensive intervention included: individualized letters and physician advice to quit smoking, motivational interviewing, behavioral counseling, education linking smoking and LEAD, help to develop a quit plan, and education about pharmacotherapy aids. The minimal intervention group received verbal advice to quit smoking from a vascular provider and a list of cessation programs and resources in their community.

There are numerous tobacco cessation aids available, but they are often underused (Ahn et al., 2008; Rooke et al., 2011). Based on a meta-analysis of 267 studies (not specific to LEAD), nonnicotinic medications (i.e., bupropion hydrochloride, varenicline, nortriptyline, cytosine) increased tobacco cessation with few adverse events (Cahill et al., 2013). Buproprion hydrochloride is available by prescription and if started a week prior to the quit date can help prevent cravings (Lindell & Reinke, 1999).

Several tobacco cessation aids are available without prescription. Based on a meta-analysis (not specific to LEAD), commercially available forms of NRT (e.g., gum, transdermal patches, nasal spray, inhaler, sublingual tablets/lozenges) increased the rate of quitting by 50% to 70% (Stead et al., 2012). Other findings from the meta-analysis were 4-mg gum was more effective than 2-mg gum for highly dependent smokers; combining a nicotine patch with a rapid delivery form of NRT was more effective than a single type of NRT; starting patches prior to the quit date might increase success; combining NRT and bupropion hydrochloride was more effective than only bupropion hydrochloride; 8 weeks of patch therapy was as effective as longer courses; and wearing the patch during waking hours (16 hours/day) was as effective as 24 hours. Side effects of NRT varied according to the type of NRT and included irritation of the skin from patches and mouth from the gum and tablets. There was no evidence that NRT increased the risk of heart attacks. Reducing risks of cardiovascular events and managing symptoms of LEAD and CLI are two main goals of therapeutic intervention. Utilization of evidence-based guidelines for prevention, diagnosis, and management of LEAD can help health care providers achieve positive patient outcomes (Kohlman-Trigoboff, 2013).

Wound Management

Assessment data are used to establish wound management goals and provide baseline information to evaluate the progress and effectiveness of interventions. Systemic support and appropriate topical therapy are necessary to maintain intact skin and promote healing. Strategies that create an environment that facilitates cellular repair and eliminates or diminishes impediments are essential to healing.

Basic principles of wound management serve as a guide for management of ischemic wounds: identification and treatment of infection, removal of necrotic tissue, insulation and protection of the wound, exudate control, maintenance of a moist wound environment, filling dead space, protection of the periwound skin, and treatment of closed wound edges. However, interventions must be tailored to the specific needs of the individual by consideration of the characteristics of the wound and degree of ischemia. For example, certain interventions such as debridement may be contraindicated depending on the nature of the wound and the perfusion status. To determine appropriate treatments, the adequacy of perfusion must be considered (WOCN, 2014). See **Table 22-6** for wound management based on interpretation of the ABI.

CLINICAL PEARL

Basic principles of wound management should be followed in management of ischemic wounds; however, modifications in "usual care" are sometimes required based on the degree of ischemia and the characteristics of the wound.

Topical Therapy/Dressings

Research has not determined if any specific dressing or topical product promotes the healing of arterial leg wounds (Nelson & Bradley, 2007). It is important to avoid cytotoxic cleansing or dressing agents (Gardner & Frantz, 2008; Gist et al., 2009).

Some experts have reported concern about the use of occlusive dressings such as hydrocolloids for ischemic wounds, although no studies are available to either support or refute this concern (Doughty, 2012; Gist et al., 2009). Occlusive dressings such as hydrocolloids are not recommended for infected wounds (Rolstad et al., 2012), and signs of infection are frequently subtle in wounds caused by LEAD; therefore, dressings that permit frequent visualization and inspection of the wound are generally recommended as opposed to opaque occlusive dressings (WOCN, 2014). If the ischemic wound is open and draining, has soft slough, necrotic material, or has exposed bones or tendons, moisture-retentive, absorbent dressings are generally of benefit; the goal is to manage exudate while preventing desiccation (Takahashi et al., 2004; WOCN, 2014). It is also recommended to avoid constrictive wraps and creams and ointments containing vasoconstrictive agents on ischemic limbs (WOCN, 2014).

CLINICAL PEARL

The goal in management of open ischemic wounds is effective management of exudate and prevention of desiccation.

Careful attention to the periwound skin is needed during dressing changes to prevent skin stripping from tape or adhesives and maceration from exudate or wet dressings. Nonadherent dressings, skin sealants, or moisture barriers may be necessary to protect fragile periwound skin (Doughty, 2012). Regardless of the type of dressing, individuals with ischemic wounds require careful monitoring to assess the response to the topical therapy and the development of any complications.

TABLE 22-6 Wound Management Based on ABI Interpretation

ABI	Interpretation	Wound Management
Unable to obliterate the pulse signal at cuff pressure > 250 mm Hg	Noncompressible arteries	• Assess toe pressure/TBI; Refer for further vascular testing/evaluation
>1.30	Elevated	• Assess toe pressure/TBI; Refer for further vascular testing/evaluation
≥1.00	Normal: Blood flow is sufficient for healing	• Provide topical therapy according to established principles of topical therapy
≤0.90	LEAD	• Provide conservative therapy (i.e., wound management that addresses all principles of care including nutrition, pressure relief, local and systemic factors) • Refer for a vascular/surgical evaluation if the wound deteriorates, or there is no response after 2 to 4 wk of conservative wound care
≤0.60 to 0.80	Borderline perfusion	• Check $TcPO_2$ if equipment available • Evaluate the need for adjunctive therapy. • Monitor the wound frequently. • Provide conservative therapy. • Refer for a vascular/surgical evaluation if the wound deteriorates, or there is no response after 2–4 wk of conservative wound care
≤0.50	Severe ischemia	• Refer for a vascular/surgical evaluation • Maintain stable, dry, black eschar
≤0.40	Critical ischemia (limb threatened)	• Refer immediately for an urgent vascular/surgical evaluation. • Maintain stable, dry, black eschar.

Reprinted with permission from Wound, Ostomy and Continence Nurses Society. (2014). *Guideline for management of wounds in patients with lower-extremity arterial disease. WOCN clinical practice guideline series 1* (p. 72). Mt. Laurel, NJ: Author.

Infection Control

Patients with ischemic wounds need careful and frequent monitoring because ischemic wounds are at increased risk for infection. Signs of infection may include increased pain and/or edema, necrosis, or periwound fluctuance. However, clinical manifestations of infection may be subtle due to reduced blood flow with only a faint halo of erythema around the wound (Doughty, 2012).

Infected wounds and/or cellulitis in patients with LEAD/CLI are limb-threatening complications that require immediate referral to an appropriate specialist for evaluation, culture-based systemic antibiotic therapy, assessment of vascular perfusion, and determination of the need for surgical intervention (Doughty, 2012; WOCN, 2014). Osteomyelitis is a concern for nonhealing wounds with exposed bone, and referral for an MRI or bone biopsy is needed for a definitive diagnosis (Stotts, 2012).

CLINICAL PEARL

Wound infection in a patient with LEAD/CLI is a limb-threatening complication that requires immediate referral to an appropriate specialist for evaluation and management.

Wound Cultures

Cultures are warranted when there are clinical indications of infection to identify the type and number of infecting organisms and guide selection of antibiotics (Bonham, 2009; Drinka et al., 2012; Spear, 2012). Blood cultures are also indicated if there are signs of systemic infection (Spear, 2012). Options and guidelines for obtaining an accurate wound culture are covered in Chapter 10, as are guidelines for appropriate management of local and invasive wound infections.

Antiseptics and Antibiotics

The use of antiseptics in open wounds is controversial because of concern over the nonselective cytotoxicity of antiseptics, especially at higher concentrations (Gardner & Frantz, 2008). Diluted antiseptics are sometimes used for short periods (e.g., 2 weeks) when critical colonization is suspected (Rolstad et al., 2012; Stotts, 2012; WOCN, 2014). Antimicrobial dressings and topical antibiotics are also sometimes used for wounds with critical colonization (Gardner & Frantz, 2008; Sieggreen et al., 2008; Stotts, 2012); all of these options are discussed in more detail in Chapter 10.

For infected ischemic wounds, culture-guided systemic antibiotics are recommended rather than topical antibiotics (Doughty, 2012; Gardner & Frantz, 2008; Sieggreen et al., 2008; WOCN, 2014). A consideration in treating patients with LEAD is that higher doses of antibiotics may be required to effectively eliminate the bacteria, because the diminished perfusion results in inadequate absorption. For example, Zammit and colleagues (2011) found that the concentration of gentamicin was significantly lower ($p = 0.01$) in foot wounds of patients with LEAD as compared to nonischemic wounds.

CLINICAL PEARL

Culture-based systemic antibiotic therapy is recommended for infected ischemic wounds; higher antibiotic doses may be required due to diminished tissue perfusion.

Debridement

For patients with LEAD, the clinician must determine if the goals of care, condition of the wound, perfusion status, and the condition of the patient warrant debridement (WOCN, 2014). Debridement should be avoided in uninfected necrotic wounds until it is determined that the wound has an adequate blood supply for healing (Gist et al., 2009; Hopf et al., 2006; WOCN, 2014). Debriding or increasing moisture in ischemic lesions can convert dry gangrene to wet gangrene and precipitate a life-threatening infection or amputation (Gist et al., 2009), and removal of eschar converts a closed wound to an open wound at increased risk for infection. Thus, clinical experts recommend keeping stable eschars intact on ischemic wounds that are dry, noninfected, and closed with fixed edges, while protecting and completely relieving pressure from the site (Doughty, 2012; WOCN, 2014). Some clinicians routinely apply an antiseptic (e.g., povidone iodine 10% solution) to the eschar and allow it to dry, with the goal of decreasing the bioburden and maintaining a dry, stable wound; however, evidence is lacking regarding effectiveness (Doughty, 2012; Thomas, 2013; WOCN, 2014). Intact, stable blisters should be maintained and monitored closely for infection or rupture (Shannon, 2013; WOCN, 2014).

CLINICAL PEARL

Clinical experts recommend maintaining stable eschar on ischemic wounds that are dry, noninfected, and closed with fixed edges.

Infected and necrotic ischemic wounds are limb threatening, and revascularization with surgical debridement is the treatment of choice in this situation (Hopf et al., 2006; WOCN, 2014). Debridement may also be indicated for wounds in which sufficient blood supply has been established. There are multiple options for debridement and a number of factors to consider in selecting the best approach for a specific patient; issues, considerations, and guidelines are discussed in detail in Chapter 9.

CLINICAL PEARL

Revascularization with surgical debridement is the treatment of choice for ischemic wounds that are infected and necrotic.

Prevention/Management of Heel Wounds

Bed and/or chairbound patients with LEAD are at high risk for heel pressure ulcers and should have their heels offloaded with products that eliminate heel pressure (Fowler et al., 2008; Langemo et al., 2008; WOCN, 2010, 2014). Ideally, off-loading devices should completely elevate the heel without creating pressure in another location, reduce friction and shear, protect from foot drop and rotation of the leg, allow for ambulation, be easy to clean, remain in place while the patient moves, decrease heat to the heel, and be cost-effective (Black, 2004; Fowler et al., 2008; Lyder, 2011). If pillows are used to elevate the heels, they should be placed longitudinally underneath the calf with the heel completely suspended in the air (Black, 2004; Langemo et al., 2008; Lyder, 2011; WOCN, 2010, 2014). Frequent monitoring is required to ensure that the pillows are positioned properly to completely suspend the heel. In addition, the heels should be assessed two to three times daily for any sign of impending pressure ulceration (WOCN, 2014).

CLINICAL PEARL

Consistent heel elevation is an essential element of care for patients with LEAD who are immobile.

Medications

Multiple medications are used for patients with LEAD in an attempt to improve arterial blood flow and walking capacity, and reduce pain. Additionally, three main types of drugs have been used to prevent progression of atherosclerotic cardiovascular disease (ASCVD) and cerebrovascular morbidity and mortality: statins, angiotensin-converting enzyme inhibitors (ACEI), and antiplatelets (Mangiafico & Mangiafico, 2011; Rooke et al., 2011).

Based on a review of data from the NHANES study, Pande and colleagues (2011) reported that treatment with two or more preventive therapies (e.g., antiplatelets, statins, ACEI) was associated with a 65% reduced risk of all-cause mortality. However, patients with LEAD are often undertreated with the recommended medications (Muller-Buhl et al., 2011; Paquet et al., 2010). Interestingly, studies have shown that patients who requested lipid-lowering medications from their physicians received more prescriptions and were more successful in achieving an LDL cholesterol level of <100 mg/dL compared to those who did not ask for the medication (McDermott et al., 2010b; McDermott et al., 2011b).

CLINICAL PEARL

Statins, antiplatelet drugs, and ACE Inhibitors are used to prevent progression of atherosclerotic vascular disease in patients with LEAD.

Statins

Statin therapy is used to lower cholesterol for both primary and secondary prevention and management of ASCVD and LEAD. Based on a meta-analysis, statins (particularly simvastatin) decreased the incidence of cardiovascular events, mortality, and stroke and increased pain-free walking distances in patients with LEAD (Aung et al., 2009). West and colleagues (2011) also reported that statin therapy effectively decreased LDL and total cholesterol in individuals with symptomatic LEAD, with the greatest reduction in individuals taking a combination of simvastatin/ezetimibe, as compared to only simvastatin.

Current guidelines from the American College of Cardiology and the American Heart Association (ACC/AHA) recommend using the maximum tolerated level of statin therapy for secondary prevention in individuals with ASCVD and LEAD, rather than treating to achieve a specific LDL cholesterol level (Stone et al., 2013). According to the ACC/AHA, high-intensity statin therapy is recommended for individuals with ASCVD/LEAD who are 75 years of age or less. Moderate-intensity therapy is recommended for individuals older than 75 years of age and for younger individuals who have contraindications or cannot tolerate high-intensity therapy. High-intensity statin therapy is a daily dose that lowers LDL cholesterol (≥50%) with drugs such as atorvastatin 40 to 80 mg or rosuvastatin 20 mg. Moderate-intensity statin therapy is a daily dose that lowers LDL cholesterol (30% to <50%) with drugs such as atorvastatin 10 mg, rosuvastatin 10 mg, simvastatin 20 to 40 mg, pravastatin 40 mg, lovastatin 40 mg, or fluvastatin 40 mg (two times per day).

CLINICAL PEARL

Current guidelines from the ACA and AHA recommend using the maximum tolerated dose of statins as opposed to treating to a certain LDL level.

Angiotensin-Converting Enzyme Inhibitors

ACEI are cost-effective drugs used to reduce the risk of cardiovascular events and increase pain-free walking distances in patients with LEAD (Hirsch et al., 2006; Norgren et al., 2007; Sigvant et al., 2011). Several studies have shown that ramipril (i.e., 10 mg/day) improved ABI, walking, and stair climbing ability (Ahimastos et al., 2006; Ahimastos et al., 2013; Ostergren et al., 2004; Shahin et al., 2013).

Antiplatelets

Antiplatelet therapy is recommended to decrease the risk of MI, stroke, and vascular death in patients with symptomatic LEAD and may benefit asymptomatic individuals with ABI < 0.90 (Rooke et al., 2011; Wong et al., 2011). Cilostazol is considered first-line therapy for patients with claudication (Mangiafico & Mangiafico, 2011). Studies have shown that cilostazol (100 mg two times per day) increased HDL cholesterol and decreased triglycerides and lipoprotein levels in patients with LEAD and intermittent claudication (Smith, 2002; Thompson et al., 2002; Wang et al., 2003), and improved pain-free walking (O'Donnell et al., 2009; Robless et al., 2008). In addition, Soga and colleagues (2011) reported an 87% limb salvage rate among individuals undergoing endovascular surgery who were treated with cilostazol compared to 75% in those who did not receive cilostazol. However, cilostazol should be avoided in patients with heart failure as it might cause fluid retention or increase ventricular arrhythmias contributing to increased morbidity (Kohlman-Trigoboff, 2013).

CLINICAL PEARL

Cilostazol is considered first-line therapy for claudication; studies demonstrate higher HDL levels, improved pain-free walking distance, higher limb salvage rates, and lower triglycerides and lipoprotein levels in patients treated with cilostazol.

Aspirin (75 mg to 325 mg daily) has been recommended as a safe and cost-effective option to reduce the risk of MI, stroke, or vascular death in patients with symptomatic LEAD (Rooke et al., 2011). Studies have shown that patients with LEAD who took aspirin, compared to no aspirin, had improved walking speeds (McDermott et al., 2003) and fewer major vascular events (Catalano et al., 2007). A meta-analysis also found that, alone or in combination with dipyridamole, aspirin therapy was associated with a reduction in nonfatal strokes (Berger et al., 2009).

Clopidogrel (75 mg/day) is considered a safe and effective drug to reduce the risk of MI, ischemic stroke, or vascular death in individuals with symptomatic LEAD (Rooke et al., 2011). Combined clopidogrel and aspirin therapy may be considered for patients who are at high risk for cardiovascular events but not at increased risk of bleeding (Rooke et al., 2011). The clinical benefits of clopidogrel must be weighed against the side effects, and combined aspirin and clopidogrel therapy should not be routinely prescribed to prevent cardiovascular disease (Squizzato et al., 2011; WOCN, 2014).

CLINICAL PEARL

Aspirin and clopidogrel, singly or in combination, are safe and effective drugs that reduce the risk of MI, ischemic stroke, or vascular death in individuals with LEAD.

Prostanoids

There is limited evidence regarding the benefits of prostaglandins (such as iloprost) in the treatment of patients with LEAD, due to variability in the trials, inconsistent results, and adverse reactions (Robertson & Andras, 2013; Rooke et al., 2011). A meta-analysis concluded that prostanoids might have some benefit for pain relief and wound healing in patients with CLI, but there were no statistically significant differences in amputations or mortality (Ruffolo et al., 2010). In addition, prostaglandins have been associated with high rates of side effects such as headache, vasodilation, diarrhea, and tachycardia (Rudisill et al., 2011).

Pentoxifylline

Pentoxifylline (400 mg three times per day) may be an option as a second-line alternative to cilostazol to improve walking distances in patients with intermittent claudication (Hirsch et al., 2006). However, a meta-analysis of patients with intermittent claudication reported inconsistent results in terms of effectiveness (Salhiyyah et al., 2012); its use should therefore be determined on an individual basis.

Hormone Replacement Therapy

Based on a review and analysis of three RCTs, there was no evidence that treating men who had LEAD or CLI with testosterone had any benefit (Price & Leng, 2012). For postmenopausal women, data from a few studies indicated a decreased risk of LEAD for women who used hormone replacement therapy (HRT) (i.e., estrogen or estrogen plus progestin). In a study of over 2,000 postmenopausal women, HRT use for 1 or more years was associated with a 52% decreased risk of LEAD (Westendorp et al., 2000). In a later study of more than 800,000 women, the women who used HRT, despite having more risk factors, had a 3.3% prevalence of LEAD compared to non-HRT users who had 4.1% prevalence (Rockman et al., 2012).

Nutrition

Adequate nutrition and hydration are necessary to maintain overall health, maintain skin integrity, and promote healing if wounds are present. Diet modification may be necessary to control or reduce weight, control lipids, and control blood sugar if the patient has diabetes. Nutritional counseling by a registered dietician is warranted for patients who have nutritional deficits.

Studies have shown that individuals with LEAD and claudication had poor nutrition with diets that were high in saturated fat, sodium, and cholesterol; and low in fiber, vitamins E, B_6, and B_{12}, and folate (de Ceniga et al., 2011; Gardner et al., 2011; Wilmink et al., 2004). Low levels of vitamin D (<30 ng/mL) have been associated with an increased prevalence of LEAD and cardiovascular risks and increased risk of amputation in patients with LEAD (Gaddipati et al., 2011; Melamed et al., 2008; van de Luijtgaarden et al., 2012). These findings underscore the importance of nutritional assessment and intervention for any patient with LEAD and especially those with ischemic wounds.

Nutritional Supplements

The specific role of individual nutrients and supplements on LEAD and clinical outcomes is uncertain. Research has not demonstrated a significant clinical benefit for patients with LEAD from supplements including alpha-lipoic acid, garlic, *Ginkgo biloba*, L-arginine, omega-3 fatty acids (fish oil, olive oil), vitamins B_6, B_9 (folic acid), B_{12}, or E; and zinc (Marti-Carvajal et al., 2013; WOCN, 2014). Although some studies have shown that folic acid is effective in reducing plasma homocysteine levels, the reduction has not resulted in any beneficial effects on cardiovascular events or the progression of LEAD (Hopf et al., 2008; Mazur et al., 2012). Studies have also reported that the addition of niacin provides no added clinical benefits over dietary interventions or statin therapy if the patient's LDL cholesterol is 40 to 80 mg/dL (Boden et al., 2011; Hiatt et al., 2010).

Mediterranean Diet

Individuals with LEAD should be encouraged to consider the benefits of a Mediterranean diet (WOCN, 2014). A recent RCT compared individuals who consumed a Mediterranean diet supplemented with extra-virgin olive oil (Group 1) or nuts (Group 2) to a control group (Group 3), who were only counseled on a low-fat diet (Ruiz-Canela et al., 2014). Compared to the control group, the risk of LEAD was 66% lower in Group 1 and 50% lower in Group 2.

CLINICAL PEARL

A Mediterranean diet supplemented with extra-virgin olive oil has been shown to reduce the risk of LEAD.

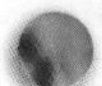 Pain Management

For patients with positional pain, keeping legs in a neutral (not elevated) or dependent position may help relieve ischemic pain. Medications such as cilostazol or pentoxifylline have provided relief for some individuals with persistent claudication pain, and cilostazol or prostanoids might benefit some patients with CLI (Ali & Carman, 2012).

Exercise

Exercise therapy is beneficial for individuals with LEAD and intermittent claudication to increase pain-free walking and maximal walking distance (Fokkenrood et al., 2013; Watson et al., 2008). Regular exercise increases circulating endothelial progenitor cells, which are bone marrow–derived cells that enhance angiogenesis and development of collateral circulation to improve blood flow (Schlager et al., 2011). Supervised exercise for 30 to 45 minutes, three times per week for a minimum of 12 weeks, improves symptoms of claudication (Fokkenrood et al., 2013; Hirsch et al., 2006; Hopf et al., 2008). There is also some early evidence that exercise may be as beneficial as angioplasty; in an RCT comparing supervised exercise therapy and percutaneous transluminal angioplasty (PTA) in 198 patients with LEAD and intermittent claudication, supervised exercise therapy provided comparable short-term benefits in walking and quality of life and was less costly (Mazari et al., 2012).

CLINICAL PEARL

Structured exercise programs have demonstrated effectiveness in relief of claudication, and there is early evidence that exercise may be as beneficial as angioplasty.

However, access to supervised exercise programs (SEP) is limited due to a lack of reimbursement (Osinbowale & Milani, 2011). In the absence of available SEP, organized home-based exercise programs (HEP) are more effective in improving functional capacity and quality of life than simply advising individuals to "go home and walk" (Makris et al., 2012). If individuals are not willing or able to participate in supervised walking programs, they should be encouraged to engage in any self-directed walking program (Scottish Intercollegiate Guidelines Network [SIGN], 2009).

Analgesics

If individuals have severe pain, analgesics may be of some benefit, although data are lacking about the effectiveness of specific analgesics for LEAD or CLI. Opiates may be prescribed to manage severe pain in patients with CLI (Doughty, 2012; Linden, 2013). Wounds due to LEAD are often painful, and it is important to assess the need for premedication prior to wound care. In cases of intractable pain that is not controlled with exercise or medications, patients who are surgical candidates should be referred for a vascular surgical evaluation, and those who are not suitable surgical candidates referred to pain specialists for management.

Adjunctive Pain Management

Pain management options for individuals with limb ischemia who have failed other treatments and are not good surgical candidates include spinal cord stimulation (SCS), lumbar sympathectomy, and peridural analgesia. SCS is provided by a percutaneous electrode or spinal cord implant. A meta-analysis of patients with CLI found that patients treated with SCS had prominent pain relief, increased $TcPO_2$, and higher rates of limb salvage than patients who received conservative care without SCS (Ubbink & Vermeulen, 2013). A 17% risk of complications occurred with SCS that included difficulty with implantation, need for reintervention to change the stimulation, and infection. Therefore, it is important to weigh the benefits of SCS against the additional cost and risk of complications. Prior to treating a patient with SCS, it is recommended to provide a 2-week trial with SCS to determine if there are improvements in the $TcPO_2$ level and pain control (Ghajar & Miles, 1998; Kumar et al., 1997; WOCN, 2014). SCS is most effective in individuals with a foot $TcPO_2$ of at least 10 to 30 mm Hg that increases more than 10 mm Hg during the trial test (Kumar et al., 1997; Ubbink & Vermeulen, 2006).

A lumbar sympathectomy or peridural analgesia might also benefit individuals with severe ischemic pain. In a study of 50 individuals with CLI, lumbar sympathectomy resulted in immediate warming of the limb and pain relief in 100% of the patients, and after 2 years, 28 (58%) of the patients had their limbs salvaged (Nemes et al., 2011). Di Minno and colleagues (2013) treated 280 patients who had CLI with peridural analgesia (i.e., a 30-day continuous infusion of a long-lasting local anesthetic, ropivacaine, via a catheter inserted into the L2 to L3 peridural space). During treatment, 261 (93.2%) participants reported reduced pain and at the 60-day follow-up (T60), pain was significantly lower than at baseline ($p < 0.001$). Also, the ABI mean values were significantly higher at T60 than at baseline (0.30 vs. 0.53; $p < 0.001$).

Edema Management for Patient with Mixed Arterial–Venous Disease

Management of individuals with LEAD and edema due to venous disease is challenging. Compression is the gold standard for managing wounds and edema due to venous disease (WOCN, 2011b). However, sustained high level compression (>30 to 40 mm Hg) is not recommended for patients with an ABI < 0.80 due to concerns over the risk of causing increased ischemia and possible tissue necrosis (Marston, 2011; WOCN, 2014).

Reduced Compression versus No Compression

For patients with mixed arterial and venous disease (ABI > 0.50 to <0.80) who have wounds and edema, reduced levels of compression applied with 23 to 30 mm Hg at the ankle can promote healing without complications (WOCN, 2014). Padding over bony prominences underneath the compression device is recommended to minimize the risk of injury (Marston, 2011). If a patient's ABI is <0.50, ankle pressure is <70 mm Hg, or toe pressure is <50 mm Hg, sustained compression should be avoided, and the patient should be evaluated for revascularization (Marston, 2011; WOCN, 2014). If the patient is revascularized, compression can then be considered to manage the edema from the venous disease (Lantis et al., 2011). In patients with advanced LEAD and significant edema who are not candidates for revascularization, dynamic compression with pump devices (intermittent pneumatic compression [IPC]) may be considered for control of edema (Dillon, 1986; Doughty, 2012).

CLINICAL PEARL

For individuals with mixed arterial–venous disease and whose ABI is >0.50 to <0.80, reduced level compression (23 to 30 mm Hg at the ankle) can reduce edema without causing ischemic complications.

To determine the appropriate method of compression, a careful assessment (i.e., patient, history, limb, and wound) is necessary. Compression wrap systems are commercially available that provide reduced levels of compression. Compression wraps should be applied according to the specific manufacturer's recommendations to achieve the desired level of pressure. Patients with mixed arterial and venous disease who are being treated with compression require close monitoring for complications or failure to heal. To avoid excessive or inadequate compression, portable, battery-operated compression monitoring systems are available that permit monitoring of interface pressures under the compression wrap, such as the PicoPress (Microlab Electtronica, Nicolo, Italy) (Partsch & Mosti, 2010). When compression is initiated, it may be necessary to change the compression more frequently to assess for complications and the patient's tolerance, particularly for patients who have neuropathy and are unable to sense pain or discomfort from the compression. Patients who fail to respond to compression therapy or who develop problems should be promptly referred for a vascular surgical evaluation.

Management Postoperative Edema

Another circumstance in which compression may be needed is for management of edema following revascularization, which occurs during the first postoperative week and lasts for about 3 months due to lymphatic and inflammatory processes (te Slaa et al., 2011). Compression is beneficial to prevent breakdown of the incision, which can cause limb-threatening wound complications, but there have been long-standing concerns about using compression after lower-extremity bypass grafts (Marston, 2011).

Methods to treat postoperative edema in these patients include constant limb elevation, IPC, limb bandaging, and compression stockings (Marston, 2011). There are limited data regarding the use of IPC to manage edema after revascularization. If IPC is used for patients with a superficial tunneled graft, compression is not applied over the graft for the first 3 days, and then the IPC device is applied distal to the endpoint of the graft (Marston, 2011). Two RCTs found that IPC applied to the foot after revascularization was no more effective than compression stockings (18 mm Hg), and in some cases, IPC increased the amount of edema compared to stockings (te Slaa et al., 2010, 2011). If patients have edema at the time of hospital discharge, compression wraps at 20 to 30 mm Hg (Marston, 2011) or stockings at 18 mm Hg can be considered (te Slaa et al., 2011).

Antiembolism Stockings

An area of concern and controversy is the use of antiembolism stockings (AES) for prevention of deep vein thrombosis (DVT) in the presence of LEAD. Several guidelines have recommended mechanical interventions (i.e., graduated compression stockings and mechanical devices such as IPC) to prevent DVT in patients who are not candidates for treatment with anticoagulant agents due to risk of bleeding (American Urological Association Education and Research, 2008; Blockley et al., 2011; Jobin et al., 2011; Kahn et al., 2012; Scottish Intercollegiate Guidelines Network [SIGN], 2010). AES (also known as graduated compression stockings) provide a low level of graduated pressure with a higher pressure at the ankle and reduced pressures toward the knee and thigh (i.e., ankle, 18 mm Hg; calf, 14 mm Hg; popliteal area, 8 mm Hg; lower thigh, 10 mm Hg, upper thigh, 10 mm Hg) and are often used to prevent DVT in immobile patients after surgery (Autar, 2009; Blockley et al., 2011; Jones, 2013). Multiple experts suggest that AES are contraindicated in patients who have LEAD, neuropathy, edema, and/or wounds on the heel/foot, ankle, or leg due to case reports of tissue damage or necrosis associated with the use of AES (Autar, 2009, 2011; Cock, 2006; Gee, 2011; Jones, 2013; Van Wicklin, 2011; Walker & Lamont, 2007). However, studies have not specifically investigated the safety and effectiveness of AES to prevent DVT in patients with LEAD.

Some studies have found that IPC devices are effective for DVT prevention, but data are lacking about their use and effectiveness in patients with LEAD (Arabi et al., 2014; Dennis et al., 2013; Ho & Tan, 2013). In addition, some manufacturers indicate that LEAD is a contraindication for their DVT prophylaxis device. Therefore, if DVT prophylaxis is indicated for a patient with LEAD, careful consideration of the risks and consultation with the primary health care provider are needed to determine what method is appropriate and safe for the patient (Gee, 2011).

Critical Limb Ischemia (CLI) Management

The primary goal in treating individuals with CLI is restoration of blood flow, which may be accomplished by surgical or endovascular interventions (Ali & Carman, 2012). However, multiple factors beyond correction of the macrovascular disease are important to consider and not all individuals are candidates for surgery. Management of individuals with CLI includes measures to reduce the risk of cardiovascular disease, strategies for pain relief, measures to promote wound healing and prevent amputations (e.g., pressure relief, aggressive treatment of infection, wound care), and interventions that enhance quality of life and promote survival (Mangiafico & Mangiafico, 2011; Slovut & Sullivan, 2008).

CLINICAL PEARL

The primary goal in treating individuals with CLI is restoration of blood flow, which may be accomplished by open surgical revascularization or by endovascular techniques.

Surgical Intervention

Surgery is indicated for patients with severe, chronic LEAD/CLI who have failed medical treatment and have tissue loss, rest pain, infected or nonhealing wounds, gangrene, and/ or intractable, lifestyle-limiting claudication pain (Bell, 2013). Prophylactic surgery is not recommended for patients with asymptomatic LEAD. Health care providers and patients considering surgery for LEAD/CLI should carefully consider the short-term and long-term benefits compared to the risks.

For patients with CLI who are able to tolerate surgery, revascularization with bypass surgery, endovascular intervention, or a combination of surgery and endovascular therapy known as hybrid therapy is a preferred intervention for limb salvage (Mangiafico & Mangiafico, 2011; Slovut & Sullivan, 2008; Varu et al., 2010). Surgical bypass, preferably with an autologous vein graft, has been the gold standard of revascularization (Conrad et al., 2011). In an observational study of 140 patients who had above-the-knee bypass surgery, the 5- and 10-year survival rates were 58% and 52%, respectively (Bosma et al., 2012).

Overall, there is insufficient evidence to support surgical bypass over percutaneous transluminal angioplasty (PTA) in terms of the effects on walking distance, amputation rates, death, complications, or progression of the disease (WOCN, 2014). Amputation rates and blood flow might be better in surgically treated patients in the short-term, but these effects may not be sustained long term (Hopf et al., 2006; WOCN, 2014). For example, in a study of 230 patients having bypass or amputation for LEAD/CLI, 107 (47%) patients expired within 6 years after surgery (Collins et al., 2010).

Endovascular treatment is increasingly being used as a first-line intervention for iliac, superficial femoral, and some infrapopliteal lesions. According to Setacci and colleagues (2011), short lesions (<5 cm) of the superficial femoral artery (SFA) may be suitable for angioplasty, PTA and stents are used for lesions 5 to 15 cm, and angioplasty with drug-coated or drug-eluting stents may be an option for short, focal infrapopliteal lesions. However, revascularization remains the gold standard for extensive lesions (Setacci et al., 2011). See Figure 22-7 for examples of vein bypass grafts.

For patients with CLI, surgery has been associated with increased complications, adverse events, and longer hospitalization stays, compared to PTA (Flu et al., 2009; Fowkes & Leng, 2008; Romiti et al., 2008; Schamp et al., 2012). As noted, endovascular management is being utilized more frequently as an alternative to open surgery (Conrad et al., 2011; Cull et al., 2010). In a study of 407 patients with CLI, the primary patency rate after PTA with stents was low, with 31% requiring reintervention; however, the 5-year limb salvage rate was good at 74% (Conrad, et al., 2011).

Angioplasty might be an alternative to primary amputation in some patients with CLI. Based on a retrospective study of 67 patients (N = 76 limbs) who were considered poor candidates for bypass surgery, limb salvage after angioplasty was achieved in 64 limbs (84%), and there were 12 major amputations (Tefera et al., 2005).

Reports from multiple meta-analyses have indicated that antiplatelet drugs (i.e., aspirin, cilostazol, clopidogrel, or dipyridamole; alone or in combination) or other antithrombotic agents (vitamin K antagonist) given before and/or after surgery promoted patency after bypass surgery or angioplasty (Belch et al., 2010; Brown et al., 2008;

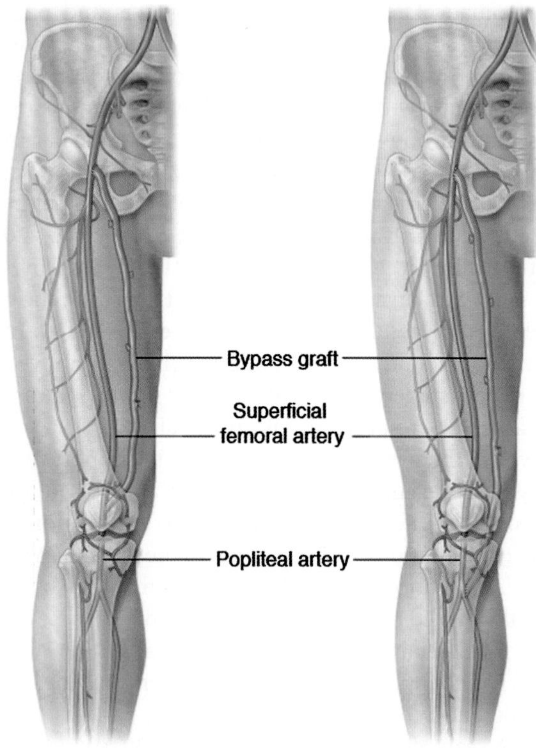

FIGURE 22-7. Examples of bypass grafts. Right leg: Common femoral to popliteal. Left leg: Common femoral to tibioperoneal.

Geraghty & Welch, 2011; Robertson et al., 2012). Other options to improve vessel patency are brachytherapy or cryoplasty. Brachytherapy is an endovascular treatment that directs radiation to the site after angioplasty or stent insertion to inhibit proliferation of smooth muscle cells (Andras et al., 2014). Multiple RCTs have demonstrated that brachytherapy along with antiplatelet therapy decreased stenosis and increased patency after angioplasty and stenting (Andras et al., 2014; Zabakis et al., 2005; Zampakis et al., 2007; Zehnder et al., 2003).

CLINICAL PEARL

Multiple studies indicate that antiplatelet drugs or other antithrombotic agents given before and/or after surgery promoted patency after bypass surgery.

Cryoplasty is performed in addition to PTA and involves application of liquid nitrous oxide to the atherosclerotic plaque, which has been shown to decrease restenosis and dissection (Silva et al., 2011). Although cryoplasty is safe and has a high rate of initial success, its usefulness is limited due to the frequent need for reintervention and high costs (Diaz et al., 2011; Gonzalo et al., 2010; Silva et al., 2011; Spiliopoulos et al., 2010).

Surgical Complications

One of the primary complications associated with surgical intervention is infection. Surgical site infections occur in 10% to 11% of bypass surgeries and 13% to 40% of major limb amputations (Coulston et al., 2012; Giles et al., 2010; O'Brien et al., 2011; Ploeg et al., 2007; Sadat et al., 2008). Risk of infection is increased with diabetes, obesity, age, steroids, CLI, below-the-knee amputations; and use of drains, skin clips, blood transfusions, and vein grafts (Coulston et al., 2012; Giles et al., 2010; O'Brien et al., 2011; Ploeg et al., 2007; Sadat et al., 2008).

Prophylactic use of systemic broad-spectrum antibiotics for 24 hours has been used successfully to reduce postoperative wound infection in patients with LEAD following revascularization (Stewart et al., 2007). However, longer courses of antibiotic therapy are recommended for patients undergoing amputation. Specifically, Sadat and colleagues (2008) found that the infection rate among patients requiring amputation was 5% in patients treated with 5 days of antibiotics (i.e., flucloxacillin or vancomycin plus gentamicin or ciproxin; metronidazole) versus 23% in those who received a 24-hour course. Additionally, the length of stay for patients who received 5 days of antibiotics was 22 days compared to 34 days for patients treated for only 24 hours. Based on results from small studies, other interventions that might reduce infections associated with vascular surgery include providing supplemental 30% oxygen (Turtianen et al., 2011) and aggressive treatment of postoperative hyperglycemia in patients with diabetes (Hirashima et al., 2012).

In addition to infection after revascularization, a review of almost 9,000 patients found that blood transfusions were associated with increased mortality, morbidity, sepsis, shock, pulmonary problems, and reoperation (O'Keeffe et al., 2010). The investigators recommended if a patient's hemoglobin is 7.0 g/dL to 9.0 g/dL, other hemodynamic and physiological parameters (e.g., BP, heart rate, urine output) should be assessed and the benefits of a blood transfusion carefully weighed against the risks.

Thrombolysis

Thrombolysis, the use of drugs or enzymes to dissolve blood clots, may be an alternative to surgery for acute limb ischemia in carefully selected patients. Compared to surgery, there have been no significant differences in limb salvage or death using thrombolytic agents to manage acute limb ischemia, but more complications have occurred with thrombolysis such as hemorrhage, stroke, or distal embolization (Berridge et al., 2013).

Indications for Amputation

Approximately 1 million individuals in the United States have lower-limb amputations and 90% are due to LEAD (Sanders & Fatone, 2011). Amputation may be required for patients with intractable pain, infection, or gangrene with limb or life-threatening sepsis. Significant predictors for amputation in patients with LEAD, diabetes, and foot infections include ABI < 0.80, gangrene, white blood cell count 15.0×10^9 or higher, and hemoglobin <10.0 g/dL

(Aziz et al., 2011). Individuals with CLI and significant necrosis on the weight-bearing portions of their feet (if ambulatory), uncorrectable flexion contractures, paralysis of the extremity, refractory ischemic rest pain, sepsis, and/or a limited life expectancy due to comorbid factors should be evaluated for primary amputation of the leg (Hirsch et al., 2006).

CLINICAL PEARL

Amputation may be required for patients with LEAD and intractable pain, infection, or gangrene with limb or life-threatening sepsis.

Preoperative Planning

When planning an amputation, assessment of the $TcPO_2$ can help determine an amputation level that will provide the best chance of healing (Arsenault et al., 2012; WOCN, 2014). Older studies have shown that a preoperative $TcPO_2$ level >20 mm Hg was associated with increased healing after amputation (Ballard et al., 1995; McMahon & Grigg, 1995; Padberg et al., 1996; Wütschert & Bounameaux, 1997). Based on a more recent meta-analysis of 14 studies, Arsenault and colleagues (2012) found that $TcPO_2$ levels <40 mm Hg were associated with a 24% increase in risk of complications following amputation, and patients with $TcPO_2$ < 10 mm Hg had almost twice the risk of failure to heal. However, the investigators concluded that overall evidence was insufficient to determine one specific optimal value to predict healing of amputations. Also, if there is an increase in $TcPO_2$ (>10 mm Hg), after an oxygen challenge, there is a greater chance of successful healing after amputation (Harward et al., 1985; Smith et al., 1996).

An amputation can be minor (i.e., removal of part or all of the foot) or major (i.e., the majority of the limb is removed) (Marshall & Stansby, 2010). A major amputation is a high-risk surgery, and it is important to optimize the patient's condition by managing comorbid conditions such as diabetes or cardiopulmonary disease. In determining the level of amputation for a patient, it is important to assess his/her current mobility and activity level, overall physical condition, presence of coexisting diseases, and the potential for successfully undergoing rehabilitation. Specific considerations for a successful residual limb and prosthetic fit include the following (Marshall & Stansby, 2010; Robinson et al., 2010):

- Individuals with severe ischemic heart disease might be unable to walk with a prosthesis due to the extra energy required.
- An above-the-knee or through-the-knee amputation might be preferable for a patient who is wheelchair bound.
- A below-the-knee amputation is not indicated for bedbound patients due to increased risk for pressure ulceration.
- A below-the-knee amputation is not advised if there is a flexion contracture of the knee that is >15 degrees.
- Surgical techniques that ensure adequate length and appropriate construction of the residual limb are essential.

Preoperative preparation to prevent complications and promote favorable outcomes includes prophylaxis for DVT and broad-spectrum antibiotic prophylaxis with coverage for anaerobes and aerobes (Marshall & Stansby, 2010). Also, when possible, it is beneficial for an individual facing an amputation to be offered an opportunity to meet with someone who has had a similar amputation to learn about what to expect following the surgery (Robinson et al., 2010).

Postoperative Care and Management

Recovery and rehabilitation after an amputation is a lengthy and multifaceted process that requires a specialized, multidisciplinary team (Robinson et al., 2010). Sanders and Fatone (2011) described four stages of postoperative recovery after an amputation:

- Acute, hospital stage: 5 to 14 days
- Postacute hospital stage: early rehabilitation that ends when wounds are healed and the patient is ready for prosthetic fitting
- Immediate recovery stage: 4 to 6 months of transition and adjustment to the initial prosthesis and ambulation and ongoing adjustments to changes in limb volume
- Stable stage: 12 to 18 months, during which time the volume and shape of the limb stabilizes to permit wearing a prosthesis for an extended period of time in preparation for a definitive prosthetic fitting.

Pain management is essential after an amputation, and pain management specialists may be needed to guide the treatment of postoperative wound pain and phantom pain. Chapman (2010) described three types of pain or sensations following an amputation:

- Phantom limb pain—a sensation of pain involving the missing limb
- Phantom limb sensation—sensation of pins and needles, tingling, or prickling in the missing limb, but not pain
- Stump pain—pain in the remaining part of the limb or stump

Analgesics such as opioids, local anesthetics, and nonsteroidal, anti-inflammatory drugs are utilized for pain control following amputation. A combination of amitriptyline and gabapentin or pregabalin may be effective for treating phantom limb pain (Marshall & Stansby, 2010; Robinson et al., 2010). Topical applications of lidocaine patches or a topical cream with lidocaine 2.5% and prilocaine 2.5% (EMLA, Akorn, Inc., Lake Forest, IL) or nonpharmacological interventions such as transcutaneous electrical nerve stimulation (TENS) might be helpful, although evidence of benefit from TENS is limited (Marshall & Stansby, 2010; Robinson et al., 2010). In some cases, nerve blocks might be effective, and if pain is due to bone spurs or neuromas, surgical intervention may be effective (Chapman, 2010).

Postamputation and Stump Care

Local complications that may occur include hematoma of the stump, flap necrosis, and/or infection. Falls resulting in injuries and stump trauma are also common after amputation due to changes in balance and center of gravity and phantom limb sensations (Robinson et al., 2010). Late postoperative complications may include formation of neuromas, osteomyelitis, bony erosions, wounds, and continued ischemia (Marshall & Stansby, 2010).

Multidisciplinary care is necessary to achieve the best rehabilitative outcomes for patients with lower-limb amputations, and occupational and physical therapists play key roles. Occupational therapists (OT) can help the patient regain his or her independence in activities of daily living such as bathing, meal preparation, and toileting. An OT can assess the home environment and determine equipment needed to facilitate self-care and independence.

Physical therapy is essential postoperatively to prevent contractures, limit edema, and facilitate mobility in and out of bed. The patient's level of function and mobility prior to the amputation are an important consideration in establishing goals for rehabilitation (Fleury et al., 2013). Under supervision of physical therapy, exercise, ambulation, and gait retraining are started early and progressively advanced using appropriate walking aids.

A variety of dressings have been used after amputation to control edema, promote wound healing and pain control, and shape the residual limb, which facilitates early prosthetic fitting and rehabilitation (Johannesson et al., 2008). There is a lack of consensus whether rigid (plaster cast), semirigid (zinc paste wrap), or soft dressings (e.g., elastic wraps; shrinker socks) are best. For below-the-knee amputations, rigid and semirigid dressings versus soft dressings have been associated with improved wound healing, volume control, and protection from trauma and reductions in knee contractures, length of hospital stays, and time to prosthetic fitting (Johannesson et al., 2008). Based on a systematic review, rigid and semirigid dressings also controlled postoperative edema and reduced limb volume more effectively than soft elastic bandages in transtibial amputations, which facilitated early prosthetic fitting (Sanders & Fatone, 2011). Factors that can limit the use of rigid dressings include the skill and time required for their application, inability to inspect the wound, and risk of pressure; and in such situations, vacuum-formed removable rigid dressings can be an effective alternative (Johannesson et al., 2008).

Despite the reported advantages of rigid and semirigid dressings, soft dressings are often used with a compressive elastic bandage or shrinker sock to absorb wound exudate, prevent edema, and help shrink and mold the shape of the stump. Elastic bandages are readily available and inexpensive but may not be as effective or might cause tissue trauma due to inconsistent application (Johannesson et al., 2008; Marshall & Stansby, 2010).

After the stump has been sufficiently molded, a cast can be made to fabricate the appropriate prosthesis. A variety of prosthetics are available depending on the type and level of amputation. Additionally, there are prosthetics designed specifically for athletic sports and activities such as golfing, running, and swimming (Marshall & Stansby, 2010). Referrals for prosthetic assessment and fitting are generally made about 1 month after surgery by the therapist who was involved in the postoperative care (Robinson et al., 2010).

Nurses play a vital role in the care of patients after a lower-limb amputation (Dowling, 2008). It is important for nurses to provide encouragement, emotional support, and education to the patient and family as they adjust to the impact of limb loss. Due to progressive ischemia, the risk of an amputation in the contralateral limb is 10% within a year and increases to 33% to 50% at 5 years (Fleury et al., 2013). Patients must be educated to monitor the remaining limb and promptly report problems to their health care provider and instructed in measures to protect the limb and prevent trauma or injury. In addition, some patients may need psychiatric or psychological counseling to help manage the emotional problems and depression that are common after an amputation including grief over loss of the limb, perceived loss of independence, and changes in body image (Fleury et al., 2013).

CLINICAL PEARL

For the patient who requires amputation, there is a 33% to 50% risk of contralateral limb amputation within 5 years; thus, it is critical to educate the patient regarding protective care for the remaining limb.

Conservative Therapy

For individuals who refuse surgery or are not good surgical candidates, conservative medical care and adjunctive therapies can sometimes be as effective as surgical intervention to promote pain relief, wound healing, and limb salvage; specific therapies include IPC, SCS, lumbar sympathectomy, and therapeutic angiogenesis with gene and cell therapy (Bunte & Shishehbor, 2013; Slovut & Sullivan, 2008; Varu et al., 2010). In a study of 74 patients with LEAD and wounds, there were no statistically significant differences in amputations or healing rates between the patients treated only with conservative wound care and those who had revascularization (McCulloch et al., 2003).

Forty-nine (53%) of the patients treated conservatively (without revascularization) retained their limbs. Marston and colleagues (2006) treated 142 patients with LEAD and wounds without revascularization, and wound closure was achieved in 25% of wounds at 6 months and in 52% at 12 months. Another study followed 49 patients with LEAD and nonhealing wounds whose $TcPO_2$ was at least 30 mm Hg; 33 (67%) patients healed completely with conservative care and without revascularization in a mean of 4.3 months (Chiriano et al., 2010). ABIs were higher in patients whose wounds healed compared to those that failed to heal (0.62 vs. 0.42), and there was a higher rate of healing if the ankle pressure was >70 mm Hg versus <70 mm Hg. The investigators concluded that conservative care should be considered for patients who are reluctant to have surgery or are poor surgical candidates if the patient's $TcPO_2$ is >30 mm Hg, ABI is at least 0.62, and the ankle pressure is >70 mm Hg.

CLINICAL PEARL

For the patient with CLI who is not a surgical candidate, conservative care and adjunctive therapies are sometimes as effective as surgery in promoting pain relief, wound healing, and limb salvage.

A study in Singapore also demonstrated benefits of conservative care. After implementation of a lower-extremity amputation prevention program in which amputations were performed only after failure of comprehensive medical care, there was a 47% reduction in amputations, 13% decrease in mortality, 5-day decrease in length of hospital stays, and cost savings of $2,566 per patient compared to outcomes during the pre-LEAP period (Tan et al., 2011).

Opioids may be necessary to manage severe pain in patients with CLI, with careful titration to achieve maximum comfort with minimal adverse effects (Woelk, 2012). Short-acting opioids may be beneficial for incident-related pain such as pain associated with dressing changes (Woelk, 2012). Some of the pain in CLI may be neuropathic and adjunctive agents such as gabapentin, ketamine, lidocaine, and tricyclic antidepressants might be helpful (Woelk, 2012). Prostanoids might also benefit some patients (Mangiafico & Mangiafico, 2011; Ruffolo et al., 2010).

Adjunctive Therapy

Adjunctive therapy may be indicated for patients with LEAD and recalcitrant wounds who have undergone vascular evaluation and determined to be "not a candidate" for revascularization. Several alternative therapies are available that have been shown to promote healing in individuals with borderline blood flow (WOCN, 2014), including hyperbaric oxygen therapy (HBOT), IPC, negative-pressure wound therapy (NPWT), and growth factor/gene therapy. In contrast, at present, there is insufficient evidence to recommend skin grafts, tissue-engineered skin, and cultured epithelial grafts until after the underlying ischemia has been corrected (Aust et al., 2008; Laurent et al., 2012; WOCN, 2014).

Hyperbaric Oxygen Therapy

Limited evidence from older studies suggests that HBOT might benefit patients with hypoxic wounds (i.e., $TcPO_2$ < 40 mm Hg) if their $TcPO_2$ levels increase to 100 mm Hg when breathing 100% pure oxygen at normobaric pressures (Cianci et al., 1988; Faglia et al., 1996; Oriani et al., 1990; Smith et al., 1996; Wattel et al., 1990). Less than a 10 mm Hg increase in $TcPO_2$ after breathing 100% oxygen predicts a lack of healing with HBOT (Grolman et al., 2001). The goal of HBOT is to resolve the tissue hypoxia, and the therapy can usually be discontinued, after the $TcPO_2$ levels have reached 40 mm Hg (WOCN, 2014).

Intermittent Pneumatic Compression

IPC therapy, also known as circulatory assist or arterial flow augmentation, may benefit patients with severe intermittent claudication or CLI who are not surgical candidates (Hopf et al., 2008). IPC devices provide intermittent compression of the calf and/or foot, which forcefully propels blood out of the foot and calf; the end result is a reduction in venous pressure, increase in arteriovenous pressure gradient, and enhanced arterial flow (Sultan, et al., 2011). Some IPC devices are cardiosynchronous and deliver compression at the end of diastole. Foot plus calf compressions (or foot compression alone) are reported to be more effective than only calf compression (Delis et al., 2002; Delis & Nicolaides, 2005). IPC is usually provided three to four times per day for 45 to 60 minutes and may be provided in the home or clinic setting as well as acute care (WOCN, 2014).

Treatment of intermittent claudication with IPC has been associated with improvement in blood flow, quality of life, walking distance, and ABI (Chang et al., 2012; Delis et al., 2002; Delis & Nicolaides, 2005; Kakkos et al., 2005; Labropoulous et al., 2002; Ramaswami et al., 2005). Some patients with CLI treated with IPC have achieved wound healing and limb salvage. In a study of 48 patients with CLI and nonhealing foot wounds treated with IPC and wound care (vs. only wound care), Kavros and colleagues (2008) reported that 58% of patients treated with IPC completely healed compared to (17%) in the control group, and limb salvage was better in the IPC group. In another study, 171 patients with CLI who were not surgical candidates were treated with IPC for 3 months (Sultan et al., 2011). Clinical improvement was achieved in 161 (94%) patients, and 94% of the patients were amputation free at 3.5 years.

Negative-Pressure Wound Therapy

Based on findings from a limited number of small, non-controlled studies, NPWT may promote healing in patients with LEAD or CLI with infected wounds or vascular grafts after surgery or debridement. Horch and colleagues (2008) used vacuum-assisted closure (VAC) therapy (V.A.C., KCI, Wiesbaden, Germany) on 21 patients with CLI who had failed conservative treatment and were not candidates for revascularization. The patients had nonhealing, infected wounds with exposed bones and tendons following radical surgical debridement. Infection control and limb salvage were achieved in 100% of the patients with debridements, NPWT, and subsequent skin grafts after bone and tendon were covered with granulation tissue. Some patients required up to three grafts (specific number not reported), and 7 months after initial limb salvage, one patient developed gangrene in his lower limb resulting in an amputation.

Nordmyr and colleagues (2009) reported healing of 80 of 121 (66%) infected wounds or vascular grafts treated with surgery and VAC therapy (Kinetic Concepts Inc., San Antonio, TX). Also, Acosta and Monsen (2012) reported that patients with infected bypass grafts who were treated with VAC therapy had a graft preservation rate of 76% (34/45), and at the 15-month follow-up, the major amputation rate was 33% and the mortality rate was 55%. Bleeding was a nonlethal complication in a small number of cases in both studies.

Growth Factors and Gene and Cell Therapy

The role of angiogenic growth factors (i.e., fibroblast growth factor, vascular endothelial growth factor) and gene therapy in the treatment of patients with LEAD or CLI remains inconclusive due to side effects and inconsistent study results (WOCN, 2014); at present, this therapy is considered investigative and is most often used in patients who have failed other treatment options and for whom amputation has been recommended (De Haro et al., 2009; Franz et al., 2009; Pearce et al., 2008). Most cell therapy utilizes autologous, bone marrow–derived, mononuclear cells (BMMNC) given as an intramuscular or intra-arterial injection (Bartsch et al., 2007; Huang et al., 2004; Moazzami et al., 2011; Pearce et al., 2008; Tateishi-Yuyama et al., 2002; Walter et al., 2011). Two meta-analyses of 13 RCTs reported less pain and improved wound healing in patients with LEAD/CLI who received BMMNC gene and cell therapy (De Haro et al., 2009; Wen et al., 2011), but a smaller meta-analysis (two studies) concluded that results of BMMNC in treatment of CLI were inconclusive (Moazzami et al., 2011).

Low-Frequency Ultrasound and Electrotherapy

Data are limited about the benefits of ultrasound and high-voltage, pulsed current (HVPC) electrotherapy for treating ischemic wounds in patients with LEAD or CLI. Results from single small studies indicated that patients who were treated with either ultrasound or HVPC electrotherapy plus standard therapy had improved healing compared to controls who received only standard care (Goldman et al., 2003; Kavros et al., 2007), but more study is needed before recommendations can be made.

Other Adjunctive Options

Other therapies that are less well known include immune modulation therapy (IMT), carbonated water immersion, and Waon therapy. IMT is the administration of autologous blood components, which have been exposed to thermal and oxidative stresses and reinjected intramuscularly into the patient (WOCN, 2014). With IMT, the patient's own blood cells are believed to down-regulate the immune and inflammatory responses involved in vascular disease (Marfella et al., 2010). An RCT of 92 patients with claudication found that compared to controls, more patients treated with IMT increased their pain-free walking distance by 50% (McGrath et al., 2002). In an RCT of 151 patients with CLI and wounds, there was a significant improvement in wound healing at 22 weeks in patients treated with IMT, compared to placebo, and at 6 months, there was complete ulcer healing in 32 of 77 (42%) patients in the IMT group (Marfella et al., 2010).

Findings from several small studies of patients with LEAD/CLI have shown that immersion of ischemic limbs (with and without wounds) into carbonated water increased blood flow and limb salvage (Dogliotti et al., 2011; Makita et al., 2006; Toriyama et al., 2002). Based on a small RCT ($N = 21$), investigators found that compared to conventional therapy (e.g., antiplatelets, statins, ACEI), after 6 weeks of Waon treatments (i.e., thermal therapy with far-infrared dry sauna at 60°C without hydration pressure), there were significant improvements in leg pain, ABI, and walking distances in the Waon group, but no improvements in the controls (Shinsato et al., 2010).

Patient Education

A key component in secondary prevention for patients with/or at risk for LEAD and wounds is education about risk reduction, disease management, and measures to enhance perfusion, prevent trauma and injuries, manage wounds, and prevent recurrence of wounds (Hopf et al., 2008; WOCN, 2014). See **Table 22-7** for key points to include in patient education for risk reduction and disease management.

CLINICAL PEARL

Patient education is a key element of effective care for any individual with or at risk for LEAD.

TABLE 22-7 Patient Education for Risk Reduction and Disease Management

Strategies for Risk Reduction and Disease Management	Patient Instructions

Modify atherosclerotic risks for coronary and cerebrovascular disease	• Adhere to prescribed medication regimen
	  • Homocysteine-lowering drugs
	  • Antiplatelet/antithrombotic drugs
	  • Lipid-lowering drugs
	  • Antihypertensive drugs

Tobacco cessation	• Develop a plan to quit smoking, including preoperative smoking cessation if surgical interventions are planned • Avoid secondhand smoke
Control hyperlipidemia	• Use the appropriate intensity of statin therapy to reduce ASCVD risks
Manage diabetes	• Maintain blood glucose control as demonstrated by HbA_{1c} <7%
Control hypertension	• Maintain BP <140/90 mm Hg to lower the risk of MI, stroke, chronic heart failure, and cardiovascular death • Use effective antihypertensive agents, which can include ACEI, beta-blockers, and thiazide diuretics

Maintain adequate nutritional and fluid intake	• Consider a Mediterranean diet to reduce risk of LEAD
	• Drink alcohol in moderation if already consuming alcohol
	• Control or reduce weight if obese to achieve goals:
	  • BMI: 18.5 to 24.9 kg/m^2
	  • Waist circumference: Women < 35 inches (89 cm); Men < 40 inches (102 cm)

Enhance arterial perfusion	• Avoid leg elevation. • If there is pain in the supine or recumbent position, place legs in a dependent position • Avoid exposure to cold • Avoid garters and constrictive clothes • Increase walking and exercise (i.e., supervised or self-directed)

Prevent chemical, thermal, and mechanical trauma or injury	• Avoid medicated corn pads, aggressive tapes and adhesives, hot water bottles, foot soaks, heating pads, and walking on hot surfaces
	• Perform proper foot care:
	  • Keep feet clean and dry: Wash daily with mild soap and water
	  • Moisturize, except between toes
	  • Avoid fragrance or irritants
	  • File calluses—use pads to protect—no cutting of callus
	• Protect feet (toes, heels):
	  • Wear well-fitting footwear at all times
	  • Do not go barefoot, even at home
	  • Wear socks or stockings with shoes to protect feet: shoes should not rub or cause pressure and should provide good support
	  • Check and empty shoes before wearing.
	  • If bedbound or chairbound, use pressure redistribution surfaces, products, or devices to offload the heels and protect toes and other bony prominences

Manage wounds properly	• Perform wound care as instructed (e.g., dressings, technique, frequency, supplies) • Observe and promptly report symptoms of complications to the health care provider (e.g., signs of infection, new or increased pain, excessive bleeding) • If compression is used for mixed arterial/venous disease, observe for signs that the compression is too tight (e.g., blue, cold, numb or tingling toes; increased pain), and promptly contact the health care provider and/ or remove the compression
Prevent recurrence	• Avoid trauma • Examine feet daily for blisters, wounds, signs of infection, and skin/nail changes • Promptly report cuts, breaks, or signs/symptoms of infection to the health care provider • Obtain routine professional care for toenails, corns and calluses • Offload pressure from feet/heels if bed/chairbound • Visit the health care provider on a regular basis

Adapted with permission from Wound, Ostomy and Continence Nurses Society. (2014). *Guideline for management of wounds in patients with lower-extremity arterial disease. WOCN clinical practice guideline series 1* (pp. 120–128). Mt. Laurel, NJ: Author.

 Conclusion

LEAD is a progressive condition due to atherosclerosis that affects large numbers of individuals in the United States and worldwide. Multiple risks and comorbid conditions are associated with LEAD, many of which are modifiable. Because of the systemic nature of atherosclerosis, individuals with LEAD are also at high risk for cardiovascular and cerebrovascular disease.

Assessment is the foundation for successful management of patients with or at risk for lower-extremity wounds due to LEAD. However, many health care providers utilize unreliable assessment methods to detect LEAD, which is often asymptomatic. Therefore, the majority of individuals with LEAD are unrecognized and/or undertreated. Early detection is the key to secondary prevention of LEAD, and measurement of the ABI is a simple and accurate noninvasive test to detect and monitor LEAD.

Comprehensive care addressing primary and secondary prevention requires interventions to reduce the risks for adverse cardiovascular or cerebrovascular events and mortality and morbidity associated with LEAD. Key preventive interventions include tobacco cessation; management of diabetes, hypertension, and lipids; increased exercise; and control or reduction of weight for individuals who are obese.

Wounds due to LEAD are challenging and complex with limb and life-threatening consequences, and care should be guided by a wound care expert. Patients may have mixed disease and multiple problems (e.g., arterial and venous; arterial and diabetes with neuropathy). Wound care must be based on accurate identification of etiology and a thorough and complete examination of the patient, limb, and wound. Preventing wounds and their recurrence is an essential component of care, and patient education is necessary for risk reduction and disease management, including specific education for leg and foot protection.

Collaborative practice and coordinated care are essential to achieve optimal outcomes for the diverse patients with LEAD and wounds. Multiple health care providers may be needed including vascular surgeons, dermatologists, dieticians, physical or occupational therapists, and infection control specialists.

CASE STUDIES

LEAD CASE STUDY

Case

Patient admitted to home health services for a nonhealing wound on the left leg.

PATIENT PROFILE

History/Risk Factors

Patient was a 96-year-old male who was a poor historian and had recently moved to live with his granddaughter. Patient/family reported a history of hypertension controlled with medication and a stroke 2 years prior to admission. The patient smoked tobacco for many years but quit smoking 30 years ago. The patient was on a regular diet, took a daily multivitamin, and his weight and albumin and protein levels were within normal limits. Other lab tests were normal (i.e., white blood cell/RBC count, hemoglobin/hematocrit). The patient was afebrile, and his blood pressure, pulse, and respirations were within normal limits.

Pain History

The patient denied pain in his legs or feet. He ambulated with a cane in the house and did not walk outside except for physician appointments. He sat up in a chair most all day and denied nocturnal pain or pain with ambulation.

Wound history

The patient had an open, draining wound on the shin of his left leg of unknown etiology and duration. The wound had been treated by the family physician with a week of oral Keflex and twice-a-day dressings (i.e., cleansed with full-strength hydrogen peroxide, applied silver sulfadiazine cream, and left open to air). After 2 1/2 months of treatment with no improvement in the wound, the physician referred the case to home health and requested a consult by a wound nurse specialist (CWCN).

INITIAL CWCN ASSESSMENT

Perfusion Status/Noninvasive Testing

On the left leg, the DP and posterior tibial pulses were palpable but diminished, capillary refill was 10 seconds, and venous refill was 26 seconds. On the right leg, pulses were palpable with normal capillary and venous refill. The left leg felt cool to touch. An ABI was performed at the bedside by the CWCN with a pocket Doppler: ABI for the left leg was 0.56 and 0.94 on the right leg. Screening with a 10-gram 5.07, Semmes-Weinstein monofilament revealed adequate protective sensation on both feet.

Ischemic Skin/Limb Changes

On both legs, there was little subcutaneous tissue, and the skin was shiny, taut, and thin; hair was absent on the toes and legs and toenails were thin. The patient visited a podiatrist for nail care. The patient used a moisturizer on the feet and legs and was instructed to omit the moisturizer between his toes and dry well between toes. Footwear was well fitting.

Wound and Periwound Characteristics

The patient had an open wound on the lower shin of his left leg and measurements were 1.7 cm length, 1.1 cm width, 0.5 cm depth, with undermining to 0.3 cm at the 12 o'clock position and 0.4 cm at the 9 o'clock position. The wound had a punched-out appearance with rolled edges (epibole), and the wound base was covered with 100% dense, yellow devitalized tissue. There was a scant amount of serous drainage, no odor, no purulence, and no pain or tenderness of the wound. The periwound skin was intact. There was no induration, erythema, or overt signs or symptoms of cellulitis and no visible exposed bones or tendons. There was no pitting edema, and the ankle and calf measured 19.9 cm and 27.3 cm in diameter, respectively.

Key Wound Problems Identified

1. Borderline perfusion to the left leg as indicated by ABI of 0.56; diminished pulses, delayed capillary refill, and prolonged venous refill.
2. Impaired skin integrity due to a nonhealing wound on the left shin, 100% covered with devitalized tissue, and scant drainage.

Initial Wound Goals

Wound to be free of devitalized tissue in 2 weeks; have 50% to 60% red, granulation tissue in 4 weeks; wound free of signs and symptoms of infection; maintain intact periwound skin.

NURSING MANAGEMENT/TREATMENT

Topical Therapy

After consultation with the physician, the devitalized tissue was carefully scored by the CWCN and silver nitrate applied to the epibole. Daily dressings with an enzymatic debriding agent were instituted, and the patient's granddaughter was instructed how to perform daily dressing changes.

Follow-Up Plans

Home health nursing visits were planned three times per week to assess and measure the wound, and a follow-up visit by the CWCN was scheduled in 2 weeks. At the 2-week follow-up by the CWCN the epibole was resolved, and the wound measurements were 1.7 cm length, 1.1 cm width, 0.5 cm depth, and undermining 0.4 cm at the 12 o'clock position and 0.5 cm at the 9 o'clock position. The wound base was covered with 95% yellow, devitalized tissue with 5% pink tissue, and a small amount of serosanguineous exudate.

Referrals/Vascular Consult

Due to the limited response of the wound, the patient was referred for further vascular studies and evaluation by a vascular surgeon. Doppler studies with segmental limb pressures and PVR were performed in the vascular laboratory. The surgeon reported that the patient had normal flow to the popliteal level on the left but had tibial stenosis and poor digital PVR. Enzymatic dressings were continued, and the surgeon referred the patient for hyperbaric oxygen therapy (HBOT).

The patient received 20 HBOT treatments ($TcPO_2$ values were not available). Upon completion of the HBOT, the wound measurements were 6 cm length, 2.4 cm width, 1.0 cm depth, and undermining 1.0 cm from the 10 to 12 o'clock position and 0.5 cm at the 6 o'clock position. The wound base was covered with 90% red and 10% yellow tissue. The wound was free of odor and pain with moderate serosanguineous drainage. The enzyme was discontinued by the surgeon, and hydrogel dressings were initiated once daily with home care nurses continuing to follow the patient twice a week.

Within 4 weeks after the HBOT, the wound began to deteriorate and the CWCN was again consulted. The wound measured 7.8 cm length, 3.2 cm width, 1.1 cm depth and was undermined 1.2 cm from the 10 to 12 o'clock and 0.7 cm at the 6 o'clock position. There was increased odor, warmth, erythema, and induration extending 2 to 4 cm around the wound, purulent exudate, and the patient complained of pain in his leg. Ankle and calf measurements on the left leg had increased to 22.4 cm and 27 cm, respectively. The clinical findings were consistent with complications of infection/cellulitis and possible osteomyelitis due to the proximity of the wound to the underlying bone. The CWCN immediately consulted the surgeon, and a bone scan was performed, which confirmed osteomyelitis. The patient was hospitalized and referred to an infectious disease (ID) specialist. A central line was placed, and the patient was begun on an intravenous antibiotic (piperacillin sodium) and moist saline dressings twice a day (BID). After a week in the hospital, the patient was discharged home and followed by the ID specialist, surgeon, and home health nurses, who continued the intravenous piperacillin and modified the topical therapy to silver hydrofiber dressings + gauze and wrap gauze changed every 2 days. After 8 weeks of the intravenous antibiotic therapy and moist wound healing, the wound completely healed, and the patient was discharged from services.

Patient Education/Discharge Planning

The patient and family received instructions regarding

- Nutrition/protein to maintain intact skin.
- Importance of taking antihypertensive medication as prescribed.
- Foot/limb protection: wash and dry feet well and moisturize except between the toes; inspect the legs and feet daily and promptly notify physician for swelling, pain, skin breakdown or wounds; wear properly fitted shoes with socks and no bare feet even in the house; check temperature of the bath water and avoid heating pads and foot soaks to prevent risk of burns, and use a pillow at night to lift heels off mattress to prevent pressure.
- Avoiding sitting up with legs dependent for prolonged periods of time.
- Continue nail care with the podiatrist.
- Keep regular physician follow-up appointments, and have ABI monitored at least annually.

KEY POINTS

This case exemplifies the importance of a thorough assessment and value of the ABI to detect LEAD in a patient with a nonhealing, lower-extremity wound. The necessity of carefully monitoring a patient's response to care and making timely referrals when a wound fails to respond or deteriorates despite appropriate care is demonstrated. The case shows that establishing specific wound care goals can help gauge progress and guide decisions regarding referrals or use of adjunctive therapies. Also, the case is an example of the importance and value of communication and collaboration among health care providers and across care settings to achieve successful outcomes.

REFERENCES

Aboyans, V., Criqui, M. H., Abraham, P., et al. (2012). Measurement and interpretation of the ankle-brachial index: A scientific statement from the American Heart Association. *Circulation, 126*, 488–492. doi:10.1161/CIR.0b013e318276fbcb.

Aboyans, V., Criqui, M., Denenberg, J., et al. (2006). Risk factors for progression of peripheral arterial disease in large and small vessels. *Circulation, 113*, 2623–2629.

Aboyans, V., Lacroix, P., Doucet, S., et al. (2008). Diagnosis of peripheral arterial disease in general practice: Can the ankle-brachial index be measured either by pulse palpation or an automatic blood pressure device? *International Journal of Clinical Practice, 62*(7), 1001–1007. doi:10.1111/j.1742-1241.2008.01784.x.

Acosta, S., & Monsen, C. (2012). Outcome after VAC®therapy for infected bypass grafts in the lower limb. *European Journal of Vascular and Endovascular Surgery, 44*, 294–299. doi:10.1016/j.ejvs.2012.06.005.

Aerden, D., Massaad, D., vonKemp, K., et al. (2011). The ankle brachial index and the diabetic foot: A troublesome marriage. *Annals of Vascular Surgery, 25*, 770–777. doi:10.1016/j.avsg.2010.12.025.

Agarwal, S. (2009). The association of active and passive smoking with peripheral arterial disease: Results from NHANES 1999-2004. *Angiology, 60*(3), 335–345. doi:10.1177/0003319708330526.

Ahimastos, A. A., Lawler, A., Reid, C. M., et al. (2006). Brief communication: Ramipril markedly improves walking ability in patients with peripheral arterial disease: A randomized trial. *Annals Internal Medicine, 144*, 660–664.

Ahimastos, A. A., Walker, P. J., Askew, C., et al. (2013). Effect of ramipril on walking times and quality of life among patients with peripheral artery disease and intermittent claudication: A randomized controlled trial. *Journal of the American Medical Association, 309*(5), 453–460. doi:10.1001/jama.2012.216237.

Ahn, C., Mulligan, P., & Salcido, R. S. (2008). Smoking-the bane of wound healing: Biomedical interventions and social influences. *Advances in Skin & Wound Care, 21*(5), 227–236; quiz 237–228. doi:10.1097/01.ASW.0000305440.62402.43.

Akhtar, B., Siddique, S., Khan, R. A., et al. (2009). Detection of atherosclerosis by ankle brachial index: Evaluation of palpatory method versus ultrasound Doppler technique. *Journal of Ayub Medical College, Abbottabad, 21*(1), 11–16.

Al-Bannawi, A., Al-Wesebai, K., Taha, S., et al. (2011). *Chlamydia pneumoniae* induces chemokine expression by platelets in patients with atherosclerosis. *Medical Principles and Practice, 20*(5), 438–443. doi:10.1159/000324553.

Ali, F. N., & Carman, T. L. (2012). Medical management for chronic atherosclerotic peripheral arterial disease. *Drugs, 72*(16), 2073–2075. doi:10.2165/11640810-000000000-00000.

Ali, Z., Sarcia, P., Mosley, T. H., et al. (2009). Association of serum myeloperoxidase with the ankle-brachial index and peripheral arterial disease. *Vascular Medicine, 14*, 215–220. doi:10.1177/1358863X08101999.

Allison, M., Aboyans, V., Granston, T., et al. (2010a). The relevance of different methods of calculating the ABI: The multiethnic study of atherosclerosis. *American Journal of Epidemiology, 171*(3), 368–376.

Allison, M. A., Peralta C. A., Wassel, C. L., et al. (2010b). Genetic ancestry and lower extremity peripheral artery disease in the multi-ethnic study of atherosclerosis. *Vascular Medicine, 15*(5), 351–359. doi:10.1177/1358863X10375586.

Alvarez, L. R., Balibrea, J. M., Surinach, J. M., et al. (2013). Smoking cessation and outcome in stable outpatients with coronary, cerebrovascular, or peripheral artery disease. *European Journal of Preventive Cardiology, 20*(3), 486–495. doi:10.1177/1741826711426090.

American Diabetes Association. (2013). Standards of medical care in diabetes—2013. *Diabetes Care, 36*(S1), S11–S66. doi:10.2337/dc13-S011.

American Heart Association. (2012). *What your cholesterol levels mean.* Retrieved July 2014 from http://www.heart.org/HEARTORG/Conditions/Cholesterol/AboutCholesterol/What-Your-Cholesterol-Levels-Mean_UCM_305562_Article.jsp

American Urological Association Education and Research, Inc. (2008). Best practice policy statement for the prevention of deep vein thrombosis in patients undergoing urologic surgery. Retrieved December 7, 2013 from http://www.guideline.gov/popups/printView.aspx?id=13433

Andras, A., Hansrani, M., Stewart, M., et al. (2014). Intravascular brachytherapy for peripheral vascular disease. *Cochrane Database of Systematic Reviews*, (1), Art. No.: CD003504. doi:10.1002/14651858.CD003504.pub2.

Aponte, J. (2011). The prevalence of asymptomatic and symptomatic peripheral arterial disease and peripheral arterial disease risk factors in the U.S. population. *Holistic Nursing Practice, 25*(3), 147–161. doi:10.1097/HNP.0b013e3182157c4a.

Arabi, Y. M., Khedr, M., Dara, S. I., et al. (2014). Use of intermittent pneumatic compression and not graduated compression stockings is associated with lower incident VTE in critically ill patients. A multiple propensity scores adjusted analysis. *Chest, 144*(1), 152–159. doi:10.1378/chest.12-2028.

Armstrong, D. W., Tobin, C., & Matangi, M. F. (2010). The accuracy of the physical examination for the detection of lower extremity peripheral arterial disease. *Canadian Journal of Cardiology, 26*(10), e346–e350.

Aronow, W. S., Ahmed, M. I., Ekundayo, O. J., et al. (2009). A propensity-matched study of the association of peripheral arterial disease with cardiovascular outcomes in community-dwelling older adults. *American Journal of Cardiology, 103*(1), 130–135. doi:10.1016/j.amjcard.2008.08.037.

Arsenault, K. A., Al-Otaibi, A., Devereaux, P. J., et al. (2012). The use of transcutaneous oximetry to predict healing complications of lower limb amputations: A systematic review and meta-analysis. *European Journal of Vascular & Endovascular Surgery, 43*, 329–336. doi:10.1016/j.ejvs.2011.12.004.

Aung, P. P., Maxwell, H., Jepson, R. G., et al. (2009). Lipid-lowering for peripheral arterial disease of the lower limb. *Cochrane Database of Systematic Reviews*, (4), Art. No.: CD000123. doi:10.1002/14651858.CD000123.pub2.

Aust, M. C., Spies, M., Guggenheim, M., et al. (2008). Lower limb revascularization preceding surgical wound coverage: An interdisciplinary algorithm for chronic wound closure. *Journal of Plastic, Reconstructive & Aesthetic Surgery, 61*, 925–933. doi:10.1016/j.bjps.2007.09.060.

Autar, R. (2009). A review of the evidence for the efficacy of anti-embolism stockings (AES) in venous thromboembolism (VTE) prevention. *Journal of Orthopaedic Nursing, 13*(1), 41–49. doi:10.1016/j.joon.2009.01.003.

Autar, R. (2011). Evidence based venous thromboprophylaxis in patients undergoing total hip replacement (THR), total knee replacement (TKR) and hip fracture surgery (HFS). *International Journal of Orthopaedic and Trauma Nursing, 15*(3), 145–154. doi:10.1016/j.ijotn.2011.01.001.

Aziz, A., Lin, W. K., Nather, A., et al. (2011). Predictive factors for lower extremity amputations in diabetic foot infections. *Diabetic Foot and Ankle, 2*, 7663. doi:10.3402/dfa.v2i0.7463.

Ballard, J. L., Eke, C. C., Bunt, T. J., et al. (1995). A prospective evaluation of transcutaneous oxygen measurements in the management of diabetic foot problems. *Journal of Vascular Surgery, 22*, 485–492.

Bangova, A. (2013). Prevention of pressure ulcers in nursing home residents. *Nursing Standard, 27*, 54–61.

Bartsch, T., Brehm, M., Zeus, T., et al. (2007). Transplantation of autologous mononuclear bone marrow stem cells in patients with peripheral arterial disease (the TAM-PAD study). *Clinical Research in Cardiology, 96*(12), 891–899. doi:10.1007/s00392-007-0569-x.

Becker, F., Robert-Ebadi, H., Ricco, J. B., et al. (2011). Chapter I: Definitions, epidemiology, clinical Presentation and prognosis. *European Journal of Vascular and Endovascular Surgery, 42*(S2), S4–S12.

Belch, J. F., Dormandy, J., & CASPAR Writing Committee. (2010). Results of the randomized, placebo-controlled clopidogrel and acetylsalicylic acid in bypass surgery for peripheral arterial disease (CASPAR) trial. *Journal of Vascular Surgery, 52*(4), 825–833. doi:10.1016/j.jvs.2010.04.027.

Bell, D. (2013). Peripheral arterial disease overview. *Podiatry Management*, 175–183. Retrieved April 15, 2014, from www.podiatrym.com/cme/CMEJan13.pdf

Bell, J. W., Chen, D., Bahls, M., et al. (2011). Evidence for greater burden of peripheral arterial disease in lower extremity arteries of spinal cord-injured individuals. *American Journal of Physiology-Heart and Circulatory Physiology, 301*(3), H766–H772. doi:10.1152/ajpheart.00507.2011.

Bennett, P. C., Lip, G. Y., Silverman, S., et al. (2010). The contribution of cardiovascular risk factors to peripheral arterial disease in South Asians and Blacks: A sub-study to the Ethnic-Echocardiographic Heart of England Screening (E-ECHOES) Study. *QJM: An International Journal of Medicine, 103*, 661–669. doi:10.1093/qjmed/hcq102.

Berger, J. S., Ballantyne, C. M., Davidson, M. H., et al. (2011). Peripheral artery disease, biomarkers, and darapladib. *American Heart Journal, 161*, 972–978. doi:10.1016/j.ahj.2011.01.017.

Berger, J. S., Krantz, M. J., Kittelson, J. M., et al. (2009). Aspirin for the prevention of cardiovascular events in patients with peripheral artery disease: A meta-analysis of randomized trials. *Journal of the American Medical Association, 301*, 1909–1919.

Bergiers, S., Vaes, B., & Degryse, J. (2011). To screen or not to screen for peripheral arterial disease in subjects aged 80 and over in primary health care: A cross-sectional analysis from the BELFRAIL study. *BMC Family Practice, 12*, 39. doi:10.1186/1471-2296-12-39.

Berridge, D. C., Kessel, D. O., & Robertson, I. (2013). Surgery versus thrombolysis for initial management of acute limb ischaemia. *Cochrane Database of Systematic Reviews*, Issue 1: Art. No.: CD002784. doi:10.1002/14651858.CD002784.pub2.

Black, J. (2004). Preventing heel pressure ulcers. *Nursing, 34*(11), 17.

Blockley, D., Large, L., & Spencer, L. (2011). Good practice guidelines for the use of antiembolic stockings. Retrieved December 11, 2013 from http://www.leicspart.nhs.uk/library/version2snp007policy-antiembolismstockingsoct09.pdf

Bloemenkamp, D. G, Mali, W. P., Tanis, B. C., Rosendaal, F. R., van den Bosch, M. A., et al. (2002). *Chlamydia pneumoniae, Helicobacter pylori* and cytomegalovirus infections and the risk of peripheral arterial disease in young women. *Atherosclerosis, 163*, 149–156.

Boden, W. E., Probstfield, J. L., Anderson, T., et al. (2011). Niacin in patients with low HDL cholesterol levels receiving intensive statin therapy. *New England Journal of Medicine, 365*(24), 2255–2267. doi:10.1056/NEJMoa1107579.

Bonham, P. A. (2009). Swab cultures for diagnosing wound infections: A literature review and clinical guideline. *Journal of Wound, Ostomy, and Continence Nursing, 36*(4), 389–395. doi:10.1097/WON.0b013e3181aaef7f.

Bonham, P. A., Cappuccio, M., Hulsey, T., et al. (2007). Are ankle and toe brachial indices (ABI-TBI) obtained by a pocket Doppler interchangeable with those obtained by standard laboratory equipment? *Journal of Wound, Ostomy, and Continence Nursing, 34*, 35–44.

Bonham, P. A., & Kelechi, T. (2008). Evaluation of lower extremity arterial circulation and implications for nursing practice. *Journal of Cardiovascular Nursing, 23*(2), 144–152.

Bonham, P. A., Kelechi, T., Mueller, M., et al. (2010). Are toe pressures measured by a portable photoplethysmograph equivalent to standard laboratory tests? *Journal of Wound Ostomy and Continence Nursing,375*(5),475–486.doi:10.1097/WON.0b013e3181eda0c5.

Bosma, J., Turkcan, K., Assink, J., et al. (2012). Long-term quality of life and mobility after prosthetic above-the knee bypass surgery. *Annals of Vascular Surgery, 26*(2), 225–232. doi:10.1016/j.avsg.2011.05.029.

Bozkurt, A. K., Tasci, I., Tabak, O., et al. (2011). Peripheral artery disease assessed by ankle brachial index in patients with established cardiovascular disease or at least one risk factor for atherothrombosis€—CAREFUL study: A national, multi-center, cross-sectional observational study. *BMC Cardiovascular Disorders, 11*, 4. doi:10.1186/1471-2261-11-4.

Brassard, A. (2009). Identification of patients at risk of ischemic events for long-term secondary prevention. *Journal of the American Academy of Nurse Practitioners, 21*(12), 677–689. doi:10.1111/j.1745-7599.2009.00444.x.

Brevetti, G., Giugliano, G., Brevetti, L., et al. (2010). Inflammation in peripheral arterial disease. *Circulation, 122*, 1862–1875. doi:10.1161/CIRCULATIONAHA.109.918417.

Brevetti, G., Schiano, V., Laurenzano, E., et al. (2008). Myeloperoxidase, but not C-reactive protein, predicts cardiovascular risk in peripheral arterial disease. *European Heart Journal, 29*, 224–230. doi:10.1093/eurheartj/ehm587.

Brooks, B., Dean, R., Patel, S., et al. (2001). TBI or not TBI: That is the question. Is it better to measure toe pressure than ankle pressure in diabetic patients? *Diabetic Medicine, 18*, 528–532.

Brown, J., Lethaby, A., Maxwell, H., et al. (2008). Antiplatelet agents for preventing thrombosis after peripheral arterial bypass surgery. *Cochrane Database of Systematic Reviews*, (4), Art. No.: CD000535. doi:10.1002/14651858.CD000535.pub2.

Bundo, M., Munoz, L., Perez, C., et al. (2010). Asymptomatic peripheral arterial disease in type 2 diabetes patients: A 10-year follow-up study of the utility of the ankle brachial index as a prognostic marker of cardiovascular disease. *Annals of Vascular Surgery, 24*, 985–993. doi:10.1016/j.avsg.2010.06.001.

Bunte, M. C., & Shishehbor, M. H. (2013). Treatment of infrapopliteal critical limb ischemia in 2013: The wound perfusion approach. *Current Cardiology Reports, 15*, 363. doi:10.1007/s11886-013-0363-5.

Cahill, K., Stevens, S., Perea, R., et al. (2013). Pharmacological interventions for smoking cessation: An overview and network meta-analysis. *Cochrane Database of Systematic Reviews*, Issue 5:Art. No.: CD009329. doi:10.1002/14651858.CD009329.pub2.

Cang, Y., Li, J., Li, Y., et al. (2012). Relationship of a low ankle-brachial index with all-cause mortality and cardiovascular mortality in Chinese patients with metabolic syndrome after a 6-year follow-up: A Chinese prospective cohort study. *Internal Medicine Journal, 51*, 2847–2856. doi:10.2169/internalmedicine.51.7718.

Carmo, G. A., Mandil, A., Nascimento, B. R., et al. (2009). Can we measure the ankle brachial index using only a stethoscope? A pilot study. *Family Practice, 26*, 22–26. doi:10.1093/fampra/cmn086.

Carter, S. (1993). Role of pressure measurements in vascular disease. In E. F. Bernstein (Ed.), *Vascular Diagnosis*, (4th ed., pp. 486–512). St. Louis, MO: CV Mosby.

Carter, S., & Lezack, J. (1971). Digital systolic pressures in the lower limb in arterial disease. *Circulation, 43*, 905–914.

Carter, S. A., & Tate, R. B. (1996). Value of toe pulse waves in addition to systolic pressures in the assessment of the severity of peripheral arterial disease and critical limb ischemia. *Journal of Vascular Surgery, 24*, 258–265.

Carter, S. A., & Tate, R. B. (2001). The value of toe pulse waves in determination of risks for limb amputation and death in patients with peripheral arterial disease and skin ulcers or gangrene. *Journal of Vascular Surgery, 33*, 708–714.

Catalano, M., Born, G., & Peto, R. (2007). Prevention of serious vascular events by aspirin amongst patients with peripheral arterial disease: Randomized, double-blind trial. *Journal of Internal Medicine, 261*, 276–284. doi:10.1111/j.1365-2796.2006.01763.x.

Chang, S., Hsu, J., Chu, C., et al. (2012). Using intermittent pneumatic compression therapy to improve quality of life for symptomatic patients with infrapopliteal diffuse peripheral obstructive disease. *Circulation Journal, 76*, 971–976.

Chaparala, R. P., Orsi, N. M., Lindsey, N. J., et al. (2009). Inflammatory profiling of peripheral arterial disease. *Annals of Vascular Surgery, 23*(2), 172–178. doi:10.1016/j.avsg.2008.06.005.

Chapman, S. (2010). Pain management in patients following limb amputation. *Nursing Standard, 25*(19), 35–40.

Cheng, C. H., Tsai, T. P., Chen, W. S., et al. (2009). Serum folate is a reliable indicator of hyperhomocysteinemia and borderline hyperhomocysteinemia in young adults. *Nutrition Research, 29*, 743–749. doi:10.1016/j.nutres.2009.09.017.

Chiriano, J., Bianchi, C., Teruya, T. H., et al. (2010). Management of lower extremity wounds in patients with peripheral arterial disease: A stratified conservative approach. *Annals of Vascular Surgery, 24*, 1110–1116. doi:10.1016/j.avsg.2010.07.012.

Cianci, P., Petrone, G., Drager, S., et al. (1988). Salvage of the problem wound and potential amputation with wound care and adjunctive hyperbaric oxygen therapy: An economic analysis. *Journal of Hyperbaric Medicine, 3*, 127–141.

Cimminiello, C., Kownator, S., Wautrecht, J. C., et al. (2011). The PANDORA study: Peripheral arterial disease in patients with non-high cardiovascular risk. *Internal and Emergency Medicine, 6*, 509–519. doi:10.1007/s11739-011-0511-0.

Clair, D., Shah, S., & Weber, J. (2012). Current state of diagnosis and management of critical limb ischemia. *Current Cardiology Reports, 14*(2), 160–170. doi:10.1007/s11886-012-0251-4.

Clegg, A., Kring, D., Plemmons, J., et al. (2009). North Carolina wound nurses examine heel pressure ulcers. *Journal of Wound, Ostomy, and Continence Nursing, 36*(6), 635–639.

Cock, K. A. (2006). Anti-embolism stockings: Are they used effectively and correctly? *British Journal of Nursing, 15*(S6), S4–S12.

Coll, B., Betriu, A., Martinez-Alonso, M., et al. (2010). Cardiovascular risk factors underestimate the atherosclerotic burden in chronic kidney disease: Usefulness of non-invasive tests in cardiovascular assessment. *Nephrology, Dialysis, Transplantation, 25*, 3017–3025. doi:10.1093/ndt/gfq109.

Collins, T. C., Nelson, D., & Ahluwalia, J. S. (2010). Mortality following operations for lower extremity peripheral arterial disease. *Vascular Health and Risk Management, 6*, 287–296.

Collins, T., Suarez-Almazor, M., & Petersen, N. (2006). An absent pulse is not sensitive for the early detection of peripheral arterial disease. *Family Medicine, 38*, 38–42.

Conen, D., Everett, B. M., Kurth, T., et al. (2011). Smoking, smoking cessation, and risk of symptomatic peripheral artery disease in women: A cohort study. *Annals of Internal Medicine, 154*(11), 719–726. doi:10.1059/0003-4819-154-11-201106070-00003.

Conrad, M. F., Crawford, R. S., Hackney, L. A., et al. (2011). Endovascular management of patients with critical limb ischemia. *Journal of Vascular Surgery, 53*(4), 1020–1025. doi:10.1016/j.jvs.2010.10.088.

Coulston, J. E., Tuff, V., Twine, C. P., et al. (2012). Surgical factors in the prevention of infection following major lower limb amputation. *European Journal of Vascular & Endovascular Surgery, 43*(5), 556–560. doi:10.1016/j.ejvs.2012.01.029.

Criqui, M. H., Fronek, A., Klauber, M. R., et al. (1985). The sensitivity, specificity, and predictive value of traditional clinical evaluation of peripheral arterial disease: Results from noninvasive testing in a defined population. *Circulation, 71*(3), 516–522.

Criqui, M. H., McClelland, R. L., McDermott, M. M., et al. (2010). The ankle-brachial index and incident cardiovascular events in the MESA (Multi-ethnic study of atherosclerosis). *Journal of the American College of Cardiology, 56*(18), 1506–1512. doi:10.1016/j.jacc.2010.04.060.

Cull, D. L., Langan, E. M., Gray, B. H., et al. (2010). Open versus endovascular intervention for critical limb ischemia: A population-based study. *Journal of the American College of Surgeons, 210*(5), 555–563. doi:10.1016/j.jamcollsurg.2009.12.019.

de Ceniga, M. V., Bravo, E., Izagirre, M., et al. (2011). Anaemia, iron and vitamin deficits in patients with peripheral arterial disease. *European Journal of Vascular & Endovascular Surgery, 41*(6), 828–830. doi:10.1016/j.ejvs.2011.01.017.

de Graaff, J. C., Ubbink, D. T., Legemate, D. A., et al. (2003). Evaluation of toe pressure and transcutaneous oxygen measurements in management of chronic critical leg ischemia: A diagnostic randomized clinical trial. *Journal of Vascular Surgery, 38*, 528–534.

De Haro, J., Acin, F., Lopez-Quintana, A., et al. (2009). Meta-analysis of randomized, controlled clinical trials in angiogenesis: Gene and cell therapy in peripheral arterial disease. *Heart and Vessels, 24*(5), 321–328. doi:10.1007/s00380-008-1140-z.

Delis, K. T., Husmann, M. J., Nicolaides, A. N., et al. (2002). Enhancing foot skin blood flux in peripheral vascular disease using intermittent pneumatic compression: Controlled study on claudicants and grafted arteriopaths. *World Journal of Surgery, 26*, 861–866. doi:10.1007/s00268-001-0297-8.

Delis, K. T., & Nicolaides, A. N. (2005). Effect of intermittent pneumatic compression of foot and calf on walking distance, hemodynamics, and quality of life in patients with arterial claudication. *Annals of Surgery, 241*, 431–441. doi:10.1097/01.sla.0000154358.83898.26.

del Rincon, I., Haas, R., Pogosian, S., et al. (2005). Lower limb arterial incompressibility and obstruction in rheumatoid arthritis. *Annals of the Rheumatic Diseases, 64*, 425–432. doi:10.1136/ard.2003.018671.

Dennis, M., Sandercock, P., Reid J., et al.; CLOTS (Clots in Legs Or sTockings after Stroke) Trials Collaboration. (2013). Effectiveness of intermittent pneumatic compression in reduction of risk of deep vein thrombosis in patients who have had a stroke (CLOTS 3): A multicentre randomised controlled trial. *Lancet, 382*(9891), 516–524. doi:10.1016/S0140-6736(13)61050-8.

Dhangana, R., Murphy, T. P., Pencina, M. J., et al. (2011). Prevalence of low ankle-brachial index, elevated plasma fibrinogen and CRP across Framingham risk categories: Data from the National Health and Nutrition Examination Survey (NHANES) 1999–2004. *Atherosclerosis, 216*, 174–179. doi:10.1016/j.atherosclerosis.2010.10.021.

Diaz, M. L., Urtasun, F., Barberena, J., et al. (2011). Cryoplasty versus conventional angioplasty in femoropopliteal arterial recanalization: 3-year analysis of reintervention-free survival by treatment received. *CardioVascular and Interventional Radiology, 34*, 911–917. doi:10.1007/s00270-010-0032-7.

Diehm, C., Allenberg, J. R., Pittrow, D., et al. (2009). Mortality and vascular morbidity in older adults with asymptomatic versus symptomatic peripheral artery disease. *Circulation, 120*, 2053–2061. doi:10.1161/CIRCULATIONAHA.109.865600.

Dieter, R. S., Tomasson, J., Gudjonsson, T., et al. (2003). Lower extremity peripheral arterial disease in hospitalized patients with coronary artery disease. *Vascular Medicine, 8*, 233–236.

Dillon, R. S. (1986). Treatment of resistant venous stasis ulcers and dermatitis with end-diastolic pneumatic compression boot. *Angiology, 37*(1), 47–56.

Di Minno, M. N., Milone, M., Russolillo, A., et al. (2013). Ropivacaine infusion in diabetics subject with peripheral arterial disease. A prospective study. *Experimental and Clinical Endocrinology & Diabetes, 121*, 91–93. doi:10.1055/s-0032-1327757.

Dogliotti, G., Galliera, E., Iorio, E., et al. (2011). Effect of immersion in CO2-enriched water on free radical release and total antioxidant status in peripheral arterial occlusive disease. *International Angiology, 30*, 12–17.

Doughty, D. (2012). Arterial ulcers. In R. Bryant & D. Nix (Eds.), *Acute & chronic wounds. Current management concepts* (4th ed., pp. 178–193). St. Louis, MO: Elsevier-Mosby.

Dowling, K. M. (2008). Patient rehabilitation following lower limb amputation. *Nursing Standard, 22*(49), 35–40.

Drinka, P., Bonham, P., & Crnich, C. (2012). Swab culture of purulent skin infection to detect infection or colonization with antibiotic resistant bacteria. *Journal of the American Medical Directors Association, 13*(1), 75–79. doi:10.1016/j.jamda.2011.04.012.

Dunkelgrun, M., Hoeks, S. E., Schouten, O., et al. (2009). Methionine loading does not enhance the predictive value of homocysteine serum testing for all-cause mortality or major adverse cardiac events. *InternalMedicine,39*,13–18.doi:10.1111/j.1445-5994.2007.01596.x.

Eiberg, J. P., Rasmussen, J. B., Hansen, M. A., et al. (2010). Duplex ultrasound scanning of peripheral arterial disease of the lower limb. *European Journal of Vascular & Endovascular Surgery, 40*, 507–512. doi:10.1016/j.ejvs.2010.06.002.

Escobar, C. E., Blanes, I., Ruiz, A., et al. (2011). Prevalence and clinical profile and management of peripheral arterial disease in elderly patients with diabetes. *European Journal of Internal Medicine, 22*, 275–281. doi:10.1016/j.ejim.2011.02.001.

Faglia, E., Favales, F., Aldeghi, A., et al. (1996). Adjunctive systemic hyperbaric oxygen therapy in treatment of severe prevalently ischemic diabetic foot ulcer: A randomized study. *Diabetes Care, 19*, 1338–1343.

Fiore, M. C., Jaen, C. R., Baker, T. B., et al. (2008). *Clinical practice guideline. Treating tobacco use and dependence: 2008 update.* U.S. Department of Health and Human Services, Public Health Service. Retrieved August 2013fromhttp://www.aafp.org/dam/AAFP/documents/patient_care/clinical_recommendations/TreatingTobaccoUseandDependence-2008Update.pdf

Fleury, A. M., Salih, S. A., & Peel, N. M. (2013). Rehabilitation of the older vascular amputee: A review of the literature. *Geriatrics & Gerontology International, 13* (2), 264–273. doi:10.1111/ggi.12016.

Flu, H. C., Lardenoye, J. H., Veen, E. J., et al. (2009). Morbidity and mortality caused by cardiac adverse events after revascularization for critical limb ischemia. *Annals of Vascular Surgery, 23*, 583–597. doi:10.1016/j.avsg.2009.06.012.

Fokkenrood, H. J., Bendermacher, B. L., Lauret, G. J., et al. (2013). Supervised exercise therapy versus non-supervised exercise therapy for intermittent claudication. *Cochrane Database of Systematic Reviews*, (8), Art. No.: CD005263. doi:10.1002/14651858.CD005263.pub3.

Fowkes, F., & Leng, G. C. (2008). Bypass surgery for chronic lower limb ischaemia. *Cochrane Database of Systematic Reviews*, (2), Art. No.: CD002000. doi:10.1002/14651858.CD002000.pub2.

Fowkes, F., Low, L., Tuta, S., et al. (2006). Ankle-brachial index and extent of atherothrombosis in 8891 patients with or at risk of vascular disease: Results of the international AGATHA study. *European Heart Journal, 27*, 1861–1867. doi:10.1093/eurheartj/ehl114.

Fowkes, F. G., Murray, G. D., Butcher, I., et al. Ankle Brachial Collaboration. (2008). Ankle brachial index combined with Framingham risk score to predict cardiovascular events and mortality: A meta-analysis, *Journal of the American Medical Association, 300*(2), 197–208. doi:10.1001/jama.300.2.197.

Fowler, E., Scott-Williams, S., & McGuire, J. B. (2008). Practice recommendations for preventing heel pressure ulcers. *Ostomy Wound Management, 54*(10), 42–57.

Franz, R. W., Parks, A., Shah, K. J., et al. (2009). Use of autologous bone marrow mononuclear cell implantation therapy as a limb salvage procedure in patients with severe peripheral arterial disease. *Journal ofVascularSurgery,50*(6),1378–1390.doi:10.1016/j.jvs.2009.07.113.

Freidank, H. M., Lux, A., Dern, P., et al. (2002). *Chlamydia pneumoniae* DNA in peripheral venous blood samples from patients with carotid artery stenosis. *European Journal of Clinical Microbiology & Infectious Diseases, 21*, 60–62.

Gaddipati, V. C., Bailey, B. A., Kuriacose, R., et al. (2011). The relationship of vitamin D status to cardiovascular risk factors and amputation risk in veterans with peripheral arterial disease. *Journal of the American Medical Directors Association, 12*, 58–61. doi:10.1016/j.jamda.2010.02.006.

Garofolo, L., Barros, N., Miranda, F. Jr., et al. (2007). Association of increased levels of homocysteine and peripheral arterial disease in a Japanese-Brazilian population. *European Journal of Vascular & Endovascular Surgery, 34*, 23–28. doi:10.1016/j.ejvs.2007.02.008.

Garcia, A. M., Marchena, P. J., Toril, J., et al. (2011). Alcohol consumption and outcome in stable outpatients with peripheral artery disease. *Journal of Vascular Surgery, 54*, 1081–1087. doi:10.1016/j.jvs.2011.03.285.

Gardner, A. W., Bright, B. C., Ort, K. A., et al. (2011). Dietary intake of participants with peripheral artery disease and claudication. *Angiology, 62*(3), 270–275. doi:10.1177/0003319710384395.

Gardner, A. W., Montgomery, P. S., & Parker, D. E. (2008). Physical activity is a predictor of all-cause mortality in patients with intermittent claudication. *Journal of Vascular Surgery, 47*, 117–122. doi:10.1016/j.jvs.2007.09.033.

Gardner, S. E., & Frantz, R. A. (2008). Wound bioburden. In S. Baranoski & E. A. Ayello (Eds.), *Wound care essentials: Practice principles* (2nd ed., pp. 93–118). Ambler, PA: Lippincott Williams & Wilkins.

Gee, E. (2011). Anti-embolism stockings. *Nursing Times, 107*(14), 18–19.

Gefen, A. (2010). The biomechanics of heel ulcers. *Journal of Tissue Viability, 19*(4), 124–131. doi:10.1016/j.jtv.2010.06.003.

Geraghty, A. J., & Welch, K. (2011). Antithrombotic agents for preventing thrombosis after infrainguinal arterial bypass surgery. *Cochrane Database of Systematic Reviews*, (6), Art. No.: CD000536. doi:10.1002/14651858.CD000536.pub2.

Ghajar, A. J., & Miles, J. B. (1998). The differential effect of the level of spinal cord stimulation on patients with advanced peripheral vascular disease in the lower limbs. *British Journal of Neurosurgery, 12*(5), 402–409.

Giles, K. A., Hamdan, A. D., Pomposelli, F. B., et al. (2010). Body mass index: Surgical site infections and mortality after lower extremity bypass from the National Surgical Quality Improvement Program 2005–2007. *Annals of Vascular Surgery, 24*(1), 48–56. doi:10.1016/j.avsg.2009.05.003.

Gist, S., Tio-Matos, I., Falzgraf, S., et al. (2009). Wound care in the geriatric client. *Clinical Interventions in Aging, 4*, 269–287.

Goessens, B. M., Visseren, F. L., Algra, A., et al. (2006). Screening for asymptomatic cardiovascular disease with noninvasive imaging in patients at high-risk and low-risk according to the European guidelines on cardiovascular disease prevention: The SMART study. *Journal of Vascular Surgery, 43*, 525–532. doi:10.1016/j.jvs.2005.11.050.

Goldman, R., Brewley, B., Zhou, L., et al. (2003). Electrotherapy reverses inframalleolar ischemia: A retrospective, observational study. *Advances in Skin & Wound Care, 16*(2), 79–89. doi:10.1097/00129334-200303000-00009.

Gonzalo, B., Solanich, T., Bellmunt, S., et al. (2010). Cryoplasty as endovascular treatment in the femoropopliteal region: Hemodynamic results and follow-up at one year. *Annals of Vascular Surgery, 24*(5), 680–685. doi:10.1016/j.avsg.2009.08.021.

Grolman, R. E., Wilkerson, D. K., Taylor, J., et al. (2001). Transcutaneous oxygen measurements predict a beneficial response to hyperbaric oxygen therapy in patients with nonhealing wounds and critical limb ischemia. *American Surgeon, 67*(11), 1072–1079.

Harward, T. R., Volny, J., Golbranson, F., et al. (1985). Oxygen inhalation-induced transcutaneous PO2 changes as a predictor of amputation level. *Journal of Vascular Surgery, 2*, 220–227.

Haslacher, H., Perkmann, T., Gruenewald, J., et al. (2012). Plasma myeloperoxidase level and peripheral arterial disease. *European Journal of Clinical Investigation, 42*(5), 463–469.

He, Y., Jiang, Y., Wang, J., et al. (2006). Prevalence of peripheral arterial disease and its association with smoking in a population-based study in Beijing, China. *Journal of Vascular Surgery, 44*, 333–338.

He, Y., Lam, T. H., Jiang, B., et al. (2008). Passive smoking and risk of peripheral arterial disease and ischemic stroke in Chinese women who never smoked. *Circulation, 118*(15), 1535–1540. doi:10.1161/CIRCULATIONAHA.108.784801.

Hebert, K., Lopez, B., Michael, C., et al. (2010). The prevalence of peripheral arterial disease in patients with heart failure by race and ethnicity. *Congestive Heart Failure, 16*(3), 118–221.

Hennrikus, D., Joseph, A. M., Lando, H. A., et al. (2010). Effectiveness of a smoking cessation program for peripheral artery disease patients:

A randomized controlled trial. *Journal of the American College of Cardiology, 56*(25), 2105–2112. doi:10.1016/j.jacc.2010.07.031.

Hiatt, W. R., Hirsch, A. T., Creager, M. A., et al. (2010). Effect of niacin ER/lovastatin on claudication symptoms in patients with peripheral artery disease. *Vascular Medicine, 15*(3), 171–179. doi:10.1177/1358863x09360579.

Hirashima, F., Patel, R. B., Adams, J. E., et al. (2012). Use of a postoperative insulin protocol decreases wound infection in diabetics undergoing lower extremity bypass. *Journal of Vascular Surgery, 56*(2), 396–402.e4. doi:10.1016/j.jvs.2012.01.026.

Hirsch, A. T., Allison, M. A., Gomes, A. S., et al. (2012). A call to action: Women and peripheral artery disease. A scientific statement from the American Heart Association. *Circulation, 125*, 1449–1472. doi:10.1161/CIR.0b013e31824c39ba.

Hirsch, A. T., Hartman, L., Town, R. J., et al. (2008). National health care costs of peripheral arterial disease in the Medicare population. *VascularMedicine, 13*(3), 209–215. doi:10.1177/1358863X08089277.

Hirsch, A. T., Haskal, Z. J., Hertzer, N. R., et al. (2006). ACC/AHA 2005 Practice Guidelines for the management of patients with peripheral arterial disease (lower extremity, renal, mesenteric and abdominal aortic): A collaborative report from the Angiography and Interventions, Society for Vascular Medicine and Biology, Society of Interventional Radiology and the ACC/AHA Task Force on Practice Guidelines (Writing Committee to Develop Guidelines for the Management of Patients With Peripheral Arterial Disease): Endorsed by the American Association of Cardiovascular and Pulmonary Rehabilitation; National Heart, Lung and Blood Institute; Society for Vascular Nursing; Trans-Atlantic Inter-Society Consensus; and Vascular Disease Foundation. *Circulation, 113*(11), e463–e654.

Ho, K. M., & Tan, J. A. (2013). Stratified meta-analysis of intermittent pneumatic compression of the lower limbs to prevent venous thromboembolism in hospitalized patients. *Circulation, 128*, 1003–1020. doi:10.1161/CIRCULATIONAHA.113.002690.

Hogh, A. L., Joensen, J., Lindholt, J. S., et al. (2008). C-Reactive protein predicts future arterial and cardiovascular events in patients with symptomatic peripheral arterial disease. *Vascular and Endovascular Surgery, 42*(4), 341–347. doi:10.1177/1538574408316138.

Hopf, H. W., Ueno, C., Aslam, R., et al. (2006). Guidelines for the treatment of arterial insufficiency ulcers. *Wound Repair and Regeneration, 14*(6), 693–710.

Hopf, H. W., Ueno, C., Aslam, R., et al. (2008). Guidelines for the prevention of lower extremity arterial ulcers. *Wound Repair and Regeneration, 16*, 175–188. Retrieved February 2013 from http://onlinelibrary.wiley.com/doi/10.1111/j.1524-475X.2008.00358.x/pdf.

Horch, R. E., Dragu, A., Lang, W., et al. (2008). Coverage of exposed bones and joints in critically ill patients: Lower extremity salvage with topical negative pressure therapy. *Journal of Cutaneous Medicine and Surgery, 12*(5), 223–229.

Hoyer, C., Sandermann, J., & Petersen, L. J. (2013). The toe-brachial index in the diagnosis of peripheral arterial disease. *Journal of Vascular Surgery, 58*(1), 231–238. doi:10.1016/j.jvs.2013.03.044.

Huang, P. P., Li, S. Z., Han, M. Z., et al. (2004). Autologous transplantation of peripheral blood stem cells as an effective therapeutic approach for severe arteriosclerosis obliterans of lower extremities. *Thrombosis and Haemostasis, 91*(3), 606–609. doi:10.1160/TH03-06-0343.

Hung, H. C., Willett, W., Merchant, A., et al. (2003). Oral health and peripheral arterial disease. *Circulation, 107*(8), 1152–1157.

Hussein, A. A., Uno, K., Wolski, K., et al. (2011). Peripheral arterial disease and progression of coronary atherosclerosis. *Journal of the American College of Cardiology, 57*(10), 1220–1225. doi:10.1016/j.jacc.2010.10.034.

Iezzi, R., Santoro, M., Marano, R., et al. (2012). Low-dose multidetector CT angiography in the evaluation of infrarenal aorta and peripheral arterial occlusive disease. *Radiology, 263*(1), 287–298. doi:10.1148/radiol.11110700.

Ix, J. H., Allison, M. A., Denenberg, J. O., et al. (2008). Novel cardiovascular risk factors do not completely explain the higher prevalence of peripheral arterial disease among African Americans: The San Diego population study. *Journal of the American College of Cardiology, 51*(24), 2347–2354. doi:10.1016/j.jacc.2008.03.022.

Ix, J. H., Biggs, M. L., Kizer, J. R., et al. (2011). Association of body mass index with peripheral arterial disease in older adults. The cardiovascular health study. *American Journal of Epidemiology, 174*(9), 1036–1043. doi:10.1093/aje/kwr228.

Ix, J. H., Katz, R., DeBoer, I. H., et al. (2009). Association of chronic kidney disease with the spectrum of ankle brachial index: The CHS (cardiovascular health study). *Journal of the American College of Cardiology, 54*(13), 1176–1184. doi:10.1016/j.jacc.2009.06.017.

Jaff, M. R., Dale, R. A., Creager, M. A., et al. (2009). Anti-chlamydial antibiotic therapy for symptom improvement in peripheral artery disease: Prospective evaluation of rifalazil effect on vascular symptoms of intermittent claudication and other endpoints in *Chlamydia pneumoniae* seropositive patients (PROVIDENCE-1). *Circulation, 119*(3), 452–458. doi:10.1161/CIRCULATIONAHA.108.815308.

Jain, A., Liu, K., Ferrucci, L., et al. (2012). The Walking Impairment Questionnaire stair-climbing score predicts mortality in men and women with peripheral arterial disease. *Journal of Vascular Surgery, 55*(6), 1662–1673.e2. doi:10.1016/j.jvs.2011.12.010.

Jalili, M. (2011). Chapter 219. Type 2 diabetes mellitus. In J. E. Tintinalli, J. Stapczynski, O. Ma, et al. (Eds.), *Tintinalli's emergency medicine: A comprehensive study guide* (7th ed.). New York, NY: Mc-Graw Hill. Retrieved April 01, 2014, from http://accessmedicine.mhmedical.com.ezproxy-v.musc.edu/content.aspx?bookid=348&Sectionid=40381702

James, P. A., Oparil, S., Carter, B. L., et al. (2014). 2014 evidence-based guideline for the management of high blood pressure in adults. Report from the panel members appointed to the Eighth Joint National Committee (JNC 8). *Journal of the American Medical Association, 311*(5), 507–520. doi:10.1001/jama.2013.284427.

Jensen, S. A., Vatten, L. J., Nilsen, T. I., et al. (2005). The association between smoking and the prevalence of intermittent claudication. *Vascular Medicine, 10*(4), 257–263.

Jobin, S., Kalliainen, L., Adebayo, L., et al. (2011). Venous thromboembolism prophylaxis. Retrieved December 7, 2013 from http://www.guideline.gov/popups/printView.aspx?id=39350

Joensen, J. B., Juul, S., Henneberg, E., et al. (2008). Can long-term antibiotic treatment prevent progression of peripheral arterial occlusive disease? A large randomized, double-blinded placebo-controlled trial. *Atherosclerosis, 196*(2), 937–942. doi:10.1016/j.atherosclerosis.2007.02.025.

Johannesson, A., Larsson, G., Oberg, T., et al. (2008). Comparison of vacuum-formed removable rigid dressing with conventional rigid dressing after transtibial amputation: similar outcome in a randomized controlled trial involving 27 patients. *Acta Orthopaedica, 79*(3):361–369. doi:10.1080/17453670710015265.

Jones, M. L. (2013). BPS2: Nursing care of patients wearing anti-embolic stockings. *British Journal of Healthcare Assistants, 7*(8), 388–390.

Jurno, M. E., Chevtchouk, L., Nunes, A. A., et al. (2010). Ankle-brachial index, a screening for peripheral obstructive arterial disease and migraine-A controlled study. *Headache, 50*(4), 626–630. doi:10.1111/j.1526-4610.2009.01536.x.

Kahn, S. R., Lim, W., Dunn, A. S., et al. (2012). Prevention of VTE in nonsurgical patients: Antithrombotic therapy and prevention of thrombosis, 9th ed.: American College of Chest Physicians evidence-based clinical practice guidelines. *Chest, 141*(S2), S195–S226. doi:10.1378/chest.11-2296.

Kakkos, S. K., Geroulakos, G., & Nicolaides, A. N. (2005). Improvement of the walking ability in intermittent claudication due to superficial femoral artery occlusion with supervised exercise and pneumatic foot and calf compression: A randomised controlled trial. *European Journal of Vascular & Endovascular Surgery, 30*(2), 164–175.

Kaperonis, E. A., Liapis, C. D., Kakisis, J. D., et al. (2006). Inflammation and *Chlamydia pneumoniae* infection correlate with the severity of peripheral arterial disease. *European Journal of Vascular & Endovascular Surgery, 31*(5), 509–515. doi:10.1016/j.ejvs.2005.11.022.

Kavros, S. J., Delis, K. T., Turner, N. S., et al. (2008). Improving limb salvage in critical ischemia with intermittent pneumatic compression: A controlled study with 18-month follow-up. *Journal of Vascular Surgery, 47*, 543–549. doi:10.1016/j.jvs.2007.11.043.

Kavros, S. J., Miller, J. L., & Hanna, S. W. (2007). Treatment of ischemic wounds with noncontact, low-frequency ultrasound: The Mayo Clinic Experience, 2004–2006. *Advances in Skin & Wound Care, 20*(4), 221–226.

Kayhan, A., Palabiyik, F., Serinsoz, S., et al. (2012). Multidetector CT angiography versus arterial duplex USG in diagnosis of mild lower extremity peripheral arterial disease: Is multidetector CT a valuable screening tool? *European Journal of Radiology, 81*(2), 542–546. doi:10.1016/j.ejrad.2011.01.100.

Khaleghi, M., Singletary, L. A., Kondragunta, V., et al. (2009). Haemostatic markers are associated with measures of vascular disease in adults with hypertension. *Journal of Human Hypertension, 23*, 530–537. doi:10.1038/jhh.2008.170.

Khan, N. A., Rahim, S. S., Anand, S. S., et al. (2006). Does the clinical examination predict lower extremity peripheral arterial disease? *Journal of the American Medical Association, 295*(5), 536–546. doi:10.1001/jama.295.5.536.

Khan, S. Z., Khan, M. A., Bradley, B., et al. (2011). Utility of duplex ultrasound in detecting and grading de novo femoropopliteal lesions. *Journal of Vascular Surgery, 54*, 1067–1073. doi:10.1016/j.jvs.2011.03.282.

Khawaja, F. J., Bailey, K. R., Turner, S. T., et al. (2007). Association of novel risk factors with ankle brachial index in African American and Non-Hispanic White populations. *Mayo Clinic Proceedings, 82*(6), 709–716. doi:10.4065/82.6.709.

Kim, E. S., Wattanakit, K., & Gornik, H. L. (2012). Using the ankle-brachial index to diagnose peripheral artery disease and assess cardiovascular risk. *Cleveland Clinic Journal of Medicine, 79*(9), 651–661. doi:10.3949/ccjm.79a.11154.

Kohlman-Trigoboff, D. (2013). Management of lower extremity peripheral arterial disease: Interpreting the latest guidelines for nurse practitioners. *The Journal for Nurse Practitioners, 9*(10), 653–660. doi:10.1016/j.nurpra.2013.08.026.

Korna, M., Eldrup, N., & Sillesen, H. (2009). Comparison of ankle-brachial index measured by an automated oscillometric apparatus with that by standard Doppler technique in vascular patients. *European Journal of Vascular & Endovascular Surgery, 38*(5), 610–615. doi:10.1016/j.ejvs.2009.07.004.

Kravos, A., & Bubnic-Sotosek, K. (2009). Ankle-brachial index screening for peripheral artery disease in asymptomatic patients between 50 and 70 years of age. *Journal of International Medical Research, 37*(5), 1611–1619. doi:10.1177/147323000903700540.

Krayenbuehl, P. A., Wiesli, P., Maly, F. E., et al. (2005). Progression of peripheral arterial occlusive disease is associated with *Chlamydia pneumoniae* seropositivity and can be inhibited by antibiotic treatment. *Atherosclerosis, 179*(1), 103–110.

Kroger, K., Stewen, C., Santosa, F., et al. (2003). Toe pressure measurements compared to ankle artery pressure measurements. *Angiology, 54*(1), 39–44.

Kumakura, H., Kanai, H., Araki, Y., et al. (2011). Sex-related differences in Japanese patients with peripheral arterial disease. *Atherosclerosis, 219*(2), 846–850. doi:10.1016/j.atherosclerosis.2011.08.037.

Kumar, K., Toth, C., Nath, R. K., et al. (1997). Improvement of limb circulation in peripheral disease using epidural spinal cord stimulation: A prospective study. *Journal of Neurosurgery, 86*(4), 662–669.

Labropoulous, N., Wierks, C., & Suffoletto, B. (2002). Intermittent pneumatic compression for the treatment of lower extremity arterial disease: A systematic review. *Vascular Medicine, 7*(2), 141–148.

Lakshmanan, R., Hyde, Z., Jamrozik, K., et al. (2010). Population-based observational study of claudication in older men: The Health in Men study. *Medical Journal of Australia, 192*(11), 641–645.

Lane, D. A., & Lip, G. Y. (2009). Treatment of hypertension in peripheral arterial disease. *Cochrane Database of Systematic Reviews*, (4), Art. No.: CD003075. doi:10.1002/14651858.CD003075.pub2.

Lane, J., Vittinghoff, E., Lane, K. T., et al. (2006). Risk factors for premature peripheral vascular disease: Results for the national health and nutritional survey, 1999–2002. *Journal of Vascular Surgery, 44*(2), 319–325.

Langemo, D., Thompson, P., Hunter, S., et al. (2008). Heel pressure ulcers: Stand guard. *Advances in Skin & Wound Care, 21*(6), 282–292.

Lantis, J. C., Boone, D., Lee, L., et al. (2011). The effect of percutaneous intervention on wound healing in patients with mixed arterial venous disease. *Annals of Vascular Surgery, 25*(1), 79–86. doi:10.1016/j.avsg.2010.09.006.

Lau, J. F., Weinberg, M. D., & Olin, J. W. (2011). Peripheral artery disease. Part 1: Clinical evaluation and noninvasive diagnosis. *Nature Reviews Cardiology, 8*, 405–418. doi:10.1038/nrcardio.2011.66.

Laurent, B., Millon, A., de Forges, M. R., et al. (2012). Pedicled flaps in association with distal bypass for lower-limb salvage. *Annals of Vascular Surgery, 26*(2), 205–212. doi:10.1016/j.avsg.2011.07.020.

Lee, Y. H., Shin, M. H., Kweon, S. S., et al. (2011). Cumulative smoking exposure, duration of smoking cessation, and peripheral arterial disease in middle-aged and older Korean men. *BMC Public Health, 11*, 94. doi:10.1186/1471-2458-11-94.

Leeper, N. J., Myers, J., Zhou, M., et al. (2013). Exercise capacity is the strongest predictor of mortality in patients with peripheral arterial disease. *Journal of Vascular Surgery, 57*(3), 728–733. doi:10.1016/j.jvs.2012.07.051.

Lezack, J. D., & Carter, S. A. (1973). The relationship of digital systolic pressures to the clinical and angiographic findings in limbs with arterial occlusive disease. *Scandinavian Journal of Clinical and Laboratory Investigation, 128*, 97–101.

Liapis, C.D., Avgerinos, E. D., Kadoglou, N. P., et al. (2009). What a vascular surgeon should know and do about atherosclerotic risk factors. *Journal of Vascular Surgery, 49*(5)1348–1354. doi:10.1016/j.jvs.2008.12.046.

Linares-Palomino, J. P., Gutierrez, J., Lopez-Espada, C., et al. (2004). Genomic, serologic and clinical case-control study of *Chlamydia pneumoniae* and peripheral artery occlusive disease. *Journal of Vascular Surgery, 40*(2), 359–366.

Lindell, K. O., & Reinke, L. F. (1999). Nursing strategies for smoking cessation. *Heart & Lung, 28*(4), 295–302.

Linden, B. (2013). Lower limb peripheral artery disease. *British Journal of Cardiac Nursing, 8*(3), 112–113.

Lockhart, P. B., Bolger, A. F., Papapanou, P. N., et al. (2012). Periodontal disease and atherosclerotic vascular disease: Does the evidence support an independent association? A scientific statement from the American Heart Association. *Circulation, 125*(20), 2520–2544. doi:10.1161/CIR.0b013e31825719f3.

Lu, B., Parker, D., & Eaton, C. B. (2008). Relationship of periodontal attachment loss to peripheral vascular disease: An analysis of NHANES 1999–2002 data. *Atherosclerosis, 200*(1), 199–205. doi:10.1016/j.atherosclerosis.2007.12.037.

Lyder, C. H. (2011). Preventing heel pressure ulcers: Economic and legal implications. *Nursing Management, 42*(11), 16–19. doi:10.1097/01.NUMA.0000406569.58343.0a.

Madu, A. J., Ubesie, A., Madu, K. A., et al. (2013). Evaluation of clinical and laboratory correlates of sickle cell ulcers. *Wound Repair and Regeneration, 21*(6), 808–812. doi:10.1111/wrr.12100.

Mahoney, E. M., Wang, K., Keo, H. H., et al. (2010). Vascular hospitalization rates and costs in patients with peripheral artery disease in the United States. *Circulation: Cardiovascular Quality & Outcomes, 3*, 642–651. doi:10.1161/CIRCOUTCOMES.109.930735.

Makisalo, H., Lepantalo, M., Halme, L., et al. (1998). Peripheral arterial disease as a predictor of outcome after renal transplantation. *Transplant International, 11*(S1), S140–S143.

Makita, S., Ohira, A., Naganuma, Y., et al. (2006). The effects on skin blood flow of immersing the ischemic legs of patients with peripheral arterial disease into artificially carbonated water. *International Journal of Angiology, 15*, 12–15. doi:10.1007/s00547-006-2063-0.

Makris, G. C., Lattimer, C. R., Lavida, A., et al. (2012). Availability of supervised exercise programs and the role of structured home-based exercise in peripheral arterial disease. *European Journal of Vascular & Endovascular Surgery, 44*(6), 569–575; discussion 576. doi:10.1016/j.ejvs.2012.09.009.

Maksimovic, M., Vlajinac, H., Radak, D., et al. (2009). Relationship between peripheral arterial disease and metabolic syndrome. *Angiology, 60*(5), 546–553. doi:10.1177/0003319708325445.

Mangiafico, R. A., & Mangiafico, M. (2011). Medical treatment of critical limb ischemia: Current state and future directions. *Current Vascular Pharmacology, 9*(6), 658–676.

Marfella, R., Luongo, C., Coppola, A., et al. (2010). Use of a non-specific immunomodulation therapy as a therapeutic vasculogenesis strategy in no-option critical limb ischemia patients. *Atherosclerosis, 208*(2), 473–479. doi:10.1016/j.atherosclerosis.2009.08.005.

Marshall, C., & Stansby, G. (2010). Amputation and rehabilitation. *Surgery, 28*(6). 284–287. doi:10.1016/j.mpsur.2010.01.017.

Marston, W. (2011). Mixed arterial and venous ulcers. *Wounds, 23*(12), 351–356.

Marston, W. A., Davies, S. W., Armstrong, B., et al. (2006). Natural history of limbs with arterial insufficiency and chronic ulceration treated without revascularization. *Journal of Vascular Surgery, 44*(1), 108–114.

Marti-Carvajal, A. J., Sola, I., Lathyris, D., et al. (2013). Homocysteine-lowering interventions for preventing cardiovascular events. *Cochrane Database of Systematic Reviews*, (1), Art. No.: CD006612. doi:10.1002/14651858.CD006612.pub3.

Masanauskiene, E., & Naudziunas, A. (2011). Comparison of ankle brachial index in patients with and without atrial fibrillation. *Medicina, 47*(12), 641–645.

Mazari, F. A., Khan, J. A., Carradice, D., et al. (2012). Randomized clinical trial of percutaneous transluminal angioplasty, supervised exercise and combined treatment for intermittent claudication due to femoropopliteal arterial disease. *British Journal of Surgery, 99*(1), 39–48. doi:10.1002/bjs.7710.

Mazur, P., Kozynacka, A., Durajski, L., et al. (2012). Nε-homocysteinyl-lysine isopeptide is associated with progression of peripheral artery disease in patients treated with folic acid. *European Journal of Vascular & Endovascular Surgery, 43*(5), 588–593. doi:10.1016/j.ejvs.2012.02.022.

McCulloch, S. V., Marston, W. A., Farber, M. A., et al. (2003). Healing potential of lower-extremity ulcers in patients with arterial insufficiency with and without revascularization. *Wounds, 15*(12), 390–394.

McDermott, M. M., Ferrucci, L., Guralnik, J. M., et al. (2010a). The ankle-brachial index is associated with the magnitude of impaired walking endurance among men and women with peripheral arterial disease. *Vascular Medicine, 15*(4), 251–257. doi:10.1177/1358863x10365181.

McDermott, M. M., Ferrucci, L., Liu, K., et al. (2011a). Women with peripheral arterial disease experience faster functional decline than men with peripheral arterial disease. *Journal of the American College of Cardiology, 57*(6), 707–714. doi:10.1016/j.jacc.2010.09.042.

McDermott, M. M., Guralnik, J. M., Albay, M., et al. (2004). Impairments of muscles and nerves associated with peripheral arterial disease and their relationship with lower extremity functioning: The InCHIANTI study. *Journal of the American Geriatrics Society, 52*(3), 405–410.

McDermott, M. M., Guralnik, J. M., Corsi, A., et al. (2005). Patterns of inflammation associated with peripheral arterial disease: The InCHIANTI study. *American Heart Journal, 150*(2), 276–281.

McDermott, M. M., Guralnik, J. M., Greenland, P., et al. (2003). Statin use and leg functioning in patients with and without lower-extremity peripheral arterial disease. *Circulation, 107*(5), 757–761.

McDermott, M. M., Liu, K., Ferrucci, L., et al. (2008). Circulating blood markers and functional impairment in peripheral arterial disease. *Journal of the American Geriatrics Society, 56*(8), 1504–1510. doi:10.1111/j.1532-5415.2008.01797.x.

McDermott, M. M., Mazor, K. M., Reed, G., et al. (2010b). Attitudes and behavior of peripheral arterial disease patients toward influencing their physician's prescription of cholesterol-lowering medication. *Vascular Medicine, 15*(2), 83–90. doi:10.1177/1358863X09353653.

McDermott, M. M., Reed, G., Greenland, P., et al. (2011b). Activating peripheral arterial disease patients to reduce cholesterol: A randomized trial. *The American Journal of Medicine, 124*(6), 557–565. doi:10.1016/j.amjmed.2010.11.032.

McDermott, M. M., Sufit, R., Nishida, T., et al. (2006). Lower extremity nerve function in patients with lower extremity ischemia. *Archives of Internal Medicine, 166*(18), 1986–1992.

McGrath, C., Robb, R., Lucas, A. J., et al. (2002). A randomized, double blind, placebo-controlled study to determine the efficacy of immune modulation therapy in the treatment of patients suffering from peripheral arterial occlusive disease with intermittent claudication. *European Journal of Vascular & Endovascular Surgery, 23*(5), 381–387.

McMahon, J. H., & Grigg, M. J. (1995). Predicting healing of lower limb ulcers. *The Australian and New Zealand Journal of Surgery, 65*(3), 173–176.

Meaume, S., & Faucher, N. (2007). Heel pressure ulcers on the increase? Epidemiological change or ineffective prevention strategies? *Journal of Tissue Viability, 17*(1), 30–33. doi:10.1016/j.jtv.2007.09.010.

Melamed, M. L., Muntner, P., Michos, E. D., et al. (2008). Serum 25-hydroxyvitamin D levels and the prevalence of peripheral arterial disease. *Arteriosclerosis, Thrombosis, and Vascular Biology, 28*, 1179–1185. doi:10.1161/ATVBAHA.108.165886.

Met, R., Bipat, S., Legemate, D. A., et al. (2009). Diagnostic performance of computed tomography angiography in peripheral arterial disease: A systematic review and meta-analysis. *Journal of the American Medical Association, 301*, 415–424. doi:10.1001/jama.301.4.415.

Mills, E., Eyawo, O., Lockhart, I., et al. (2011). Smoking cessation reduces postoperative complications: A systematic review and meta-analysis. *American Journal of Medicine, 124*(2), 144–154 e148. doi:10.1016/j.amjmed.2010.09.013.

Moazzami, K., Majdzadeh, R., & Nedjat, S. (2011). Local intramuscular transplantation of autologous mononuclear cells for critical lower limb ischemia. *Cochrane Database of Systematic Reviews*, Issue 12:Art. No.: CD008347. doi:10.1002/14651858.CD008347.pub2.

Mogelvang, R., Pedersen, S. H., Flyvbjerg, A., et al. (2012). Comparison of osteoprotegerin to traditional atherosclerotic risk factors and high-sensitivity C-reactive protein for diagnosis of atherosclerosis. *American Journal of Cardiology, 109*(4), 515–520. doi:10.1016/j.amjcard.2011.09.043.

Mohamad, T. N., Afonso, L. C., Ramappa, P., et al. (2013). Primary and secondary prevention of coronary artery disease. *Medscape Reference*. Retrieved May 2014 from http://emedicine.medscape.com/article/164214-overview#aw2aab6b3

Monreal, M., Alvarez, L., Vilaseca, B., et al. (2008). Clinical outcome in patients with peripheral artery disease. Results from a prospective registry (FRENA). *European Journal of Internal Medicine, 19*(3), 192–197. doi:10.1016/j.ejim.2007.09.003.

Mukamal, K. J., Kennedy, M., Cushman, M., et al. (2008). Alcohol consumption and lower extremity arterial disease among older adults. The cardiovascular health study. *American Journal of Epidemiology, 167*(1), 34–41. doi:10.1093/aje/kwm274.

Muller-Buhl, U., Laux, G., & Szecsenyi, J. (2011). Secondary pharmacotherapeutic prevention among German primary care patients with peripheral arterial disease. *Internal Journal of Vascular Medicine, 2001*:316496. doi:10.1155/2011/316496.

Nelson, E. A., & Bradley, M. D. (2007). Dressings and topical agents for arterial leg ulcers. *Cochrane Database of Systematic Reviews*, Issue 1:Art. No.: CD001836. doi:10.1002/14651858.CD001836.pub2.

Nemes, R., Surlin, V., Chiutu, L., et al. (2011). Retroperitoneoscopic lumbar sympathectomy: Prospective study upon a series of 50 consecutive patients. *Surgical Endoscopy, 25*(9), 3066–3070. doi:10.1007/s00464-011-1671-8.

Nicolai, S. P., Kruidenier, L. M., Rouwet, E. V., et al. (2009). Ankle brachial index in primary care: Are we doing it right? *British Journal of General Practice, 59*(563), 422–427. doi:10.3399/bjgp09X420932.

Nicolai, S. P., Kruidenier, L. M., Rouwet, E. V., et al. (2008). Pocket Doppler and vascular laboratory equipment yield comparable results for ankle brachial index measurement. *BMC Cardiovascular Disorders, 8*, 26. doi:10.1186/1471-2261-8-26.

Nordmyr, J., Svensson, S., Bjorck, M., et al. (2009). Vacuum assisted wound closure in patients with lower extremity arterial disease. *International Angiology, 28*(1), 26–31.

Norgren, L., Hiatt, W. R., Dormandy, J. A., et al. (2007). Inter-society consensus for the management of peripheral arterial disease (TASC II). *Journal of Vascular Surgery, 45*(S1), S5–S67. doi:10.1016/j.jvs.2006.12.037.

Norgren, L., Hiatt, W. R., Dormandy, J. A., et al. (2010). The next 10 years in the management of peripheral artery disease: Perspectives from the PAD 2009 conference. *European Journal of Vascular & Endovascular Surgery, 40*(3), 375–380. doi:10.1016/j.ejvs.2010.05.005.

O'Brien, R., Pocock, N., & Torella, F. (2011). Wound infection after reconstructive arterial surgery of the lower limbs: Risk factors and consequences. *The Surgeon, 9*(5), 245–248. doi:10.1016/j.surge.2010.10.005.

O'Donnell, M. E., Badger, S. A., Sharif, M. A., Makar, R. R., et al. (2009). The effects of cilostazol on exercise-induced ischaemia-reperfusion injury in patients with peripheral arterial disease. *European Journal of Vascular & Endovascular Surgery, 37*(3), 326–335. doi:10.1016/j.ejvs.2008.11.028.

O'Hare, A. M., Glidden, D. V., Fox, C. S., & Hsu, C. Y. (2004). High prevalence of peripheral arterial disease in persons with renal insufficiency: Results from the national health and nutrition examination survey 1999-2000. *Circulation, 109*(3), 320–323.

Ohtake, T., Oka, M., Ikee, R., et al. (2011). Impact of lower limbs' arterial calcification on the prevalence and severity of PAD in patients on hemodialysis. *Journal of Vascular Surgery, 53*(3), 676–683. doi:10.1016/j.jvs.2010.09.070.

Okamoto, K., Oka, M., Maesato, K., et al. (2006). Peripheral arterial occlusive disease is more prevalent in patients with hemodialysis: Comparison with the findings from multidetector-row computed tomography. *American Journal of Kidney Diseases, 48*(2), 269–276.

O'Keeffe, S. D., Davenport, D. L., Minion, D. J., Sorial, E. E., et al. (2010). Blood transfusion is associated with increased morbidity and mortality after lower extremity revascularization. *Journal of Vascular Surgery, 51*(3), 616–621.e3. doi:10.1016/j.jvs.2009.10.045.

Oriani, G., Meazza, D., Favales, F., et al. (1990). Hyperbaric oxygen therapy in diabetic gangrene. *Journal of Hyperbaric Medicine, 5*(3), 171–175.

Osinbowale, O. O., & Milani, R. V. (2011). Benefits of exercise therapy in peripheral arterial disease. *Progress in Cardiovascular Diseases, 53*(6), 447–453. doi:10.1016/j.pcad.2011.03.005.

Ostergren, J., Sleight, P., Dagenais, G., et al. (2004). Impact of ramipril in patients with evidence of clinical or subclinical peripheral arterial disease. *European Heart Journal, 25*(1), 17–24.

Otsubo, S., Kitamura, M., Wakaume, T., et al. (2012). Association of peripheral artery disease and long-term mortality in hemodialysis patients. *International Urology and Nephrology, 44*(2), 569–573. doi:10.1007/s11255-010-9883-8.

Ouriel, K., & Zarins, C. K. (1982). Doppler ankle pressure: An evaluation of 3 methods of expression. *Archives of Surgery, 117*(10), 1297–1300.

Ousey, K. (2009). Heel ulceration – An exploration of the issues. *Journal of Orthopaedic Nursing, 13*(2), 97–104. doi:10.1016/j.joon.2009.06.001.

Ouwendijk, R., deVries, M., Stijnen, T., et al. (2008). Multicenter randomized controlled trial of the costs and effects of noninvasive diagnostic imaging in patients with peripheral arterial disease: The DIPAD Trial. *American Journal of Roentgenology, 190*(5), 1349–1357. doi:10.2214/AJR.07.3359.

Padberg, F. T., Back, T. L., Thompson, P. N., et al. (1996). Transcutaneous oxygen (TcPO2) estimates probability of healing in the ischemic extremity. *Journal of Surgical Research, 60*(2), 365–369.

Palacios, R., Alonso, I., Hidalgo, A., et al. (2008). Peripheral arterial disease in HIV patients older than 50 years of age. *AIDS Research and Human Retroviruses, 24*(8), 1043–1046. doi:10.1089/aid.2008.0001.

Pande, R. L., Perlstein, T. S., Beckman, J. A., et al. (2011). Secondary prevention and mortality in peripheral artery disease: National health and nutrition examination study, 1999 to 2004. *Circulation, 124*, 17–23. doi:10.1161/CIRCULATIONAHA.110.003954.

Paneni, F., Beckman, J. A., Creager, M. A., et al. (2013). Diabetes and vascular disease: Pathophysiology, clinical consequences, and medical therapy. Part I. *European Heart Journal, 34*(31), 2436–2446. doi:10.1093/eurheartj/eht149.

Paquet, M., Pilon, D., Tetrault, J. P., et al. (2010). Protective vascular treatment of patients with peripheral arterial disease: Guideline adherence according to year, age and gender. *Canadian Journal of Public Health, 101*(1), 96–100.

Partsch, H., & Mosti, G. (2010). Comparison of three portable instruments to measure compression pressure. *International Angiology, 29*(5), 426–430.

Pearce, W. H., Burt, R., & Rodriguez, H. E. (2008). The use of stem cells in the treatment of inoperable limb ischemia. *Perspectives in Vascular Surgery and Endovascular Therapy, 20*(1), 45–47. doi:10.1177/1531003507313300.

Planas, A., Clara, A., Marrugat, J., et al. (2002). Age at onset of smoking is an independent risk factor in peripheral artery disease development. *Journal of Vascular Surgery, 35*(3), 506–509.

Ploeg, A., Lange, C., Lardenoye, J. W., et al. (2007). Nosocomial infections after peripheral arterial bypass surgery. *World Journal of Surgery, 31*(8), 1687–1692. doi:10.1007/s00268-007-9130-3.

Powell, T. M., Glynn, R. J., Buring, J. E., et al. (2011). The relative importance of systolic versus diastolic blood pressure control and incident symptomatic peripheral artery disease in women. *Vascular Medicine, 16*(4), 239–246. doi:10.1177/1358863X11413166.

Price, J., & Leng, G. C. (2012). Steroid sex hormones for lower limb atherosclerosis. *Cochrane Database of Systematic Reviews*, (10), Art. No.:CD000188. doi:10.1002/14651858.CD000188.pub2.

Qadan, L. R., Ahmed, A. A., Safar, H. A., et al. (2008). Prevalence of metabolic syndrome in patients with clinically advanced peripheral vascular disease. *Angiology, 59*(2), 198–202. doi:10.1177/0003319707304582.

Ramaswami, G., D'Ayala, M., Hollier, L. H., et al. (2005). Rapid foot and calf compression increases walking distance in patients with intermittent claudication: Results of a randomized study. *Journal of Vascular Surgery, 41*(5), 794–801.

Regensteiner, J. G., Hiatt, W. R., Coll, J. R., et al. (2008). The impact of peripheral arterial disease on health-related qualify of life in the peripheral arterial disease awareness, risk, and treatment: New resources for survival (PARTNERS) program. *Vascular Medicine, 13*(1), 15–24. doi:10.1177/1358863X07084911.

Resnick, H. E., Lindsay, R. S., McDermott, M. M., et al. (2004). Relationship of high and low ankle brachial index to all-cause and cardiovascular disease mortality. *Circulation, 109*, 733–739. doi:10.1161/01.CIR.0000112642.63927.54.

Robertson, L., & Andras, A. (2013). Prostanoids for intermittent claudication. *Cochrane Database of Systematic Reviews*, (4), Art. No.: CD000986. doi:10.1002/14651858.CD000986.pub3.

Robertson, L., Ghouri, M. A., & Kovacs, F. (2012). Antiplatelet and anticoagulant drugs for prevention of restenosis/reocclusion following peripheral endovascular treatment. *Cochrane Database of Systematic Reviews*, (8), Art. No.:CD002071. doi:10.1002/14651858.CD002071.pub3.

Robinson, V., Sansam, K., Hirst, L., et al. (2010). Major lower limb amputation —what, why and how to achieve the best results. *Orthopaedics and Trauma, 24*(4), 276–285.

Robless, P., Mikhailidis, D., & Stansby, G. P. (2008). Cilostazol for peripheral arterial disease. *Cochrane Database of Systematic Reviews*, (1), Art. No.: CD003748. doi:10.1002/14651858.CD003748.pub3.

Rockman, C. B., Maldonado, T. S., Jacobowitz, G. R., et al. (2012). Hormone replacement therapy is associated with a decreased prevalence of peripheral arterial disease in postmenopausal women. *Annals of Vascular Surgery, 26*(3), 411–418. doi:10.1016/j.avsg.2011.10.012.

Rolstad, B. S., Bryant, R. A., & Nix, D. P. (2012). Topical management. In R. A. Bryant & D. P. Nix (Eds.), *Acute & chronic wounds. Current management concepts* (4th ed., pp. 289–306). St. Louis, MO: Elsevier-Mosby.

Romiti, M., Albers, M., Brochado-Neto, F. C., et al. (2008). Meta-analysis of infrapopliteal angioplasty for chronic critical limb ischemia. *Journal of Vascular Surgery, 47*(5), 975–981.e1. doi:10.1016/j.jvs.2008.01.005.

Rooke, T. W., Hirsch, A. T., Misra, S., et al. (2011). 2011 ACCF/AHA focused update of the guideline for the management of patients with peripheral artery disease (updating the 2005 guideline): A report of the American College of Cardiology Foundation/American Heart Association Task Force on Practice Guidelines. *Journal of the American College of Cardiology, 58*(19), 2020–2045. doi:10.1016/j.jacc.2011.08.023.

Roy, M. S., & Peng, B. (2008). Complications. Six-year incidence of lower extremity arterial disease and associated risk factors in Type 1 diabetic African-Americans. *Diabetic Medicine, 25*(5), 550–556. doi:10.1111/j.1464-5491.2008.02434.x.

Rudisill, H., Kelsberg, G., & Safranek, S. (2011). Effective therapies for intermittent claudication. *American Family Physician, 84*(6), 702–704.

Ruffolo, A. J., Romano, M., & Ciapponi, A. (2010). Prostanoids for critical limb ischemia. *Cochrane Database of Systematic Reviews,* (1), Art. No.: CD006544. doi:10.1002/14651858.CD006544.pub2.

Ruiz-Canela, M., Estruch, R., Corella, D., et al. (2014). Association of Mediterranean diet with peripheral artery disease: The PREDIMED randomized trial. *Journal of the American Medical Association, 311*(4), 415–417. doi:10.1001/jama.2013.280618.

Rumwell, C., & McPharlin, M. (2009). *Vascular technology* (4th ed.). Pasadena, CA: Davies Publishing, Inc.

Sadat, U., Chaudhuri, A., Hayes, P. D., et al. (2008). Five day antibiotic prophylaxis for major lower limb amputation reduces wound infection rates and the length of in-hospital stay. *European Journal of Vascular & Endovascular Surgery, 35*(1), 75–78. doi:10.1016/j.ejvs.2007.07.016.

Sahli, D., Eliasson, B., Svensson, M., et al. (2004). Assessment of toe blood pressure is an effective screening method to identify diabetes patients with lower extremity arterial disease. *Angiology, 55*(6), 641–651.

Salhiyyah, K., Senanayake, E., Abdel-Hadi, M., et al. (2012). Pentoxiphylline for intermittent claudication. *Cochrane Database of Systematic Reviews,* (1), Art. No.: CD005262. doi:10.1002/14651858.CD005262.pub2.

Sana, G., Alesso, D., Mediati, M., et al. (2011). Prevalence of peripheral arterial disease in subjects with moderate cardiovascular risk: Italian results from the PANDORA study data from PANDORA (prevalence of peripheral arterial disease in subjects with moderate CVD risk, with no overt vascular diseases nor diabetes mellitus). *BMC Cardiovascular Disorders, 11*(59). doi:10.1186/1471-2261-11-59.

Sanders J. E., & Fatone, S. (2011). Residual limb volume change: Systemic review of measurement and management. *Journal of Rehabilitation Research & Development, 48*(8), 949–986. doi:10.1682/JRRD.2010.09.0189.

Scanlon, C., Park, K., Mapletoft, D., et al. (2012). Interrater and intrarater reliability of photoplethysmography for measuring toe blood pressure and toe-brachial index in people with diabetes mellitus. *Journal of Foot and Ankle Research, 5*(13). doi:10.1186/1757-1146-5-13.

Schamp, K. B., Meerwaldt, R., Reijnen, M. M., et al. (2012). The ongoing battle between infrapopliteal angioplasty and bypass surgery for critical limb ischemia. *Annals of Vascular Surgery, 26*(8), 1145–1153. doi:10.1016/j.avsg.2012.02.006.

Schlager, O., Amighi, J., Haumer, M., et al. (2009). Inflammation and adverse cardiovascular outcome in patients with renal artery stenosis and peripheral artery disease. *Atherosclerosis, 205*(1), 314–318. doi:10.1016/j.atherosclerosis.2008.12.022.

Schlager, O., Giurgea, A., Schuhfried, O., et al. (2011). Exercise training increases endothelial progenitor cells and decreases asymmetric dimethylarginine in peripheral arterial disease: A randomized controlled trial. *Atherosclerosis, 217*(1), 240–248. doi:10.1016/j.atherosclerosis.2011.03.018.

Scottish Intercollegiate Guidelines Network (SIGN). (2009). *Diagnosis and management of peripheral arterial disease. A national clinical guideline.* Retrieved December 2012 from http://guidelines.gov/content.aspx?id=9924

Scottish Intercollegiate Guidelines Network (SIGN). (2010). *Prevention and management of venous thromboembolism A national guideline.* Retrieved December 7, 2013 from http://guidelines.gov/content.aspx?id=25639

Selvin, E., & Erlinger, T. P. (2004). Prevalence of and risk factors for peripheral arterial disease in the United States: Results from the national health and nutritional examination survey, 1999–2000. *Circulation, 110*(6), 738–743.

Setacci, C., de Donato, G., Teraa, M., et al. (2011). Chapter IV: Treatment of critical limb ischemia. *European Journal of Vascular and Endovascular Surgery, 42*(S2), S43–S59.

Shahin, Y., Cockcroft, J. R., & Chetter, I. C. (2013). Randomized clinical trial of angiotensin-converting enzyme inhibitor, ramipril, in patients with intermittent claudication. *British Journal of Surgery, 100*(9), 1154–1163. doi:10.1002/bjs.9198.

Shannon, M. M. (2013). A retrospective descriptive study of nursing home residents with heel eschar or blisters. *Ostomy Wound Management, 59*(1), 20–27.

Shinsato, T., Miyata, M., Kubozono, T., et al. (2010). Waon therapy mobilizes CD34+ cells and improves peripheral arterial disease. *Journal of Cardiology, 56*(3), 361–366. doi:10.1016/j.jjcc.2010.08.004.

Sieggreen, M. Y., Kline, R. A., & Sibbald, R. G. (2008). Arterial ulcers. In S. Baranoski & E. A. Ayello (Eds.), *Wound care essentials: Practice principles* (2nd ed., pp. 317–337). Ambler, PA: Lippincott Williams & Wilkins.

Signorelli, S. S., Stivala, A., Bonaccorso, C., et al. (2010). High frequency of *Chlamydophila pneumoniae* infections: Patients with peripheral arterial disease and those with risk factors for cardiovascular diseases compared to normal subjects. *Journal of Chemotherapy, 22*(6), 392–396.

Signorelli, S. S., Stivala, A., Di Pino, L., et al. (2006). Chronic peripheral arteriopathy is associated with seropositivity to *Chlamydia pneumoniae. Journal of Chemotherapy, 18*(1), 103–106.

Sigvant, B., Henriksson, M., Lundin, F., et al. (2011). Asymptomatic peripheral arterial disease: Is pharmacological prevention of cardiovascular risk cost effective. *European Journal of Cardiovascular Prevention & Rehabilitation, 18*(2), 254–261. doi:10.1177/1741826710389368.

Silva, G. V., Fernandes, M. R., Cardoso, C. O., Miranda, W. R., et al. (2011). Cryoplasty for peripheral artery disease in an unselected patient population in a tertiary center. *Texas Heart Institute Journal, 38*(2), 122–126.

Silvestro, A., Diehm, N., Savolainen, H., et al. (2006). Falsely high ankle-brachial index predicts major amputation in critical limb ischemia. *Vascular Medicine, 11*(2), 69–74.

Slovut, D. P., & Sullivan, T. M. (2008). Critical limb ischemia: Medical and surgical management. *Vascular Medicine, 13*(3), 281–291. doi:10.1177/1358863X08091485.

Smith, J. A. (2002). Measuring treatment effects of cilostazol on clinical trial endpoints in patients with intermittent claudication. *Clinical Cardiology, 25*(3), 91–94.

Smith, B. M., Desvigne, L. D., Slade, J. B., et al. (1996). Transcutaneous oxygen measurements predict healing of leg wounds with hyperbaric therapy. *Wound Repair and Regeneration, 4*(2), 224–229.

Smolderen, K. G., Aquarius, A. E., de Vries, J., et al. (2008). Depressive symptoms in peripheral arterial disease: A follow-up study on prevalence, stability, and risk factors. *Journal of Affective Disorders, 110*(1), 27–35. doi:10.1016/j.jad.2007.12.238.

Soga, Y., Iida, O., Hirano, K., et al. (2011). Impact of cilostazol after endovascular treatment for infrainguinal disease in patients with critical limb ischemia. *Journal of Vascular Surgery, 54*(6), 1659–1667. doi:10.1016/j.jvs.2011.06.024.

Sorensen, L. T. (2012). Wound healing and infection in surgery. The clinical impact of smoking and smoking cessation: A systematic review and meta-analysis. *Archives of Surgery, 147*(4), 373–383. doi:10.1001/archsurg.2012.5.

Soto-Barreras, U., Olvera-Rubio, J. O., Loyola-Rodriguez, J. P., et al. (2013). Peripheral arterial disease associated with caries and periodontal disease. *Journal of Periodontology, 84*(4), 486–494. doi:10.1902/jop.2012.120051.

Spear, M. (2012). Best technique for obtaining wound cultures. *Plastic SurgicalNursing,32*(1),34–36.doi:10.1097/PSN.0b013e31824a7e53.

Spiliopoulos, S., Katsanos, K., Karnabatidis, D., et al. (2010). Cryoplasty versus conventional balloon angioplasty of the femoropopliteal artery in diabetic patients: Long-term results from a prospective randomized single-center controlled trial. *Cardiovascular and Interventional Radiology, 33*(5), 929–938. doi:10.1007/s00270-010-9915-x.

Squizzato, A., Keller, T., Romualdi, E., et al. (2011). Clopidogrel plus aspirin alone for preventing cardiovascular disease. *Cochrane Database of Systematic Reviews,* (1), Art. No.: CD005158. doi:10.1002/14651858.CD005158.pub3.

Stamatelopoulos, K. S., Kitas, G. D., Papamichael, C. M., et al. (2010). Subclinical peripheral arterial disease in rheumatoid arthritis. *Atherosclerosis, 212*(1), 305–309. doi:10.1016/j.atherosclerosis.2010.05.007.

Stead, L. F., Perera, R., Bullen, C., et al. (2012). Nicotine replacement therapy for smoking cessation. *Cochrane Database of Systematic Reviews,* (11), Art. No.: CD000146. doi:10.1002/14651858.CD000146.pub4.

Stein, R., Hrijac, I., Halperin, J. L., et al. (2006). Limitation of the resting ankle-brachial index in symptomatic patients with peripheral arterial disease. *Vascular Medicine, 11*(1), 29–33. doi:10.1191/1358863x06vm663oa.

Stewart, A. H., Eyers, P. S., & Earnshaw, J. J. (2007). Prevention of infection in peripheral arterial reconstruction: A systematic review and meta-analysis. *Journal of Vascular Surgery, 46*(1), 148–155. doi:10.1016/j.jvs.2007.02.065.

Stone, N. J., Robinson, J., Lichtenstein, A. H., et al. (2013). 2013 ACC/AHA guideline on the treatment of blood cholesterol to reduce atherosclerotic cardiovascular risk in adults: A report of the American College of Cardiology/American Heart Association Task Force on Practice Guidelines. *Circulation.* doi:10.1161/01.cir.0000437738.63853.7a.

Stotts, N. A. (2012). Wound infection: Diagnosis and management. In R. A. Bryant & D. P. Nix (Eds.), *Acute & chronic wounds. Current management concepts* (4th ed., pp. 270–278). St. Louis, MO: Elsevier-Mosby.

Subramaniam, T., Nang, E. E., Lim, S. C., et al. (2011). Distribution of ankle-brachial index and the risk factors of peripheral artery disease in a multi-ethnic Asian population. *Vascular Medicine, 16*(2), 87–95. doi:10.1177/1358863X11400781.

Sultan, S., Hamada, N., Soylu, E., et al. (2011). Sequential compression biomechanical device in patients with critical limb ischemia and nonreconstructible peripheral vascular disease. *Journal of Vascular Surgery, 54*(2), 440–447. doi:10.1016/j.jvs.2011.02.057.

Sumner, A. D., Khali, Y. K., & Reed, J. F. (2012). The relationship of peripheral arterial disease in metabolic syndrome prevalence in asymptomatic US adults 40 years and older: Results from the National Health and Nutrition Examination Survey (1999–2004). *Journal of Clinical Hypertension,14*(3),144–148.doi:10.1111/j.1751-7176.2011.00580.x.

Szeberin, Z., Fehervari, M., Krepuska, M., et al. (2011). Serum fetuin-A levels inversely correlate with the severity of arterial calcification in patients with chronic lower extremity atherosclerosis without renal disease. *International Angiology, 30*(5), 474–550.

Takahashi, P. Y., Kiemele, L. J., & Jones, J. P. (2004). Wound care for elderly patients: Advances and clinical applications for practicing physicians. *Mayo Clinic Proceedings, 79*(2), 260–267.

Tan, M. L., Feng, J., Gordois, A., et al. (2011). Lower extremity amputation prevention in Singapore: Economic analysis of results. *Singapore Medical Journal, 52*(9), 662–668. Retrieved April 2013 from http://www.cgh.com.sg/Research/Documents/Radiology_Lower%20extremity%20amputation%20prevention%20in%20Singapore.pdf

Tanaka, M., Ishii, H., Aoyama, T., et al. (2011). Ankle brachial pressure index but not brachial-ankle pulse wave velocity is a strong predictor of systemic atherosclerotic morbidity and mortality in patients on maintenance hemodialysis. *Atherosclerosis, 219*(2), 643–647. doi:10.1016/j.atherosclerosis.2011.09.037.

Tapp, R. J., Balkau, B., Shaw, J. E., et al. (2007). Association of glucose metabolism, smoking and cardiovascular risk factors with incident peripheral arterial disease: The DESIR study. *Atherosclerosis, 190*(1), 84–89. doi:10.1016/j.atherosclerosis.2006.02.017.

Tateishi-Yuyama, E., Matsubara, H., Murohara, T., et al. (2002). Therapeutic angiogenesis for patients with limb ischaemia by autologous transplantation of bone-marrow cells: A pilot study and a randomized controlled trial. *The Lancet, 360*(9331), 427–435. doi:10.1016/S0140-6736(02)09670-8.

Tefera, G., Hoch, J., & Turnipseed, W. D. (2005). Limb-salvage angioplasty in vascular surgery practice. *Journal of Vascular Surgery, 41*(6), 988–993.

Tekin, N., Baskan, M., Yesilkayali, T., et al. (2011). Prevalence of peripheral arterial disease and related risk factors in Turkish elders. *BMC Family Practice, 12,* 96. doi:10.1186/1471-2296-12-96.

te Slaa, A., Dolmans, D. E., Ho, G. H., et al. (2010). Evaluation of A-V impulse technology as a treatment for oedema following polytetrafluoroethylene femoropopliteal surgery in a randomized controlled trial. *European Journal of Vascular & Endovascular Surgery, 40*(5), 635–642. doi:10.1016/j.ejvs.2010.06.011.

te Slaa, A., Dolmans, D. E., Ho, G. H., et al. (2011). Prospective randomized controlled trial to analyze the effects of intermittent pneumatic compression on edema following autologous femoropopliteal bypass surgery. *World Journal of Surgery, 35*(2), 446–454. doi:10.1007/s00268-010-0858-9.

Thomas, D. R. (2013). Managing peripheral disease and vascular ulcers. *Clinics in Geriatric Medicine, 29* (2), 425–431. doi:10.1016/j.cger.2013.01.010.

Thompson, P. D., Zimet, R., Forbes, W. P., et al. (2002). Meta-analysis of results from eight randomized, placebo-controlled trials on the effect of cilostazol on patients with intermittent claudication. *American Journal of Cardiology, 90*(12), 1314–1319.

Tivesten, A., Mellstrom, D., Jutberger, H., et al. (2007). Low serum testosterone and high serum estradiol associate with lower extremity peripheral arterial disease in elderly men. The MrOS study in Sweden. *Journal of the American College of Cardiology, 50*(11), 1070–1076. doi:10.1016/j.jacc.2007.04.088.

Toriyama, T., Kumada, Y., Matsubara, T., et al. (2002). Effect of artificial carbon dioxide foot bathing on critical limb ischemia (Fontaine IV) in peripheral arterial disease. *International Angiology, 21*(4), 367–373.

Turtianen, J., Saimanen, E. I., Partio, T. J., et al. (2011). Supplemental postoperative oxygen in the prevention of surgical wound infection after lower limb vascular surgery: A randomized controlled trial. *World JournalofSurgery,35*(6),1387–1395.doi:10.1007/s00268-011-1090-y.

Ubbink, D. T., & Vermeulen, H. (2006). Spinal cord stimulation for critical leg ischemia: A review of effectiveness and optimal patient selection. *Journal of Pain and Symptom Management, 31*(S4), S30–S35.

Ubbink, D. T., & Vermeulen, H. (2013). Spinal cord stimulation for non-reconstructable chronic critical leg ischaemia. *Cochrane Database of Systematic Reviews,* (2), Art. No.: CD004001. doi:10.1002/14651858.CD004001.pub3.

Ustunsoy, H., Sivrikoz, C., Sirmatel, F., et al. (2007). Is *Chlamydia pneumoniae* a risk factor for peripheral atherosclerosis? *Asian Cardiovascular & Thoracic Annals, 15*(1), 9–13.

Vahl, A. C., Geselschap, J., van Swijndregt, A. D., et al. (2008). Contrast enhanced magnetic resonance angiography versus intra-arterial digital subtraction angiography for treatment planning in patients with peripheral arterial disease: A randomized controlled diagnostic trial. *European Journal of Vascular and Endovascular Surgery, 35*(5), 514–521. doi:10.1016/j.ejvs.2007.12.002.

Vainas, T., Stassen, F. R., Schurink, G. W., et al. (2005). Secondary prevention of atherosclerosis through *Chlamydia pneumoniae* eradication (Space Trial): A randomised clinical trial in patients with peripheral arterial disease. *European Journal of Vascular & Endovascular Surgery, 29*(4), 403–411.

van de Luijtgaarden, K. M., Voute, M. T., Hoeks, S. E., et al. (2012). Vitamin D deficiency may be an independent risk factor for arterial disease. *European Journal of Vascular & Endovascular Surgery, 44*(3), 301–306. doi:10.1016/j.ejvs.2012.06.017.

Van Wicklin, S. A. (2011). Implementing AORN recommended practices for prevention of deep vein thrombosis. *AORN Journal, 94*(5), 443–451. doi:10.1016/j.aorn.2011.07.018.

Varu, V. N., Hogg, M. E., & Kibbe, M. (2010). Critical limb ischemia. *Journal of Vascular Surgery, 51*(1), 230–241. doi:10.1016/j.jvs.2009.08.073.

Veeranna, V., Zalawadiya, S. K., Niraj, A., et al. (2011). Homocysteine and reclassification of cardiovascular risk. *Journal of the American College of Cardiology, 58*(10), 1025–1033. doi:10.1016/j.jacc.2011.05.028.

Verbeck, W. J., Kollias, A., & Stergiou, G. S. (2012). Automated oscillometric determination of the ankle-brachial index: A systematic review and meta-analysis. *Hypertension Research, 35*, 883–891. doi:10.1038/hr.2012.83.

Vidula, H., Tian, L., Liu, K., et al. (2008). Biomarkers of inflammation and thrombosis as predictors of near-term mortality in patients with peripheral arterial disease: A cohort study. *Annals of Internal Medicine, 148*(2), 85–93.

Vouyouka, A. G., Egorova, N. N., Salloum, A., et al. (2010). Lessons learned from the analysis of gender effect on risk factors and procedural outcomes of lower extremity arterial disease. *Journal of Vascular Surgery, 52*(5), 1196–1202. doi:10.1016/j.jvs.2010.05.106.

Wahlgren, C. M., & Magnusson, P. K. (2011). Genetic influences on peripheral arterial disease in a twin population. *Arteriosclerosis, Thrombosis, and Vascular Biology, 31*(3), 678–682.

Walker, L., & Lamont, S. (2007). The use of antiembolic stockings. Part 1: A literature review. *British Journal of Nursing, 16*(22), 1408–1412.

Walter, D. H., Krankenberg, H., Balzer, J. O., et al. (2011). Intraarterial administration of bone marrow mononuclear cells in patients with critical limb ischemia: A randomized-start, placebo-controlled pilot trial (PROVASA). *Circulation. Cardiovascular Interventions, 4*(1), 26–37. doi:10.1161/CIRCINTERVENTIONS.110.958348.

Wang, T., Elam, M. B., Forbes, W. P., et al. (2003). Reduction of remnant lipoprotein cholesterol concentrations by cilostazol in patients with intermittent claudication. *Atherosclerosis, 171*(2), 337–342.

Wassel, C. L., Loomba, R., Ix J. H., et al. (2011). Family history of peripheral artery disease is associated with prevalence and severity of peripheral artery disease: The San Diego population study. *Journal of the American College of Cardiology, 58*(13), 1386–1392. doi:10.1016/j.jacc.2011.06.023.

Watson, C., & Alp, N. J. (2008). Role of *Chlamydia pneumoniae* in atherosclerosis. *Clinical Science, 114*(8), 509–531. doi:10.1042/CS20070298.

Watson, L., Ellis, B., & Leng, G. C. (2008). Exercise for intermittent claudication. *Cochrane Database of Systematic Reviews*, (4), Art. No.:CD000990. doi:10.1002/14651858.CD000990.pub2.

Wattel, F., Mathieu, D., Coget, J. M., et al. (1990). Hyperbaric oxygen therapy in chronic vascular wound management. *Angiology, 41*(1), 59–65.

Wen, Y., Meng, L., & Gao, Q. (2011). Autologous bone marrow cell therapy for patients with peripheral arterial disease: A meta-analysis of randomized controlled trials. *Expert Opinion on Biological Therapy, 11*(12), 1581–1589. doi:10.1517/14712598.2011.626401.

West, A. M., Anderson, J. D., Epstein, F. H., et al. (2011). Low-density lipoprotein lowering does not improve calf muscle perfusion, energetics, or exercise performance in peripheral arterial disease. *Journal of the American College of Cardiology, 58*(10), 1068–1076. doi:10.1016/j.jacc.2011.04.034.

Westendorp, I. C., in't Veld, B. A., Grobbee, D. E., et al. (2000). Hormone replacement therapy and peripheral arterial disease: The Rotterdam study. *Archives of Internal Medicine, 160*(16), 2498–2502.

Wiesli, P., Czerwenka, W., Meniconi, A., et al. (2002). Roxithromycin treatment prevents progression of peripheral arterial occlusive disease in *Chlamydia pneumoniae* seropositive men: A randomized, double-blind, placebo-controlled trial. *Circulation, 105*(22), 2646–2652.

Willigendael, E. M., Tejink, J. A., Bartelink, M. L., et al. (2005). Smoking and the patency of lower extremity bypass grafts: A meta-analysis. *Journal of Vascular Surgery, 42*(1), 67–74.

Wilmink, A. B., Welch, A. A., Quick, C. R., et al. (2004). Dietary folate and vitamin B6 are independent predictors of peripheral arterial occlusive disease. *Journal of Vascular Surgery, 39*(3), 513–516.

Woelk, C. J. (2012). Management of critical limb ischemia. *Canadian Family Physician, 58*, 960–963.

Wong, P. F., Chong, L. Y., Mikhaildis, D. P., et al. (2011). Antiplatelet agents for intermittent claudication. *Cochrane Database of Systematic Reviews*, (11), Art. No.: CD001272. doi:10.1002/14651858.CD001272.pub2.

Wound, Ostomy and Continence Nurses Society. (2010). *Guideline for prevention and management of pressure ulcers*. Mt. Laurel, NJ: Author.

Wound, Ostomy and Continence Nurses Society. (2011a). *Ankle brachial index: Quick reference guide for clinicians*. Mt. Laurel, NJ: Author.

Wound, Ostomy and Continence Nurses Society. (2011b). *Guideline for management of wounds in patients with lower-extremity venous disease. WOCN clinical practice guideline series 4*. Mt. Laurel, NJ: Author.

Wound, Ostomy and Continence Nurses Society. (2012). *Guideline for management of wounds in patients with neuropathic disease. WOCN clinical practice guideline series 3*. Mt. Laurel, NJ: Author.

Wound, Ostomy and Continence Nurses Society. (2014). *Guideline for management of wounds in patients with lower-extremity arterial disease. WOCN clinical practice guideline series 1*. Mt. Laurel, NJ: Author.

Wütschert, R., & Bounameaux, H. (1997). Determination of amputation level in ischemic limbs: Reappraisal of the measurement of TcPo2. *Diabetes Care, 20*(8), 1315–1318.

Wütschert, R., & Bounameaux, H. (1998). Predicting healing of arterial leg ulcers by means of segmental systolic pressure measurements. *VASA: European Journal of Vascular Medicine, 27*(4), 224–228.

Xu, D., Li, J., Zou, L., et al. (2010). Sensitivity and specificity of the ankle-brachial index to diagnose peripheral artery disease: A structured review. *Vascular Medicine, 15*(5), 361–369. doi:10.1177/1358863X10378376.

Yamada, T., Ohta, T., Ishibashi, H., et al. (2008). Clinical reliability and utility of skin perfusion pressure measurement in ischemic limbs-Comparison with other noninvasive diagnostic methods. *Journal of Vascular Surgery, 47*(2), 318–323. doi:10.1016/j.jvs.2007.10.045.

Yao, S. T., Hobbs, J. T., & Irvine, W. T. (1969). Ankle systolic pressure measurements in arterial disease affecting the lower extremities. *British Journal of Surgery, 56*(9), 676–679.

Zabakis, P., Kardamakis, D. M., Siablis, D., et al. (2005). External beam radiation therapy reduces the rate of re-stenosis in patients treated with femoral stenting: Results of a randomized study. *Radiotherapy & Oncology 74*(1), 11–16.

Zammit, M. C., Fiorentino, L., Cassar, K., et al. (2011). Factors affecting gentamicin penetration in lower extremity ischemic tissues with ulcers. *International Journal of Lower Extremity Wounds, 10*(3), 130–137. doi:10.1177/1534734611418571.

Zampakis, P., Karnabatidis, D., Kalogeropoulou, C., et al. (2007). External beam irradiation and restenosis following femoral stenting: Long-term results of a prospective randomized study. *Cardiovascular and Interventional Radiology, 30*(3), 362–369. doi:10.1007/s00270-004-0275-2.

Zehnder, T., von Briel, C., Baumgartner, I., et al. (2003). Endovascular brachytherapy after percutaneous transluminal angioplasty of recurrent femoropopliteal obstructions. *Journal of Endovascular Therapy, 10*(2), 304–311.

QUESTIONS

1. A wound nurse specialist is counseling patients with lower-extremity arterial disease (LEAD). Which statement accurately describes a characteristic of the condition?
A. LEAD is an acute disease caused by uncontrolled hypertension.
B. LEAD is associated with increased risk of MI, stroke, and vascular death.
C. LEAD causes progressive fibrosis and softening of the arterial walls.
D. As LEAD progresses, dilation occurs in response to tissue demands.

2. A wound nurse specialist learns that a patient's atherosclerosis and plaque formation have advanced to the third stage of development. What condition characterizes this stage?
A. Fatty streaks form
B. Advanced lesion develops
C. initial lesion develops
D. Atheroma develops

3. Which patient condition would the wound nurse specialist associate with increased risk for lower-extremity arterial disease (LEAD)?
A. A patient with low levels of fibrinogen
B. A patient with low homocysteine levels
C. A patient with elevated C-reactive protein
D. A patient with increased high-density lipoprotein [HDL]

4. A patient is diagnosed with infrapopliteal disease. In what area of the body would the wound nurse specialist expect the patient to complain of pain?
A. The foot
B. The buttocks
C. The calf
D. The thigh

5. What is the initial classic type of pain that is associated with lower-extremity arterial disease (LEAD)?
A. Positional pain
B. Intermittent claudication
C. Resting pain
D. Continuous pain

6. The wound specialist nurse is assessing a patient with acute limb ischemia. Which of the following is a hallmark sign of this condition?
A. Sudden onset of the six "Ps"
B. Chronic ischemic rest pain
C. Development of collateral vessels
D. ABI of 0.40 or less

7. The wound specialist nurse is assessing the limbs of a patient with ischemia. What common clinical characteristic might the nurse document?
A. Rubor on elevation of legs
B. Early capillary refill
C. Moist, dull, loose skin
D. Prolonged venous refill time

8. The wound specialist nurse is measuring and calculating the ABI of a patient with lower-extremity arterial disease (LEAD). Which step of the procedure has the nurse performed correctly?
A. The nurse performs the ABI in a quiet, cool environment on a patient who has a full bladder.
B. The nurse places the patient in a flat, supine position with one small pillow placed behind the patient's head for comfort.
C. The nurse places the pressure cuff with the bottom of the cuff approximately 5 to 7 cm above the cubital fossa on the arm.
D. The nurse divides the lower of the dorsalis pedis or posterior tibial systolic pressure by the higher of the right or left brachial pressures to obtain ABI.

9. A wound specialist nurse documents a patient's ABI as 0.90. What is the interpretation of this finding?
A. Elevated
B. Normal
C. LEAD
D. Borderline perfusion

10. A patient with lower-extremity arterial disease (LEAD) presents with the following: toe pressure <30 mm Hg, and TBI < 0.64. What complication would the wound specialist nurse suspect?
A. Nonhealing wounds
B. Infection
C. Wet gangrene
D. Intractable rest pain

ANSWERS: 1.**B**, 2.**D**, 3.**C**, 4.**A**, 5.**B**, 6.**A**, 7.**D**, 8.**B**, 9.**C**, 10.**A**

CHAPTER 23

Lower Extremity Neuropathic Disease

Myra Varnado

OBJECTIVES

1. Compare and contrast arterial, venous, neuropathic, and mixed ulcers in terms of risk factors, pathology, clinical presentation, and management guidelines.
2. Describe critical parameters to be included in assessment of the individual with a lower extremity ulcer.
3. Demonstrate the procedure for sensory testing using Semmes-Weinstein monofilaments and tuning fork.
4. Interpret findings from sensory testing and identify implications for patient education and management.
5. Use assessment data to determine causative and contributing factors for a lower extremity ulcer and to develop individualized management plans that are evidence based.
6. Identify options and guidelines for effective "off-loading" of plantar surface ulcers.
7. Explain why debridement is contraindicated in a noninfected ischemic ulcer covered with dry eschar.
8. Describe clinical characteristics and management options for Charcot fracture.
9. Describe indications for referral to vascular surgeon, podiatrist, orthotist, and orthopedic surgeon.
10. Identify indications that a lower extremity ulcer is "atypical" and requires additional diagnostic workup and/or medical–surgical intervention.

Topic Outline

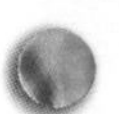
Introduction

Etiology and Pathology of LEND

Acquired Neuropathic Disorders
- Systemic Diseases
- Trauma
- Infectious or Autoimmune Disorders
- Other Causes

Inherited Neuropathic Disorders
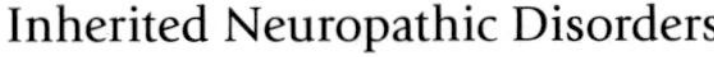

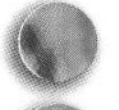
Prevalence and Incidence

Pathology, Classification, and Manifestations of Peripheral Neuropathy
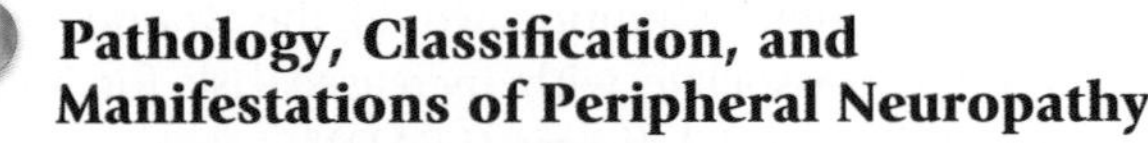

Sensory Neuropathy
Motor Neuropathy
Autonomic Neuropathy

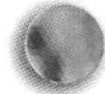
Diagnosis of LEND

History
Diagnostic Tests
Comprehensive Foot Exam
- Overview
- Sensory Testing with 10-g Monofilament
- Vibratory Sense Testing
- Position Sense Testing
- Reflex Testing
- Assessment of Musculoskeletal/Biomechanical Status
- Shoe Condition/Wear Patterns
- Vascular Assessment
- Dermal Temperature Assessment for Soft Tissue Inflammation
- Skin, Nail, Soft Tissue Assessment

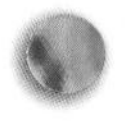
Assessment/Classification of Neuropathic Foot Ulcer

Wagner Classification System
University of Texas Diabetic Foot Classification System

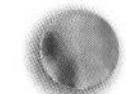
Management Neuropathic Ulcers

Wound Bed Preparation

Introduction

Lower extremity neuropathic disease (LEND), also known as peripheral neuropathy (PN), is caused by an acquired or inherited disorder that interferes with the normal neurologic function of the lower extremities. LEND involves damage to the peripheral nervous system, the extensive communication network that conveys information between the central nervous system (brain and spinal cord) and other parts of the body, such as the feet. With normal function, any trauma to the feet activates sensory nerves that send a message to the brain and spinal cord, and the brain and spinal cord respond by coordinating movement to withdraw from the painful stimulus (National Institutes of Neurological Disorders [NIH], 2014; Wound, Ostomy and Continence Nurses Society [WOCN], 2012). The individual with LEND sustains damage to structures within the peripheral nervous system that interfere with this vital communication system. The neurologic structures typically affected are the axon, cell body, and/or the myelin sheath (NIH, 2014; WOCN, 2012).

CLINICAL PEARL

Lower extremity neuropathic disease involves damage to the system that communicates information between the brain and spinal cord and the lower legs and feet.

LEND is a common feature of many systemic diseases and may lead to autonomic dysfunction, motor disability, and a loss of sensation to the lower extremities, especially the feet. Sensory loss, motor damage causing foot deformities, and changes in blood flow related to autonomic dysfunction place the individual at risk for a foot wound, which may go unrecognized for some time due to the lack of pain. Infection and ischemia frequently complicate neuropathy, and neuropathic and neuroischemic ulcers are the most common reasons for foot amputations and the associated morbidity and mortality (Centers for Disease Control and Prevention [CDC], 2011; NIH, 2014; WOCN, 2012).

CLINICAL PEARL

Neuropathic and neuroischemic ulcers are the most common reasons for foot amputations and the associated morbidity and mortality.

Etiology and Pathology of LEND

There are a number of conditions that can cause peripheral neuropathy; they are commonly grouped into *acquired neuropathic disorders* and *inherited neuropathic disorders*.

Acquired Neuropathic Disorders

Acquired peripheral neuropathies are grouped into three categories: those caused by systemic disease, those caused by trauma, and those caused by infectious or autoimmune disorders. Neuropathies with no known cause are classified as idiopathic neuropathies (NIH, 2014; WOCN, 2012).

Systemic Diseases

Systemic diseases affect the entire body and are a common cause of peripheral neuropathy. Any disease state that compromises the body's ability to convert nutrients into energy, to adequately perfuse the tissues, to process and eliminate metabolic waste products, and/or to support tissue repair can cause nerve damage (CDC, 2011; NIH, 2014; WOCN, 2012). Diabetes mellitus, and the associated chronic hyperglycemia, is a leading cause of peripheral neuropathy in the United States and is the systemic disease state most researched and referenced in regard to LEND and LEND wounds (WOCN, 2012). However, diabetes is not the only systemic condition that results in neuropathy. Other systemic conditions include kidney disease, which can result in abnormally high levels of toxic metabolic end products that severely damage nerve tissue (CDC, 2011, 2014; NIH, 2014; WOCN, 2012). Hormonal imbalances, such as hypothyroidism or increased production of growth hormone, can also cause peripheral neuropathy. The reduced metabolic rate associated with hypothyroidism leads to fluid retention and edema, which exerts pressure on peripheral nerves. Overproduction of growth hormone can lead to acromegaly, a condition characterized by abnormal enlargement of the bones and joints; the nerves running through the affected joints can become mechanically entrapped (NIH, 2014; WOCN, 2012). Another systemic condition resulting in sensory and motor neuropathy is B_{12} deficiency, such as occurs with pernicious anemia. Neurologic symptoms vary and may be nonspecific but commonly include feelings of numbness, tingling, weakness, lack of coordination, and clumsiness. Both sides of the body are typically affected equally, and the legs are affected more than the arms. A severe deficiency can result in more serious neurologic symptoms, such as paralysis (NIH, 2014; WOCN, 2012).

CLINICAL PEARL

Diabetes, and the associated hyperglycemia, is a leading cause of neuropathy in the United States, but is not the only condition that results in neuropathy.

Trauma

Physical trauma is the most common cause of mechanical injury to the peripheral nervous system. Trauma resulting from motor vehicle accidents, falls, or sports-related activities can cause partial or total disruption, compression, crushing, or stretching of the nerves. The most severe example of trauma-related neuropathy is spinal cord injury, which typically results in partial or complete paraplegia or quadriplegia (NIH, 2014; WOCN, 2012).

Infectious or Autoimmune Disorders

Lyme disease, diphtheria, and Hansen's disease (leprosy) are bacterial diseases characterized by extensive peripheral nerve damage. Viral and bacterial infections can also cause indirect nerve damage by provoking autoimmune disorders, in which specialized cells and antibodies of the immune system attack the body's own tissues, including the nervous system (CDC, 2011; NIH, 2014; WOCN, 2012).

Other Causes

Certain cancer drugs and antiretroviral agents (used to treat HIV/ AIDS) are associated with irreversible peripheral nerve damage, as are selected anticonvulsants, antiviral agents, and antibiotics. When medications cause neuropathic symptoms, the decision to continue use of that drug is based upon a benefit-to-risk comparison, that is, the potential for worsening and irreversible neuropathy versus the potential risk of disease progression if the medication is discontinued.

Vitamin deficiencies and alcoholism can also cause widespread damage to nerve tissue. Vitamins E, B_1 (thiamine), B_6, and B_{12} and niacin are essential to healthy nerve function. Thiamine deficiency is common among people with alcoholism because these individuals commonly have poor dietary habits, and thiamine deficiency can cause a painful sensory neuropathy involving the extremities. Some neuropathic research indicates that excessive alcohol consumption may contribute directly to nerve damage, a condition referred to as alcoholic neuropathy (CDC, 2011; WOCN, 2012). Excessive alcohol consumption and cigarette smoking are also known to increase the risk of LEND among individuals with diabetes (CDC, 2011; WOCN, 2012).

Inherited Neuropathic Disorders

Inherited neuropathic disorders, also known as familial neuropathies, are caused by inborn genetic anomalies or genetic mutations. Some genetic errors lead to mild neuropathies with symptoms that begin in early adulthood and result in little, if any, significant impairment. More severe hereditary neuropathies often appear in infancy or childhood and may lead to reduced life expectancy due to wounds, fractures, and other unrecognized health issues (NIH, 2014).

Examples of inherited or familial neuropathies are congenital insensitivity to pain and a group of neuropathies collectively known as Charcot-Marie-Tooth disease. These neuropathies result from genetic flaws that cause impairments in the neuron and/or myelin sheath tissue and result in sensory and motor neuropathies, respectively (NIH, 2014; WOCN, 2012).

Prevalence and Incidence

Of non–diabetes-related causes of peripheral neuropathy and neuropathic wounds, Hansen's disease (leprosy) is the primary worldwide cause of treatable peripheral neuropathy. Worldwide, 1 to 2 million persons are permanently disabled as a result of Hansen's disease; while the infection can be treated and individuals receiving antibiotic treatment are considered free of active infection, the nerve damage remains and must be recognized and treated (NIH, 2014; WOCN, 2012).

CLINICAL PEARL

Hansen's disease (leprosy) is the primary cause of treatable peripheral neuropathy worldwide.

In the United States, diabetes affects 23.6 million individuals, with approximately 17 million persons being over 20 years of age. Of significance, 15% of these 23.6 million individuals are unaware they have the disease. The prevalence and incidence of diabetes is rising, as evidenced by the fact that the diagnosis of diabetes among adults increased 49% from 1990 to 2000. Diabetes-related neuropathy is the most common cause of foot ulceration in the diabetic population; complications of neuropathy account for more hospitalizations than all other diabetic complications combined (e.g., three times as many patients are admitted to the hospital for neuropathic foot ulceration than for ischemic ulceration). Neuropathy with loss of protective sensation (LOPS) occurs in 40% of the population with diabetes in industrialized nations; 15% of the individuals with neuropathy will develop foot ulceration, and 14% to 24% of those who develop an ulceration will require amputation (CDC, 2011, 2014; NIH, 2014; WOCN, 2012). The overall prevalence of lower extremity neuropathy, as reported by the Centers for Disease Control and Prevention (CDC), is 2.4 per 100,000 US individuals; the prevalence is highest among older individuals (9 per 100,000) (CDC, 2014; NIH, 2014; WOCN, 2012). In the United States, the cost of diabetes care averages $174 billion annually, with $116 billion related to direct care. As noted, the management of neuropathic wounds accounts for a substantial component of the direct care costs. According to the CDC, patients with diabetic neuropathy and wounds have a relapse rate of 66% over 5 years, and 12% of neuropathic wounds result in amputation (CDC, 2011, 2014; WOCN, 2012).

CLINICAL PEARL

Complications of neuropathy account for more hospitalizations than all other diabetic complications combined.

Diabetes complicated by peripheral neuropathy is responsible for 50% to 70% of all nontraumatic amputations in the United States, and 85% of these amputations are preceded by a foot ulcer (CDC, 2011, 2014; NIH, 2014; WOCN, 2012). In 2010, about 73,000 nontraumatic lower limb amputations were performed in adults aged 20 years or older with diagnosed diabetes. Amputation is particularly common among the African American population, who are up to four times more likely to have an amputation than White Americans, irrespective of age or socioeconomic status (CDC, 2011; NIH, 2014; WOCN, 2012). In 2009, the age-adjusted lower extremity amputation (LEA) rate was highest for toe amputation (1.8 per 1,000 diabetic population), followed by below-the-knee amputation (0.9 per 1,000 diabetic population), foot amputation (0.5 per 1,000 diabetic population), and above-the-knee amputation (0.4 per 1,000 diabetic population) (CDC, 2011, 2014; WOCN, 2012). The immediate mortality rate among patients undergoing above-the-knee amputations is 5%; and 50% to 84% will undergo subsequent amputation of the other limb within 2 to 3 years. These figures are highly significant since the 5-year survival rate for patients with bilateral amputations is <50% (CDC, 2011; NIH, 2014; WOCN, 2012).

CLINICAL PEARL

Diabetes complicated by peripheral neuropathy is responsible for 50% to 70% of all nontraumatic amputations in the United States, and 85% of these amputations are preceded by a foot ulcer.

Most importantly, at least 50 % of all amputations due to neuropathy are preventable with early intervention (CDC, 2014; NIH, 2014; WOCN, 2012). Thus, the focus of this chapter will be on the pathology, prevention, and early management of neuropathic wounds.

CLINICAL PEARL

At least 50% of all amputations due to neuropathy are preventable with early intervention.

Pathology, Classification, and Manifestations of Peripheral Neuropathy

More than 100 specific types of peripheral neuropathy have been identified, and each has a characteristic pattern of development, symptomatology, and prognosis. However, the type and severity of functional impairment and symptoms depend on the type and severity of nerve damage and can be broadly categorized as sensory neuropathy, motor neuropathy, autonomic neuropathy, and mixed neuropathy (NIH, 2014). Sensory neuropathy results in paresthesias and LOPS, motor neuropathy results in foot deformities and abnormal weight bearing, and autonomic neuropathy causes very dry skin and may contribute to osteopenia and fractures of the bones of the foot. Neuropathic changes often result in a foot ulcer, which is frequently complicated by infection and ischemia; these conditions collectively account for the morbidity and amputations associated with neuropathic ulcers (Birke & Sims, 1986; CDC, 2011, 2014; NIH, 2014; WOCN, 2012).

CLINICAL PEARL

Neuropathic changes often result in a foot ulcer, which is frequently complicated by infection and ischemia; these conditions collectively account for the morbidity and amputations associated with neuropathic ulcers.

Sensory Neuropathy

Sensory nerves transmit messages related to touch, position, pressure, temperature, and pain, such as the feeling of light touch or the pain caused by stepping on a sharp object. Sensory nerve damage causes a complex array of symptoms because sensory nerves have a diverse and

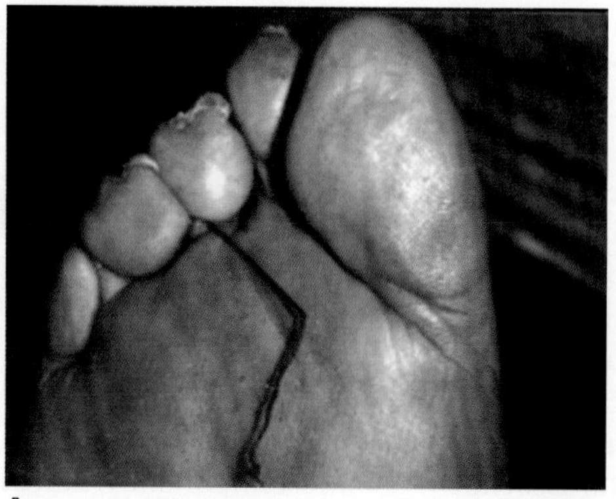
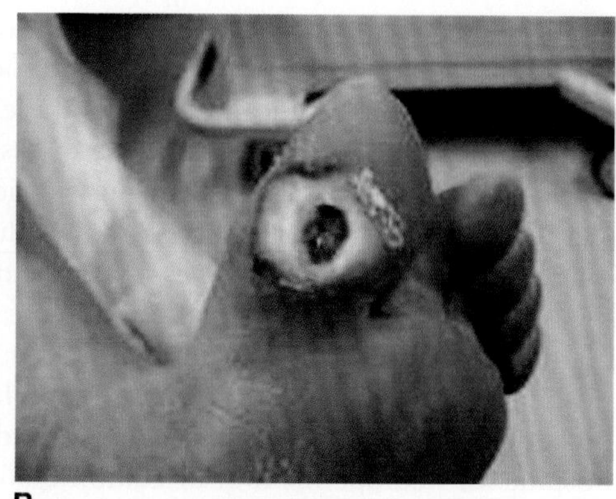

FIGURE 23-1. Injury/ulceration due to sensory neuropathy. **A.** Direct injury from a sewing needle. **B.** Repeated pressure from walking.

highly specialized range of functions, from detecting temperature and pain to detecting pressure and foot position. Patients with sensory nerve damage are typically unable to coordinate complex movements like walking or maintaining balance when their eyes are shut and are at increased risk of falling (WOCN, 2012).

Paresthesias are a very painful form of sensory neuropathy; the damaged nerves produce exquisite pain that is usually described as tingling, pins and needles, electric shock, burning and/or stabbing in nature. Individuals with paresthesias frequently report that the pain is worse at night. They may also report severe itching; increased sensitivity to normally painless stimuli, as in the bed sheets touching their feet (allodynia); or an abnormally exaggerated response to painful stimuli (hyperalgesia) (Armstrong et al., 1997a; NIH, 2014; WOCN, 2012). Patients with paresthesias should be referred to a neurologist for evaluation and treatment, which typically involves anticonvulsant medications such as gabapentin or pregabalin.

CLINICAL PEARL

Paresthesias are a very painful form of sensory neuropathy; these patients require referral to a neurologist for evaluation and treatment.

Sensory neuropathy also causes progressive anesthesia and loss of proprioceptive sense, which accounts for most of the neuropathic ulcers and for the increased risk of falling. Individuals with progressive anesthesia may report numbness that begins distally and progresses up the foot; the neuropathy typically occurs in a "stocking and glove" pattern, with patients feeling as though they are wearing stockings and gloves, although they are not. Many patients cannot recognize the shapes of small objects or distinguish among different shapes, just by touching. More significantly, individuals with progressive sensory neuropathy lose the ability to recognize minor (and eventually major) trauma to the feet. For example, the individual with sensory loss would not recognize a poorly fitting shoe or the resultant blister and would not recognize small objects in the shoe, such as a pebble. Individuals with advanced sensory loss may step on a needle or piece of glass without experiencing pain; as a result, they continue to walk on the foot and the object becomes embedded, eventually resulting in major infection. Individuals with advanced disease can also sustain major burns from hot water without recognition. Loss of proprioceptive sense means the individual does not recognize situations in which the foot is on the edge of a step or on rough terrain and does not make adjustments in posture; as a result, they are at high risk for falls (NIH, 2014; WOCN, 2012) (Figs. 23-1 and 23-2).

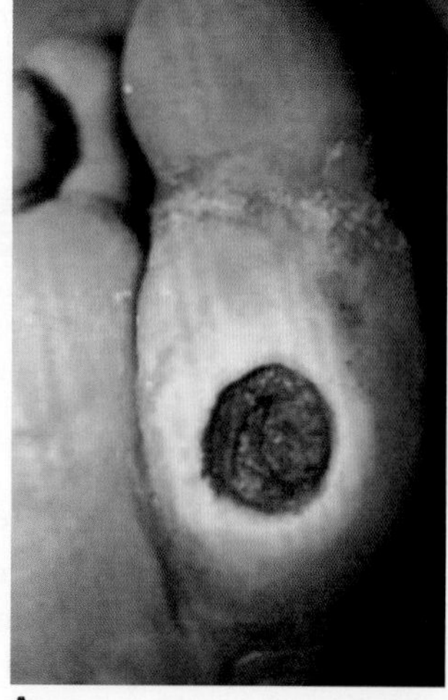
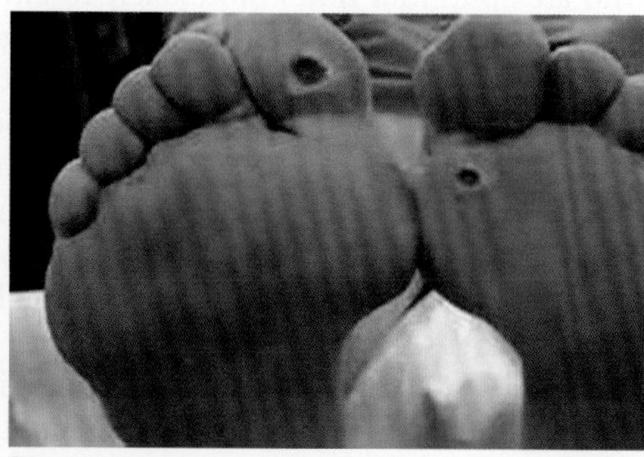

FIGURE 23-2. Injury/ulceration due to sensory neuropathy. **A.** Metatarsal head wound with periwound callus. **B.** IP joint wound of great toe from hallux rigidus.

CLINICAL PEARL

Sensory neuropathy causes progressive anesthesia and loss of proprioception, which places the individual at risk for unrecognized trauma and for falls.

Motor Neuropathy

Motor nerves control movement and tone of the muscles of the foot and affect foot contours, weight bearing, and gait. Damage to the motor nerves alters the contours of the foot, resulting in foot deformities, abnormal weight-bearing patterns, and altered gait. For example, abnormal rigidity of the toes and ankles due to atrophy of the intrinsic muscles is a common manifestation of motor neuropathy and causes increased plantar foot pressure when walking. Soft tissue glycosylation can result in shortening of the Achilles tendon, which causes deformities such as abnormally prominent metatarsal heads and claw toes. The abnormal prominence of the metatarsal heads causes abnormal weight bearing and increased exposure of the metatarsal heads to pressure and shear, which is manifest initially by callus formation and eventually by ulcer formation. Damage to the motor nerves can also result in foot drop (Birke & Sims, 1986; NIH, 2014; WOCN, 2012) (Figs. 23-3 and 23-4 for illustrations of the effects of motor neuropathy).

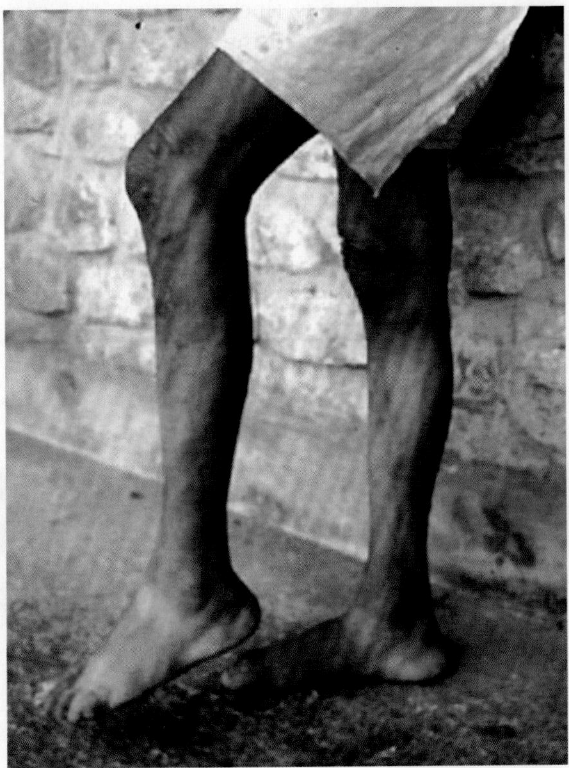

FIGURE 23-3. Changes characteristic of motor neuropathy: foot drop related to loss of anterior tibialis muscle function.

CLINICAL PEARL

Motor neuropathy alters the contours of the foot, resulting in foot deformities, abnormal weight-bearing patterns, and altered gait.

Autonomic Neuropathy

Autonomic nerves regulate biologic activities that are not under conscious control, such as thermal regulation and sweating, and blood vessel tone and diameter. Loss of autonomic control of the sweat glands commonly manifests as severely dry skin (anhidrosis) that may result in partial-thickness or full-thickness fissures; these wounds then permit invasion of pathogens that can cause serious soft tissue infections. Autonomic neuropathy can also cause persistent vasodilation of the arterial vessels in the foot, due to loss of sympathetic innervation, which normally provides for partial constriction when the foot is at rest. Persistent high-volume blood flow is thought to contribute to demineralization of the bones in the foot over time, eventually producing thin fragile bones (osteopenia) that are vulnerable to fracture. If a fracture is sustained but promptly recognized and appropriately managed with off-loading, the bone normally heals and there is no loss of structure. However, in many cases, the fracture is unrecognized due to coexisting sensory loss. If the fracture is unrecognized and the individual continues to walk on the damaged foot, additional fractures may occur with progressive damage to the bony structure of the foot. The end result can be total collapse of the normal architecture of the foot, with development of a rocker bottom foot that is high risk for plantar surface ulcerations. This defect is known as Charcot neuroarthropathy. Autonomic involvement may also compromise the function of other body systems, causing complications such as urinary retention due to loss of detrusor contractility, gastroparesis and

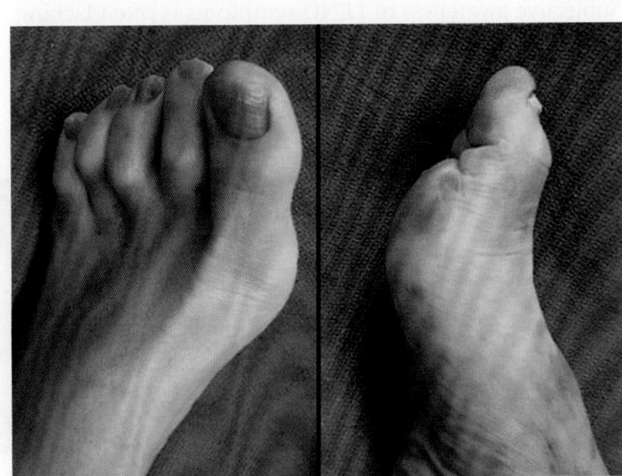

FIGURE 23-4. Changes characteristic of motor neuropathy. Prominent metatarsal heads and claw toe deformity.

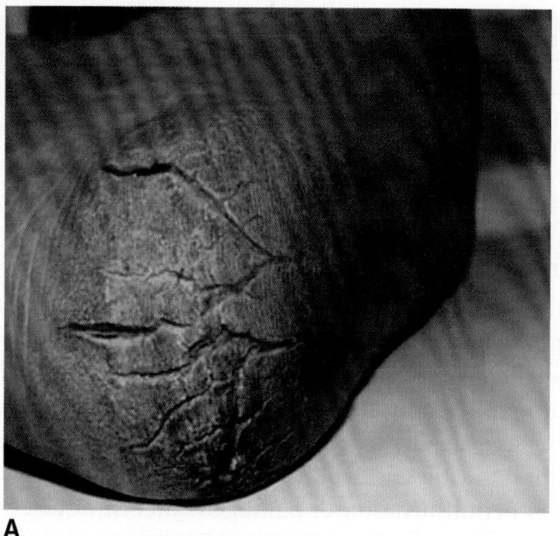

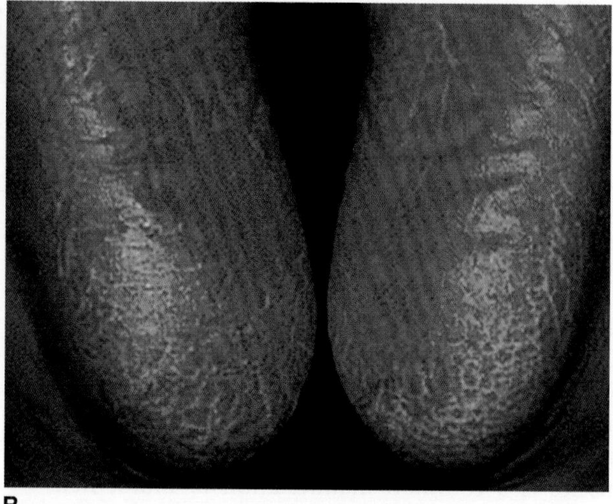

FIGURE 23-5. Changes characteristic of autonomic neuropathy: dry cracked feet and fissures due to autonomic neuropathy. **A.** Heel fissures. **B.** Anhidrosis.

persistent vomiting due to loss of gastric motility, or lower extremity edema due to cardiovascular compromise (NIH, 2014; WOCN, 2012) (Figs. 23-5 and 23-6).

CLINICAL PEARL

Autonomic neuropathy causes altered function of the sweat glands, causing very dry feet; it may also cause high-volume blood flow that results in osteopenia and increased risk for fractures.

Patients may have a combination of different types of neuropathy concomitantly, such as sensory–autonomic or sensory–motor neuropathy (NIH, 2014; WOCN, 2012). See **Table 23-1** for a comparison of sensory, motor, and autonomic neuropathy.

Diagnosis of LEND

Subjective awareness of LEND symptoms is often lacking, as symptoms may be subtle (particularly at the onset of the disease process), and the absence of sensation is more difficult to recognize than the occurrence of pain. The diagnosis is also complicated by the fact that symptoms are highly variable.

History

Prompt diagnosis is dependent on a thorough history and physical exam and the performance of simple noninvasive tests to evaluate sensory, vibratory, and proprioceptive function. The history should include the patient's medical and surgical history, with a focus on chronic conditions known to cause neuropathy, the patient's symptoms, work environment, social habits (including past and current alcohol intake), exposure to toxins, known HIV disease (or risk factors), history of infectious diseases associated with neuropathy, family history of neurologic disease, and past or present use of medications associated with neuropathy (NIH, 2014; WOCN, 2012).

Diagnostic Tests

Related diagnostic tests (e.g., CBC, CMP, HbA_{1c}, thyroid profile, B_{12} levels) should be ordered as needed, for example, when the cause of the neuropathy is unclear, or for monitoring of a known disease process such as diabetes. Blood tests can be used to diagnose diabetes,

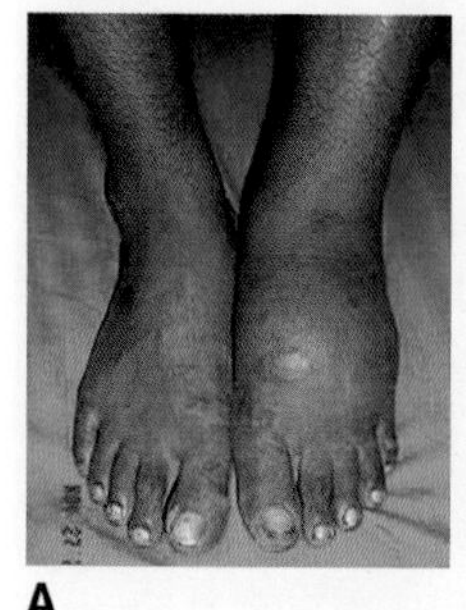

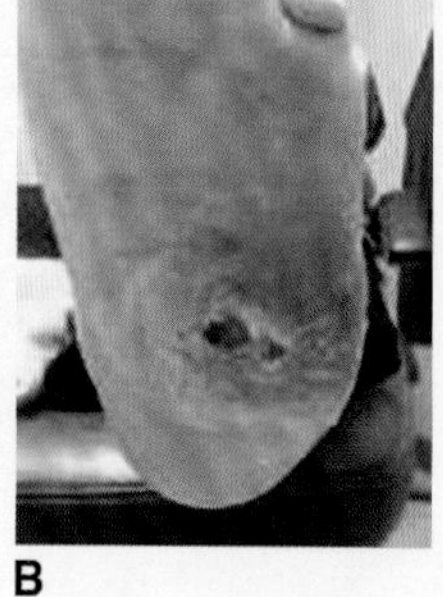

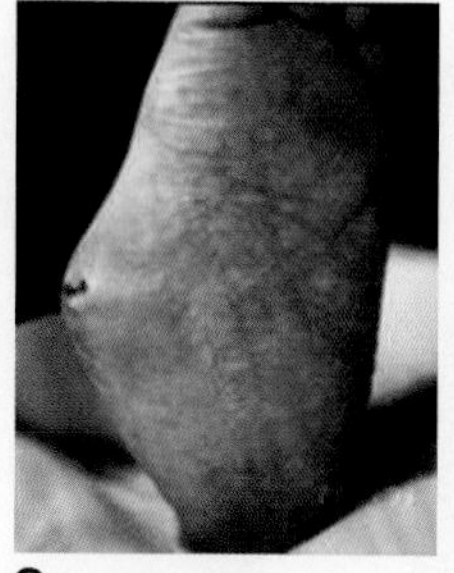

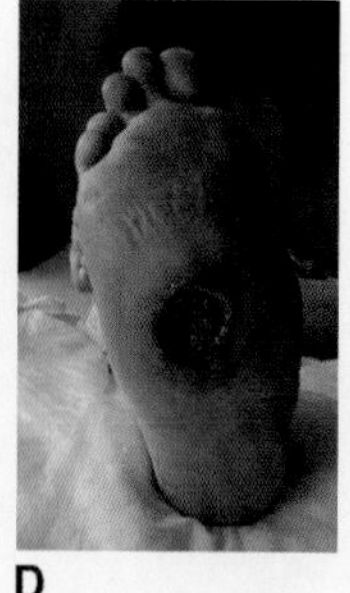

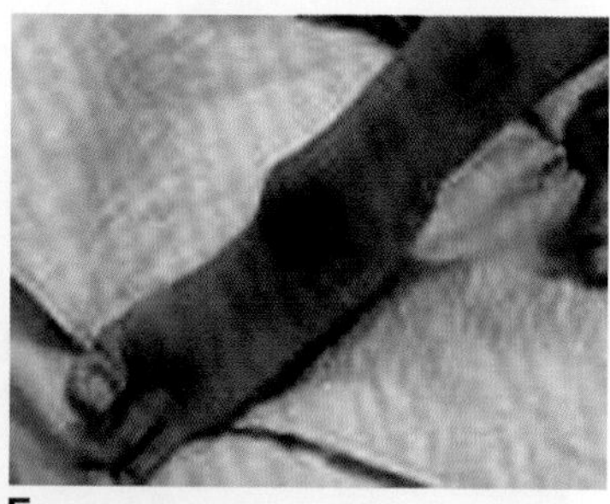

FIGURE 23-6. Changes characteristic of autonomic neuropathy. **A.** Forefoot Charcot. **B and C.** Midfoot Charcot. **D.** Hindfoot Charcot. **E.** Ankle Charcot.

TABLE 23-1 Comparison of Sensory, Motor, and Autonomic Neuropathy

Neuropathic Component	Pathophysiology	Assessment Tools	Manifestation
Sensory	• Myelin sheath is disrupted by hyperglycemia • Segmental demyelinization causes slowing of nerve conduction and impairment of sensory perception	• Sensory perception testing using a 10-g* (5.07 Semmes-Weinstein) monofilament, to identify LOPS • Vibratory perception (using a tuning fork) • Position sense testing	• Loss of protective sensation/ increased risk for painless trauma • Sensory ataxia and increased risk of falls • Insensate lesions • Insensate injury • Charcot neuroarthropathy
Motor	• Atrophy of intrinsic muscles of the foot • Subluxation of metatarsophalangeal joints	• Gait assessment • Range of motion • Muscle testing • Deep tendon reflex testing • Observation for deformities, callus formation	• Callus • Claw/hammer toes • Muscle weakness • Contracture of Achilles tendon
Autonomic	• Loss of vasomotor control • Arterial–venous shunting • Bone blood flow hyperemia • Impaired microvascular skin perfusion	Thorough skin and nail assessment of: • Skin of LE and feet (observe for abnormal dryness and/or fissures) • Interdigital spaces • Evidence of fungal infections • LE hair growth	• Anhidrosis • Callus • Interdigital or plantar surface fissures • Onychomycosis (fungal skin and toenails) • Peripheral edema • Charcot neuroarthropathy

From Birke and Sims (1986), CDC (2014), NIH (2014), Pecoraro et al. (1990), WOCN (2012).

vitamin deficiencies, liver or kidney dysfunction, and other hormonal or metabolic disorders and to identify signs of abnormal immune system activity (CDC, 2011, 2014; NIH, 2014; WOCN, 2012). For the patient with diabetes, the HbA1c provides very helpful information regarding glycemic control during the 3 months preceding the test.

Based on the results of the patient history, foot exam, tests of peripheral neurologic function, and any previous screening or testing, additional testing and referral to a neurologist may be required to help determine the nature and extent of the neuropathy and to develop a management plan (NIH, 2014).

Comprehensive Foot Exam

A comprehensive foot exam (CFE) should be performed for at-risk patient populations to promptly identify changes in neurologic or vascular status that increase the risk for neuropathic foot wounds and amputations (Birke & Sims, 1986; CDC, 2011; NIH, 2014; WOCN, 2012). The American Diabetes Association includes an annual CFE as a standard of care for individuals with diabetes (CDC, 2011, 2014; WOCN, 2012).

CLINICAL PEARL

An annual comprehensive foot exam is standard of care for individuals with diabetes.

Overview

The foot exam should be performed on both feet and should include general foot inspection (status of skin, hair, and nails; presence of callus; presence, severity, and distribution of edema), palpation for increased or decreased temperature, assessment of foot pulses (Fig. 23-7), assessment of muscle strength at ankles and toes, observation for foot deformities (e.g., claw toes, prominent metatarsal heads, midfoot arch collapse, misshapened foot), testing for LOPS using the 10-g Semmes-Weinstein monofilament, testing for vibratory sense, and testing for position sense (Birke & Sims, 1986; Bonham & Kelechi, 2008; CDC, 2011; WOCN, 2012).

An in-depth assessment provides very complete data regarding current foot status and risk factors for development of neuropathy and its complications; however, in some settings, an in-depth assessment is not feasible. In those settings, a modified assessment can be conducted using validated tools such as Inlow's 60-second Diabetic Foot Screen. This tool has been designed to allow the clinician to screen persons with diabetes for diabetes-related foot ulcers and/or risk factors for ulceration and other limb-threatening complications. Positive findings on the 60-second Foot Screen mandate follow-up and provide guidance as to needed interventions (Fig. 23-8) (Canadian Association of Wound Care [CAWC], 2014).

Sensory Testing with 10-g Monofilament

The 10-g nylon monofilaments are constructed to buckle when a 10-g force is applied. Most monofilament exams call for filament application at four to ten sites: 1st, 3rd,

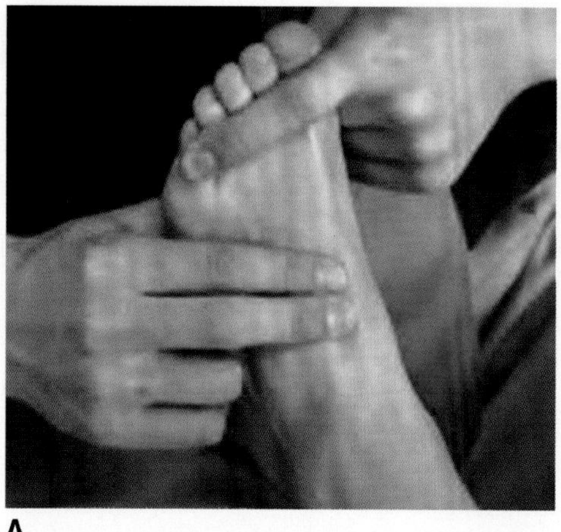

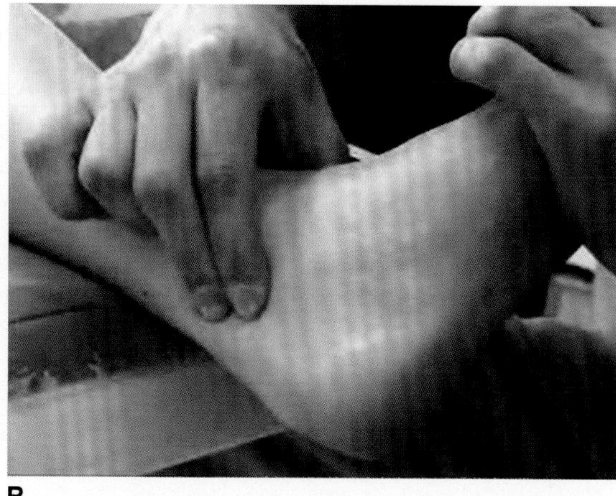

FIGURE 23-7. Pulse palpation. **A.** Dorsalis pedis. **B.** Posterior tibilais.

and 5th toes and metatarsal heads, medial and lateral midfoot, and dorsal surface between great toe and 2nd toe. The 10-point exam includes testing of the heel; however, many clinicians use the 9-point exam, which excludes the heel, due to the high occurrence of false-negative readings at the heel as a result of callus and thickened skin. If the individual has a callus at any of the testing sites, the filament should be applied proximal to the callus.

The inability to detect 10 g of pressure at one or more anatomic sites on the plantar surface of the foot is considered to be LOPS. LOPS places the individual at high risk for ulceration due to unrecognized repetitive trauma; the risk of ulceration is 9.9 times higher, and the risk of amputation among those with an ulceration is 17 times greater among individuals with LOPS as compared to those with intact sensation. Therefore, any individual who fails to respond to all test sites must receive intensive education and counseling regarding foot protection and daily foot inspection (Birke & Sims, 1986; NIH, 2014; Pecoraro et al., 1990; WOCN, 2012). See Boxes 23-1 to 23-3 and Table 23-2.

CLINICAL PEARL

Sensory function is tested with a 10-g monofilament; failure to recognize 10 g of pressure represents loss of protective sensation (LOPS), which places the individual at risk for unrecognized repetitive trauma.

Vibratory Sense Testing

While monofilament testing is widely accepted as the most critical objective measure of sensory perception, vibratory sense testing is also a reliable and validated indicator of sensory perception, and data suggest that loss of vibratory sense typically occurs prior to LOPS. Thus, vibratory sense testing may enable the clinician to detect neuropathy at an earlier point and to intervene with education and counseling regarding the importance of tight glycemic control. To conduct vibratory sense testing, the clinician uses a 128-Hz tuning fork; the tip of the vibrating fork is placed over the base of the great toe at the first metatarsal bone bilaterally, and the individual is asked to report the point at which vibration ceases. An abnormal response is defined as the individual's loss of vibratory sensation while the examiner still perceives it.

Position Sense Testing

Proprioception is the accurate detection of the foot's spatial position in relation to its environment and the rest of the body, without the benefit of visual input. Loss of normal proprioception places the individual at increased risk for falls. To test for proprioceptive sense, the person is asked to close her/his eyes; the clinician then moves the great toe in different directions (up, down, medially, and laterally) and asks the person to tell in which direction the toe is pointing. Inability to consistently identify the direction in which the toe is pointing is considered loss of position sense.

CLINICAL PEARL

To test for proprioceptive sense, the individual is asked to close his/her eyes; the clinician then moves the great toe in different directions and asks the individual to state in which direction the toe is pointing.

Reflex Testing

Ankle reflexes can be tested with the patient either kneeling or resting on a couch/table. The Achilles tendon is stretched until the ankle is in a neutral position; the clinician then strikes the tendon with the reflex hammer and observes for plantar flexion. Total absence of ankle reflex is regarded as an abnormal result (NIH, 2014; WOCN, 2012).

Assessment of Musculoskeletal/Biomechanical Status

Motor neuropathy causes loss of foot muscle strength and shortening of the Achilles tendon; these changes result in altered foot structure and abnormal gait as well as muscle wasting throughout the foot (NIH, 2014; WOCN, 2012).

INLOW'S

60-second Diabetic Foot Screen

Canadian Association of Wound Care  Association canadienne du soin des plaies

www.cawc.net

SCREENING TOOL

Patient Name: **Clinician Signature:**

ID number: **Date:**

Look – 20 seconds	Score: Left Foot	Score: Right Foot	Care Recommendations
1. Skin 0 = intact and healthy 1 = dry with fungus or light callus 2 = heavy callus build up 3 = open ulceration or history of previous ulcer			
2. Nails 0 = well-kept 1 = unkempt and ragged 2 = thick, damaged, or infected			
3. Deformity 0 = no deformity 2 = mild deformity 4 = major deformity			
4. Footwear 0 = appropriate 1 = inappropriate 2 = causing trauma			
Touch – 10 seconds	**Left Foot**	**Right Foot**	**Care Recommendations**
5. Temperature – Cold 0 = foot warm 1 = foot is cold			
6. Temperature – Hot 0 = foot is warm 1 = foot is hot			
7. Range of Motion 0 = full range to hallux 1 = hallux limitus 2 = hallux rigidus 3 = hallux amputation			
Assess – 30 seconds	**Left Foot**	**Right Foot**	**Care Recommendations**
8. Sensation – Monofilament Testing 0 = 10 sites detected 2 = 7 to 9 sites detected 4 = 0 to 6 sites detected			
9. Sensation – Ask 4 Questions: i. Are your feet ever numb? ii. Do they ever tingle? iii. Do they ever burn? iv. Do they ever feel like insects are crawling on them? 0 = no to all questions 2 = yes to any of the questions			
10. Pedal Pulses 0 = present 1 = absent			
11. Dependent Rubor 0 = no 1 = yes			
12. Erythema 0 = no 1 = yes			
Score Totals =			

Screening for foot ulcers and/or limb-threatening complications. Use the highest score from left or right foot.

Score = 0 to 6 → recommend screening yearly
Score = 7 to 12 → recommend screening every 6 months
Score = 13 to 19 → recommend screening every 3 months
Score = 20 to 25 → recommend screening every 1 to 3 months

Comments:

FIGURE 23-8. Inlow 60-second screening tool.

Instructions for Use

General Guidelines: This tool is designed to assist in screening persons with diabetes to prevent or treat diabetes-related foot ulcers and/or limb-threatening complications. The screen should be completed on admission of any person with diabetes and then repeated as directed by risk and clinical judgment. **Do not confuse patient visits with patient screening.** Your patient may require frequent and regular visits for routine care but complete the screening as indicated or as relevant based on clinical judgment.

Specific Instructions:

Step 1: Explain screening to the patient and have them remove their shoes, socks from both feet.
Step 2: Remove any dressings or devices that impair the screening.
Step 3: Review each of the parameters for each foot as listed in the Inlow's 60-second Diabetic Foot Screen and select the appropriate score based on patient's status. (An amputation may affect the score on the affected limb.)
Step 4: Once the screen is completed determine care recommendations based on patient need, available resources and clinical judgement.
Step 5: Use the highest score from either the left or right foot to determine recommended screening intervals.
Step 6: Set up an appointment for the next screening based on screening score and clinical judgement.

Parameter Review

1. Skin

Assess the skin on the foot: top, bottom and sides including between the toes.

0 = skin is intact and has no signs of trauma. No signs of fungus or callus formation
1 = skin is dry, fungus such as a moccasin foot or interdigital yeast may be present. Some callus build-up may be noted
2 = heavy callus build-up
3 = open skin ulceration present

2. Nails

Assess toenails to determine how well they are being managed either by the patient or professionally.

0 = nails well-kept
1 = nails unkempt and ragged
2 = nails thick, damaged or infected

3. Deformity

Look for any bony changes that can put the patient at significant risk and prevent the wearing of off-the-shelf footwear

0 = no deformity detected
2 = may have some mild deformities such as dropped metatarsal heads (MTHs) (the bones under the fat pads on the ball of the foot). Each MTH corresponds to the toe distal to it, so there is a 1st MTH at the base of the first toe etc. Bunions/Charcot may also be considered a deformity as well as deformities related to trauma.
4 = Amputation

4. Footwear

Look at the shoes that the patient is wearing and discuss what he or she normally wears.

0 = shoes provide protection, support and fit the foot. On removal of the footwear there are no reddened areas on the foot
1 = shoes are inappropriate do not provide protection or support for the foot.
2 = shoes are causing trauma (redness or ulceration) to the foot either through a poor fit or a poor style (eg., cowboy boots).

5. Temperature – cold

Does the foot feel colder than the other foot or is it colder than it should be considering the environment? This can be indicative of arterial disease.

0 = foot is of "normal" temperature for environment.
1 = foot is cold – compared to other foot or compared to the environment

6. Temperature – hot

Does the foot feel hotter than the other foot or is it hotter than it should be considering the environment? This can be indicative of an infection or Charcot changes.

0 = foot is of "normal" temperature for environment
1 = foot is hot – compared to other foot or compared to the environment

7. Range of Motion

Move the first toe back and forth – plantar flex and dorsiflex.

0 = first toe (hallux) is easily moved
1 = hallux has some restricted movement
2 = hallux is rigid and cannot be moved
3 = hallux amputated

8. Sensation – Monofilament testing

Using the 5.07 monofilament, test the sites listed. Do not test over heavy callus.

- digits: 1st, 3rd, 5th
- MTH: 1st, 3rd, 5th
- midfoot: Medial, Lateral
- heel
- top (dorsum) of foot

And then score out of 10:

0 = 10 out of 10 sites detected
2 = 7 to 9 out of 10 sites detected
4 = 0 to 6 out of 10 sites detected

9. Sensation – Questions

Ask the following four questions:

i. Are your feet ever numb?
ii. Do they ever tingle?
iii. Do they ever burn?
iv. Do they ever feel like insects are crawling on them?

0 = answered No to all four questions
2 = answered Yes to one or more of the four questions

10. Pedal pulses

Palpate (feel) the dorsalis pedis pulse located on the top of the foot. If unable to feel the pedal pulse feel for the posterior tibial pulse beneath the medial malleolus.

0 = pulse present
1 = pulse absent

11. Dependent rubor

Pronounced redness of the feet when the feet are down and pallor when the feet are elevated. This can be indicative of arterial disease.

0 = no dependent rubor
1 = dependent rubor present

12. Erythema

Look for redness of the skin that does not change when the foot is elevated. This can be indicative of infection or Charcot changes.

0 = no redness of the skin
1 = redness noted

Reminder: Strategies for the prevention and management of diabetic foot ulcers need to consider more than just the results from a foot screen. It is important that the health-care professional completes a holistic assessment that also monitors lipids, hypertension, glucose and patient activity and exercise. **Persons with diabetes who are cognitively impaired or have diseases such as end-stage renal disease are at higher risk and may need more frequent screening than indicated.**

FIGURE 23-8. *(Continued)*

Interpreting Results

Inlow's 60-second Diabetic Foot Screen has been designed to allow the clinician to screen persons with diabetes to prevent or treat diabetes-related foot ulcers and/or limb-threatening complications. By combining the results from different parameters identified with Inlow's 60-second Diabetic Foot Screen, the clinician can identify pathologies and/or care deficits.

Parameters												
1	2	3	4	5	6	7	8	9	10	11	12	Indications
												Self Care Parameters:
												High scores in parameters 1, 2 and 4 → indicative of self care deficit.
												Integument Parameters:
												Moderate scores in parameters 4 and 7 → indicative of callous formation.
												High scores in parameters 1, 6 and 12 → indicative of infected ulcer.
												High scores in parameters 2, 6 and 12 → indicative of infected nails.
												Arterial Flow Parameters:
												High scores in parameters 5, 10 and 11 → indicative of peripheral arterial disease.
												Sensation Parameters:
												High scores in parameters 8 and 9 → indicative of loss of protective sensation or neuropathy.
												Boney Changes Parameters:
												High scores in parameters 3, 8 and 9 → indicative of Charcot changes.

Determining Risk

Inlow's 60-second Diabetic Foot Screen can also assist in determining patient risk. By reviewing the results from Inlow's 60-second Diabetic Foot Screen, the clinician can use the International Working Group on the Diabetic Foot (IWGDF) – Risk Classification System to identify a risk category for their patients.

Step 1: Complete Inlow's 60-second Diabetic Foot Screen by assessing both feet on every patient with diabetes.

Step 2: Using the IWGDF Risk Classification System, identify which category your patients falls into.

International Working Group on the Diabetic Foot (IWGDF) – Risk Classification System (Modified[1])

Risk category	Criteria
0	Normal – no neuropathy
1	Loss of protective sensation
2a	LOPS and deformity
2b	Peripheral arterial disease
3a	Previous hx of ulceration
3b	Previous hx of amputation

1. Lavery LA, Peters EJG, Williams JR, Murdoch JR, Hudson A, Lavery DC. Reevaluating the Way We Classify the Diabetic Foot. Restructuring the diabetic foot risk classification system of the International Working Group on the Diabetic Foot. *Diabetes Care* 31:154–156, 2008.

Considerations Based on Clinical Settings

1. **Acute Care:** Due to the high turnover of patients in acute care, clinicians needs to ensure that the initial assessment goes with the patient to their next level of care.
2. **Long Term or Residential Care:** Patients with diabetes may have mobility issues and are in bed or wheelchairs. Feet still may become traumatized by the use of inappropriate footwear even if they are non-weight bearing.
3. **Dialysis Unit:** Some dialysis units may wish to augment this tool with toe pressures and blood work, depending on their clinical support.
4. **Home or Community Care:** Clinicians can use this tool for communication with their patients, each other or other departments, such as specialized clinics.
5. **Foot Clinic:** Foot clinic standards of assessment will be at a higher standard. However, this document is a good communication tool with other clinicians who may be caring for the person with diabetes.

More Information

For more information on the assessment and management of the diabetic foot, refer to:

1. *Best Practice Recommendations for the Prevention, Diagnosis and Treatment of Diabetic Foot Ulcers*: Update 2010 at www.cawc.net
2. RNAO Best Practice Guideline *Reducing Foot Complications for Persons with Diabetes* at www.rnao.org
3. RNAO Best Practice Guideline *Assessment and Management of Foot Ulcers for People with Diabetes* at www.rnao.org
4. *The International Working Group on the Diabetic Foot* at www.iwgdf.org
5. *Diabetes, Healthy Feet and You* at www.cawc.net/index.php/public/feet/

FIGURE 23-8. *(Continued)*

BOX 23-1.
Diabetes Foot Screen Instructions

Section 1

The twelve questions can be answered in the "R" (right foot) or "L" (left foot) blank with a "Y" or "N" to indicate a positive or negative finding. Fill in all blanks.

Question 1: Is there a history of foot ulcer?

Question 2: Is there a foot ulcer now?

The purpose of these questions is to determine if the patient currently has or has ever had an ulcer on the foot. History of a foot ulcer places the patient at an increased risk of developing another foot ulcer and increases the potential of future amputation. The patient with a past or present foot ulcer is considered permanently in Risk Category 3.

Question 3: Is there toe deformity?

Question 4: Is there an abnormal shape of the foot?

This is determined by inspecting the general shape of the patient's foot. Conditions to consider include prominent bony areas, partial or complete amputations of the foot or toes, clawed toes, prominent metatarsal heads, bunions, or "Charcot foot."

A Charcot foot is a neuropathic foot that may present with swelling, increased temperature, and *little or no pain.* Advanced cases show progressive signs of deformity into what is referred to as a "rocker bottom" or "boat-shaped" foot. A patient with a Charcot foot is permanently in Risk Category 3.

Question 5: Are the toenails thick or ingrown?

Identify mycotic, significantly hypertrophic, or ingrown nails.

Question 6: Is there callus buildup?

Identify focal and/or heavy callus.

Question 7: Is there swelling?

Swelling may stem from a variety of causes such as a Charcot fracture, infection, venous insufficiency, or CHF.

Question 8: Is there elevated skin temperature?

Elevated, localized skin temperature can indicate excessive mechanical stress, bone fracture, or an infection and requires further evaluation. Skin temperature can be measured by a commercially available thermometer or by touch. A temperature elevation of greater than 2°C on the thermometer or a noticeable difference by touch when compared with the contralateral foot is considered clinically significant.

Question 9: Is there muscle weakness?

A manual muscle test of foot and great toe dorsi and plantar flexion.

Question 10: Can the patient see the bottom of his/her feet?

Obesity and/or lack of knee and hip flexibility can prevent a patient from seeing his/her feet. Self-inspection and foot care are difficult with these limitations often requiring family or outside assistance.

Question 11: Is the patient wearing improperly fitted shoes? Does the patient wear footwear appropriate for her/his category of risk?

An improperly fitted shoe may create foot pressures that lead to further complications. Patients with sensory loss often wear shoes that are too short and/or narrow resulting in ischemic ulcers on the medial or lateral metatarsal heads or the toes of a foot with claw toe deformity. Properly sized added depth shoes with soft custom-molded insoles are usually indicated for patients with loss of sensation and deformity to prevent ulceration.

Question 12: Is there an absent pedal pulse?

See risk and management categories.

Section 2

Examine the foot and record problems identified on the Foot Screen form. Draw calluses, preulcerative lesions (a closed lesion, i.e., blister or hematoma), or open ulcers as accurately as possible using the appropriate "pattern" to indicate what type of condition is present. Label areas that are red as "R," warm "W" (warmer than the other parts of the foot or the opposite foot), dry "D," or macerated "M" (friable, moist, soft tissue) on the corresponding location of the foot drawing provided on the screen form.

A sensory exam using the 10-g monofilament is performed as indicated on the foot drawing. Responses are recorded in the appropriate circles. A positive response is recorded in the corresponding circle with a "+" if the patient is able to feel the filament and a negative response is recorded with a "−" if the patient cannot feel the filament.

Section 3

The accurate placement of patients into their respective Risk Category is a key element in the Foot Screen. The higher the Risk Category, the higher the risk a patient has of recurrent foot ulceration, progressive deformity, and, ultimately, amputation of the foot. All patients, regardless of category, should be rescreened annually and should be given basic patient education.

A detailed description of the Risk Category is available in the document "Risk and Management Categories for the Foot."

Another common change in foot structure is displacement and thinning of the plantar surface fat pads, due to motor neuropathy, the effects of aging, or both; this results in abnormally prominent metatarsal heads (LaBorde, 2009; Maluf et al., 2004). Changes in muscle tone and muscle function can also cause a variety of foot deformities; for example, the "claw toe" deformity occurs as a result of hyperextension at the metatarsophalangeal joint combined with flexion contractures at the proximal and distal interphalangeal joints. The claw toe deformity usually affects all of the toes, though the great toe contracture is typically the most severe. This deformity places the individual at high risk for ulcerations involving both the plantar and dorsal surfaces; this is because the hyperextension causes the dorsum of the toe to point upward and the flexion contractures cause the distal toe to point downward, meaning that the individual will require extradepth shoes and protection of the distal toe pad. In addition, the bony prominences are exposed to repetitive high pressure with every step (CDC, 2011; WOCN, 2012).

CLINICAL PEARL

To assess for motor neuropathy, the clinician should observe for foot deformities, callus formation, or altered gait/weight bearing and should assess for range of motion and muscle strength.

BOX 23-2.

Diabetes Foot Screen

Name (Last, First, MI) ______________ Date: ___/___/___

Fill in the following blanks with a "Y" or "N" to indicate findings of the right or left foot

	R	L
Is there a history of a foot ulcer?	_____	_____
Is there a foot ulcer now?	_____	_____
Is there toe deformity?	_____	_____
Is there swelling or an abnormal foot shape?	_____	_____
Are the toenails long, thick, or ingrown?	_____	_____
Is there heavy callus buildup?	_____	_____
Is there swelling?	_____	_____
Is there elevated skin temperature?	_____	_____
Is there foot or ankle muscle weakness?	_____	_____
Can the patient see the bottom of their feet?	_____	_____
Are the shoes appropriate in style and fit?	_____	_____
Is there limited ankle dorsiflexion?	_____	_____
Is there an absent pedal pulse?	_____	_____

Note the level of sensation in the circles:
+ = Can feel the 5.07 filament; – = Can't feel the 5.07 filament

RIGHT LEFT

Skin conditions on the foot or between the toes:

Draw in: Callous ▤, Preulcer ▦, Ulcer ■ (note length and width in cm)

Label with: **R**, redness; **M**, maceration; **D**, dryness; **T**, tinea

Risk Category:

___0 No loss of protective sensation

___1 Loss of protective sensation

___2 Loss of protective sensation with <u>either</u> high pressure (callus/deformity) or poor circulation

___3 History of plantar ulceration, neuropathic fracture (Charcot foot), or amputation

Rev 03/22/12 LSUHSC Diabetes Foot Program Performed by:_______________

BOX 23-3.

Filament Application Instructions

Note: The sensory testing device used with the Diabetes Foot Screen is a nylon filament mounted on a holder that has been standardized to deliver a 10-g force when properly applied. Research has shown that a patient who can feel the 10-g filament in the selected sites has "protective sensation" and has a reduced risk of developing plantar ulcers.

1. Use the 10-g filament to test for "protective sensation."
2. Test the sites indicated on the Diabetes Foot Screen.
3. Apply the filament perpendicular to the skin's surface (see diagram A).
4. The approach, skin contact, and departure of the filament should be 1½ seconds.
5. Apply sufficient force to cause the filament to bend (see diagram B).

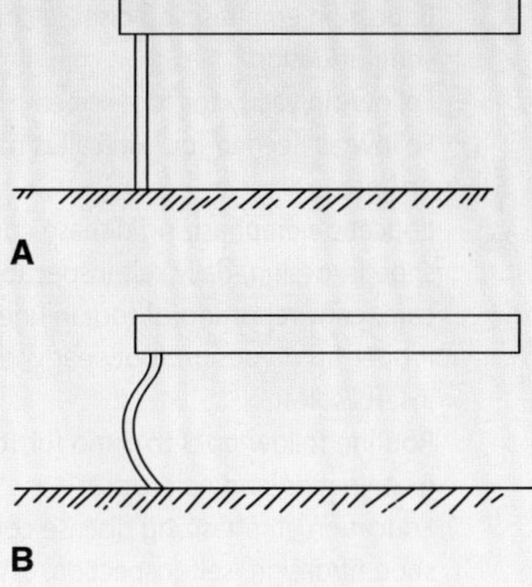

6. Do not allow the filament to slide across the skin or make repetitive contact at the test site.
7. Randomize the selection of test sites and time between successive tests to reduce patient guessing.
8. Ask the patient to respond "Yes" when the filament is felt and record the response on the Diabetes Foot Screen Form.
9. Apply the filament along the margin of and NOT on an ulcer, callus, scar, or necrotic tissue. DO NOT touch feet with hands-only filament.
10. Have the patient close their eyes while the filament test is being performed.

REV 9/12

Musculoskeletal assessment includes inspection of the contours of the foot and identification of any deformities. As noted, abnormally prominent metatarsal heads and claw toe deformity are common abnormalities; other potential deformities include hammertoes, overlapping toes, and midfoot or hindfoot deformities, which suggest possible Charcot foot. Callus formation at the site of the deformity is common, due to repetitive trauma. The skin and soft tissue over bony deformities are at high risk for ulceration caused by repetitive exposure to pressure and

TABLE 23-2 Diabetes Foot Program

Risk Category	Description
Risk and management categories for the foot	
0	Diabetes, but no loss of protective sensation in feet
1	Diabetes, loss of protective sensation (LOPS) in feet
2	Diabetes, loss of protective sensation in feet with *either* high pressure (callus/deformity) or poor circulation
3	Diabetes, history of plantar ulceration or neuropathic fracture
Note: "loss of protective sensation" is assessed using a 5.07 monofilament at 10 locations on each foot	
Category	**Management Category**
Lower extremity amputation prevention program	
0	Education emphasizing disease control, proper shoe fit/design Follow-up yearly for foot screen Follow as needed for skin/callus/nail care or orthoses
1	Education emphasizing disease control, proper shoe fit/design, daily self-inspection, skin/nail care, early reporting of foot injuries Proper fitting/design footwear with soft inserts/soles Routine follow-up 3 to 6 mo for foot/shoe examination and nail care
2	Education emphasizing disease control, proper shoe fit/design, self-inspection, skin/nail/callus care, early reporting of foot injuries Depth-inlay footwear, molded/modified orthoses; modified shoes as needed Routine follow-up 1 to 3 mo for foot/activity/footwear evaluation and callus/nail care
3	Education emphasizing disease control, proper fitting footwear, self-inspection, skin/nail/callus care and early reporting of foot injuries Depth-inlay footwear, molded/modified orthoses; modified/custom footwear, ankle–foot orthoses as needed Routine follow-up 1 to 12 weeks for foot/activity/footwear evaluation and callus/nail care

Diabetes Foot Clinic visit frequency may vary based on individual patient needs.

shear; the cumulative damage is typically unrecognized due to the effects of coexisting sensory neuropathy (CDC, 2011, 2014; WOCN, 2012) (Fig. 23-9).

The musculoskeletal assessment should also include muscle strength testing and gait evaluation. To assess muscle strength, the nurse should place her/his hand against the plantar and then dorsal surface of the foot and should ask the individual to push down or up against her/his hand. The nurse should also assess range of motion and should be alert to any obvious signs of muscle weakness, such as foot drop or visible atrophy. The nurse should ask the individual to stand and walk and should note any patterned gait abnormalities; in addition, the nurse should use a Harris Mat if available to identify abnormalities in patterns of weight bearing. It is also helpful to assess footwear for common wear patterns that can indicate gait abnormality and elevated stepping pressure and to observe for callus formation over the plantar surface, since callus formation is indicative of repetitive exposure to friction and superficial shear (Birke & Sims, 1986; WOCN, 2012; Zimny et al., 2004).

Shoe Condition/Wear Patterns

The nurse should assess the individual's footwear for general condition, wear patterns along the outer soles and heels, and bottomed out areas in the insoles and interior shoe lining; all of these findings are indicative of abnormal pressure points and gait abnormalities. It is also essential for the nurse to assess the footwear in regard to appropriateness of fit and design in relation to the size and shape of the patient's foot (Health Resources and Services Administration [HRSA], 2011; NIH, 2014; WOCN, 2012). Providing patients with a tracing pattern of their feet offers an objective tool to identify appropriateness of shoe design and sizing. The tracing should be made with the individual in a standing position and with weight equally distributed over both feet. The individual's shoes should then be placed over the tracing; if the foot tracing extends beyond the shoe margins, the shoes are not appropriate for that individual to wear (HRSA, 2011; NIH, 2014; WOCN, 2012).

CLINICAL PEARL

Providing patients with a tracing pattern of their feet offers an objective tool to identify appropriateness of shoe design and sizing.

Pressure mapping is used to identify high pressure points; it is first performed with the individual standing with weight equally distributed and then with "step in motion," which identifies any abnormal pressure points as the individual progresses through the gait cycle. Pressure mapping capability is now available in commercial settings (local pharmacies and shoe stores that offer over-the-counter insoles and shoes without a prescription) and is also used by orthotists/pedorthists to identify insoles that provide even weight distribution (WOCN, 2012) (Fig. 23-10).

Vascular Assessment

Lower extremity vascular assessment is a key element of neuropathic foot workup, because 30% of patients with neuropathic disease have coexisting arterial disease, and this has a profound impact on management and prognosis. The critical elements of vascular assessment include general inspection of the skin, hair, and nails to

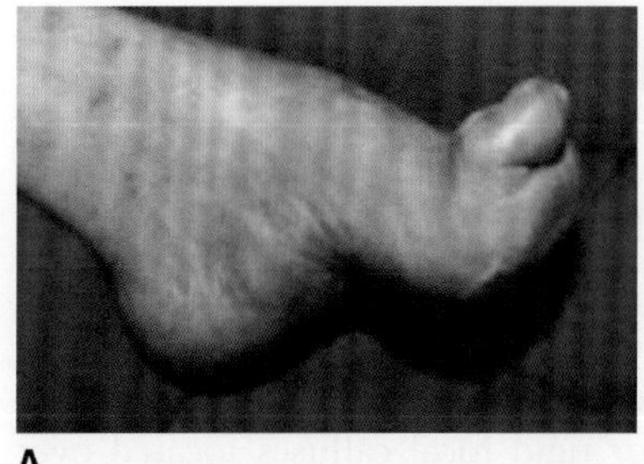
A

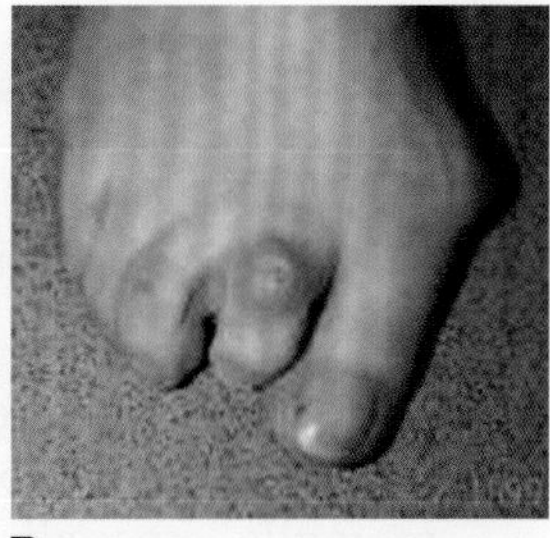
B

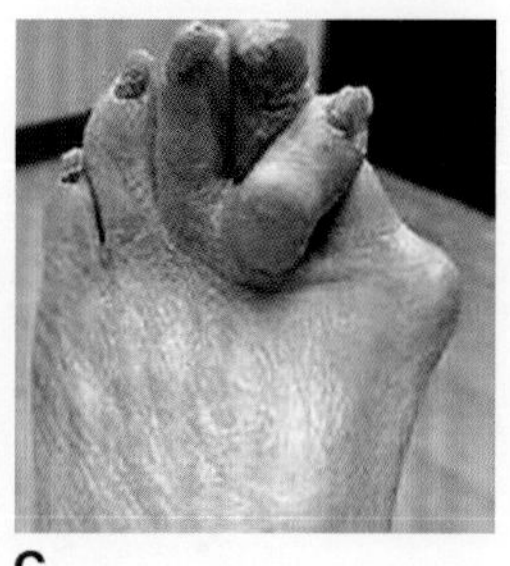
C

FIGURE 23-9. Common foot deformities. **A.** Prominent metatarsal heads. **B.** Bunion deformity and claw toes. **C.** Crossed toes.

identify atrophic changes; assessment of pedal pulses and capillary refill; and measurement of ABI. For a detailed description of the parameters and processes included in a comprehensive vascular exam, please refer to Chapter 22.

CLINICAL PEARL

Vascular assessment is a critical element of the comprehensive foot exam; 30% of patients with neuropathic disease also have lower extremity arterial disease, and this has a profound effect on management and prognosis.

Dermal Temperature Assessment for Soft Tissue Inflammation

Dermal temperature measurement with an infrared, noncontact thermometer has been identified by the International Working Group on the Diabetic Foot as one of the most promising technological developments for the objective measurement of inflammation. An increase in temperature of >2°C at a particular site, as compared to the same site on the contralateral foot or to adjacent areas of the same foot, is considered to be positive for inflammation (Armstrong et al., 2007; Armstrong & Lavery, 1997; Lavery et al., 2004; WOCN, 2012). Dermal temperature assessments are performed at sites of bony deformity and, if applicable, at sites of previous ulceration. This simple measurement can be a very powerful addition to the comprehensive foot assessment and can also be used to assess the efficacy of offloading measures throughout and following healing. Data indicate that 82% of neuropathic foot wounds are preceded by inflammation and callus, which means that the observation of either callus formation or temperature elevation should prompt the clinician to implement preventive care such as improved pressure redistribution and very close monitoring of the involved area (Armstrong et al., 2007; Lavery et al., 2004; Lavery et al., 1997; Sage et al., 2001; WOCN, 2012). Infrared dermal thermometers are currently available from a variety of

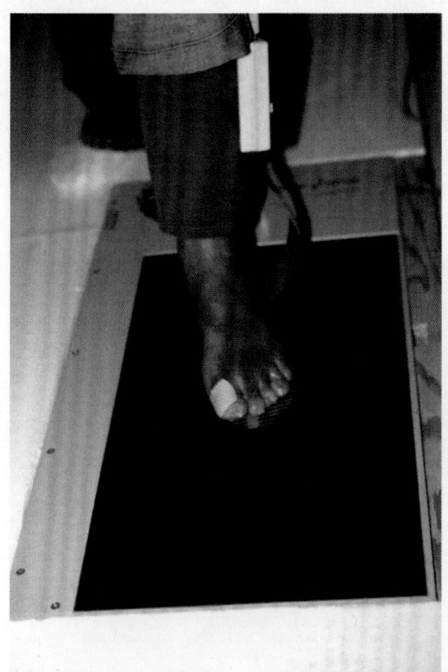
A

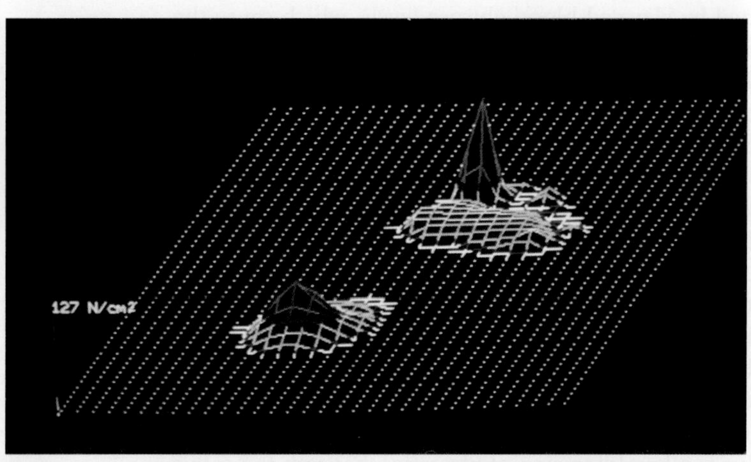

B

FIGURE 23-10. A and B. Pressure mapping.

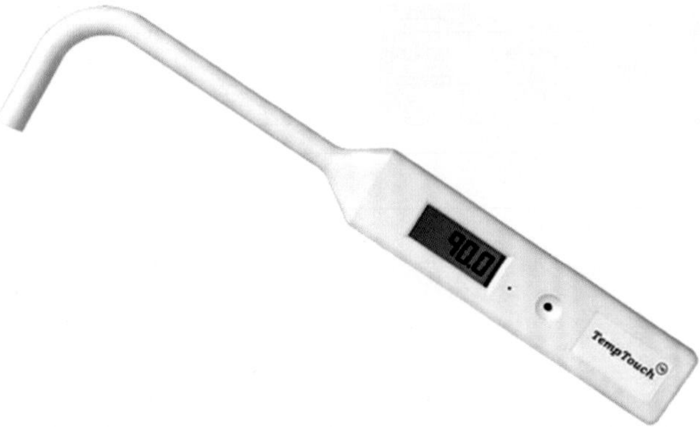

FIGURE 23-11. TempTouch dermal thermometer.

medical equipment providers and range in price from $40 to $800. In a study comparing nine commercially available infrared thermometer options, the lesser priced options performed as well as the higher priced options, in terms of detecting a *temperature difference* (Foto et al., 2009) (Fig. 23-11).

CLINICAL PEARL

Dermal temperature measurement can be used to detect inflammation, which is indicated by an increase in temperature of >2°C at any site as compared to adjacent skin or the contralateral foot.

Skin, Nail, and Soft Tissue Assessment

The nurse should assess the skin for color, texture, and turgor, with particular attention to the presence, location, and distribution of any calluses, and to skin hydration and the presence of fissures. A callus is a thickened area of skin that occurs in response to repeated exposure to friction, shear, and pressure; calluses develop over sites of abnormally high pressures associated with altered foot contours and gait (Fig. 23-12). Callus development is further supported by elevated blood glucose levels, which cause the tissue to become rigid, inflexible, and more resistant to collagenase digestion. Calluses can be generalized, as is frequently seen over the heel, or focal, as is frequently seen over the metatarsal heads. Focal calluses are particularly destructive lesions, because the callus itself increases the pressure and shear exerted on the underlying tissue during walking. A very common scenario includes abnormal gait and weight bearing leading to callus formation, which leads to development of an ulcer in the tissue beneath the callus. Because the individual frequently has sensory as well as motor neuropathy, there is no discomfort associated with either the callus or the ulcer; thus, the ulcer may go unrecognized for a period of time. Hemorrhage into a callus is a heralding sign of ulceration beneath the callus (Sage et al., 2001; WOCN, 2012).

CLINICAL PEARL

Focal calluses are particularly destructive lesions, because the callus itself increases the pressure and shear exerted on the underlying tissues during walking.

In conducting the foot examination, the nurse should observe for and palpate any calluses and should intervene promptly, especially for rigid focal calluses located over bony prominences. Interventions include paring of the callus and recommendations regarding pressure redistributing footwear and insoles.

Skin hydration is another critical assessment parameter. As noted, autonomic neuropathy adversely affects the function of the sweat glands; the most common outcome is very dry skin (xerosis), which may result in fissure formation, typically over the heels. However, overhydration of the skin occasionally occurs, which also increases the risk for fissure formation; fissure formation due to overhydration usually involves the interdigital spaces. Thus, the nurse should assess for either overly dry or overly wet skin and for fissure formation. In assessing the skin, the nurse should also be alert to any lesions and any evidence of fungal infections, which are common among the diabetic population. Tinea pedis is the most common fungal infection involving the foot, and there are different clinical presentations based on the specific organism. It may manifest as very dry, scaly, circular lesions on the plantar surface, with no itching or pain, or as an acute infection involving the dorsal surface, with erythema, blistering, and pain. Tinea infections can also cause interdigital fissures (Sage et al., 2001; WOCN, 2012) (Fig. 23-13).

The nurse should also assess the status of the nails, with particular attention to evidence of ingrown nails, cuticle infection (paronychia), or fungal infection of the nails (onychomycosis), which is evidenced by thickened, discolored, or abnormally crumbly nails (WOCN, 2012).

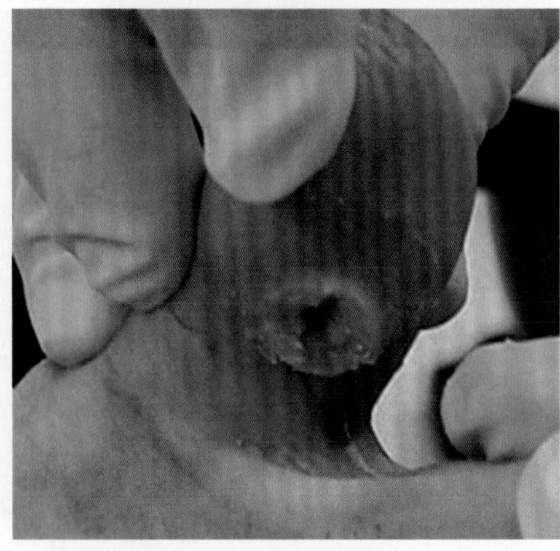

FIGURE 23-12. Interdigital callus.

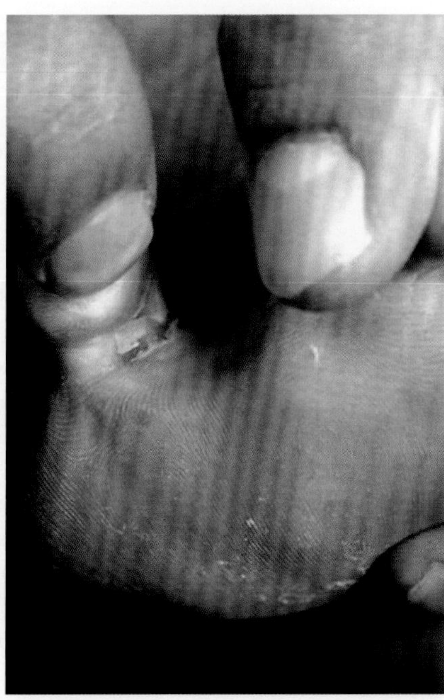

FIGURE 23-13. Interdigital tinea from moisture.

Finally, the nurse should assess for lower extremity edema, noting the type and severity and whether the edema is unilateral or bilateral. Edema may be related to comorbid conditions such as heart failure, nephropathy, or venous insufficiency. Unilateral edema may be a heralding sign of Charcot deformity (i.e., neuropathic fracture), particularly if the edema is accompanied by increased warmth and bounding pulses (Seidel, 2006; WOCN, 2012). A detailed description of venous edema, lymphedema, and lipedema is provided in Chapter 21.

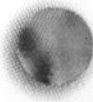

Assessment/Classification of Neuropathic Foot Ulcer

If the individual presents with a foot ulcer, the nurse should conduct a comprehensive assessment of wound status (Seidel, 2006; WOCN, 2012). (See Chapter 3 for parameters to be included in wound assessment, and see Table 23-3 for clinical characteristics of neuropathic ulcers.)

Several wound classification systems have been developed to assist the clinician in classifying and synthesizing assessment data related to foot ulcers in the diabetic population. The systems provide a consistent approach and a common language among health professionals, present a clear picture of the neuropathic wound, direct and validate treatment decisions, and may promote appropriate reimbursement for care.

Wagner Classification System

The Wagner Classification System was originally developed as a treatment guideline, to provide direction for level of surgical intervention (Wagner, 1981; WOCN, 2012) (Box 23-4). It is now also used to objectively identify wounds for which treatment with hyperbaric oxygen therapy (HBOT) would be appropriate; for example, a Wagner Grade 3 diabetic foot ulcer qualifies for HBOT. Limitations of this system include limited focus on perfusion status and the presence/severity of neuropathy.

TABLE 23-3 Clinical Characteristics of Neuropathic Ulcers

Wound Feature	Description
Shape	Usually are rounded or oblong and found over bony prominence May initially be covered with callus tissue May resemble laceration, puncture, or blister, if from direct trauma, shearing, or heat
Wound base	May be necrotic, pink, or pale Depth varies from partial thickness to deep bone involvement
Wound edge	Typically well-defined and smooth edges May or may not have undermining
Periwound	Callus formation around the wound is common when the individual is walking/weight bearing on wound Continued development of callus after serial debridement may indicate inadequate off-loading of pressure Erythema and induration may indicate infection and/or cellulitis Maceration may be present
Exudate	Drainage is usually small to moderate in amount Large amounts of exudate may indicate complicating factors, including venous insufficiency, heart failure, renal failure or insufficiency, or infection Color is usually serous or clear Foul odor and purulence are common indicators of infection
Location	The majority of neuropathic/diabetic foot wounds are located at pressure points and bony deformities on the plantar surface of the forefoot Most common sites are the interphalangeal joint of the great toe and 1st and 5th metatarsal heads

From Falanga (2005), Pecoraro et al. (1990), Sage et al. (2001), Weir (2010), WOCN (2012), Zimny et al. (2004).

CLINICAL PEARL

Classification systems for foot ulcers in the diabetic population include the Wagner Classification System and the University of Texas Diabetic Foot Classification System.

BOX 23-4. Wagner Classification System

0: At-risk foot, preulcer, no open lesions, skin intact; may have deformities, callus, or cellulitis
1: Superficial ulcer with partial- or full-thickness tissue loss
2: Probing to ligament, tendon, or joint capsule with soft tissue infection
3: Deep ulcer with abscess, osteomyelitis, or joint sepsis
4: Gangrene localize to toes or forefoot
5: Ulcer with gangrene involving entire foot, beyond salvage

University of Texas Diabetic Foot Classification System

The University of Texas Diabetic Foot Classification System (Box 23-5) classifies the wound by grade and by stage; grade captures the depth of the wound and staging captures complications affecting healing, specifically infection and ischemia (Lavery et al., 1996; WOCN, 2012). The classification system has been validated through a retrospective analysis of 360 diabetic patients in an outpatient diabetic foot clinic; the validation study demonstrated that wound outcomes deteriorated as the grade and stage of wounds increased. In addition, healing time has been shown to correlate positively with grade of ulcer ($P > 0.05$); there is a direct relationship between higher stage and greater time to healing and increased risk of amputation (Lavery et al., 1996). Thus, one advantage of this system is its predictive value.

Management of Neuropathic Ulcers

Wound management for neuropathic foot wounds includes a focus on basic wound bed preparation tenets as well as management of systemic conditions affecting wound healing (tight glycemic control) and correction of neuropathic wound etiology, which is chiefly related to off-loading, that is, relief of repetitive pressure and shear stress.

BOX 23-5. University of Texas Diabetic Foot Classification System

Grading
0: Pre- or postulcer with epithelization
1: Superficial wound not involving tendon, bone, or capsule
2: Ulcer penetrates to tendon or capsule.
3: Ulcer penetrates to bone or joint.

Staging
A: Neuropathic wound: noninfected/nonischemic
B: Acute Charcot joint: infection present
C: Infected diabetic foot with ischemia
D: Ischemic limb with infection

CLINICAL PEARL

Management of neuropathic wounds must include attention to relief of repetitive pressure and shear (off-loading), tight glycemic control, and basic wound bed preparation tenets.

Wound Bed Preparation

Wound bed preparation is the process of identifying common impediments to healing chronic wounds and implementing corrective management strategies to promote closure. The process is orderly and based upon well-demonstrated scientific evidence, using the TIME Model (Tissue integrity, Inflammation/Infection, Moisture balance, Edge progression). These principles have been addressed in detail in Chapter 7; thus, this discussion will be limited to considerations and interventions of particular significance in management of the individual with diabetes and/or a neuropathic ulcer (Falanga, 2005; Schultz et al., 2003; Weir, 2010; WOCN, 2012).

Tissue Integrity

Necrotic tissue is a known risk factor for wound infection and for delayed healing; thus, prompt and complete debridement of all necrotic debris, both visible and nonvisible, is essential to the establishment of a clean wound bed that supports repair. There are multiple approaches to wound debridement, including surgical, CSWD (conservative sharp wound debridement), enzymatic, autolytic, mechanical, and biologic. Surgical debridement is typically recommended for management of neuropathic foot ulcers, as this approach has been shown in limited studies to reduce the risk of infection and promote healing (Steed et al., 1996). If the patient is not initially a candidate for surgical debridement, the nurse should initiate noninstrumental debridement with products that eliminate necrotic tissue while also controlling bacterial loads. (See Chapter 9 for in-depth discussion of debridement options.)

CLINICAL PEARL

Surgical debridement is typically recommended for the management of neuropathic foot ulcers, as this approach has been shown in limited studies to reduce the risk of infection and promote healing.

Periwound callus is a common complication of plantar surface neuropathic wounds and is indicative of continued repetitive pressure and shear (i.e., weight bearing) on the neuropathic wound. In addition, callus actually increases soft tissue trauma from pressure and shear if the patient continues to walk, and calloused wound edges prevent epithelial resurfacing. Thus, callus should be routinely removed by means of paring. It is essential to provide adequate off-loading following removal of periwound callus (WOCN, 2012).

Inflammation and Infection

High bacterial counts and/or prolonged inflammation leads to high levels of inflammatory cytokines and protease activity and decreased growth factor activity, all of which impair wound healing. Removal of infected debris and use of topical antimicrobials and systemic antibiotics are frequently required to reverse inflammation, balance wound bacterial loads, reduce cytokine and protease activity, and restore wound healing potential. Tight glycemic control is also essential, since hyperglycemia interferes with normal white blood cell function.

Moisture Balance

Moisture balance is essential to promote granulation tissue formation and epithelial migration across the wound surface. Excessive wound moisture creates edematous hypergranulation tissue and macerates wound edges, which delays wound healing. Inadequate wound moisture, desiccation, removes the fluids that support wound healing and cell migration and causes cell death. Thus, effective wound management must include exudate management and maintenance of a moist wound surface.

Epithelial Edge Advancement

An open epithelial wound edge is essential for keratinocyte migration, epithelial resurfacing, and wound closure. Effective healing requires the reestablishment of an intact epithelium and restoration of skin function. Wounds with extensive undermining of the wound edge may require surgical debridement, and surface wounds that fail to epithelialize may require skin grafts or skin substitutes (Falanga, 2005; Schultz et al., 2003; Weir, 2010; WOCN, 2012).

Neuropathic Foot and Wound Off-Loading

Routine activities, such as walking, can result in repetitive stress and pressure over bony prominences, especially when there are foot deformities and limitations in joint mobility that result in altered gait and abnormal weight bearing. This repetitive stress is a significant component in the pathway to ulcerations in the neuropathic foot. Once an ulcer develops, the continued exposure to pressure and shear prevents healing and contributes to wound deterioration, sometimes to bone. Effective off-loading is a key component of a comprehensive prevention program and an essential element of a comprehensive neuropathic wound management plan (Caselli et al., 2002; WOCN, 2012).

CLINICAL PEARL

Routine activities, such as walking, can result in repetitive stress and pressure over bony prominences, especially in patients with altered gait and abnormal weight bearing. Once an ulcer develops, continued exposure to pressure and shear prevents healing and contributes to deterioration.

Off-loading is defined as the removal of focal pressure from a specific foot site/area and subsequent redistribution of that pressure over the larger foot surface. The practice of off-loading is discussed widely in medical literature as a key intervention utilized throughout all phases of neuropathic/diabetic foot and wound management. Effective off-loading is not typically accomplished with use of "off-the-shelf"/self-selected shoes or therapeutic/diabetic shoes. In contrast, inexpensive "Med-Surg shoes" *do* optimize off-loading and promote wound healing; these shoes are designed to permit customization and accommodation of the patient's foot wound, by simple means, and for any site (from toes to heel and either dorsal or plantar surface). A readily available, reasonably priced, off-the-shelf "Med-Surg" shoe system with excellent pressure mapping data is made and distributed by Darco International. The Darco system for providing customized pressure relief involves the following steps: a transparent film dressing is placed over the wound and the wound site is marked with lipstick; the patient is then asked to step onto the insole, which transfers the marked site onto the insole; the clinician then removes pegs from the insole in the marked area to create "off-loading" of the wound site during weight bearing. Additional accommodative shoe options are available for forefoot ulcers (Ortho wedge); forefoot, midfoot, and some Charcot foot ulcers (Darco wound healing shoe); and heel ulcers (Heel wedge) (Birke et al., 2000, 2002; WOCN, 2012). All of these options have simple customization procedures and simple instructions (Figs. 23-14 and 23-15).

CLINICAL PEARL

Off-loading is defined as the removal of focal pressure from a specific foot site/area and subsequent redistribution of that pressure over the larger foot surface.

Off-Loading and Soft Tissue Management

Off-loading provides for tissue load management of the foot, just as a support surface provides for effective tissue load management across the resting surface of the body. The goal of tissue load management is to maintain soft tissue viability, support the bony architecture, and promote wound healing by protecting the affected site(s) against pressure and shear. Off-loading devices used for *prevention* are designed to eliminate peak pressures by providing *even pressure distribution*, thus reducing the risk of ulceration; off-loading devices used for *treatment* are designed to *totally eliminate shear and pressure* in the affected area to optimize healing.

CLINICAL PEARL

Products that provide *even distribution of plantar surface pressures* (such as customized insoles) can be used for *prevention* of neuropathic ulcers; in contrast, *treatment* of plantar surface ulcers requires use of products that completely *off-load* the ulcerated area (such as a total contact cast).

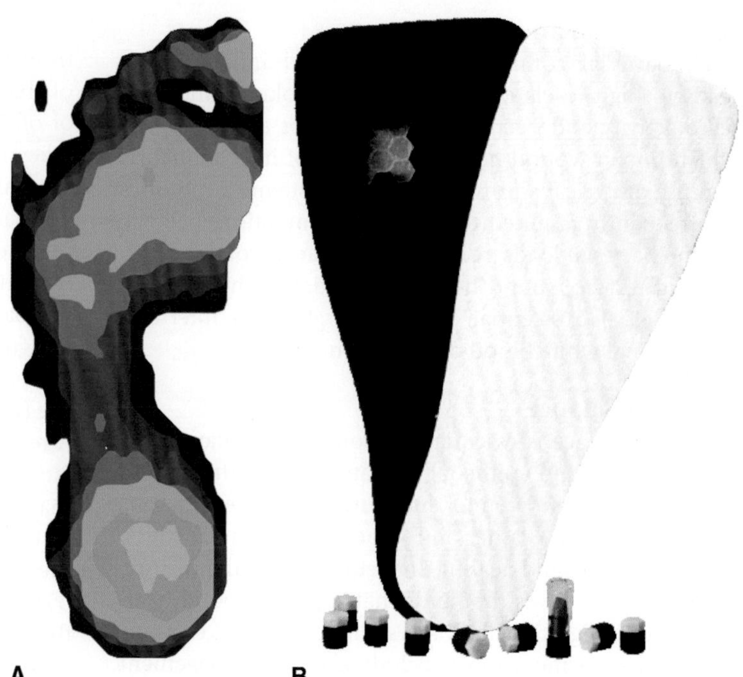

FIGURE 23-14. Pressure mapping with DARCO Med–Surg shoe with Peg-Assist insole. **A.** Pressure mapping. **B.** Pegs can be removed in areas of high pressure or ulceration to provide offloading. (Courtesy Darco International. http://www.darcointernational.com).

A B

Effective off-loading requires a basic understanding of plantar surface biomechanics and the complex nature of foot-to-ground interactions. The two mechanical forces that contribute most significantly to neuropathic ulcerations are pressure and shear. Peak plantar pressures are highest in the forefoot and midfoot, compared with the rear or hindfoot; when the metatarsal heads are abnormally prominent, the forefoot pressures are further increased. Charcot foot deformity also causes a marked increase in plantar surface pressures, most commonly in mid- and forefoot pressures. Shear forces are affected by friction exerted against the plantar foot surface during walking and by gait velocity and muscle strength. Studies are ongoing in regard to the relative roles played by pressure and shear, with the goal of developing a clinical model that can be used to develop footwear that provides better protection against plantar surface ulceration (Yavuz et al., 2007, 2008; WOCN, 2012).

Gait abnormalities are common among individuals with neuropathy, and these abnormalities play a major role in development of plantar surface ulcers. For example, patients frequently exhibit a conservative gait strategy characterized by slower walking speed and wider gait base, which results in prolonged foot support (increased pressure) and increased shearing of plantar soft tissue during walking. In addition, glycosylation of soft tissues associated with hyperglycemia causes shortening of the plantar surface tendons; this causes reduced flexibility of ankle, subtalar, and first metatarsophalangeal joints, which has been shown to result in high focal plantar surface pressures and increased risk of ulceration. Finally, motor neuropathy can cause loss of anterior tibialis muscle strength and tone, which results in foot drop and further derangement in gait and pressure distribution. Fortunately, assistive devices such as ankle foot orthotics (AFOs) and braces can provide at least partial correction of foot drop and resultant gait abnormalities. Physical therapists should be routinely consulted for evaluation and management of gait abnormalities. In addition, all prefabricated off-loading devices must be carefully assessed to assure effective accommodation for the size and shape of the patient's foot, even pressure distribution, and, ideally, reduction in shear force (Birke et al., 2000, 2002; WOCN, 2012).

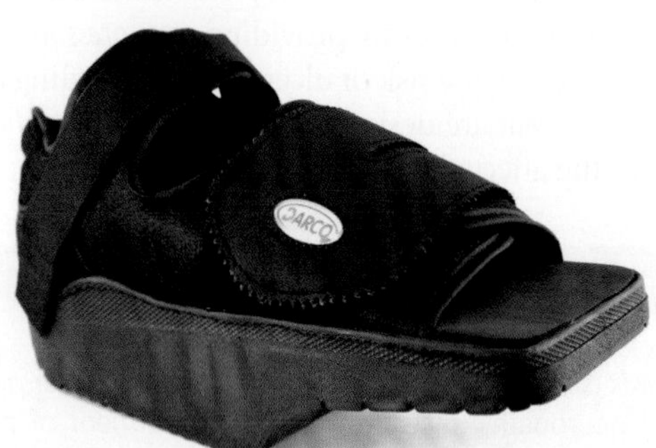

FIGURE 23-15. DARCO Ortho Wedge. (Courtesy Darco International. http://www.darcointernational.com)

Off-Loading Modalities for Treatment of Neuropathic Ulcers

Total Contact Casting (TCC) is considered the "gold standard" for off-loading neuropathic foot wounds. Studies of the TCC have demonstrated healing rates as high as 95% at 12 weeks (Lewis & Lipp, 2013). A TCC is minimally padded and molded carefully to the shape of the foot; a rocker bottom walking plate is then attached to allow limited ambulation while completely off-loading the forefoot

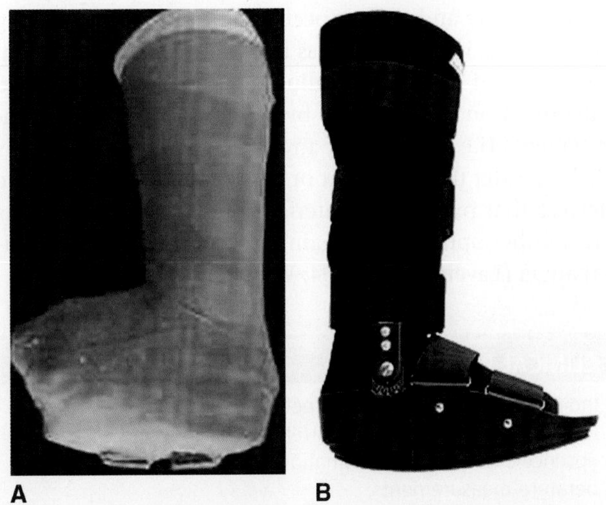

FIGURE 23-16. **A.** Total contact cast. **B.** Removable cast walker.

until the ulcer heals (Fig. 23-16). The TCC is closed at the distal foot (toes) to provide protection; it is initially changed every 5 to 7 days, but once the ulcer stabilizes and the exudate and edema are controlled, it can be changed every 1 to 2 weeks.

CLINICAL PEARL

Total contact casting (TCC) is considered the "gold standard" for off-loading neuropathic foot wounds and is associated with healing rates as high as 95% at 12 weeks.

TCCs have fixed ankle support and a rigid rocker sole (typically); this prevents forward motion of the tibia during midstance, limits forward propulsion during stepping, and redistributes some of the pressure/shear forces to the device itself. The rocker bottom sole prevents focal pressure during stepping and allows the foot to glide through the stepping phases, totally protecting the forefoot. Ankle high TCCs are not recommended as they do not provide enough casting material and support to transfer pressure and shear forces to the cast. Not all patients with diabetes and foot ulcers are good candidates for TCC; contraindications include documented LEAD, active wound infection or a sinus tract with deep extension into the foot that requires daily access for wound care, unstable gait, fluctuating edema, or active skin disease, restless leg syndrome, cast claustrophobia or known nonadherence to treatment plan, and lack of adequately trained staff to apply the TCC (Armstrong et al., 2005; Lewis & Lipp, 2013; WOCN, 2012).

Safe and effective application of a TCC requires a skilled provider; inappropriate application creates the risk of additional ulcers that are unrecognized until the cast is changed (due to sensory neuropathy). Newer products are being developed that provide for simplified application (e.g., Total Contact Cast EZ; Derma Sciences). Another approach is to place the patient in a removable cast walker (RCW) and then to wrap the RCW with cast material to render it nonremovable; this is known as instant total contact cast (iTCC). Some clinicians use the iTCC until the wound is 50% healed and then omit the cast wrapping, converting the device back to an RCW. If healing stalls (likely due to incomplete adherence to off-loading), the clinician can reinstitute the iTCC. Limitations of the iTCC and RCW involve the application of a prefabricated, fixed device to feet that may be misshapen and are typically insensate. Great care must be taken to ensure that the fixed device will accommodate the size and shape of the patient's foot and will not cause pressure injury in the absence of the patient's pain warning system (Armstrong et al., 2005; Nabuurs-Franssen et al., 2005; WOCN, 2012).

The TCC and other nonremovable devices are associated with the highest healing rates because they eliminate the problem of patient nonadherence often encountered when using a removable device. Modification of a standard RCW to increase patient adherence to off-loading (iTCC) may increase both the proportion of ulcers that heal and the rate of healing for diabetic neuropathic wounds. However, the care team must ensure that the fixed RCW is appropriately sized and fitted. Otherwise, device-related injury can occur to the foot that may be undetected due to the sensory deficit (Armstrong et al., 2005; Nabuurs-Franssen et al., 2005; WOCN, 2012).

CLINICAL PEARL

The TCC and other nonremovable devices are associated with the highest healing rates because they eliminate the problem of patient nonadherence often encountered with removable devices.

There are a variety of off-loading options that are referenced in the medical literature; however, none provide the same rate and degree of healing as the nonremovable TCC and iTCC (Armstrong et al., 2005). In clinical situations when TCC or iTCC is not available, or when the wound and neuropathic issues (e.g., deformity, gait issues) are minimal, other off-loading options may be feasible. For example, as already explained, selected systems are commercially available that are relatively inexpensive and that allow for customization, that is, elimination of pressure at the specific wound sites (e.g., Darco Peg Assist System). Another option is to use accommodative dressings, such as adhesive felt pads and crest pads, in combination with off-loading shoes (Birke et al., 2002; Katz et al., 2005; WOCN, 2012).

One simple and inexpensive approach to off-loading that can be used for patients who are not candidates for the TCC, RCW, or iTCC involves use of adhesive felt pads. The adhesive felt is cut to the shape of the foot with a cut out that accommodates the wound site; the felt is then applied directly to the skin surface and secured with a conformable gauze dressing. The patient is then placed in a "Med-Surg" shoe that accommodates the dressing. The pad remains on the foot and is changed at least weekly by the clinician. This approach has demonstrated excellent off-loading of plantar surface wounds located over the metatarsal heads (Fig. 23-17).

Devices such as "crest pads" can be used to reduce pressure on the distal toes for patients with claw toes. These devices are made of rolled gauze covered with moleskin, with a cutout in the moleskin for toe placement (Beuker et al., 2005; Birke et al., 2002; WOCN, 2012). See Fig. 23-18, which illustrates the crest pad procedure. See **Table 23-4** for off-loading options.

Assessment of Effective Off-Loading

The wound nurse managing the patient with a neuropathic ulcer must continually evaluate the effectiveness of the management plan, and this includes evaluation of the ability of the off-loading device to sufficiently protect the ulcer from pressure and shear. Specific indicators of off-loading effectiveness include progress in wound healing, minimal recurrence of periwound callus, and absence of localized inflammation as indicated by dermal temperature measurements (i.e., absence of any sites where temperature is >2°C greater than adjacent or contralateral sites). In-shoe devices that provide for interface pressure measurements are another option that is gaining recognition in the clinical arena (Lavery et al., 2004; WOCN, 2012).

CLINICAL PEARL

Indicators of off-loading effectiveness include progress in wound healing, minimal recurrence of periwound callus, and absence of localized inflammation as indicated by dermal temperature measurements.

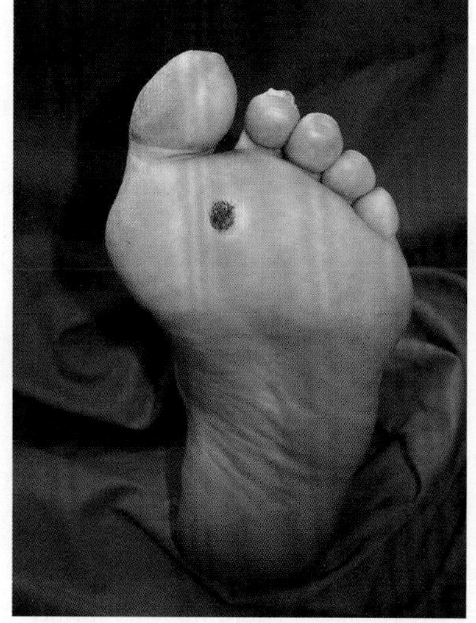

A

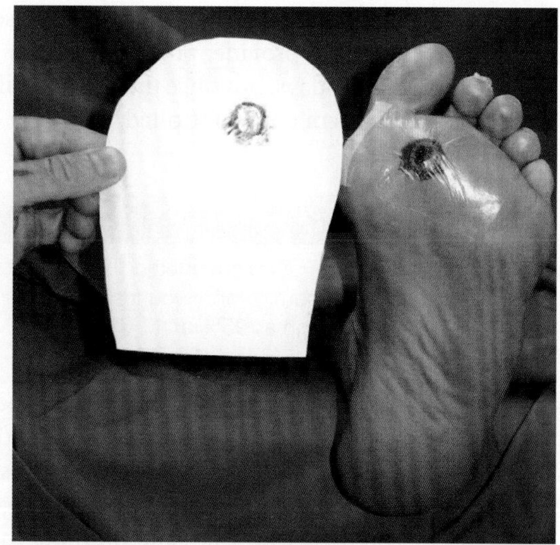

B

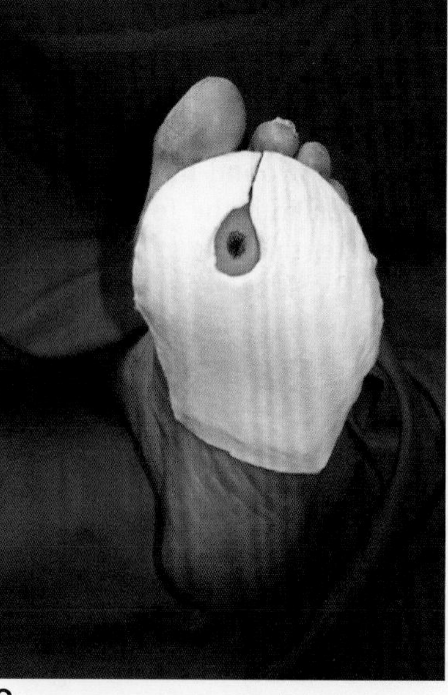

C

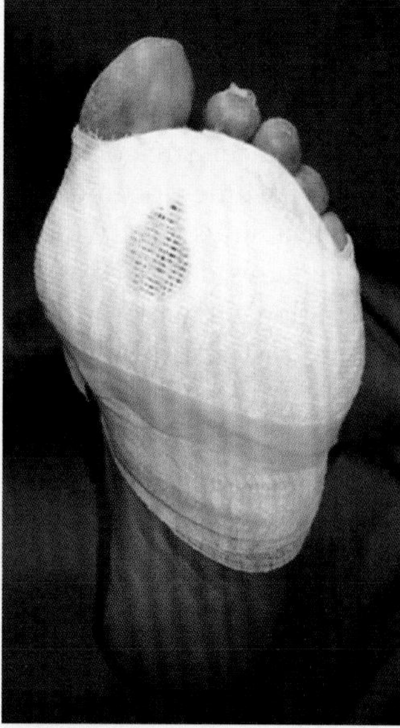

D

FIGURE 23-17. Steps of procedure for construction of off-loading adhesive felt pad. **A.** Individual with a second metatarsal head preulceration suitable for off-loading with an adhesive felt relief pad. **B.** The lesion is covered with a transparent dressing and the lesion is marked with lipstick. The mark is transferred to the back of the ¼ inch adhesive felt pad. **C.** Skin Prep is applied to the foot and the felt pad is cut out and attached insuring that the relief hole is directly over the lesion area. **D.** The pad is wrapped with a Kling gauze dressing and secured with tape. **E.** The foot with the relief pad is placed in an OrthoWedge shoe, and the patient is instructed in a heel weight-bearing gait.

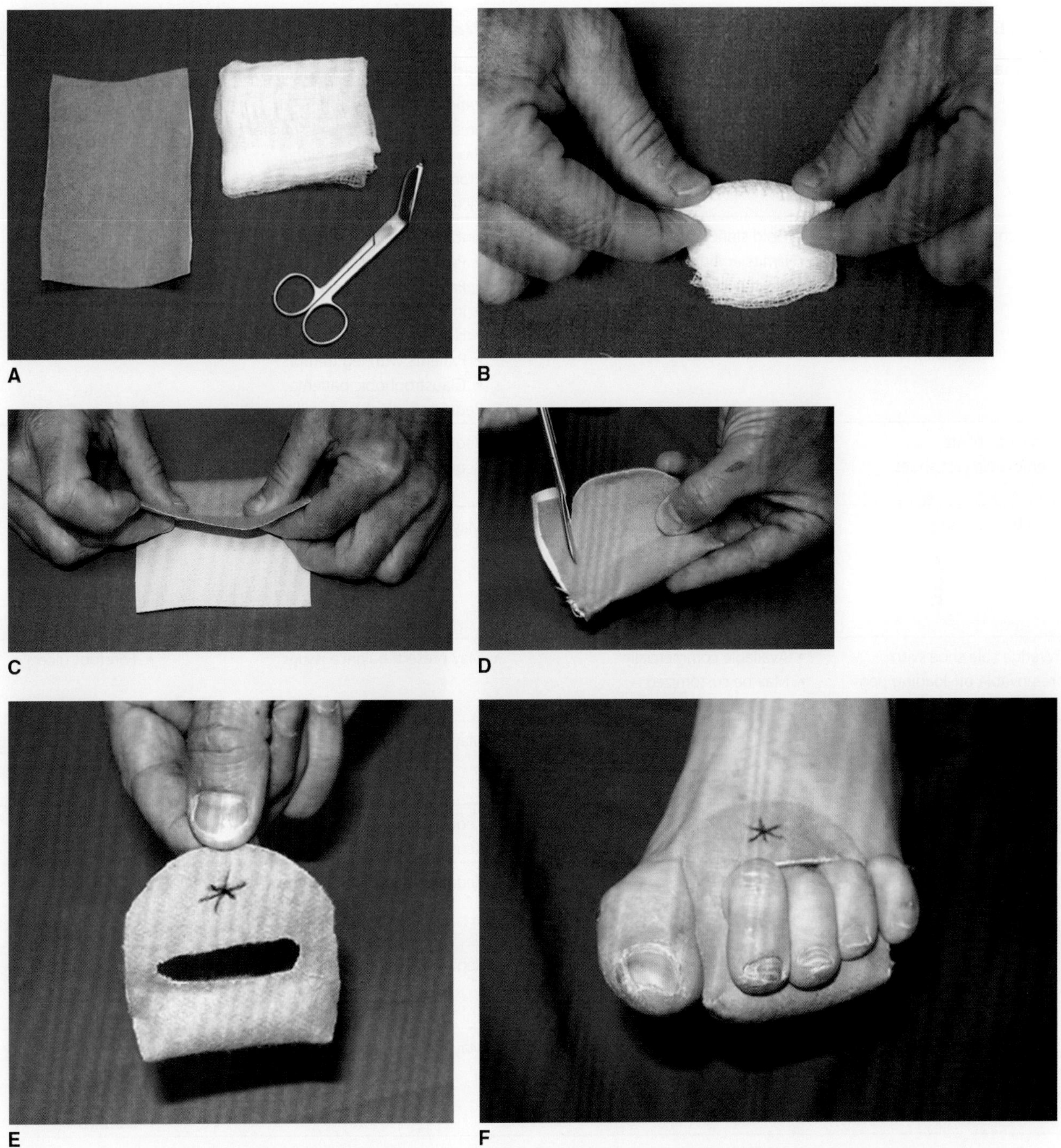

FIGURE 23-18. Crest pad construction for claw toe deformity. **A.** Materials used to fabricate a crest pad: moleskin, gauze, scissors. **B.** Cut three to four gauze sponges to size and roll tightly. **C.** Fold moleskin tightly over roll of gauze. **D.** Trim Moleskin as shown. **E.** Finished crest pad with hole cutout for toes. **F.** Crest pad fit to the patient with claw toe deformity and preulcerative callus over the second and third toes.

Off-Loading for Ulcer Prevention

There is limited literature addressing the efficacy of off-loading for prevention of wounds. A Cochrane Review of four off-loading for prevention randomized controlled trials (RCT) found that in-shoe orthotics are of benefit. Other pressure-relieving interventions such as running shoes are widely used but have not been adequately evaluated scientifically, and removable casts or foam inlays do not appear to have been evaluated at all in randomized controlled studies (Cavanagh & Bus, 2011; Spencer, 2000; Yavuz et al., 2008; WOCN, 2012). In identifying patients who may benefit from preventive off-loading, the wound

TABLE 23-4 Off-Loading Options for the Management of Wounds due to LEND

Off-loading Method	Advantages	Disadvantages	Wound Sites
Bedrest	• TOTAL non–weight bearing	• Patient adherence is difficult • Presents quality of life issues for patients • Promotes hyperglycemia • Promotes patient debilitation • Increases risk for posterior heel pressures	• All wound sites

Total contact cast	• Gold standard
	• Limits ambulation
	• Irremovable: forces patient compliance
		• Not advisable to use for:
		  • Patients with LEAD
		  • Patients with unstable gait
		  • Infected wounds
		  • Highly exudative wounds
		  • Patients with leg tremors
		  • Claustrophobic patients
		• Requires high clinical skill to apply
			• All wound sites

Walking splints Removable cast shoes	• Provides daily wound surveillance and care • Good option for infected wounds	• Requires strict patient adherence • Requires assistive ambulating device	• All wound sites
Football dressing	• Simple to make • Inexpensive • Ease of use with dressings • Irremovable: forces patient compliance	• May present balance issues	• Forefoot ulcers
Wedge sole shoe with removable off-loading pegs	• Available commercially • May be customized • Inexpensive	• May present balance issues	• Forefoot ulcers
Heel sole shoe with removable off-loading pegs	• Available commercially • May be customized • Inexpensive	• May present balance issues	• Plantar/posterior heel ulcers
Custom modified healing shoe with extradepth toe box	• Provides pressure relief specific to wound location	• Requires specialized equipment • Requires specialized skill to make	• All wound sites
Adhesive felt pad	• Simple to make • Inexpensive • Ease of use with dressings	• Requires at least weekly replacement	• Metatarsal head ulcers
Felted foam pads	• Simple to make • Inexpensive • Ease of use with dressings	• Requires every 3- to 4-day replacement	• Claw toes
Interdigital pads (silicone or foam), Lamb's wool padding	• Available commercially • May be used for wound prevention or during healing	• May increase forefoot width	• Crowded toes • Crossed toes • Interdigital wounds
Padded socks	• Available commercially	• May cause local foot ischemia and/or constriction if shoe fit does not allow for increased padding	• Bony deformities
Ball and ring shoe stretcher	• Available commercially • Simple to use • Provides pressure relief on leather shoes at specific sites of bony foot deformity	• Does not work with nonleather shoes	• Bony deformities

Adapted from information in Beuker et al. (2005), Birke et al. (2002), Bus et al. (2008), Cavanagh and Bus (2011), Frykberg et al. (2006), Steed et al. (2006).

nurse should be aware that risk factors for neuropathic ulceration include the following:

- Loss of protective sensation (LOPS) demonstrated by a 10-g monofilament exam
- Bony deformity of toes or foot (claw toes, prominent metatarsal heads, Charcot foot, etc.)
- Rigid interphalangeal and/or ankle joints
- Compromised arterial perfusion (ABI <0.9 or >1.3)
- Focal callus formation
- History of previous foot ulceration or amputation. Individuals who are unable to visualize the entire foot due to poor eyesight (e.g., due to diabetic retinopathy) or to limited hip/knee joint flexion that makes it difficult to bring the foot within the visual field are also at risk (NIH, 2014; WOCN, 2012)

CLINICAL PEARL

Individuals at risk for plantar surface ulcerations (those with LOPS, LEAD, bony deformities, or history of ulceration) require prevention; in-shoe orthotics are of proven benefit, and running shoes are widely used though they have not been scientifically evaluated.

Current recommendations for preventive off-loading in patients with an at-risk foot are as follows:

- Teaching patients to avoid walking barefoot or in stocking feet indoors or out of doors.
- Regular callus removal provided by a skilled health care professional.
- Therapeutic footwear, including a custom-molded insole in a shoe with adequate depth toe box (for individuals at significant risk of ulceration, such as those with foot deformities or history of ulceration); therapeutic footwear should be worn during both indoor and outdoor walking (Cavanagh & Bus, 2011).
- Some "off-the-shelf" athletic shoe designs are acceptable as a shoe option for patients who do not have severe foot deformities. A "Shoe List" that indicates shoes that can be obtained from local stores can be of great benefit to patients who would benefit from a properly designed "off-the-shelf" shoe. It is essential for nurses to investigate appropriate shoe options within their own communities so that patients have a reliable guide to shoes that are both appropriate and available. (See Fig. 23-19 for a sample "Shoe List.")

Commercially Available Shoes

Individuals with intact sensation and no deformities can wear commercially available shoes so long as they meet the following criteria for correct "fit":

1. Allow for ½ inch space beyond the longest toe.
2. Allow adequate width and depth to accommodate for toe spread and clearance.
3. Ensure adequate width at the ball of the foot.
4. Assure adequate fit from heel to ball of foot.
5. Assure that the shape of the shoe matches the shape of the foot.

When purchasing shoes, individuals should be counseled to adhere to the following guidelines:

- Size and purchase shoes in the afternoon to accommodate foot edema.
- Stand and walk when sizing and purchasing new shoes.
- Wear socks or stockings that would normally be worn with the shoes during sizing and fitting of new shoes.
- Measure both feet and size shoes to fit the larger foot.
- Gradually increase wear time for new shoes, that is, by 2-hour increments each day, with routine foot inspection following each wearing.

Therapeutic Footwear

All individuals with any degree of LOPS should have their footwear professionally fitted, because their sensory deficits preclude recognition of problems with the fit of their shoes. Appropriately fitting footwear is critical for indoor as well as outdoor use for all individuals, and especially those who lack normal protective sensation. Individuals with LOPS and foot deformities, callus, impaired perfusion, or history of ulceration or amputation require therapeutic, customized shoes that are sized correctly, effectively accommodate any deformities, and provide even pressure distribution. Therapeutic footwear is a benefit allowed by many insurers in the United States for individuals with diabetes who meet established criteria. At the time of this writing, this benefit does not apply to individuals with neuropathy caused by disease processes other than diabetes. Criteria that qualify patients for therapeutic footwear include the following:

1. Diabetes diagnosis
2. One or more of the following:
   - History of partial or complete foot amputation
   - History of previous foot ulceration
   - Current foot ulceration
   - Foot deformity
   - History of preulcerative callus formation
   - Documented neuropathy with evidence of callus formation
   - Poor or impaired circulation (CMS, 2011)

CLINICAL PEARL

Individuals with LOPS and foot deformities, callus, impaired perfusion, or history of ulceration or amputation require therapeutic customized footwear that accommodate any deformities and provide even distribution of plantar surface pressures.

Therapeutic footwear include the following features: (1) extradepth toe box; (2) constructed of leather or suede (preferably); (3) cushioned outer soles;

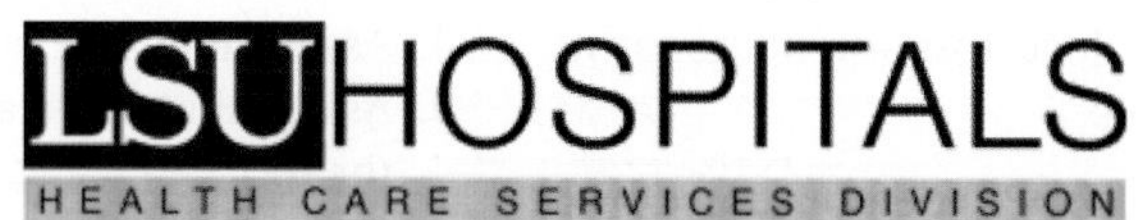

Approved Shoe List

Bring your shoes to your appointment and we will evaluate the fit before you wear them.

Men's Footwear

Maker	Model	Style	Sizes	Price	Vendor	Comments
Dr. Scholl's	"Stabilizer"	Walker	6 ½ - 13 Med/Wide	$25.00	Wal-mart	L,Wh,Bk,Lc
Athletic Works	"Jogger"	Walker Jogger	6 ½ - 14 Med/Wide	$10.00-$25.00	Wal-mart	NL, L, Wh, Bl, S, Lc, Vel
Volt	"Corey V"	Athletic	6 ½ - 14 Med/Wide	$15.00-$20.00	Wal-mart	L, Wh, Lc, *
Etonic	"Trans Am"	Walker	6 ½ - 15 D – 4E	$40.00+	Academy	L, Wh, Bk, Lc
New Balance	"571"	Walker	6 ½ - 15 D – 4E	$40.00+	Academy	L, Wh, Bk, Lc
Reebock	"DMX"	Walker	6 ½ - 15 D – 2E	$70.00+	Academy	L, Wh, Bk, Lc, *
SAS	"Time out"	Casual Dress	6 - 15 NN-WW	$110.00	SAS	L, Assorted colors, Lc, Vel
Sand & Sun	Water/shower footwear	Slip on stretch	5-12	$8.00	Wal-mart	Assorted colors

Women's Footwear

Maker	Model	Style	Sizes	Price	Vendor	Comments
Athletic Works	"Jogger"	Jogger	5 ½ - 10 Med/Wide	$10.00-$25.00	Wal-mart	NL, L, Wh, Bl, S, Lc, Vel
Etonic	"Trans"	Walker	5-10, B-D	$40.00+	Academy	L, Wh, Bk, Lc, Vel
New Balance	"571"	Walker	5-10, B-2E	$40.00+	Academy	L, Wh, Bk, Lc
Reebock	"DMX"	Walker	5-10, B-D	$70.00+	Academy	L, Wh, Bk, Lc, *
SAS	"Free Time"	Casual Dress	5-12 NN,-WW	$100.00	SAS	L, Assorted colors, Lc, Vel
Sand & Sun	Water/shower footwear	Slip on stretch	5-12	$8.00	Wal-mart	Assorted colors

Uppers: L –leather, NL- non-leather
Colors: Wh- white, Bk- black, S- silver, Br- brown, Bl- blue
Closure: Lc- laces, Vel- Velcro
Sole modifications: *- cannot be modified

LSU Diabetes Foot Program
Baton Rouge, LA

FIGURE 23-19. Sample "Shoe List."

(4) customizable insole cushioning that provides pressure redistribution/relief of pressure at common pressure points, in addition to shear reduction; and (5) option to customize as needed with rocker bottom soles or heel flares. Rocker bottom soles prevent focal pressure to plantar surface sites because they allow the foot to glide through the step without pressure at any point during stepping. Shoes with flared heels provide extra stability for people who strike the ground at midfoot or forefoot (WOCN, 2012).

Customizable insoles that provide even pressure redistribution and shear reduction are a critical feature of therapeutic footwear. As noted earlier, pressure mapping is being increasingly used by orthotists and pedorthists to identify high-pressure areas as a basis for insole customization. A recent study evaluated the ability of custom insoles designed to match the patient's foot and weightbearing patterns to reduce plantar surface pressures; 20 patients with 70 high-pressure areas were evaluated, and pressure was effectively reduced in 64/70 sites. The investigators concluded that use of pressure mapping to develop custom insoles provides for positive outcomes in the majority of cases (Owings et al., 2008).

Another study compared a shear-reducing insole with "standard therapy" (i.e., extradepth shoes with molded insoles designed to reduce vertical pressure) in the management of 299 diabetic patients with severe neuropathy or a history of previous ulcer or amputation; patients also received podiatrist evaluation, sensorimotor and vascular assessment, and diabetes education. The shear-reducing insole was constructed of two viscoelastic layers, with two intervening thin sheets of a low friction material; this design was shown to reduce peak shear force (but not vertical pressure) by 57%, as compared to three other multilayer viscoelastic insoles that did not have the intervening layers. Among those with a previous ulcer, there was a relative 90% reduction in ulcers (13/38 vs. 1/40). Thus, at least in patients with a history of a foot ulcer, reducing shear stress in addition to standard reduction of vertical forces resulted in 90% reduction in foot ulcer recurrence. No benefit was found in patients without a previous plantar foot ulcer (Lavery et al., 2005).

CLINICAL PEARL

Emerging evidence suggests that insoles designed to reduce shear force as well as pressure may be beneficial in reducing the incidence of recurrent ulceration in individuals who have a history of plantar surface ulcers.

Topical Wound Care

Topical therapy and dressing selection for management of neuropathic ulcers are based on the principles of moist wound healing, specifically exudate management, maintenance of a moist wound surface, and protection of the periwound skin; these principles and guidelines have been addressed in detail in Chapters 7 and 8. The discussion in this chapter will be limited to considerations and evidence unique to neuropathic ulcers.

Dressings

Dressings must be compatible with the off-loading devices in use; for example, patients being off-loaded with a TCC require dressings that are designed for weekly dressing changes. Dressings with lower moisture vapor transmission rates have been associated with faster healing than those with higher moisture vapor transmission rates; in a study involving 36 diabetic patients and 10 Hansen's disease patients, 80% healed in 10 weeks with consistent off-loading using a TCC and moisture retentive dressings (Bolton, 2007).

Advanced Wound Therapies

A variety of skin substitutes and dermal tissue replacements are available for use with diabetic foot wounds and have demonstrated accelerated wound healing when used in combination with adequate wound off-loading. These biologic dressings provide a matrix or scaffolding that promotes cell migration and cellular activities associated with wound healing. They also provide a variety of growth factors, stem cells, and other substances that promote healing and are typically missing in the chronic wound environment. Advanced biologic dressings are intended for use during the proliferative phase of repair and should not be used until the wound bed is completely clean and infection has been controlled.

Management Bacterial Loads

As noted throughout this text, heavy bacterial loads prolong the inflammatory phase and prevent the proliferative processes required for wound healing. Individuals with diabetes are at high risk for infectious complications, especially if their glucose levels are poorly controlled and/or they have coexisting ischemic disease. *Staphylococcus aureus* is the predominant pathogen in diabetic foot infections, but the microbiology of diabetic foot infections typically includes increased incidence of MDRO (multidrug-resistant organism) infections, such as MRSA, and MRSA has been associated with a higher rate of treatment failure. Predisposing factors to MDRO infections include prolonged duration of the wound (chronicity), previous hospitalizations, chronic kidney disease, and nasal colonization with MRSA. Foot wounds with ischemia or gangrene may have anaerobic pathogens. Thus, effective management of the patient with a neuropathic wound includes continual monitoring for indicators of wound infection and prompt and effective treatment of any infection that does occur, in order to reduce the risk of serious infections progressing to limb loss. There is no evidence to support the use of prophylactic antibiotic therapy.

CLINICAL PEARL

Effective management of the patient with a neuropathic wound includes continual monitoring for indicators of wound infection and prompt and effective management of any infection that does occur, in order to reduce the risk of serious infections progressing to limb loss.

As addressed in detail in Chapter 10, all open wounds are contaminated with bacteria, and simple contamination or colonization does not interfere with healing and does not require treatment. However, surface infection (critical colonization) and invasive infection (cellulitis) do require treatment and must be promptly recognized. The laboratory diagnosis of infection includes bacterial counts $>10^5$ CFU/g of tissue and/or the presence of beta hemolytic strep. However, the initial diagnosis of wound infection is typically made clinically. The classic signs of invasive infection include periwound erythema, induration, and pain, increased volumes of exudate, purulent drainage, foul odor, and possibly fever, tachycardia, and malaise. When there is involvement of the bone or joint or anaerobic infection of the soft tissues, there may be exposed bone, tunneling, abscess formation, tissue necrosis (gangrene), and/or crepitus.

CLINICAL PEARL

The initial diagnosis of wound infection is typically made clinically; the nurse must be aware that signs of infection may be subtle in the diabetic patient, especially if there is coexisting ischemia and sensory neuropathy.

The nurse must be aware that the signs of infection may be subtle in the diabetic patient, especially when there is coexisting ischemia and sensory neuropathy; thus, the nurse must be alert to mild erythema and limited induration with or without complaints of pain or tenderness. The nurse must also be aware that surface infection (critical colonization) manifests primarily as deterioration in the quality and quantity of granulation tissue, failure to progress, and indicators of persistent inflammation (such as persistent high-volume exudate).

Aggressive intervention is required for infections characterized by deep abscess, extensive bone or joint involvement, crepitus, substantial necrosis (gangrene), or necrotizing fasciitis. An infectious disease consult may be indicated, in addition to systemic antibiotic therapy (ideally culture based) and surgical debridement of all necrotic tissue. Severe infections will progress to necrosis without aggressive treatment, and wet necrosis requires intravenous antibacterials and surgical debridement. Wet necrosis in a foot complicated by ischemia also requires vascular reconstruction.

CLINICAL PEARL

Aggressive intervention (infectious disease consult and systemic antibiotic therapy) is indicated for deep abscesses, extensive bone or joint involvement, crepitus, substantial necrosis, or necrotizing fasciitis.

Systemic antibiotic therapy is an essential element of management for infection involving the periwound tissues, bones, or joints; in order to assure the use of the appropriate agent, a wound culture should be obtained prior to the initiation of antibiotic therapy whenever there is viable tissue exposed in the wound bed. Tissue obtained by biopsy, ulcer curettage, or aspiration is preferable to wound swab specimens and is considered the gold standard for confirming a diagnosis of infection in diabetic, neuropathic ulcers. (Transcutaneous bone biopsies are considered the most accurate approach to diagnosis of osteomyelitis.) While tissue culture is ideal, in many settings, this is not an option and the nurse must obtain a swab culture; in this case, the culture should be obtained using the Levine technique. This technique is described in detail in Chapter 10.

Surface infection can usually be managed with topical antimicrobial agents (antiseptics and/or antibiotics). However, in the patient with diabetes and increased risk of limb-threatening sepsis, systemic antibiotic therapy may be required in addition to topical agents to prevent progression to invasive infection. For example, topical mupirocin may be given short term (typically <2 weeks) in conjunction with systemic antibiotics. Use of topical antimicrobials should be based upon culture results as each has a defined bactericidal spectrum.

There is lack of consensus about the use of topical antimicrobial therapy in addition to systemic antibiotic therapy for infected neuropathic ulcers, especially those complicated by ischemia; however, topical agents may help to eradicate multidrug-resistant organisms and to promote healing and should generally be considered for at least a 2-week trial in wounds that are responding poorly to systemic agents alone. Topical treatments may also be helpful in the removal of biofilms, which have been implicated in persistent infections. However, there are no specific tests that have been standardized and approved by any official oversight agency for evaluating the efficacy of topical agents; thus, at this time, their use is based on anecdotal reports of benefit. In addition, topical antimicrobials can cause sensitivity reactions, so patients must be monitored closely for any adverse reaction. Another approach to delivery of antibiotics is local implantation of antibiotic beads and gels following surgical debridement of necrotic tissue; these agents have proven useful in promoting wound cleansing, limb salvage, and earlier surgical closure.

CLINICAL PEARL

A 2-week trial of adjuvant topical antimicrobial therapy should be considered for wounds responding poorly to systemic antibiotics alone.

See Chapter 10 for an in-depth discussion of assessment and management of both surface (localized) and invasive infection.

In summary, evaluation of the neuropathic foot with a wound should involve a thorough examination of the extremity for clinical signs of infection, along with laboratory and imaging studies. (See **Table 23-5** for laboratory and imaging indicators of infection.) In patients with foot ulcers and diabetes, laboratory markers may or may not be elevated in the presence of infection; normal lab results do not preclude infection. Invasive infection requires culture-based antibiotic therapy and prompt removal of any necrotic tissue; an infectious disease consult may be required and, when there is bone or joint involvement, an orthopedic consult may also be needed. Surface infection can usually be managed with topical antibacterial agents (WOCN, 2012).

TABLE 23-5 Laboratory and Radiologic Indicators of Infection

Imaging Study	Benefits	Comments
Useful imaging studies for diagnosing wound infection		
Plain x-rays	Can detect foot abnormalities such as osteomyelitis, fractures, Charcot foot, soft tissue gas, foreign bodies or structural foot deformity	The sensitivity of plain x-rays is variable and may be attributable to timing of the radiograph in relation to the chronicity of the ulcer
Magnetic resonance imaging (MRI)	Considered the gold standard in diagnosing osteomyelitis	Selective for soft tissue lesions with good sensitivity and specificity: sensitivity 90% and specificity 79%
Technetium-99 phosphate bone scan	Demonstrates moderate accuracy for diagnosis of infection in the toes and forefoot	
Indium-111 (leukocyte scan)	Demonstrates moderately good discrimination characteristics for diagnosing infection and has a low-to-moderate accuracy for osteomyelitis	Usually available in most facilities and at a lower cost than MRI/CT
Positron emission tomography (PET)	PET scans can demonstrate the difference between Charcot foot and florid osteomyelitis	Other more cost-effective options are available, such as plain x-rays

Osteomyelitis

Osteomyelitis is an infectious complication of particular importance in the management of diabetic foot ulcers because there are multiple bones in each foot and very little soft tissue; thus, surface infection can rapidly progress to deep soft tissue and bone infection. In addition, diabetes is associated with three comorbid conditions that increase the risk of bone infection: immunocompromise, neuropathy, and arterial disease. *Staphylococcus aureus* is the predominant pathogen, but *streptococcal* infections are also common, and either pathogen can result in necrotizing fasciitis. Osteomyelitis should be suspected with any tunneling wound and any wound with exposed bone and must be ruled out when there is evidence of Charcot osteoarthropathy. MRI has demonstrated the highest sensitivity and specificity for evaluating soft tissue and bone pathology in patients with diabetes and foot ulcers; granulocyte scanning is also utilized and is helpful in differentiating between osteoarthropathy and bone infection. When osteomyelitis is determined to be present, bone biopsy with culture is recognized as the gold standard for determining the specific pathogen and its sensitivities. Resection of necrotic bone and long-term systemic antibiotic therapy are required for treatment; limited evidence suggests that oral agents may be as effective as systemic antibiotics (WOCN, 2012).

CLINICAL PEARL

Osteomyelitis is a complication of particular significance in the management of diabetic ulcers; resection of necrotic bone and long-term systemic antibiotic therapy are required for treatment.

Adjunctive Therapies

Neuropathic ulcers that fail to heal with standard therapy may require the use of adjunctive therapies; in addition to biologic wound dressings (discussed earlier in this chapter), HBOT, negative pressure wound therapy (NPWT), monochromatic infrared energy, and electrical stimulation have been shown to be of potential benefit in the management of these wounds.

Hyperbaric Oxygen Therapy

HBOT has been shown to reduce the number of major amputations in people with diabetes and chronic foot ulcers. However, there is a need for high-quality RCT that objectively demonstrates the benefits of HBOT for this patient population, especially since HBOT is a costly therapy. See Chapter 11 for further discussion of HBOT.

Negative Pressure Wound Therapy

In a well-designed RCT comparing NPWT to advanced moist wound therapy (AMWT) in the treatment of 342 patients with diabetes and foot ulcers, there was a statistically significant improvement in healing rates among individuals receiving NPWT (43.2% complete closure for NPWT compared to 28.9% complete closure for AMWT, $P = 0.007$). In addition, NPWT was associated with significantly faster closure ($P = 0.001$). There was no significant difference between the groups in rates of infection, cellulitis, or osteomyelitis (Blume et al., 2008).

Ultrasound Therapy

Ennis et al. (2005) demonstrated in a double-blind, randomized, controlled, multicenter study that therapeutic ultrasound increased the rate of healing of recalcitrant diabetic foot ulcers. However, further study is needed before definitive recommendations can be made.

Monochromatic Infrared Energy (Nitric Oxide)

Nitric oxide is produced by monochromatic infrared energy therapy and has been shown to improve sensory perception, at least temporarily, in patients with diabetes. In a retrospective study of 2,239 diabetic patients with established neuropathy, MIRE was shown to reduce both LOPS and neuropathic pain; 93% demonstrated LOPS prior to treatment, as compared to 53% posttreatment, and neuropathic pain was reduced by 67% (Harkless et al., 2006). MIRE is also thought to potentially enhance wound healing due to the cellular effects of nitric oxide. Boykin (2010) suggests that inadequate levels of nitric oxide contribute to the impaired healing seen in many diabetic foot wounds, and preliminary studies indicate that nitric oxide (NOx) levels in wound fluid may predict wound healing. Further study is needed to determine the potential role of NOx and MIRE in diabetic wound management (Boykin, 2010).

Electrical Stimulation

In a small study, 10 patients with diabetes and 10 without diabetes, all with stages III and IV wounds, were treated with biphasic electrical stimulation for 30 minutes, three times per week for 4 weeks in a 32°C room. Blood flow increased in the diabetes group at the periphery of the wound, and the healing rate in the diabetes group over 4 weeks was 70%. The evidence suggested that the use of electrical stimulation in a warm room significantly increased healing and skin blood flow. However, more study is needed since this was a small study with no control arm. Studies have failed to demonstrate any benefit of electrical stimulation in the treatment of diabetic peripheral neuropathy (Lawson & Petrofsky, 2007; Petrofsky et al., 2007).

CLINICAL PEARL

Nonhealing neuropathic ulcers require advanced therapies; hyperbaric oxygen therapy, negative pressure wound therapy, monochromatic infrared energy, and electrical stimulation are of potential benefit.

 Surgical Intervention

Multiple surgical procedures have been developed to treat diabetic neuropathic and neuroischemic ulcers with varying levels of success. Goals of surgery are to achieve limb salvage, prevent ulceration/reulceration, and promote optimal functionality of the lower extremity. True randomized clinical trials comparing operative procedures and techniques are not available.

Procedures to Correct Structural Deformities

Surgical procedures of particular benefit in the management of the diabetic foot are those designed to correct deformities, thus eliminating high-pressure areas and reducing the risk of ulcer development (or promoting repair of existing ulcers). Tenotomy and exostectomy are the procedures most commonly performed; claw toe corrections and arthrodesis are less commonly performed. Tenotomy (also known as tendon release, tendon lengthening, and heel cord release) involves lengthening of the Achilles tendon, which reduces forefoot pressures in patients with limited dorsiflexion, and may promote healing of ulcers involving the metatarsal heads and toes. Exostectomy involves removal of bony deformities that cause pain, prevent functional shoe fitting, and contribute to ulceration of the soft tissue by increasing pressure and shear forces during walking. It is important to retain enough of the bone to maintain stability of the joint and to immobilize the foot with a cast for at least 6 to 8 weeks postoperatively (WOCN, 2012).

Arthrodesis (fusion) involves surgical reconstruction of Charcot foot. This procedure is recommended only when there is significant deformity or ulceration that prevents effective off-loading with orthotic devices and is performed in <25% of individuals with Charcot osteoarthropathy. The goals of surgery are to resect and smooth bony prominences, correct deformity, and achieve a stable and level foot that can be appropriately fitted with shoes and protected by accommodative footwear that supports ambulation. Because the bones are soft and fragmented, fusion of one or more joints is usually required. The chronic inflammation of the bone makes this a very difficult procedure with potential for multiple complications; however, with proper patient selection, 65% to 70% of patients heal with a stable foot. Ideally, surgery is delayed until any plantar surface ulcers have healed (Dalla Paola et al., 2007; Sayner & Rosenblum, 2005; Sohn et al., 2010; Wang, 2003; Zgonis et al., 2008). Positive outcomes may be further supported by the adjunctive use of an implantable bone growth stimulator (Hockenbury et al., 2007).

Nerve Decompression Procedures

Unrecognized nerve entrapment may coexist with peripheral neuropathy in diabetic patients with foot ulcers.

Surgical decompression of the nerves is hypothesized to reduce the incidence of ulcer recurrence. However, a Cochrane Review of RCTs related to decompressive surgery failed to identify a single RCT or any other well-designed prospective study that showed improvements in predefined end points after decompressive surgery. The results of this review suggest that the role of decompressive surgery for diabetic symmetric distal neuropathy is unproven and that further well-designed RCTs are warranted (Chaudhry et al., 2008).

CLINICAL PEARL

Surgical procedures of particular benefit in the management of the diabetic foot are those designed to correct deformities, thus eliminating high-pressure areas and reducing the risk of ulcer development.

Surgical Correction of LEAD

Adequate perfusion is obviously critical to wound healing, and the patient with advanced LEAD may require endovascular procedures or bypass to promote repair. However, it is essential to consider the risks versus short-term and long-term benefits. Short-term outcomes may be better in surgically treated patient, but these effects may not be sustained long term. Surgical options for revascularization include angioplasty with or without stent placement and bypass grafting. There is no evidence to support bypass over angioplasty or other treatments in terms of the effects on walking distance, disease progression, amputation rates, complications, or death. In addition, while there may be multiple occlusions involving the vessels supplying the foot, treating the most occluded vessel may improve blood flow sufficiently to promote ulcer healing. See Chapter 22 for more information about surgical treatment of LEAD.

Amputation

The subsequent natural history for the patient with a high-level amputation is poor: various studies have reported a 5-year mortality rate of 40% to 70%. This can be partly attributed to changes in the patient's lifestyle, which becomes more sedentary and restricted, adversely affecting overall health. However, there are situations in which amputation is essential, either to prevent spread of infection and salvage unaffected tissue or to provide for relief of ischemic pain and improved quality of life. When amputation is required, all efforts should be made to carry out the lowest-level amputation possible so that the patient can walk with or without a prosthesis. For example, partial foot amputation, if feasible, is preferable to below-the-knee amputation. The most commonly performed partial foot amputations are ray amputations, transmetatarsal amputation, and Syme's amputation (amputation of the foot through the articulation of the ankle with removal of the malleoli of the tibia and fibula). Ray amputation is performed when necrosis has spread through the base of the toes; transmetatarsal amputation is necessary when the forefoot is involved. Removal of the metatarsals alters weight bearing of the forefoot and increases the risk for development of ulcers under the remaining metatarsals; therefore, therapeutic footwear is particularly critical for these individuals. Fortunately, 90% of patients with partial foot amputations will be able to use a prosthesis and remain mobile, compared to 75% of those with below-the-knee amputations and only 25% of those requiring above-the-knee amputations (Caputo, 2008).

CLINICAL PEARL

90% of patients with partial foot amputations will be able to use a prosthesis, as compared to 75% of those with below-the-knee amputations and 25% of those with above-the-knee amputations.

Charcot Neuropathic Osteoarthropathy

Any condition that causes sensory and/or autonomic neuropathy can lead to a Charcot joint, also known as neuropathic osteoarthropathy. Today, this pathology is most commonly due to diabetes, but it can also be caused by syphilis, chronic alcoholism, Hansen's disease, spinal cord injury, renal failure and dialysis, and congenital insensitivity to pain (WOCN, 2012). Charcot foot deformity is caused by an insidious, noninfectious destruction of the bones and joints of the foot, which results in pathologic fractures, joint dislocations, and loss of normal foot structure. Predisposing factors include bone hyperemia, osteopenia, joint instability, and sensorimotor deficits. Charcot foot deformity increases the risk for plantar surface ulceration and also significantly increases the risk for amputation (Armstrong et al., 1997b; Nielson, & Armstrong, 2008; Sella, 2009; Verity et al., 2008).

CLINICAL PEARL

Risk factors for Charcot foot deformity include bone hyperemia, osteopenia, joint instability, and sensorimotor deficits.

Pathology

There are two main theories as to the pathology of Charcot foot deformity.

The first theory is labeled the neurotraumatic theory and suggests that sensory neuropathy leaves the individual unable to recognize traumatic injury and that recurrent unrelieved mechanical stress results in progressive destruction of the bones and joints of the foot. The second theory is the neurovascular theory, which states that autonomic neuropathy results in loss of sympathetic tone to the vessels, which in turn causes persistent dilatation of the vessels supplying the soft tissues and bony structures; the resulting hyperemia causes osteopenia, which leaves the bones much more susceptible to fracture and trauma from walking (Armstrong & Peters, 2002; Jude & Boulton, 2002; Nielson & Armstrong, 2008). In many cases, the damage is probably caused by some combination of unrecognized trauma and increased blood flow (see Fig. 23-6).

Clinical Presentation

Prevention of Charcot foot deformity requires prompt recognition of the initial injury and inflammation, which is manifest by the following: unilateral swelling, which may be significant; increased local skin temperature (3°C to 7°C) as compared to adjacent unaffected sites; erythema, bounding pulses; and possibly complaints of mild pain, which is disproportionate to the severity of the underlying injury. During this acute inflammatory stage, it is sometimes difficult to differentiate between fracture, cellulitis, and osteomyelitis, and laboratory studies commonly used to diagnose infection (e.g., WBC count, sedimentation rate) may also be misleading since they will rise in response to the acute inflammatory process. Plain radiographs (AP, lateral, and oblique views) do provide a definitive diagnosis once bony involvement has occurred. MRI provides definitive diagnosis of osteomyelitis, which is infection of the bone typically associated with a penetrating ulcer/wound (Armstrong & Peters, 2002; Nielson & Armstrong, 2008; Nube et al., 2002). Late stages of Charcot foot are manifest as significant foot deformity, which most commonly involves the forefoot (45%) or midfoot (35%). Specific changes include unusual bony prominences, unstable joints, collapse of the midfoot structures, and development of rocker bottom foot (Armstrong, & Peters, 2002; Nielson & Armstrong, 2008; Nube et al., 2002; Saunders & Mrdjencovich, 1991). See Figures 23-6 and 23-20.

CLINICAL PEARL

Prevention of Charcot foot deformity requires prompt recognition and appropriate management of any injury; appropriate management involves off-loading until inflammation subsides and bony healing has occurred.

Phases

Charcot foot development progresses through several phases, which include the acute inflammatory phase, the subacute coalescence phase, and the resolution (consolidation) phase (Table 23-6). The acute phase represents the phase immediately postinjury and is characterized by severe inflammation; the coalescence phase represents early healing and beginning formation of bone callus; and the consolidation phase represents final healing with stabilization and remodeling of the bone.

CLINICAL PEARL

Indicators of injury include increased local skin temperature (3°C to 7°C) as compared to adjacent unaffected sites; erythema, bounding pulses, and possibly complaints of mild pain, which is disproportionate to the severity of the underlying injury.

Impact

Sohn et al. (2010) performed a retrospective review of VA patients with Charcot arthropathy and/or a diabetic foot ulcer in 2002 and who were followed for 5 years thereafter. Among the patients with Charcot foot, 59% (538) were treated for foot ulcers during the 5-year period following development of Charcot foot; 66% (354) of those developed a foot ulcer immediately before or at the time of development of Charcot arthropathy, and the remaining

Pathology Charcot Foot

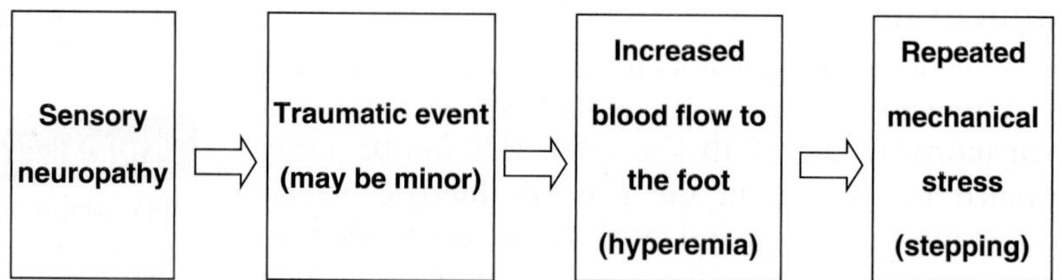

1. Loss of protective sensation (sensory neuropathy)
2. Traumatic event: May simply be a misstep (misplaced or awkward step) or twisting of the foot and/or the ankle causing inflammation
3. Increased blood flow (hyperemia) related to inflammatory response and arterio-venous shunting (autonomic neuropathy) from walking on an injured foot-causes demineralization of foot/ankle bones.
4. Repeated Mechanical Stress: Continued ambulation on injured foot (continued, repeated high pressures), which lead to collapse of supportive foot architecture.

FIGURE 23-20. Charcot foot development.

TABLE 23-6 Eichenholtz Classification of Charcot Foot Healing: Clinical Presentation and Phases

Clinical Presentation	Dissolution Phase	Coalescence Phase	Consolidation Phase
Edema	May be profound	Decreased	Decreased
Erythema	May be severe	Generally absent	Generally absent
Temperature (compare affected site to unaffected site with dermal thermometer)	May be 3°C–7°C increased	Generally >2°C increased	Generally <2°C increased
X-ray image	May demonstrate fractures, dislocations, and subluxations *May NOT show abnormality during the earliest, acute phase of injury*	May demonstrate early consolidation, formation of bone callus	Demonstrates bone consolidation, stability

Adapted from information in Eichenholtz (1966), McCrory et al. (1998).

34% developed the ulcer as a complication of Charcot deformity. Individuals with ulcers but no Charcot deformity were seven times more likely to require amputation than those who had Charcot deformity but no ulcers. Those over 65 years of age who had both an ulcer and Charcot deformity had 12 times higher risk of amputation than those with Charcot deformity only. The results of this study suggest that Charcot deformity, in and of itself, does not pose a serious amputation risk; it is the development of plantar surface ulceration that causes increased risk of amputation. Thus, prevention of ulceration is of paramount importance in the management of these individuals.

Management

Nonsurgical management during the acute phase of Charcot foot is focused on reducing inflammation through non–weight bearing, usually with a TCC or walking splint that is changed every 1 to 2 weeks. Non–weight bearing should be continued until the temperature of the affected foot is within 2°C of the temperature of the unaffected foot, and bone callus consolidation is visible on x-ray. Dermal thermometry assessment should be conducted with every office visit, and serial x-rays should be obtained monthly (Armstrong & Lavery, 1997; Jude & Boulton, 2002; McGill et al., 2000). If the patient is unable to adhere to total non–weight bearing, partial weight bearing with use of an assistive walker or crutches is acceptable in moderation. Surgery is never considered during the acute phase due to the impaired integrity of the bony tissue (Armstrong & Peters, 2002; Edmonds, 2006).

Once the acute inflammation has resolved, the cast can be removed, but the patient should wear a brace to protect the foot, for example, patellar tendon-bearing brace, accommodative footwear with a modified AFO, a Charcot restraint orthotic walker (CROW), or double metal upright AFO (Verity et al., 2008).

Long-term management must include lifelong protection and monitoring for the involved limb as well as optimal diabetes management. Specific measures include appropriately fitted footwear, as discussed earlier in this chapter; the patient with bony deformities should have custom shoes and orthoses fitted by a certified pedorthist (C-Ped). Management also includes professional foot care on a routine and "as-needed" basis and intensive patient education. Specifically, patients should be educated regarding the serious nature of Charcot deformity and increased risk for ulceration and eventual amputation, the importance of daily foot inspection and dermal temperature monitoring, and a PLAN for response to any evidence of foot inflammation: prompt reporting of problems to health care professional; limiting ambulation; change to healing shoe or customized walking splint; continued monitoring of dermal temperature; and access to diabetic foot clinic (Armstrong et al., 2007; Lavery et al., 2004; Jude & Boulton, 2002).

CLINICAL PEARL

Long-term management of the patient with Charcot osteoarthropathy includes protection and monitoring for the involved limb as well as optimal diabetes management.

Surgery is performed in fewer than 25% of patients with Charcot deformity (Armstrong & Peters, 2002; Edmonds, 2006).

Fungal Skin and Nail Infections

An infectious complication of particular significance to the diabetic population is fungal skin and nail infections. Skin infections are of particular concern, since they can result in blistering or fissures that permit bacterial entry, which can lead to lymphangitis or cellulitis. Clinical presentation, diagnosis, and management of fungal infections (Kelechi & Lukacs, 1997; Singal & Khanna, 2011) are discussed in detail in Chapter 27; instructions critical to the diabetic patient include the following:

- Dry feet well after bathing, especially between toes.
- Apply an antifungal powder or cream (e.g., miconazole 2% powder) to the feet daily until symptoms are gone.
- Utilize toe spacers to prevent interdigital crowding and maceration.

Nutritional Management

Basic principles of nutritional management for the patient with diabetes mellitus (i.e., control of serum glucose, hyperlipidemia, and hypertension) should be applied to the patient who has developed a neuropathic foot ulcer. Nutrition therapy should be individualized with consideration given to usual food and eating habits, metabolic profile, treatment goals, and desired outcomes. Nutritional assessment and management has been discussed in detail in Chapter 6; thus, this discussion will be limited to factors of particular importance to the diabetic patient.

Glycemic Control

Tight glycemic control is of critical importance, as hyperglycemia is known to adversely affect all phases of wound repair. The most recent ADA treatment guidelines (2014) state that HbA1c should be maintained at <7% in order to reduce the risk of microvascular complications and neuropathy. This level of glycemic control is also needed to support repair. This level of glycemic control requires consistent commitment from the patient; thus, the nurse must educate and counsel the patient, emphasize the importance of glycemic management, and discuss and agree on treatment goals. Goals should be set that are consistent with the patient's comorbid conditions, preferences, and ability to manage the treatment regime, and HbA1c goals must be individualized for each patient. For example, the ADA suggests less stringent goals for individuals with limited life expectancy, multiple comorbidities, and/or a history of severe hypoglycemia (American Diabetes Association [ADA], 2014).

CLINICAL PEARL

Nutritional management of the patient with diabetes and neuropathy includes tight glycemic control (HbA1c < 7.0%); in addition, there is increasing evidence that supplementation with alpha-lipoic acid (ALA) may slow progression or even partially reverse the symptoms of neuropathy.

Alpha-Lipoic Acid Supplementation

There is increasing evidence that supplementation with the micronutrient ALA may slow the progression of neuropathy or even partially reverse the symptoms of neuropathy. In an RCT comparing outcomes for 233 diabetic patients who received ALA once daily for 4 years to 227 diabetic patients who received placebo, the individuals receiving ALA showed clinical improvement and nonprogression of neuropathic symptoms, as measured by both the Neuropathy Impairment Score (NIS) ($P = 0.013$) and the Neuropathy Impairment Score—Lower Leg (NIS-LL) ($P = 0.025$). These results are consistent with the results of a meta-analysis of 4 RCTs involving 1,258 patients, in which 600-mg ALA per day (given IV) significantly reduced symptoms of neuropathy and improved neuropathic deficits (Ziegler et al., 2011). Similarly, the Symptomatic Diabetic Neuropathy 2 trial demonstrated significant improvement in neuropathic symptoms and deficits in 181 diabetic patients treated with variable dosages of ALA (as compared to those receiving placebo) (Casellini & Vinik, 2007). Finally, the Sidney 2 trial evaluated the results of variable dosages of ALA (600 mg vs. 1,200 mg vs. 1,800 mg daily) compared to placebo over 5 weeks and found significant reduction in neuropathic pain in all ALA groups; they also found a dose-dependent increase in side effects and concluded that 600 mg/day offers the best risk/benefit balance (Ziegler, 2006).

Other Micronutrient Supplements

One small study compared L-arginine (a precursor to endothelial-derived nitric oxide) to placebo and found no effect on endothelial dysfunction, $TcPO_2$ levels, or clinical indicators of neuropathy (Jude et al., 2010).

Thirteen randomized trials have addressed the potential benefits of vitamin B_1 (thiamine) on symptoms of diabetic or alcoholic neuropathy; however, the trials were small and the overall evidence suggests that vitamin B_1 is less effective than ALA, cilostazol, or cytidine triphosphate in providing short-term improvement in clinical outcomes and nerve conduction (Ang et al., 2008).

One study evaluated the potential benefits of vitamin B_{12} (cobalamin) supplementation in community-dwelling diabetic patients found to have B_{12} deficiency (as determined by methylmalonic acid [MMA] levels and cobalamin levels) and demonstrated improved MMA levels and reduced neuropathy in 88% of the subjects (Solomon, 2011).

Vitamin D deficiency, characterized as <30 ng/mL, is associated with self-reported peripheral neuropathy symptoms even after adjusting for demographic factors, obesity, comorbidities, use of medications for neuropathy, and diabetes duration and control. Soderstrom et al. (2011) studied results from the 2001 to 2004 National Health and Nutrition Examination Survey for adults over 40 years of age with diabetes and self-reported peripheral neuropathy and found that vitamin D deficiency was correlated with symptoms of peripheral neuropathy, including LOPS. This suggests that testing for vitamin D deficiency and providing supplementation when indicated may help prevent or improve neuropathy in some individuals (Soderstrom et al., 2011). In addition, diabetic patients with autonomic neuropathy frequently exhibit reduced bone quality; individuals who have additional fracture risks should receive aggressive treatment for osteoporosis (Okazaki, 2011).

Neuropathic Pain Management

Approximately 10% to 20% of the diabetic population suffer from disabling pain due to neuropathy. The pain can be severe, have a significant impact on quality of life and activities of daily living, and be difficult to treat particularly if complicated by a neuropathic wound. Depression, anxiety, sleep disturbances, and other adverse effects of neuropathic pain should be monitored, and appropriate referrals should be made to assure optimal management (Dworkin et al., 2007).

A variety of medications are available for the treatment of neuropathic pain in patients with LEND. Medications for the relief of specific sensory symptoms are recommended, as they improve the quality of life for the patient (**Table 23-7**).

TABLE 23-7 Suggested Pharmacological Interventions for the Treatment of Neuropathic Pain in Patients with LEND

Pain Description	Medication	Comments
Dysesthesia described as a "burning sensation," "sunburn-like," or "skin tingles;" allodynia	Capsaicin cream (Topical)	Dose: 0.025% and 0.075% topically applied very sparingly 3–4×/d, in mapped areas (indicating sites of greatest neuropathic pain) May provide pain relief in those who fail to respond to other therapies. Skin irritation may lead to nonadherence. Systemic effects are rare
	Gabapentin (oral) (Neurontin)	Dose: High dosing of 1,200 to 3,600 mg in divided doses over 24 h may be necessary. Low doses may not be effective Provides high-level pain relief in 1/3 of those with painful neuropathic pain Adverse advents include dizziness, somnolence, edema, and gait disturbance
	Pregabalin (oral) (Lyrica)	Pregabalin dose: 100 mg 3× daily. Increase gradually to maximum of 600 mg daily. Demonstrated effectiveness in patients with painful diabetic neuropathy. Individual, personalized treatment is needed to maximize pain relief and minimize adverse events.
	Selective serotonin reuptake inhibitors (SSRIs): fluoxetine, paroxetine (oral)	Dose: 20 to 40 mg/d; increase and taper doses gradually SSRIs may be better tolerated by patients but limited evidence for relief in neuropathic pain, and more high-quality studies are required
	Serotonin and noradrenergic reuptake inhibitors (SSNaRI): Duloxetine (Cymbalta) Venlafaxine (oral)	Duloxetine, (Cymbalta) (oral) Dose: 60–120 mg/d; increase and taper doses gradually Six trials ($N = 2,220$) demonstrated effects of duloxetine on diabetic neuropathic pain with 50% pain improvement at 12 weeks at a dose of 60 and 120 mg daily. Minor side effects are common at therapeutic doses. Serious side effects are rare. Direct comparisons of duloxetine to other drugs shown to be effective in neuropathic pain are needed 58 patients received duloxetine and amitriptyline in a randomized, double-blind crossover, active-control trial. Significant improvement in pain was achieved with both treatments compared to baseline values ($P < 0.001$ for both) Venlafaxine dose: 75–150 mg/d Evidence supports similar effectiveness to tricyclic antidepressants
Paresthesia described as "pins and needles," "electric-like," "numb aching feet," or "as if my feet have been in ice water," "knife-like," shooting pains, or lancinating pains	Tricyclic antidepressants: imipramine, amitriptyline (oral)	Dose: 50 mg qhs; may be increased to 150 mg by mouth, with lower dosing for elderly Tricyclic antidepressants are effective for moderate pain relief in neuropathic pain, except HIV neuropathy Antidepressants, including tricyclics, duloxetine, and venlafaxine, should be considered for the treatment of patients with painful DPN
	Analgesics (opioids) Tramadol (Ultram) (oral)	Tramadol dose: 100–400 mg q6h Tramadol is an effective symptomatic treatment for peripheral neuropathic pain, particularly for paresthesia, allodynia, and touch-evoked pain.
	Opioids	Short-term studies provided mixed results in effectiveness of opioids for neuropathic pain Intermediate-term studies demonstrate that opioids are effective for any etiology of neuropathic pain over placebo. Further randomized controlled trials are needed to establish long-term efficacy, safety, and effects on quality of life Opiate analgesia in combination with gabapentin should be considered for the treatment of patients with painful DPN, which cannot be controlled with monotherapy.
Other pharmacological interventions	Analgesics (systemic administration of local anesthetic agents: intravenous lidocaine, mexiletine, lidocaine plus mexiletine, mexiletine, tocainide, and flecainide) (oral analogs)	32 RCTs demonstrated parenteral lidocaine and its oral analogs (i.e., mexiletine, tocainide, flecainide) were safe and superior to placebo in decreasing the intensity of neuropathic pain. Limited data showed there were no differences in efficacy or adverse effects of lidocaine or its analogs compared to carbamazepine, amantadine, gabapentin, or morphine
	Lidoderm patch (topical)	A Lidoderm patch (lidocaine 5%) can reduce the intensity of common neuropathic pain. The patch is applied topically to the wound site or affected neuropathic area for 12 h. The patch should be left off for 12 h before reapplying to reduce risk of toxicity

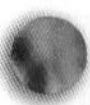

Exercise Programs and Health Promotion

Patients should be encouraged to participate in regular exercise programs, with modifications to accommodate any comorbidities and ulcerations. Specifically, patients should be instructed to obtain medical advice and clearance before beginning any routine exercise; this is particularly important for individuals who exhibit resting tachycardia and/or lack of heart rate variability during deep breathing or exercise, since these findings may be indicative of autonomic neuropathy and high risk of coronary artery disease. Individuals with neuropathic ulcers should be instructed to avoid weight-bearing exercises and to focus instead on non–weight-bearing exercises such as swimming, water aerobics, bicycling, rowing, chair, and upper body exercises. Individuals with neuropathy but no active ulcers may pursue weight-bearing exercises with medical clearance, but must be educated to wear well-fitting shoes and socks (WOCN, 2012).

The overall goal of management for any individual is improved overall health status. For the person with diabetes, this is particularly critical. Key elements of health maintenance include management of modifiable risk factors: smoking cessation, weight loss, blood pressure control, and limited intake of alcohol.

CLINICAL PEARL

Key elements of health maintenance for the individual with diabetes include smoking cessation, weight loss, blood pressure control, and limited intake of alcohol.

As noted earlier, appropriate goals for glucose control should be established based on the individual's comorbidities, life expectancy, and self-care goals, and appropriate education and counseling should be provided to assist the individual in meeting those goals. Similarly, the individual who is considering smoking cessation, weight loss, or other lifestyle modifications should be provided with education, support, and referrals as indicated. Vitamin B_{12} levels should be monitored on a routine basis with supplementation as indicated. All individuals should be provided with intensive and specific education regarding preventive foot care and the critical importance of daily foot inspection and skin temperature monitoring. Individuals who smoke, have LOPS and foot deformities, or have a history of ulceration or other lower extremity complications should be referred to foot specialists for ongoing preventive care and lifelong surveillance.

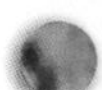

Prevention Recurrent Ulceration

Primary and secondary prevention are key areas of focus for the wound care nurse. An analysis of the cost-effectiveness of foot care based on published guidelines found that preventive care can improve survival, reduce ulceration and amputation rates, is cost-effective, and can even save on long-term costs when compared with standard care.

As is true of pressure ulcer prevention programs, neuropathic ulcer prevention begins with identification of "at-risk" individuals; major risk factors for neuropathic ulceration include loss of protective sensation (LOPS), lower extremity arterial disease (LEAD), a history of previous ulceration or amputation, gait abnormalities and high plantar surface pressures, rigid foot deformities, poor glycemic control (as evidenced by HbA1c > 9%), longstanding diabetes (>10 years), diabetic nephropathy (especially individuals on dialysis), smoking, and visual disturbances (Lavery et al., 1998).

The wound care nurse can then use the individual's risk profile to develop an individualized program for preventive foot care and surveillance based on their risk level (Table 23-2). For example, as noted earlier, patients who smoke, have LOPS and structural abnormalities, or have a history of lower extremity complications should be referred to foot care specialists for ongoing preventive care and lifelong surveillance. A multidisciplinary approach is recommended for optimal management of these high-risk individuals.

CLINICAL PEARL

Individuals at risk for neuropathic ulceration (those with LOPS, foot deformities, LEAD, gait abnormalities, poor glycemic control) should be placed on an individualized program for preventive foot care and surveillance based on his/her level of risk.

All at-risk individuals should receive periodic foot screening to identify neuropathic changes, deformities, areas of impending ulceration, and indications of vascular compromise; education and referrals should be based on the findings. The Lower Extremity Amputation Prevention (LEAP) program includes five major prevention interventions: (1) foot screening; (2) patient education; (3) appropriate footwear selection; (4) daily foot inspection by the patient; and (5) management of simple foot problems (to prevent deterioration into more significant problems).

The patient and his/her family are the individuals responsible for daily foot care, foot protection, and foot inspection; thus, individualized patient education programs are integral to prevention of neuropathic ulcers. A 2010 Cochrane Review found that educating patients about preventive foot care seemed to improve their foot care knowledge and behavior short term, and one RCT involving patients with previous diabetic foot disease suggested that intensive education may be effective in preventing recurrent ulceration or amputation; however, further study is needed to determine whether education alone, without additional preventive measures, is sufficient to reduce the incidence of ulcers and/or amputations. At present, education is considered one element of a comprehensive prevention program; periodic surveillance, with frequency based on level of risk, is the other major component (Dorresteijn et al., 2010).

Patient education should include instruction regarding the individual's risk factors and interventions to help ameliorate their specific risk factors, such as therapeutic footwear for individuals with deformities. All patients must be instructed in the following:

- Routine self-care measures (e.g., never going barefoot, inspecting feet daily, breaking shoes in gradually)
- Early recognition and prompt reporting of potential foot problems
- Routine foot surveillance by health care providers
- Individual footwear requirements

In addition, all individuals with neuropathy should have ready access to specialized foot care whenever they detect a potential problem.

Current evidence also strongly supports incorporation of routine skin temperature testing into standard preventive care. One study compared outcomes for diabetic patients in risk categories 2 and 3 (neuropathy and foot deformity, or previous history of ulceration or partial/complete foot amputation) who were randomized to either standard therapy or enhanced therapy. Standard therapy included therapeutic footwear, diabetic foot education, and regular evaluation by a podiatrist; the enhanced therapy also included skin temperature testing at pressure points or previous problematic areas with a dermal thermometer morning and night. Any sites with elevated temperature (>4°F or >2.2°C) were considered to be inflamed, and subjects were instructed to reduce activity and contact the study nurse. Over the 6-month study period, the enhanced therapy group had significantly fewer diabetic foot complications (enhanced therapy group 2% vs. standard therapy group 20%; 7 ulcers and 2 Charcot fractures among standard therapy patients vs. 1 ulcer in the enhanced therapy group) (Lavery et al., 2004).

Another 15-month multicenter study compared individuals with a prior history of diabetic foot ulceration assigned to one of three groups: standard care, standard care + structured foot examination, and enhanced therapy. All subjects received therapeutic footwear, diabetes foot education, and regular foot and nail care. Subjects in the standard care + structured exam group performed a structured foot inspection daily and recorded their findings in a logbook. Subjects in the enhanced therapy group measured skin temperature at 6-foot sites each day. Individuals in the standard therapy and the standard care + structured exam groups were instructed to contact the study nurse immediately for any identified foot abnormalities, and subjects in the enhanced therapy group were instructed to report temperature differences and to reduce activity until temperatures returned to normal. Subjects in the enhanced therapy group had fewer foot ulcers than those in the standard therapy and standard therapy + structured foot examination groups (8.5% in enhanced therapy group vs. 29.3% in the standard therapy group and 30.4% in the standard therapy + structured foot examination group) (Armstrong et al., 2007).

Consistent use of properly fitted footwear is a critical element of preventive care for the individual with neuropathy; shoes that are correctly fitted and that have appropriate insoles provide protection against traumatic injury and can also help to normalize gait and pressure distribution, thus reducing the size of existing calluses and preventing new callus formation. One study ($n = 78$) demonstrated a reduction in callus size that was directly proportional to the amount of time spent wearing running shoes (Singh et al., 2005).

Commercially available shoes are generally appropriate for patients who do not have bony deformities (e.g., prominent metatarsal heads, inflexible great toe [hallux rigidus], or Charcot foot deformity) or LOPS. These shoes are ideally selected according to the following criteria: (1) constructed of natural materials (e.g., leather or suede); (2) shape and size of shoe matches shape and size of foot (rounded or squared toe box); (3) outer soles are cushioned and inner soles are removable; (4) the toe box has sufficient depth to permit the individual to pinch up the exterior shoe material at the toe box; and (5) shoes are secured with Velcro or laces. Individuals should be taught to use their foot tracings to assure that the shoes accommodate their feet.

Individuals with LOPS require professionally fitted footwear since they will be unable to recognize any problems with fit, such as abnormally tight shoes or shoes that rub. Individuals with foot deformities, history of ulceration, or partial foot amputations require custom fit therapeutic footwear and insoles and should be routinely referred to an orthotist or pedorthist.

In teaching individuals with LOPS or ischemia about appropriate use of protective footwear, the nurse should emphasize the importance of wearing protective footwear at all times when out of bed and the importance of shaking the shoes out before donning to assure that there are no foreign bodies.

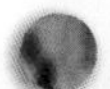 Conclusion

LEND and wounds associated with LEND continue to be the most significant precedent for nontraumatic LEA in the United States. Direct and indirect health care costs associated with LEND and LEND wounds consume nearly $200 billion annually. LEND results in long-term disability and high mortality within 5 years of incident amputation.

The goal in management of the diabetic patient with neuropathy is prevention of ulceration and amputation, which requires appropriate footwear, daily foot care, and daily foot inspection. In addition, current evidence strongly supports the benefit of skin temperature checks with a dermal infrared thermometer to promptly identify areas of inflammation, coupled with off-loading measures and professional evaluation. Effective management of neuropathic ulcers requires attention to off-loading, glycemic control, aggressive debridement to eliminate necrotic tissue, and systemic and topical therapies to control bacterial loads.

Patient education and patient involvement is critical to success in management and requires mutual goal setting and ongoing patient involvement.

REFERENCES

American Diabetes Association. (2014). Standards of Medical Care in diabetes—2014 *Diabetes Care, 37*(Suppl 1), 317–321. doi: 10.2337/dc14.

Ang, C. D., ALviar, M. J. M., Dans, A. L., et al. (2008). Vitamin B for treating peripheral neuropathy. *Cochrane Database of Systematic Reviews,* (*3*), CD004573. doi: 10.1002//14651858.CD004573.pub2.

Armstrong, D. G., Holtz-Neiderer, K., Wendel, C., et al. (2007). Skin temperature monitoring reduces the risk for diabetic foot ulceration in high-risk patients. *American Journal of Medicine, 120*(12), 1042–1046.

Armstrong, D. G., & Lavery, L. A. (1997). Monitoring healing of acute Charcot's arthropathy with infrared dermal thermometry. *Journal of Rehabilitation Research and Development, 34*(3), 317–321.

Armstrong, D. G., Lavery, L. A., Fletschrit J, et al. (1997a). Is electrical stimulation effective in reducing neuropathic pain in patients with diabetes? *Journal of Foot and Ankle Surgery, 36*(4), 260–263.

Armstrong, D. G., Lavery, L. A., Wu, S., et al. (2005). Evaluation of removable and irremovable cast walkers in the healing of diabetic foot wounds: A randomized controlled trial. *Diabetes Care, 28,* 551–554.

Armstrong, D. G., & Peters, E. J. (2002). Charcot's arthropathy of the foot. *Journal of the American Podiatric Medical Association, 92*(7), 390.

Armstrong, D. G., Todd, W. F., Lavery, L. A., et al. (1997b). The natural history of acute Charcot's arthropathy in a diabetic foot specialty clinic. *Journal of American Podiatric Medical Association, 87*(6), 272–278.

Beuker, B., VanDeursen, R. W., Price, P., et al. (2005). Plantar pressure in off-loading devices used in diabetic ulcer treatment. *Wound Repair Regeneration, 13,* 537–542.

Birke, J. A., Patout C. A., Jr., & Foto, J. G. (2000). Factors associated with ulceration and amputation in the neuropathic foot. *Journal of Orthopaedic and Sports Physical Therapy, 30*(2), 91–97.

Birke, J. A., Pavich, M. A., Patout, C. A., et al. (2002). Comparison of forefoot ulcer healing using alternative offloading methods in patients with diabetes mellitus. *Advances in Skin & Wound Care, 15,* 210–215.

Birke, J. A., & Sims, D. S. (1986). Plantar sensory threshold in the ulcerated foot. *Leprosy Review, 57*(3), 261–267.

Blume, P. A., Walters, J., Payne, W., et al. (2008). Comparison of negative pressure wound therapy using vacuum-assisted closure with advanced moist wound therapy in the treatment of diabetic foot ulcers. *Diabetes Care, 31,* 631–636.

Bolton, L. (2007). Operational definition of moist wound healing. *Journal of Wound, Ostomy, and Continence Nursing, 34*(1), 23–29. Evidenced-Based Report Card.

Bonham, P., & Kelechi, T. (2008). Evaluation of lower extremity arterial circulation and implications for nursing practice. *Journal of Cardiovascular Nursing, 23*(2), 144–152.

Boykin, J. V., Jr. (2010). Wound nitric oxide bioactivity: A promising diagnostic indicator for diabetic foot ulcer management. *Journal of Wound, Ostomy, and Continence Nursing, 37*(1), 25–32.

Bus, S. A., Valk, G. D., van Deursen, R. W., et al. (2008). Specific guidelines on footwear and offloading. *Diabetes/Metabolism Research Reviews, 24*(Suppl 1), S192–S193.

Canadian Association of Wound Care (CAWC). Inlow's 60 second diabetic foot exam. Retrieved September 30, 2014, from http://cawc.net/index.php/resources/60-second-diabetic-foot-screen/

Caputo, W. (2008). Surgical management of the diabetic foot. *Wounds, 20*(3), 74–83.

Caselli, A., Pham, H., Giurini J. M., et al. (2002). The forefoot-to-rearfoot plantar pressure ratio is increased in severe diabetic neuropathy and can predict foot ulceration. *Diabetes Care, 25*(6), 1006.

Casellini, C., & Vinik, A. (2007). Clinical manifestations and current treatment options for diabetic neuropathies. *Endocrine Practice, 13*(5), 550–566. © 2007 American Association of Clinical Endocrinologists.

Cavanagh, P. R., & Bus, S. A. (2011). Offloading the diabetic foot for ulcer prevention and healing. *Plastic and Reconstructive Surgery, 127*(Suppl 1), 248S–256S.

Center for Disease Control and Prevention (CDC) Department of Health and Human Services, National Estimates on Diabetes. (2014). Retrieved July 22, 2014 from http://www.cdc.gov/diabetes/pubs/references07.htm

Centers for Disease Control and Prevention. (2011). *National diabetes fact sheet: General information and national estimates on diabetes in the United States, 2011.* Atlanta, GA: US Department of Health and Human Services.

Centers for Medicare and Medicaid Services (CMS). (2011). Medicare's Coverage of Diabetic Supplies and Services. www.medicare.gov/Pubs/pdf/11022.pdf

Chaudhry, V., Russell, J., & Belzberg, A. (2008). Decompressive surgery of lower limbs for symmetrical diabetic peripheral neuropathy. *Cochrane Database of Systematic Reviews,* (*3*), CD006152. doi: 10.1002/14651858.CD006152.pub2.

Dalla Paola, L., Volpe, A., Varotto, D., et al. (2007). Use of retrograde nail in ankle arthrodesis in Charcot neuroarthropathy: A limb salvage procedure. *Foot and Ankle International, 28*(9), 967–970.

Dorresteijn, J. A., Kriegsman, N., Didi, M. W., et al. (2010). Complex interventions for preventing diabetic foot ulceration. *Cochrane Database of Systematic Reviews,* (*1*), CD007610. doi: 10.1002/14651858.CD007610.

Dworkin, R. H., O'Connor, A. B., Backonja, M., et al. (2007). Pharmacologic management of neuropathic pain: Evidence-based recommendations. *Pain, 132*(3), 237–251.

Edmonds, M. (2006). Diabetic foot ulcers: Practical treatment recommendations. *Drugs, 66*(7), 913–929.

Eichenholtz, S. N. (1966). *Charcot joints.* Vol. 227. Springfield, IL: Charles C. Thomas.

Ennis, W., Foremann, P., Mozen, N., et al. (2005). Ultrasound therapy for recalcitrant diabetic foot ulcers: A randomized, double-blind, controlled, multicenter study. *Ostomy Wound Management, 51*(9), 14.

Falanga, V. (2005). Wound healing and its impairment on the diabetic foot. *The Lancet, 366*(9498), 1736–1743.

Foto, J., Brasseaux, D., Hupp, D., et al. (2009). A comparison of different handheld infrared thermometers for measuring dermal skin temperature. *Diabetes Professional Resources Online.* Abstract # 1100-P. Accessed November 28, 2014.

Frykberg, R. G., Zgonis, T., & Armstrong D. G., et al. (2006). Diabetic foot disorders: a clinical practice guideline (2006 revision). *Journal of Foot and Ankle Surgery, 45*(5 Suppl), S1–S66.

Harkless, L. B., de Lellis, S., Carnegie, D. H., et al. (2006). Improved foot sensitivity and pain reduction in patients with peripheral neuropathy after treatment with monochromatic infrared photo energy—MIRE. *Journal of Diabetes and its Complications, 20*(2), 81–87.

Health Resources and Services Administration (HRSA). (2011). *LEAP Resources.* Retrieved July 30, 2014, from http://www.hrsa.gov/hansensdisease/leap/index.htm

Hockenbury, R. T., Gruttadauria, M., & McKinney, I. (2007). Use of implantable bone growth stimulation in Charcot ankle arthrodesis. *Foot and Ankle International, 28*(9), 971–976.

Jude, E. B., & Boulton, A. J. (2002). Medical treatment of Charcot's arthropathy. *Journal of the American Podiatric Medical Association, 92*(7), 381.

Jude, E. B., Dang, C., & Boulton, A. J. (2010). Effect of L-arginine on the microcirculation in the neuropathic diabetic foot in type 2 diabetes mellitus: A double blind, placebo-controlled study. *Diabetic Medicine, 27*(1), 113–116.

Katz, I., Harlan, A., Miranda-Polma, B., et al. (2005). A randomized trial of two irremovable off-loading devices in management of plantar neuropathic diabetic foot ulcers. *Diabetes Care, 28,* 555–559.

Kelechi, T. J., & Lukacs, K. S. (1997). Patient with dystrophic toenails, calluses, and heel fissures. *Journal of Wound Ostomy Continence Nursing, 24*(4), 237–242.

Laborde, M. (2009). Midfoot ulcers treated with gastrocnemius–soleus recession. *Foot and Ankle International, 30*(9), 842–846.

Lavery, L. A., Armstrong, D. G., & Harkless, L. B. (1996). Classification of diabetic foot wounds. *Journal of Foot and Ankle Surgery, 35,* 528–531.

Lavery, L. A., Armstrong, D. G., Vela, S., et al., (1998). Practical criteria for screening patients at high risk for diabetic foot ulceration. *Archives of Internal Medicine, 158*(2), 157–162.

Lavery, L. A., Armstrong, D. G., & Walker, S. C. (1997). Healing rates of diabetic foot ulcers associated with midfoot fracture due to Charcot's arthropathy. *Diabetic Medicine, 14*(1), 46–49.

Lavery, L. A., Higgins, K. R., Lanctot, D. R., et al. (2004). Home monitoring of foot skin temperatures to prevent ulceration. *Diabetes Care, 27*(11), 2642–2647.

Lavery, L., Lanctot, D., Constantinides, G., et al. (2005). Wear and biomechanical characteristics of a novel shear-reducing insole with implications for high-risk persons with diabetes. *Diabetes Technology & Therapeutics, 7*(4), 638–646.

Lawson, D., & Petrofsky, J. S. (2007). A randomized control study on the effect of biphasic electrical stimulation in a warm room on skin blood flow and healing rates in chronic wounds of patients with and without diabetes. *Medical Science Monitor, 13*(6), CR258–CR263.

Lewis, J., & Lipp, A. (2013). Pressure-relieving interventions for treating diabetic foot ulcers. *Cochrane Database of Systematic Reviews*, (3), 1–1: CD002302. doi: 10.1002/14651858.CD002302.pub2.

Maluf, K. S., Mueller, M. J., Strube, M. J., et al. (2004). Tendon Achilles lengthening for the treatment of neuropathic ulcers causes a temporary reduction in forefoot pressure associated with changes in plantar flexor power rather than ankle motion during gait. *Journal of Biomechanics, 37*, 897–906.

McCrory, J., Morag, E., Norkitis, A., et al. (1998). Healing of Charcot fractures: Skin temperature and radiographic correlates. *The Foot, 8*, 158–165.

McGill, M., Molyneaux, L., Bolton, T., et al. (2000). Response of Charcot's arthropathy to contact casting: Assessment by quantitative techniques. *Diabetologia, 43*(4), 481–484.

Nabuurs-Franssen, M. H., Sleegers, R., Huijberts, M. S., et al. (2005). Total contact casting of the diabetic foot in daily practice: A prospective follow-up study. *Diabetes Care, 28*, 243–247.

National Institutes of Neurological Disorders and Stroke. Peripheral neuropathy fact sheet. Retrieved July 22, 2014, from http://www.ninds.nih.gov/disorders/peripheralneuropathy/detail_peripheralneuropathy.htm

Nielson, D. L., & Armstrong, D. G. (2008). The natural history of Charcot's neuroarthropathy. *Clinics in Podiatric Medicine and Surgery, 25*(1), 53–62.

Nube, V. L., McGill, M., Molyneaux, L., et al. (2002). From acute to chronic: Monitoring the progress of Charcot's arthropathy. *Journal of the American Podiatric Medical Association, 92*(7), 384.

Okazaki, R. (2011). Diabetes mellitus and bone metabolism. *Clinical Calcium, 21*(5), 669–675.

Owings, T. M., Woerner, J. L., Frampton, J. D., et al. (2008). Custom therapeutic insoles based on both foot shape and plantar pressure measurement provide enhanced pressure relief. *Diabetes Care, 31*(5), 839–844.

Pecoraro, R. E., Reiber, G. E., & Burgess, E. M. (1990). Pathways to diabetic limb amputation: Basis for prevention. *Diabetes Care, 13*, 513–521.

Petrofsky, J. S., Schwab, E., Lo, T., et al. (2007). The thermal effect on the blood flow response to electrical stimulation. *Medical Science Monitor, 13*(11), 498–504.

Sage, R. A., Webster, J. K., & Fisher, S. G. (2001). Outpatient care and morbidity reduction in diabetic foot ulcers associated with chronic pressure callus. *Journal of the American Podiatric Medical Association, 91*(6), 275–279.

Saunders, L. J., & Mrdjencovich, D. (1991). Anatomical patterns of bone and joint destruction in neuropathic diabetics. *Diabetes, 40*, 529A.

Sayner, L. R., & Rosenblum, B. I. (2005). External fixation for Charcot foot reconstruction. *Current Surgery, 62*(6), 618–623.

Schultz, G. S., Sibbald, R. G., Falanga, V., et al. (2003). Wound bed preparation. *Wound Repair and Regeneration, 11*(Suppl 1), S1–S28.

Seidel, H. M. (2006). Blood vessels. In H. M. Seidel (Ed.), *Mosby's guide to physical examination* (6th ed.). St. Louis, MO: Mosby, Elsevier Science.

Sella, E. J. (2009). Current concepts review: Diagnostic imaging of the diabetic foot. *Foot and Ankle International, 30*(6), 568–576.

Singal, A., & Khanna, D. (2011). Onychomycosis: Diagnosis and management. *Indian Journal of Dermatology, 77*(6), 659–672.

Singh, N., Armstrong, D. H., & Lipsky, B. (2005). Preventing foot ulcers in patients with diabetes. *Journal of American Medical Association, 293*(2), 217–228.

Soderstrom, L. H., Johnson, S. P., dia, V. A., et al. (2011). Association between vitamin D and diabetic neuropathy in a nationally representative sample: Results from 2001–2004 NHANES. *Diabetes Medicine, 29*(1), 50–55. doi: 10.111. j.1464-5491.2011.03379.x. (Epub ahead of print).

Sohn, M. W., Stuck, R. M., Pinzur, M., et al. (2010). Lower-extremity amputation risk after charcot arthropathy and diabetic foot ulcer. *Diabetes Care, 33*(1), 98–100.

Solomon, L. R. (2011). Diabetes as a cause of clinically significant functional cobalamin deficiency. *Diabetes Care, 34*(5), 1077–1080. (Epub 2011 Mar 18).

Spencer, S. A. (2000). Pressure relieving interventions for preventing and treating diabetic foot ulcers. *Cochrane Database of Systematic Reviews*, (3), CD002302. doi: 10.1002/14651858.CD002302.

Steed, D. L., Attinger, C., Colaizzi, T., et al. (2006). Guidelines for the treatment of diabetic ulcers. *Wound Repair and Regeneration, 14*(6), 680–692.

Steed, D. L., Donohoe, D., Webster, M. W., et al. (1996). Effect of extensive debridement and treatment on the healing of diabetic foot ulcers. *Journal of the American College of Surgery, 183*, 61–64.

Verity, S., Sochocki, M., Embil, J. M., et al. (2008). Treatment of Charcot foot and ankle with a prefabricated removable walker brace and custom insole. *Foot and Ankle Surgery, 14*(1), 26–31.

Wagner, F. W. (1981). The dysvascular foot: A system for diagnosis and treatment. *Foot and Ankle, 2*(2), 64–122.

Wang, J. C. (2003). Use of external fixation in the reconstruction of the Charcot foot and ankle. *Clinics in Podiatric Medicine and Surgery, 20*(1), 97–117.

Weir, G. (2010). Diabetic foot ulcers—Evidence-based wound management. *Continuing Medical Education, 28*(40), 76–80.

Wound, Ostomy and Continence Nurses Society (WOCN). (2012). *Guideline for management of wounds in patients with lower-extremity neuropathic disease.* Mt. Laurel, NJ: Wound Ostomy and Continence Nurses Society (WOCN), 100. (WOCN clinical practice guideline series; no. 3).

Yavuz, M., Erdemir, A., Botek, G., et al. (2007). Peak plantar pressure and shear locations: Relevance to diabetic patients. *Diabetes Care, 30*(10), 2643–2645.

Yavuz, M., Tajaddinia, A., Botekc, G., et al. (2008). Temporal characteristics of plantar shear distribution: Relevance to diabetic patients. *Journal of Biomechanics, 3*, 556–559.

Zgonis, T., Stapleton, J., Jeffries, L., et al. (2008). Surgical treatment of Charcot neuroarthropathy. *AORN Journal, 87*, 971–990.

Ziegler, D. (2006). Treatment of diabetic polyneuropathy: Update 2006. *Annals of the New York Academy of the Sciences, 1084*, 250–266.

Ziegler, D., Low, P. A., Litchy, W. J., et al. (2011). Efficacy and safety of antioxidant treatment with a α-lipoic acid over 4 years in diabetic polyneuropathy: The NATHAN 1 trial. *Diabetes Care, 34*(9), 2054–2060. (Epub 2011 Jul 20).

Zimny, S., Schatz, H., Pfohl, M. (2004). The role of limited joint mobility in diabetic patients with an at-risk foot. *Diabetes Care, 27*, 942–946.

QUESTIONS

1. The wound care nurse is assessing a patient who has developed a "rocker bottom" foot with plantar surface ulcerations. What condition would the nurse document?
   A. Charcot neuroarthropathy
   B. Foot drop
   C. Progressive anesthesia and loss of proprioception
   D. Paresthesia

2. The wound care nurse provides testing of lower extremity sensory function for patients at risk for lower extremity neuropathic disease (LEND). Which statement accurately describes this testing?
   A. A 5-g monofilament should be used to test for sensory function and loss of protective sensation.
   B. Loss of vibratory sense typically occurs after LOPS; therefore, vibratory sense testing is not as reliable a test as monofilament testing.
   C. Inability to consistently identify the direction in which the toe is pointing is considered loss of position sense.
   D. Foot deformities such as hammertoes are indicative of sensory neuropathy.

3. The wound care nurse palpates a callus on the heel of a diabetic patient. What interventions would the nurse recommend?
   A. Off-loading involving bedrest
   B. Paring of the callus
   C. Skin hydration
   D. Removing shoes in the home setting

4. Which of the following accurately describes a clinical characteristic of a neuropathic ulcer?
   A. Edges are typically poorly defined and rough.
   B. The ulcer is typically located on the plantar surface, most commonly over a metatarsal head.
   C. The wound is necrotic, red, or deep purple.
   D. Erythema and induration are classic indicators of callus formation.

5. The wound care nurse documents a patient's wound risk category as 2 as outlined in the Diabetes Foot Program guidelines. Along with education emphasizing disease control and proper shoe fit, what follow-up schedule would be recommended for this patient?
   A. Yearly for foot screen
   B. 3 to 6 months for foot/shoe examination and nail care
   C. 1 to 3 months for foot/activity/footwear examination and nail care
   D. 1 to 12 weeks for foot/activity/footwear evaluation and callus/nail care

6. The wound care nurse is conducting a filament application using the diabetes foot screen. Which step of the procedure is performed accurately?
   A. The filament is applied perpendicular to the skin's surface.
   B. The approach, skin contact and departure of the filament, is 5 seconds.
   C. The filament is slid across the skin to achieve repetitive contact at test site.
   D. The filament is applied directly on an ulcer, callus, scar, or necrotic tissue.

7. The wound care nurse is classifying a diabetic foot ulcer using the Wagner Classification System. What number would the nurse use to document a deep ulcer with joint sepsis?
   A. 1
   B. 2
   C. 3
   D. 4

8. The wound care nurse grades a patient's foot ulcer as a 3 on the University of Texas Diabetic Foot Classification System. Which characteristics warrant this classification?
   A. Pre- or postulcer with epithelization
   B. Superficial; not involving tendon, bone, or capsule
   C. Ulcer penetrates through to tendon or capsule
   D. Ulcer penetrates to bone or joint

9. The wound care nurse is preparing a management plan for a patient with a neuropathic foot ulcer. Which intervention is recommended for these types of wounds?
   A. Surgical debridement of any necrotic tissue
   B. Softening of callus with moisture therapy
   C. Maintenance of a dry wound surface
   D. Off-loading with therapeutic/diabetic shoes

10. Which off-loading option is considered to be the "gold standard" for management of plantar surface ulcers in the diabetic patient?
    A. Removable cast walker with rocker bottom
    B. Total contact cast
    C. Customized diabetic shoe
    D. Heel sole shoe with removable off-loading pegs

11. Which lab result is an indicator of infection in the patient with a diabetic foot ulcer?
    A. Erythrocyte sedimentation rate (ESR) 15 mm/h
    B. Fasting blood glucose 98 mg/dL
    C. C-reactive protein (CRP) 4.5 mg/L
    D. HbA_{1c} (hemoglobin A_{1c}) 7%

12. Which imaging study is the gold standard in diagnosing osteomyelitis?
A. Plain x-rays
B. Magnetic resonance imaging (MRI)
C. Technetium-99 phosphate bone scan
D. Positron emission tomography (PET)

13. Which characteristic would the wound care nurse recognize as a sign of Charcot foot healing that is in the coalescence phase of the Eichenholtz Classification System?
A. Edema is increased.
B. Erythema is severe.
C. Temperature in involved area slightly higher than surrounding area (>2°C).
D. X-ray image demonstrates fracture, dislocation, or subluxation.

14. Which pharmacological intervention would the wound care nurse typically recommend for a patient with pain described as "dysesthesia"?
A. Capsaicin cream
B. Tricyclic antidepressant
C. Analgesics
D. Opioids

15. Which off-loading device is associated with the highest healing rates?
A. Walking splints
B. Adhesive felt pads
C. Padded socks
D. Total contact cast

16. The wound care nurse is teaching a patient with intact foot sensation how to purchase and wear commercial shoes to lower the risk of skin damage. Which of the following is a recommended guideline?
A. Allow for ¼ inch space beyond the longest toe.
B. Size and purchase shoes in the morning before edema sets in.
C. Measure both feet and size shoes to the smaller foot.
D. Gradually increase wear time for new shoes by 2-hour increments daily.

ANSWERS: 1.**A**, 2.**C**, 3.**B**, 4.**B**, 5.**C**, 6.**A**, 7.**C**, 8.**D**, 9.**A**, 10.**B**, 11.**C**, 12.**B**, 13.**C**, 14.**A**, 15.**D**, 16.**D**

CHAPTER 24

Differential Assessment of Lower Extremity Wounds

Dorothy Doughty and Laurie L. McNichol

OBJECTIVES

1. Compare and contrast arterial, venous, neuropathic, and mixed ulcers in terms of risk factors, pathology, clinical presentation, and management guidelines.
2. Describe critical parameters to be included in assessment of the individual with a lower extremity ulcer.
3. Use assessment data to determine causative and contributing factors for a lower extremity ulcer and to develop individualized management plans that are evidence based.
4. Describe indications for referral to vascular surgeon, podiatrist, orthotist, and dermatologist.
5. Identify indications that a lower extremity ulcer is "atypical" and requires additional diagnostic workup and/or medical–surgical intervention.

Topical Outline

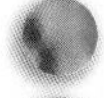
Introduction

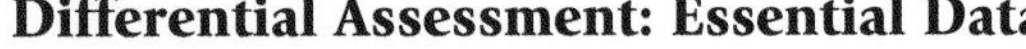
Differential Assessment: Essential Data

Assessment of Risk Factors
Ulcer History
Pain History
Physical Examination
  Circulatory Status
  Sensorimotor Status
  Ulcer Assessment

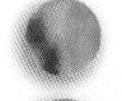
Differential Assessment: Data Synthesis

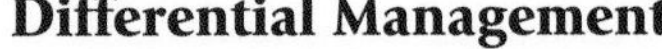
Differential Management

Ischemic Ulcer Complicated by Venous Insufficiency and 2+ Edema
Venous Ulcer in Patient with Mixed Arterial–Venous Disease and ABI <0.8
Neuropathic Ulcer Complicated by Arterial Insufficiency
Referrals

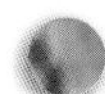
Conclusion

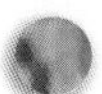

Introduction

Previous chapters in this text have addressed general principles related to wound healing, wound assessment, and wound management, and the preceding chapters in this section have described the pathology, clinical presentation, and management of lower extremity wounds, including venous ulcers, arterial ulcers, and neuropathic ulcers. Chapter 25 will address the pathology and management of common "atypical" lower extremity wounds.

Lower extremity wounds are very common, especially in the older adult population, due to the increasing prevalence of the underlying disease processes associated with development of these ulcers. Venous ulcers are the most common type of lower extremity wound, affecting up to 1% of the population at some point in their lifetime (Jones et al., 2013); however, the incidence of arterial and neuropathic ulcers is rising, due in part to the increasing prevalence of poorly controlled diabetes. Current estimates suggest that >8% of the US population is affected by diabetes (Markova & Mostow, 2012), and these numbers are expected to rise with the continued increase in the number and percent of adults and children who are obese or morbidly obese.

Lower extremity wounds present a major burden to the health care system; they are costly to treat, frequently refractory to standard wound care, and high risk for recurrence

(Markova & Mostow, 2012). Thus, comprehensive and evidence-based management is essential, as are ongoing patient education and routine follow-up to minimize the risk of recurrence.

CLINICAL PEARL

Lower extremity wounds are costly to treat, frequently refractory, and at high risk for recurrence; thus, comprehensive and evidence-based management is essential, as are ongoing patient education and routine follow-up.

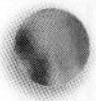

Differential Assessment: Essential Data

The critical "first step" in effective management of any wound is accurate determination of the etiologic factors followed by interventions to correct those factors. This step is of particular importance in management of lower extremity ulcers, because interventions that are essential to effective management of a venous ulcer (leg elevation and compression therapy) are typically *contraindicated* with an arterial ulcer and of no benefit in management of a neuropathic ulcer. Thus, accurate differential assessment is an essential skill for the wound care nurse.

CLINICAL PEARL

A critical "first step" in effective wound management is accurate identification and correction of causative factors; this is particularly important in lower extremity ulcer care, since interventions that are essential to management of one type of ulcer are commonly contraindicated or of no benefit in management of others.

Assessment of Risk Factors

Accurate differential assessment begins with the patient interview (history) and physical examination. In conducting the patient interview, the nurse must ask specific questions related to known risk factors for venous insufficiency, arterial insufficiency, and neuropathy. For example, DVT, obesity, a sedentary lifestyle, and paralysis of the calf muscle are known risk factors for venous insufficiency, while coronary artery disease, hyperlipidemia, hypertension, diabetes, and tobacco use are the primary risk factors for arterial insufficiency and, in the United States, longstanding diabetes and metabolic disorders are the most common risk factors for neuropathy. The nurse should be aware that many individuals, especially elder adults, will have risk factors for all types of lower extremity wounds; thus, the history is insufficient, in and of itself, to determine the etiology of the wound.

CLINICAL PEARL

Many individuals will have risk factors for all types of lower extremity wounds; thus, the history is insufficient, in and of itself, to determine the etiology of the wound.

Ulcer History

Additional elements of the patient history of particular benefit to differential assessment are medications, which provide additional clues regarding the individual's comorbid conditions and risk factors, and ulcer history, to include onset, triggering factors, and previous treatment and response. The patient with a venous ulcer may report that the ulcer began with a small cut or insect bite, while the patient with an arterial ulcer may report spontaneous necrosis of the toes or a traumatic injury that failed to heal and developed into a steadily worsening ulcer. The patient with a neuropathic ulcer may be unaware as to when and how the ulcer began due to loss of normal sensation. ("I just noticed I had drainage on my sock and started looking and found it.") Response to previous treatment also provides important clues; for example, the patient who states his leg was "wrapped up" and that the wrap caused his pain and ulcer to worsen is unlikely to have a venous ulcer (WOCN, 2011; WOCN, 2012; WOCN, 2014).

Pain History

One of the assessment parameters most critical to differential assessment is the pain history; the nurse should carefully query the patient as to the location, severity, and characteristics of any wound-related pain, and about exacerbating and relieving factors. Classic descriptors of pain for each type of ulcer are as follows:

- *Venous ulcers*: pain is typically described as "aching, heavy, and dull" and typically involves the entire leg. Severity is variable. Pain is usually worsened by dependency and edema and relieved by elevation. Many patients state they "feel good in the morning" (after their legs have been elevated all night) and that the pain gets steadily worse throughout the day (WOCN, 2011).
- *Arterial ulcers*: pain is typically described as "intense, cramping, and throbbing" and typically involves the calf, lower leg, and foot. Severity is variable and typically progressive; early in the disease process, pain occurs only with significant activity and is fairly rapidly relieved by rest and dependency (intermittent claudication), while advanced disease causes pain when the legs are placed in a horizontal and neutral position (such as for sleeping) and eventually persists even when the legs are dependent. Pain is worsened by activity and elevation and at least partially relieved by rest and dependency. Patients may report having to sleep in their recliners so that they can keep their legs down (WOCN, 2014).
- *Neuropathic ulcers*: pain is typically described as "pins and needles," stinging, burning, and "electric shock" in nature and is sometimes worse at night, when the individual is trying to sleep. Severity is variable. Pain may be reduced by walking, which helps to "drown out" the abnormal signals generated by the damaged nerves

("I get up and walk it off, but it starts again when I go back to bed and try to sleep"); many individuals require pharmaceutical pain management (WOCN, 2012).

CLINICAL PEARL

Data obtained from patient history of particular importance to differential assessment include medications (which provide clues as to significant comorbidities), ulcer onset and history (to include treatment to date and response), and pain history (particularly the exacerbating and relieving factors).

Physical Examination

The next step in patient assessment is the physical examination of the lower extremities, which should include in-depth assessment of circulatory status, sensorimotor function, and ulcer status.

Circulatory Status

The nurse must assess for indicators of normal versus compromised arterial perfusion and normal versus compromised venous return. Both limbs should be assessed, with comparison of the affected to the unaffected limb. Parameters to be included in vascular assessment include status of skin, hair, and nails; skin color at rest and changes with elevation and dependency; skin temperature; capillary refill time; lower limb pulses, with particular attention to the dorsalis pedis and posterior tibialis pulses; ankle brachial index measurement; observation for varicose veins and/or prominent ankle veins; and assessment of edema, to include distribution, type (pitting vs. nonpitting), and severity (WOCN, 2011; WOCN, 2014).

CLINICAL PEARL

Physical assessment of an individual with a leg ulcer must include vascular assessment, sensorimotor assessment, and wound assessment.

Indicators of arterial compromise include trophic changes in the skin, hair, and nails, such as thin shiny skin, diminished or absent hair growth, and thin ridged nails (which may not be visible in the patient with coexisting fungal infection of the nails); elevational pallor or ashen tone to the skin; dependent rubor; coolness of the distal limb and foot; prolonged capillary refill time (>3 seconds); diminished or absent pedal pulses; and Ankle Brachial Index (ABI) <0.9 or >1.3 (severe arterial disease is typically manifest by ABI <0.5). The patient who keeps his or her legs down in response to ischemic pain frequently also has some degree of dependent edema (WOCN, 2014).

Indicators of venous insufficiency include hemosiderin staining of the lower leg, pitting edema extending from the ankle to the knee, presence of varicosities and prominent ankle veins, fibrotic changes in the skin and soft tissue (lipodermatosclerosis), and venous dermatitis (erythema, pruritis, and dermatitic changes involving the gaiter ["sock"] area of the leg) (WOCN, 2011).

Indicators of lymphedema include edema (either pitting or nonpitting) extending from the toes to the groin, cobblestone texture to the skin, and, with advanced disease, papillomatous lesions.

Sensorimotor Status

The nurse must also screen for changes in sensorimotor status indicative of neuropathy. This includes assessment of sensory function using a 10-g Semmes-Weinstein monofilament; assessment of vibratory sense at the base of the great toe or medial aspect of the first metatarsophalangeal joint; assessment of proprioceptive (position) sense; observation of gait and footwear, to include appropriateness of the shoe in relation to the size and contours of the foot and abnormal wear patterns; assessment for foot deformities and callus formation; and assessment of skin hydration. Assessment of plantar surface skin temperature is also very helpful; skin temperature should be measured at multiple sites using a dermal infrared thermometer, and any site at which the temperature is >4.0°F higher than the surrounding skin must be further assessed for inflammatory changes and possible impending ulceration (WOCN, 2012).

Indicators of neuropathy include loss of protective sensation (LOPS), as evidenced by failure to sense the 10-gram monofilament at one or more sites; loss of vibratory sense, which frequently precedes LOPS; loss of position sense; abnormal gait and wear patterns in footwear; foot deformities, such as hammertoes, claw toes, or Charcot deformity; very dry skin with fissure formation (or very wet skin); and possibly "hot spots" (areas of elevated temperature) (WOCN, 2012).

Once the nurse has completed the history and physical assessment, she/he should be able to determine whether the patient has arterial, venous, and/or neuropathic disease. However, as noted, many individuals have risk factors and physical manifestations of more than one pathologic process (e.g., mixed arterial–venous disease, mixed neuropathic ischemic disease, or mixed venous and neuropathic disease), and it is possible that one person could present with all three disease processes (arterial, venous, and neuropathic). Thus, assessment of the ulcer itself, along with the predominant pain pattern, is essential to accurate identification of the primary etiology of the wound.

CLINICAL PEARL

Assessment of the ulcer itself (particularly location, appearance of wound bed, and exudate), along with predominant pain pattern, is essential to accurate identification of the primary etiology of the wound.

Ulcer Assessment

The nurse should always conduct a comprehensive assessment of ulcer status, to include location, shape, dimensions and depth, presence and extent of any tunneling or undermining, type of tissue in the wound bed, status of wound edges, status of surrounding tissue, exudate (volume, color, consistency, and odor), and any signs and symptoms of infection. However, the parameters most critical to differential assessment are **location, wound bed appearance,** and **exudate**. Arterial wounds are usually located distally (toes and forefoot) because those are the areas most distal to the heart; arterial wounds may also present as nonhealing traumatic injuries (because there is insufficient perfusion to support healing). Most commonly, arterial wounds have a punched out appearance, with a pale or necrotic wound bed and limited exudate. In contrast, venous ulcers are typically located between the ankle and knee, are shallow and irregular in appearance, and have large volumes of exudate; the wound bed is usually dark red and may have a layer of yellow film due to high bacterial loads. Neuropathic wounds are located on the plantar surface of the foot or on areas of the foot in contact with the shoe (such as tips or tops of toes); these wounds are red and wet unless there is coexisting ischemia and are commonly located in the center of a callus (WOCN, 2011; WOCN, 2012; WOCN, 2014).

CLINICAL PEARL

Wound location is a major clue as to etiology: arterial wounds are usually located distally (toes and forefoot) or in areas of traumatic injury that failed to heal; venous ulcers are almost always located between the ankle and the knee (most commonly around the medial malleoli); and neuropathic ulcers are located over the foot in areas in contact with the shoe (most commonly the plantar surface).

Differential Assessment: Data Synthesis

Determination of primary etiology is based on **predominant pain pattern, ulcer location, ulcer appearance,** and **exudate** and supported by a review of the vascular and sensorimotor assessment data.

For example, if the patient presented with complaints of severe cramping pain that was worsened by activity and partially relieved by rest and dependency, and assessment revealed a nonhealing wound on the anterior lower shin that began with a small cut and progressively worsened, and assessment further revealed a wound bed that was 50% necrotic and 50% very pale pink, with minimal exudate, the wound nurse should establish a preliminary assessment of an ischemic wound. However, the nurse should then review the vascular assessment to assure consistency with the preliminary assessment and would expect to find trophic changes, diminished pulses, and abnormal ABI. The nurse might also find that the patient exhibited LOPS at 8/10 sites tested, along with loss of vibratory sense and loss of position sense. This would establish an additional nursing diagnosis of neuropathic changes but would not change the determination regarding primary wound etiology. In this situation, the patient would be determined to have an ischemic ulcer with coexisting neuropathy (WOCN, 2012; WOCN, 2014).

In another example, the patient presents with complaints of a nonhealing wound located just above the inner ankle that she thinks began with a small nick and has enlarged considerably over the past 8 weeks, despite daily application of antibiotic ointment. On assessment, the ulcer bed is 70% dark red and 30% yellow; there is a moderately large volume of exudate and dark gray discoloration over the lower extremity consistent with hemosiderin staining, along with 2+ edema. The patient describes two types of pain: a dull aching pain that is worse at the end of the day and worse when the edema is worse and that improves with leg elevation and occasional cramping pain in the calf and lower leg that occurs only when she walks significant distances and is relieved by sitting down for 5 to 10 minutes. A review of the vascular and sensorimotor data reveals normal sensorimotor function, 1+ pulses on the involved leg, 2+ edema on the involved leg, and an ABI of 0.7. This patient has mixed arterial–venous disease, but the ulcer is due to venous insufficiency, as indicated by ulcer location, primary pain pattern, and ulcer appearance. Thus, management will be based on the primary etiology, with modifications as indicated for an individual with coexisting arterial disease (WOCN, 2011; WOCN, 2014).

See **Table 24-1** for the classic presentation of arterial, venous, and neuropathic ulcers.

Differential Management

Once the differential assessment and classification have been completed, the wound nurse proceeds with development of an individualized management plan based on the primary etiology with modifications based on any coexisting pathology. If there is no coexisting pathology, the management plan is determined by ulcer classification, for example, leg elevation and compression therapy for venous ulcers, measures to improve perfusion for arterial ulcers, and offloading for neuropathic ulcers. However, when there is additional coexisting pathology, the "usual" management plan may need to be modified. Common types of "mixed disease" requiring modifications include the following: ischemic ulcer in patient with mixed arterial–venous disease and 2+ edema, venous ulcer in patient with mixed arterial–venous disease and ABI < 0.8, and neuropathic ulcer complicated by arterial insufficiency.

CLINICAL PEARL

Wound management is based on the primary etiology of the wound, with modifications as indicated based on any coexisting pathology.

TABLE 24-1 Differential Assessment Arterial, Venous, and Neuropathic Ulcers

	Pain Pattern	Location	Appearance	Associated Findings
Arterial	• Cramping, throbbing • Worsened by activity and elevation • Relieved by rest and dependency	• Distal foot • Nonhealing traumatic injury	• Punched out • Pale or necrotic wound bed • Minimal exudate	• Diminished pulses, abnormal ABI, trophic changes • Infection common (S/S of infection may be muted)
Venous	• Dull, aching, "heavy" • Worsened by dependency • Relieved by elevation	• Ankle to knee	• Shallow with irregular edges • Wound bed dark red; may have yellow film • Highly exudative	• Edema and hemosiderin staining common • Venous dermatitis or periwound maceration common
Neuropathic	• "Pins and needles," burning, "electric shock" • Partially relieved by walking	• Plantar surface of foot • Area of foot in contact with shoe	• Red unless there is coexisting ischemia • Exudative	• LOPS and foot deformities common • Callus common (may be macerated)

Ischemic Ulcer Complicated by Venous Insufficiency and 2+ Edema

In this case, initial management strategies would include measures to improve perfusion, such as revascularization, medical management, and smoking cessation. Topical therapy would be determined by the characteristics of the ulcer and the potential for healing; for example, a very poorly perfused wound covered with dry eschar and no signs of infection would be left open to air or covered with dry gauze, while an open wound in a patient with an ABI of 0.55 would be managed according to moist wound healing principles, with particular attention to prevention of infection. Management of edema would also be determined by the degree of arterial insufficiency; in the patient with very advanced disease in which there is no potential for healing, any form of elevation or compression would be contraindicated and edema management would not be appropriate. In contrast, if the wound is open and perfusion is borderline (e.g., ABI 0.5), edema management *would* be indicated, since edema is a known impediment to tissue oxygenation and wound healing. In this case, very simple and conservative measures to reduce edema (leg elevation) should be undertaken along with monitoring for any worsening of ischemic pain; as noted in the chapter on arterial ulcers, dynamic compression therapy is also sometimes beneficial for the patient with mixed disease (WOCN, 2011; WOCN, 2014).

Venous Ulcer in Patient with Mixed Arterial–Venous Disease and ABI <0.8

In this case, the "usual" therapy involves leg elevation and therapeutic-level compression therapy; however, therapeutic-level compression is contraindicated in a patient whose ABI is <0.8. If the ABI is >0.5 and <0.8, as in the patient example provided above, modified compression therapy (light compression) should be initiated with 23 to 30 mm Hg compression at the ankle. If this is poorly tolerated, the nurse should consider dynamic compression therapy (WOCN, 2011; WOCN, 2014).

Neuropathic Ulcer Complicated by Arterial Insufficiency

In this case, management is dictated by the degree of arterial insufficiency and the characteristics of the ulcer (open vs. closed and infected vs. noninfected). If there is advanced arterial insufficiency with ABI <0.5 and very limited potential for healing, and the wound is closed and uninfected, the wound should be left open to air or covered with dry gauze and monitored for signs of infection until perfusion is improved to a point to support healing. Offloading should be maintained to prevent worsening of the existing ulcer or development of new ulcers. If there is borderline perfusion and/or the wound is open, the principles of moist wound healing should be followed, along with consistent offloading and medical and behavioral strategies to maximize perfusion (WOCN, 2012; WOCN, 2014).

Referrals

Referrals are frequently required for individuals with lower extremity ulcers and should be initiated in the following situations: (1) when comprehensive assessment reveals that the patient history and ulcer characteristics are inconsistent with ulcers caused by venous, arterial, neuropathic, or mixed disease; (2) when the assessment reveals mixed arterial–venous disease, but the severity of the arterial disease and potential for healing is unclear; (3) when additional expertise is required for optimal management, for example, total contact casting for neuropathic plantar surface ulcer or customized footwear for diabetic patient with foot deformities; and/or (4) when medical–surgical intervention is required to promote healing. In situations where wound etiology is unclear, a dermatology referral is frequently indicated, as dermatologists specialize in difficult cutaneous wounds and they are usually the ones best prepared to provide differential diagnosis and management of atypical wounds. In situations involving mixed arterial–venous disease or mixed neuroischemic disease, a vascular consult is most appropriate.

CLINICAL PEARL

Referrals are indicated when the etiology of the wound is unclear, when the wound fails to respond to initial management, or when additional expertise or medical–surgical intervention is required for management.

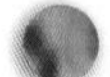

Conclusion

Lower extremity wounds are common, and effective management is critical to wound healing and prevention of recurrence. The first step in effective wound management is accurate identification of the causative and contributing factors. This can be a challenge since many patients present with wounds of mixed etiology. Thus, a comprehensive assessment and accurate synthesis of the assessment data are critical to positive outcomes and must be based on vascular assessment parameters, sensorimotor parameters, pain pattern, and the location and characteristics of the ulcer. Treatment is then based on primary etiology, with modifications as indicated based on contributing factors and comorbidities. Whenever the wound etiology is unclear, or for wounds that are refractory to initial management, appropriate referrals are mandatory.

CASE STUDY

A 67-year-old black female referred to wound clinic for nonhealing ulcer of left leg.

Relevant medical history: type 2 diabetes mellitus × 20 years currently managed with Glucotrol XL and diet; last HbA_{1C} 7.2; hypertension managed with Lotensin; no history of cardiac or cerebrovascular disease; history of "blood clot in the left leg" following cholecystectomy 2 years ago

Social history: lives alone; cognitively intact; no tobacco or alcohol abuse

Vascular assessment: no elevational pallor or dependent rubor; pulses palpable but somewhat diminished; ABI on right 0.84; ABI on left 0.76; 2+ edema left leg; capillary refill 3 seconds bilaterally

Sensorimotor assessment: no response to 5.07 monofilament on either foot; hammertoes 2nd to 4th toes bilaterally; marked callus first metatarsal heads bilaterally; dry feet

Pain assessment: minimal in AM; worse at end of day; described as "aching"; relieved by elevation and ibuprofen; also reports occasional "burning" pain in legs at night

Ulcer assessment: location medial malleolus left leg; 8.5 cm × 6.6 cm × 0.0 cm; ulcer bed 80% red and 20% yellow film; large amounts serous exudate; surrounding skin macerated

DATA ANALYSIS

- "+" risk factors for arterial, venous, and neuropathic
- Ulcer location/characteristics, volume of exudate, and pain pattern consistent with venous
- "Standard" management venous ulcer: compression + elevation (surgery?)
- Review of vascular assessment data to rule out contraindications to compression: ABI <0.8 but >0.5 so need modified ("light") compression
- Topical therapy: need protection for periwound skin and absorptive antimicrobial dressing (e.g., alginate and/or foam with silver or other antimicrobial) + light compression
- Review of sensorimotor assessment: needs aggressive "foot care" education, correctly fitted footwear, tight glucose control, careful daily inspection, and dermal temperature checks to prevent neuropathic ulcers

REFERENCES

Jones, J. E., Nelson, E. A., & Al-Hity, A. (2013). Skin grafting for venous leg ulcers: Update of Cochrane Database. *Cochrane Database of Systematic Reviews, 1*, CDOO1737.

Markova, A., & Mostow, E. (2012). US skin disease assessment: Ulcer and wound care. *Dermatologic Clinics, 30*(1), 107–111.

Wound Ostomy Continence Nurses Society. (2014). *Guideline for management of wounds in patients with lower extremity arterial disease.* Mt. Laurel, NJ: WOCN Society.

Wound Ostomy Continence Nurses Society. (2012). *Guideline for management of wounds in patients with lower extremity neuropathic disease.* Mt. Laurel, NJ: WOCN Society.

Wound Ostomy Continence Nurses Society. (2011). *Guideline for management of wounds in patients with lower extremity venous disease.* Mt. Laurel, NJ: WOCN Society.

QUESTIONS

1. The wound care nurse assesses a patient for known risk factors for venous insufficiency. These factors include:
A. Coronary artery disease
B. Hyperlipidemia
C. Obesity
D. Diabetes

2. A patient with a leg ulcer describes his pain as a "stinging sensation" that gets worse at night. What type of ulcer would the nurse suspect?
A. Neuropathic
B. Arterial
C. Venous
D. Peripheral

3. Upon assessment of a patient with leg ulcers, the wound care nurse documents venous insufficiency. What is a sign of this condition?
A. Thin, shiny skin
B. Elevational pallor
C. Prolonged capillary refill time
D. Pitting edema

4. The wound care nurse is assessing vibratory sense at the base of a patient's great toe using a tuning fork. This test is used to assess for:
A. Lymphedema
B. Neuropathy
C. Venous deficiency
D. Arterial deficiency

5. The wound care nurse is assessing a wound on the great toe of a patient. The wound presents with a "punched-out appearance with a necrotic wound bed and limited exudate." What type of wound would the nurse most likely document?
A. Neuropathic
B. Arterial
C. Venous
D. Peripheral

6. What is the most common location of neuropathic ulcers?
A. Around the medial malleoli
B. Toes
C. Plantar surfaces
D. Forefoot

7. The wound care nurse is assessing a wound on a patient's ankle that has the appearance of a venous ulcer. Which characteristic would likely be present?
A. Pale wound bed
B. Shallow wound with irregular edges
C. Minimal exudate
D. Necrotic wound bed

8. What pain pattern would most likely be assessed in a patient with an arterial wound?
A. Dull, aching, heavy
B. Pins and needles
C. Cramping, throbbing
D. Burning, electric shock

9. In which type of ulcer would callus (possibly macerated) be a common associated finding?
A. Neuropathic
B. Arterial
C. Venous
D. Peripheral

10. A patient presents with an ischemic ulcer complicated by venous insufficiency and pitting edema. The wound is covered with dry eschar, and there are no signs of infection. What would be an initial management strategy for this patient?
A. Moist wound healing
B. Vascular consult
C. Therapeutic-level compression therapy
D. Prophylactic antibiotics

ANSWERS: 1.**C**, 2.**A**, 3.**D**, 4.**B**, 5.**B**, 6.**C**, 7.**B**, 8.**C**, 9.**A**, 10.**B**

CHAPTER 25

Atypical Lower Extremity Wounds

Barbara Pieper

OBJECTIVES

1. Describe critical parameters to be included in the assessment of an individual with a lower extremity ulcer.
2. Use assessment data to determine causative and contributing factors for a lower extremity ulcer and to develop individualized management plans that are evidence based.
3. Identify indications that a lower extremity ulcer is "atypical" and requires additional diagnostic workup and/or medical–surgical intervention.
4. Describe pathology, clinical presentation, and management for each of the following: vasculitic ulcers, pyoderma gangrenosum, calciphylaxis, sickle cell ulcer, basal cell carcinoma, squamous cell carcinoma, and factitious ulcers.

Topic Outline

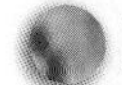 Introduction

As discussed in previous chapters, the most common types of lower extremity ulcers are venous ulcers, neuropathic ulcers, and arterial (ischemic) ulcers. However, there are a number of other pathologic conditions that can result in lower extremity ulcers, and the most common of those conditions are the focus of this chapter, that is, vasculitis, sickle cell disease, pyoderma gangrenosum (PG), calciphylaxis, squamous and basal cell carcinoma, and factitious ulcers. While these ulcers are often considered less common, Tang et al. (2012) examined 350 wound biopsies sent for diagnoses to a wound pathology service and found that 29.7% were "atypical" causes. The majority of the specimens were neoplasms with the most common being squamous cell carcinoma; neoplasms were followed by PG and vasculitis (Tang et al., 2012). Effective management of the wounds presented in this chapter primarily involves treatment of the underlying condition versus specific dressings used for wound care; thus, the focus is on the pathology, clinical presentation, diagnosis, and management of the underlying pathology.

CLINICAL PEARL

A number of lower extremity ulcers are caused by pathologies other than venous, arterial, and neuropathic disease; thus, the wound nurse must always be alert to indicators of atypical wounds and must complete a thorough assessment in order to identify etiology.

 Vasculitis and Ulceration

Prevalence and Incidence

Vasculitis is an autoimmune connective tissue disease that leads to inflammation and potential damage to vital organs (Brown, 2012) and is characterized by damage or destruction of blood vessels. Cutaneous and systemic vasculitis is uncommon, and there are limited epidemiologic data. The estimated annual incidence of cutaneous vasculitis is reported as 38.6 cases per million (de Araujo & Kirsner, 2001). Some authors state that it is more common in women (de Araujo & Kirsner, 2001); others say it appears more commonly in men than in women, although women are diagnosed at a younger age (Brown, 2012). Authors agree that vasculitis is more common among older individuals, and Brown specifies 65 to 74 as the most common age range (Brown, 2012; de Araujo & Kirsner, 2001).

The nomenclature for vasculitis can be confusing. Vasculitis is defined as an autoimmune connective tissue inflammatory disease that targets blood vessels. In contrast, vasculopathy is a noninflammatory condition characterized by excessive thrombus formation in the microcirculation (Kerk & Goerge, 2013a, 2013b). In some conditions, the terms are used interchangeably; for example, livedoid vasculopathy, also called livedoid vasculitis, is characterized by painful purpuric lesions of the lower extremities that frequently ulcerate and leave white, stellate atrophic scars (atrophie blanche) with dyspigmentation and telangiectasia (de Araujo & Kirsner, 2001; Kerk & Goerge, 2013a, 2013b). Although livedoid vasculitis clinically resembles a vasculitis, it is a vasculopathy, not a vasculitis; namely, it is a thrombotic phenomenon without inflammation.

Pathology

The etiology of vasculitis is most likely multifactorial, with a combination of predisposing factors and triggering factors. Predisposing factors include genetic makeup, ethnicity, environmental exposure, and gender (de Araujo & Kirsner, 2001), while triggering factors include infectious causes (most common), drugs (about 10% of cases), malignancy (less common and most likely to involve lymphoproliferative malignancies), connective tissue diseases, and cryoprotein disorders, among others. In some patients, the definitive etiologic agent for cutaneous vasculitis cannot be identified.

Vasculitis may be recurrent or intermittent with new lesions appearing over time (Brown, 2012; de Araujo & Kirsner, 2001). Because of similarities to other clinical conditions, histologic confirmation is essential (de Araujo & Kirsner, 2001). de Araujo and Kirsner (2001) note that cutaneous vasculitis involves the postcapillary venules and is characterized by the following: endothelial cell swelling, neutrophilic invasion of blood vessel walls, presence of disrupted neutrophils (often called leukocytoclasia), extravasation of red blood cells (RBCs), and fibrinoid necrosis of the blood vessel walls. This constellation of findings is known as cutaneous necrotizing vasculitis.

For further information on the etiology and pathology of vasculitis, the reader is referred to the American College of Rheumatology website (http://www.rheumatology.org/Practice/Clinical/Patients/Diseases_And_Conditions/Vasculitis/) as well as the BSR and BHPR Guideline for the Management of Adults with ANCA-associated Vasculitis (Ntatsaki et al., 2014).

Clinical Presentation

Vasculitis commonly presents as palpable purpura (raised areas of nonblanchable erythema), which signifies extravasation of RBCs outside of the blood vessel into the surrounding tissue (de Araujo & Kirsner, 2001). The clinical presentation varies and may include red macules, wheals, papules, nodules, ulcers, vesicles, and blisters (de Araujo & Kirsner, 2001). The size of the blood vessel affected determines the clinical picture; for example, if large vessels are affected, the lesions may be widespread. The lesions are most commonly located on the lower legs and are symmetrical but can occur anywhere on the body. Some cutaneous lesions may heal quickly (in 1 to 4 weeks), but ulcerative lesions frequently have a prolonged healing course. Scarring and hyperpigmentation may occur (de Araujo & Kirsner, 2001). Figure 25-1 shows a vasculitic ulcer on the lower extremity with purpura and necrosis.

The severity of the disease process can be assessed with the Birmingham Vasculitis Activity Score (BVAS) (http://www.epsnetwork.co.uk/BVAS/bvas_flow.html); currently in use is version 3 (Suppiah et al., 2011). The scale is divided into sections reflecting new-onset or worsening disease in

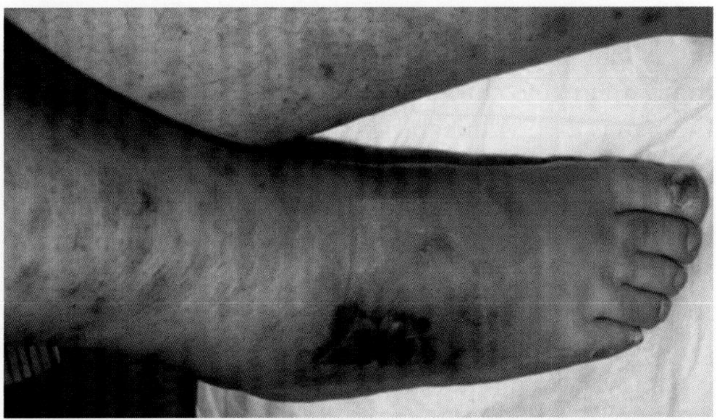

FIGURE 25-1. A vasculitic ulceration that has occurred in a patient who has leukocytoclastic vasculitis. (Reprinted with permission from Goodheart, H. P. (2003). *Goodheart's photoguide of common skin disorders* (2nd ed.). Philadelphia, PA: Lippincott Williams & Wilkins.)

nine organ systems: general, cutaneous, mucous membrane/eyes, ENT, chest, and the cardiovascular, abdominal, renal, and nervous system. A total score is calculated and is used to guide treatment decisions and other disease activity assessments (Mukhtyar et al., 2009).

Diagnosis

Diagnosis of vasculitis lesions begins by eliminating other causes/conditions, namely with a thorough history, physical examination, and laboratory data. The aim is to identify the triggering factor if possible and to determine the presence and severity of organ system involvement (Brown, 2012; de Araujo & Kirsner, 2001). Some of the laboratory tests include antinuclear antibodies, complement levels, cryoglobulins, antistreptolysin O antibodies, hemocult testing, antibodies for viral hepatitis, rheumatoid factor, and urinalysis to assess for renal involvement. Various radiographs may be done to diagnose respiratory tract or neurologic disease. A biopsy of the lesion for histological evaluation is crucial. Even if the patient is known to have a condition associated with vasculitis, the clinician cannot assume that the ulcer is due to vasculitis; a thorough workup and histologic evaluation must always be performed. For example, Seitz et al. (2010) examined the causative factors for leg ulcers in 36 persons with rheumatoid arthritis and found the following: 3 patients had necrotizing vasculitis, 2 had PG, 8 had venous ulcers, 4 had arterial ulcers, 3 had combined venous/arterial ulcers, 5 had pressure ulcers, and 11 were due to other causes. These findings underscore the fact that vasculitic ulcers are less common and that a thorough workup is necessary to determine the cause of the patient's wound.

CLINICAL PEARL

Vasculitic ulcers are acutely painful wounds that require treatment with anti-inflammatory medications; diagnosis is based on clinical assessment, laboratory studies, and biopsy.

Management

If a triggering factor for vasculitis is identified, initial management should focus on management of that disease process or triggering agent. If the disease process involves multiple organ systems, the management approach must address all involved systems. Disease limited to the skin may require only treatment of the skin lesions and is based on the characteristics of the lesions. For example, lower extremity lesions accompanied by edema may necessitate leg elevation and compression in addition to topical therapy. If the disease process and/or lesions are widespread, systemic corticosteroids may be used; the dose of corticosteroids is determined by the severity of the disease activity. Sometimes corticosteroids are combined with other immunosuppressive agents (such as cyclophosphamide). Other immunosuppressive therapies may be used depending upon the number of organ systems involved, relapse rates, and side effect profile (Brown, 2012).

In discussing vasculitis in general, Brown (2012) presented the following as priorities for nursing management: (a) general patient education and information about vasculitis; (b) information and discussion regarding medication regimens; (c) discussion of side effects of medications and implications for monitoring and reporting; (d) assessment for complications of drug therapy, to include blood work monitoring; (e) provision of information about patient support groups; (f) advice regarding self-care such as regular exercise, rest, and positive life style choices; (g) informed consent and patient agreement to adhere to complex drug regimens; (h) involvement of family and friends in care if the patient desires; (i) if vasculitis affects work, advice regarding how to inform the work environment; (j) measures to promote quality of life; and (k) advice as to when the patient should seek advice and support. If the person with vasculitis has open wounds, the dressing should be selected to fit the area of the body involved, to manage any exudate and maintain a moist surface, and to prevent traumatic removal by limiting the application of adhesive to the skin. The dressing should be one that the patient can apply, and the patient's insurance coverage for the dressing needs to be considered. Some patients experience marked pain with vasculitis. Pain should be treated with appropriate analgesics taking into consideration the patient's overall health status and prescribed medications.

Sickle Cell Ulcers

Prevalence and Incidence

Sickle cell disease is a single amino acid molecular disorder of hemoglobin that leads to a number of pathological changes; these include changes in the shape and rigidity of the RBC that cause obstruction of the microcirculation with subsequent tissue ischemia and infarction (Kato et al., 2009; Minniti et al., 2010). Sickle cell disease is the most common inherited hematologic disorder and is chronic (Jenerette et al., 2014). It affects about 100,000 persons in the United States with most of them being African American (Hassell, 2010). Leg ulcers are a common and often disabling complication of sickle cell disease; interestingly, the first patient described with sickle cell disease in the United States in 1910 had leg ulcers (Minniti et al., 2010). The prevalence of leg ulcers varies, but they are uncommon in children <10 years of age (Minniti et al., 2010). There is insufficient evidence to link sickle cell trait with leg ulcers (Tsaras et al., 2009).

Pathology

As noted, sickle cell disease is a genetic disorder involving abnormal hemoglobin. A child born with sickle cell disease has two genes for hemoglobin S, one from each parent. The abnormal hemoglobin causes RBCs to develop a crescent (sickle) shape and to become stiff and sticky; these altered RBCs are unable to pass normally through the smaller blood vessels and instead obstruct the blood vessels, thus causing acute ischemia of the involved tissues or organs. In contrast to sickle cell disease (designated as HbSS to indicate two genes for hemoglobin S), the child born with sickle cell trait has only one abnormal gene; the other hemoglobin gene is normal (HbAS). These children do not develop sickle cell disease, but they can pass the sickle cell gene on to their children. There is also a condition known as HbSC, which is a more common and milder sickling disorder associated with lower incidence of complications such as leg ulcers (Madu et al., 2013).

The pathology of sickle cell anemia is marked by repeated episodes of vascular occlusion, reperfusion injury, hypoxemia, and vascular inflammation (Jenerette et al., 2014). This process results in unpredictable episodes of "sickle cell crisis"; these episodes are acutely painful and may result in organ or tissue damage due to the ischemic nature of the underlying pathology. Leg ulcers are more common in patients with homozygous sickle cell disease (HbSS) and less common in those with the milder HbSC disease (Delaney et al., 2013; Minniti et al., 2010). The geographic distribution of leg ulcers among patients with sickle cell disease varies as well; for example, 75% of patients with sickle cell disease (HbSS) in Jamaica have leg ulcers, while only 8% to 10% of patients with sickle cell disease in North America are affected with leg ulcers (Minniti et al., 2010).

The pathogenesis of leg ulcers in sickle cell disease is complex and includes a combination of factors: vascular obstruction by dense sickled red cells, venous incompetence, bacterial infections, excessive vasoconstriction when in a dependent position, in situ thrombosis, anemia resulting in decreased oxygen carrying capacity, and decreased nitric acid bioavailability (Minniti et al., 2010). Nitric oxide (NO) is produced by the endothelium and is a critical regulator of normal vascular function and vasodilation (Kato et al., 2009). Intravascular hemolysis, such as occurs during sickle cell crises, releases hemoglobin into the plasma, and hemoglobin acts as a potent scavenger of NO. Chronic NO depletion may contribute to vasoconstriction and further tissue ischemia (Kato et al., 2009; Morris, 2008). Sickle cell ulcers may be caused by an acute ischemic episode or by minor trauma to chronically ischemic tissues; any break in the skin is then vulnerable to secondary infection.

Minniti et al. (2014) examined the microcirculation of the tissues in and around sickle cell leg ulcers. They found the highest blood flow within the ulcer bed with reduced blood flow in the immediate periwound area. They also found evidence of venous stasis, inflammation, and thrombotic changes that were consistent with the pathology of chronic venous ulcers in non–sickle cell disease individuals.

Clinical Presentation

Sickle cell ulcers usually occur in areas with minimal subcutaneous tissue, thin skin, and decreased blood flow. The most common sites are the medial and lateral malleoli of the lower leg (Minniti et al., 2010) (Fig. 25-2). Less common sites include the anterior tibia, dorsum of the foot, and Achilles tendon. The ulcers are typically painful, indolent, intractable, and very slow to heal. Having a sickle cell leg ulcer is also associated with priapism and pulmonary hypertension, and all are markers of advanced sickle vasculopathy (Minniti et al., 2010).

CLINICAL PEARL

Sickle cell ulcers are painful ulcers that are very slow to heal, prone to recurrence, and commonly associated with venous insufficiency; management involves moist wound healing, edema management, and pain control.

Halabi-Tawi et al. (2008) presented a 20-case series of patients with sickle cell anemia and current or past leg ulcers; they completed chart reviews, interviewed the patients, and conducted clinical examinations. The clinical

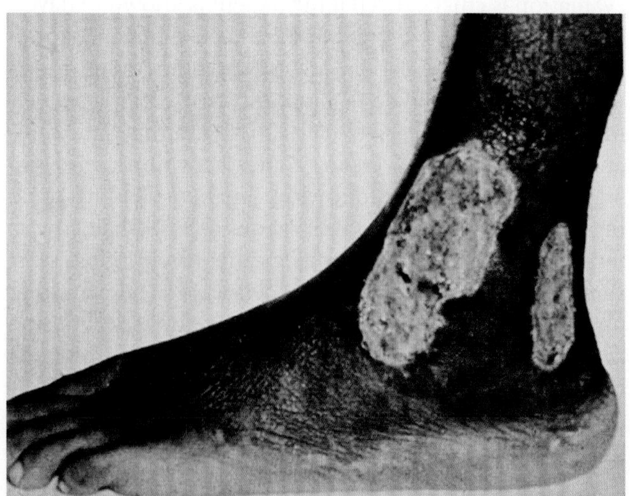

FIGURE 25-2. Chronic leg ulcers in an adult patient with sickle cell anemia (SCA). (Reprinted with permission from Greer, J. P., et al. (2013). *Wintrobe's clinical hematology* (13th ed.). Philadelphia, PA: Wolters Kluwer Health.)

features they identified included: median ulcer area, 12 cm^2; median ulcer time, 29.5 months; 85% had local/regional infection; 50% had ankle stiffness; 85% had mood disorders; and median age of ulcer onset was 21 years. These patients had many additional physical conditions such as priapism in 50% of males; acute chest syndrome, 50%; proteinuria, 35%; retinopathy, 30%; osteonecrosis, 30%; pulmonary hypertension, 22%; and stroke, 10%.

Diagnosis

The diagnosis is generally made based on the history of sickle cell disease and the clinical presentation (Madu et al., 2013). As with any ulceration, a biopsy may be done to rule out other causes.

Management

Management involves treatment of the underlying disease process, pain control, and topical therapy based on ulcer characteristics. Systemic treatment commonly involves either hydroxyurea, which increases the production of fetal (normal) hemoglobin, or blood transfusions to temporarily correct anemia and provide normal RBCs (Delaney et al., 2013). Current data indicate that pain is an issue for most patients; Halabi-Tawi and colleagues found that 90% of patients needed analgesics for management of ulcer pain, and many used more than one type of analgesic. Topical therapy is based on the principles addressed throughout this text: establishment of a clean wound bed, management of exudate, maintenance of a moist wound bed, and protection from infection and trauma. Because venous insufficiency is common in patients with sickle cell ulcers, compression wraps are commonly indicated. Debridement is essential if there is necrotic tissue, and osteomyelitis should be ruled out whenever a wound is slow to heal. Studies indicate that systemic infection, amputation, and death due to leg ulcers are uncommon in patients with sickle cell disease (Minniti et al., 2010).

A variety of treatment strategies have been suggested for nonhealing sickle cell ulcers, including skin grafts, hyperbaric oxygen therapy, arginine butyrate, growth factor therapy, zinc sulfate, and herbal agents; however, Minniti et al. (2010) concluded that there has been little improvement in the efficacy of management and clinical outcome in leg ulcers related to sickle cell disease over the last 100 years. Similarly, Marti-Carvajal et al. (2012) performed a Cochrane review of six randomized controlled trials including 198 participants with 250 ulcers related to sickle cell disease. Four of the studies were done in Jamaica and two in the United States. Study treatments included topical agents to the ulcer and systemic medications. The authors concluded that the evidence for use of interventions to treat people with sickle cell ulcers is not strong and all trials had a high risk of bias.

Obviously, a primary goal of management for individuals with sickle cell disease is ulcer prevention. This involves overall disease management, to reduce the incidence of vasoocclusive episodes, and prevention of trauma, which is commonly the precipitating factor for ulcer development. Prevention strategies include use of protective wraps, shin guards, or orthotic devices, especially during activities that could cause injury to the lower leg; strict avoidance of venipunctures to the lower extremity; and management of venous insufficiency and edema (Minniti et al., 2010).

Pyoderma Gangrenosum

Prevalence and Incidence

PG is a rare chronic inflammatory skin disease that affects 3 to 10 patients per million population per year. It typically begins with an acutely painful nodule or pustule that breaks down to form a progressively enlarging ulcer (Ruocco et al., 2009). It can occur at any age but is most common between 20 and 50 years of age and is slightly more common among women than among men. About 50% of patients have coexisting systemic inflammatory diseases, with the most common being inflammatory bowel disease (ulcerative colitis and Crohn's disease); about 2% to 12% of patients with PG also have IBD. Other inflammatory conditions that have been associated with PG include arthritis (seronegative arthritis, spondylitis of inflammatory bowel disease, and rheumatoid arthritis) and lymphoproliferative disorders (myelogenous leukemia, hairy cell leukemia, myelofibrosis, and monoclonal gammopathy) (Ratnagobal & Sinha, 2013; Ruocco et al., 2009). The mortality rate for pyoderma can be as high as 30%; negative prognostic indicators include male gender, advanced age at onset, and bullous PG associated with malignant hematologic conditions.

Pathology

Although the etiology is unknown and the pathogenesis not well understood, PG does not appear to be an infectious process as was theorized in 1930 and is not associated with lymphangitis or lymphadenopathy (Ruocco et al., 2009). Because it is associated with systemic conditions with a suspected autoimmune pathogenesis, the most commonly held theory is that it represents an autoimmune process targeting the skin. Another theory suggests that PG is caused by a dysfunction of the neutrophils, specifically either a hyperreactive response or a defect in chemotaxis (Wollina, 2007). However, the disease is idiopathic in 25% to 50% of patients, underscoring the fact that we do not yet understand either the etiology or the pathology of PG (Fraccalvieri et al., 2012; Ratnagobal & Sinha, 2013; Ruocco et al., 2009).

Clinical Presentation

The hallmark of PG is an ulcer with a raised dusty red or violaceous (purplish) border that is inflamed and frequently undermined and a boggy, necrotic base (Ruocco et al., 2009) (Fig. 25-3). The base may appear perforated, and light pressure frequently produces purulent drainage. There is typically a bright halo of erythema extending about 2 cm from the ulcer border.

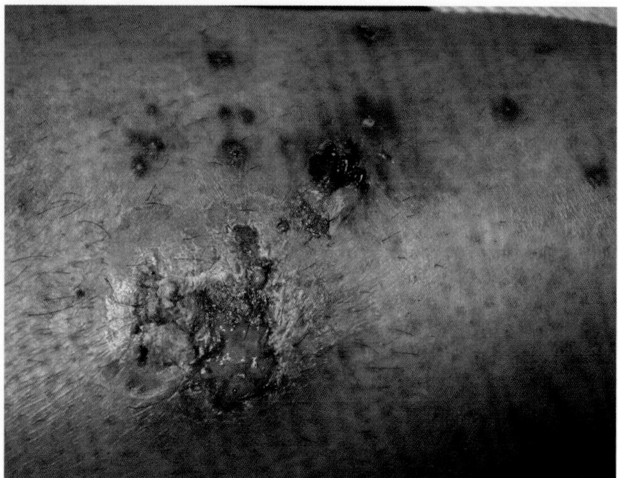

FIGURE 25-3. Pyoderma gangrenosum, with early pustules and ulcerations on the shin. (Reprinted with permission from Gorroll, A. H., & Mulley, A. G. (2009). *Primary care medicine* (6th ed.). Philadelphia, PA: Wolters Kluwer Health.)

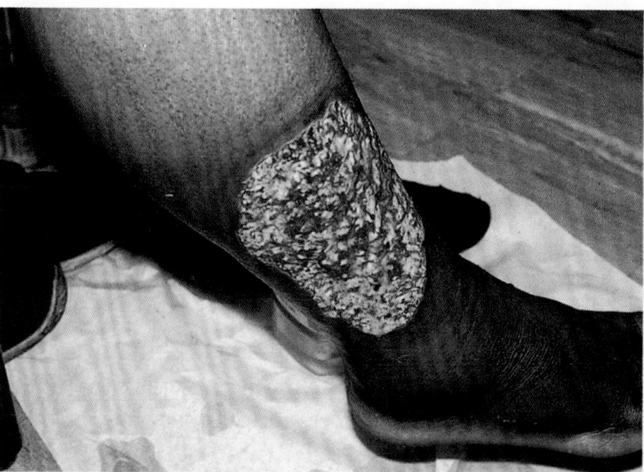

FIGURE 25-4. This large pyoderma gangrenosum ulceration is located on the lower extremity and shows beginning healing with a crater-like (cribriform) scar. (Reprinted with permission from Goodheart, H. P. (2003). *Goodheart's photoguide of common skin disorders* (2nd ed.). Philadelphia, PA: Lippincott Williams & Wilkins.)

CLINICAL PEARL

Pyoderma gangrenosum ulcers are caused by an autoimmune process that causes full-thickness skin loss; the ulcers are painful and may exhibit pathergy (acute exacerbation in response to minor trauma).

The ulcer starts as a deep, painful nodule or a superficial hemorrhagic pustule; it may develop spontaneously or in response to minimal trauma (Ruocco et al., 2009). Ulcers often expand rapidly in one direction and slowly in another resulting in a serpiginous pattern. Ulcers can enlarge through extension of the undermined border or through development of new hemorrhagic pustules, either singular or multiple. PG ulcers can be confined to the dermis but often extend into the fat or fascia. Although they can develop on any area of the body, the ulcers most commonly occur on the lower extremities or trunk (Fig. 25-4).

The progression and long-term outcome of PG are unpredictable. The clinical course may involve an explosive onset and rapid spread of the lesions or an indolent progression with gradually spreading ulcers. In the explosive version, the individual usually experiences pain, fever, hemorrhagic blisters with purulent drainage, extensive necrosis, and a soggy ulcer border with a marked inflammatory halo. The indolent version is characterized by slowly enlarging and acutely painful ulcers that frequently exhibit granulation tissue within the ulcer bed and crusting and hyperkeratosis at the border (Ruocco et al., 2009). The ulcers may heal in one area, only to recur in the same area or at another site. Trauma, either accidental trauma or surgical trauma, may precipitate ulcer development; this is known as Koebner's phenomenon. In addition, even minor trauma can precipitate an exacerbation of existing lesions, a phenomenon known as pathergy.

PG has variant forms, one of which is peristomal and is classified as a rare subset, accounting for 0.6% of peristomal skin problems (Hanley, 2011; Ruocco et al., 2009). Patients with ulcerative colitis or Crohn's disease who have undergone ileostomy or colostomy are potentially at risk for peristomal PG. The lesions appear in the peristomal area 2 months to 25 years after the surgery and may be triggered or worsened by trauma to the skin from leakage of stool or adhesive trauma caused by repetitive removal of the appliance.

Diagnosis

The diagnosis is based primarily on the history and clinical presentation. A detailed history is important to rule out other potential causes of the skin lesions and to determine if there is a treatable associated systemic disorder. A biopsy is typically done to rule out other causes such as malignancy, vasculitis, and infection. The histopathologic findings are nonspecific and include an undermined ulcer border with edema, neutrophilic inflammation, and engorgement and thrombosis of small and medium blood vessels; neutrophilic inflammation is the cytologic hallmark (Ratnagobal & Sinha, 2013; Ruocco et al., 2009). Other studies may be indicated to rule out associated systemic disorders; for example, laboratory studies may be done to rule out hematologic malignancies and arthritis syndromes, and colonoscopy should be done for the patient who has signs and symptoms of inflammatory bowel disease.

Management

Treatment is empiric since the etiology and pathology of PG are not well understood (Ruocco et al., 2009). Treatment is dependent upon the severity of the lesions, associated diseases, overall health status of the patient, and risk of prolonged treatment. Goals of care are to (a) reduce inflammation and promote healing; (b) reduce pain; and (c) control any underlying disease process, while minimizing adverse effects (Ruocco et al., 2009). Systemic corticosteroids and cyclosporine are effective, but the severity of the PG lesions must justify the risks of using these medications. Effective treatment of the underlying systemic disease (when present) usually results in healing or improvement of the ulcers.

Although debridement may be needed to eliminate necrosis and prevent bacterial overgrowth, invasive surgical debridement is discouraged as it may trigger new lesions (Ruocco et al., 2009); autolytic or enzymatic debridement is a much safer approach for these patients. Should surgery be required for a patient with a history of PG, the surgeon should always be made aware so that he or she can limit the size of incisions and can make every attempt to minimize tissue trauma. Some surgeons use prophylactic systemic corticosteroids or cyclosporine perioperatively to reduce the risk of development of PG ulcers.

Systemic treatment is usually needed to control the inflammatory process, and corticosteroids are often considered the gold standard in treatment (Ratnagobal & Sinha, 2013). Doses may be initially high (e.g., 100 to 200 mg/day of prednisone) in order to establish remission; pulsed therapy with methylprednisone 1 g/day for 5 consecutive days is another approach that is frequently used. Guidelines are lacking on the frequency or timing of pulse doses (Sinha & Bagga, 2008). Once the inflammation is under control, the dose can be tapered. Any patient being treated with corticosteroids must be monitored and treated for the side effects of steroid therapy. Alternatives to corticosteroid therapy include other anti-inflammatory drugs, such as sulfasalazine, dapsone, and sulfapyridine; these drugs may be given as solo therapy or may be given in combination with corticosteroids. Other systemic agents mentioned in the literature include steroid-sparing immunosuppressives, cyclosporine, methotrexate, intravenous immunoglobulins, and infliximab (Agarwal & Andrews, 2013; Ratnagobal & Sinha, 2013; Ruocco et al., 2009; Wollina, 2007).

Local therapy includes dressings to manage the exudate and maintain a moist wound bed; antimicrobial dressings are sometimes used to control bacterial loads and reduce inflammation. Because pain is a major issue for these patients, dressings should provide for atraumatic removal; around the clock analgesics may be needed as well. Topical and intralesional corticosteroids have also been used (Ruocco et al., 2009).

When PG lesions are located adjacent to a stoma, the wound ostomy continence nurse needs to consider both treatment of the ulcers and fit of the ostomy appliance. Topical agents should provide for exudate management and should be applied in accordance with manufacturers' recommendations. Although a convex appliance may improve the pouch seal and help to prevent leakage of effluent, the associated peristomal pressure may exacerbate the peristomal PG; thus, a flexible version may be needed as opposed to a rigid product (Hanley, 2011). The contracted, cribriform scarring that results from healing of peristomal PG necessitates careful appliance selection (Hanley, 2011).

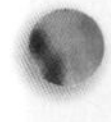 Calciphylaxis (Calcific Uremic Arteriolopathy)

Prevalence and Incidence

Calciphylaxis, also called calcific uremic arteriolopathy, occurs most commonly in patients with chronic kidney disease on hemodialysis, though it has also been reported in nonuremic individuals. The reported annual incidence among individuals with chronic kidney disease is 1% and the prevalence is 4%, but there are concerns that these numbers may rise as a result of the increasing prevalence of chronic kidney disease in the United States (Feeser, 2011; Hayashi, 2013; Markova et al., 2012; Ross, 2011). Calciphylaxis is more common in women and Caucasians; obesity, diabetes, hypercoagulability, warfarin therapy, hyperparathyroidism, hypoalbuminemia, and trauma are additional risk factors (Vedvyas et al., 2012). The mean age of patients is 48 years (Markova et al., 2012), and the disease is associated with severe pain and a 2-year mortality rate of 50% to 80% (Meissner et al., 2006; Ong & Coulson, 2012; Ross, 2011). Risk of mortality is affected by the site of the calciphylaxis lesions; proximal disease (lesions affecting the abdomen, thighs, and buttocks) is associated with a higher mortality rate than distal disease (lesions affecting the lower limbs) (Vedvyas et al., 2012).

Pathology

The pathogenesis of calciphylaxis is unclear and controversial (Hayashi, 2013). Contributing factors seem to include hypercalcemia, hyperphosphatemia, and high calcium–phosphate product levels, and these findings have led to recommendations that patients with chronic kidney disease may benefit from low-calcium dialysate and careful attention to both calcium and phosphorus levels. Histopathologic findings in patients with active disease include intimal proliferation, medial calcification, and thrombosis of the small vessels in the dermis and subcutaneous tissue and calcium deposits in the soft tissues; these pathologic changes cause progressive tissue ischemia and subcutaneous tissue necrosis (Hayashi, 2013; Markova et al., 2012; Meissner et al., 2006; Vedvyas et al., 2012).

Clinical Presentation

As noted, calciphylaxis is characterized by thrombosis of the small vessels in the dermis and subcutaneous fat leading to cutaneous ischemia, tissue infarction, and necrosis (Markova et al., 2012; Meissner et al., 2006). The lesions are described as violaceous (purple-hued) reticulated plaques progressing to nonhealing, deep, stellate (star-shaped) ulcers that usually become gangrenous (Markova et al., 2012) (Fig. 25-5). They are extremely painful, and pain management may be the patient's greatest concern. The most common location is the lower leg, but lesions

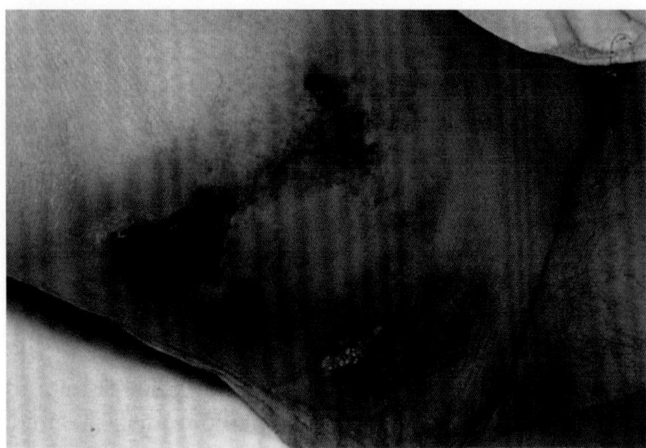

FIGURE 25-5. This calciphylaxis leg ulcer presented on an elderly female with end-stage renal disease and elevated parathyroid hormone level; she developed widespread induration of the lower extremities, which led to purpuric and necrotic ulcerations.

can also occur on the abdomen, buttocks, thighs, pannus, breasts, and penis; there may be internal organ involvement as well. Lesions are usually multiple. The ulcers predispose the patient to secondary infection and sepsis, which are contributing factors to the high mortality rate associated with this disease (Meissner et al., 2006).

CLINICAL PEARL

Calciphylaxis is commonly seen in patients with renal failure; effective management requires treatment of the underlying disease process, measures to prevent and manage infection, and pain control.

Diagnosis

There is no single definitive diagnostic study for calciphylaxis; the diagnosis is based primarily on the patient's history and clinical manifestations and supported by laboratory values (e.g., elevated calcium, phosphorus, and calcium–phosphorus product levels) (Feeser, 2011). The differential diagnosis must rule out other conditions that result in painful necrotic skin ulcers, such as diabetic gangrene, skin necrosis due to heparin-induced thrombocytopenia, warfarin skin necrosis, scleroderma, and PG (Hayashi, 2013; Ng & Peng, 2011). Hayashi (2013) proposed diagnosis based on the following: on hemodialysis for chronic kidney disease or glomerular filtration rate (GFR) of <15 mL/min/173 m^2 and the presence of painful, nontreatable skin ulcers with concomitant painful purpura. Feeser (2011) suggested the use of various noninvasive radiographic techniques and ultrasonography to detect vessel calcification and the presence of calciphylaxis lesions. Both Feeser and Hayashi recommend biopsy only if necessary to confirm the diagnosis since it is invasive and can potentially cause worsening of the skin lesions. When biopsy is done, a wedge biopsy may be preferred to a punch biopsy to assure adequate sampling (Markova et al., 2012). Biopsy findings include (a) calcific deposits in the medial layer of small to medium blood vessels of the reticular dermis and subcutaneous fat, (b) intramural fibrin thrombi in the dermis and subcutaneous tissue, and (c) lobular fat necrosis with increased neutrophils, lymphocytes, and foamy histiocytes (Markova et al., 2012; Ong & Coulson, 2012).

Management

There are few effective treatments, and at present, care is primarily supportive. Ross (2011) noted that traditional care has focused on management of the calcium–phosphate–PTH axis: minimizing calcium intake and use of calcimimetics, cautious use of vitamin D supplements, strict phosphate control, and, if necessary, surgical parathyroidectomy. Other suggested strategies include: (a) avoidance of trauma (e.g., avoidance of subcutaneous injections, skin trauma, biopsies); (b) avoidance of warfarin and use of alternative anticoagulants; (c) systemic management to include aggressive pain control, treatment of sepsis, anemia management, and appropriate nutrition; and (d) meticulous wound care, to include strategies for optimizing perfusion and preventing hypotension. In general, instrumental debridement should be avoided due to the risk of poor healing, though limited evidence supports surgical debridement for selected patients (Vedvyas et al., 2012). Some authors recommend hyperbaric oxygen therapy, noting that HBOT may improve tissue oxygenation and may help to prevent wound infection (Feeser, 2011; Meissner et al., 2006; Ross, 2011). Local or systemic corticosteroids are not used (Hayashi, 2013).

Newer approaches to treatment include intravenous sodium thiosulfate (STS) and bisphosphonates (Ross, 2011; Vedvyas et al., 2012). Intravenous STS is thought to improve outcomes for calciphylaxis patients via several mechanisms of action, including antioxidative effects, vasodilation, and chelation. Its ability to promote vasodilation is thought to explain the rapid resolution of pain that has been reported by a number of calciphylaxis patients. STS can also complex with calcium salts to form calcium thiosulfate, which is much more soluble and much easier to clear via hemodialysis. Intravenous STS is administered after a hemodialysis treatment. It has limited use in peritoneal dialysis. Intravenous STS is considered benign and relatively low cost and has been used for more than 70 years as an antidote to poisoning from cyanide and nitrogen mustard compounds (Meissner et al., 2006; Ross, 2011; Vedvyas et al., 2012). Bisphosphonates' mechanisms of action include inhibition of osteoclast activity, mobilization of intravascular calcium, and suppression of inflammatory cytokines, which is thought to be the primary mechanism underlying the rapid pain relief reported by some patients (Ross, 2011; Vedvyas et al., 2012). While FDA guidelines currently recommend that bisphosphonates be avoided in patients with chronic kidney disease, the predominant opinion is that they are cleared effectively through hemodialysis and are therefore probably safe for these patients (Ross, 2011; Vedvyas et al., 2012). Currently, there are no randomized controlled trials to either support or refute the use of STS or bisphosphonates in management of calciphylaxis (Vedvyas et al., 2012).

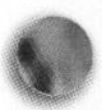

Malignant Wounds: Squamous Cell Carcinoma and Basal Cell Carcinoma

Prevalence and Incidence

Basal cell carcinoma and squamous cell carcinoma are commonly diagnosed nonmelanoma skin cancers, affecting about 1 million Americans each year (Council, 2013). Basal cell carcinoma is the most common form of skin cancer (Schnirring-Judge & Belpedio, 2010). Sun exposure is a critical variable in development of both basal cell and squamous cell carcinoma; a recent meta-analysis documented a significantly higher risk of squamous cell carcinoma among persons who work outdoors and a less significant but increased risk for basal cell carcinoma as well (Fartasch et al., 2012). There is a growing concern about nonmelanoma skin cancers in the elderly because of the increasing numbers of older adults, greater longevity, and the impact of lifetime sun exposure. Other groups at risk for squamous cell carcinoma are immunosuppressed patients, especially those who have received a transplant, and cigarette smokers (Davies, 2009).

Squamous and basal cell skin cancers can also occur in chronic leg ulcers. Performing punch biopsies on 144 patients with 154 chronic leg ulcers, Senet et al. (2012) reported a 10.4% skin cancer frequency in chronic leg ulcers; of the 16 skin cancers, 9 were squamous cell and 5 were basal cell. In this study, factors associated with skin cancer were older age, abnormal excessive granulation tissue at the wound edge, high clinical suspicion of cancer, and number of biopsies (Senet et al., 2012). Chronic wounds can undergo malignant transformation, and these wounds are known as Marjolin's ulcers; while malignant transformation of a leg ulcer remains rare (Schnirring-Judge & Belpedio, 2010), the diagnosis should be considered whenever a leg ulcer presents as a vegetating lesion, which is common for Marjolin's leg ulcers (Combemale et al., 2007). Factors that increase the risk for malignant transformation of a chronic wound include exposure to the cytotoxic by-products of chronic inflammation, impairments in the cell reproduction (mitotic) cycle, epidermal implantation resulting in a dermal foreign body reaction, immunologic factors, and epithelial cell mutations (Schnirring-Judge & Belpedio, 2010; Sharma et al., 2011). Combemale et al. (2007) examined malignant transformation in leg ulcers, 80% of which were venous ulcers. Important findings were abnormal granulation tissue, absence of healing, and unusual patterns of ulcer enlargement/extension. Pathology revealed that 98% of the tumors were squamous cell carcinoma and 82% were very well or well differentiated. The overall death rate was 32% and was higher among patients with lymph node or visceral metastases (Combemale et al., 2007).

Pathology

Ultraviolet (UV) rays in sunlight damage the DNA in skin cells (Davies, 2009). Of the UV types, UVB rays are the most harmful and are the main cause of nonmelanoma skin cancer.

Clinical Presentation

Figure 25-6 provides a comparison of basal cell carcinoma, squamous cell carcinoma, and malignant melanoma. Basal cell carcinoma often appears as a nonhealing sore or a pearly pink papule (Council, 2013) with a rolled, well-rounded border and adjacent crusting (Schnirring-Judge & Belpedio, 2010) (Fig. 25-7). The lesion most typically occurs in a sun-exposed area but can also occur in an area of minimal exposure. Basal cell carcinoma has four subtypes: superficial multifocal, nodular (most common type), morpheaform/infiltrative, and basosquamous (metatypical).

CLINICAL PEARL

SCC and BCC can be mistaken for chronic wounds; a biopsy is indicated for any wound that fails to respond to appropriate therapy.

Squamous cell carcinoma has a precursor state known as actinic keratosis; these lesions appear as scaly pink papules, commonly on the head, face, and dorsal hands/forearms (Council, 2013) (Fig. 25-8). Davies (2009) stated that patients typically describe the lesions as starting as a pimple and increasing in size to a thickened lesion (see Fig. 25-8). On the lip and genitalia, the squamous cell lesion presents as a fissure or small erosion that bleeds, fails to heal, and may be tender (Davies, 2009). Invasive squamous cell carcinoma presents as a nonhealing or wart-like growth. These lesions tend to develop where there is evidence of sun damage, such as thickened, wrinkled skin; hyperkeratotic skin; telangiectasia; and irregular pigmentation (Davies, 2009). About 5% of squamous cell carcinomas metastasize, usually to the nearest lymph node; factors affecting the risk for metastasis include the size of the tumor, rate of growth, and anatomical location (Davies, 2009).

Diagnosis

Tissue biopsy is the gold standard for diagnosis. Schnirring-Judge and Belpedio (2010) stated that the biopsy should be taken from the proximal or leading edge of the wound and should include 50% of wound and 50% adjacent tissue. This is done so the interface between the pathology and surrounding tissue can be described. A second specimen should be taken in the middle of the wound. Specimens need to be carefully labeled and described. The biopsy provides information about the histopathological subtype, degree of differentiation, histologic grade, and presence or absence of perineural vascular or lymphatic invasion

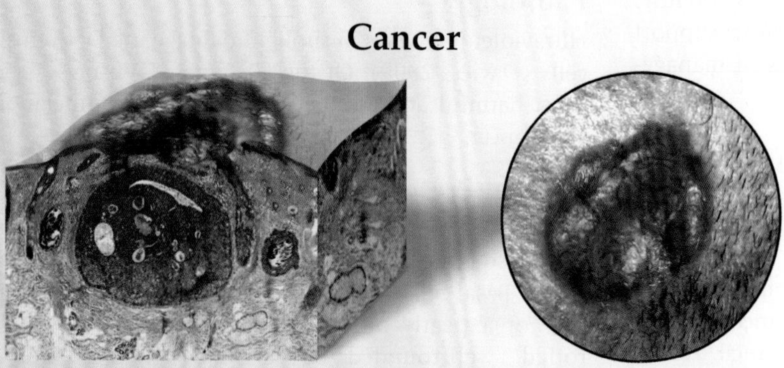

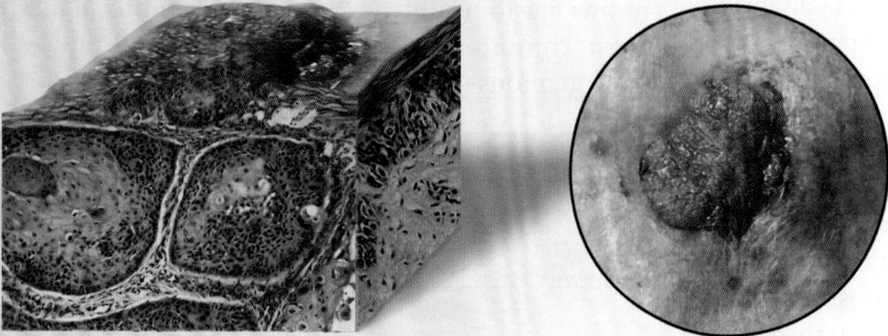

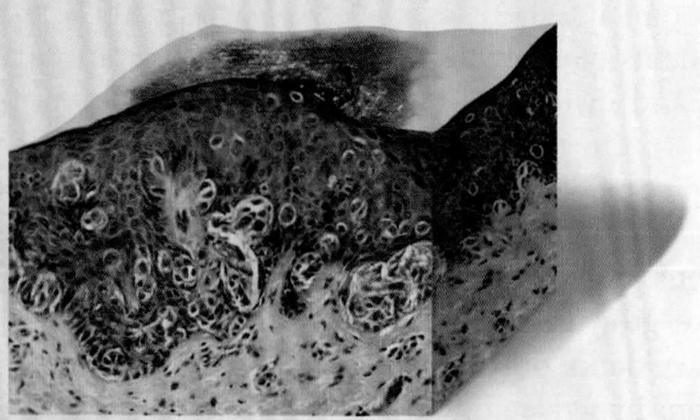

FIGURE 25-6. Comparison of basal cell, squamous cell, and malignant melanoma. (Courtesy Anatomical Chart Company.)

(Momen & Al-Niaimi, 2013). Nonmelanoma skin cancers are staged according to the TNM staging system. Imaging with magnetic resonance imaging (MRI) or computed tomography (CT) is used to assess the anatomical degree of invasion (Momen & Al-Niaimi, 2013).

The differential diagnosis of squamous cell carcinoma includes basal cell carcinoma, malignant melanoma, actinic keratosis, pyogenic granulomas, seborrheic warts, warts, and other wounds (Momen & Al-Niaimi, 2013). Kricker et al. (2014) examined growth rates and patterns for basal and squamous cell carcinomas. Basal cell carcinomas increased in size over time; there was no consistent evidence that squamous cell carcinomas demonstrated progressive enlargement. Larger basal cell carcinomas were independently associated with older age, male gender, no skin checks by a physician, aggressive tumor type, ulceration, and lesions associated with scar tissue, whereas squamous cell carcinoma was associated with male gender, location on an extremity, and skin checks by a physician (Kricker et al., 2014).

Management

The aim of treatment is to remove the primary tumor and any metastases (if possible) (Momen & Al-Niaimi, 2013);

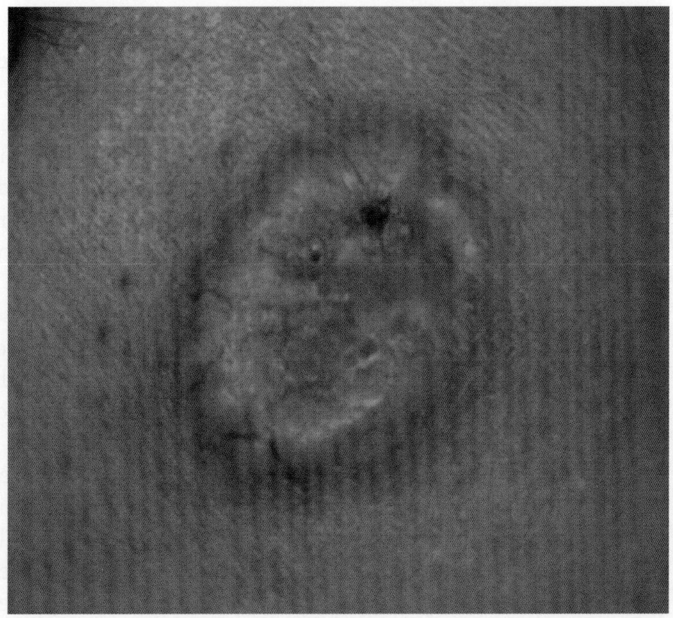

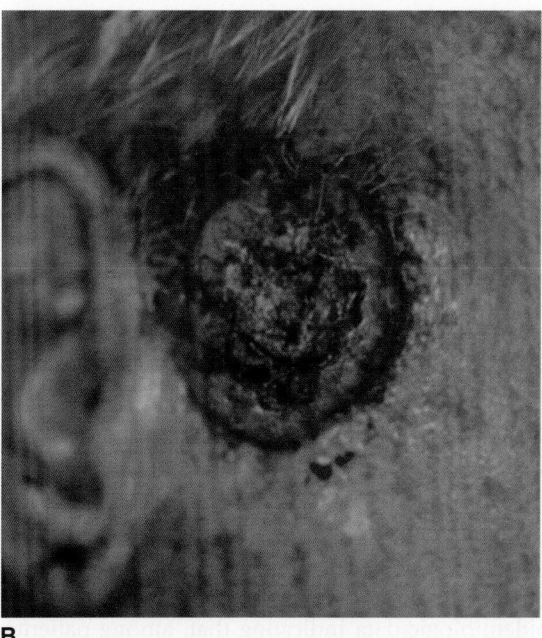

FIGURE 25-7. Nodular basal cell carcinoma. **A.** A red, translucent nodule with rolled border, as seen here, is a classic presentation of nodular basal cell carcinoma. **B.** Nodular basal cell carcinoma demonstrating ulceration. (Reprinted with permission from DeVita, V. T., Lawrence, T. S., & Rosenberg, S. A. (2008). *DeVita, Hellman, and Rosenberg's cancer principles & practice of oncology* (8th ed.). Philadelphia, PA: Wolters Kluwer Health.)

some advanced tumors cannot be removed. Surgical excision of nonmelanoma skin cancers is the primary method of treatment; Mohs micrographic surgery may be selected because it allows preservation of normal tissue and complete resection of the tumor. Excision of basal cell carcinoma has a cure rate of 95% (Council, 2013). While the goal in treatment is to minimize tissue loss while maximizing potential for cure, Combemale et al. (2007) reported that 57% (29/51) of their participants required leg amputation irrespective of histologic differentiation. Cure rates for squamous cell carcinoma are reported by extensiveness and treatment, that is, metastatic squamous cell carcinoma has a 5-year cure rate at 34%; Mohs surgery, 95%; and radiotherapy, 90% (Momen & Al-Niaimi, 2013).

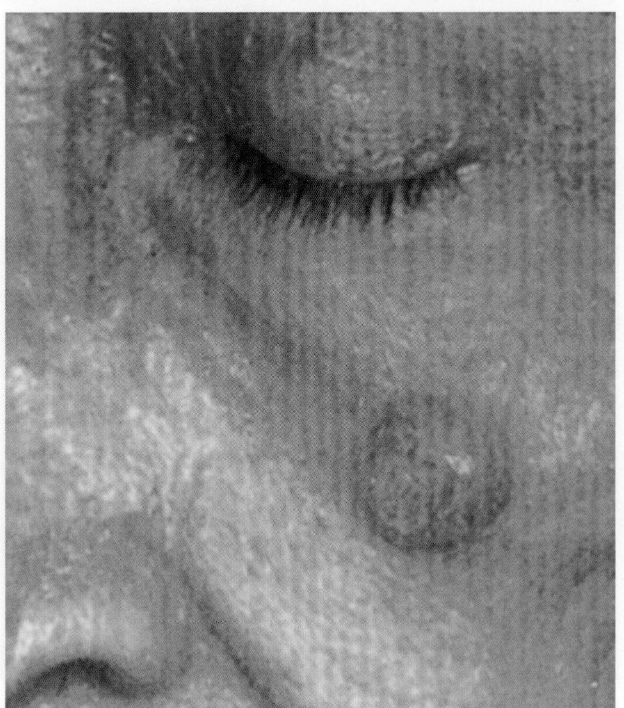

FIGURE 25-8. Squamous cell carcinoma usually appears on sun-exposed skin of fair-skinned adults over 60. It may develop in an actinic keratosis. The face and the back of the hand are often affected, as shown here. (Reprinted with permission from Hall, J. C. (2000). *Sauer's manual of skin diseases* (8th ed.). Philadelphia, PA: Lippincott Williams & Wilkins.)

Cryotherapy is commonly used to treat actinic keratosis. Imiquimod (applied five times weekly for 6 weeks) and 5-fluorouracil (applied twice daily for 6 to 12 weeks) are topical therapies used for precancerous actinic keratosis and also FDA approved for treatment of basal cell carcinoma (Council, 2013). Bath-Hextall et al. (2014) reported results from a randomized controlled trial that indicated imiquimod was inferior to surgery for basal cell carcinoma; however, it may still be an option for small low-risk superficial or nodular basal cell carcinomas. Radiation therapy is used to treat advanced, inoperable basal and squamous cell carcinomas, and definitive radiation may also be recommended for curative intent in patients who are not candidates for surgical treatment (Fecher, 2013). For basal cell carcinoma that is unresectable, cisplatin-based chemotherapy has shown the most activity alone and in combination with other cytotoxic agents; many therapies are in development (Fecher, 2013).

Patient teaching in terms of safe sun exposure is important for prevention. This teaching may include avoiding/

minimizing sun exposure from 10 AM to 4 PM, which is the time for peak UVB; sunscreen with a solar protection factor (SPF) of 15; protective clothing, hats, and sunglasses; and avoidance of tanning beds (1.5 times greater risk of basal cell carcinoma and 2.5 times greater risk of squamous cell carcinoma) (Davies, 2009; Firnhaber, 2012; Momen & Al-Niaimi, 2013).

It is important to consider the patient's quality of life when providing education and counseling. Mathias et al. (2014) examined quality of life in persons with advanced basal cell carcinoma. The most commonly reported and problematic symptoms were hair loss (79%), loss of taste (79%), bleeding (57%), and oozing or open wounds (50%). They reported feeling anxious, depressed, unable to concentrate, and worried about future surgery and procedures.

After diagnosis and treatment, patients need to be regularly followed. The follow-up period is 2 to 5 years for squamous cell carcinoma (Davies, 2009); this is based on epidemiologic data indicating that, among patients with recurrence, 58% had recurrence in the first year and 95% within the first 5 years (Davies, 2009). The majority of squamous cell carcinomas have low risk for metastasis; however, some grow aggressively and have a 2% to 6% risk of metastasis (Momen & Al-Niaimi, 2013). Metastatic sites for squamous cell carcinomas include regional lymph nodes, liver, and lung; metastatic lesions have a 5-year cure rate of 34% (Momen & Al-Niaimi, 2013). In contrast, metastatic basal cell carcinoma is rare with an incidence of <1% (Mathias et al., 2014).

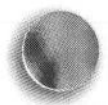

Factitious Ulcers: Dermatitis Artefacta

Prevalence and Incidence

Factitious means artificially created or developed. Factitious disorder refers to a mental disorder in which a person deliberately produces, feigns, or exaggerates symptoms as if having a physical or mental illness when, in fact, the person has consciously created their symptoms. Within factitious disorders, dermatitis artefacta is a psychocutaneous condition where the person creates skin lesions to satisfy a psychological need (Choudhary et al., 2009; Gattu et al., 2009; Koblenzer, 2000). The person is fully aware of the actions (Holt et al., 2013). Unconscious motivating factors (bereavement, divorce, unemployment, debt, bullying, and abuse) are often responsible for this self-destructive behavior (Holt et al., 2013). The highest incidence occurs in late adolescence to early adulthood; most affected are women (female–male ratios range from 3:1 to 20:1) who have a personality disorder (Gregurek-Novak et al., 2005; Koblenzer, 2000; Shah & Fried, 2006). It is considered a rare condition. The incidence is not known, but the prevalence is 33% in patients diagnosed with anorexia and bulimia (Gattu et al., 2009; Koblenzer, 2000).

Pathology

The pathology relates to the source of the ulcers as they can be caused by any mechanical or irritant factors (Fig. 25-9). For example, one woman placed cotton threads and needles under the skin to cause keloids and other changes (Choudhary et al., 2009). Cohen and Vardy (2006) reported a case series of 14 soldiers with acute contact dermatitis with systemic symptoms, that is, acute erythematous rash with numerous papules and pustules in a linear pattern (arms, abdomen, and thighs), fever, malaise, and headache. All were dissatisfied with military service but denied intentionally inflicting the skin lesions; eight admitted to exposure to inflicting agents such as plants or blankets.

Histopathology of the ulcer may rule out organic causes. The diagnosis must be carefully made in order to avoid missing significant pathology. For example, a 20-year-old woman presented with itchy, edematous, livid crusted lesions on the right upper extremity, which were diagnosed as dermatitis artefacta. The histopathologic, immunohistochemical staining, and other studies revealed a rare subcutaneous panniculitis-like T-cell lymphoma (Soylu et al., 2010).

Clinical Presentation

The ulcers/wounds are located on body locations that are easily reached by the dominant hand (Gregurek-Novak et al., 2005; Motherway et al., 2008). The ulcers or skin lesions are produced through mechanical means (fingernails, sharp or blunt objects, etc.) (see Fig. 25-9) or the application of irritants (chemicals, burning cigarettes, etc.) (Choudhary et al., 2009; Cohen & Vardy, 2006). The person typically denies the self-inflicted cause (Choudhary et al., 2009). The prognosis for cure is poor, and the condition tends to wax and wane with life circumstances and events (Koblenzer, 2000; Motherway et al., 2008).

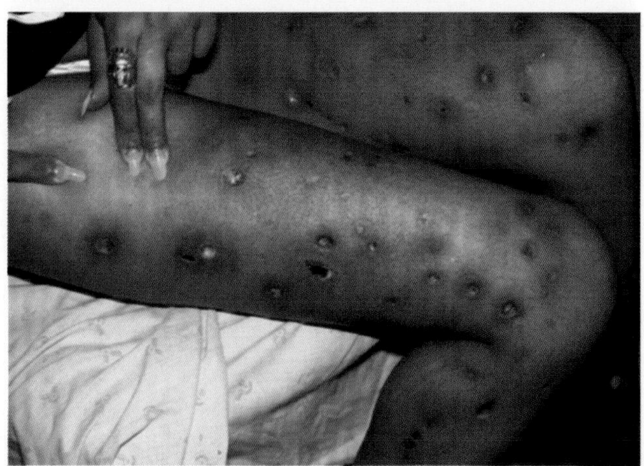

FIGURE 25-9. Neurotic excoriations (factitia). The self-induced ulcers are seen in a patient convinced that she was infested with lice. (Reprinted with permission from Goodheart, H. P. (2003). *Goodheart's photoguide of common skin disorders* (2nd ed.). Philadelphia, PA: Lippincott Williams & Wilkins.)

Factitial dermatoses can occur in children; in this population, the most common manifestations are trichotillomania (compulsive urge to pull out one's hair), neurotic excoriations (repetitive scratching), and acne excoriee (picking acne) (Shah & Fried, 2006).

Diagnosis

Dermatitis artefacta is difficult to diagnosis by clinical findings (Kwon et al., 2006). Diagnostic clues include denial, amnesia, or indifference to the symptoms or how the lesions occurred (Choudhary et al., 2009). The diagnosis is usually made by exclusion or when the person is discovered inflicting the lesion. Lesions do not conform to known dermatoses, are located on easily reached body locations, and have bizarre, clear-cut or linear morphological features (Choudhary et al., 2009; Cohen & Vardy, 2006; Gregurek-Novak et al., 2005). Examples of locations may include the inguinal region, under the breasts, face, arms, and legs (Gregurek-Novak et al., 2005).

Management

The wound care/dermatology practitioner needs to work closely with the mental health provider. The mental disorder needs to be treated. Medications such as selective serotonin reuptake inhibitors, low-dose antipsychotic medications, and antidepressant medications have been used (Choudhary et al., 2009; Koblenzer, 2000). For example, Kwon et al. (2006) and Motherway et al. (2008) presented case studies of women with recurrent skin lesions and abscesses; treatment of the mental health problem markedly improved the skin disease. The person may deny psychiatric distress and have negative feelings toward the provider for raising such an issue. Creating an accepting, empathic, and nonjudgmental relationship is important (Koblenzer, 2000). Even after the lesions have healed, it is sometimes helpful to continue to see the patient for supervision and to offer support (Koblenzer, 2000). The lesions tend to heal when covered. Therefore, selection of a dressing that fits the location and characteristics of the ulcers/lesions and that provides coverage is appropriate.

Children's treatment needs are similar to that of the adult. The treatment includes a nonjudgmental care provider, avoiding accusations and blame, observation of the parent–child interaction, screening for other psychiatric conditions, and psychotherapy if necessary (Shah & Fried, 2006). Although antidepressants are beneficial for the adult, they must be carefully considered in children in terms of the potential for short- and long-term side effects and safety (Shah & Fried, 2006).

Conclusion

Although often considered lesser diagnosed wounds, atypical lower extremity ulcers need to be considered when examining wounds on the lower extremities. Although this chapter focused on the lower extremity, many of these wounds can occur on other areas of the body. Vasculitic, PG, sickle cell anemia, calciphylaxis, squamous and basal cell carcinomas, and factitious ulcers are examples of atypical ulcers. The assessment of these ulcers includes a detailed history and possibly a wound biopsy. Although the wound dressing is an important aspect of care, generally the underlying pathology is the crucial focus of treatment. These wounds can be excruciatingly painful and result in deformities/scarring of the skin. Thus, pain needs to be managed and quality of life and psychosocial issues dealt with. Patient/family teaching is critical due to the long-term follow-up and intensive treatment required.

REFERENCES

Agarwal, A., & Andrews, J. M. (2013). Systematic review: IBD-associated pyoderma gangrenosum in the biologic era, the response to therapy. *Alimentary Pharmacology and Therapeutics, 38*(6), 563–572.

American College of Rheumatology, Vasculitis. http://www.rheumatology.org/Practice/Clinical/Patients/Diseases_And_Conditions/Vasculitis/

Bath-Hextall, F., Ozolins, M., Armstrong, S. J., et al.; on behalf of the Surgery versus Imiquimod for Nodular and Superficial Basal Cell Carcinoma (SINS) Study Group. (2014). Surgical excision versus imiquimod 5% cream for nodular and superficial basal-cell carcinoma (SINS): A multicentre, non-inferiority, randomized controlled trial. *Lancet Oncology, 15*, 96–105.

Birmingham Vasculitis Activity Score (version 3). http://www.epsnetwork.co.uk/BVAS/bvas_flow.html

Brown, S. (2012). Vasculitis: Pathophysiology, diagnosis and treatment. *Nursing Standard, 27*(12), 50–57.

Choudhary, S., Khairkar, P., Singh, A., et al. (2009). Dermatitis artefacta: Keloids and foreign body granuloma due to overvalued ideation of acupuncture. *Indian Journal of Dermatology, Venereology and Leprology, 75*(6), 606–608.

Cohen, A. D., & Vardy, D. A. (2006). Dermatitis artefacta in soldiers. *Military Medicine, 171*(6), 497–499.

Combemale, P., Bousquet, M., Kanitakis, J.; the Angiodermatology Group of the French Society of Dermatology. (2007). Malignant transformation of leg ulcers: A retrospective study of 85 cases. *Journal of the European Academy of Dermatology and Venereology, 21*(7), 935–941.

Council, M. L. (2013). Common skin cancers in older adults: Approach to diagnosis and management. *Clinics in Geriatrics Medicine, 29*(2013), 361–372.

Davies, A. (2009). The effective management of squamous cell carcinoma. *British Journal of Nursing, 18*(9), 539–543.

de Araujo, T. S., & Kirsner, R. S. (2001).Vasculitis. *Wounds, 13*(3), 23–34.

Delaney, K. M., Axelrod, K. C., Buscetta, A., et al. (2013). Leg ulcers in sickle cell disease: Current patterns and practices. *Hemoglobin, 37*(4), 325–332.

Fartasch, M., Diepgen T. L., Schmitt, J., et al. (2012). The relationship between occupational sun exposure and non-melanoma skin cancer. *Deutsches Arzteblatt International, 109*(43), 715–720.

Fecher, L. A. (2013). Systemic therapy for inoperable and metastatic basal cell cancer. *Current Treatment Options in Oncology, 14*(2), 237–248.

Feeser, D. L. (2011). Calciphylaxis: No longer rare; no longer calciphylaxis? A paradigm shift for Wound, Ostomy and Continence Nursing. *Journal of Wound Ostomy Continence Nursing, 38*(4), 379–384.

Firnhaber, J. M. (2012). Diagnosis and treatment of basal cell and squamous cell carcinoma. *American Family Physician, 86*(2), 161–168.

Fraccalvieri, M., Fierro, M. T., Salomone, M., et al. (2012). Gauze-based negative pressure wound therapy: A valid method to manage pyoderma gangrenosum. *International Wound Journal, 11*(2), 164–168.

Gattu, S., Rashid, R. M., & Khachemoune, A. (2009). Self-induced skin lesions: A review of dermatitis artefacta. *Cutis, 84*(5), 247–251.

Gregurek-Novak, T., Novak-Bilic, G., & Vucic, M. (2005). Dermatitis artefacta: Unusual appearance in an older woman. *Journal of the European Academy of Dermatology and Venereology, 19*(2), 223–225.

Halabi-Tawi, M., Lionnet, F., Girot, R., et al. (2008). Sickle cell leg ulcers: A frequently disabling complication and a marker of severity. *British Journal of Dermatology, 158*, 339–344.

Hanley, J. (2011). Effective management of peristomal pyoderma gangrenosum. *British Journal of Nursing, 20*(7), S12–S17.

Hassell, K. L. (2010). Population estimates of sickle cell disease in the U.S. *American Journal of Preventive Medicine, 38*(4 Suppl), S512–S521.

Hayashi, M. (2013). Calciphylaxis: Diagnosis and clinical features. *Clinical Experimental Nephrology, 17*(4), 498–503.

Holt, P., El-Dars, L., Kenny, A., et al. (2013). Serial photography and Wood's light examination as an aid to the clinical diagnosis of dermatitis artefacta. *Journal of Visual Communication in Medicine, 36*(1–2), 31–34.

Jenerette, G. M., Brewer, C. A., Edwards, L. J., et al. (2014). An intervention to decrease stigma in young adults with sickle cell disease. *Western Journal of Nursing Research, 36*(5), 599–619.

Kato, G. J., Hebbel, R. P., Steinberg, M. H., et al. (2009). Vasculopathy in sickle cell disease: Biology, pathophysiology, genetics, translational medicine, and new research directions. *American Journal of Hematology, 84*(9), 618–625.

Kerk, N., & Goerge, T. (2013a). Livedoid vasculopathy—Current aspects of diagnosis and treatment of cutaneous infarction. *Journal of the German Society of Dermatology, 11*, 407–410.

Kerk, N., & Goerge, T. (2013b). Livedoid vasculopathy—A thrombotic disease. *Vasa, 42*, 317–322.

Koblenzer, C. S. (2000). Dermatitis artefacta. Clinical features and approaches to treatment. *American Journal of Clinical Dermatology, 1*(1), 47–55.

Kricker, A., Armstrong, B., Hansen, V., et al. (2014). Basal cell carcinoma and squamous cell carcinoma growth rates and determinants of size in community patients. *Journal of the American Academy of Dermatology, 70*(3), 456–464.

Kwon, E., Dans, M., Koblenzer, C., et al. (2006). Dermatitis artefacta. *Journal of Cutaneous Medicine and Surgery, 10*(2), 108–113.

Madu, A. J., Ubesie, A., Madu, K. A., et al. (2013). Evaluation of clinical and laboratory correlates of sickle leg ulcers. *Wound Repair and Regeneration, 21*(6), 808–812.

Markova, A., Lester, J., Wang, J., et al. (2012). Diagnosis of common dermapathies in dialysis patients: A review and update. *Seminars in Dialysis, 25*(4), 408–418.

Marti-Carvajal, A. J., Knight-Madden, J. M., & Martinez-Zapata, M. J. (2012). Interventions for treating leg ulcers in people with sickle cell disease (review). *Cochrane Database Systematic Review, 11*, CD008394. doi: 10.1002/14651858.CD008394.pub2.

Mathias, S. D., Chren, M-M., Colwell, H. H., et al. (2014). Assessing health-related quality of life for advanced basal cell carcinoma and basal cell carcinoma nevus syndrome: Development of the first disease-specific patient-reported outcome questionnaire. *Journal of the American Medical Association Dermatology, 150*(2), 169–176.

Meissner, M., Gille, J., & Kaufmann, R. (2006). Calciphylaxis: No therapeutic concepts for a poorly understood syndrome? *Journal der Deutschen Dermatologischen Gesellschaft, 4*, 1037–1044.

Minniti, C. P., Delaney, K. M., Gorbach, A. M., et al. (2014). Vasculopathy, inflammation, and blood flow in leg ulcers of patients with sickle cell anemia, *American Journal of Hematology, 89*(1), 1–6.

Minniti, C. P., Eckman, J., Sebastiani, P., et al. (2010). Leg ulcers in sickle cell disease. *American Journal of Hematology, 85*(10), 831–833.

Momen, S., & Al-Niaimi, F. (2013). Squamous cell carcinoma—Aetiology, presentation and treatment options. *Dermatological Nursing, 12*(2), 14–20.

Morris, C. R. (2008). Mechanisms of vasculopathy in sickle cell disease and thalassemia. *Hematology/the Education Program of the American Society of Hematology*, 177–185, doi: 10.1182/asheducation-2008.1.177.

Motherway, L., Gallagher, D., Guerandel, A., et al. (2008). Dermatitis artefacta: An unusual diagnosis in psychodermaology. *Irish Journal of Psychological Medicine, 25*(2), 71–72.

Mukhtyar, C., Lee, R., Brown, D., et al. (2009). Modification and validation of the Birmingham Vasculitis Activity Score (version 3). *Annals of the Rheumatic Diseases, 68*(12), 1827–1832.

Ng, A. T., & Peng, D. H. (2011). Calciphylaxis. *Dermatologic Therapy, 24*(2), 256–262.

Ntatsaki, E., Carruthers, D., Chakravarty, K., et al. (2014). BSR and BHPR guideline for the management of adults with ANCA-associated vasculitis *Rheumatology (Oxford), 53*, 2306–2309. www.rheumatology.oxfordjournals.org, doi: 10.1093/rheumatology/ket445.

Ong, S., & Coulson, I. H. (2012). Diagnosis and treatment of calciphylaxis. *Skinmed, 10*(3), 166–170.

Ratnagobal, S., & Sinha, S. (2013). Pyoderma gangrenosum: Guideline for wound practitioners. *Journal of Wound Care, 22*(2), 68–72.

Ross, E. A. (2011). Evolution of treatment strategies for calciphylaxis. *American Journal of Nephrology, 34*(5), 460–467.

Ruocco, E., Sangiuliano, S., Gravina, A. G., et al. (2009). Pyoderma gangrenosum: An updated review. *Journal of the European Academy of Dermatology and Venereology, 23*, 1008–1017.

Schnirring-Judge, M., & Belpedio, D. (2010). Malignant transformation of a chronic venous stasis ulcer to basal cell carcinoma in a diabetic patient: Case study and review of pathophysiology. *Journal of Foot and Ankle Surgery, 49*(2010), 75–79.

Seitz, C. S., Berens, N., Brocker, E. B., et al. (2010). Leg ulceration in rheumatoid arthritis—An underreported multicausal complication with considerable morbidity: Analysis of thirty-six patients and review of the literature. *Dermatology, 220*(3), 268–273.

Senet, P., Combemale, P., Debure, C., et al.; for the Angio-Dermatology Group of the French Society of Dermatology. (2012). Malignancy and chronic leg ulcers. *Achieves of Dermatology, 148*(6), 704–708.

Shah, K. N., & Fried, F. G. (2006). Factitial dermatoses in children. *Current Opinion in Pediatrics, 18*(4), 403–409.

Sharma, A., Schwartz, R. A., & Swan, K. G. (2011). Marjolin's warty ulcer. *Journal of Surgical Oncology, 103*(2), 193–195.

Sinha, A., & Bagga, A. (2008). Pulse steroid therapy. *Indian Journal of Pediatrics, 75*(10), 1057–1066.

Soylu, S., Gul, U., Kilic, A., et al. (2010). A case with an indolent course of subcutaneous panniculitis-like T-cell lymphoma demonstrating Epstein-Barr virus positivity and simulating dermatitis artefacta. *American Journal of Clinical Dermatology, 11*(2), 147–150.

Suppiah, R., Mukhtyar, C., Flossmann, O., et al. (2011). A cross-sectional study of the Birmingham Vasculitis Activity Score version 3 in systemic vasculitis. *Rheumatology, 50*(5), 899–905.

Tang, J. C., Vivas, A., Rey, A., et al. (2012). Atypical ulcers: Wound biopsy results from a university wound pathology service. *Ostomy Wound Management, 58*(6), 20–29.

Tsaras, G., Owusu-Ansah, A., Boateng, F. O., et al. (2009). Complications associated with sickle cell trait: A brief narrative review. *American Journal of Medicine, 122*(6), 507–512.

Vedvyas, C., Winterfield, L. S., & Vleugels, R. A. (2012). Calciphylaxis: A systematic review of existing and emerging therapies. *Journal of the American Academy of Dermatology, 67*(6), e253–60. doi: 10.1016/j.jaad.2011.06.009.

Wollina, U. (2007). Pyoderma gangrenosum—A review. *Orphanet Journal of Rare Diseases, 2*, 19. doi: 10.1186/1750-1172-2-19.

QUESTIONS

1. From what data would a definitive diagnosis of vasculitis be derived?
A. Patient history
B. Presence of comorbid conditions
C. Blood testing
D. Histologic evaluation of the lesion

2. A patient presents with sickle cell ulcers. On what site are these ulcers most commonly seen?
A. Medial and lateral malleoli of the lower leg
B. Anterior tibia
C. Dorsum of the foot
D. Achilles tendon

3. A wound nurse is managing the leg ulcers of a patient with sickle cell disease. Which intervention is NOT normally recommended as therapy?
A. Use of hydroxyurea to increase production of fetal hemoglobin
B. Blood transfusions to provide normal RBCs
C. IV morphine for pain management
D. Compression wraps to prevent venous insufficiency

4. Which patient would the wound nurse consider to be at higher risk for the development of pyoderma gangrenosum?
A. A patient with diabetes mellitus
B. A patient with Crohn's disease
C. A patient with sickle cell anemia
D. A patient with lupus

5. A patient presents with a leg ulcer that is characterized by thrombosis of the small vessels in the dermis and subcutaneous fat, leading to cutaneous ischemia, tissue infarction, and necrosis. Which type of atypical leg ulcer would the wound nurse suspect?
A. Sickle cell ulcers
B. Calciphylaxis
C. Vasculitis
D. Pyoderma gangrenosum

6. The wound nurse is assessing a patient with calciphylaxis. What management regimen would the nurse recommend?
A. Use of debridement at bedside to eliminate necrosis and prevent bacterial overgrowth
B. Skin grafts, hyperbaric oxygen therapy, and zinc sulfate
C. Corticosteroids combined with other immunosuppressive agents
D. Supportive care until underlying disease process is under control

7. A patient presents with a skin lesion that appears as a scaly pink papule on his or her head, which according to the patient, "started as a pimple and got bigger and thicker with time." What diagnosis would the wound nurse suspect?
A. Basal cell carcinoma
B. Squamous cell carcinoma
C. Malignant melanoma
D. Actinic keratosis

8. A patient is scheduled for a tissue biopsy to diagnose squamous cell carcinoma. What is a step in the procedure for obtaining these specimens?
A. The biopsy should be taken from the proximal edge of the wound.
B. The biopsy should include 25% of wound and 25% of adjacent tissue.
C. A second specimen should be taken from the lateral side of the wound.
D. A third specimen should be taken from the skin adjacent to the wound.

9. A patient is diagnosed with actinic keratosis. What type of therapy is commonly used to treat this condition?
A. Surgical excision of the lesions
B. Mohs micrographic surgery
C. Cryotherapy
D. Use of selective serotonin reuptake inhibitors

10. The wound nurse is assessing an adolescent patient who is diagnosed with dermatitis artefacta on her arms. What is a diagnostic characteristic of these lesions?
A. Bizarre, clear-cut or linear morphological features
B. Nonhealing pearly pink papules
C. Cutaneous ischemia, tissue infarction, and necrosis
D. Palpable purpura (raised areas of nonblanchable erythema)

ANSWERS: 1.**D**, 2.**A**, 3.**C**, 4.**B**, 5.**B**, 6.**D**, 7.**B**, 8.**A**, 9.**C**, 10.**A**

CHAPTER 26

Foot and Nail Care

Michele (Shelly) Burdette-Taylor and Lynn Fong

OBJECTIVES

1. Identify goals and objectives for a structured comprehensive foot and nail program.
2. Describe factors to be included in a comprehensive lower extremity assessment, to include client history, vascular assessment, sensorimotor assessment, skin and nail assessment, wound assessment, and pain assessment.
3. Describe common pathologic conditions affecting the foot and nails, and implications for the foot and nail care nurse.
4. Outline guidelines for foot and nail care, to include the following: management of hypertrophic nails, management of hypertrophic skin and cuticles, management of corns and calluses, and prevention and management of ingrown nails.
5. Describe infection control issues and implications for the foot care nurse.
6. Discuss the role of the foot care nurse in patient education and appropriate referrals.

Topic Outline

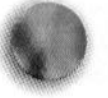 **Guidelines for Foot and Nail Care**

Assessment
Management Hypertrophic Nails
Management of Hypertrophic Skin and Cuticles
Management of Corns and Calluses
Equipment and Policies/Procedures

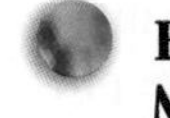 **Education, Prevention, and Routine Management**

Follow-up
Off-loading and Padding
Routine Foot Care
Footwear and Foot Inspection
Compression Socks or Stockings
Walking and Exercise
Smoking Cessation
Glycemic Control

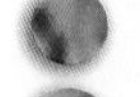 **Multidisciplinary Teams**

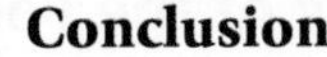 **Conclusion**

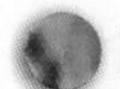 Introduction

As noted throughout this text, the primary goal for all wound care clinicians is to prevent skin and tissue breakdown whenever possible and to promote healing when wounds occur. This is particularly important when caring for individuals with lower extremity arterial disease (LEAD) or lower extremity neuropathic disease (LEND), since they are very high risk for ulceration, impaired healing, and amputation (Markova & Mostow, 2012). There are over one hundred thousand limbs amputated each year in the United States, which equates to over 2,000 limbs amputated per week. Amputation renders the individual vulnerable to fear and anxiety, depression, limited mobility, and increased risk of mortality (Barshes et al., 2013; Mustapha et al., 2013).

Foot and nail care, screening, and education are key responsibilities for the certified wound care nurse (CWCN) and certified foot and nail care nurse (CFCN); both specialty certifications are offered through the Wound Ostomy Continence Nursing Certification Board (WOCNCB). Three out of four Americans experience serious foot problems in their lifetime, and foot care nurses are prepared to assist with prevention and management (Crawford & Fields-Varnado, 2013; Gallagher, 2012). The knowledgeable foot and wound care nurse can play a key role in reducing the complications and cost of care for people with diabetes and LEAD, specifically by preventing injuries and wounds, assuring appropriate footwear, providing education, and initiating prompt and appropriate referrals. Research has shown that implementation of a foot care program incorporating effective assessment tools and evidence-based procedures for foot and nail care reduces foot-related pain and injury and also reduces the number of amputations (Fujiwara et al., 2011; Sheridan, 2012; Weck et al., 2013; Woo et al., 2013). In addition, the CFCN can establish an independent practice as an entrepreneur or incorporate skills into his or her present practice as an intrapreneur.

CLINICAL PEARL

The knowledgeable foot and nail care nurse can reduce complications and cost for individuals with diabetes and LEND or LEAD, by preventing injuries and wounds, assuring appropriate footwear, providing education, and initiating prompt and appropriate referrals.

The purpose of this chapter is to provide guidelines for foot and nail assessment, vascular and sensorimotor screening, basic foot and nail care, and appropriate and timely referrals. The specific objectives of a comprehensive foot and nail care program are listed in Box 26-1 (Jacobson, 1933).

Appropriate foot and nail care has a significant impact on quality of life, specifically by promoting mobility, maintaining comfort, and preventing wounds, amputations, and falls (Lavery et al., 2013). Painful corns, calluses, and deformities increase the risk of falls in the older population (Ricci, 2011), and toenails that have not been trimmed appropriately or in a timely manner increase the risk for injury in both older and neuropathic individuals (Reich & Szepietowski, 2011). Raynaud's, arthritis, gout, diabetes with LEND, lower extremity venous disease (LEVD), and cardiovascular disease with LEAD are common conditions that compromise the individual's ability to safely care for the feet and nails and thereby increase the risk of inadvertent injury (Mustapha et al., 2013). Any wound in the individual with LEND or LEAD places the person at risk for amputation, and, as noted, chronic wounds and amputations lead to depression, limited mobility, pain, morbidity, and increased risk of mortality (Alvarsson et al., 2012; Kimmel & Robin, 2013).

BOX 26-1. Objectives of Foot and Nail Care Program

- Reduce injury and ulceration that may lead to amputation
- Prevent or minimize development or progression of foot deformities and compensate for existing deformities through appropriate footwear modifications
- Encourage walking
- Facilitate proper use of footwear and over-the-counter compression socks
- Increase knowledge and referrals
- Save Medicare/other payers money by reducing hospital readmissions and identifying minor issues earlier
- Assist with monitoring and education to help individuals maintain target hemoglobin A1c levels
- Conduct comprehensive foot and nail assessment
- Identify high-risk individuals and refer appropriately
- Develop an individual plan of action based on findings
- Increase patient satisfaction
- Reduce falls

CLINICAL PEARL

Any wound in the individual with LEND or LEAD places the person at risk for amputation.

 Foot and Nail Care: Overview

A key responsibility of the foot and nail care nurse is to conduct a comprehensive lower extremity assessment; this must include vascular status, sensorimotor status, skin and nail status and presence of any wounds, ability to heal, and appropriateness of footwear and foot care. The objective is to promptly identify any individual with or at risk for ulceration and to intervene appropriately to prevent injury and/or to promote healing and prevent amputation.

CLINICAL PEARL

A key responsibility of the foot care nurse is to conduct a comprehensive lower extremity assessment, to include vascular status, sensorimotor status, skin and nail status, presence and status of any wounds, ability to heal, and appropriateness of footwear and foot care.

The risk of ulceration is highest among people with LEND and loss of protective sensation (LOPS) (Crawford & Fields-Varnado, 2013). Peripheral polyneuropathy is common among people with diabetes, Hansen's disease, alcoholism, and those with a spinal cord injury or multiple sclerosis. LOPS creates risk for unrecognized injury; the injury initiates an inflammatory response but, because there is no pain, the person does not recognize the injury and thus fails to provide appropriate care (Woo et al., 2013). Wounds may go unnoticed for days or weeks and are often recognized only when infection has developed; at that point, there is a marked reduction in the potential for healing and a significant increase in the risk for amputation (Lipsky et al., 2012).

As stated, vascular assessment is a key component of lower limb assessment for all individuals, because adequacy of perfusion is a key determining factor in outcomes for any individual with a wound; those with adequate perfusion are generally able to heal, while those with poor perfusion are at high risk for failure to heal and resultant amputation. The risk of amputation is highest among people with cardiovascular disease and LEAD (Kohlman-Trigoboff, 2013; Mills et al., 2014; Talarico, 2013; WOCN, 2008). Diminished or absent blood flow significantly compromises the ability to heal and increases the risk of infection, and may eventually result in amputation. Chronic limb ischemia worsens over time, but signs and symptoms are frequently insidious and unrecognized until a wound is sustained that fails to heal and/or deteriorates rapidly (Mustapha et al., 2013).

CLINICAL PEARL

Adequacy of perfusion is a key determining factor in outcomes for any individual with a wound; those with adequate perfusion are generally able to heal, while those with poor perfusion are at high risk for failure to heal and resultant amputation.

Prevention of unrecognized trauma and amputation in the high-risk individual requires skilled foot and nail care provided by an appropriately educated professional. Patient and family education and referrals are required to maximize perfusion, minimize sensorimotor loss, and assure appropriate protective footwear (McCulloch, 2012; Wu et al., 2014). With the aging population and increasing incidence of obesity and diabetes, foot and nail care should be recognized and incorporated as a standard component of quality health care in every setting (Amaeshi, 2012; Brechow et al., 2013; Gallagher, 2012; Meaney, 2012; Moakes, 2012; Woo et al., 2013).

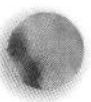 Anatomy and Physiology of the Foot and Nails

The foot is a complicated part of the body because of its location in relation to the heart, and the number of bones, joints, and tendons and ligaments. The anatomy and function of the feet change over time, and these changes are accelerated by age, pregnancy, and trauma. The bony prominences of the plantar surface are prone to stress fractures; in addition, the fat pads on the plantar surface gradually thin, the feet get longer and wider, and the arch has a tendency to flatten. The joints and skin also undergo structural and physiological degeneration with age. These are all normal age-related changes in the feet.

There are 26 bones, 33 joints, 107 ligaments, and 19 muscles in each foot. There are three anatomical sections of the foot: forefoot, midfoot, and hindfoot (Fig. 26-1). The multiple bones, joints, ligaments, nerves, and muscles work together to enable effective weight bearing and locomotion throughout the activities of daily living. Normal structure and function of the bones, muscles, joints, and connective tissue are essential for normal gait and for protection against abnormal pressure and shear forces. The skin provides protection against bacterial and fungal invasion, and maintenance of intact skin is a major concern for the foot care clinician. The nails function to protect the distal digit. The nail unit consists of the nail matrix, nail bed, hyponychium, and proximal and lateral nail folds (Fig. 26-2). These structures are described briefly, and nail-related terms are included in the glossary for this section of the core curriculum.

CLINICAL PEARL

Normal structure and function of the bones, muscles, joints, and connective tissue are essential for normal gait and for protection against abnormal pressure and shear forces.

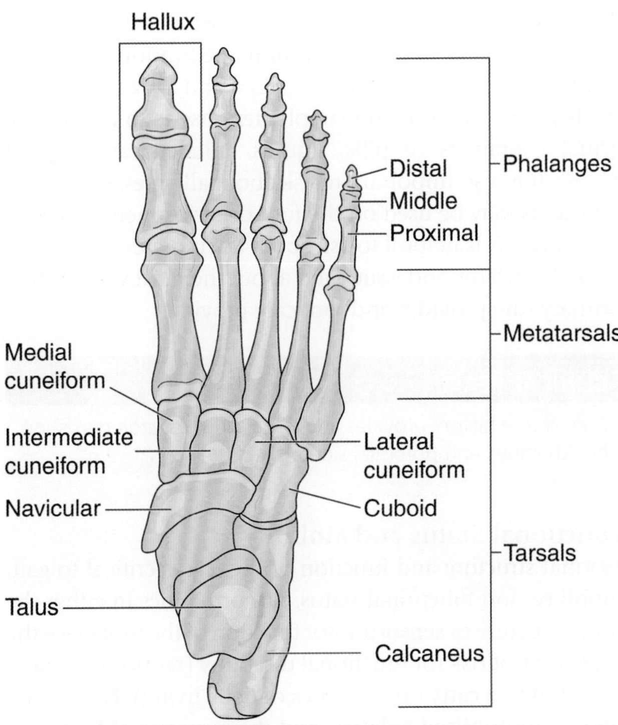

FIGURE 26-1. Anatomical sections of the feet.

The **nail plate** (toenail) is comprised of three overlapping layers of keratinized epithelial cells; as noted, the nail plate functions to protect the distal digit against friction and pressure. The water content of the nail plate is normally 10% to 30%; lower water content results in brittle nails, and higher water content results in nails that are soft and prone to splitting. The **nail bed** refers to the epithelium that lies directly beneath the nail plate and interlocks with the nail plate to provide tight adherence. The **nail matrix** is the reproductive layer of the nail bed and the source of new nail; it extends from a point about 8 mm proximal to the cuticle to the distal edge of the lunula (the white crescent-shaped area at the base of the nail). Normal time frame for development of a new toenail is 12 to 18 months. The **nail folds** are the folds of skin adjacent to the nail; the proximal nail fold is continuous with the cuticle, which seals and protects the nail bed against microorganisms. The **hyponychium** is the junction between the free nail border (distal nail that is not attached to the nail bed) and the adherent nail (nail plate attached to the underlying epithelium); it is sometimes referred to as the "quick."

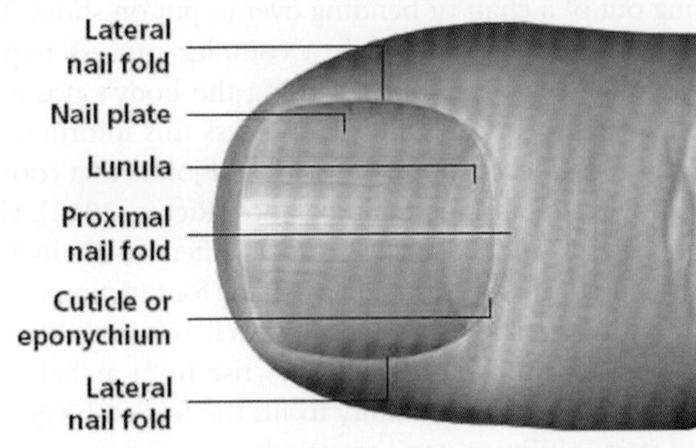

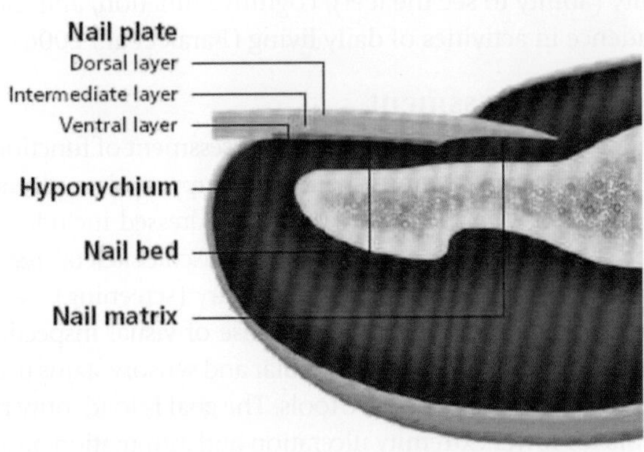

FIGURE 26-2. Nail unit.

In providing foot and nail care, the clinician must be alert to indicators of systemic conditions affecting perfusion and sensorimotor function and must be knowledgeable regarding conditions unique to the feet and nails. As noted earlier, the most common pathologic conditions of the legs, feet, toes, and nails are related to LEAD, LEND, and LEVD; these conditions have been covered in detail in previous chapters (Chapters 21, 22, and 23). Fungal skin infections involving the skin and nails are common as well. Conditions unique to the foot include bony deformities, stress fractures, and neuromas. Common pathologic conditions unique to the nail and surrounding skin include onychomycosis, onychogryphosis, subungual hemorrhage, paronychia, and onychocryptosis. These conditions are discussed in greater detail later in this chapter.

Assessment Guidelines

Effective foot and nail care requires the clinician to conduct a focused health and medication history and physical examination (Gallagher, 2012).

Client History

The goal in obtaining a client history is to determine the social, familial, and health history and to assess cognitive and functional status. The medication history is an important element of the client history and should be obtained prior to conducting any clinical intervention; it provides clues regarding conditions, diseases, and symptoms that may not have been reported during the history and alerts the clinician to medications that would affect foot and nail care (such as anticoagulants or chemotherapeutic agents). The history should also include lifestyle issues such as smoking history and current patterns of tobacco use, exercise, foot hygiene, weight, body mass index, and nutritional intake (Crawford & Fields-Varnado, 2013). Throughout the process of collecting the history, the clinician must be alert to issues that require client education and necessary referrals.

CLINICAL PEARL

Throughout the process of collecting the history, the clinician must be alert to issues that require client education and necessary referrals.

Social History

It is important to learn as much as possible about the individual's daily routines and resources. Appropriate questions to ask include the following: Where do you live (home, apartment, assisted living facility, car, etc.)? (Muirhead et al., 2011) Do you live alone and provide your own care, or do you have a caregiver? Are you on a fixed income? Can you afford to purchase new shoes and other care items? Do you drive yourself, or do you have someone who can take you to the doctor's office or to other appointments? How do you manage foot and nail care at present, and what concerns do you have about your foot and nail care? How is your vision, and can you see your feet? Can you put on and take off your shoes and socks? When asking these questions, the clinician should also assess the individual's affect, indicators of depression or hopelessness, and evidence of a helpful versus toxic support system (Gallagher, 2012).

Family History

A brief family history is helpful in assessing the individual's risk for LEAD, LEVD, and LEND. The clinician can briefly query the individual as to whether or not they have any immediate relatives with early-onset cardiovascular disease, diabetes, leg ulcers caused by LEAD or LEVD, or other circulatory problems (Kimmel & Robin, 2013; Kohlman-Trigoboff, 2013; Wellborn & Moceri, 2014; WOCN, 2008).

Health History

The clinician should query the individual regarding any medical problems or surgical history. Most individuals over the age of 50 have one or more comorbidities that may affect perfusion, mobility, or sensorimotor status. Specific questions regarding arthritis, diabetes, circulatory problems, and problems with nerve damage/neuropathy are particularly relevant (Boulton, 2013). For the individual with diabetes, it is important to ask about usual management, blood glucose levels, and the last HbA1c results. The individual should be asked about foot and leg pain and, if present, should be queried further in regard to characteristics, severity, and exacerbating and relieving factors. The individual should also be asked about recent changes in the feet or nails and any problems with footwear or foot care.

CLINICAL PEARL

Most individuals over the age of 50 have one or more comorbidities that may affect perfusion, mobility, or sensorimotor status.

Medication History

As noted, it is very important to ask about medications, since this provides additional clues regarding existing health issues and potential side effects; this is particularly important when assessing an older individual, since it is common for older individuals to take 10 or more medications each day. The best way to determine prescribed and over-the-counter medication, vitamin, and supplement use is to ask for the actual containers of pills, liquids, inhalers, and topical agents. It is also important to ask about allergies, since topical agents may be used on the foot or recommended to the individual. It is helpful to ask about the individual's health-related concerns and issues and about their last visit to their primary care provider and foot care provider.

CLINICAL PEARL

Medication history provides additional clues regarding existing health issues and potential side effects.

Functional Status and Mobility

Normal structure and function of the feet is critical to gait, mobility, and functional status. Abnormalities in either the bony structure or sensorimotor function of the foot place the individual at risk for functional disability (reduced mobility and ability to carry out activities of daily living). Foot weakness, compromised balance, and the presence of foot pain are risk factors for mobility issues and falls (Eckles, 2012). Three quarters of active older adults complain of foot pain, and loss of mobility is a frequently verbalized concern for these individuals. Functional disability is common among individuals with poor foot health or foot pain, including an increased incidence of falls (Eckles, 2012; Richie, 2012). Normal balance is vital to activities of daily living, such as getting out of a chair or bending over to put on shoes. The ability to maintain balance is a complex process requiring accurate sensory input regarding the body's position, normal cerebrocortical ability to process this information, and normal function of the muscles and joints that coordinate movement and maintain balance (Richie, 2012). Gait abnormalities and balance disorders often result in falls and fractures (Eckles, 2012). In assessing for functional ability, the clinician should ask about the client's mobility and ambulatory stability (e.g., ability to rise from a chair and walk to another point), ability to lift the feet and legs and climb stairs, ability to stand erect with correct posture, visual acuity (ability to see the feet), cognitive function, and independence in activities of daily living (Barak et al., 2006).

Physical Assessment

In addition to a focused history and assessment of functional status, the foot nurse must conduct an appropriate physical examination. The specific areas to be addressed include vascular status, sensorimotor function, musculoskeletal issues, and status of the skin and nails. Primary (screening) assessment is accomplished through the use of visual inspection, palpation, and evaluation of vascular and sensory status using noninvasive and inexpensive tools. The goal is to identify risk factors for lower extremity ulceration and amputation and to use the assessment data to construct an individualized plan of care for education and management that promotes limb preservation. (Jones et al., 2012) (See Fig. 26-3 for sample screening form.)

Research has shown that implementation of a foot care program using effective assessment tools, policies, and procedures reduces pain and injuries among people at risk for limb loss (Alavi et al., 2012; Woo et al., 2013).

Vascular Assessment

Diminished blood flow is the single most significant risk factor for amputation (Kohlman-Trigoboff, 2013; WOCN, 2008). Blood flow to the lower extremity can be classified as adequate, diminished, or severely diminished; early detection of compromised blood flow allows for prompt medical treatment and less invasive surgical procedures to eradicate blockages (Burland 2012; Kohlman-Trigoboff, 2013). The foot care nurse should conduct a noninvasive vascular assessment of the lower extremity to detect indicators of arterial or venous disease that require referral. Assessment parameters include the following:

- General inspection of the skin, hair, and nails to determine the presence of atrophic changes such as thin shiny skin, diminished or absent hair growth, and/or thinning and ridging of the nails (WOCN, 2008). Visible muscle atrophy is another potential indicator of arterial insufficiency, as is "clubbing" of the toes and nails.
- Assessment for color changes in the lower extremity with elevation and dependency. The individual should be placed in the supine position, and the leg should be raised above the level of the heart for 10 to 20 seconds. The nurse should observe for color changes, such as development of pallor (light skin) or a cyanotic or gray tone (dark skin). The individual should then be placed in a sitting position with the foot and leg hanging down, and the nurse should observe for dependent rubor (a purple red discoloration of the distal leg and foot) (WOCN, 2008).
- Palpation of lower extremity pulses, both the posterior tibialis and the dorsalis pedis. Findings should be documented as absent, 0; diminished, 1; normal, 2; or strong and bounding, 3 (Kohlman-Trigoboff, 2013). A handheld Doppler can be used to auscultate the pulses; this is particularly important when the pulses are difficult to palpate or nonpalpable.
- Palpation of the legs and feet for temperature changes, using the back of the hand and comparing the temperature of one foot and leg to the contralateral foot and leg and temperature of the distal leg and foot to the proximal leg. Findings should be recorded as hot, warm, cool, or cold.
- Assessment of capillary refill. The nurse should apply firm pressure with her or his thumb to the pad of the great toe for 2 seconds. When pressure is released, the color should return to normal within 2 to 3 seconds. Capillary refill time > 3 seconds is an indicator of possible LEAD. (Although capillary refill is commonly evaluated using the nail bed, the nails are often discolored and thickened due to onychomycosis; thus, the toe pad should be used instead of the nail bed.)
- Ankle–brachial index (ABI), also known as ankle–brachial pressure index (ABPI). This is the most objective noninvasive measure of perfusion to the lower extremity and is a critical element of the vascular assessment. In order to get valid results, it is critical to follow evidence-based guidelines for ABI measurement and interpretation; see Chapter 22.
- Assessment for edema. Edema can be caused by a number of pathologic conditions, including cardiovascular or renal disease, severe malnutrition, lower extremity venous disease, lymphatic disorders, and a condition known as lipedema (see Chapter 21). The foot care nurse should note whether the edema is generalized or limited to the legs and feet, whether it is unilateral or bilateral, and whether there are other indicators of venous disease, lymphedema, or lipedema. Individuals with evidence of venous or lymphatic disorders require referral to a vascular specialist or lymphedema specialist, while individuals with generalized edema should be referred to their primary care physician, cardiologist, or nephrologist.
- Assessment for indicators of venous disease. Early indicators of venous disease include pitting edema of variable severity, varicosities, dilated ankle and foot veins, and hemosiderosis (Crawford & Fields-Varnado, 2013; WOCN, 2011). Venous dermatitis is another possible indicator; this is manifested as dermatitis (dry scaly skin, pruritis, and erythema) involving the lower leg. Manifestations of venous disease are discussed in detail in Chapter 21 and, as noted, mandate referral to a vascular specialist.

Sensorimotor Assessment

Diabetes is a common comorbid condition among older individuals and those seeking foot care services, and long-standing or poorly controlled diabetes significantly increases the risk for both LEAD and LEND (Marston, 2006; WOCN, 2012). In addition, there are many conditions other than diabetes that increase the risk for neuropathic disease. Neuropathy places the individual at risk for LOPS resulting in painless trauma, loss of position sense resulting in falls, altered gait resulting in plantar surface ulcers, and Charcot foot deformity. Neuropathy is a major contributing factor to nontraumatic lower limb amputations. Thus, the screening assessment for any individual seeking foot care must include assessment for sensory and motor function. The critical elements of a screening assessment are discussed briefly in this chapter; Chapter 23 provides an in-depth discussion of the pathology, assessment, and management of LEND and neuropathic ulcers.

CLINICAL PEARL

Long-standing or poorly controlled diabetes significantly increases the risk for both LEAD and LEND, both of which increase the risk of ulceration and possible amputation.

Annual Comprehensive Diabetes Foot Exam Form

Name: ______________________ Date: __________ ID#: __________

I. Presence of Diabetes Complications

1. Check all that apply.

❑ Peripheral Neuropathy
❑ Nephropathy
❑ Retinopathy
❑ Peripheral Vascular Disease
❑ Cardiovascular Disease
❑ Amputation *(Specify date, side, and level)*

Current ulcer or history of a foot ulcer? Y___ N___

For Sections II & III, fill in the blanks with "Y" or "N" or with an "R," "L," or "B" for positive findings on the right, left, or both feet.

II. Current History

1. Is there pain in the calf muscles when walking that is relieved by rest? Y___ N___
2. Any change in the foot since the last evaluation? Y ___ N___
3. Any shoe problems? Y__ N___
4. Any blood or discharge on socks or hose? Y___ N___
5. Smoking history? Y__N__
6. Most recent hemoglobin A1c result ____% _____ *date*

III. Foot Exam

1. Skin, Hair, and Nail Condition

Is the skin thin, fragile, shiny and hairless? Y __ N__

Are the nails thick, too long, ingrown, or infected with fungal disease? Y __ N__

Measure, draw in, and label the patient's skin condition, using the key and the foot diagram below.

C=Callus U=Ulcer PU=Pre-Ulcer
F=Fissure M=Maceration R=Redness
S=Swelling W=Warmth D=Dryness

2. Note Musculoskeletal Deformities

❑ Toe deformities
❑ Bunions (Hallus Valgus)
❑ Charcot foot
❑ Foot drop
❑ Prominent Metatarsal Heads

3. Pedal Pulses Fill in the blanks with a "P" or an "A" to indicate present or absent.

Posterior tibial Left____ Right____
Dorsalis pedis Left____ Right____

4. Sensory Foot Exam *Label sensory level with a "+" in the five circled areas of the foot if the patient can feel the 5.07 (10-gram) Semmes-Weinstein nylon monofilament and "-" if the patient cannot feel the filament.*

Notes

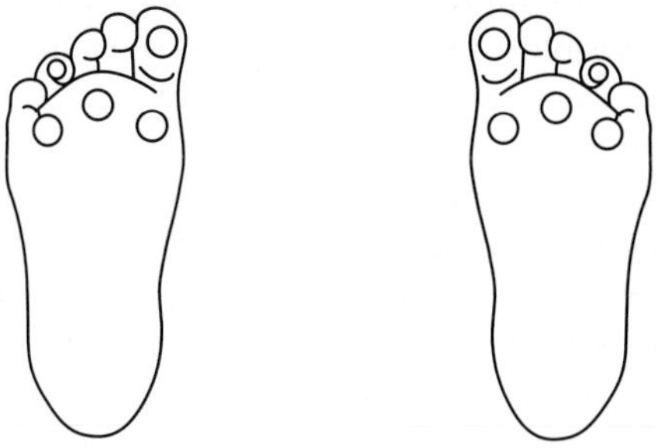

Right Foot

Left Foot

Notes

IV. Risk Categorization *Check appropriate box.*

❑ **Low Risk Patient**
All of the following:
❑ Intact protective sensation
❑ Pedal pulses present
❑ No deformity
❑ No prior foot ulcer
❑ No amputation

❑ **High Risk Patient**
One or more of the following:
❑ Loss of protective sensation
❑ Absent pedal pulses
❑ Foot deformity
❑ History of foot ulcer
❑ Prior amputation

V. Footwear Assessment *Indicate yes or no.*

1. Does the patient wear appropriate shoes? Y__ N __
2. Does the patient need inserts? Y __ N __
3. Should corrective footwear be prescribed? Y __ N __

VI. Education *Indicate yes or no.*

1. Has the patient had prior foot care education? Y _N_
2. Can the patient demonstrate appropriate foot care? Y_N_
3. Does the patient need smoking cessation counseling? Y_N_
4. Does the patient need education about HbA1c or other diabetes self-care? Y_N_

Provider Signature ______________________

VII. Management Plan *Check all that apply.*

1. Self-management education:

Provide patient education for preventive foot care. Date: ____
Provide or refer for smoking cessation counseling. Date: ____
Provide patient education about HbA1c or other aspect of self-care. Date: ____

2. Diagnostic studies:

❑ Vascular Laboratory
❑ Hemoglobin A1c (at least twice per year)
❑ Other: ____

3. Footwear recommendations:

❑ None
❑ Athletic shoes
❑ Accommodative inserts
❑ Custom shoes
❑ Depth shoes

4. Refer to:

❑ Primary Care Provider
❑ Diabetes Educator
❑ Podiatrist
❑ RN Foot Specialist
❑ Pedorthist
❑ Orthotist
❑ Endocrinologist
❑ Vascular Surgeon
❑ Foot Surgeon
❑ Rehab. Specialist
❑ Other: ______

5. Follow-up Care:

Schedule follow-up visit. Date: ______

FIGURE 26-3. Screening form.

Monofilament Testing of Sensory Function

This test should be done using the Semmes-Weinstein 5.07 monofilament instrument (WOCN, 2012), a nylon filament (fishing line) mounted on a holder and standardized to deliver 10 g of force when pressed against the skin with enough force to bend the monofilament into a C-shape. This tool is recommended by both the International Diabetes Federation and the World Health Organization (WHO) for screening of sensory function (Atkins, 2010; Plucknette et al., 2012; Woo et al., 2013). The nurse asks the client to close their eyes and to report each time he or she senses touch on his or her foot; the nurse then tests 4 to 10 sites on the plantar surface and dorsum of the foot. If the individual senses touch at all sites, she or he has intact protective sensation; inability to sense touch at any site denotes LOPS. LOPS has immediate implications for education and counseling; for example, the individual with any degree of LOPS must be counseled to have footwear professionally fitted since she or he will be unable to accurately detect discomfort from shoes that are rubbing against the foot. (See Fig. 26-4A and B for typical neuropathic wounds, i.e., loss of the 5th toe and damage to the great toe due to poorly fitted shoes.) The individual with LOPS must also be consistently educated and reminded to wear protective footwear whenever she or he is out of bed in order to prevent trauma, to check bathwater temperature to prevent burns, and to visually inspect the feet each day to identify areas of impending or actual ulceration. (See Chapter 23 for further information regarding monofilament testing.)

CLINICAL PEARL

LOPS has immediate implications for education and counseling; for example, the individual with LOPS must be educated to wear protective footwear, to check bathwater temperature, and to visually inspect the feet every day for evidence of impending or actual ulceration.

Vibratory Sense Testing

The use of a tuning fork delivering 128 cps is another cost-effective and reliable method of testing for sensory neuropathy (O'Brien & Karem, 2013). The nurse strikes the tuning fork on an object or her or his hand, places the handle of the fork to the base of the great toe or the medial aspect of the first metatarsophalangeal joint, and records the individual's ability to perceive the vibration and point at which the vibration ceases. If the individual cannot accurately report vibratory sense or the point at which the vibration stops (either spontaneously or as a result of the nurse squeezing the prongs of the tuning fork), she or he is considered to have loss of vibratory sense and early-onset sensory neuropathy.

Position Sense Testing

As noted, individuals who lose position sense are at increased risk for falls because they fail to recognize when their foot is at the edge of a step or on rough terrain and therefore fail to compensate by adjusting their posture and gait appropriately (Aliberti, 2012). A simple test for proprioception is to have the individual close his or her eyes; the nurse then moves the great toe up, down, medially, and laterally and asks the individual to report the direction in which the toe has been moved. Inability to reliably report position of the great toe is documented as loss of position sense and requires client education to hold onto stair rails and to watch their feet when walking on rough terrain.

CLINICAL PEARL

Individuals who lose position sense are at increased risk for falls and should be counseled accordingly.

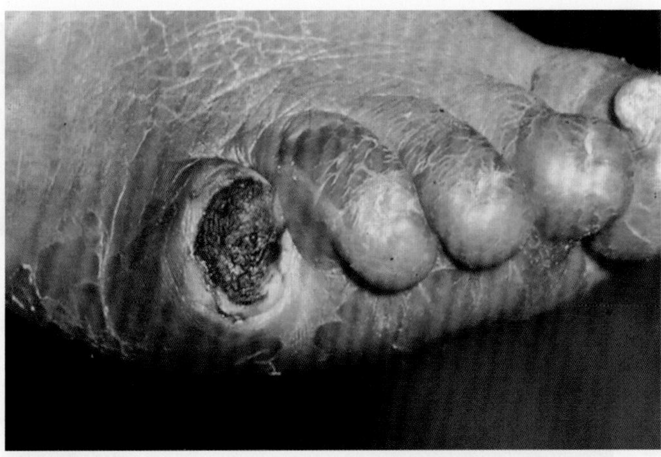
A

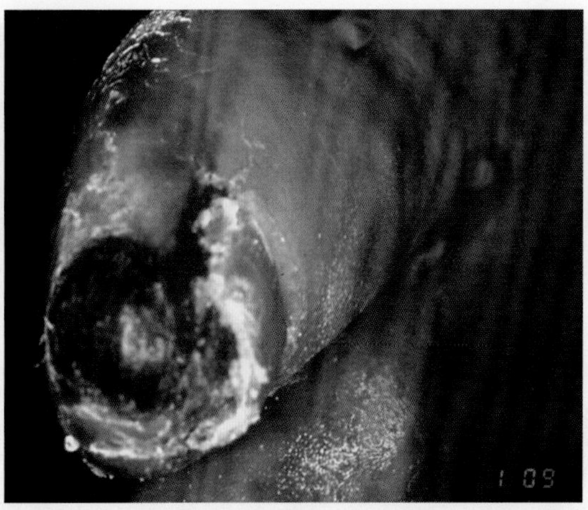
B

FIGURE 26-4. A and B. Neuropathic wounds (loss of the 5th toe and damage to the great toe due to poorly fitted shoes).

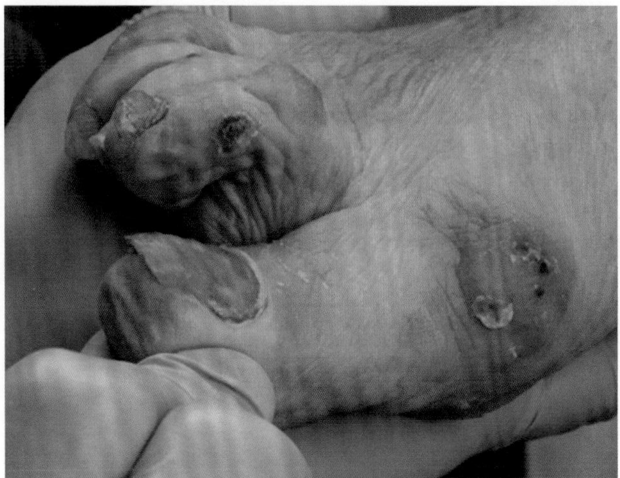

FIGURE 26-5. Corn/callus.

Inspection for Deformities Caused by Motor Neuropathy

Damage to the motor nerves causes impaired function of the muscles that are responsible for maintenance of normal foot contours, gait, and weight bearing. Motor neuropathy leads to muscle imbalance, anatomic changes, and functional disorders (Kelechi & Johnson, 2012; WOCN, 2012). Deformities caused by motor neuropathy include hammer toes, overlapping toes, foot drop, hallux valgus (deviation of the great toe away from midline, also known as bunion), hallux varus (deviation of the great toe toward midline), displacement of the plantar surface fat pads, abnormally prominent metatarsal heads, and an abnormally prominent 5th metatarsophalangeal joint, also known as a tailor bunion or bunionette. These deformities increase the risk of friction damage (e.g., corns and calluses) (Fig. 26-5) and ulcers from poorly fitted footwear (Fig. 26-6). Other visual indicators of motor neuropathy include signs of abnormal weight bearing (e.g., callus formation and abnormal wear patterns in footwear).

Altered Weight Bearing and Plantar Surface Pressure Points

This is a simple test that provides very helpful information regarding plantar surface pressures during weight bearing; it requires a pressure mapping device such as a Harris Mat or digital imprint device. The patient is asked to stand on the device, and this provides an "ink print" (Harris Mat) or digital imprint that visibly displays any areas of high pressure. The presence of high-pressure areas (also known as "hot spots") mandates referral to an orthotist or pedorthist for fitting with weight redistributing insoles and therapeutic shoes.

CLINICAL PEARL

The presence of high-pressure areas (per pressure mapping devices) mandates referral to an orthotist or pedorthist for fitting with appropriate insoles and footwear.

Foot Tracing

This allows the nurse and client to evaluate the fit of the current footwear. The individual stands on a sheet of paper and the nurse traces the outline of each foot while the individual is in a weight-bearing position. The individual's shoes are then placed over the tracings; if the shoes do not fit within the lines of the tracings, it provides visual evidence that the footwear is not correctly fitted.

Assessment of Muscle Strength and Range of Motion

Range of motion is assessed by asking the individual to move the foot up and down and back and forth

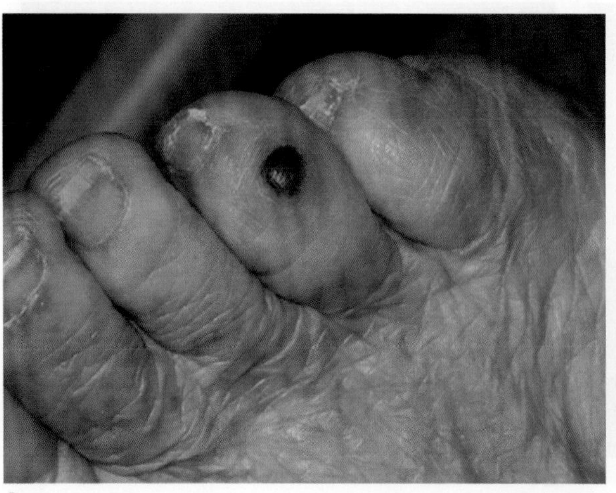

A

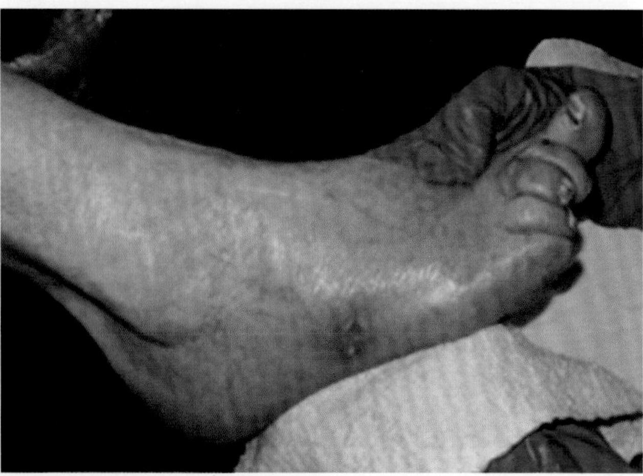

B

FIGURE 26-6. **A and B.** Injury/ulcer due to poorly fitted shoes.

(active range of motion). Muscle strength is assessed by placing the examiner's hand against the foot and asking the person to push the foot down against the examiner's hand. Both extremities are evaluated, and one side is compared to the other (WOCN, 2008, 2012). Reduced strength and/or range of motion are indicators of motor neuropathy.

Assessment for Autonomic Neuropathy

Autonomic neuropathy involves damage to the nerves that control sweat gland function and appropriate vasoconstriction of the arteries in the lower extremity. Damage to these nerves is evidenced by dry cracked skin with or without fissure formation, an abnormally warm pink foot, and, in severe cases, development of Charcot neuroarthropathy, also known as Charcot foot (Fig. 26-7) (Game, 2012; Hovaguimian, 2012). Whenever an individual presents with an abnormally warm pink foot, it is important to rule out an infectious process by assessing for fever, elevated white blood cell (WBC) count, and hyperglycemia (Madan & Pai, 2013; Milne et al., 2013). An x-ray may be needed to rule out an acute fracture and to differentiate among acute arthritic conditions (e.g., gout), chronic arthritis, and early-onset Charcot neuroarthropathy (Milne et al., 2013; WOCN, 2012).

CLINICAL PEARL

Whenever an individual presents with an abnormally warm and pink foot, it is necessary to rule out Charcot neuroarthropathy via x-ray and laboratory tests.

Charcot neuroarthropathy (also known as Charcot osteoarthropathy) is a complex complication resulting from a combination of autonomic neuropathy, sensory neuropathy, and possibly motor neuropathy. Autonomic neuropathy results in persistent vasodilation of the pedal arteries, which is thought to cause, over time, demineralization of the small bones in the foot (osteopenia); these fragile bones are at increased risk for fracture as a result of minor trauma, and the risk is even greater if the individual also has motor neuropathy resulting in abnormal gait and weight bearing. If the fracture is recognized promptly and the foot is appropriately off-loaded until the fracture heals, the architecture of the foot is preserved. However, because of sensory neuropathy and LOPS, the fracture(s) may not be recognized; in this case, the fracture is untreated and the individual continues to walk on the fractured foot, resulting in additional fractures over time and eventual collapse of the

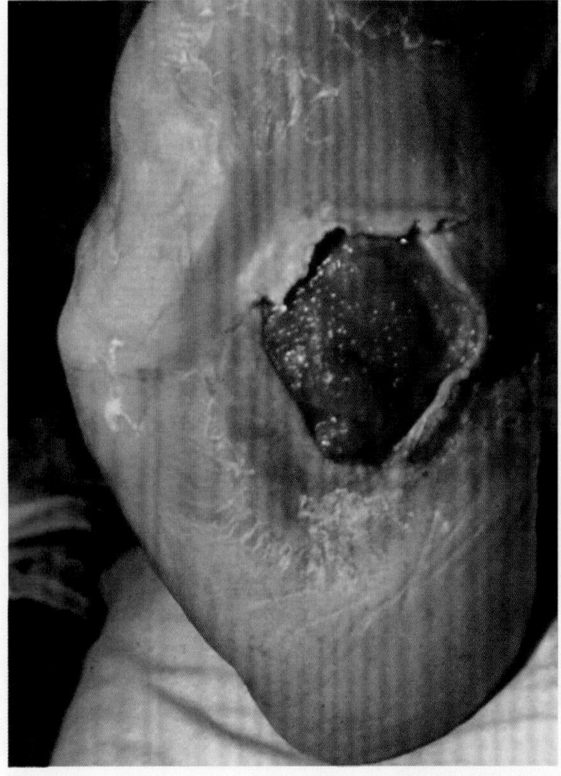

A

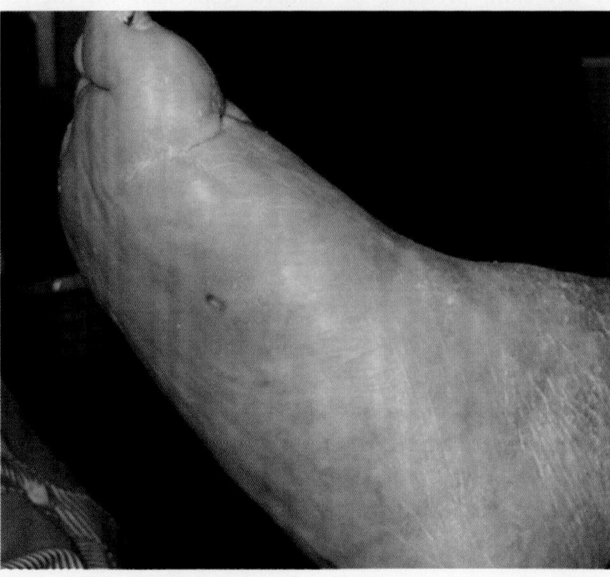

B

FIGURE 26-7. **A,B.** Examples of Charcot neuroarthropathy.

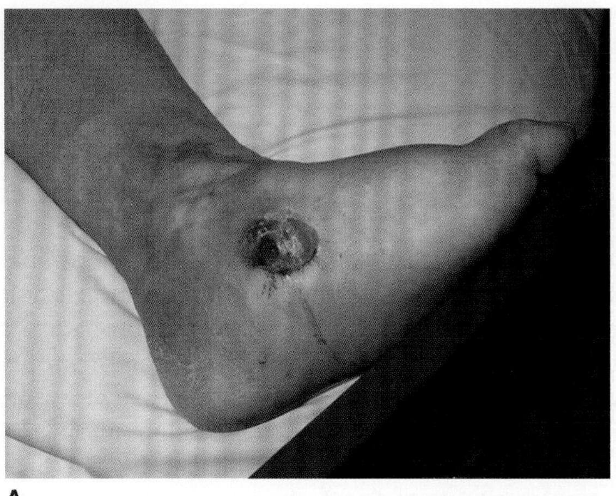

A

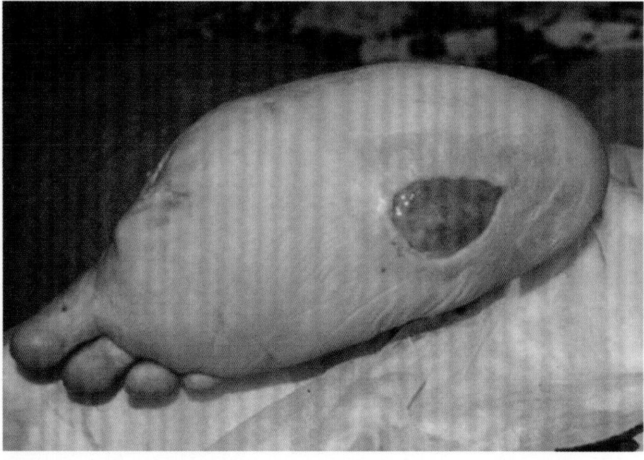

B

FIGURE 26-8. **A and B.** Rocker-bottom foot.

normal architecture of the foot (Milne et al., 2013; Pupp & Kolvunen, 2011; Sanchez et al., 2013). The loss of normal foot architecture results in a "rocker-bottom foot" with high midfoot pressures and higher risk of ulceration and possible amputation (Pupp & Kolvunen, 2011) (Fig. 26-8). A Charcot joint is most common in the midfoot but can involve the great toe, knee, or other jointed area (Madan & Pai, 2013).

Assessment of Skin Status

The condition of the skin of the lower extremity and foot is an important indicator of any underlying condition and usual foot care and hygiene. The foot care nurse should carefully inspect the skin of the lower leg, foot, and web spaces for texture, hydration, and cleanliness. The nurse should be alert to the following: thin atrophic skin; excessively dry skin; presence of fissures (especially on the heels); presence of corns and calluses (including interdigital corns); maceration of web spaces and any lesions or fissures involving the web spaces; evidence of tinea pedis (athlete's foot), which may present as dry scaly lesions on the plantar surface or as moist painful desquamation of the plantar surface and painful fissures between the toes (Erwin et al., 2013; Habif et al., 2006); and evidence of plantar warts (verruca plantaris), which are caused by the human papillomavirus. The foot care nurse must be aware that, in addition to these commonly occurring conditions, there are a myriad of dermatologic conditions that may cause foot lesions, including psoriasis, contact dermatitis, and melanomas (Bristow et al., 2010; Johnson & Taylor, 2012; Mechem & Zafren, 2014; Watkins, 2011). Any suspicious or unknown lesion mandates prompt referral to a dermatologist (Johnson & Taylor, 2012).

Presence and Characteristics of Any Wounds

Any lesions or wounds on the feet and legs should be noted and appropriate referrals made. If the individual is being managed in a comprehensive foot and wound care center, the wound/foot care nurse can provide an in-depth wound assessment and management and can involve other specialists as indicated (Snyder et al., 2010). If the individual is being seen in a center limited to foot care, she or he should be referred to a wound treatment center or the appropriate specialist. See Chapters 21, 22, and 23 for an in-depth discussion of the pathology, presentation, and management of lower extremity wounds caused by LEAD, LEND, and LEVD. (Figs. 26-9 to 26-11 depict ulcers of arterial, neuropathic, and venous etiology.)

Condition of the Toenails and Cuticles

Toenails should remain relatively the same throughout the life span, though both old and new injuries may affect the shape, size, and rate of growth of the nail. The cuticle is the hardened skin at the base and edge of the

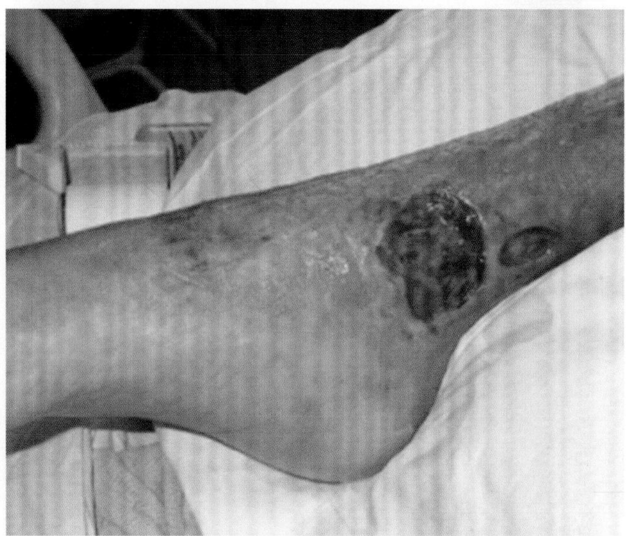

FIGURE 26-9. Arterial ulcer.

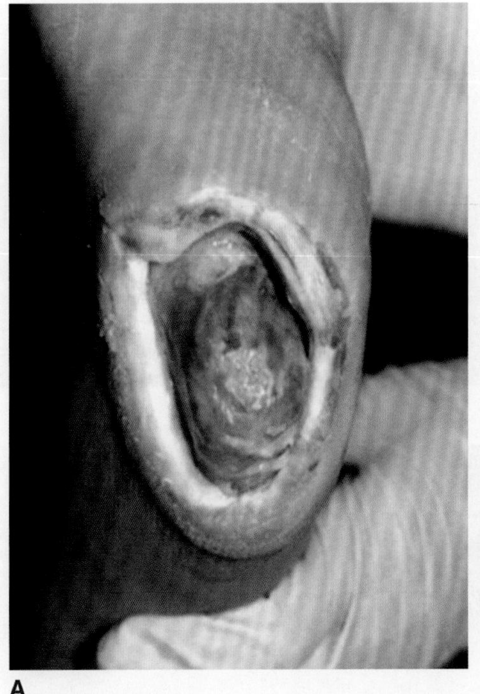

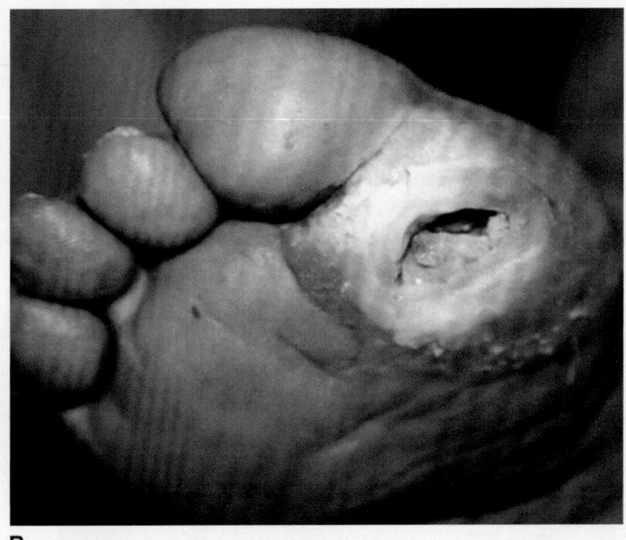

A B

FIGURE 26-10. **A and B.** Neuropathic ulcers.

nail that serves to seal and protect the nail matrix from invasion of pathogens (see Fig. 26-2). Critical factors to include in assessment of the nails and cuticles include the following: thickness, color, and brittleness of the nails; nail deformities (e.g., incurvated nails; "ram's horn" nails, also known as onychogryphosis; or thickened deformed nails, also known as onychodystrophy); evidence of fungal infection (onychomycosis), such as nails that are discolored, flaking, brittle, or thickened; integrity of the cuticle; evidence of ingrown nails (onychocryptosis); and evidence of inflammation and infection around the toenail (paronychia), which is commonly associated with damage to the cuticle or presence of onychocryptosis (Erwin, 2013; Goldstein, 2014; Habif et al., 2006) (Figs. 26-12A–E).

CLINICAL PEARL

Critical factors to include in assessment of the nails and cuticles include thickness, color, and brittleness of the nails, nail deformities, evidence of fungal infection, integrity of the cuticle, evidence of ingrown nails, and evidence of inflammation around the nail.

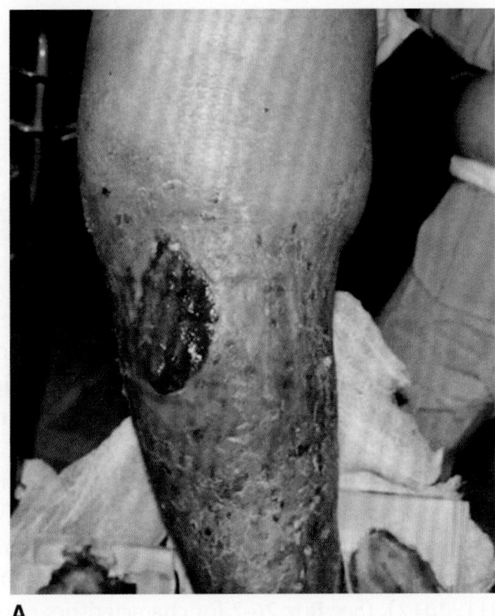

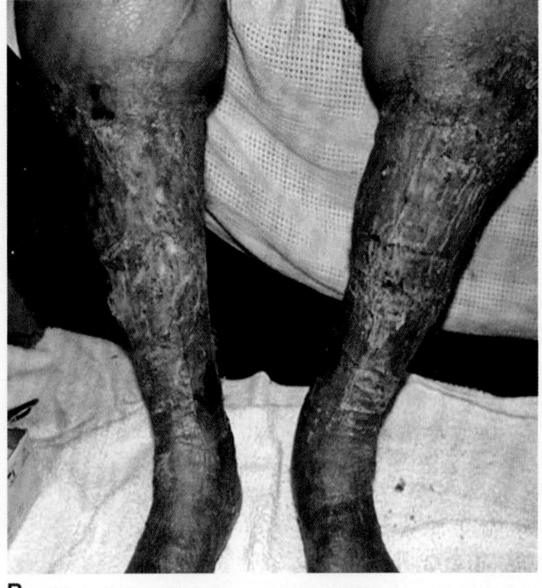

A B

FIGURE 26-11. **A and B.** Venous ulcers.

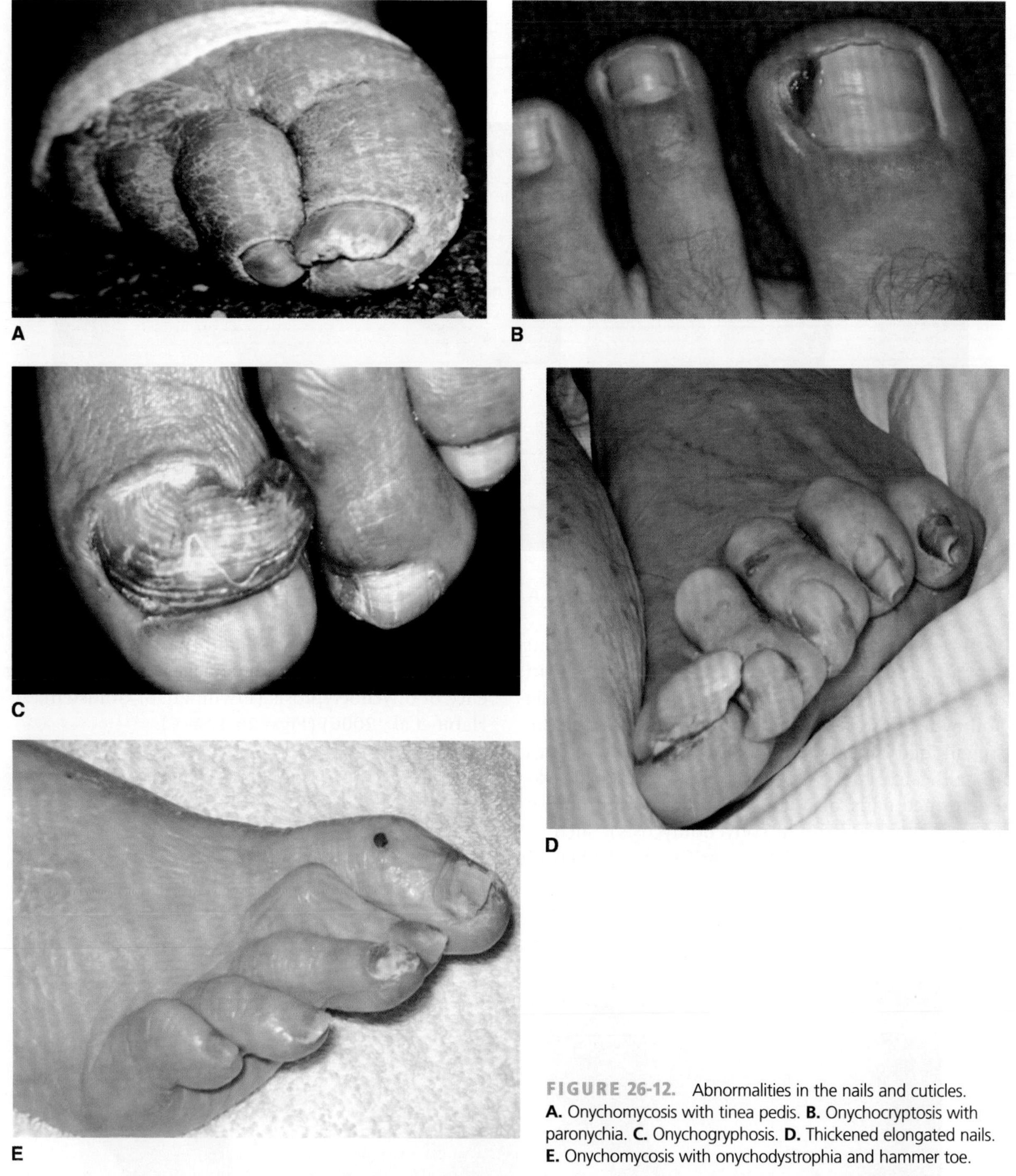

FIGURE 26-12. Abnormalities in the nails and cuticles. **A.** Onychomycosis with tinea pedis. **B.** Onychocryptosis with paronychia. **C.** Onychogryphosis. **D.** Thickened elongated nails. **E.** Onychomycosis with onychodystrophia and hammer toe.

The information gathered during the physical assessment allows the foot care nurse to develop an individualized plan of care for education and counseling that addresses self protection during activities of daily living, as well as indicated referrals for further evaluation, follow-up, and management.

Assessment of Lower Extremity Pain

Pain has been defined as "an unpleasant sensory and emotional experience associated with actual or potential tissue damage or disease" (Garnett, 2005). Pain is a common symptom of many disorders involving the lower extremities, including LEAD, LEND, LEVD, musculoskeletal conditions (such as arthritis or plantar fasciitis), and nerve damage (such as interdigital neuroma). Pain is subjective, and no confirmatory physical or laboratory examination can substantiate the presence or severity; thus, pain assessment involves a careful history that includes the following: intensity of pain using established pain scale, frequency of occurrence and time of occurrence, characteristics, and exacerbating and relieving factors (Wellborn & Moceri, 2014; WOCN, 2008, 2011, 2012). (See Box 26-2 for characteristics of pain associated with arterial, neuropathic, and venous disease.)

BOX 26-2. Characteristics of Arterial, Neuropathic, and Venous Pain

LEAD (arterial pain)
- Characteristics
  - Intermittent claudication
  - Sharp
  - Shooting
  - May occur at night (nocturnal pain)

LEND (neuropathic pain)
- Altered sensation not described as pain
  - Numbness
  - Warm/cool
  - Prickling
  - Tingling
  - "Stocking glove" pattern
- Characteristics of pain
  - Burning, itching
  - Shooting, "electrical shock"
  - Paresthesias
  - Unrelenting

LEVD (venous pain)
- Characteristics
  - Throbbing/aching of variable severity
  - May be relieved by leg elevation and compression
  - End of the day—achy leg syndrome—heavy legs

Common Pathologic Nail Conditions

Onychomycosis

Onychomycosis is a common fungal infection of the nail plate, nail bed, or both and accounts for over 50% of common nail disorders in older adults (Figs. 26-12A and 26-13). The most common causative organism is *Trichophyton rubrum;* other organisms are dermatophyte fungi, nondermatophyte fungi, and yeast (Gupta et al., 2011). Toenails are 25 times more likely than fingernails to develop onychomycosis, and the first and second toes are the most susceptible, probably due to repeated trauma that weakens the seal between the nail plate and nail bed, thus permitting entry of the pathogen (Kelechi & Johnson, 2012). The infection easily spreads to other toe nails (Parrish et al., 2005) and is difficult to treat due to the difficulty in penetrating the nail (Elewski & Tosti, 2014).

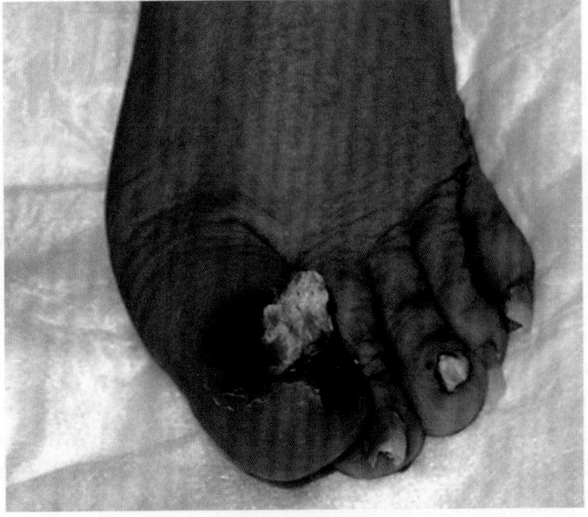

FIGURE 26-13. Onychomycosis with hypertrophic nail and C-shaped nails.

CLINICAL PEARL

Onychomycosis is a common fungal infection that accounts for over 50% of common nail disorders in older adults; it is usually more of an aesthetic issue than health issue.

There is a strong correlation between close quarter living environments (nursing homes, boarding schools, and military living quarters) and transmission of onychomycosis. People of all ages can be affected by onychomycosis, but older and adolescent populations are most at risk (Gazes & Zeichner, 2013). While onychomycosis is in general more of an aesthetic issue than a health issue, there is evidence that diabetic patients with onychomycosis are at increased risk for diabetic foot ulcers (Elewski & Tosti, 2014; Takehara et al., 2011).

The signs and symptoms of onychomycosis include: (1) discoloration of the nail plate (white, brown, yellow patches or streaks), (2) subungual hyperkeratosis (thickening and deformity of the toenails), (3) onycholysis (separation of nail plate from nail bed), and (4) brittle and crumbly nails. In addition to the cosmetic issues, some individuals with onychomycosis report tenderness and trauma to the lateral skin folds of the affected nail(s).

If systemic treatment is being considered, the diagnosis must be confirmed prior to initiation of therapy (Parrish et al., 2005). The diagnosis typically involves examination of nail scrapings obtained from the undersurface of the nail, top of the nail, or nail bed proximal to the affected portion of the nail. Specimens, direct microscopy, and cultures may be performed. There are benefits and drawbacks to the procedures for differential diagnosis and to systemic intervention.

Systemic treatment and topical solutions are utilized either separately or concurrently, although the most common method is a combination of both; this is because systemic treatment is more effective than topical treatment in penetrating hyperkeratotic layers of the nail. The treating physician must consider the causative organism, potential adverse events, drug interactions, patient compliance, and cost (Parrish et al., 2005). Liver toxicity is a potential adverse effect; therefore, it is necessary to monitor liver function at baseline and throughout treatment (Kelechi & Johnson, 2012). Allylamines and azoles are the most commonly used systemic antifungal agents; reported cure rates range from 35% to 70%, but recurrence is common. Treatment can take up to 1 year because it is difficult for the drugs to penetrate the keratin layers, due to the lack of blood vessels (Westerberg & Voyack, 2013).

Topical antifungals have low incidence of drug–drug interactions and few contraindications; this makes them appealing to many older patients, especially those taking multiple medications and those for whom oral antifungals are contraindicated (Parrish et al., 2005). If <50% of the nail bed is affected, some clinicians may opt to use topical therapy alone (Kelechi & Johnson, 2012), even in individuals for whom systemic therapy would be an option. Ciclopirox 8% lacquer is a topical agent that can be applied daily up to 7 days; it should then be removed using nail polish remover.

CLINICAL PEARL

Topical antifungals have limited contraindications and drug–drug interactions and are therefore appealing to the patient taking multiple medications and those for whom oral agents are contraindicated.

Some clinicians use a 20% to 40% urea compound to reduce hyperkeratosis, either as a solo treatment or followed by nail debridement (Kelechi & Johnson, 2012). Menthol vapor rub and tea tree oil have also been used to treat onychomycosis. Daily application around the cuticle is typically recommended for one full year to allow complete regrowth of the toenail, since these agents primarily affect the developing nail. The mechanism of action remains unclear, but anecdotal outcomes have been very good, and these agents are low cost and low risk in addition to being of potential great benefit. Topical agents also serve as a deodorizer.

Up to 50% of individuals with onychomycosis develop recurrent infections within 1 year after treatment (Elewski & Tosti, 2014); thus, it is important for the foot and nail care nurse to educate patients on strategies to reduce the risk of infection or reinfection (Pariser et al., 2013). These include the following:

- Avoid walking barefoot in public places such as pools, spas, gyms, and lockers where moisture is abundant and fungal organisms can thrive.
- Bring your own nail clippers and files to the nail salon.
- Wear properly fitting shoes made of natural materials with a toe box high enough to accommodate thickened nails and any toe deformities.
- Trim the nails according to the shape of the end of the toe (either curved or straight across) to avoid nail trauma that could cause breaks in the skin.
- File the nails with a course nail or emery board to smooth the edges after trimming.
- Wash the feet and dry between the toes daily (Kelechi & Johnson, 2012).
- Treat tinea pedis promptly, because fungal skin infections are thought to cause onychomycosis due to the proximity of the skin and nails (Elewski & Tosti, 2014).
- For individuals with onychomycosis, wash or replace shoes and inserts regularly.

CLINICAL PEARL

Up to 50% of individuals with onychomycosis develop recurrent infections within 1 year after treatment; thus, it is important to educate patients on strategies to reduce the risk of infection or reinfection.

Onychocryptosis

Onychocryptosis (ingrowing or ingrown toenail) affects 20% of the population, with older adults and adolescents being most affected (see Fig. 26-12B). Adolescents are at increased risk because their feet are growing at a rapid rate and they perspire more heavily. This creates a moist environment that makes the nails more susceptible to splitting. Older people who have difficulty caring for their feet and nails due to loss of visual acuity or physical mobility may develop an overgrowth of skin and nails that increases risk for ingrown nails (Heidelbaugh & Lee, 2009).

Onychocryptosis occurs when the lateral edge of the nail splinters and invades the periungual space, producing pain and reducing mobility and activity (Cohen & Scher, 2005); the resulting inflammation at the site can lead to infection (Heidelbaugh & Lee, 2009). The great toe is the most common site, although ingrown toenails can involve any nail (Heidelbaugh & Lee, 2009).

Factors contributing to onychocryptosis include improper nail trimming or tearing of the nails, excessive pressure during ambulation, repetitive or accidental trauma, tight shoes, C-shaped pattern of nail growth (incurvated nails), and obesity. All of these factors can add additional pressure to the nail and increase the risk for toe and nail injury. Proper nail trimming is an important element of care in prevention of onychocryptosis (Nandedkar-Thomas & Scher, 2005).

One form of conservative treatment involves placing a sliver of an alcohol prep pad between the edge of the nail and the skin/cuticle of the affected area to prevent the nail from growing into the periungual space (Heidelbaugh & Lee, 2009). Gutter splint, a surgical intervention, involves partial nail avulsion of the affected lateral edge of the nail bed followed by chemical matricectomy (removal of part or all of the nail).

CLINICAL PEARL

One conservative approach to management of ingrown nails is to place a sliver of an alcohol prep pad between the edge of the nail and the skin to prevent the nail from growing into the periungual space.

Onychogryphosis

Onychogryphosis is described as abnormally thickened nails with the appearance of an oyster shell or ram's horn (see Fig. 26-12C). The nail plate can be uneven, thickened, brown, or opaque and may curve toward the other nails. The main risk factor for this condition is inadequate nail care, due to self-neglect or inability to perform nail care due to limited mobility, lack of dexterity, poor eyesight, and/or insufficient professional nursing services. The older populations are most affected. It is also prevalent in the homeless and cognitively impaired populations. Proper nail trimming and filing is a key preventive measure (Nandedkar-Thomas & Scher, 2005). Management requires thinning of the nail followed by appropriate trimming, that is, reducing the height and length of the nail using nippers and a sturdy file.

Common Skin Disorders of the Foot and Lower Extremity

As noted previously, the older population and people with diabetes are at increased risk for LEAD, LEVD, and LEND; thus, the foot care nurse must be knowledgeable regarding these conditions and must be able to recognize and manage wounds caused by these pathologies (or make appropriate referrals). In addition, the foot care nurse must be able to identify and manage common skin conditions, for example, xerosis, fissures, and tinea pedis. Finally, the foot care nurse must be alert to indicators of skin malignancies (squamous cell carcinoma, basal cell carcinoma, and melanoma) and must assure prompt referral to dermatology for any abnormal lesions or suspected malignancies.

The goal in provision of foot and nail care is to prevent seemingly simple conditions that can be managed and treated from leading to a life of wounds and limb loss. For example, maintenance of normal nail thickness and length can optimize mobility and comfort and prevent traumatic injuries to the adjacent toes. Prompt identification of early ischemic or neuropathic changes with appropriate referrals and education can prevent ulcerations that could progress to amputation. Similarly, appropriate management of an ingrowing toenail can reduce pain, risk of infection, and ulceration that could lead to greater problems or even eventual amputation.

CLINICAL PEARL

The goal in provision of foot and nail care is to prevent seemingly simple conditions that can be managed and treated from leading to a life of wounds and limb loss.

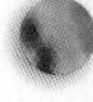

Systemic Conditions and Implications for Foot Care Nurses

Some of the systemic conditions that commonly affect the legs, feet, and nails are osteoarthritis, gout, LEAD, LEND, LEVD, and Raynaud's.

Osteoarthritis

Osteoarthritis is the most common type of arthritis, especially among the older population; rheumatoid arthritis is less common but causes greater morbidity. Osteoarthritis produces pain and stiffness, while rheumatoid arthritis causes deformity and loss of function in addition to pain. Any form of arthritis limits the individual's ability to provide his or her own foot care. Care goals include relief of pain, improvement in joint function, and enhanced ability to perform activities of daily living (Fischer et al., 2011; Hendry et al., 2013; Riskowki et al., 2011). Interventions include foot care, gentle massage, use of therapeutic shoes, over-the-counter compression socks (when indicated for management of edema), exercises, smoking cessation and weight loss if indicated, and orthotics when needed (Riskowki et al., 2011).

Gout

Gout is a less common form of arthritis that usually affects the joint of the great toe but may also present in the ankles and knees. It is caused by the accumulation of urate crystals in joints; this triggers an acute inflammatory response and severe pain. Gout is more common in males and is triggered by high levels of uric acid; thus, treatment involves measures to reduce uric acid levels, that is, avoiding alcoholic beverages, losing weight, and eating smaller amounts of purine-rich foods such as asparagus, mushrooms, mussels, and organ meats (Rome et al., 2013). The foot care nurse may assess individuals and assist in diagnosis, intervention, therapeutic foot and nail care, and footwear selection (Rome et al., 2013).

CLINICAL PEARL

Any form of arthritis limits the individual's ability to provide his or her own foot care.

Lower Extremity Arterial Disease

LEAD is manifest by changes in the skin and nails as well as abnormal ABI, diminished pulses, and prolonged capillary refill time. In addition to assuring that the patient is referred to a vascular specialist, the nurse must take every precaution to avoid any trauma to the skin during foot and nail care and must educate the patient regarding measures to improve perfusion (e.g., smoking cessation) and to prevent traumatic injury to the leg and foot during activities that increase the risk for trauma (e.g., use of protective footwear and shin guards) (WOCN, 2008). Foot and nail care is essential on a regular basis to monitor progression of disease and to prevent wounds that could lead to an amputation. In addition, ongoing communication with the primary and cardiovascular providers is critical to limb preservation.

CLINICAL PEARL

The individual with evidence of LEAD should be referred to a vascular specialist; in addition, the nurse must take every precaution to avoid any trauma to the skin during foot and nail care and must educate the patient regarding measures to prevent trauma and improve perfusion.

Lower Extremity Venous Disease

Lower extremity venous disease (LEVD) is manifest by edema, hemosiderosis, and/or venous dermatitis (Paul et al., 2011). Calf pump muscle dysfunction is a key contributing factor to LEVD and chronic lower extremity venous ulcers. The foot and nail nurse should assure that the individual is being followed by a vascular specialist and should reinforce the importance of leg elevation, consistent use of compression stockings, and adherence to walking/exercise programs (Kelechi & Johnson, 2012; O'Brien et al., 2012).

CLINICAL PEARL

The individual with edema or evidence of LEVD should be educated regarding the importance of leg elevation and routine use of compression socks or stockings.

Lower Extremity Neuropathic Disease

LEND is usually manifest by diminished sensory awareness, foot deformities, altered weight bearing, and dry skin. Some individuals report paresthesias (pins and needles sensation, burning pain, and/or "electric shock" sensations); these individuals require prompt referral to a neurologist for further assessment and pain management (WOCN, 2012). Foot care nurses play a critical role in management of patients with LEND, specifically in monitoring for changes in sensorimotor status, perfusion status, or HbA1c; in addition, they are responsible for ongoing education and counseling regarding protective footwear, foot care, and daily foot inspection. Provision of professional nail care that maintains the nails at a safe length and thickness, and prompt intervention for potential problems such as an ingrowing nail or callus formation are additional critical responsibilities (Aalaa et al., 2012). For the individual with diabetes, appropriate care also involves reinforcement of the importance of tight glycemic control (Christman et al., 2011; Sacks & John, 2014).

CLINICAL PEARL

Foot care nurses play a critical role in management of patients with LEND, specifically monitoring for changes in sensorimotor function and education regarding glycemic control, protective footwear, and routine foot inspection.

Raynaud's

Raynaud's phenomenon is a vasoconstrictive condition that results in decreased blood flow to the hands and feet in response to cold or stress (Fischer et al., 2011). The foot care nurse should intervene by educating the patient to avoid cold and to slowly and gently warm the hands and feet.

 Common Foot Malformations

The most common malformations and disorders of the foot are hallux valgus (bunion), hallux varus, hallux rigidus/limitus, bunionette (tailor bunion), Charcot foot (neuroarthropathy, osteoarthropathy), neuroma, flat feet (pes planus), high arch (pes cavus), plantar fasciitis, and heel spurs. Malformations of the toes, feet, and ankles lead to an increased risk of corns, calluses, falls, pain, wounds, and amputations.

Hallux Valgus

Hallux valgus (bunion) is an abnormal prominence (outgrowth) of the joint between the big toe and the foot (first metatarsophalangeal joint) (Fig. 26-14A and B). Hallux valgus is a very common deformity; it can be minor or major and may or may not cause pain but can cause a serious balance and mobility issue later in life. It is the most common foot deformity and is related to genetics, previous footwear, and trauma. Clinical presentation includes bulging of the first metatarsophalangeal joint medially and away from the foot. The hallux (great toe) tilts toward the 2nd toe and may push up or under it. Calluses may form due to ill-fitting shoes or because of pressure, shear, or friction caused by the deformity and the resulting abnormal gait. Walking may become difficult and dangerous due to pain and balance issues. An x-ray can identify the skeletal changes including any changes due to osteoarthritis. Wearing proper shoes may reduce symptoms; it is critical to provide a wider forefoot and toe box to accommodate the deformity. It may also be helpful to refer the patient to an orthotist or pedorthist for inserts and therapeutic shoes; if the patient has intractable symptoms or is interested in surgical intervention, the foot care nurse should initiate a referral to an orthopedic surgeon.

CLINICAL PEARL

Corns and calluses form due to ill-fitting shoes and/or pressure, shear, and friction caused by bony abnormalities and abnormal weight bearing.

Hallux Varus

Hallux varus is characterized by a medial deviation of the great toe (hallux) from its straight axis; the toe begins to point toward the other foot. This deformity often develops after a previous surgery for hallux valgus, usually due to overcorrection. Other known causes include trauma, rheumatoid arthritis, and psoriasis. Taping the great toe toward the little toe for 3 months may help. Depending on the length of time the deformity has been present and other comorbidities; surgery may be indicated. To prevent injury, the individual should be counseled to wear shoes that have a wider toe box and are made of soft moldable materials.

Hallux Rigidus/Hallux Limitus

Hallux rigidus and hallux limitus are both great toe joint issues in which movement of the hallux becomes restricted (see Fig. 26-14C). With hallux limitus joint movement is restricted during weight bearing but is otherwise normal; this condition is characterized by intact cartilage and little or no arthritis. With hallux rigidus, the great toe becomes arthritic with associated cartilage loss, resulting in bone-on-bone motion and pain. Hallux rigidus/limitus is the result of trauma and hyperglycemia and most commonly occurs in people with diabetes. Clinical presentation includes stiffness of the great toe, which "sticks up" and leads to major problems when the toe box of the shoe is too shallow or narrow. Pain is caused by excessive flexion of the great toe; it may also occur during standing, due to pronation and rolling of the big toe joint that causes

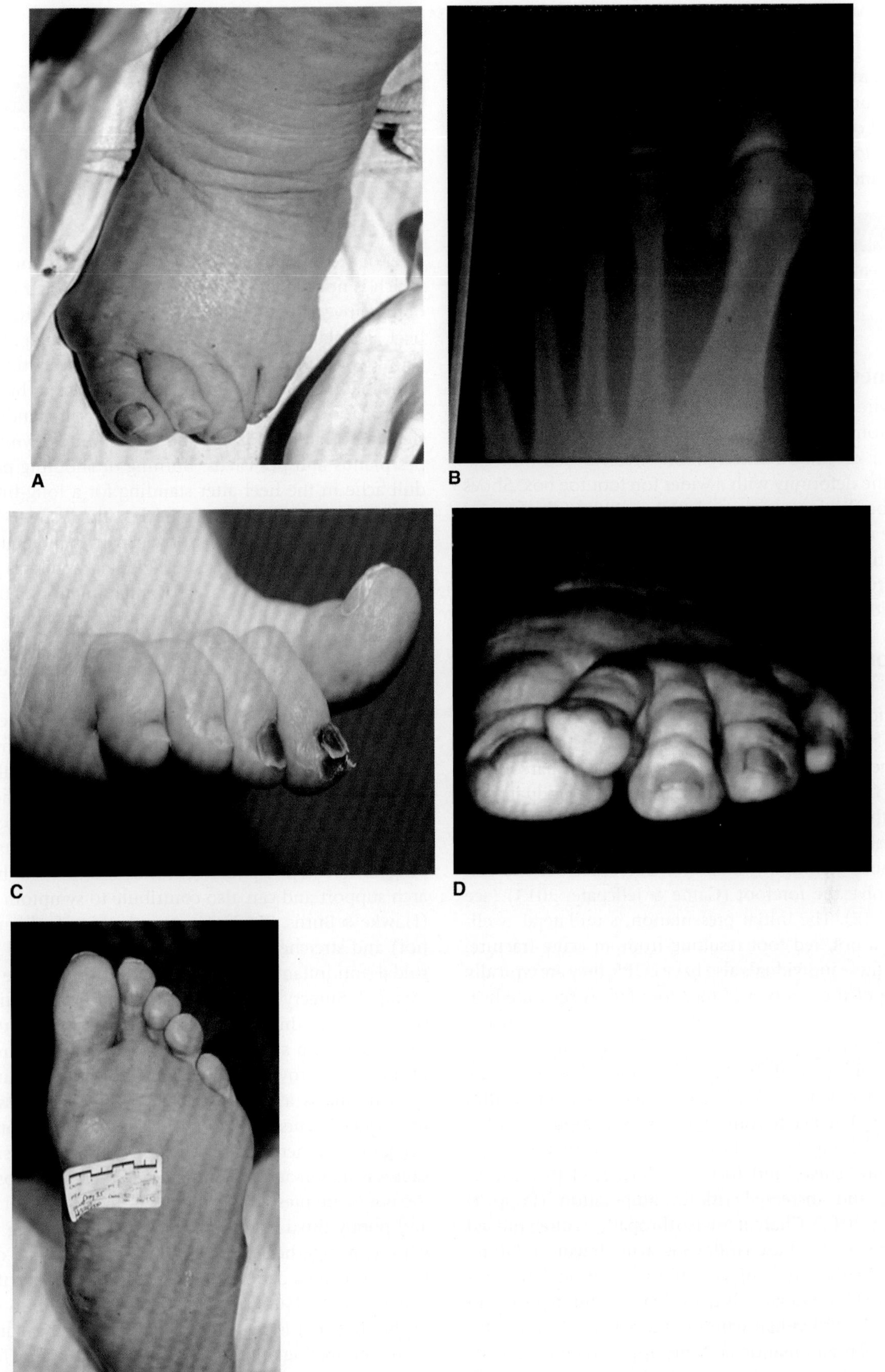

FIGURE 26-14. Common toe and foot deformities. **A.** Hallux valgus (bunion). **B.** X-ray of bunion. **C.** Hallux rigidus with claw toes and subungual hematoma. **D.** Overlapping toes. **E.** Charcot neuroarthropathy.

restricted motion. Surgery is often times required to correct the structural problem. Like most foot and toe malformations and conditions, wearing the appropriate footwear is essential to prevent pressure, shear, and friction causing calluses and wounds.

CLINICAL PEARL

The patient with plantar surface calluses should be referred to an orthotist or pedorthist for pressure-redistributing insoles (inserts) and therapeutic shoes.

Bunionette

Bunionette (tailor bunion) is a bulge caused by an abnormally prominent 5th metatarsal joint. The deformity can be major or minor. Intervention involves accommodation of the deformity with a wider forefoot toe box. Shoes should be sized to accommodate the width of the foot; to alleviate any pressure, shear, and friction; and to off-load any existing wounds. Surgery is rarely indicated; when the deformity cannot be managed with conservative measures, referral to a podiatrist or orthopedic surgeon is indicated.

Charcot Foot

Charcot foot (osteoarthropathy, neuroarthropathy) is a gross deformity of the foot directly related to poor glucose control. Nearly 13% of individuals with diabetes who have LOPS and/or autonomic neuropathy develop Charcot foot disease (CFD) (Hanson, 2011). CFD involves gradual thinning of the bones (osteopenia), fractures, deformities, and abnormalities in weight bearing; the midfoot is the segment most commonly involved, but exacerbations can also involve the forefoot (Game & Jeffcoate, 2013) (see Fig. 26-14E). The initial presentation is unilateral swelling and a hot, red foot resulting from an acute fracture. Because these individuals also have LOPS, they are typically unaware of the injury and therefore fail to seek medical care and continue to put weight on the foot. This creates an environment of continued inflammation, additive damage, and gradual settling of the bones into a chronic (cold) Charcot joint. With severe deformity, difficulties in gait and balance become a major issue, along with fall issues. The bony deformities result in abnormal increases in pressure, shear, and friction, which lead to calluses, wounds, and increased risk of amputation (Pupp & Kolvunen, 2011). Charcot osteoarthropathy is often missed during the acute phase (following acute fracture); failure to recognize the initial injury results in additional fractures because the individual fails to off-load the injured foot. In contrast, the individual who monitors his or her feet for evidence of inflammation and who appropriately off-loads the foot in response to evidence of injury can prevent additional injury and deformity and the potential for subsequent amputation. Recognizing the initial presentation and responding with prompt referrals and follow-up is essential for this serious and frequently missed condition.

CLINICAL PEARL

Charcot foot disease (CFD) involves gradual thinning of the bones (osteopenia), fractures, deformities, and abnormalities in weight bearing.

Conditions Causing Heel/Arch Pain

Heel or arch pain may be due to thinning of the fat pads, which is normal with aging or which can occur as a result of repetitive activity that increases pressure on the arch and heel. Pes planus (flat foot) and pes cavus (high arch foot) should be seriously considered when evaluating symptoms that include pain on the bottom, edge, or back of the heel or foot. Sharp pain that occurs upon standing after sleeping or sitting for a while is a common symptom of pes planus and pes cavus. Burning or shooting pain or a dull ache in the heel after standing for a long time on a hard surface are all signs of a heel or arch issue.

The most common cause of heel pain is an outgrowth of the bone also known as a spur. Plantar fasciitis is another common cause and is caused by inflammation of the plantar fascia and/or Achilles tendon, oftentimes due to poor foot mechanics (American College of Physicians, 2012). Other causes include tendonitis, which is usually related to repetitive activity, and arthritic conditions such as rheumatoid arthritis or gout. X-rays are important for determining the underlying problem and to rule out stress fractures, osteoarthritis, and other inflammatory or skeletal issues. Treatment is based on the underlying problem; however, footwear modifications to support normal foot mechanics can frequently help to reduce pain. Night splints, strapping, orthotics, and padding may be indicated for heel and arch support and can also contribute to symptom control (Hawke & Burns, 2012). Contrast bathing (cold and then hot) and stretches may help to reduce pain, and nonsteroidal anti-inflammatory drugs (NSAIDs) may be recommended. Surgery or injections are additional options for some patients; thus, the wound care nurse should refer any individual with significant or refractory symptoms to the primary care provider, podiatrist, or orthopedic surgeon.

Neuroma is a painful overgrowth of nerve tissue that most often occurs between the 3rd and 4th toe bones. The overgrowth of nerves is triggered by bony compression that causes irritation and inflammation of the nerve; most often, the bones are pressed together by footwear that is too tight and poorly fitted. Neuromas are common among women who wear high-heeled shoes and nurses who are on their feet for extended periods of time. Most commonly, the individual reports sharp, burning, or shooting pain in the ball of the foot that is triggered or worsened by walking; others report tingling or numbness or the sensation of having a stone in the shoe. Treatment recommendations include footwear modifications and the addition of orthotics. Padding and taping, physical therapy, and medication may be indicated. The individual with severe or refractory symptoms should be referred to a podiatrist for injections or surgery.

Common Toe Deformities/ Malformations

Hammer toes, claw toes, and mallet toes are deformities caused by contractures of the interphalangeal joints (see Fig. 26-12E). A hammer toe involves contracture of the proximal interphalangeal joint, a mallet toe involves contracture of the distal interphalangeal joint, and a claw toe involves contractures of both the proximal and distal interphalangeal joints. All of these deformities cause the interphalangeal joints to protrude upward and the distal toe to point downward. Causative factors include ill-fitting shoes, hyperglycemia, and previous trauma. The adverse results can be as minor as an unsightly deformity that detracts from the appearance of the foot to the development of recurrent corns and calluses that cause pain with ambulation (due to pressure, shear, and friction that occurs with walking). People with toe deformities benefit from footwear with a toe box that is made of flexible material and that is wide enough and high enough to accommodate the deformity. Surgery may be indicated and would necessitate referral to a podiatrist or orthopedic surgeon. Other deformities include webbed toes, six toes, and 2nd or 3rd toes that are longer than the first. Any foot or toe deformity must be taken into consideration when providing recommendations, education, or referrals regarding footwear.

CLINICAL PEARL

Hammer toes, claw toes, and mallet toes are deformities caused by contractures of the interphalangeal joints. Conservative management involves modifications in footwear to accommodate the deformities; definitive management requires surgery to correct the deformity.

Guidelines for Foot and Nail Care

Foot and nail care must be provided with caution and appropriate equipment. The overall goals of care are to reduce the length and height of the nails to within normal range, maintain intact cuticles, and pare or file corns and calluses. Ideally, hygienic care is provided first; for example, bathing the feet in warm water with or without a mild cleanser assures that the feet and nails are clean. Bathing the feet also softens the nails and cuticles (thus facilitating nail and cuticle care).

CLINICAL PEARL

The goals of foot and nail care are to reduce the length and height of the nails to within normal range, maintain intact cuticles, and pare or file corns and calluses.

Assessment

At the initial visit, a comprehensive lower extremity assessment should be conducted. Follow-up visits require general inspection for evidence of any lesions or ulcers, assessment of dorsalis pedis and posterior tibialis pulses, observation for dependent rubor, and assessment for LOPS. The patient should also be queried regarding any foot-related pain or concerns.

The feet should be inspected for corns or calluses and for any lesions or maceration of the interdigital spaces. The foot care nurse should use a nail curette, spatula, or orange wood stick to remove debris from beneath the nails and to assess the free nail border (Etnnyre et al., 2011; Gallagher, 2012). During this process, the nurse also assesses the nails for length and thickness. If there is callus obscuring the distal end of the toe and the free nail border the callus should be removed either by paring (with a scalpel or rasper) or by filing with an emery board.

Management Hypertrophic Nails

If the nail is abnormally thickened, it should be thinned prior to trimming. This may be done with use of a large coarse grain emery board or with an electric grinder. (If an electric grinder is used, the clinician must be aware of the potential for aerosolizing mycotic and bacterial organisms and must implement appropriate CDC infection control guidelines.) (Abramson, 1990; Burrow & McLarnon, 2006; Etnnyre et al., 2011)

Due to concerns regarding aerosolization of organisms, many clinicians elect not to use a grinder and instead use alternative methods for thinning hypertrophic nails. One approach is to apply a 2 × 2 gauze or cotton ball soaked with mineral oil, warm water, or saline to the nail for 5 minutes to soften the nail and then to reduce the nail with a nipper (cutting from top down), followed by filing with a coarse grain emery board. The nail should not be trimmed until it has been adequately thinned and the free nail border has been established. The nail should be trimmed in a side-to-side fashion, and the general rule of thumb is to follow the contours of the nail and toe, while taking into consideration any specific needs or requests reported by the patient. Some individuals request that the nail be trimmed as short as possible while others prefer the nail left a little longer; when honoring a request for "short nails," the nurse must be careful to trim only the nail beyond the free nail border. The nail should always be filed after trimming to eliminate any sharp edges that could cause trauma or predispose the toe to an ingrowing nail.

CLINICAL PEARL

The nail should not be trimmed until it has been adequately thinned and the free nail border has been established; the nail should always be filed after trimming to eliminate sharp edges.

Management of Hypertrophic Skin and Cuticles

Excessive skin around the nail should be trimmed with extreme caution; it is frequently safer to file rough skin with an emery board or to remove excess skin with a rasper or paring scalpel. A pterygium blade is an acceptable and safe instrument for reduction of overgrown cuticles. Cuticles should be manipulated with caution, and the nurse should avoid pushing the cuticles back or clipping the skin around the cuticles, as injury to the cuticles creates the potential for bacterial invasion and infection.

Management of Corns and Calluses

Corns or calluses should be carefully pared or filed from "top down" using a rasper, scalpel, or file, and the individual should be asked whether he or she prefers the callus or corn to be totally removed or whether he or she prefers that a thin layer be left. (Some individuals experience acute tenderness if the callus or corn is completely removed; this is particularly true of the homeless population.) When caring for an individual with corns or calluses, the nurse must determine the source of recurrent friction; the individual with plantar surface calluses should be referred to an orthotist for appropriate insoles and may benefit from a thin protective glycerine-based gel dressing, while the individual with corns needs to be educated regarding the need for a deeper and wider toe box and use of a protective toe sleeve, mole skin, corn pad, or lambswool (available from podiatric supply centers).

CLINICAL PEARL

Corns or calluses should be pared or filed from "top down" using a rasper, scalpel, or file.

Equipment and Policies/Procedures

Having the right equipment and established policies and procedures for foot and nail care are of critical importance (Box 26-3). Nippers, clippers, curettes, orange sticks, pterygium blades, files of a variety of coarseness, and nail raspers are commonly used tools; a list of commonly used pieces of equipment, supplies, and tools is provided in Box 26-4 and illustrated in Figure 26-15. Infection control is essential for protection of both the provider and recipient of foot care. Tools and equipment must be effectively disinfected using cold disinfection protocols, disinfecting solutions, steam, or autoclave (Box 26-5). It is equally important for the foot care nurse to use appropriate personal protective equipment (PPE), including use of a mask, gown, apron, scrubs, gloves, and eye protection. Disinfecting surfaces with bleach or lysol wipes, disinfecting diagnostic instruments with isopropyl alcohol, and regular use of sanitizing gel and hand washing are all essential for reducing the risk of cross-contamination.

CLINICAL PEARL

Infection control is essential for protection of both the provider and recipient of foot care.

Education, Prevention, and Routine Management

Education and referrals are an essential element of the foot nurse role. Clients and caregivers must be taught the basics of foot care, signs and symptoms that require follow-up, and the importance of appropriate footwear and activity. In addition, individuals should be referred to an orthotist or pedorthist for properly fitted footwear and insoles when indicated (Ahroni & Scheffler, 2006; Malemute et al., 2011).

Follow-up

Frequency of follow-up is individualized based on the patient's risk status, which is determined by the presence or absence of protective sensation and foot deformities, perfusion status, and presence or history of ulcerations or amputations. As explained earlier in the chapter, a base line assessment should be done at the point of entry into the foot care practice. The frequency of in-depth follow-up assessment is based on results of the initial assessment. If the individual is high risk, follow-up assessments should be done in 3 to 6 months; an individual at lower risk requires in-depth assessment less frequently (e.g., annually). Limited assessment (to include pulse palpation, inspection for dependent rubor, and inspection of the feet, web spaces, and nails) is performed at each visit. The objective is to monitor the individual closely enough to prevent an insult or injury that could lead to a wound, especially a nonhealing wound due to LEAD or LEND. The nurse should be particularly attentive in assessing individuals over 50 years of age with a history of cardiovascular disease; those over 60 years of age with a history of smoking, cardiovascular disease, or diabetes; and all individuals over 70 years of age (these populations represent individuals at high risk for compromised blood flow or LOPS) (WOCN, 2012).

CLINICAL PEARL

Frequency of follow-up is individualized based on the patient's risk status, which is determined by the presence or absence of protective sensation and foot deformities, perfusion status, and presence or history of ulcerations or amputations.

Off-loading and Padding

Off-loading and padding are important for people with diabetes, those over the age of 70, those with osteoarthritis, and individuals with foot deformities, plantar surface callus, or previous injuries or ulcerations (Armstrong et al., 2014; Caselli, 2011; Cheskin, 2013). Reduction in plantar surface pressures can be achieved with orthotics, inserts, moleskin or glycerine gel pads, felted foam, and/or total contact casting (Huppin, 2011; McGuire, 2010; Rizzo et al., 2012). (Total contact casting is usually limited to treatment of plantar surface ulcers and acute Charcot osteoarthropathy and is not used for prevention.) The foot care nurse can use simple

BOX 26-3. **Your Institutional or Company Name**

Nursing Practice Manual

Guidelines for Foot and Nail Care to Include Hygiene, Assessment, and Intervention (HAI)

The care of the hands/feet and finger/toenails is part of daily personal hygiene. Assessment of the lower extremity helps in detection of infection, wounds, nail/skin integrity issues, and/or other complications associated with overall health.

Purpose

To guide the practice of certified foot and nail care nurses (CFCN) who, within their scope of practice and specialty training, incorporate foot and nail care to meet nursing and patient goals of health promotion, patient education, health risk reduction, and promotion of comfort and safety.

CFCN's provide foot and nail care based on theoretical knowledge of:

1. Anatomy and physiology of the lower extremity
2. Structure and function of the feet and nails
3. Common pathology of the foot and related nursing interventions
4. Normal aging-related changes of the feet and hands
5. Abnormal changes of the feet and hands due to underlying conditions or life style behaviors
6. Lower extremity assessment to include peripheral neuropathy, perfusion, dermatologic conditions, and musculoskeletal deformities
7. Use of nail care instruments
8. Universal precautions and instrument disinfection

Equipment/Supplies:

1. Nail and cuticle clipper and nipper
2. Rasper, curettes, and nail files/emery boards
3. Wash cloths and towels
4. Monofilament and Doppler
5. Skin care products, e.g., moisturizer, antifungal powder

Precautions

1. A lower extremity assessment will be conducted specifically for peripheral neuropathy and perfusion prior to intervention.
2. Individuals with diabetes, peripheral vascular disease (PVD), or thickened or otherwise abnormal toenails may be referred to a DPM, PCP, and/or Vascular Surgeon.

Steps	Key Points
1. Wash the hands before and after the procedure	1. Standard universal precaution
2. Explain the procedure to the patient	2. Relieve patient anxiety and use as an opportunity to educate
3. Apply nonsterile gloves	3. Universal precautions
4. Provide hand/foot hygiene	4. Basic personal hygiene
5. Dry thoroughly, especially between the toes	5. Moisture between the toes can lead to maceration, irritation, and increased susceptibility to fungus
6. Debride nails—reduce length and height (you may refer to Medicare Codes here for Foot and Nail Care)	6. Nails should extend slightly beyond the end of the fingers or toes. Debride nails according to the shape of the finger or toe
7. Smooth rough edges with a nail file or emery board	7. To prevent further injury
8. Reduce hyperkeratotic lesions with rasper or file	8. Helps to reduce increasing pressure, shear, or friction and possible wound or lesion
9. Apply moisturizer to the feet and hands, may apply antifungal powder to web spaces	9. Keep the skin moist, web spaces dry—reduce maceration
10. Educate and refer as needed for proper foot and nail care for individuals with personal hygiene problems, diabetes, peripheral neuropathy, and vascular disease	10. Use adult learning principles with simple to complex concepts and continuous reinforced instruction and praise

APPROVED BY:
EFFECTIVE DATE: REVIEWED:
SUPERCEDES: New
PREPARED BY:

References:

Aalaa, M., Malazy, O. T., Sanjari, M., et al. (2012). Nurses' role in diabetic foot prevention and care; a review. *Journal of Diabetes and Metabolic Disorders, 11*, 24. Retrieved December 10, 2012, from www.jdmdonline.com

Bakker, K., Apelqvist, J., & Schaper, N. C. (2012). Practical guidelines on the management and prevention of the diabetic foot 2011. *Diabetes/Metabolism Research and Reviews, 28*(Suppl 1), 225–231.

Chan, H., Lee, D., Leung, E., et al. (2012). The effects of a foot and toenail care protocol for older adults. *Geriatric Nursing, 33*, 6, 1–9. Retrieved December 10, 2012, from www.nursingconsult.com

Smith, F., Duell, D., Martin, B. (2008). *Clinical nursing skills basic to advanced* (p. 905). Upper Saddle, NJ: Pearson.

strategies such as moleskin padding or glycerine-based gel pads. Clients with significant callus formation or deformities should be referred to an orthotist or pedorthist for construction of custom-molded toe lifts (for individuals with hammer toes) or customized insoles or inserts for plantar surface calluses or pressure points (Lavery et al., 2012).

Routine Foot Care

Routine foot care includes hygiene, skin care, and nail care. Hygiene should be conducted daily. The individual should be taught to gently lather a cleanser on the skin of the feet and between the toes, to use a cloth to reduce hyperkeratotic lesions and cuticle overgrowth around the nails, and

BOX 26-4. Foot and Nail Care Equipment, Supplies, Tools, and Accessories

- Basin or no-rinse disposable cloths
- Heavy-duty car wash paper towels
- Nail nippers (4.5- to 5.5-inch spring barrel type)
- Pterygium blade
- Emery boards or files
- Orange sticks
- Curettes—small for dental and nails
- Emollients
- Gloves
- Gauze pads—for flossing toes
- Goggles, gown, mask (refer to institutional policy regarding safety and infection control)
- Disinfectant solution—dimethyl benzyl ammonium chloride—Barbicide/Marvicide—fungicide, bactericide, germicide
- Alcohol prep pads
- Bleach
- Tea tree—antibacterial, antifungal
- Vapor rub
- Variety of corn, callus, toe pads, lambswool for accommodating deformities, etc.
- Instruments for lower extremity assessment—blood pressure cuff, Doppler, Semmes-Weinstein monofilament, tape measure, tuning fork, Plexor

BOX 26-5. Disinfection of Foot and Nail Equipment

CDC.GOV Guidelines for Sterilization and Disinfecting of Foot and Nail Care Instruments

A. Heat sterilization, including steam or hot air (see manufacturer's recommendations, steam sterilization processing time from 3 to 30 minutes)
B. Glutaraldehyde-based formulations (>2% glutaraldehyde, caution should be exercised with all glutaraldehyde formulations when further in-use dilution is anticipated); glutaraldehyde (1.12%) and 1.93% phenol/phenate. One glutaraldehyde-based product has a high-level disinfection claim of 5 minutes at 35°C.
C. Hydrogen peroxide 7.5% (will corrode copper, zinc, and brass)
D. Hypochlorite, single-use chlorine generated on-site by electrolyzing saline containing >650 to 675 active free chlorine (will corrode metal instruments)
E. Sodium hypochlorite (5.25% to 6.15% household bleach diluted 1:500 provides >100 ppm available chlorine)
F. Phenolic germicidal detergent solution (follow product label for use—dilution)
G. Iodophor germicidal detergent solution (follow product label for use—dilution)

Disinfecting solutions commonly used are Barbicide and Marvicide.

Instruments must be cleaned and disinfected between clients.

www.Cdc.gov

to rinse the feet well prior to drying them. The nurse should emphasize the importance of special attention to web spaces, heels, and cuticles, especially for older individuals and those with diabetes, who are at high risk for dry skin (Terrie, 2013; Woodbury et al., 2013). Clients should be taught to moisturize the feet with a small amount of a gentle fragrance-free cream or lotion but to avoid putting cream between the toes. If the web spaces tend to be moist, the nurse should consider recommending use of an over-the-counter antifungal powder, such as miconazole. A swipe of the finger between the toes after the powder application allows for just enough powder to be applied to the skin of the web space without caking. Individuals with recurrent calluses or corns should be taught to use a pumice stone to those areas after bathing; three swipes each day (until the callus is reduced) are usually sufficient (Chan et al., 2012). Nail care between provider visits includes use of a file or emery board to smooth the nail edges and observation for any injury, ingrowing nails, or signs of paronychia (infection in or around the nail).

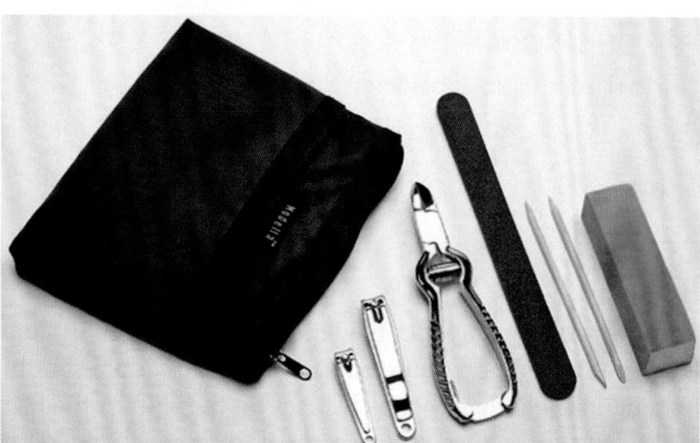

FIGURE 26-15. Foot care tools.

CLINICAL PEARL

If web spaces tend to be moist, an over-the-counter antifungal powder may be recommended; a swipe of the finger between the toes following powder application prevents caking.

Footwear and Foot Inspection

Proper therapeutic footwear and daily foot inspection are two of the most important interventions in preventing injuries that lead to wounds, pain, and amputations (www.leap.gov). Medicare has defined a therapeutic shoe as one that is long enough, wide enough, and high enough to accommodate the foot and any deformities, that has a rubber nonskid sole, and that can be secured with Velcro, laces, or a hook and latch closure (Cheskin, 2013; Huppin, 2011). Since 2005, Medicare coverage has included therapeutic footwear for beneficiaries with diabetes and one other related complication (such as LOPS, compromised blood flow, foot deformity, prior ulcer, or amputation) (Cheskin, 2013). Unfortunately, only 9% of the beneficiaries have taken advantage of this benefit; barriers include lack of awareness of the benefit; difficulty in obtaining the prescription; the time required for fitting, ordering, and refitting the shoes and inserts; and challenges in obtaining reimbursement (DiSantostefano, 2011; Huppin, 2011). In addition to consistent use of therapeutic shoes, the nurse must teach the client the importance of daily foot inspection to assure that there are no signs of injury or inflammation and the importance of promptly reporting any evidence of pathology (LEAP, 2013; Woodbury et al., 2013).

CLINICAL PEARL

Proper therapeutic footwear and daily foot inspection are two of the most important interventions in preventing injuries that lead to wounds, pain, and amputations.

It is common for an individual's feet to differ in size; the nurse should teach the client to base shoe measurements and purchases on the larger foot (Cheskin, 2013; Huppin, 2011). In addition, clients should be taught to break new shoes in gradually, for example, to increase wear time by 2 hours each day and to inspect the feet carefully for any indicators of pressure or trauma. It is also important to instruct clients to wear shoes with socks or hosiery of appropriate thickness. When shopping for shoes, the individual should wear the socks or hosiery that he or she will routinely wear with the shoes (WOCN, 2012; Kimmel & Robin, 2013).

Compression Socks or Stockings

Individuals who have edema and/or lower leg discomfort should be taught to wear low-dose over-the-counter (OTC) graduated compression socks or stockings; the level of compression should be determined by the severity of the edema and the underlying venous insufficiency (Roseler-Velderrain et al., 2013). Low-dose OTC graduated compression socks begin at 12 to 16 mm Hg; individuals with limited edema may obtain satisfactory results with this level or may require socks or stockings with 15 to 20 mm Hg. Individuals with significant edema due to LEVD typically require at least 20 to 30 mm Hg and may require 30 to 40 mm Hg (Clarke-Moloney et al., 2012; Farrow, 2010; Kelechi & Johnson, 2012; WOCN, 2011). Edema and lymphedema are common lower extremity conditions that interfere with activities of daily living and comfort; these conditions also increase the risk for ulceration and impaired healing.

Walking and Exercise

Walking and other exercise, with or without the use of mobility aids, is critical to maintenance of strength, endurance, and independence in activities of daily living (WOCN, 2008, 2011, 2012). Use of mobility aids may be indicated for safe and effective ambulation, and a referral to physical therapy may be indicated to ensure that the individual is using the mobility device correctly (Nagi et al., 2011; Tofthagen et al., 2012). There are various types of exercises that can be incorporated into activities of daily living for improved mobility and quality of life. Activities that enhance endurance, strength, balance, and flexibility are recommended for older individuals and those with diabetes. The nurse should be aware that inactivity is a major contributing factor to disease and death. In contrast, walking is associated with reduced incidence of falls, higher self-esteem, better posture and balance, and improved socialization. Walking on a regular basis is also associated with weight maintenance and stronger muscles and bones (Kreider et al., 2011; Kruse et al., 2010; Richie, 2012; Sebastian & Long, 2014; Swann, 2011). The nurse should encourage individuals to incorporate exercise into their daily activities and should consider suggesting that the individual use a pedometer to measure their activity each day. Measuring and logging steps or distance is an objective method of helping clients to see results and motivating them to continue their efforts, with the ultimate goal of preventing falls and foot issues (Huebschmann et al., 2011).

CLINICAL PEARL

Walking and other exercise, with or without the use of mobility aids, is critical to maintenance of strength, endurance, and independence in activities of daily living; inactivity is a major contributor to disease and death.

Smoking Cessation

Smoking significantly increases the risk of LEAD and amputation. Thus, smoking cessation is essential for healthy feet and prevention of LEAD. It has been known since before 1951 and documented by over 1,400 authorities from over 14 countries that smoking is an extremely dangerous habit (WOCN, 2008). It immediately constricts the blood vessels throughout the body, causes arterial damage and thickening of the vessel walls, and increases the cardiac workload. Smoking affects all organs but most especially the peripheral arteries. The nurse must educate patients regarding the impact of smoking and should refer clients committed to smoking cessation to a comprehensive program that utilizes approved medications and patches as well as counseling and supportive group therapy.

Glycemic Control

Nurses specializing in foot and nail care can also play a critical role in helping clients to attain tight glucose control, by teaching, reteaching, encouraging, and motivating individuals to adhere to management protocols and to maintain HbA1c at accepted levels. In addition, the foot nurse can assist the client with management of other comorbidities, such as hypertension, hyperlipidemia, hypercholesteremia, nutritional compromise, and obesity (Hamdy & Colberg, 2014). Creative use of adult learning principles and motivational strategies and a client-centered approach increases the chances that the nurse will be able to assist the client to achieve a higher level of health (Gravely et al., 2011). A weekly telephone call has been shown to improve client–nurse relationships and client cooperation with foot and nail care and tight glucose control (Cyrus et al., 2014).

CLINICAL PEARL

Education and counseling regarding smoking cessation and glycemic control are critical elements of the foot care nurse role.

 Multidisciplinary Teams

Improved health outcomes long term will require a multidisciplinary approach, a commitment to evidence-based practice, and education for all involved. Multidisciplinary teams that include surgeons, nurses, podiatrists, pedorthists, orthotists, diabetes educators, wound and foot care experts, and dieticians should be part of the think tank to develop policies, protocols, and algorithms based on research (Sanders et al., 2013). The foot care nurse can play a critical role in monitoring and management of the lower extremity, with specific goals including lower extremity preservation and improved overall foot care health and quality of life.

 Conclusion

Professional foot and nail care is a critical element of any lower extremity amputation prevention program. Nurses knowledgeable in foot and nail care are prepared to provide ongoing monitoring of vascular status, sensorimotor status, and foot and nail issues and to provide preventive care, education, and referrals to optimize perfusion and to prevent limb loss associated with painless trauma and preventable lesions. In addition to monitoring and education, the foot and nail care nurse is prepared to thin and trim hypertrophic nails, to pare corns and calluses, to identify common foot and nail pathology, and to provide referrals for appropriate footwear and foot care.

 Acknowledgment

The authors would like to thank the contributions of N. Jean Donnan, Cynthia Kolenda, Olenn Lekovish, and Thomas Lekovish.

REFERENCES

Aalaa, M., Malazy O. T., Sanjari, M., et al. (2012). Nurses' role in diabetic foot prevention and care; a review. *Journal of Diabetes and Metabolic Disorders, 11*(24), 1–6. Retrieved December 10, 2012, from www.jdmdonline.com

Abramson, C. (1990). Inhalation of nail dust: A podiatric hazard. In D. J. McCarthy, C Abramson. & M. J. Rupp (Eds.), *Infectious diseases of the lower extremity* (pp. 293–298). Baltimore, MD: Williams & Williams.

Ahroni, J. H., & Scheffler, N. M. (2006). *101 tips on foot care for people with diabetes*. Alexandria, VA: American Diabetes Association.

Alavi, A., Ayello, E. A., Botros, M., et al. (2012). Screening for the high-risk diabetic foot: A 60-second tool. *Advances in Skin and Wound Care, 25*(10), 465–476.

Aliberti, E. (2012). *The domino effect: Risk of falls in older adults with diabetes*. Philips Lifeline. Retrieved March 5, 2013, from www.lifelinessystems.com

Alvarsson, A., Sandgren, B., Wendel, C., et al. (2012). A retrospective analysis of amputation rates in diabetic patients: Can lower extremity amputations be further prevented? *Cardiovascular Diabetology, 11*(18), 1–11.

Amaeshi, I. J. (2012). Exploring the impact of structured foot health education on the rate of lower extremity amputation in adults with type 2 diabetes. A systematic review. *Diabetic Foot Journal (Clinical Review), 15*, 1–8.

American College of Physicians. (2012). Plantar fasciitis. *Annals of Internal Medicine*, ITC1-2-14.

Armstrong, D., Adam, I., Bevilacqua, N. T., et al. (2014). Offloading foot wounds in people with diabetes. *Wounds, 26*(1), 13–20.

Atkins, C. (2010). Evidence-based foot care in patients with diabetes. *Lower Extremity Review Magazine. August*, Retrieved March 5, 2012, from www.lowerextremityreview.com

Bakker, K., Apelqvist, J., & Schaper, N. C. (2012). Practical guidelines on the management and prevention of the diabetic foot 2011. *Diabetes/Metabolism Research and Reviews, 28*(Suppl 1), 225–231.

Barak, Y., Wagneaar, R. C., & Holt, K. G. (2006). Gait characteristics of elderly people with a history of falls: A dynamic approach. *Physical Therapy, 86*(11), 1501–1510.

Barshes, N. R., Sigireddi, M., Wrobel, J. S., et al. (2013). The system of care for the diabetic foot: Objectives, outcomes, and opportunities. *Diabetic Foot and Ankle, 4*, 21847. http://ddx.doi.org/10.3402/dfa.v4iO.21847

Boulton, A. J. M. (2013). The pathway to foot ulceration in diabetes. *Medical Clinic of North America, 97*, 775–790.

Brechow, A., Slesaczeck, T., Munch, D., et al. (2013). Improving major amputation rates in multicomplex diabetic foot patient: Focus on the severity of peripheral artery disease. *Therapeutic Advances in Endocrinology and Metabolism*. Retrieved March 5, 2014, from http://tae.sagepub.com

Bristow, I. R., deBerker, D., Acland, K. M., et al. (2010). Clinical guidelines for the recognition of melanoma of the foot and nail unit. *Journal of Foot and Ankle Research, 3*, 25.

Burland, P. (2012). Vascular disease and foot assessment in diabetes. *Practice Nursing, 23*(4), 187–193.

Burrow, J. G., & McLarnon, N. A. (2006). World at work: Evidence-based risk management of nail dust in chiropodists and podiatrists. *Occupational and Environmental Medicine, 63*(10), 713-716.

Caselli, M. A. (2011). Prescription shoes for foot pathology. *Podiatry Management, October*, 165–178.

Centers for Medicare and Medicaid Services, Part B, NHIC Foot Care Billing Guide, April 2013, J14 A/B MAC, CMS Corp, 1–32.

Chan H., Lee D., Leung E., et al. (2012). The effects of a foot and toenail care protocol for older adults. *Geriatric Nursing, 33*(6), 446–453.

Christman, A. L., Selvin, E., Margolis, D. J., et al. (2011). Hemoglobin A1c is a predictor of healing rate in diabetic wounds. *Journal of Investigational Dermatology, 131*, 2121–2137.

Cheskin, M. (2013). Sizing up footwear. *Podiatry Management*. Retrieved March 5, 2014, from www.podiatrym.com

Clarke-Moloney, M., Keane, N., O'Conner, V., et al. (2012). Randomized controlled trial comparing European standard class 1 to class 2 compression stockings for ulcer recurrence and patient compliance. *International Wound Journal, 11*, 404–408.

Crawford, P. E., & Fields-Varnado, M. (2013). Guideline for the management of wounds in patients with lower-extremity neuropathic disease. *Journal of Wound Ostomy Continence Nursing, 40*(1), 34–45.

Cyrus, O., Vanderstrasse, A., Gilliss, C. L., et al. (2014). Improving diabetes self-management through telephonic education: A quality improvement study. *Practical Diabetology, March/April*, 6–11.

DiSantostefano, J. (2011). Medicare foot care coverage guidelines. *Journal of Nurse Practitioners, 7*(10), 1–3. Retrieved March 5, 2012, from www.cms.gov/MLNMattersArticles/downloads/SE1113.pdf

Eckles, R. (2012). The biomechanics of aging. *Podiatry Management, 31*, 147–157. Retrieved January 18, 2013, from www.podiatrym.com

Elewski, B. E., & Tosti, A. (2014). Tavaborole for the treatment of onychomycosis. *Expert Opinion on Pharmacotherapy, 15*(10), 1439–1448.

Erwin, B. L., Styke, L. T., & Kyle, J. A. (2013). Fungus of the feet and nails. *US Pharmacist, 38*(6), 51–54.

Etnnyre, A., Zarate-Abbott, P., Roehrick, L. et al. (2011). The role of certified foot and nail care nurses in prevention of lower extremity amputation. *Journal of Wound Ostomy Continence Nurses Society, 38*(3), 1–10.

Farrow, W. (2010). Phlebolymphedema—A common underdiagnosed and undertreated problem in the wound care clinic. *Journal of the American College of Certified Wound Specialists, 2*, 14–23.

Fischer, A., Swigris, R. E., Lampner, C., et al. (2011). Rheumatoid arthritis: A practical guide for the primary care provider, 1–22. Retrieved March 5, 2012, from www.medscape.org/viewarticle/745566

Fujiwara, Y., Kishida, K., Terao, M., et al. (2011). Beneficial effects of foot care nursing for people with diabetes mellitus: An uncontrolled before and after intervention study. *Journal of Advanced Nursing, 67*(9), 1952–1962.

Gallagher, D. (2012). The certified foot care nurse and the importance of comprehensive foot assessments. *Journal of Wound Ostomy Continence Nurses', 39*(2), 194–196.

Game, F. (2012). Choosing life or limb: Improving survival in the multi complex diabetic foot patient. *Diabetes/Metabolism Research Reviews, 28*(Suppl 1), 97–100.

Game, R., & Jeffcoate, W. (2013). The Charcot foot: Neuropathic osteoarthropathy. *Advances in Skin and Wound Care, 26*(9), 421–428.

Garnett, W. R. (2005). Optimizing antiepileptic drug therapy in the elderly. *Annals of Pharmacotherapy, 39*(11), 1852–1860.

Gazes, M. I., & Zeichner, J. (2013). Onychomycosis in close quarter living: Review of the literature. *Mycoses, 56*(6), 610–613.

Goldstein, A. O. (2014). Onychomycosis, 1–13. Retrieved March 5, 2014, from www.uptodate.com/contents/onychomycosis

Gravely, S. S., Hensley, B. K., & Hagood-Thompson, C. (2011). Comparison of three types of diabetic foot ulcer education plans to determine patient recall of education. *Journal of Vascular Nursing, 29*(3), 1–8.

Gupta, A. K., Drummond-Main, C., Cooper, E. A., et al. (2011). Systematic review of nondermatophyte mold onychomycosis: Diagnosis, clinical types, epidemiology, and treatment. *American Academy of Dermatology, 66*(3), 494–502.

Habif, T. P., Campbell, J. L., Chapman, M. S., et al. (2006). *Dermatology*. Philadelphia, PA: Mosby, Elsevier.

Hamdy, O., & Colberg, S. (2014). 10 keys to long-term weigh loss for adults with diabetes. *Diabetes Self-Management*, October, 64–67.

Hanson, E. (2011). *Diabetic foot care*. Hobart, NY: Hatherleigh Press.

Hawke, F., & Burns, J. (2012). Brief Report: Custom foot orthoses for foot pain: what does the evidence say? *Foot & Ankle International, 33*(12), 1161–1163.

Heidelbaugh, J. J., & Lee, H. (2009). Management of the ingrown toenail. *American Family Physician, 79*(4), 303–308.

Hendry, G. J., Gibson, K. A., Pile, K., et al. (2013). "They just scraped off the calluses": A mixed methods exploration of foot care access and provision for people with rheumatoid arthritis in southwestern Sydney, Australia. *Journal of Foot and Ankle Research, 6*(34), 1–11. Retrieved March 5, 2014, from www.jfootankleres.com

Hovaguimian, A. (2012). Diagnosis and treatment of diabetic neuropathy for the non-neurologist. *Practical Diabetology*, May/Jun, 8–12.

Huebschmann, A. M., Crane, L. A., Belansky, E. S., et al. (2011). Patients with diabetes walk less, fear injury. *Diabetes Care*. Retrieved March 5, 2012, from www.medscape.com

Huppin, L. (2011). Evidence-based medicine (EBM) and orthotic therapy. *Podiatry Management, 86*, 97–102.

Johnson, S. R., & Taylor, M. A. (2012). Identification and management of malignant skin lesions among older adults. *Journal of Nurse Practitioners, 6*(8), 1–8.

Jones, N. J., Chess, J., Cawley, S., et al. (2012). Prevalence of risk factors for foot ulceration in a general haemodialyisis population. *International Wound Journal*, 683–688, doi: 10.1111/j.1742-481X.2012.01044.x.

Kelechi, T. J., & Johnson, J. J. (2012). Guideline for the management of wounds in patients with lower extremity venous disease. *Journal of Wound Ostomy Continence Nurses, 39*(6), 598–606.

Kimmel, H. M., & Robin, A. L. (2013). An evidence-based algorithm for treating venous leg ulcers utilizing the Cochrane database of systematic reviews. *Wounds, 25*(9), 242–250.

Kohlman-Trigoboff, D. (2013). Management of lower extremity peripheral arterial disease interpreting the latest guidelines for nurse practitioners. *Journal of Nurse Practitioners, 9*(10), 653–668.

Kreider, R. B., Serra, M., Beavers, K. M., et al. (2011). A structured diet and exercise program promotes favorable changes in weight loss, body composition, and weight maintenance. *Journal of American Dietetic Association, 111*(6), 828–843.

Kruse, R. L., LeMaster, J. W., & Madsen, R. W. (2010). Fall and balance outcomes after an intervention to promote leg strength, balance, and walking in people with diabetic peripheral neuropathy: "Feet first" randomized controlled trial. *Physical Therapy, 90*(11), 1568–1579.

Lavery, L. A., La Fontaine, J., Higgins, K. R., et al. (2012). Shear-reducing insoles to prevent ulceration in high-risk diabetic patients. *Advances in Skin & Wound Care, 25*(11), 519–524.

Lavery, L. A., La Fontaine, J., & Kim, P. J. (2013). Preventing the first or recurrent ulcers. *Medical Clinics of North America, 97*, 807–820.

Lipsky, B. A., Berendt, A. R., Cornia, P. B., et al. (2012). 2012 Infectious diseases society of America clinical practice guideline for diagnosis and treatment of diabetic foot infections. *Clinical Infectious Disease, 54*(12), 132–173.

Lower Extremity Amputation Prevention (LEAP). (2013). Retrieved March 5, 2013, from Health Resources and Services Administration, www.hrsa.gov/hansensdiease/leap

Madan, S. S., & Pai, D. R. (2013). Charcot neuroarthropathy of the foot and ankle. *Orthopaedic Surgery, 5*, 86–93.

Malemute, C. L., Shultz, J. A., Ballejos, M., et al. (2011). Goal setting education and counseling practices of diabetes educators. *Diabetes Educator, 37*(4), 549–563.

Markova, A., & Mostow, E. N. (2012). US skin disease assessment: Ulcer and wound care. *Dermatology Clinic, 30*, 107–111.

Marston, W. A.; Dermagraft Diabetic Foot Ulcer Study Group. (2006). Risk factors associated with healing chronic diabetic foot ulcers: the importance of hyperglycemia. *Ostomy Wound Management, 52*(3), 26–32.

McCulloch, D. K. (2012). Patient information: Foot care in diabetes mellitus (Beyond the Basics), 1–13. Upto Date, Retrieved 18 January, 2013, from www.uptodate.com

McGuire, J. (2010). Transitional off-loading: An evidence-based approach to pressure redistribution in the diabetic foot. *Advances in Skin and Wound Care, 23*(4), 175–190.

Meaney, B. (2012). Diabetic foot care: prevention is better than cure. *Journal of Renal Care, 38*(Suppl 1), 90–98.

Mechem, C. C., & Zafren, K. (2014). Frostbite, 1–11. Retrieved January 5, 2014, from www.uptodate.com/contents/frostbite

Mills, J. L., Conte, M. S., Armstrong, D. G., et al. (2014). The society of vascular surgery lower extremity threatened limb classification system: Risk stratification based on wound, ischemia, and foot infection. *Journal of Vascular Surgery, 59*(1), 220–234.

Milne, T. E., Rogers, J. R., Kinnear, E. M., et al. (2013). Developing an evidence-based clinical pathway for the assessment, diagnosis, and management of acute Charcot neuro-arthropathy: A systematic review. *Journal of Foot and Ankle Research, 6*(30), 1–12.

Moakes, H. (2012). An overview of foot ulceration in older people with diabetes. *Nursing Older People, 24*(7), 14–19.

Muirhead, L., Roberson, A. J., & Secrest, J. (2011). Utilization of foot care services among homeless adults: Implications for advanced practice nurses. *Journal of American Academy of Nurse Practitioners, 23*, 209–215.

Mustapha, J. A., Heaney, C., Clark, M., et al. (2013). Building a successful amputation prevention program. *Endovascular Today, May*, 44–50.

Nagi, K., Inoue, T., Yamada, Y., et al. (2011). Effects of toe and ankle training in older people: A cross-over study. *Geriatrics Gerontology International, 11*, 246–255.

Nandedkar-Thomas, M. A., & Scher R. K. (2005). An update on disorders of the nails. *Journal of American Academy of Dermatology, 52*(5), 877–887.

O'Brien, J. A., Edwards, H. E., Finlayson, K. J., et al. (2012). Understanding the relationships between calf muscle pump, ankle range of motion, and healing for adults with venous leg ulcers: A review of the literature. *Wound Practice & Research, 20*(2), 80–85.

O'Brien, T., & Karem, J. (2013). Relative sensory sparing in the diabetic foot implied through vibration testing. *Diabetic Foot & Ankle, 4*, 21278. Retrieved May, 5, 2013, from http://dx.doi.org/10.3402/dfa.v410.21278

Paul, J. C., Pieper, B., & Templin, T. N. (2011). Itch: Association with chronic venous disease, pain, and quality of life. *Journal of Wound Ostomy Continence Nurses, 38*(1), 46–54.

Pariser, D., Scher, R. K., Elewski, B., et al. (2013). Promoting and maintaining or restoring healthy nails: practical recommendations for clinicians and patients. *Seminars in Cutaneous Medicine and Surgery, 32*(2 Suppl 1), S13–S14.

Parrish, C. A., Sobera, J. O., & Elewski, B. E. (2005). Modification of the Nail Psoriasis Severity Index. *Journal of American Academy of Dermatology, 53*(4), 745–747.

Plucknette, B. F., Brogan, M. S., Anain, J. M., et al. (2012). Normative values for foot sensation: Challenging the 5.07 monofilament. *Journal of Diabetic Foot Complications, 4*(1), 16–25.

Pupp, G., & Kolvunen, R. (2011). Limb salvage and the Charcot foot: What the evidence Shows. *Podiatry Today*, March, 68–72.

Reich, A., & Szepietowski, J. C. (2011). Health-related quality of life in patients with nail disorders. *American Journal of Clinical Dermatology, 12*(5), 313–320.

Ricci, E. (2011). Managing common foot problems in older people. *Nursing and Residential Care, 13*(12), 1–6.

Richie, D. H. (2012). Preventing falls in the elderly. *Podiatry Today, September*, 38–51.

Riskowki, J., Dufour, A. B., & Hannan, M. T. (2011). Arthritis, foot pain, and shoe wear: Current musculoskeletal research on feet. *Current Opinion Rheumatology, 23*(2), 148–155.

Rizzo, L., Tedeschi, A., Fallani, E., et al. (2012). Custom-made orthesis and shoes in a structured follow-up program reduces the incidence of neuropathic ulcers in high-risk diabetic foot patients. *International Journal of Lower Extremity Wounds, 11*(1), 59–64.

Rome, K., Stewart, S., Vandal, A. C., et al. (2013). The effects of commercially available footwear on foot pain and disability in people with gout. *BMC Musculoskeletal Disorders, 14*(278), 1–16.

Rosales-Velderrain, A., Padilla, M., Choe, C. H., et al. (2013). Increased microvascular flow and foot sensation with mild continuous external compression. Retrieved March 5, 2014, from www.ncbi.nlm.nih.gov/pmc/articles/PMC3970751/

Sacks, D. B., & John, W. G. (2014). Interpretation of hemoglobin A1c values. *Journal of American Medical Association, 311*(22), 2271–2272.

Sanders, A. P., Stoeldraaijers, L., Pero, M., et al. (2013). Patient and professional delay in the referral trajectory of patients with diabetic foot ulcers. *Diabetes Research and Clinical Practice, 102*, 105–111.

Sanchez, J. A., Lazaro-Martinez, J. L., Quintana-Marrero, Y., et al. (2013). Charcot neuroarthropathy triggered and complicated by osteomyelitis. How limb salvage can be achieved. *Diabetic Medicine, 30*, e229–e232.

Sebastian, A., & Long, T. (2014). Exercise for health and fitness. Nurse.com WEST, 28–33.

Sheridan, S. (2012). The need for a comprehensive foot care model. *Nephrology Nursing Journal, 39*(5), 387–401.

Snyder, R. J., Kirsner, R. S., Warriner, R. A., et al. (2010). Consensus recommendations on advancing the standard of care for treating neuropathic foot ulcers in patients with diabetes. *Wounds*(Suppl), 1–23.

Swann, J. I. (2011). Preventing falls by reducing risks and encouraging activity. *British Journal of Healthcare Assistants, 5*(9), 436–439.

Talarico, R. (2013). Preventing diabetic foot amputations: Podiatry, protocols, and perfusion. *Podiatry Management*, November–December, 127–134.

Takehara, K., Oe, M., Tsunemi, Y., et al. (2011). Factors associated with presence and severity of toenail onychomycosis in patients with diabetes: A cross-sectional study. *International Journal of Nursing Studies, 48*, 1101–1108.

Terrie, Y. C. (2013). Diabetic foot care: The importance of routine care. Retrieved December 5, 2013, from www.pharmacytimes.com/publications/issue/2013/October2013/diabetic-foot-care on

Tofthagen, C., Visovsky, C., & Berry, D. L. (2012). Strength and balance training in adults with peripheral neuropathy and high risk of fall: Current evidence and implications for future research. *Oncology Nursing Forum, 39*(5), E416–E424.

Watkins, J. (2011). Early identification of skin problems in older patients. *British Journal of Healthcare Assistants, 5*(9), 424–428.

Weck, M., Slesaczeck, T., Paetzold, H., et al. (2013). Structured health care for subjects with diabetic foot ulcers results in a reduction of major amputation rates. *Cardiovascular Diabetology, 12*(45). Retrieved May 5, 2013, from www.ncbi.nlm.nih.gov/pmc/articles?PMC3627905

Wellborn, J., & Moceri, J. T. (2014). The lived experiences of persons with chronic venous insufficiency and lower extremity ulcers. *Journal of Wound Ostomy & Continence Nursing, 41*(2), 122–126.

Westerberg, D. P., & Voyack, M. J. (2013). Onychomycosis: Current trends in diagnosis and treatment. *American Family Physician, 88*(11), 762–770.

Woo, K. Y., Santos, V., & Gamba, M. (2013). Understanding diabetic foot. *Nursing*. Retrieved March 5, 2014, from www.nursing2013.com on

Woodbury, M. G., Botros, M., Kuhnke, J. L., et al. (2013). Evaluation of a peer-led self-management programme PEP talk: Diabetes, healthy feet and you. *International Wound Journal, 10*(6), 703–710.

Wound Ostomy Continence Nurses' (WOCN) Society. (2008). *Best practice guidelines management of wounds in patients with lower-extremity arterial disease*. Laurel, NJ.

Wound Ostomy Continence Nurses' Society. (2011). *Best practice guidelines management of wounds in patients with lower-extremity venous disease*. Laurel, NJ.

Wound Ostomy Continence Nurses' Society. (2012a). *Best practice guidelines management of wounds in patients with lower-extremity neuropathic disease*. Laurel, NJ.

Wound Ostomy Continence Nurses' Society. (2012b). Ankle brachial index: Quick reference guide for clinicians. *Journal of Wound Ostomy & Continence, 39*(25), S21–S29.

Wu, S. V., Tung, H. H., Liang, S. Y., et al. (2014). Differences in perceptions of self-care, health education barriers, and educational needs between diabetes patients and nurses. *Contemporary Nurse, 46*(2), 187–196.

QUESTIONS

1. The wound care nurse is assessing a patient's legs and feet for arterial or venous disease. Which statement describes a properly performed assessment?
   A. To assess for color changes, place the patient in the supine position and raise the leg above heart level for 10 to 20 seconds.
   B. Use the palm of the hand to compare the temperature of one foot and leg to the contralateral foot and leg.
   C. Apply firm pressure with the thumb to the pad of the great toe for 2 seconds to assess for edema.
   D. Press the nail bed to assess for capillary refill; when pressure is released, the color should return to normal within 5 seconds.

2. The wound care nurse assessing a patient's lower extremities for sensorimotor function asks the patient to close her eyes and moves the great toe up, down, medially, and laterally, asking the individual to state the direction of movement. What assessment is being performed by the nurse?
   A. Plantar surface pressure
   B. Range of motion
   C. Sensory neuropathy
   D. Proprioception

3. The CFCN is initiating pharmacologic therapy for a patient with onychomycosis. For what adverse condition would the nurse monitor the patient related to this therapy?
   A. High glucose levels
   B. Liver toxicity
   C. Irregular heartbeat
   D. Onychocryptosis

4. The wound care nurse assessing a patient's toenails notes that the nails have an oyster shell appearance. What nail alteration would the nurse suspect?
   A. Onychocryptosis
   B. Onychomycosis
   C. Ingrown toenails
   D. Onychogryphosis

5. What type of arthritis is the most common form producing pain, stiffness, and limited mobility?
   A. Rheumatoid arthritis
   B. Gout
   C. Osteoarthritis
   D. Fibromyalgia

6. The wound care nurse is assessing patients for lower extremity arterial disease (LEAD) and lower extremity venous disease (LEVD). What is a symptom denoting LEVD?
   A. Hemosiderosis
   B. Abnormal ABI
   C. Diminished sensory awareness
   D. Prolonged capillary refill time

7. A patient describes pain in his lower extremities as an "electric shock" sensation. What disease would the wound care nurse suspect is occurring?
   A. LEND
   B. LEAD
   C. LEVD
   D. Raynaud's phenomenon

8. For which foot deformity might the CFCN recommend taping the great toe toward the little toe for 3 months?
   A. Hallux valgus
   B. Hallux rigidus
   C. Hallux varus
   D. Charcot

9. Charcot is a severe deformity of the foot directly related to:
   A. Osteoarthritis
   B. Poor glucose control
   C. Bunionettes
   D. Neuroma

10. The CFCN assesses the toes of a patient and notes a toe with one bent joint causing the toe to point downward. What condition would the nurse document?
    A. Claw toe
    B. Hammer toe
    C. Bunion
    D. Webbed toe

11. Which statement accurately describes a recommended guideline for proper foot and nail care?
    A. Soak the feet of the diabetic patient.
    B. Remove excessive skin around the nail with a rasper.
    C. Use a nipper to reduce nail height.
    D. Avoid clipping the skin around the cuticles.

12. Which lifestyle habit significantly increases the risk of lower extremity arterial disease and amputation?
    A. Smoking
    B. Alcohol use
    C. Obesity
    D. Limited physical activity

ANSWERS: 1.**A**, 2.**D**, 3.**B**, 4.**D**, 5.**C**, 6.**A**, 7.**A**, 8.**C**, 9.**B**, 10.**B**, 11.**D**, 12.**A**

CHAPTER 27

Wounds Caused by Infectious Processes

Freya Van Driessche

OBJECTIVES

1. Describe the pathology, presentation, and management of the following: herpes simplex lesions; varicella-zoster lesions; dermatophyte lesions; deep fungal infections; impetigo; ecthyma; ecthyma gangrenosum; hidradenitis suppurativa; cellulitis; necrotizing fasciitis; folliculitis; mycobacterial infection.
2. Identify indications and contraindications to wound cultures for the patient with cellulitis.
3. Explain the significance of prompt diagnosis of necrotizing fasciitis, and early indicators of the condition.

Topic Outline

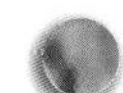 Introduction

Infection is not commonly considered to be a major cause of wounds; however, because infectious organisms are so common worldwide, they are one of the most common etiologic factors for skin wounds. Despite being so common, these wounds are rarely seen in wound clinics; they are most commonly managed by primary care providers. Because of their frequency, all health care providers should be familiar with these wounds and their treatment.

CLINICAL PEARL

Because infectious organisms are so common worldwide, they are one of the most common etiologic factors for skin wounds.

Many types of pathogens can cause wounds, including viral, fungal, and bacterial microorganisms. Wounds caused by infectious processes vary in severity from minor, limited skin disease to ulcers that can be life threatening. This chapter describes the majority of infections that cause wounds in the United States and briefly addresses a few of the less common infectious organisms known to cause wounds throughout the world.

Viral Infections Causing Wounds

The herpes virus family is a group of 8 viruses that cause an array of disease in humans. Following primary infection, these viruses become latent within cells, which means they are a lifelong threat with the potential to reactivate and cause recurrent disease. These viruses include cytomegalovirus, which can cause congenital birth defects; the Epstein-Barr virus, which causes infectious mononucleosis; and human herpes virus 8, which is implicated in the pathogenesis of Kaposi's sarcoma. Two very common viruses, herpes simplex virus (HSV) and the varicella–zoster virus (VZV), can cause skin wounds.

CLINICAL PEARL

Herpes viruses become latent within cells following primary infection, meaning they are a lifelong threat with the potential to cause recurrent disease.

Herpes Simplex

One of the most common infections in humans is caused by the HSV. Most infections are subclinical; that is, the majority of those infected do not know they have the disease. When clinical disease does occur, it presents as recurrent outbreaks of vesicles and ulcerative lesions of the skin and mucous membranes. HSV type 1 (HSV-1) is the main cause of orolabial herpes, commonly known as "cold sores" or "fever blisters." HSV type 2 (HSV-2) is the main cause of genital herpes. The US prevalence of positive serology is around 54% for HSV-1 and about 16% for HSV-2 (Bradley et al., 2014). The diagnosis of these conditions is most commonly made on an empiric basis but can be confirmed by a number of methods, one of which is the Tzanck smear. This is a bedside or in-office diagnostic procedure that involves lancing an intact blister and obtaining cellular material from the base of the deroofed blister that is then stained and examined under the microscope. HSV infection is evidenced by the presence of multinucleated giant cells. However, this is a nonspecific test, because VZV can also cause these cytologic changes and Tzanck testing cannot distinguish HSV-1 from HSV-2. Thus, the value of the test lies primarily in confirmation that the lesions are caused by HSV-1, HSV-2, or VZV. When possible, it is helpful to also send the contents of the blisters for viral culture and polymerase chain reaction (PCR), which provides more sensitive results (Nahass et al., 1992).

CLINICAL PEARL

HSV-1 is the main cause of orolabial herpes, and HSV-2 is the main cause of genital herpes.

HSV-1

Primary HSV-1 infection is frequently subclinical; clinically evident disease is manifest by herpetic gingivostomatitis, characterized by numerous broken vesicles on the gingiva, mouth, and lips and accompanied by fever, malaise, and lymphadenopathy. The eroded areas are often covered by a white membrane. Gingivostomatitis usually occurs in children and young adults, which is the age at which most patients contract the virus (though, as noted, most infected individuals do not have clinical signs of infection). Symptomatic primary infections can cause severe odynophagia and resultant dehydration and are therefore often treated with antivirals such as acyclovir, famciclovir, or valacyclovir in addition to analgesics and IV hydration. The majority of patients will experience occasional recurrences with minor symptoms; these recurrences are unlikely to involve fever or systemic symptoms, and, typically, the only treatment needed is topical anesthetic agents. The recurrences primarily involve lesions known as herpes labialis ("cold sores"); they present as a localized grouping of painful vesicles on an erythematous base that may eventually erode, most commonly on the vermilion border of the lips (Fig. 27-1). These outbreaks tend to be associated with a 24-hour prodrome of stinging, itching, or burning where the outbreak will appear. For recurrences of greater severity, episodic treatment with oral antivirals initiated during the prodromal phase has been shown to reduce time to healing of the lesions, in contrast to topical antivirals, which have not shown effectiveness with more severe outbreaks (Cernik et al., 2008). Daily, chronic suppressive therapy with antivirals is reserved for those with very severe or very frequent recurrences of herpes labialis.

CLINICAL PEARL

Mild orolabial herpes (HSV-1) can be treated with topical antiviral agents; moderate-to-severe disease should be treated with systemic antivirals initiated during the prodromal phase; and very severe disease may require chronic suppressive therapy.

Less commonly, HSV-1 can cause disease on other areas of the body. Herpetic whitlow is HSV-1 infection of the finger or nail folds. It can occur via autoinoculation but can also develop in a health care worker whose finger comes in contact with an active oral lesion of a patient. Lesions involving the hair follicle, most commonly the beard, are known as herpes sycosis. These tend to present as erosions, and the area of involvement may be extensive. Herpes

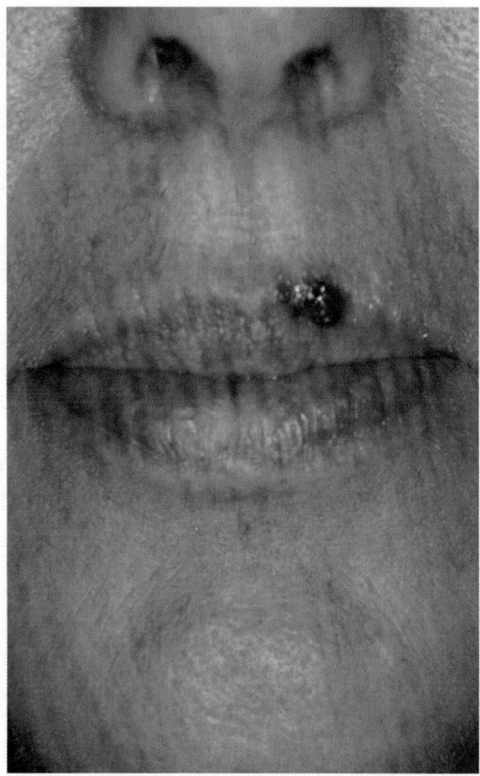

FIGURE 27-1. A recurrence of HSV-1 infection, "herpes labialis." As shown here, these recurrences tend to be localized to the vermilion border of the lip and are grouped vesicles on an erythematous base.

gladiatorum refers to herpetic lesions involving the lateral neck, forearms, and face that develop in wrestlers after a match with an infected wrestler. The presence of vesicles and/or erosions on these parts of the body should thus prompt the provider to consider HSV-1 as a possible etiology (Usatine & Tinitigan, 2010).

HSV-2

Though HSV-1 is an increasingly common cause of genital herpes, HSV-2 remains the primary etiology. The virus causes the same types of lesions as HSV-1, but HSV-2 has a specific tropism for the tissues in the genital region and is transmitted sexually. Clinically, the lesions appear as grouped vesicles on an erythematous base that can erode and ulcerate and can occur on the cervix, vagina, skin of the vulva, penis, and/or the anogenital region (Fig. 27-2). The primary infection can be severe, with extremely painful genital ulcers, fever, malaise, inguinal lymphadenopathy, and dysuria (Corey et al., 1983). Primary infections should be treated with oral antiviral medication to reduce the duration of the initial episode and to decrease the risk of serious sequelae, including meningitis. Medication choices include acyclovir, valacyclovir, and famciclovir, which should be administered promptly upon diagnosis of primary genital herpes. These lesions are partial thickness wounds and should be treated as such, with occlusion and a moist wound-healing environment, in addition to topical or systemic antibiotic therapy if needed.

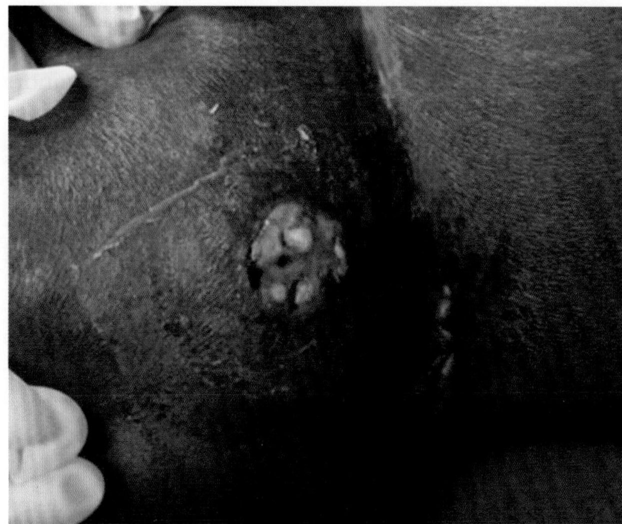

FIGURE 27-2. Anogenital ulceration caused by HSV-2.

In contrast, some patients are completely asymptomatic upon primary infection, especially individuals who are seropositive for HSV-1 at the time of HSV-2 acquisition (Langenberg et al., 1999). These individuals frequently still shed the virus even though they are asymptomatic, which means they can easily transmit the virus to others.

CLINICAL PEARL

Herpes lesions are partial thickness wounds and should be treated with moist wound healing principles.

Recurrent episodes of genital herpes tend to be less severe, with a shorter disease course and a lack of systemic symptoms. As with orolabial herpes, a prodrome may occur before eruption. Symptoms include shooting pain and tingling in the legs and genital region. Recurrences of genital herpes are more common with HSV-2 infection than with HSV-1. Most patients with HSV-2 will experience recurrences, even if the primary infection was asymptomatic. With time, the number of recurrences per year decreases. Treatment varies depending on the severity and number of recurrences per year. For those with severe outbreaks occurring more than six times per year, chronic daily suppressive therapy with one of the aforementioned antivirals can be given. For those with less than six recurrences per year, or those with mild or moderate recurrences, antiviral treatment limited to periods of recurrent disease is recommended. In those with limited disease or very infrequent recurrences, treatment may not be necessary (Cernik et al., 2008).

Varicella–Zoster Virus

VZV is one virus that causes two distinct diseases, varicella (commonly known as "chicken pox") and zoster (commonly known as "shingles"). Before the advent of the varicella vaccine in 1995, varicella was a very common self-limiting childhood disease. The virus is spread by aerosolized nasopharyngeal droplets of an actively infected individual and is extremely contagious. Clinical presentation includes fever, malaise, pharyngitis, and a pruritic vesicular rash. Following primary infection, the virus becomes dormant in the nerve ganglion. When the virus reactivates at a later time and begins to travel down the nerve to the skin, the clinical syndrome that develops is termed zoster. Classically, the infection begins as an area of pain and skin discomfort confined to a unilateral dermatomal configuration. The most commonly affected dermatome is the thoracic, but lumbar and sacral dermatomes can also be involved. If a cranial dermatome is affected, zoster is more severe; serious sequelae may occur, including herpes zoster ophthalmicus, depending on the exact nerve affected. Shortly after the onset of pain and discomfort in the involved area, red macules appear and quickly evolve into bullae that follow the dermatomal configuration. These bullae may rupture, leaving the patient with wounds in the form of erosions and ulcers (Fig. 27-3). These wounds may become secondarily infected. However, the classic progression of lesions is from bullae/vesicles to pustules to crusted lesions. Once the lesions have entered the crusted phase, they are no longer contagious. Individuals who have never had varicella or the VZV vaccine and who therefore lack immunity to the virus can be infected by an individual with zoster; a nonimmune individual who becomes infected following exposure to zoster will develop varicella, not zoster (because zoster by definition is the recurrent form of varicella). The diagnosis of zoster involves the same techniques as are used for diagnosing HSV: the Tzanck smear, viral culture, PCR, and direct fluorescence antibody testing. The clinical progression of zoster is essentially the same as for varicella: bullous lesions that erupt, crust, and close. In some individuals with zoster, the pain continues for months to years following resolution of the rash; this syndrome is termed postherpetic neuralgia. It generally affects about 34% of those with zoster, but 60% to 70% of individuals over age 60 (Weinberg, 2007).

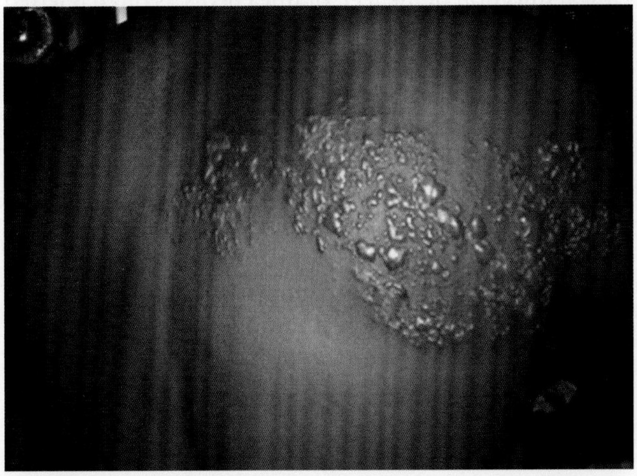

FIGURE 27-3. A herpes zoster outbreak in a T2 dermatomal distribution.

CLINICAL PEARL

VZV is one virus that cause two distinct infections, varicella (chicken pox) and herpes zoster (shingles); the virus is spread by nasopharyngeal droplets from an infected individual and is extremely contagious.

Ten to twenty percent (10% to 20%) of individuals will develop zoster at some point in their lives. Zoster is most commonly seen in late middle-aged and elderly individuals, most likely due to the age-related decrease in cellular immunity, which allows the VZV to replicate and cause disease. For this reason, immunosuppression due to HIV/AIDS, malignancy, and transplant surgery is also associated with increased risk for developing zoster. In immunosuppressed individuals, the rash may be more ulcerative and necrotic, frequently extends far beyond the dermatomal region, and may become disseminated. Treatment of zoster is similar to treatment of HSV, with a choice of acyclovir, famciclovir, or valacyclovir for 7 days; treatment is ideally initiated within 72 hours of the appearance of lesions. Local wound care (occlusion and a moist environment) and proper antibiotic therapy should be instituted if there are extensive or infected ulcerations. Analgesia may be needed for associated pain. There is a zoster vaccine now available that is recommended for individuals over 60 years of age. It reduces the incidence of zoster and postherpetic neuralgia (Cohen et al., 2013).

CLINICAL PEARL

Herpes infections should be treated with antivirals and with the principles of moist wound healing; analgesia may be needed for associated pain relief.

Fungal Infections Causing Wounds

Fungal infections are more likely to cause rashes than wounds; however, severe fungal infections may cause areas of erosions and ulceration. In addition, fungal infections commonly occur in the periwound or perineal area; therefore, the wound nurse must be able to recognize and recommend treatment for common fungal infections. The most common fungal infections of the skin include the dermatophytes and *Candida albicans*, which can cause a variety of clinical presentations. Less common is infection with a fungus called *Sporothrix schenckii*, which can cause wounds with a unique clinical picture. Some systemic mycoses, such as coccidioidomycosis, histoplasmosis, and North American blastomycosis, are endemic to the United States and can disseminate to the skin, causing lesions that may ulcerate.

CLINICAL PEARL

Fungal infections cause rashes, and severe infections may cause areas of erosion and ulceration. These infections are common in the periwound and perineal area—therefore, the wound nurse must be able to recognize these infections and make appropriate treatment recommendations.

Dermatophytes

The dermatophytes are fungi that subsist on keratin, a protein that is found in the superficial skin, nails, and hair. The diseases that they cause include, but are not limited to, tinea capitis, tinea barbae, and tinea pedis. These three are discussed in more detail as these forms of tinea can lead to wounds in certain cases.

Tinea Capitis

Commonly known as "ringworm of the scalp," tinea capitis is a fairly common childhood disease in the United States. Most cases occur in school age, preadolescent African-American boys. About 90% of cases are caused by *Trichophyton tonsurans* (Mirmirani & Tucker, 2013), which invades the hair shaft and causes a scaly, red rash on the involved area of the scalp. The rash is comprised of papules in an annular configuration. The hairs in the affected areas break off near the surface of the scalp, leaving areas of alopecia. Diagnosis of tinea capitis requires use of a scalpel to take a scraping of the scalp that includes some hair follicles and scale; the scraping is treated with potassium hydroxide ("KOH prep") and is examined for presence of fungal features under the microscope. A minority of cases of tinea capitis are due to *Microsporum* species; these cases can be diagnosed with use of Wood's lamp, which emits ultraviolet light and causes the affected area to fluoresce a greenish yellow color. However, since *Microsporum* is a minor cause of tinea capitis in the United States, a negative Wood's lamp examination does not exclude the diagnosis of tinea capitis.

CLINICAL PEARL

Dermatophytes are fungi that live on keratin; they cause infections such as tinea capitis (ringworm), tinea barbae, and tinea pedis (athletes' foot).

If the immune response to the fungus is exaggerated, a kerion may form at the affected area, which presents as a painful, boggy, inflamed nodule that is often mistaken for an abscess due to the pustules and crusts on the surface (Fig. 27-4). Removal of the crust can help with relief of pain; the erosions revealed by crust removal should be treated with moist wound healing and, in the event of a secondary bacterial infection, with antibiotics. Treatment should also involve an oral antifungal (e.g., terbinafine or griseofulvin) to eliminate the dermatophyte.

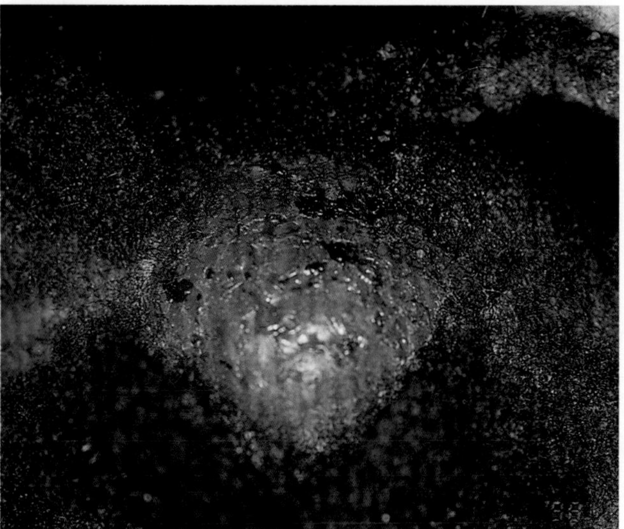

FIGURE 27-4. A tinea capitis infection with formation of a painful, boggy nodule known as a kerion. (Reprinted with permission from Fleisher, G. R., Ludwig, S., & Baskin, M. N. (2004). *Atlas of pediatric emergency medicine*. Philadelphia, PA: Lippincott Williams & Wilkins).

Tinea Barbae

Tinea barbae is another fungal infection that affects the hair follicle; in this case, the target organ is the hair of the beard and mustaches of men. The fungi that cause this pathology are the zoonotic fungi *Trichophyton mentagrophytes* and *Trichophyton verrucosum*; cattle and horses are the usual source of the fungus, and the infection is therefore most common in men working in the agricultural business. It usually presents as a very red and highly inflamed kerion-like lesion; pustules or crusting with erosions may be seen as well. The hairs within the lesion are easily and painlessly removed. These wounds may result in secondary bacterial infections that require systemic antibiotics. The diagnosis and treatment are the same as for tinea capitis, as both infect the hair follicle; the wound nurse should be aware that topical antifungals are nontherapeutic.

Tinea Pedis

Fungal infection of the feet, or tinea pedis, is often referred to as "athlete's foot." It is extremely common, affecting about 15% of the population (Bell-Syer et al., 2012). *Trichophyton rubrum* and *T. mentagrophytes* are common causes. Infection can cause a variety of presentations. The commonly seen chronic form of tinea pedis presents as a mildly erythematous background rash with associated scale and a "moccasin" distribution over the feet. The moccasin distribution means that the rash covers the areas of the foot covered by a shoe (moccasin) and is due to the tendency of fungal organisms to grow in moist, warm, occluded areas covered by shoes. Chronic tinea pedis does not cause secondary wounds and is usually treated with topical antifungal agents.

Acute tinea pedis has a strikingly different presentation, with both bullous and ulcerative forms. *Trichophyton mentagrophytes* infection typically causes inflammatory bullae and vesicles on the plantar arch of the feet; the lesions cause extreme burning discomfort that is relieved by unroofing the blister. Unroofing usually leaves erosions, which are often complicated by cellulitis and lymphangitis.

Acute ulcerative tinea pedis is more commonly seen in diabetics and immunosuppressed patients and presents as erosions and ulcers, most commonly involving the third and fourth web spaces. Diagnosis involves examination of skin scrapings for fungal elements under the microscope, as described previously for the diagnosis of other forms of tinea. While treatment of chronic tinea pedis usually involves topical antifungal medications, treatment of acute tinea pedis (both bullous and ulcerative forms) requires oral antifungals. However, it is important to provide proper wound care to the areas involved in acute tinea pedis in addition to providing systemic antifungals. An occlusive environment is usually contraindicated, as is the use of ointment products, because the fungi tend to thrive in moist, occlusive settings (which explains their prevalence among patients who wear tight, occlusive footwear). Wound care should be directed at debriding any necrotic material (in ulcerative acute tinea pedis), absorbing exudate, and keeping the wound base moist and the surrounding skin dry. If the patient is diabetic, care should be taken to offload the feet in order to prevent chronic ulceration in the area.

CLINICAL PEARL

Chronic tinea pedis is manifest by a mildly erythematous scaly rash that causes minimal or no symptoms; in contrast, acute tinea pedis is manifest by acute inflammation, erosions, and ulcers, typically involving the 3rd and 4th web spaces.

Candida albicans

Although a component of the "normal flora" for humans, the fungus *C. albicans* can become pathogenic under certain conditions. *Candida* can cause a wide array of human pathology, from minor skin infections to invasive systemic disease. Wound care providers should be knowledgeable regarding intertrigo, a condition that develops due to accumulation and "trapping" of moisture in the skin folds; intertrigo is particularly common in the obese, those with diabetes, and those who wear diapers or other occlusive dressings in skin folds. Commonly affected areas include the inframammary area, axillary area, natal cleft, area at the base of the pannus, and the gluteal fold. As stated, moisture and heat become trapped in the skin fold, resulting in maceration and possibly skin loss due to friction or mechanical stretch. These areas are also conducive to both bacterial and fungal growth, and secondary superinfections can occur, often with *C. albicans*.

Clinically, candidal intertrigo presents as "beefy-red" macerated plaques and patches, often with peripheral scaling and smaller satellite lesions. Due to continued friction, eroded areas are often seen. However, intertrigo may be secondarily infected with organisms other than *Candida*, and it is important to determine the causal pathogen to direct treatment. When superinfection is present and the causative agent is not clear, diagnostic workup is required and should include examination of KOH-treated scale samples under the microscope to examine for fungal features, use of a Wood's lamp to determine if certain bacteria are present, and skin culture. Wood's lamp is used to diagnose or "rule out" infection with *Corynebacterium minutissimum*; if the organism is present, the area of affected skin will fluoresce a coral-red color. This bacterial infection is known as erythrasma, which presents clinically with erythematous patches or plaques in intertriginous folds that can look like *Candida* intertrigo.

CLINICAL PEARL

Fungal and bacterial superinfections are common in patients with intertrigo; common causative organisms are *C. albicans and C. minutissimum*.

For candidal intertrigo, treatment involves topical antifungals such as nystatin along with measures to keep the affected area dry and cool (Kalra et al., 2014). Oral fluconazole is occasionally required for treatment of resistant candidiasis. Erythrasma should be treated with oral medications such as erythromycin or clarithromycin (Avci et al., 2013). Superficial wounds should be treated with dressings that keep the wound surface moist, the surrounding skin dry, and the skin folds separated (to eliminate friction). See Chapter 17 for further discussion regarding pathology, prevention, and management of intertrigo.

Deep Fungal Infections

Sporotrichosis

Often fungal organisms in the environment can be inoculated in the skin, with resultant disease. One example is sporotrichosis, a condition caused by the dimorphic fungus, *S. schenckii*. Epidemiologically, it is seen most often in South and Central America, but outbreaks and isolated cases are seen all over the world, including the United States. *Sporothrix schenckii* is a saprophyte found in wood, rose thorns, shrubs, and straw and occasionally on animals such as cats and armadillos. It most commonly causes disease when it is directly inoculated into the skin, classically when the thorn of a rose bush traumatically pierces a gardener's skin. Those with occupational exposure, such as carpenters, landscapers and gardeners are at greatest risk of acquiring the condition. Less commonly, the conidia of the fungus can be inhaled with resultant systemic disease, but this is only seen in immunocompromised individuals.

Lymphocutaneous sporotrichosis begins at the site of inoculation; it initially presents as a small, indurated papule, which subsequently grows in size to form a nodule, which frequently ulcerates. The infection spreads through the lymphatics, and new papules form proximal to the inoculation site along the lymphatic pathway; these new lesions then also progress to nodules and ulcerations. A less common form of this infection is fixed cutaneous sporotrichosis; these lesions present as verrucous plaques or ulcers, but there is no lymphocutaneous spread (De Araujo et al., 2001).

Diagnosis of sporotrichosis is made via clinical history and the characteristic evolution and spread of the lesions. However, to confirm the diagnosis, material from the lesion should be cultured in Sabouraud agar. Histologic examination may not reveal the causal organism, as they are often low in number. Although spontaneous resolution has been observed, sporotrichosis is usually treated with systemic medications, including saturated solution of potassium iodide, itraconazole, and amphotericin B. Oral potassium iodide is a low cost treatment that is mainly used in developing nations. Itraconazole is the preferred treatment for lymphocutaneous and fixed cutaneous cases, with few side effects and a high cure rate. Amphotericin B is used in disseminated cases. Topically applied heat is a treatment option for those who are intolerant to antifungal medications, as the organism grows at low temperatures (Ramos-e-Silva et al., 2007).

CLINICAL PEARL

Deep fungal infections are less common and usually occur when the causative organism is inoculated into the skin via traumatic injury with a contaminated object (e.g., when a rose thorn pierces a gardener's thumb).

Chromoblastomycosis

Chromoblastomycosis is a subcutaneous mycosis that can be caused by numerous different pigmented fungi. Chromoblastomycosis can be chronic and difficult to treat. It is caused by direct inoculation of the skin with one of the following: *Fonsecaea pedrosoi, Fonsecaea compacta, Phialophora verrucosa, Cladosporium carrionii,* or *Rhinocladiella aquaspersa*. It is most common among agricultural workers living in tropical climates. Most cases are in Brazil and Madagascar, though it can be seen in rural areas of North America. Given that chromoblastomycosis is mostly seen in people working in agriculture, it is predominantly seen in middle-aged men (Ameen, 2009).

Clinically, chromoblastomycosis occurs at a site of fungus inoculation years after the original trauma. The lesion begins as a small red papule that eventually progresses to a verrucous-appearing nodule that spreads and can create cauliflower-like lesions, usually on the lower extremities. Black dots, representing fungal organisms, can be seen on the surface of the lesions. The surface can ulcerate and crust, and, though rare, neoplastic transformation has been reported. In some cases, elephantiasis may develop due to lymphatic invasion and damage.

Diagnosis of the lesion can be made with a KOH test, which is best performed by taking a sample from an area with a black dot. Microscopically, a signature "Medlar body" will be seen, which looks like a copper penny and represents sclerotic cells. Diagnosis can also be made by histology and fungal culture. Treatment may involve surgical excision of small lesions; however, lesions may recur. Oral antifungal agents such as itraconazole, terbinafine, and Amphotericin B can be used. Oral flucytosine has also been used in combination with antifungal agents with good results (Lopez Martinez & Mendez Tovar, 2007).

Coccidioidomycosis

A second type of deep fungal infection that may cause cutaneous disease is a systemic mycosis, such as coccidioidomycosis. Two different types of fungi, *Coccidioides immitis* and *Coccidioides posadasii,* can cause coccidioidomycosis, an infection that can present in a variety of ways depending on host factors. In the United States, *C. immitis* is endemic to the soil of California's San Joaquin River Valley, and *C. posadasii* is found in other areas of the southwest. Both organisms cause the same types of clinical manifestations. The most common route of infection is via inhalation of the organism's spores. Most cases are subclinical (60%); if symptoms do occur, they are similar to a flu-like illness with fever, fatigue, sore throat, and cough. This is known as "Valley fever" and can persist for up to a few weeks. A minority of patients with Valley fever will develop cutaneous manifestations, such as erythema nodosum or erythema multiforme (Borchers & Gershwin, 2010).

Some individuals are at risk for developing disseminated disease upon inhalation of the spores; these individuals include those with immunosuppression due to HIV/AIDS or immunosuppressive medications, women who are pregnant, the elderly, and infants. Dissemination occurs hematogenously and causes granulomatous infection in the bones, skin, and meninges, although virtually any organ can be infected. Skin lesions often appear on the face, classically the nasolabial fold, though they can occur on the extremities as well. They can begin as a verrucous papule or nodule and may eventually ulcerate. Rarely, localized cutaneous disease develops as a result of direct inoculation of the skin; these lesions present as nodules that ulcerate and may be complicated by lymphangitis.

Though rare, coccidioidomycosis must be considered by health care providers when patients present with ulcerations in atypical locations. A detailed medical history and attention to recent travel are important to an accurate diagnosis. To confirm a diagnosis of coccidioidomycosis, culture and histology must be performed. Treatment for disseminated disease or solitary skin lesions typically involves itraconazole or fluconazole for 3 to 6 months.

Histoplasmosis

Classically caused by *Histoplasma capsulatum,* histoplasmosis is another infection that is contracted via inhalation of spores. It can be entirely asymptomatic or it can cause pulmonary disease, with rare dissemination to other organs, including the skin. *H. capsulatum* is endemic to the

Mississippi and Ohio River Valley in the United States and is frequently found in bat and bird droppings. Disseminated disease can cause indurated plaques within the oronasopharynx, which may ulcerate. Dissemination to the skin can present in a variety of ways, including papules, nodules, and ulcerated plaques. Primary (direct inoculation) skin infection is exceedingly rare but has been reported as a penile chancre (Chang & Rodas, 2012). In disseminated and severe disease, especially in those who are immunocompromised, Amphotericin B therapy is recommended for treatment. Itraconazole can be used in patients with less severe disease.

North American Blastomycosis

Blastomyces dermatitidis is a dimorphic fungus endemic to North America, specifically the Southeast and the Great Lakes area. The fungus is transmitted through inhalation of aerosolized spores of the organism. Most affected patients are middle aged to elderly males. As is true of other systemic mycoses, clinical presentation can vary from asymptomatic, to a mild pulmonary flu-like disease, to severe and disseminated disease. The lungs are the most common site of the infection, and the skin is the second most common site of involvement. Skin lesions begin as papules or nodules that evolve into verrucous lesions with irregular but clearly defined borders; the lesions vary in color from gray to violaceous. The lesions may form crusts; removal of the crust reveals underlying erosion. The diagnostic process is similar to that for other systemic mycoses and includes microscopic examination of KOH-stained sputum for fungal elements, histology, and culture, with culture being the gold standard. After a diagnosis is made, itraconazole for 6 months is the recommended therapy (Lopez-Martinez & Mendez-Tovar, 2012). Ulcerated lesions typically resolve as the infection is treated.

CLINICAL PEARL

Though rare, systemic fungal infections such as coccidioidomycosis must be considered by health care providers when patients present with ulcerations in atypical locations. A detailed medical history and attention to recent travel are important to an accurate diagnosis.

 Bacterial Infections Causing Wounds

Though commonly thought of as agents that infect existing wounds, bacteria can also be the very reason a wound exists; wounds caused by bacterial infections range in severity from mild to life threatening.

Impetigo

Impetigo is a common skin infection among children; in fact, it is one of the top skin disorders seen by general practitioners in the pediatric population (Mohammedamin et al., 2006). The average age of patients presenting with impetigo is between 1 and 8 years (Koning et al., 2006). *Staphylococcus aureus* is the main causal pathogen, but it

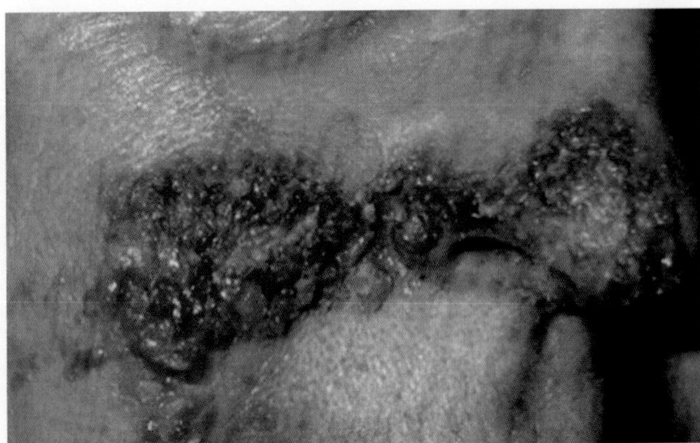

FIGURE 27-5. Impetigo on the face. Note the characteristic honey-colored crusting.

can also be caused by *Streptococcus pyogenes*; both are gram-positive organisms. The disease usually manifests on areas of the body that are not covered by clothing, such as the face, arms, hands, and neck. Lesions begin as red macules that progress to vesicles that rupture and leave a classic "honey-colored" crust (Fig. 27-5). The crusts are easily removed, leaving erosions. These wounds are infectious; the fluid that forms on them can be transferred to others, to other areas of the body, and to fomites.

Bullous impetigo is a more severe variant of impetigo. It is caused by a strain of *S. aureus* that produces an exfoliative toxin, which attacks cell adhesion molecules in the skin and causes the formation of bullae. It is usually seen in newborn infants, where it can be life threatening, but adults can develop the condition as well. The trunk is commonly affected, and when the bullae burst, the result is open erosions or crusted lesions.

Ecthyma

Ecthyma is a condition similar to impetigo in that it is caused by *S. pyogenes*, and the initial clinical presentation is similar to that of impetigo, with vesicles overlying a red skin base. However, the lesions are deeper, extending into the dermis, and have thicker crusts, which, if removed, reveal ulcers (Fig. 27-6). Because the lesions extend into the deep dermis, they usually heal with scarring. It is therefore of utmost importance to provide proper wound care in addition to treatment of the infection itself. The lesions should be kept moist and occluded to accelerate the healing process. These lesions are most commonly seen in patients with poor hygiene, those who are immunosuppressed, and elderly patients who are not well cared for.

In nonbullous impetigo, bullous impetigo, and ecthyma, the diagnosis is made on clinical appearance. If the patient does not respond to empiric treatment, the lesions can be cultured to determine the causative organism, which determines the treatment course. For limited, nonbullous disease, topical antibiotics such as mupirocin or retapamulin are sufficient. In ecthyma, bullous disease, and extensive nonbullous disease, oral antibiotic therapy

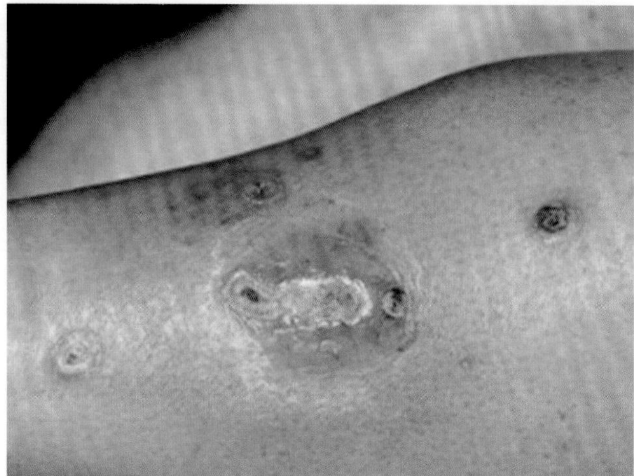

FIGURE 27-6. Ecthyma of the lower extremity. Note the yellow-gray thick crust. It is harder and thicker than the crust of impetigo.

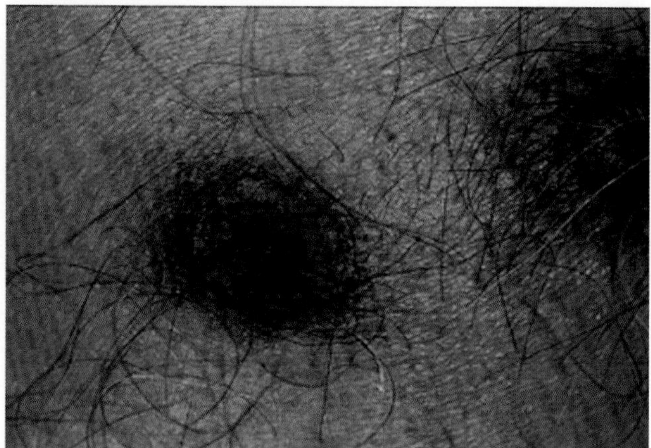

FIGURE 27-7. Ecthyma gangrenosum. Note the central gray-black eschar surrounded by an erythematous halo.

should be provided with agents such as cephalexin, dicloxacillin, or clindamycin (Stevens et al., 2014).

> **CLINICAL PEARL**
>
> Impetigo, bullous impetigo, and ecthyma are diagnosed clinically and treated empirically, with topical or systemic antibiotics that are effective against *S. aureus and S. pyogenes.*

Ecthyma Gangrenosum

Not to be confused with ecthyma, ecthyma gangrenosum is an infection most commonly caused by the gram-negative bacterium *Pseudomonas aeruginosa;* however, there are case reports of ecthyma gangrenosum caused by other pathogens as well (Pathak et al., 2013). It is particularly common in individuals with serious chronic health conditions, such as immunodeficiency or malignant disease, and it may be the first sign of a malignancy or HIV. Although it can present at all ages, it is more common in children.

While ecthyma gangrenosum is an uncommon condition, it is important for the clinician to recognize it when it occurs because it is usually an indicator of bacteremia and actual or impending sepsis. Because the condition is most common in individuals with *Pseudomonas* bacteremia, the infection is usually spread hematogenously. The initial clinical presentation involves vesicles surrounded by a pink halo, which become violaceous and hemorrhagic and begin to necrose. The final lesions are ulcers with black edges and/or centers and an erythematous border (Fig. 27-7). The clinical presentation and evolution is explained by bacterial invasion of the cutaneous blood vessels, which causes a necrotizing vasculitis.

> **CLINICAL PEARL**
>
> While ecthyma gangrenosum is an uncommon condition, it is important for the clinician to recognize it when it occurs because it is usually an indicator of bacteremia and actual or impending sepsis.

A nonbacteremic form of ecthyma gangrenosum exists that is characterized by development of lesions at the site of *Pseudomonas* inoculation; while initially a local infection, untreated lesions can progress to bacteremia and eventual sepsis. For example, this is sometimes seen in otherwise healthy infants with diaper dermatitis; the macerated occlusive environment leads to superficial breaks in the skin that permit *Pseudomonas* inoculation (Goolamali et al., 2009). Any site of trauma in a neutropenic patient can serve as a portal of entry for the pathogen; thus, oncology patients (especially children) are at risk for ecthyma gangrenosum. Treatment involves prompt administration of intravenous antipseudomonal antibiotics. If the lesions do not respond to antibiotic therapy, surgical debridement is required to prevent further seeding and spread of the bacterium.

Hidradenitis Suppurativa

Hidradenitis suppurativa (HS) is characterized by follicular occlusion in areas of the body with apocrine glands, which leads to subsequent inflammation, infection, and abscess formation. The lesions present clinically as painful nodules that occur most commonly in the axillae and inguinal areas. These lesions can become secondarily infected and can also rupture to form shallow erosions and ulcerations. Over time, there is progression to interconnecting sinus tracts and cord-like scarring in affected areas, causing the patient pain, embarrassment, and disfigurement. The exact pathogenesis remains unknown, but studies have suggested that an abnormal immune response is to blame. The prevalence of the disease is around 1%. HS is more common in women, smokers, and those who are overweight/obese. It most commonly occurs in adults aged 20 to 40, and the increased androgen levels in this age group are thought to play a potential contributing role.

Treatment begins with addressing lifestyle factors such as smoking, weight loss, and wearing loose clothing to avoid friction to the involved areas. Medical management includes washing the affected areas with antiseptic solutions to reduce commensal bacteria, daily oral doxycycline or minocycline, and daily topical clindamycin. If treatment is unsuccessful, or there is scar development, oral clindamycin 300 mg twice daily and oral rifampicin 300 mg twice daily for 10 weeks can be tried. Biologics such as infliximab, adalimumab, and ustekinumab can be considered in severe disease. Isotretinoin can be used for severe disease as well but is less efficacious than when used for treatment of acne. Intralesional corticosteroids can be used for acute flares. Surgery should be reserved for those who have failed lifestyle/medical interventions and is performed to remove active foci of disease or areas of severe scarring/sinus tract formation. Despite therapy, the usual course of disease is chronic, often lasting around 20 years. Routine follow-up with a dermatologist, surgeon, and/or wound specialist is recommended.

CLINICAL PEARL

Hidradenitis suppurativa is a chronic condition of the hair follicles and apocrine glands (typically in the axillae and perineum) that causes significant pain and scarring; treatment involves hygienic care, topical and systemic antibiotics and anti-inflammatory agents, and sometimes surgical excision of the involved area.

Cellulitis

Cellulitis is a very common bacterial infection of the skin, involving the deep dermis and subcutaneous fat. It most commonly involves the lower extremity but can occur anywhere on the body. Usually, cellulitis causes local symptoms, but patients can develop systemic symptoms such as fever and chills, indicating bacteremia. Early clinical indicators include erythema, swelling, tenderness, and increased warmth of the affected area. Blistering, erosions, and ulcers may also be present. It is usually caused by *S. pyogenes* (most common) and *S. aureus*.

Multiple conditions predispose to cellulitis, including preexisting skin lesions such as eczema, fungal infections, lymphedema, surgical wounds, traumatic wounds, and venous disease and ulcerations (Phoenix et al., 2012). The diagnosis is a clinical one. Taking culture swabs from intact skin is not helpful or recommended but should be taken in the setting of cellulitis with any purulence. Blood cultures are indicated only for severe infection, signs and symptoms of sepsis, and for patients with underlying immunodeficiency or malignancy. Treatment for cellulitis involves systemic antibiotic therapy with an agent that covers MRSA; if a culture is obtained, the results should be used to assure that the antibiotic selected is effective against the infecting organism. If there is no purulence and a valid culture cannot be obtained, the antibiotic selected should provide coverage for MSSA and beta-hemolytic streptococcus. Those with no evidence of purulence should undergo treatment for MSSA or beta-hemolytic streptococcus.

CLINICAL PEARL

Cellulitis may occur in the absence of any visible wound or purulent drainage; in this case, cultures are of no benefit, and antibiotics should be prescribed that eradicate MSSA and beta-hemolytic streptococcus.

Necrotizing Fasciitis

Though uncommon, necrotizing fasciitis (necrotizing soft tissue infection) is a life-threatening infection that involves rapid spread of inflammation and necrosis throughout the skin, subcutaneous fat, and fascia, resulting in massive tissue loss and very large wounds (Fig. 27-8). The incidence is reported to be around 0.4 per 100,000 (Salcido, 2007). Mortality rates have declined significantly over the past 10 to 20 years, due primarily to increased awareness, earlier diagnosis, and prompt intervention; reported mortality rates are now around 10%. The most important factor affecting mortality is the time between onset and debridement of the lesions, so it is important for health care providers to immediately recognize and accurately diagnose this condition (Bellapianta et al., 2009).

Types

Necrotizing fasciitis typically begins after minor or major trauma to the skin that permits bacterial inoculation, such as insect bites, cuts, surgical incisions, ulcers, or burns. Many types of bacteria can cause the infection, and necrotizing fasciitis is divided into three major types based on the infecting organism(s). Type 1 is the most common and is due to a polymicrobial infection, involving as many as 4 to 5 different organisms. These include non–group A *Streptococcus*, anaerobes, and even fungi. Type 2 is due to *S. pyogenes*, with or without *Staphylococcus* coinfection. Type 3 is caused by marine bacteria, most commonly *Vibrio vulnificus*, which occurs when a break in the skin is inoculated by seawater or a marine insect bite. Risk factors for necrotizing fasciitis

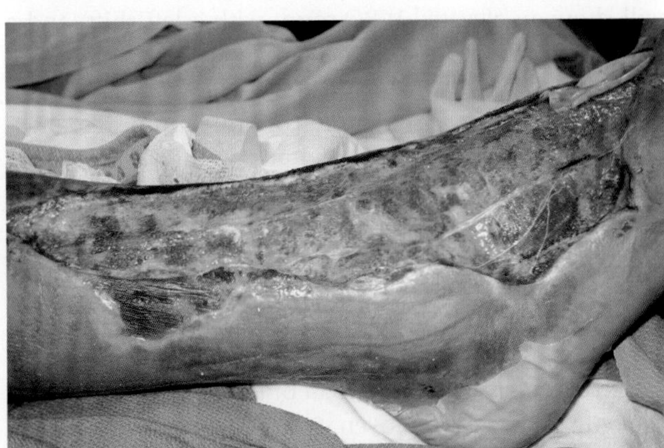

FIGURE 27-8. Necrotizing fasciitis of the lower extremity. There is loss of the epidermis, dermis, and subcutaneous tissue. Note how the fascia is easily visible. (Reprinted with permission from *Wound Care: An Incredibly Visual! Pocket Guide (Incredibly Easy! Series)*. Philadelphia, PA: Lippincott Williams & Wilkins, 2010.)

are numerous; the most common include diabetes, obesity, malignancy, burns, AIDS, and other conditions associated with immunosuppression (Kihiczak et al., 2006).

CLINICAL PEARL

Necrotizing fasciitis is a life-threatening and rapidly progressing infection that can cause massive tissue loss; prompt detection and early aggressive debridement are essential to positive outcomes.

Clinical Presentation

The lesions typically begin as erythematous, painful, edematous areas on the skin and are often mistaken for cellulitis. The most common site of involvement is an extremity, but perianal lesions and trunk wounds are also common, and head and facial wounds have been reported. An early clue that the lesion may be necrotizing fasciitis is pain that is out of proportion to the early physical findings. The other major indicator is the rapid progression of the area of involvement; the erythematous border can advance as rapidly as 2.5 cm/hour, and within hours to days, the involved skin becomes dusky and serosanguinous blisters begin to form. The reason the infection spreads so rapidly along the fascia is because fascia has a relatively poor blood supply. The infection damages and destroys the cutaneous nerves as well as the soft tissues and the skin, resulting in anesthesia of the involved skin and necrosis of the soft tissues and the skin in the involved area. Patients become progressively more toxic as the disease progresses, with fever, chills, unstable vital signs and eventually vascular collapse and multiorgan failure.

Diagnosis

The diagnosis of necrotizing fasciitis is made clinically and requires a high index of suspicion. It is helpful to use a marker to indicate the area of initial involvement and to closely monitor the site for rapid progression. Lab values will show an elevated WBC count with a left shift, and a normochromic, normocytic anemia may also be seen. In addition, the ESR will be high. CT, MRI, or plain radiographs can be used to identify (or "rule out") free air in the tissues; if present, this is an indicator of gas-producing organisms (Trent & Kirsner, 2002).

Treatment

When necrotizing fasciitis is suspected, an urgent surgical consult is required because, as already noted, the most important aspect of treatment is early and aggressive surgical debridement to eliminate all of the infected tissue. It is the only intervention proven to decrease mortality. Broad-spectrum antibiotic therapy should also be instituted after cultures have been obtained; although penetration to the fascia is low due to the poor blood supply, broad spectrum antibiotic therapy does decrease bacterial loads and levels of bacterial toxins and can reduce the risk of multiorgan failure (Bellapianta et al., 2009). Hyperbaric oxygen has also been reported to be of benefit in controlling bacterial loads and is sometimes used as adjunctive therapy in addition to wide surgical debridement and systemic antibiotics. Supportive care is of course essential and includes IV fluids, vasopressors if indicated, nutritional support, and management of comorbidities. Once a clean wound bed is established, negative pressure wound therapy is initiated to promote rapid ingrowth of healthy granulation tissue; flaps and grafts are typically required for final wound closure.

Vibrio vulnificus

Vibrio vulnificus, a type of bacteria found in marine environments, can cause serious septicemia in certain individuals who eat raw shellfish in which the organism lives and can also cause localized cutaneous disease. *Vibrio vulnificus* is endemic in the United States off the Atlantic and Gulf Coast (Horseman & Surani, 2011). Cutaneous infection occurs when the bacterium is inoculated through breaks or cuts in the skin barrier, usually during water sports, fishing, or boating. Since *V. vulnificus* is found in raw shellfish, a common portal of entry is through small breaks in the skin caused by opening oysters.

In most individuals, cutaneous infection with the organism results in a mild cellulitis. The skin lesions begin to form within days of exposure and are limited to the site of inoculation. They begin as painful areas of erythema and edema, which can progress to hemorrhagic bullae that result in crusted erosions when they rupture. In a small subset of vulnerable patients, the lesions can progress to necrotizing fasciitis and septicemia.

Systemic *V. vulnificus* sepsis caused by oral ingestion of the organism is most likely to develop in individuals with liver disease, diabetes mellitus, and/or immunodeficiencies. The mortality rate for sepsis caused by this organism exceeds 50%. The characteristic bullous lesions can develop on the skin in patients with systemic disease, even though the bacterium was not contracted via a wound infection. The skin lesions can present anywhere on the body but are usually seen on the lower extremities. The lesions associated with systemic *V. vulnificus* can progress to ulcers and, at worst, necrotizing fasciitis (Horseman & Surani, 2011).

CLINICAL PEARL

Vibrio vulnificus, a type of bacteria found in marine environments, can cause serious septicemia in certain individuals who eat raw shellfish in which the organism lives and can also cause localized cutaneous disease.

Both systemic sepsis and severe localized wound infections caused by *V. vulnificus* are treated with a combination of oral minocycline or doxycycline and intravenous cefotaxime or ceftriaxone. Cases of necrotizing fasciitis are treated with aggressive surgical debridement, antibiotic therapy, supportive care, and appropriate wound care. Minor wound infections in healthy hosts can be treated with oral antibiotics and local wound care.

Bacterial Folliculitis

Folliculitis is a superficial infection of the skin that is limited to the area around hair follicles. Folliculitis usually begins with trauma to the hair follicle; the trauma renders the hair follicle vulnerable to pathogen invasion. Both bacteria and fungi can cause folliculitis, though the most common pathogen is *S. aureus*. The lesions present as multiple pruritic, red, pustular lesions involving the hair follicles. When several infected hair follicles coalesce into a single, inflamed area or nodule, it is known as a carbuncle. If the infection involves the dermis or subcutaneous fat, the entity is termed a furuncle. Though folliculitis is very common, the true incidence is not known; this is because most cases are minor and resolve quickly and do not require professional intervention.

Certain conditions predispose patients to folliculitis, including immunosuppression, existing dermatoses, diabetes mellitus, obesity, use of heavy emollients, and living in a humid climate. One of the most important risk factors is frequent shaving; in fact, folliculitis is often seen on the face of men in the beard and mustache area, which is also known as "sycosis barbae." The rash is extremely pruritic and usually starts around the nose and upper lip area. The pustules that develop have hair protruding from the center. Shaving and facial cleansing can cause the pustules to burst, with a resultant spread of the infection. The pustular lesions can be eroded by continued shaving, and the persistent trauma and infection can eventually lead to scarring and alopecia of the area.

CLINICAL PEARL

Folliculitis is characterized by a pustular rash with hair protruding from the center of the lesions; treatment involves atraumatic hair removal and topical antibacterial/antibiotic agents.

Staphylococcal folliculitis can occur on any hair-bearing area, but the face, buttocks, legs, and axillae are the sites most commonly affected. Treatment with topical antibiotics such as mupirocin is usually sufficient; in addition, the individual needs to be counseled regarding atraumatic approaches to hair removal (Luelmo-Aguilar & Santandreu, 2004).

Gram-negative folliculitis can be caused by the bacterial species *Proteus*, *Klebsiella*, *Enterobacter*, and *Serratia*. This is most common in patients who are taking long-term antibiotic therapy (often for acne vulgaris). Because this condition is common in patients with acne, gram-negative folliculitis can be confused for an acne flare. The lesions are usually around the nose and chin. Samples of the drainage from the pustules should be sent for Gram stain and culture to confirm the diagnosis, and the condition should be treated with oral antibiotics and/or isotretinoin.

Pseudomonas aeruginosa folliculitis is a specific type of gram-negative folliculitis that presents in patients who have recently been in a whirlpool, and it is colloquially known as "hot-tub folliculitis." It can also be seen in patients who have worn a wet suit for prolonged periods of time. The lesions are papular and pustular and located around the hair follicles in areas occluded by swimwear. The infection is self-limiting but may leave areas of erosions and hypopigmentation. No treatment is indicated.

Mycobacterial Infection (Leprosy)

Caused by *Mycobacterium leprae* and also known as "Hansen's disease", leprosy is an infection that affects the skin and peripheral nervous system. *Mycobacterium leprae* is a mycobacterium that grows extremely slowly, making it very hard to culture. Similar to *Mycobacterium tuberculosis*, it is an acid-fast bacillus and is an obligate intracellular organism. According to the National Hansen Disease Registry, in 2009, there were 213 new cases of leprosy in the United States; most of the cases involved immigrants from areas where leprosy is endemic, such as Asia, Africa, and Latin America. Since the disease is now very rare, especially in the United States, there is often a long lag time between development of the disease and diagnosis.

The mechanism by which the bacterium is transmitted has not been fully elucidated; it most likely spreads via the respiratory route and less commonly through direct skin inoculation. Interestingly, most people do not develop Hansen's disease after exposure to the bacillus. One large study revealed that those who live with someone with leprosy have a higher chance of developing the disease than neighbors or other individuals. Genetic susceptibility also appears to be a key factor. Other risk factors include increasing age and exposure to an individual with the lepromatous form of the disease (Moet et al., 2006).

Hansen's disease varies in severity, from the least severe tuberculoid form to the most severe and widespread lepromatous form. The type that manifests depends on the immunity of the patient to the organism. In those with a high level of cellular immunity to the bacterium, tuberculoid leprosy develops. Clinically, this appears as a few well-demarcated lesions with areas of central anesthesia and hypopigmentation, sometimes with associated hair loss. Histologically, there are granulomas with very little, if any, acid-fast bacilli seen in the specimen. Lepromatous leprosy occurs in patients with little or no immunity and is characterized by diffuse, ill-defined plaques all over the body; the lesions often give the patient a characteristic facial appearance that is described as "leonine." Patients often lose their eyebrows and develop nodules on their ears. On histology, foamy macrophages with abundant bacilli are noted.

In individuals who are closer to the tuberculoid end of the disease spectrum, sensory and/or motor nerve damage can occur under the skin lesions; this may be caused by the

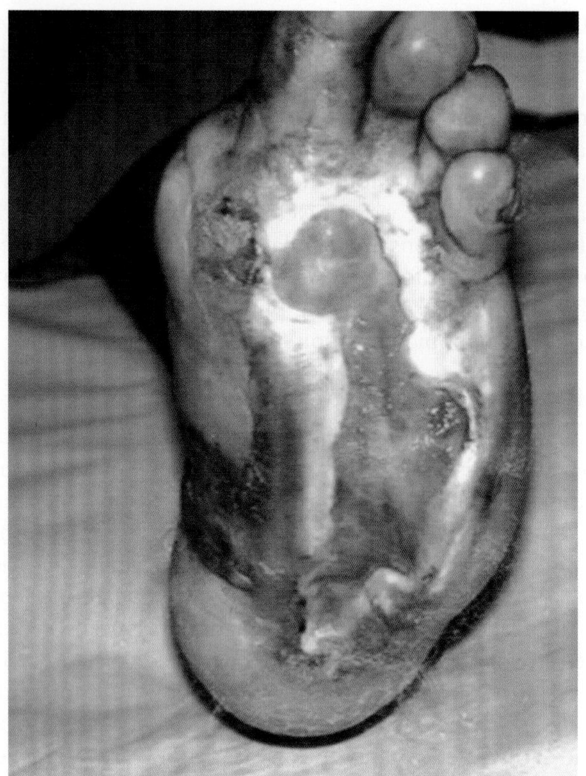

FIGURE 27-9. Tuberculoid leprosy. The patient has nerve involvement, leading to a loss of sensation in the foot in this case, and a large area of ulceration.

patient's immunologic response to the pathogen, with the nerve damage caused by the resulting inflammation. The nerve damage causes the areas to become hypoesthetic, which renders the individual more vulnerable to injury such as cuts or severe burns. The affected individual may present to the provider with localized areas of nonhealing ulcers. In lepromatous leprosy, the nerve damage is due to bacterial infiltration of nerves and is not limited to the area of skin lesions. Patchy areas of sensory and/or motor loss can develop; painful neuropathy can develop as well. In the United States, this neuropathy is often mistaken for diabetic neuropathy. Ulcers may develop on the feet due to the loss of sensation and may be mistaken for diabetic foot ulcers (Fig. 27-9).

The diagnosis of Hansen's disease usually requires skin biopsy and PCR testing of the tissue for *M. leprae*. Similar to treatment for *M. tuberculosis*, treatment of leprosy involves a multidrug regimen. For tuberculoid forms, treatment for 12 months with dapsone and rifampin is recommended, while for lepromatous forms, 24 months are required and clofazimine should be added to the regimen (Anderson et al., 2007).

Conclusion

Infectious wounds are a very common cause of wounds worldwide. Viruses, bacteria, and fungi can all cause wounds. Infections range in severity from very commonplace wounds, such as herpes labialis, to very severe and life-threatening wounds, such as necrotizing fasciitis. Though many infections do not cause chronic wounds, some infections can cause great damage to the skin and underlying tissues, resulting in lasting morbidity and disability even when the infection has resolved. It is important for the clinician to be aware of the history and physical findings associated with wounds caused by infectious processes, and to assure accurate diagnosis, because effective treatment of the underlying infection is the first essential step in resolving the cutaneous manifestations.

REFERENCES

Ameen, M. (2009). Chromoblastomycosis: Clinical presentation and management. *Clinical and Experimental Dermatology, 34*(8), 849–854. doi: 10.1111/j.1365-2230.2009.03415.x.

Anderson, H., Stryjewska, B., Boyanton, B. L., et al. (2007). Hansen disease in the United States in the 21st century: A review of the literature. *Archives of Pathology and Laboratory Medicine, 131*(6), 982–986. doi: 10.1043/1543-2165(2007)131[982:hditus]2.0.co;2.

Avci, O., Tanyildizi, T., & Kusku, E. (2013). A comparison between the effectiveness of erythromycin, single-dose clarithromycin and topical fusidic acid in the treatment of erythrasma. *The Journal of Dermatological Treatment, 24*(1), 70–74. doi: 10.3109/09546634.2011.594870.

Bell-Syer, S. E., Khan, S. M., & Torgerson, D. J. (2012). Oral treatments for fungal infections of the skin of the foot. *Cochrane Database of Systematic Reviews, 10*, CD003584. doi: 10.1002/14651858.CD003584.pub2.

Bellapianta, J. M., Ljungquist, K., Tobin, E., et al. (2009). Necrotizing fasciitis. *Journal of the American Academy of Orthopaedic Surgeons, 17*(3), 174–182.

Borchers, A. T., & Gershwin, M. E. (2010). The immune response in coccidioidomycosis. *Autoimmunity Reviews, 10*(2), 94–102. doi: 10.1016/j.autrev.2010.08.010.

Bradley, H., Markowitz, L. E., Gibson, T., et al. (2014). Seroprevalence of herpes simplex virus types 1 and 2—United States, 1999–2010. *Journal of Infectious Diseases, 209*(3), 325–333. doi: 10.1093/infdis/jit458.

Cernik, C., Gallina, K., & Brodell, R. T. (2008). The treatment of herpes simplex infections: an evidence-based review. *Archives of Internal Medicine, 168*(11), 1137–1144. doi: 10.1001/archinte.168.11.1137.

Chang, P., & Rodas, C. (2012). Skin lesions in histoplasmosis. *Clinics in Dermatology, 30*(6), 592–598. doi: 10.1016/j.clindermatol.2012.01.004.

Cohen, K. R., Salbu, R. L., Frank, J., et al. (2013). Presentation and management of herpes zoster (shingles) in the geriatric population. *Pharmacy and Therapeutics, 38*(4), 217–227.

Corey, L., Adams, H. G., Brown, Z. A., et al. (1983). Genital herpes simplex virus infections: Clinical manifestations, course, and complications. *Annals of Internal Medicine, 98*(6), 958–972.

De Araujo, T., Marques, A. C., & Kerdel, F. (2001). Sporotrichosis. *International Journal of Dermatology, 40*(12), 737–742.

Goolamali, S. I., Fogo, A., Killian, L., et al. (2009). Ecthyma gangrenosum: An important feature of pseudomonal sepsis in a previously well child. *Clinical and Experimental Dermatology, 34*(5), e180–e182. doi: 10.1111/j.1365-2230.2008.03020.x.

Horseman, M. A., & Surani, S. (2011). A comprehensive review of *Vibrio vulnificus*: An important cause of severe sepsis and skin and soft-tissue infection. *International Journal of Infectious Diseases, 15*(3), e157–e166. doi: 10.1016/j.ijid.2010.11.003.

Kalra, M. G., Higgins, K. E., & Kinney, B. S. (2014). Intertrigo and secondary skin infections. *American Family Physician, 89*(7), 569–573.

Kihiczak, G. G., Schwartz, R. A., & Kapila, R. (2006). Necrotizing fasciitis: A deadly infection. *Journal of the European Academy of Dermatology and Venereology, 20*(4), 365–369. doi: 10.1111/j.1468-3083.2006.01487.x.

Koning, S., Mohammedamin, R. S., van der Wouden, J. C., et al. (2006). Impetigo: Incidence and treatment in Dutch general practice in 1987 and 2001—Results from two national surveys. *British Journal of Dermatology, 154*(2), 239–243. doi: 10.1111/j.1365-2133.2005.06766.x.

Langenberg, A. G., Corey, L., Ashley, R. L., et al. (1999). A prospective study of new infections with herpes simplex virus type 1 and type 2. Chiron HSV Vaccine Study Group. *New England Journal of Medicine, 341*(19), 1432–1438. doi: 10.1056/nejm199911043411904.

Lopez Martinez, R., & Mendez Tovar, L. J. (2007). Chromoblastomycosis. *Clinics in Dermatology, 25*(2), 188–194. doi: 10.1016/j.clindermatol.2006.05.007.

Lopez-Martinez, R., & Mendez-Tovar, L. J. (2012). Blastomycosis. *Clinics in Dermatology,30*(6),565–572.doi:10.1016/j.clindermatol.2012.01.002.

Luelmo-Aguilar, J., & Santandreu, M. S. (2004). Folliculitis: Recognition and management. *American Journal of Clinical Dermatology, 5*(5), 301–310.

Mirmirani, P., & Tucker, L. Y. (2013). Epidemiologic trends in pediatric tinea capitis: A population-based study from Kaiser Permanente Northern California. *Journal of the American Academy of Dermatology, 69*(6), 916–921. doi: 10.1016/j.jaad.2013.08.031.

Moet, F. J., Pahan, D., Schuring, R. P., et al. (2006). Physical distance, genetic relationship, age, and leprosy classification are independent risk factors for leprosy in contacts of patients with leprosy. *Journal of Infectious Diseases, 193*(3), 346–353. doi: 10.1086/499278.

Mohammedamin, R. S., van der Wouden, J. C., Koning, S., et al. (2006). Increasing incidence of skin disorders in children? A comparison between 1987 and 2001. *BMC Dermatology, 6*, 4. doi: 10.1186/1471-5945-6-4.

Nahass, G. T., Goldstein, B. A., Zhu, W. Y., et al. (1992). Comparison of Tzanck smear, viral culture, and DNA diagnostic methods in detection of herpes simplex and varicella-zoster infection. *JAMA, 268*(18), 2541–2544.

Pathak, A., Singh, P., Yadav, Y., et al. (2013). Ecthyma gangrenosum in a neonate: Not always pseudomonas. *BMJ Case Report.* doi: 10.1136/bcr-2013-009287.

Phoenix, G., Das, S., & Joshi, M. (2012). Diagnosis and management of cellulitis. *BMJ, 345*, e4955. doi: 10.1136/bmj.e4955.

Ramos-e-Silva, M., Vasconcelos, C., Carneiro, S., et al. (2007). Sporotrichosis. *Clinics in Dermatology, 25*(2), 181–187. doi: 10.1016/j.clindermatol.2006.05.006.

Salcido, R. S. (2007). Necrotizing fasciitis: Reviewing the causes and treatment strategies. *Advances in Skin & Wound Care, 20*(5), 288–293; quiz 294–285. doi: 10.1097/01.ASW.0000269317.76380.3b.

Stevens, D. L., Bisno, A. L., Chambers, H. F., et al. (2014). Executive summary: Practice guidelines for the diagnosis and management of skin and soft tissue infections: 2014 Update by the infectious diseases society of america. *Clinical Infectious Diseases, 59*(2), 147–159. doi: 10.1093/cid/ciu444.

Trent, J. T., & Kirsner, R. S. (2002). Diagnosing necrotizing fasciitis. *Advances in Skin & Wound Care, 15*(3), 135–138.

Usatine, R. P., & Tinitigan, R. (2010). Nongenital herpes simplex virus. *American Family Physician, 82*(9), 1075–1082.

Weinberg, J. M. (2007). Herpes zoster: Epidemiology, natural history, and common complications. *Journal of the American Academy of Dermatology, 57*(6 Suppl), S130–S135. doi: 10.1016/j.jaad.2007.08.046.

QUESTIONS

1. The wound care nurse is devising a treatment plan for a patient diagnosed with moderately severe orolabial herpes (HSV-1). Which therapy is recommended?

A. Topical antiviral agents alone
B. Systemic antivirals initiated during the prodromal phase
C. Chronic suppressive therapy
D. Systemic antivirals and chronic suppressive treatment

2. The wound care nurse is teaching new nurses how to recognize and treat herpes lesions. Which statement accurately describes this disease process and the recommended treatment?

A. Herpes lesions are full-thickness wounds that should be kept dry.
B. Herpes lesions should be treated with moist wound healing principles.
C. Recurrent episodes of genital herpes tend to be more severe.
D. Recurrences of genital herpes are more common with HSV-1 infection than with HSV-2.

3. Which patient would the wound care nurse place at higher risk for contracting zoster (shingles)?

A. A 32-year-old patient who has never had chickenpox
B. A 47-year-old patient who has active genital herpes
C. A 12-year-old patient who was immunized for varicella–zoster virus
D. A 79-year-old patient who had chicken pox as a child

4. The wound care nurse is assessing a patient who presents with a very red and inflamed kerion-like lesion in the beard area, with hair that is easily removed. The patient states his occupation as "cattle farmer." What disease state would the nurse suspect?

A. Tinea barbae
B. Tinea pedis
C. *Candida albicans*
D. Candidal intertrigo

5. Which medication has few side effects and a high cure rate and is the preferred treatment for lymphocutaneous and fixed cutaneous cases of sporotrichosis?

A. Potassium iodide
B. Amphotericin B
C. Itraconazole
D. Terbinafine

6. A pediatric nurse is assessing a rash on the face of a 4-year-old patient. The rash contains red macules and vesicles that have ruptured and caused a "honey-colored" crust. What common childhood skin infection would the nurse suspect?

A. Ecthyma gangrenosum
B. Impetigo
C. Tinea capitis
D. Cellulitis

7. Which skin condition requires immediate recognition by the clinician, as it is usually an indicator of bacteremia and actual or impending sepsis?

A. Ecthyma gangrenosum
B. Hidradenitis suppurativa
C. Cellulitis
D. Bullous impetigo in adult

8. Which skin infection is diagnosed clinically and treated with topical or systemic antibiotics effective against *S. aureus and S. pyogenes*?

A. Histoplasmosis
B. Chromoblastomycosis
C. Hidradenitis suppurativa
D. Bullous impetigo

9. The wound care nurse is developing a treatment plan for a patient with hidradenitis suppurativa. Which measure is recommended for this chronic condition?

A. Maintaining tight glycemic control
B. Wearing tighter clothing to protect against bacterial invasion
C. Daily oral doxycycline or minocycline
D. Atraumatic hair removal and topical antibacterial/antibiotic agents

10. The wound care nurse is planning treatment for a patient diagnosed with mild cellulitis. Which action is recommended?

A. Taking culture swabs from intact skin
B. Systemic antibiotic therapy with an agent that covers MRSA
C. Ordering blood cultures
D. Surgical debridement of the lesions

11. The wound care nurse documents type 2 necrotizing fasciitis on a patient chart. What is the typical causative factor for this type of infection?

A. Non-group A *Streptococcus*
B. *Streptococcus pyogenes*
C. *Vibrio vulnificus*
D. *Streptococcus pyogenes* and *S. aureus*

ANSWERS: 1.**B**, 2.**B**, 3.**D**, 4.**A**, 5.**C**, 6.**B**, 7.**A**, 8.**D**, 9.**C**, 10.**B**, 11.**B**

CHAPTER 28

Wounds Caused by Dermatologic Conditions

Ashwin Agarwal and Adela Rambi G. Cardones

OBJECTIVES

1. Describe the pathology, clinical presentation, and management of blistering skin diseases such as pemphigus vulgaris and bullous pemphigoid.
2. Differentiate between Stevens-Johnson syndrome and toxic epidermal necrolysis and outline management guidelines for either/both of these conditions.
3. Explain the basic pathology and management of psoriasis.
4. Explain the difference in pathology and presentation of irritant contact dermatitis and allergic contact dermatitis and discuss management guidelines.

Topic Outline

Introduction

Throughout this text, we have emphasized correction of etiologic factors as a critical "first step" in effective wound management. Some wounds are caused by dermatologic conditions that cause acute inflammation of the epidermal and dermal layers, or epidermal loss. The wound care nurse needs to be knowledgeable regarding dermatologic conditions that can cause skin and tissue loss and should assure appropriate workup and treatment when there is any reason to suspect that dermatologic pathology is causing or contributing to the wound. This chapter focuses on dermatologic conditions associated with skin and tissue loss.

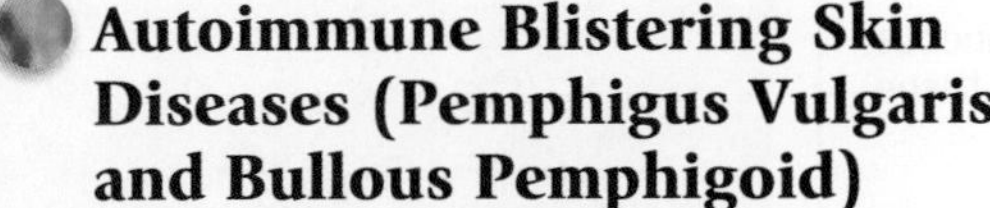

Autoimmune Blistering Skin Diseases (Pemphigus Vulgaris and Bullous Pemphigoid)

Pemphigus vulgaris (PV) is the most common form of the pemphigus category of cutaneous diseases. It is a potentially life-threatening autoimmune blistering disorder,

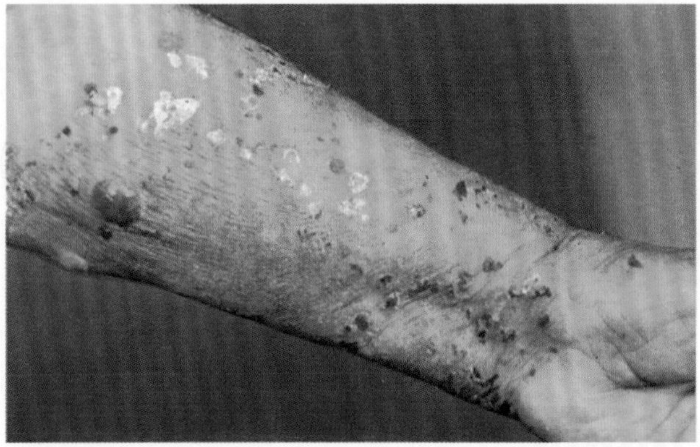

FIGURE 28-1. Pemphigus vulgaris skin blisters. Pemphigus vulgaris blisters on the forearm. (Reprinted with permission from Smeltzer, S., & Bare, B. (2000). *Brunner and Suddarth's textbook of medical-surgical nursing* (9th ed.). Philadelphia, PA: Lippincott Williams & Wilkins.)

characterized by the formation of *flaccid intraepithelial skin layer blisters* (Fig. 28-1) and the loss of skin cell adhesion in the epidermal layer of the skin as well as the mucous membranes (Fig. 28-2). The underlying pathology involves development of self-antibodies to cell adhesion molecules. This triggers an immune reaction, which causes destruction of cell-to-cell connections and results in separation of cells and cell layers. PV itself is a rare disease, with an incidence reported between 0.1% and 0.5% per 100,000 people per year, although rates are higher among those of Jewish ancestry and those from Southeast Europe, India, and the Middle East (Kneisel & Hertl, 2011). The average age of onset is between 40 to 60 years, with a reported equivalent or close to equivalent sex ratio (Joly & Litrowski, 2011).

CLINICAL PEARL

The pathology of blistering pemphigoid skin disorders is development of antibodies to cell adhesion molecules, which causes breakdown of cell-to-cell and skin layer–to–skin layer connections and results in blister formation.

Bullous pemphigoid (BP) is another major autoimmune blistering skin disease that is characterized by *tense subepithelial blisters* of the skin and erosive mucous membrane lesions (Fig. 28-3). The blisters and erosions are caused by the deposition of autoantibodies within the basement membrane, which is located below the epidermis but above the dermis; the dermal papillae lie just under this membrane (see Fig. 28-2). Just as with pemphigus, there is a subsequent immune system–mediated activation and destruction of skin cells bound to the antibodies. It is a disease of older adults, usually over the age of 60 years, with incidence rates cited as 4 to 22 cases per million individuals per year (Joly et al., 2012; Marazza et al., 2009). It is the most common autoimmune blistering skin disease in Europe but may be seen more in countries such as Malaysia and Thailand

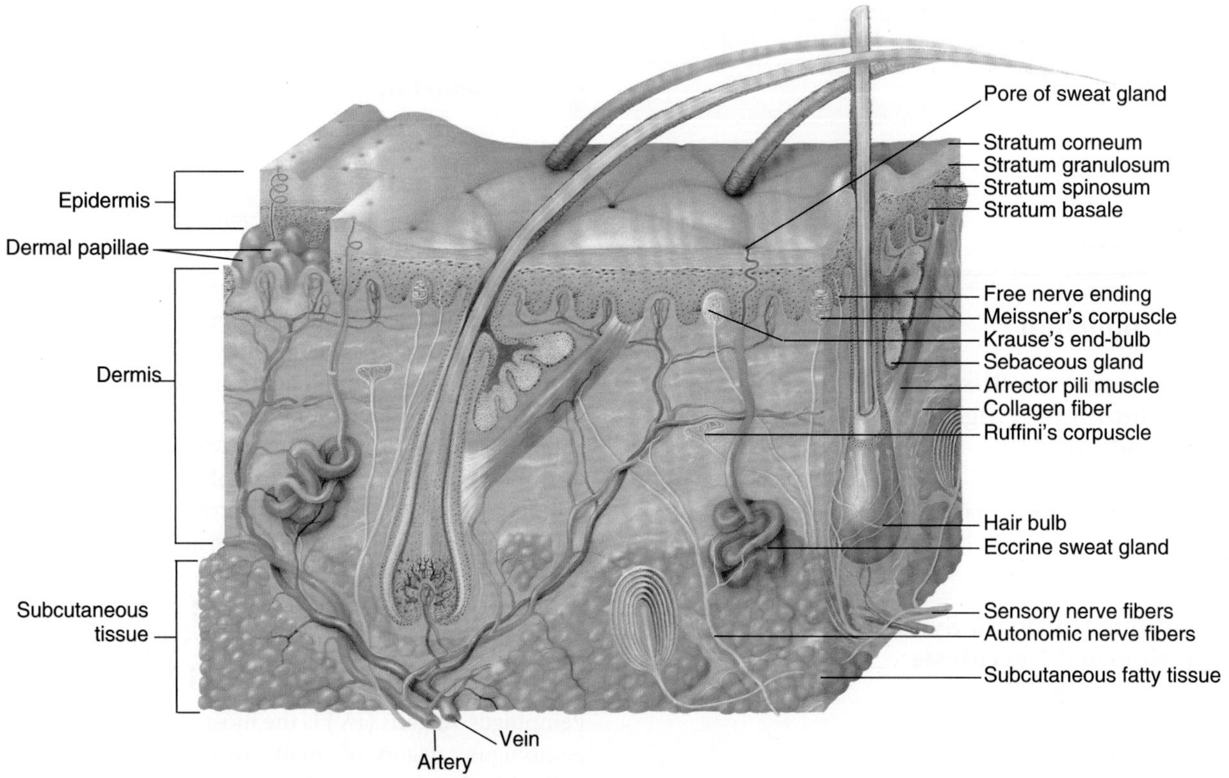

FIGURE 28-2. Layers of the skin graphic. Layers of the skin (epidermis and dermis), associated adnexa, and underlying subcutaneous tissue.

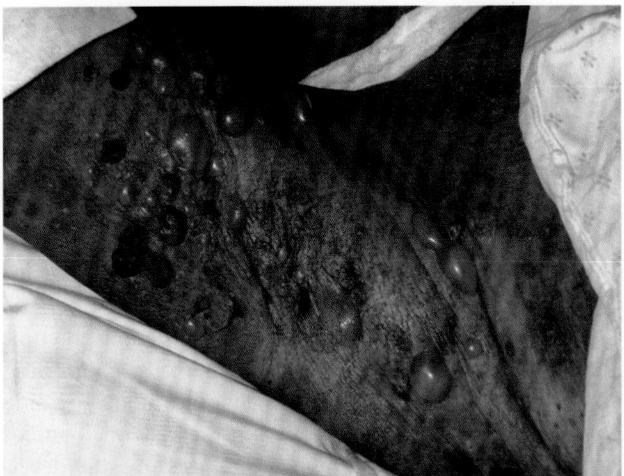

FIGURE 28-3. Bullous pemphigoid skin blisters. Axilla bullae in bullous pemphigoid.

(Kulthanan et al., 2011). Data suggest a slight female predominance in BP, although the reason is unknown (Marazza et al., 2009).

CLINICAL PEARL

PV causes destruction of cell-to-cell connections within the epidermis and causes flaccid intraepithelial blisters; BP causes separation between the epidermal and dermal layers and results in formation of tense blisters.

Pathology

PV is mediated by IgG autoantibodies that target protein components of desmosomes, which are critical in maintaining epidermal cell-to-cell adhesion and skin integrity; specific targets include the desmoglein-1 (Dsg1) and/or desmoglein-3 (Dsg3) components of desmosomes (Amagai et al., 1999). With BP, the IgG autoantibodies target two major hemidesmosomal proteins: bullous pemphigoid antigen 180 (BP 180) and bullous pemphigoid antigen 230 (BP 230). These proteins normally function to maintain tight adherence between epithelial cells and the underlying basement membrane layer (Kasperkiewicz et al., 2012). Understanding the pathology and the specific proteins targeted by the autoantibodies helps to explain differences in clinical presentation among patients with PV and those with BP. Patients with PV demonstrate flaccid, *intraepithelial* blisters since the proteins targeted are those that maintain cell-to-cell adhesion of epidermal cells. In contrast, patients with BP present with tense, *subepithelial* blisters because the autoantibodies target the proteins that maintain adhesion between the epidermis and basement membrane layers.

Clinical Presentation

Patients with PV present with flaccid bullae, skin erosions, and possibly mucous membrane erosions. Most PV patients

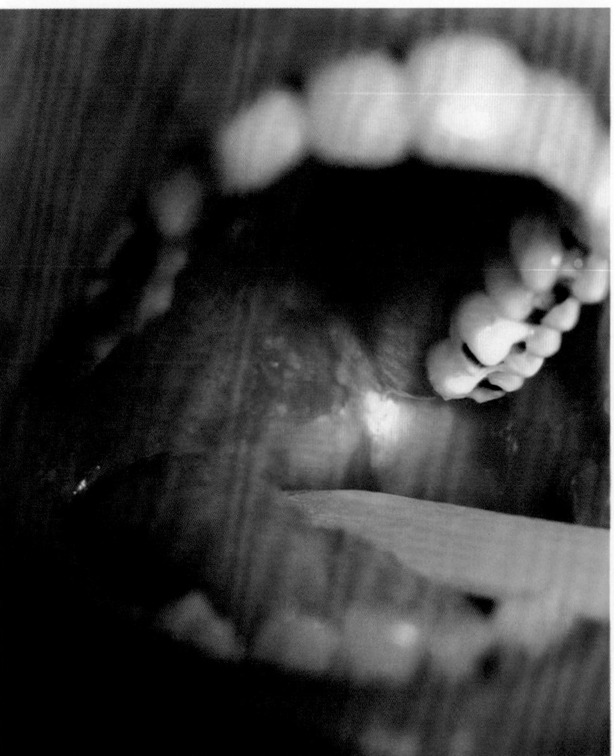

FIGURE 28-4. Pemphigus vulgaris oral lesions. Oral mucosal pemphigus vulgaris lesion.

do develop mucosal involvement, and these lesions most commonly occur in the oral cavity (Fig. 28-4). Other sites include the conjunctivae, nose, esophagus, vulva, vagina, cervix, and anus. There can be significant pain associated with PV lesions, and oral lesions can compromise chewing and swallowing, resulting in poor dietary intake and weight loss. Patients with oral lesions may also complain of hoarseness. Intact PV blisters are flaccid and easily ruptured, and these patients typically have a positive Nikolsky sign, that is, mechanical pressure applied to normal skin or the edge of blisters results in new blister formation or extension of the existing blister and sloughing of the epidermis (Venugopal & Murrell, 2011). The end result is painful erosions that bleed easily.

BP may begin with a prodromal phase of weeks to months preceding blister appearance; this phase is characterized by a pruritic, eczema-like skin rash or urticarial plaques (Kasperkiewicz et al., 2012). The classic blisters are tense bullae on an erythematous or urticarial base; they are numerous, widely distributed, 1 to 3 cm in diameter (see Fig. 28-3), and often associated with intense itching. The blisters eventually rupture, resulting in weeping erosions with crust formation; the lesions resolve without scarring (Fig. 28-5). The most commonly involved areas include the trunk, the underarm and groin areas, and extremity flexures (Yancey & Egan, 2000). Mucosal erosions are seen in about 10% to 30% of patients with BP (Kneisel & Hertl, 2011) and present as erosive gingivitis or inflammation of

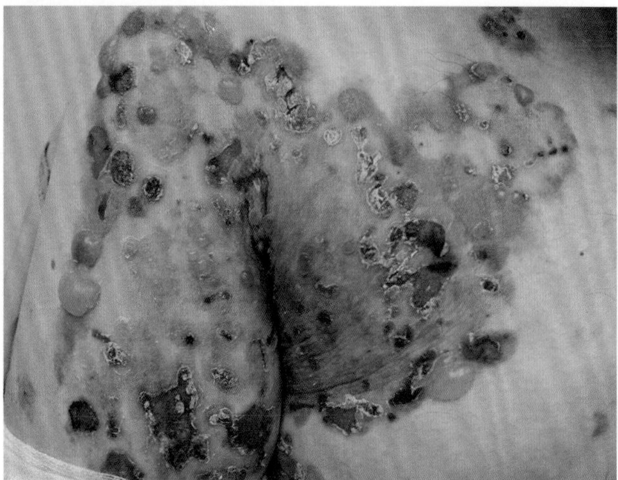

FIGURE 28-5. Bullous pemphigoid crusts/weeping erosions from burst bullae. Bullous pemphigoid lesions seen in various stages of development including tense bullae, weeping erosions, and crusts.

the mucosa. Localized forms of BP occur in up to 30% of patients, with lesions found on the lower legs, sites of trauma, or the anogenital region (Tran & Mutasim, 2005).

CLINICAL PEARL

Most patients with PV and some patients with BP develop mucosal lesions, most commonly oral lesions.

The typical clinical course for both PV and BP is one of chronicity, characterized by recurrent episodes of relapse and remission over months to years, with lesions at varying stages depending on the level of disease control. However, BP patients have reported remission rates of up to 50% following 3 years of treatment (Venning & Wojnarowska, 1992).

CLINICAL PEARL

The typical clinical course for both PV and BP is one of chronicity, characterized by recurrent episodes of relapse and remission over months to years.

Diagnosis

The gold standard for diagnosing PV or BP remains direct immunofluorescence (DIF) of the adjacent, unaffected skin. Patients with PV will demonstrate a characteristic interepithelial IgG deposition, whereas patients with BP demonstrate linear IgG and C3 complement in the basement membrane (Jordan et al., 1971). A 4-mm punch biopsy at the edge of a blister or erosion can also aid in the diagnosis. Histologic findings characteristic of PV include detachment of epithelial cells but retention of the basal layer of the epidermis, which resembles a "row of tombstones." In contrast, BP is characterized by *detachment* of the basal epidermal layer from the basement membrane separating the epidermis and dermis. The infiltrate in BP tends to be eosinophil rich, sometimes forming small abscesses. In the urticarial phase, significant dermal edema may also be present (Lever et al., 2009).

Management

PV varies in severity from relatively mild to life threatening, and therapy must be tailored to the severity of the disease as well as the patient's age and comorbidities (Hooten et al., 2014). For mild disease, therapy with topical corticosteroids is usually sufficient. For moderate to severe disease, systemic corticosteroid therapy (prednisone 1 to 1.5 mg/kg/d) is highly effective in controlling active disease. However, there are significant adverse side effects and risks associated with chronic systemic corticosteroid therapy including high blood pressure, the development of diabetes mellitus, osteoporosis, increased risk of infection, gastrointestinal ulcers, weight gain, and bone necrosis. For this reason, long-term therapy should involve adjuvant or, when possible, primary therapy with steroid-sparing agents such as azathioprine and mycophenolate mofetil (Hooten et al., 2014). More recently, rituximab immunotherapy has been reported to be effective in treating refractory disease (Hooten, et al., 2014; Kasperkiewicz et al., 2011; Martin et al., 2011). Similar principles apply to the treatment of BP. First-line therapy for mild to moderate disease is topical therapy, whereas moderate to severe disease often requires systemic immunomodulation. Even in the presence of extensive disease, therapy with high-potency topical steroids (such as clobetasol 0.05% ointment) can be attempted. This can be as effective as systemic corticosteroid therapy, but with fewer associated side effects (Joly et al., 2002). Systemic anti-inflammatory agents such as tetracyclines can also be helpful for some patients. Adjuvant long-term steroid-sparing agents such as azathioprine, mycophenolate mofetil, and methotrexate are recommended to minimize the risk of adverse effects from chronic steroid therapy. Biologic agents such as rituximab and intravenous immunoglobulin are additional options for treatment of refractory disease.

Evidence-based wound care is critical to promote wound healing and to reduce infection risk for patients with either PV or BP. It is appropriate to puncture and drain large blisters in a sterile environment; however, the epithelial roof should be left intact after drainage to provide wound coverage. Open wounds should be managed with principles of moist wound healing; dressings should be selected with the goals of managing any exudate, maintaining a moist wound surface, and providing atraumatic removal. Adhesive dressings are usually contraindicated due to the potential for further epidermal trauma with removal; nonadhesive contact layer dressings, foam dressings, or gel dressings are generally preferred and should be secured with wrap gauze, binders, or other alternatives to adhesive securement. Twice-daily application of high-potency topical corticosteroids such as clobetasol propionate ointment or gel may be used as adjunct to systemic therapy and has been shown to promote healing of erosions (Bystryn & Rudolph, 2005). It is important to maintain a high clinical "index of suspicion" for bacterial or viral superinfection of PV wounds, which is more likely due to immunosuppression, and is most likely to be caused by herpes simplex. Should superinfection occur, it should be treated appropriately, either with oral antibiotics or with antiviral therapy, because superinfection can delay healing and worsen existing lesions (Caldarola et al., 2008).

CLINICAL PEARL

Management of blistering skin conditions involves topical and systemic corticosteroids; open wounds should be managed with principles of moist wound healing, specifically management of exudate, maintenance of a moist wound surface, and avoidance of further trauma with dressing removal.

Stevens-Johnson Syndrome/Toxic Epidermal Necrolysis

Stevens-Johnson syndrome (SJS) and toxic epidermal necrolysis (TEN) are severe, life-threatening immune system–mediated skin and mucous membrane disorders characterized by significant epidermal necrosis and detachment and often resulting from a drug reaction. They are considered as two variants of the same skin disease and are differentiated by disease severity and the percentage of body surface area (BSA) affected by the associated erosions and blisters. SJS is characterized by skin fragility, detachment, and denudation involving >10% BSA in addition to widespread macules or flat atypical targetoid lesions; lesions typically involve the trunk and face. Mucous membrane involvement is also present in over 90% of patients (Figs. 28-6 and 28-7) (Bastuji-Garin et al., 1993). TEN is considered more severe, with a proposed definition of skin detachment involving >30% BSA (Bastuji-Garin et al., 1993). In addition to large areas of epidermal denudation, patients present with widespread erythematous macules or flat targetoid lesions and with mucous membrane involvement (Fig. 28-8). Furthermore, both SJS and TEN typically cause systemic symptoms that include fever and respiratory distress.

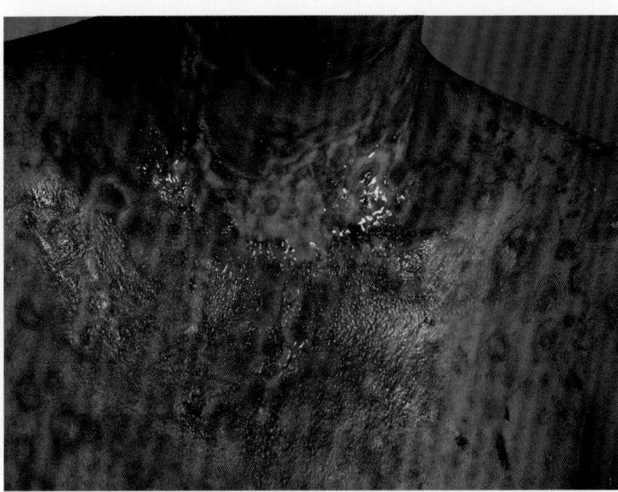

FIGURE 28-6. SJS skin lesions. SJS targetoid, dusky plaques with ulceration.

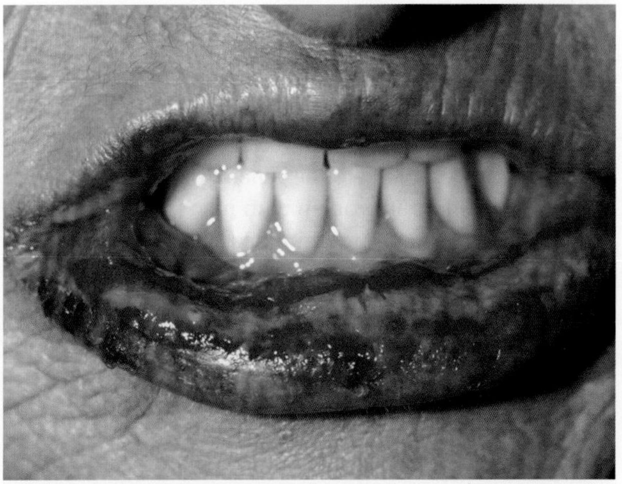

FIGURE 28-7. SJS mucosal lesions. Ulcerations on the lower lip mucosal surface in SJS.

CLINICAL PEARL

SJS and TEN are frequently caused by a drug reaction and are characterized by skin fragility, epidermal detachment, and extensive denudation; mucous membrane involvement is present in >90% of cases. TEN is the more severe form, with >30% BSA involvement.

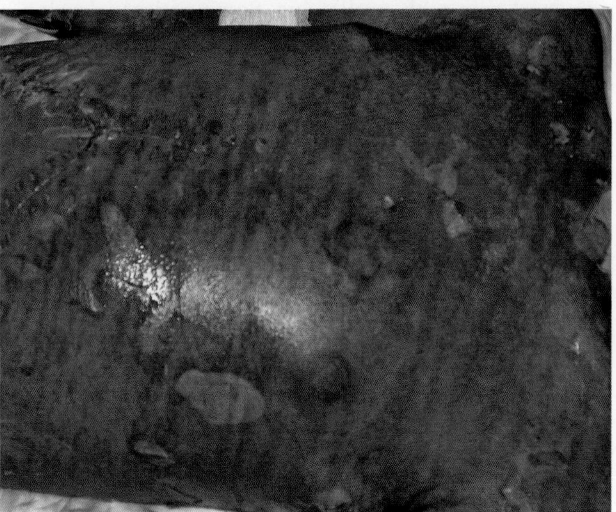

FIGURE 28-8. TEN skin lesions. Scalded skin with diffuse redness and sloughing between lesions in this patient with TEN. (Reprinted with permission from Mulholland, M. W., Ronald V. Maier, R. V., et al. (2006). *Greenfield's surgery scientific principles and practice* (4th ed.). Philadelphia, PA: Lippincott Williams & Wilkins.)

The estimated incidence of SJS/TEN ranges from 2 to 7 cases per million people per year, with SJS being more common; the ratio of SJS to TEN is approximately 3 cases to 1 (Chan et al., 1990). These conditions are more than one hundred times more common among HIV-infected individuals as compared to the general population and are also more common in women than men (Mittmann et al., 2012). Mortality rates are estimated to be approximately 10% for SJS and more than 30% for TEN (Sekula et al., 2013).

Pathology

Although not fully understood, SJS and TEN are thought to be mediated by a T-cell–mediated destruction of skin epithelial cells. Once activated by a particular drug or infection, an inflammatory cascade ensues that leads to epithelial cell death, blistering, and partial to full necrosis of the epidermis (Nassif et al., 2004). Various T-cell protein mediators of cell death are elevated in patients with SJS and TEN, lending further support to the hypothesis that these conditions are autoimmune in origin. For example, the blister fluid level of granulysin, a cytotoxic protein secreted by killer T cells, has been shown to be elevated in these patients and correlates with disease severity (Chung et al., 2008). In addition, soluble Fas ligand, a protein involved in a different cell death pathway, is also found in high concentration in the blister fluid of these patients (Murata et al., 2008).

Clinical Presentation

The prodromal phase is manifest by fever (usually >38°C) and influenza-like symptoms including malaise, muscle pains, and aches; these symptoms occur 1 to 3 days before the onset of skin lesions. During this phase, patients may also complain of visual problems, itching or burning of the eyes, and pain with swallowing. Some patients develop a nonspecific and diffuse red rash prior to appearance of the classic SJS/TEN lesions. It is critical to suspect SJS/TEN whenever patients present with fever >38°C, mucosal inflammation, skin tenderness, and blistering (Bircher, 2005). When the reaction is caused by a medication, the cutaneous lesions usually appear within the first 8 weeks of treatment in both children and adults. The most commonly implicated medication is allopurinol; other drugs commonly associated with SJS/TEN include anticonvulsants (e.g., phenobarbital, carbamazepine, lamotrigine), sulfonamide drugs, nevirapine, and NSAIDs (Halevy et al., 2008).

CLINICAL PEARL

Drugs commonly associated with SJS/TEN include allopurinol, anticonvulsants, sulfonamides, nevirapine, and NSAIDs.

The skin lesions initially present either as confluent, red oval macules or as papules with pruritic centers or as diffuse erythema (atypical target lesions) (see Figs. 28-6 and 28-8). The lesions are associated with significant tenderness and pain that is out of proportion to the findings on the skin exam. The lesions usually start on the face and trunk and spread symmetrically to other areas; the scalp, palms, and soles are usually spared. More classic target lesions with dusky, dark centers are also sometimes seen, followed by formation of vesicles (clear fluid-filled blisters <1 cm in diameter) and bullae (fluid-filled blisters >1 cm in diameter).

CLINICAL PEARL

Early SJS/TEN lesions present as confluent macules or papules or as diffuse erythema and are associated with significant tenderness and pain that is out of proportion to the findings on the skin exam.

Patients with TEN may also experience sudden onset of extensive skin sloughing in the absence of an erythematous rash; in these situations, the clinical picture often resembles extensive thermal injury (Fig. 28-9). These patients also demonstrate a positive Nikolsky sign (Lyell, 1956). The large areas of denudation gradually reepithelialize, but resurfacing may take up to 4 weeks (Jordan et al., 1991). Patients with SJS are more likely to experience a morbilliform eruption as part of the clinical picture.

Painful ocular, nasal, and oral mucosal erosions and crusts are seen in most patients with SJS/TEN in addition to the skin lesions (see Fig. 28-7). Ocular lesions usually involve purulent conjunctivitis, bullae, or corneal ulcerations and are seen in around 80% of patients (Morales et al., 2010). Oral lesions typically present as hemorrhagic erosions with inflammation. In women, vulvovaginal erosions, bullae, or ulcers may be seen along with other pathology.

Diagnosis

A large (>4 mm) punch biopsy or deep shave biopsy is helpful in confirming the diagnosis through histologic analysis. DIF can be used to rule out other immune-mediated

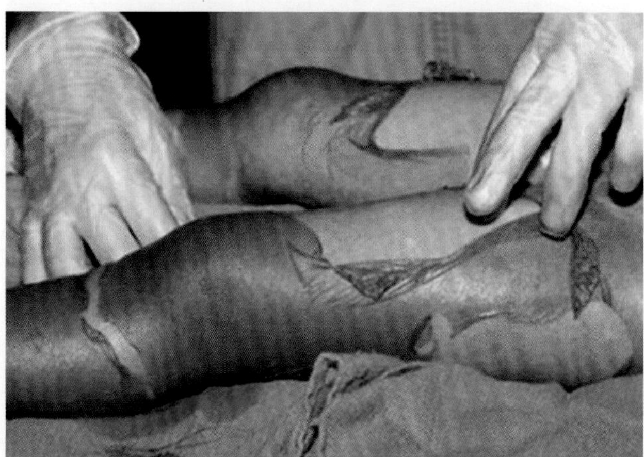

FIGURE 28-9. SJS/TEN skin denudation. This patient demonstrates confluent epidermal sloughing, which is easily removed with gentle pressure (the Nikolsky sign).

blistering disorders. Skin biopsy may reveal subepidermal bullae, complete epidermal necrosis, and T cells in the dermis. Soluble Fas ligand and granulysin proteins are elevated in SJS/TEN; thus, studies are ongoing regarding their usefulness as diagnostic serum studies (Abe et al., 2009; Murata et al., 2008).

Management

Patients who are thought to have early signs of SJS/TEN should have any suspected culprit drug discontinued immediately. Early discontinuation has been shown to reduce the risk of death; specifically, mortality risk is reduced by 30% for every day preceding development of blisters and erosions (Garcia-Doval et al., 2000). Patients should be admitted to an inpatient facility and to an intensive care or burn unit depending on the extent of skin involvement or other diseases. It is critical to monitor for significant fluid loss in patients with extensive skin sloughing; severe hypovolemia may result in low-volume state shock, systemic infection, and multiorgan dysfunction. For this reason, care of the patient with TEN should resemble major burn care with ongoing attention to wound management, fluid and electrolyte supplementation, nutritional support, infection monitoring, and pain control. Ophthalmologic consultation should be obtained to monitor for eye inflammation and to assure appropriate ocular care, and gynecologic examination should be performed on all female patients to prevent complications. While the principles of supportive care are clear, definitive treatment for SJS and TEN is not well defined (Worswick & Cotliar, 2011). Some authors recommend high-dose IVIG as standard therapy, but the evidence for this remains controversial (Worswick & Cotliar, 2011). The use of systemic steroids is equally contended. Some authors recommend corticosteroids for patients with SJS but not those with TEN, and there is some evidence of increased mortality when corticosteroids are used to treat TEN patients. Cyclosporine has recently shown promise as a systemic agent, with decreased mortality compared to IVIG (Kirchhof et al., 2014). Plasmapheresis and anti–tumor necrosis factor (TNF) monoclonal antibodies are other therapeutic options that have been used, though concrete evidence of their efficacy is still lacking.

CLINICAL PEARL

Patients who are thought to have early signs of SJS/TEN should have any suspected culprit drug discontinued immediately to reduce mortality.

The extent of skin sloughing should be evaluated regularly. Debridement is not recommended, as this results in extensive denudation. Patients who were treated with IVIG and conservative skin management had a dramatically lower mortality rate compared to patients who were treated with aggressive debridement (Stella et al., 2007). Topical therapy should follow the principles of moist wound healing, as discussed previously in the section on PV and BP; specifically, dressings should be selected that absorb excess exudate, maintain a moist wound surface, and prevent trauma with removal. Petrolatum and other nonadherent contact layer dressings are commonly used; nonadherent gauze impregnated with nanocrystalline silver is another commonly used approach. A comparison of the two methods does not exist. Of note, the nanocrystalline silver dressing can be left in place for up to 7 days, which may improve patient comfort and reduce pain associated with dressing changes (Fong & Wood, 2006). Wrap gauze and other nonadhesive options should be used to secure the primary contact layer dressing in place, in order to prevent further trauma with dressing removal.

CLINICAL PEARL

Management of the patient with SJS/TEN requires intensive systemic support (fluid and electrolyte replacement, nutritional support, pain management), ophthalmologic and gynecologic consults, infection prevention, and evidence-based wound care.

Psoriasis

Psoriasis is a chronic skin disorder characterized most often by well-circumscribed, erythematous plaques with silver scales (Fig. 28-10). The incidence of psoriasis is estimated to be around 100 cases per 100,000 individuals,

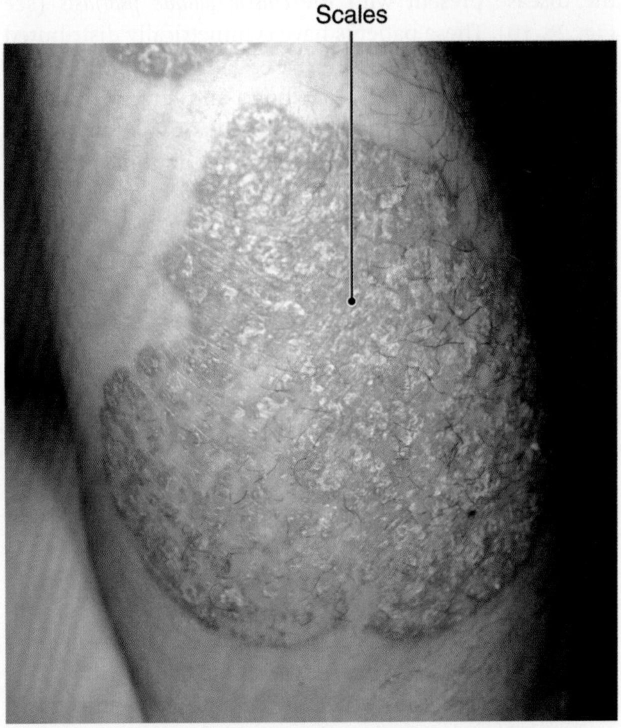

Scales

FIGURE 28-10. Psoriasis skin plaques. A large, erythematous plaque with secondary silvery scaling in this patient with plaque psoriasis.

with reported prevalence ranging from 0.91% to 8.5% of the population, and no clear gender bias (Parisi et al., 2013). Psoriasis appears to have two age peaks of onset: one between ages 30 and 39 and a second between the ages of 50 and 59. Genetic predisposition is a major risk factor; up to 40% of patients with psoriasis have first-degree relatives with the disorder (Gladman et al., 1986). However, there are also a number of environmental factors that appear to be risk factors for psoriasis, including smoking, obesity, and alcohol consumption (Higgins, 2000; Li et al., 2012; Setty et al., 2007).

CLINICAL PEARL

Genetic predisposition is a major risk factor for psoriasis; other risk factors include smoking, obesity, and alcohol consumption.

Pathology

Psoriasis is currently considered to be an immune system–mediated disease resulting in hyperproliferation and abnormal differentiation of the epidermis, leading to redness and scaling (Nickoloff & Nestle, 2004). Individuals with psoriasis manifest a larger number of epidermal stem cells, more cells undergoing mitosis, and shorter epidermal turnover time.

Clinical Presentation

Patients with psoriasis can exhibit different phenotypes (Callen et al., 2003). Up to 80% of adult patients with the disease present with the *classic plaque psoriasis* (see Fig. 28-10). These patients have symmetrically distributed erythematous plaques with silver scale on the scalp, back, and extensor surfaces of the elbows and knees (Tollefson et al., 2010). They may also have lesions involving the intergluteal cleft, external ear canal, and umbilical region. The lesions can be pruritic, although this is not always the case. Psoriasis can also present in an *inverse form*, affecting the inguinal, perineal, genital, intergluteal, axillary, and inframammary regions. In the inverse form, the plaques may lack the characteristic silvery white scaling and may instead present as well-demarcated erythematous plaques with inverse distribution. *Guttate psoriasis* is manifest by numerous small (<1 cm), drop-like, red, and scaly papules that are located primarily on the trunk (Fig. 28-11). This type of psoriasis is frequently associated with a precipitating factor, such as a recent streptococcal throat infection. *Pustular psoriasis* is a severe form of the disease that can be life threatening; these patients present with acute widespread erythema, scaling, and sheets of pustules and erosions (Fig. 28-12). The cutaneous manifestations may be accompanied by fever, liver dysfunction, and diarrhea. This form of psoriasis is associated with pregnancy, infections, and withdrawal of oral corticosteroid therapy. A subset of patients with psoriasis have limited *palmoplantar* involvement. Although the actual BSA involved in these cases is

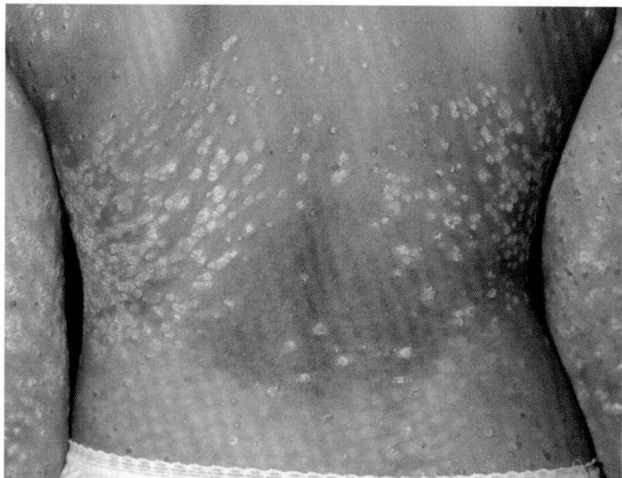

FIGURE 28-11. Guttate psoriasis lesions. Small drop-like spots of guttate psoriasis may be seen during different stages of the disease, especially during an acute flare.

limited, the location of the plaques and papules can make this condition debilitating. Finally, patients with psoriasis can present with *erythroderma*, or redness and scaling involving >30% total body surface area (TBSA). These patients require supportive treatment to prevent excessive loss of fluid and protein and often require systemic therapy.

CLINICAL PEARL

80% of adult patients present with plaque psoriasis, which most commonly involves the scalp, back, and extensor surfaces of the elbows and knees. Less common forms of psoriasis include inverse psoriasis, guttate psoriasis, and pustular psoriasis, which can be life threatening.

Nail plate involvement can be an important clue in diagnosis of psoriasis. Nail changes seen with psoriasis include pitting, brown color changes, small hemorrhages, and nail

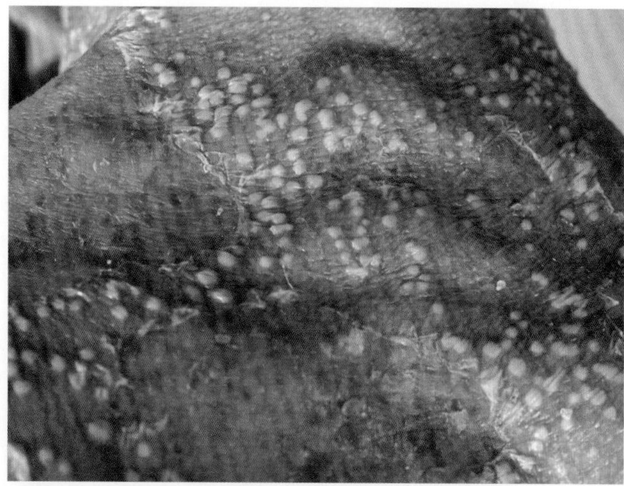

FIGURE 28-12. Pustular psoriasis lesions. Pustular psoriasis lesions seen here with lakes of pus.

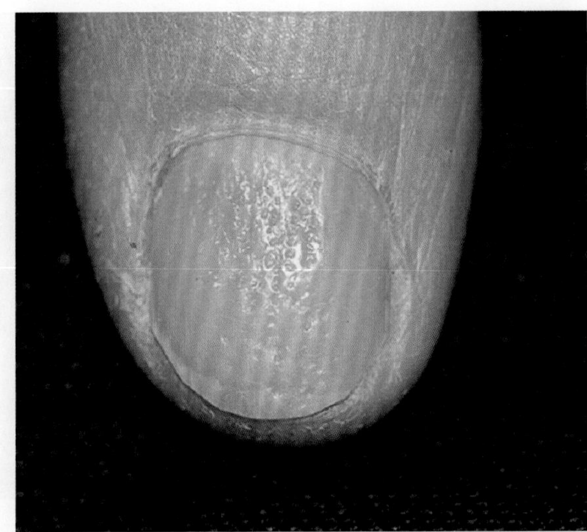

FIGURE 28-13. Psoriasis nail pitting. Nail pitting in psoriasis. Onycholysis and "oil spots" (not shown here) can also be seen.

bed thickening (Fig. 28-13). Another potential diagnostic clue is joint pain; anywhere from 7% to 48% of patients with psoriasis also have arthritis, and this can precede or follow onset of the skin manifestations (Reich et al., 2009).

The clinician caring for the patient with psoriasis should be aware that exacerbating factors include bacterial and viral infections and a number of drugs, including beta blockers, lithium, antimalarial agents such as hydroxychloroquine, antegrade continence enema (ACE) inhibitors, and NSAIDs.

Diagnosis

The diagnosis of psoriasis is made by a thorough history and characteristic findings on physical examination. A 4-mm punch skin biopsy is helpful in ruling out other pathologic conditions with similar presentations. Histologic findings include psoriasiform hyperplasia or thickening of the epidermis, retention of cell nuclei in the topmost layer of epidermis, neutrophils in the epidermis, and sometimes microabscesses.

Management

Limited, mild to moderate disease (<5% to 10% of BSA) is often managed with emollients, supportive therapy, and topical agents. Topical corticosteroids remain the mainstay of therapy for limited disease. The vehicle and potency of the corticosteroid can be varied depending on the patient's preference, severity of disease, and the body site. For example, a liquid solution or foam would be a better choice for the scalp, whereas an ointment or cream would be better for glabrous (hairless) skin. High-potency topical steroids such as clobetasol 0.05% can be used on thick plaques on the trunk, but lower-potency steroids such as hydrocortisone 2.5% would be more appropriate for facial or intertriginous involvement. Nonsteroidal alternatives such as calcipotriene and topical tacrolimus or pimecrolimus can be used as steroid-sparing agents for facial or intertriginous areas to minimize skin atrophy. Other commonly used alternatives are topical retinoids (e.g., once daily tazarotene 0.05% cream). Keratolytics such as topical salicylic acid preparations can also be used to help remove scaling and increase the effectiveness of other topical agents.

CLINICAL PEARL

Topical corticosteroids remain the mainstay of therapy for limited psoriatic disease; phototherapy and biologic agents may be required for more extensive disease.

Phototherapy, most frequently with narrow band UVB, can be utilized for more extensive disease. Moderate to severe disease necessitates systemic therapies including retinoids, methotrexate, and cyclosporine. Several biologic agents are now available as treatment options for moderate to severe psoriasis. Anti-TNF agents are effective and safe therapies. To date, there are five FDA-approved anti-TNF medications available in the United States: etanercept, adalimumab, infliximab, certolizumab, and golimumab. Other biologic agents such as ustekinumab have recently been gaining popularity for patients who fail conventional treatment. It is of utmost importance that the side effects and appropriateness of each therapy be reviewed before it is initiated. Any monitoring guidelines need to be addressed as well.

Referral to dermatology is recommended when the diagnosis is unclear, initial topical therapy is inadequate, the provider is unfamiliar with treatment modalities, or the patient has widespread disease. Rheumatology referral is important if joint disease is suspected.

Irritant and Allergic Dermatitis

Irritant contact dermatitis (ICD) is a local inflammatory skin reaction to various chemical or physical agents. It is caused by a direct, irritant-induced cell death effect and is not a primary immune-mediated phenomenon, in contrast to allergic contact dermatitis (ACD). ICD comprises up to 80% of occupation-related contact dermatitis (Clark & Zirwas, 2009) and is most commonly seen among professionals in food handling, health care, mechanical industry, and the cleaning industry. Other predisposing factors include age (with highest reactivity found among infants and decreased reactivity with increasing age); sex (women at greater risk possibly due to their involvement in high-risk occupations, a phenomenon also seen with ACD); family history of eczema; and environmental conditions such as higher temperature and humidity (Schwindt et al., 1998; Thyssen et al., 2010). Common culprit agents include detergents, solvents (e.g., benzene, acetone), oxidizing agents (bleach, benzoyl peroxide), acids (sulfuric acid), alkaline agents (soap, soda, cement, ammonia), metals, fiberglass, wood, plants, paper, and soil. These agents act to disrupt the skin barrier and to cause cell damage (Dickel et al., 2002).

ACD is a T-cell immune system–mediated delayed hypersensitivity reaction to external agents, which leads to a cutaneous reaction. An eczematous dermatitis is the most common reaction; manifestations include redness, blister formation, itching, and skin thickening isolated to the site of contact. The most common inciting stimuli include poison ivy, oak, and sumac, latex materials, nickel, soaps, fragrances, hair care and makeup products, rubber, plastics, cleansers, resins, acrylics, and protective equipment (Davis et al., 2008). Unlike ICD, the incidence of ACD increases with age.

CLINICAL PEARL

ICD is a local skin reaction caused by direct cellular damage from a chemical agent and is the most common form of contact dermatitis; in contrast, ACD is a T-cell immune system–mediated hypersensitivity reaction.

Pathology

ICD develops when the topmost (stratum corneum) layer of the epidermis is disrupted by chemical or physical agents, leading to a loss of the skin barrier and damage to epidermal cells. The damaged cells then release cytokines that attract immune cells such as macrophages to clear the dead and damaged epidermal cells. ACD is characterized by swelling of the epidermal cells and vesicle (blister) formation and by histopathologic evidence of lymphocytes and eosinophils within the epidermal skin layer.

Clinical Presentation

ICD is characterized by skin redness, dryness, and an eczema-like skin reaction and can result in a chemical burn. Acute ICD can occur from a single exposure to an irritating substance and may present with swelling, vesicles, bullae, oozing, redness, burning, and pain limited to the site of contact (Fig. 28-14). Chronic ICD, on the other hand, is caused by repeated exposure to mild- or low-concentration irritants and is manifest by redness, scaling, thickening of the skin, and fissure formation, typically on the face, fingertips, digit webspaces, and the dorsum of the hands (Fig. 28-15). With both ICD and ACD, patients may complain of stinging, itching, and generalized skin discomfort and pain.

Acute ACD lesions are usually well demarcated and scaly, red, and hardened (Fig. 28-16); they may also present as weepy vesicles and bullae on an edematous base, especially when the lesions involve the eyelids, lips, or genitalia. Patients may complain of itching, burning, pain, and stinging. In chronic disease resulting from continued exposure, the skin is scaly but thicker, dry, and fissured with swelling and crusting. In both acute and chronic ACD, the lesions are usually confined to sites of contact with the inciting stimulus and are therefore frequently seen on the hands and face; if the allergen is a lotion, detergent, body wash, or other "general use" product, the lesions may exhibit widespread distribution.

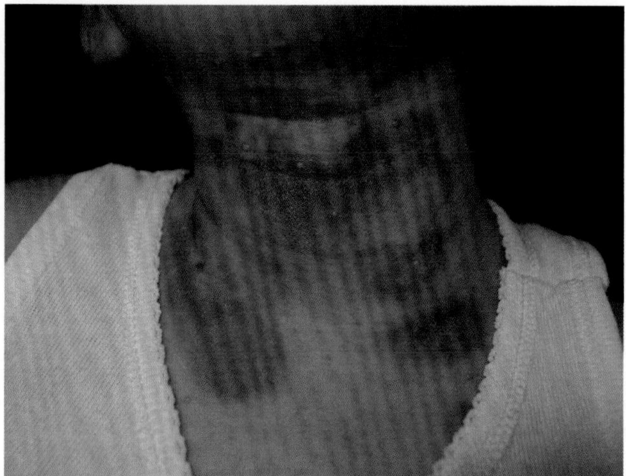

FIGURE 28-14. Acute ICD rash with vesicles. This patient demonstrated a localized irritant dermatitis to imiquimod therapy used for molluscum of neck. (Image provided by Stedman's.)

Diagnosis

The diagnosis of ICD or ACD is based on a thorough history and detailed physical examination. The history should focus on any exposure to occupational, chemical, or physical agents commonly associated with ICD and ACD and specifically on agents to which the involved areas have been exposed. The physical examination involves meticulous inspection of the skin and the affected areas, with attention to the location and morphology of the lesions, which can help to elucidate possible etiologies. It is necessary to rule out ACD via patch testing, which should be done via outpatient dermatology consultation. A skin biopsy is also important to exclude other skin pathologies

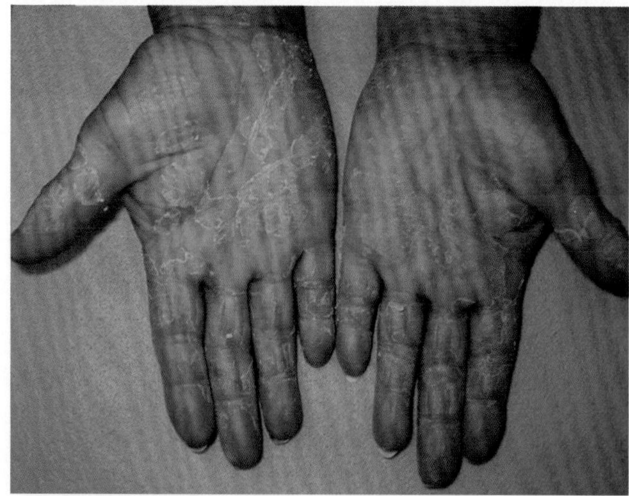

FIGURE 28-15. Chronic irritant contact dermatitis. ICD seen on the hands of this health care worker, with scaling, thickened skin. (Image provided by Stedman's.)

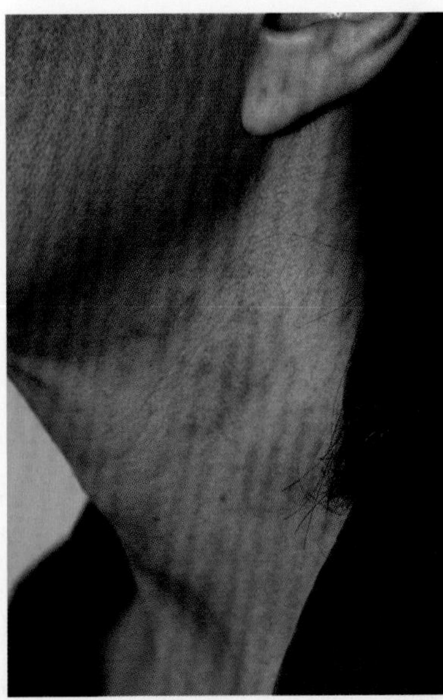

FIGURE 28-16. Allergic contact dermatitis. Acute ACD from poison ivy exposure. The patient's dog had rubbed her neck and face.

such as psoriasis or other inflammatory dermatoses. A KOH preparation and culture swabs of scaling can rule out a fungal or bacterial infection.

Management

The primary goal of therapy for both ICD and ACD is to identify and eliminate contact with the inciting stimulus, followed by treatment of the inflamed skin to allow for healing and reestablishment of the skin barrier. Topical corticosteroid ointments and emollients such as petroleum jelly are used empirically as first-line therapy and act to reduce inflammation and to protect the affected skin (Bourke et al., 2009). For mild ICD, high-potency corticosteroids such as clobetasol 0.05%, fluocinonide 0.05%, or betamethasone dipropionate 0.05% ointments are preferred, once to twice daily for several weeks. For facial and intertriginous ICD and ACD involvement, low-medium potency corticosteroids are advised, such as hydrocortisone 2.5% ointment once to twice daily for several weeks. For severe acute ICD and ACD or chronic ICD with skin thickening, a very high-potency topical corticosteroid can be used such as clobetasol 0.05% ointment. For chronic ACD, medium-potency topical corticosteroids such as triamcinolone 0.1% ointment or cream can be used.

CLINICAL PEARL

The primary goal of therapy for both ICD and ACD is to identify and eliminate contact with the inciting stimulus, followed by treatment of the inflamed skin to allow for healing and reestablishment of the skin barrier.

Topical calcineurin inhibitors like tacrolimus 0.01% and pimecrolimus 1% twice daily can be used as an alternative to topical corticosteroids for chronic ACD, localized ACD unresponsive to corticosteroids, and ACD of the face or intertriginous regions. For ACD involving >20% of BSA or for acute ACD affecting the face, hands, feet, and genitalia, oral corticosteroids (e.g., prednisone taper starting at 0.5 to 1 mg/kg/d, maximum 60 mg daily) are first line for a rapid response (Beltrani et al., 2006). Phototherapy can also be used in chronic ACD unresponsive to topical and oral corticosteroids.

Emollients, moisturizers, and colloidal oatmeal packs are beneficial in the treatment of both ICD and ACD as they soften the skin, reduce water loss, decrease irritation, and improve skin barrier function; they should be applied multiple times per day. For a weeping dermatitis, dermatologists often recommend a drying agent such as aluminum acetate soaks. Caregivers and patients should be aware that skin barrier recovery may take up to 4 weeks after irritant exposure, while skin hyperreactivity can last for more than 10 weeks (Lee et al., 1997).

Conclusion

Common dermatologic conditions are likely to be encountered by the wound care professional. Blistering conditions such as autoimmune blistering disorders and severe drug reactions can be life-threatening and require both supportive and systemic therapy. Because these disorders can result in erosions, appropriate wound care is an integral part of their treatment. Other papulosquamous disorders such as psoriasis and contact dermatitis are not associated with the development of ulcerations or wounds; however, these are conditions commonly encountered in clinical practice, and the wound nurse should be able to recognize them and to make appropriate referrals.

REFERENCES

Abe, R., Yoshioka, N., Murata, J., et al. (2009). Granulysin as a marker for early diagnosis of the Stevens-Johnson syndrome. *Annals of Internal Medicine, 151*(7), 514–515.

Amagai, M., Tsunoda, K., Zillikens, D., et al. (1999). The clinical phenotype of pemphigus is defined by the anti-desmoglein autoantibody profile. *Journal of the American Academy of Dermatology, 40*(2), 167–170.

Bastuji-Garin, S., Rzany, B., Stern, R. S., et al. (1993). Clinical classification of cases of toxic epidermal necrolysis, Stevens-Johnson syndrome, and erythema multiforme. *Archives of Dermatology, 129*(1), 92–96.

Beltrani, V. S., Bernstein, I. L., Cohen, D. E., et al. (2006). Contact dermatitis: A practice parameter. *Annals of Allergy, Asthma, and Immunology, 97*(3 Suppl 2), S1–38.

Bircher, A. J. (2005). Symptoms and danger signs in acute drug hypersensitivity. *Toxicology, 209*(2), 201–207, doi: 10.1016/j.tox.2004.12.036.

Bourke, J., Coulson, I., & English, J. (2009). Guidelines for the management of contact dermatitis: An update. *The British Journal of Dermatology, 160*(5),946–954,doi:10.1111/j.1365-2133.2009.09106.x.

Bystryn, J. C., & Rudolph, J. L. (2005). Pemphigus. *Lancet, 366*(9479), 61–73, doi: 10.1016/s0140-6736(05)66829-8.

Caldarola, G., Kneisel, A., Hertl, M., et al. (2008). Herpes simplex virus infection in pemphigus vulgaris: Clinical and immunological considerations. *European Journal of Dermatology, 18*(4), 440–443, doi: 10.1684/ejd.2008.0439.

Callen, J. P., Krueger, G. G., Lebwohl, M., et al. (2003). AAD consensus statement on psoriasis therapies*. *Journal of the American Academy of Dermatology, 49*(5), 897–899, doi: 10.1016/S0190-9622(03)01870-X.

Chan, H. L., Stern, R. S., Arndt, K. A., et al. (1990). The incidence of erythema multiforme, Stevens-Johnson syndrome, and toxic epidermal necrolysis. A population-based study with particular reference to reactions caused by drugs among outpatients. *Archives of Dermatology, 126*(1), 43–47.

Chung, W. H., Hung, S. I., Yang, J. Y., et al. (2008). Granulysin is a key mediator for disseminated keratinocyte death in Stevens-Johnson syndrome and toxic epidermal necrolysis. *Nature Medicine, 14*(12), 1343–1350, doi: 10.1038/nm.1884.

Clark, S. C., & Zirwas, M. J. (2009). Management of occupational dermatitis. *Dermatologic Clinics, 27*(3), 365–383, vii-viii, doi: 10.1016/j.det.2009.05.002.

Davis, M. D., Scalf, L. A., Yiannias, J. A., et al. (2008). Changing trends and allergens in the patch test standard series: A mayo clinic 5-year retrospective review, January 1, 2001, through December 31, 2005. *Archives of Dermatology, 144*(1), 67–72, doi: 10.1001/archdermatol.2007.2.

Dickel, H., Kuss, O., Schmidt, A., et al. (2002). Importance of irritant contact dermatitis in occupational skin disease. *American Journal of Clinical Dermatology, 3*(4), 283–289.

Fong, J., & Wood, F. (2006). Nanocrystalline silver dressings in wound management: A review. *International Journal of Nanomedicine, 1*(4), 441.

Garcia-Doval, I., LeCleach, L., Bocquet, H., et al. (2000). Toxic epidermal necrolysis and Stevens-Johnson syndrome: Does early withdrawal of causative drugs decrease the risk of death? *Archives of Dermatology, 136*(3), 323–327.

Gladman, D. D., Anhorn, K. A., Schachter, R. K., et al. (1986). HLA antigens in psoriatic arthritis. *The Journal of Rheumatology, 13*(3), 586–592.

Halevy, S., Ghislain, P.-D., Mockenhaupt, M., et al. (2008). Allopurinol is the most common cause of Stevens-Johnson syndrome and toxic epidermal necrolysis in Europe and Israel. *Journal of the American Academy of Dermatology, 58*(1), 25–32.

Higgins, E. (2000). Alcohol, smoking and psoriasis. *Clinical and Experimental Dermatology, 25*(2), 107–110.

Hooten, J. N., Hall III, R. P., & Cardones, A. R. (2014). Updates on the Management of Autoimmune Blistering Diseases. *Skin Therapy Letter, 19*(5), 1–6.

Joly, P., & Litrowski, N. (2011). Pemphigus group (vulgaris, vegetans, foliaceus, herpetiformis, brasiliensis). *Clinics in Dermatology, 29*(4), 432–436.

Joly, P., Roujeau, J. C., Benichou, J., et al. (2002). A comparison of oral and topical corticosteroids in patients with bullous pemphigoid. *The New England Journal of Medicine, 346*(5), 321–327, doi: 10.1056/NEJMoa011592.

Joly, P., Baricault, S., Sparsa, A., et al. (2012). Incidence and mortality of bullous pemphigoid in France. *The Journal of Investigative Dermatology, 132*(8), 1998–2004, doi: 10.1038/jid.2012.35.

Jordan, R. E., Triftshauser, C. T., & Schroeter, A. L. (1971). Direct immunofluorescent studies of pemphigus and bullous pemphigoid. *Archives of Dermatology, 103*(5), 486–491.

Jordan, M. H., Lewis, M. S., Jeng, J. G., et al. (1991). Treatment of toxic epidermal necrolysis by burn units: Another market or another threat? *The Journal of Burn Care & Rehabilitation, 12*(6), 579–581.

Kasperkiewicz, M., Shimanovich, I., Ludwig, R. J., et al. (2011). Rituximab for treatment-refractory pemphigus and pemphigoid: A case series of 17 patients. *Journal of the American Academy of Dermatology, 65*(3), 552–558.

Kasperkiewicz, M., Zillikens, D., & Schmidt, E. (2012). Pemphigoid diseases: Pathogenesis, diagnosis, and treatment. *Autoimmunity, 45*(1), 55–70, doi: 10.3109/08916934.2011.606447.

Kirchhof, M. G., Miliszewski, M. A., Sikora, S., et al. (2014). Retrospective review of Stevens-Johnson syndrome/toxic epidermal necrolysis treatment comparing intravenous immunoglobulin with cyclosporine. *Journal of the American Academy of Dermatology*, doi: 10.1016/j.jaad.2014.07.016.

Kneisel, A., & Hertl, M. (2011). Autoimmune bullous skin diseases. Part 1: Clinical manifestations. *JDDG: Journal der Deutschen Dermatologischen Gesellschaft, 9*(10), 844–857.

Kulthanan, K., Chularojanamontri, L., Tuchinda, P., et al. (2011). Prevalence and clinical features of Thai patients with bullous pemphigoid. *Asian Pacific Journal of Allergy and Immunology, 29*(1), 66–72.

Lee, J. Y., Effendy, I., & Maibach, H. I. (1997). Acute irritant contact dermatitis: Recovery time in man. *Contact Dermatitis, 36*(6), 285–290.

Lever, W. F., Elder, D. E., Elenitsas, R., et al. (2009). *Lever's histopathology of the skin*. Philadelphia, PA: Lippincott Williams & Wilkins.

Li, W., Han, J., Choi, H. K., et al. (2012). Smoking and risk of incident psoriasis among women and men in the United States: A combined analysis. *American Journal of Epidemiology, 175*(5), 402–413, doi: 10.1093/aje/kwr325.

Lyell, A. (1956). Toxic epidermal necrolysis: An eruption resembling scalding of the skin. *The British Journal of Dermatology, 68*(11), 355–361.

Marazza, G., Pham, H. C., Scharer, L., et al. (2009). Incidence of bullous pemphigoid and pemphigus in Switzerland: A 2-year prospective study. *The British Journal of Dermatology, 161*(4), 861–868, doi: 10.1111/j.1365-2133.2009.09300.x.

Martin, L. K., Werth, V. P., Villaneuva, E. V., et al. (2011). A systematic review of randomized controlled trials for pemphigus vulgaris and pemphigus foliaceus. *Journal of the American Academy of Dermatology, 64*(5), 903–908.

Mittmann, N., Knowles, S. R., Koo, M., et al. (2012). Incidence of toxic epidermal necrolysis and Stevens-Johnson Syndrome in an HIV cohort: An observational, retrospective case series study. *American Journal of Clinical Dermatology, 13*(1), 49–54, doi: 10.2165/11593240-000000000-00000.

Morales, M. E., Purdue, G. F., Verity, S. M., et al. (2010). Ophthalmic Manifestations of Stevens-Johnson Syndrome and Toxic Epidermal Necrolysis and Relation to SCORTEN. *American Journal of Ophthalmology, 150*(4), 505–510e501, doi: 10.1016/j.ajo.2010.04.026.

Murata, J., Abe, R., & Shimizu, H. (2008). Increased soluble Fas ligand levels in patients with Stevens-Johnson syndrome and toxic epidermal necrolysis preceding skin detachment. *The Journal of Allergy and Clinical Immunology, 122*(5), 992–1000, doi: 10.1016/j.jaci.2008.06.013.

Nassif, A., Bensussan, A., Boumsell, L., et al. (2004). Toxic epidermal necrolysis: Effector cells are drug-specific cytotoxic T cells. *The Journal of Allergy and Clinical Immunology, 114*(5), 1209–1215, doi: 10.1016/j.jaci.2004.07.047.

Nickoloff, B. J., & Nestle, F. O. (2004). Recent insights into the immunopathogenesis of psoriasis provide new therapeutic opportunities. *The Journal of Clinical Investigation, 113*(12), 1664–1675, doi: 10.1172/jci22147.

Parisi, R., Symmons, D. P., Griffiths, C. E., et al. (2013). Global epidemiology of psoriasis: A systematic review of incidence and prevalence. *The Journal of Investigative Dermatology, 133*(2), 377–385, doi: 10.1038/jid.2012.339.

Reich, K., Kruger, K., Mossner, R., et al. (2009). Epidemiology and clinical pattern of psoriatic arthritis in Germany: A prospective interdisciplinary epidemiological study of 1511 patients with plaque-type psoriasis. *The British Journal of Dermatology, 160*(5), 1040–1047, doi: 10.1111/j.1365-2133.2008.09023.x.

Schwindt, D. A., Wilhelm, K. P., Miller, D. L., et al. (1998). Cumulative irritation in older and younger skin: A comparison. *Acta Dermato-Venereologica, 78*(4), 279–283.

Sekula, P., Dunant, A., Mockenhaupt, M., et al. (2013). Comprehensive survival analysis of a cohort of patients with Stevens-Johnson syndrome and toxic epidermal necrolysis. *The Journal of Investigative Dermatology, 133*(5), 1197–1204, doi: 10.1038/jid.2012.510.

Setty, A. R., Curhan, G., & Choi, H. K. (2007). Obesity, waist circumference, weight change, and the risk of psoriasis in women: Nurses' Health Study II. *Archives of Internal Medicine, 167*(15), 1670–1675, doi: 10.1001/archinte.167.15.1670.

Stella, M., Clemente, A., Bollero, D., et al. (2007). Toxic epidermal necrolysis (TEN) and Stevens–Johnson syndrome (SJS): Experience with high-dose intravenous immunoglobulins and topical conservative approach: A retrospective analysis. *Burns, 33*(4), 452–459.

Thyssen, J. P., Johansen, J. D., Linneberg, A., et al. (2010). The epidemiology of hand eczema in the general population—prevalence and main findings. *Contact Dermatitis, 62*(2), 75–87, doi: 10.1111/j.1600-0536.2009.01669.x.

Tollefson, M. M., Crowson, C. S., McEvoy, M. T., et al. (2010). Incidence of psoriasis in children: A population-based study. *Journal of the American Academy of Dermatology, 62*(6), 979–987, doi: 10.1016/j.jaad.2009.07.029.

Tran, J. T., & Mutasim, D. F. (2005). Localized bullous pemphigoid: A commonly delayed diagnosis. *International Journal of Dermatology, 44*(11), 942–945, doi: 10.1111/j.1365-4632.2004.02288.x.

Venning, V., & Wojnarowska, F. (1992). Lack of predictive factors for the clinical course of bullous pemphigoid. *Journal of the American Academy of Dermatology, 26*(4), 585–589.

Venugopal, S. S., & Murrell, D. F. (2011). Diagnosis and clinical features of pemphigus vulgaris. *Dermatologic Clinics, 29*(3), 373–380.

Worswick, S., & Cotliar, J. (2011). Stevens-Johnson syndrome and toxic epidermal necrolysis: A review of treatment options. *Dermatologic Therapy, 24*(2), 207–218, doi: 10.1111/j.1529-8019.2011.01396.x.

Yancey, K. B., & Egan, C. A. (2000). Pemphigoid: Clinical, histologic, immunopathologic, and therapeutic considerations. *The Journal of the American Medical Association, 284*(3), 350–356.

QUESTIONS

1. The wound care nurse differentiates pemphigus vulgaris from bullous pemphigoid when planning care for patients. Which statement accurately describes a characteristic of these diseases?

A. Bullous pemphigoid causes destruction of cell-to-cell connections within the epidermis causing flaccid intraepithelial blisters.
B. Pemphigus vulgaris causes separation between the epidermal and dermal layers of the skin.
C. Patients with bullous pemphigoid present with flaccid bullae, skin erosions, and possibly mucous membrane erosions.
D. Bullous pemphigoid may begin with a prodromal phase of weeks to months characterized by a pruritic, eczema-like skin rash or urticarial plaques.

2. The wound care nurse is preparing a treatment plan for a patient with severe pemphigus vulgaris. Which of the following is a recommended treatment measure?

A. Therapy with topical corticosteroids
B. Systemic corticosteroid therapy
C. Topical corticosteroids plus antibiotic therapy
D. Systemic corticosteroids plus adjuvant therapy with steroid-sparing agents

3. The wound care nurse is planning evidence-based wound care for a patient with bullous pemphigoid. Which intervention is recommended?

A. Puncture and drain large blisters in a sterile environment.
B. Remove the epithelial roof of blisters that have been punctured.
C. Select dressings with the goal of managing bleeding.
D. Select adhesive dressing to manage exudate.

4. What is the most frequent etiology for Steven-Johnson syndrome (SJS) and toxic epidermal necrolysis (TEN)?

A. Burns
B. Electric shock
C. Drug reactions
D. Influenza

5. The wound care nurse is assessing a patient who presents with fever (38.5°C), visual disturbances, itching of the eyes, and pain upon swallowing. The patient is currently taking allopurinol for chronic gout. What skin condition would the nurse suspect?

A. Bullous pemphigoid
B. Pemphigus vulgaris
C. Steven-Johnson syndrome
D. Psoriasis

6. What should be the focus of care management for a patient with severe SJS/TEN?

A. Continuing current medication regimen
B. Care resembling major burn care
C. Therapy with topical corticosteroids
D. Use of surgical debridement

7. Psoriasis is considered to be an immune system–mediated disease. Which of the following is a characteristic of psoriasis?

A. Large number of epidermal stem cells
B. Fewer cells undergoing mitosis
C. Longer epidermal turnover time
D. Asymmetrical ulcer development on scalp, back, elbows, and knees

8. The wound care nurse is assessing the skin of a patient presenting with numerous small (<1 cm), drop-like, red, and scaly papules that are located primarily on the trunk. The patient states she had recently been diagnosed with a streptococcal throat infection. What form of psoriasis would the nurse suspect?
   A. Plaque psoriasis
   B. Inverse psoriasis
   C. Guttate psoriasis
   D. Pustular psoriasis

9. A patient with which of the following types of psoriasis would require supportive treatment to prevent excessive loss of fluid and possibly systemic therapy?
   A. Plaque psoriasis
   B. Psoriasis with erythroderma involving > 30% total body surface area (TBSA)
   C. Guttate psoriasis
   D. Psoriasis with widespread palmoplantar involvement

10. Which of the following is a mainstay of therapy for limited psoriatic disease?
   A. Topical corticosteroids
   B. Phototherapy
   C. Biologic agents
   D. Immunosuppressant therapy

11. A patient presents with skin redness, dryness, an eczema-like skin reaction, and a resultant chemical burn. The patient states that the rash occurred after he used a new cleanser to clean his bathroom. What type of skin infection would the nurse suspect?
   A. Psoriasis
   B. Allergic dermatitis
   C. Pemphigus vulgaris
   D. Contact dermatitis

ANSWERS: 1.**D**, 2.**D**, 3.**A**, 4.**C**, 5.**C**, 6.**B**, 7.**A**, 8.**C**, 9.**B**, 10.**A**, 11.**D**

CHAPTER 29

Oncology-Related Skin and Wound Care

Carole Bauer

OBJECTIVES

1. Describe the pathology and presentation of radiodermatitis and current guidelines for prevention and management.
2. Describe common skin reactions associated with targeted chemotherapies and implications for prevention and management.
3. Outline strategies and resources for management of extravasation injuries.
4. Identify common challenges and patient concerns related to malignant fungating wounds and options for management.
5. Describe presentation and management for each of the following: palmar–plantar erythrodysesthesia, cutaneous T-cell lymphoma, and graft versus host disease.

Topic Outline

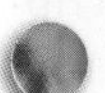 **Introduction**

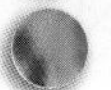 **Radiation Dermatitis**
- Prevalence/Incidence
- Pathology
- Radiation Recall
- Risk Factors
  - Treatment Factors
  - Patient Factors
- Clinical Presentation
- Diagnosis
- Prevention
- Treatment
  - Dry Desquamation
  - Wet Desquamation
  - Late Radiation Toxicity

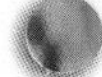 **Extravasation**
- Risk Factors
- Pathology
- Clinical Presentation
- Diagnostics
- Management

Targeted Chemotherapy Skin Reactions
- Prevalence/Incidence
- Risk Factors
- Pathology
- Clinical Presentation
  - Rash
  - Hand-Foot Skin Reaction
  - Xerosis
  - Pruritis
  - Paronychia
- Management
  - Rash
  - Hand-Foot Skin Reaction
  - Xerosis
  - Pruritis
  - Paronychia

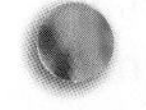 **Palmar–Plantar Erythrodysesthesia (Hand-Foot Syndrome)**
- Prevalence/Incidence
- Risk Factors
- Pathology
- Clinical Presentation
- Prevention and Management

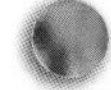 **Cutaneous T-Cell Lymphoma (Mycosis Fungoides and Sézary Syndrome)**
- Prevalence/Incidence
- Risk Factors

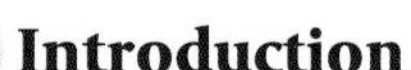

Introduction

In 2014, the American Cancer Society reports that there will be an estimated 1,665,540 new cases of cancer diagnosed. In addition, there will be 585,540 cancer deaths in the United States. This makes cancer the second most common cause of death in the United States, accounting for nearly one of every four deaths (American Cancer Society, 2014). These statistics emphasize the importance of understanding skin and wound conditions unique to the cancer patient. Wounds in oncology patients can provide distinctive challenges to the wound care nurse. Not only must the wound care nurse consider all of the "traditional" wounds and their causes, but skin disorders related to the cancer itself or to the treatment being provided must also be considered. This chapter will address skin lesions that are manifestations of the malignant process as well as disorders resulting from the effects of treatments to eliminate or control the disease.

Radiation Dermatitis

Radiation therapy is the use of high-energy waves, rays, or particles to shrink or kill cancer cells. There are several types of radiation beams currently used in the treatment of cancer, including gamma rays, x-rays, and proton beams. Radiation therapy can be delivered externally in the form of a beam delivered to the targeted areas through the skin, or internally, via implantation of a radioactive source. Internal radiation therapy, also known as brachytherapy, can be provided in many forms, such as placing the radioactive source into temporary catheters, tubes, or balloons or implanting the radioactive energy into the body in the form of seeds or pellets. Radiation works by altering the DNA structure of the cancer cell, which either kills the cell or prevents the cell from replicating. Radiation also affects normal cells within the radiation field that are reproducing, such as skin cells. Thus, for the patient undergoing external beam radiation, skin changes can be expected (National Cancer Institute, n.d. b).

Prevalence/Incidence

Radiation therapy is a commonly used modality in the treatment of cancer. It is estimated that at least 50% of patients diagnosed with cancer will receive radiation therapy during the course of their treatment. No true incidence has been recorded for radiation dermatitis; however, Feight et al. (2011) report that up to 95% of patients who receive radiation will experience some type of skin reaction.

CLINICAL PEARL

Up to 95% of patients who receive radiation will experience some type of skin reaction.

Pathology

As noted, radiation therapy delivers high-energy particles to the treatment field; these particles damage the cells' DNA, which disrupts replication and causes cell death. This explains the therapeutic benefit in treatment of cancer; the radiation damages rapidly proliferating tumor cells. Unfortunately, other rapidly proliferating cells in the treatment field, including the skin, are also affected. A number of terms have been used to describe radiation dermatitis, including radiation dermatitis, radiodermatitis, radiation skin reaction, and even radiation "burns." Today, the term radiation "burn" is no longer used as a description for the skin changes caused by radiation therapy and rather is reserved for those persons who are involved in radiation accidents.

In 1990, Hopewell was the first to describe the radiation-induced changes in the skin. These changes occur over time and are described as: "1.) A transient early erythema, seen within a few hours of irradiation, which subsides after 24 – 48 hours; 2.) the main erythematous reaction, reflecting indirectly a varying severity of loss of epidermal basal cells; either a dry or moist desquamatory response may be seen after 3 – 6 weeks; 3.) a late phase of erythema associated with dermal ischemia and possibly necrosis, seen after 8 – 16 weeks; and 4.) the appearance of late skin damage, i.e., dermal atrophy (>26 weeks), telangiectasia and necrosis (>52 weeks)" (Hopewell, 1990, p. 756).

On a cellular level, radiation affects the structures of both the dermis and the epidermis. Radiation dermatitis is caused by depletion of stem cells in the basal layer of the epidermis. The basal layer of the skin is comprised of a single layer of replicating cells, and a reduction in basal cell density is evident by the time the patient has received 20 to 25 grays of radiation. Repetitive doses of radiation cause a progressive loss of basal cells that reaches a nadir at approximately 21 days. There is complete regeneration of the epidermis at all dose fractions up to 45 Gy (Archambeau et al., 1995).

CLINICAL PEARL

Repetitive doses of radiation cause a progressive loss of basal epidermal cells that reaches a nadir at approximately 21 days; there is complete regeneration of the epidermis at all dose fractions up to 45 Gy.

The total dose of radiation prescribed is divided into fractions or smaller portions of the total dose given over a set period of time. Each subsequent exposure results in inflammatory cell recruitment to the radiation field. This results in inhibition of normal granulation tissue, fibrogenesis, and angiogenesis. The damage that occurs is a result of multiple factors including damage to stem cells, endothelial cell changes, inflammation, apoptosis, and necrosis (Hymes et al., 2006).

In addition to the acute damage described above, radiation therapy can produce late effects in the skin and soft tissue that may become evident months or years following therapy. Late toxicity is defined as those changes that occur beyond 90 days after the completion of radiation therapy and include subcutaneous induration, hyperpigmentation, hypopigmentation, telangiectasia, photosensitivity, xerosis, atrophy, fibrosis, ulceration, and impaired healing (McQuestion, 2010; Wong et al., 2013). The skin and soft tissue changes seen with late radiation toxicity are the result of progressive changes to the vasculature and the soft tissue, primarily progressive damage to the dermal vessels, loss of normal fibroblasts and collagen, and progressive fibrosis of the soft tissues. These changes make the tissue more vulnerable to breakdown and less likely to heal. Radiation necrosis can be related to several factors including high-dose treatment, acute dermatitis that has never resolved, and dermal ischemia. Management of wounds in previously radiated tissue is difficult due to the persistent dermal ischemia; research is ongoing in this area (Hymes et al., 2006).

CLINICAL PEARL

The skin and soft tissue changes seen with late radiation toxicity are the result of progressive changes to the blood vessels and the soft tissues (e.g., loss of normal fibroblasts and collagen and progressive fibrosis of the soft tissue). These changes make the tissue more vulnerable to breakdown and less likely to heal.

Radiation Recall

Radiation recall is defined as a skin reaction that occurs after the administration of certain chemotherapeutic drugs in an area where radiation has previously been administered. Little is known about the incidence, pathogenesis, or treatment of this condition. This leaves health care providers and the patient with only two options: discontinue the chemotherapeutic agent, which may adversely affect overall prognosis, or continue the agent despite the risk of further skin reaction. Symptoms of radiation recall dermatitis are the same as those for radiation dermatitis and include erythema, desquamation, edema, vesiculation, necrosis, ulceration, and hemorrhage (Bauer & Bauer, 2009).

CLINICAL PEARL

Radiation recall is a skin reaction that occurs after administration of certain chemotherapeutic drugs in a previously irradiated area.

Risk Factors

Although little is known about the specific risk factors related to radiation dermatitis, it is hypothesized that both treatment-related factors and patient-related factors can affect the development of radiation dermatitis. Treatment-related factors have undergone the most scrutiny.

Treatment Factors

The risk of skin damage is related to the total dose as well as the fraction dose, the type of radiation energy used (photon and electrons deliver a higher dose to the skin), and the volume and surface area of skin exposed. If the fraction is >2 Gy per treatment, the time to onset of skin damage is reduced and there is an increased risk for the development of a more severe skin reaction. Today, radiation therapy is most often delivered via linear accelerators or megavoltage units, which are skin sparing. These units deliver the radiation to target the tissues 1.5 to 3 cm below the skin surface. Electron beams, which have a shorter wave length, are often used to deliver what is sometimes called a boost for treatment of lymph nodes that lie close to the skin surface; thus, electron beam therapy is associated with more severe skin reactions. Cobalt 60, an older type of treatment unit, is used to target tissues only 0.5 cm below the skin surface and is associated with increased risk of skin damage. In addition to the type of energy, fraction dose, and total dose delivered, the duration of therapy also affects the onset and severity of radiation dermatitis. Those patients who undergo a longer treatment course are at greater risk for severe dermatitis as compared to those who have a shorter treatment course (McQuestion, 2011). Several other treatment-related factors can affect the development and severity of radiation dermatitis. If the patient's treatment field includes the head and neck region, breast, axilla, perineum, or areas with skin folds, they are at risk for earlier onset and greater severity of skin reactions.

The size of the treatment field also affects risk; larger treatment areas are associated with earlier onset and greater severity of skin reactions.

CLINICAL PEARL

The risk of skin damage is related to the total radiation dose, fraction dose, type of radiation used, the volume and surface area of exposed skin, skin integrity at baseline, skin care provided during therapy, and whether or not the involved area involves body folds resulting in skin-to-skin contact.

If a tangential field is used or a bolus is given, the patient is at greater risk for significant radiation dermatitis (McQuestion, 2010). With a bolus (boost) dose, overlapping fields may receive increased radiation at the skin level. Tissue expanders such as those used with breast cancer patients also present a unique problem related to the development of radiation dermatitis because of the thin skin over the area of the tissue expander. Finally, patients undergoing concurrent chemotherapy, immunotherapy, or targeted therapy are at increased risk for radiation dermatitis.

Patient Factors

Several patient-specific factors also affect the risk for radiation dermatitis. These factors are similar to those known to result in impaired wound healing and include smoking, poor nutritional status, older age, obesity, race, comorbid conditions (e.g., diabetes, renal failure), and problems with skin integrity prior to initiation of radiation therapy. Previous sun exposure and normal skin care routines (e.g., use of harsh soaps, perfumed soap, or lotions or scrubbing the skin) can also affect the risk for radiation dermatitis. Additionally, if the patient is receiving treatment to an area where there is skin to skin contact such as in the axilla, under the breast, or in the perineal area, there is an increased risk for the development of radiation dermatitis.

Genetic factors can also affect risk for development of radiation dermatitis. Diseases that reduce the ability to repair DNA such as ataxia telangiectasia, Fanconi's anemia, and Blooms' syndrome are associated with increased risk for the development of radiation skin reactions. Familial polyposis, Gardner's syndrome, hereditary malignant melanoma, and dysplastic nevus syndrome may also be associated with a greater risk for skin reactions. It is also thought that individual differences in DNA may explain the increased severity of reactions in some patients, even when there is no known genetic disorder. At this time, there are no diagnostic tests to screen for these differences although researchers continue to search for ways to predict increased radiosensitivity (Hymes et al., 2006).

Patients who have a connective tissue disorder or autoimmune disease (e.g., scleroderma, systemic lupus erythematosus and perhaps rheumatoid arthritis) may also be at increased risk for the development of radiation dermatitis. It is thought that these conditions are associated with lymphocytes that are more radiosensitive than those in the general population. Thus, there is a relative contraindication to administration of radiation therapy for these individuals; treatment decisions must be individualized and must involve a comprehensive risk–benefit assessment (Hymes et al., 2006). Patients who are infected with the HIV virus also demonstrate increased risk; skin reactions tend to develop at an earlier point and tend to be more severe in this patient population (Hymes et al., 2006).

Clinical Presentation

As noted, transient erythema frequently develops following the first treatment and typically disappears within a few hours but returns following subsequent treatments. Persistent erythema, warmth, and a rashy appearance to the skin may develop during the first 2 weeks of therapy, assuming 1.8 to 2 Gy per treatment (single-dose fraction). Hyperpigmentation may develop at weeks 2 to 4 due to overactivity of the melanocytes. When the total dose reaches 20 Gy or more, dryness, pruritus, flaking, and dry desquamation may occur. Moist desquamation may develop once the total dose reaches 45 to 60 Gy (Fig. 29-1). Moist desquamation results in partial-thickness skin loss with exposure of the dermis; the

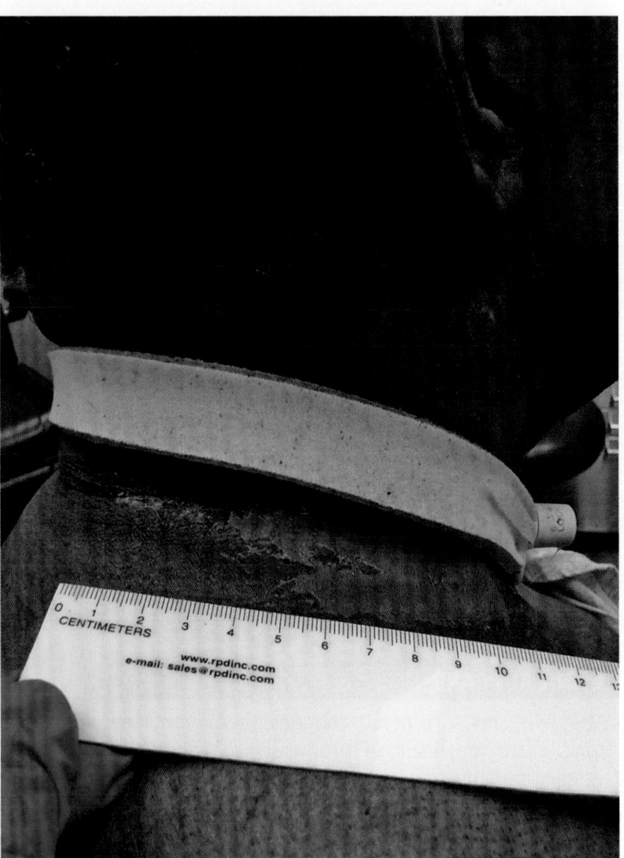

FIGURE 29-1. Radiodermatitis with moist desquamation.

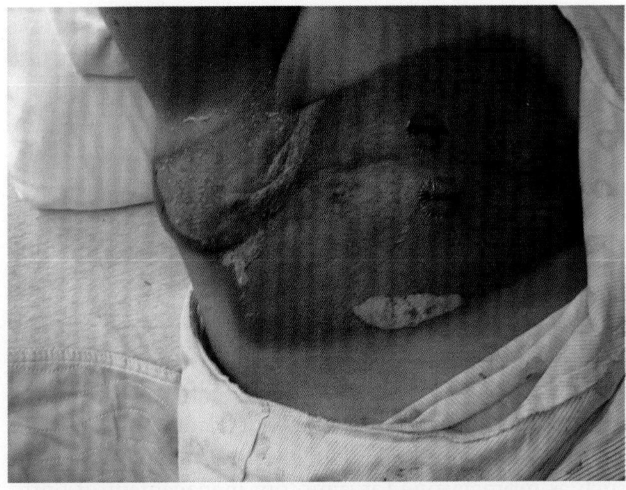

FIGURE 29-2. Moist desquamation with crusting.

involved areas are moist, red, and painful. The volume of exudate is variable; if the lesions are exposed to air and the exudate is allowed to dry on the surface of the wound, there is crusting (Fig. 29-2) (McQuestion, 2011).

Patients may complain of sensations of skin tightness, dryness, pruritus, pain, general distress, and negative impact on activities of daily living (ADL) and quality of life. If symptoms are severe, patients may have difficulty with self-care activities. The patient may experience financial burden related to radiation dermatitis if they are unable to work or must purchase wound care supplies (Feight et al., 2011). Finally, severe skin reactions may cause the patient to discontinue therapy.

There are several scales that are used for assessment and classification of radiation dermatitis; the most widely used is the Common Terminology Criteria for Adverse Events (Table 29-1) (CTCAE) (Chen et al., 2012; Feight et al., 2011). Although this is the scale most often used, no reliability or validity data have been published. There are several other scales for grading skin reactions: Radiation Therapy Oncology Group (RTOG) Acute Radiation Morbidity Scoring Criteria, Radiation Oncology Group/European Organization for Research and Treatment of Cancer Toxicity Criteria, Skin Toxicity Assessment Tool (STAT), and Radiation-Induced Skin Reaction Assessment Scale (RISRAS).

Both the RISRAS and the STAT tools have published validity and reliability scores, and the RISRAS is the one tool that includes patient symptoms as well as objective signs of skin damage; however, at present, neither of these are widely used (Berthelet et al., 2004; Feight et al., 2011; Noble-Adams, 1999).

Diagnosis

Diagnosis of radiation dermatitis is based on thorough history and physical exam and is typically straightforward. However, the examining clinician should consider the following in the differential diagnosis: skin infection, contact dermatitis, eczema, and cutaneous hypersensitivity syndromes. If the cause of the skin reaction is not clear based on physical exam and history, the patient should be referred to a dermatologist.

Prevention

While it would be preferable for prevention measures to be instituted prior to the development of radiation dermatitis, there is little evidence to support the use of any one product for the prevention of radiation dermatitis. Feight et al. (2011) state, "although avoidance of skin reactions caused by radiation therapy would be preferred, it often is not possible" (p. 481). More recently, Wong et al. (2013) convened an international multidisciplinary group of experts with the objective to develop an evidence-based guideline on prevention and treatment of both acute and late toxicities of radiation therapy. This guideline, supported by those of the Skin Toxicity Study Group of the Multinational Association for Supportive Care in Cancer (MASCC), further expounds upon the guideline developed by Feight and colleagues in 2011 for the Oncology Nursing Society. The recommendations by both groups include the following:

- Bathing/shampooing with mild soap/shampoo and water was associated with lower incidence and severity of radiation dermatitis (Bauer et al., in press; Feight et al., 2011; Roy et al., 2001; Wong et al., 2013).
- Use of antiperspirants was found to be safe for women undergoing radiation for breast cancer (Lewis et al., in press; Wong et al., 2013).

TABLE 29-1 Common Terminology Criteria for Adverse Events v4.0: Radiation Dermatitis

Adverse Event	1	2	3	4	5
Dermatitis, radiation	Faint erythema or dry desquamation	Moderate to brisk erythema; patchy moist desquamation, mostly confined to skin folds and creases; moderate edema	Moist desquamation in areas other than skin folds and creases; bleeding induced by minor trauma or abrasion	Life-threatening consequences; skin necrosis or ulceration of full-thickness dermis; spontaneous bleeding from involved site; skin graft indicated	Death

Used with permission from Chen, A. P., Setser, A., Anadkat, M. J., et al. (2012). Grading dermatologic adverse events of cancer treatments: The common terminology criteria for adverse events version 4.0. *Journal of the American Academy of Dermatology, 67*(5), 1025–1039.

- Topical corticosteroids such as mometasone were found to reduce discomfort, burning, and itching; the recommendation is to begin therapy prior to the first treatment (Wong et al., 2013).
- A weak recommendation was made for use of silver sulfadiazine cream to reduce severity of radiation dermatitis among women receiving radiation for breast cancer (Wong et al., 2013).

CLINICAL PEARL

There is very limited evidence-based guidance for prevention of radiodermatitis; current guidelines endorse routine bathing with gentle cleansers, routine use of antiperspirants, and preventive use of topical corticosteroids to reduce discomfort, burning, and itching.

Feight et al. (2011) also recommend the following skin care regimen for patients receiving radiation therapy, based primarily on expert opinion:

1. Instruct patients undergoing radiation therapy to clean the skin twice daily with pH-balanced cleansers paying particular attention to areas with skin-to-skin contact. Pat the skin dry; do not rub.
2. Use only an electric razor in the treatment field.
3. Do not apply topical moisturizers, gels, or emulsions before treatment. Moisturizers are recommended twice daily but should be applied after treatment to the treatment field. These moisturizers should be plain, nonscented, lanolin-free, hydrophilic creams.
4. If itching or irritation develops, initiate low-dose corticosteroid creams (if not already in use).
5. Avoid the following:
   - Swimming in lakes and pools and use of hot tubs or saunas
   - Tapes and adhesives in the treatment field
   - Use of ice or heating pads
   - Exposure to sun; the skin should be protected against sunlight and against cold

Both Feight et al. (2011) and Wong et al. (2013) recommend against the use of many products including aloe vera, silver leaf dressings, and trolamine based on current evidence. They additionally state that the current evidence is too weak or contradictory to permit any recommendations regarding for or against the use of sucralfate and its derivatives, hyaluronic acid or hyaluronic acid–based combinations, silver dressings, ascorbic acid, LED (light-emitting diode lasers), petroleum-based ointments, Theta-Cream, dexpanthenol, oral proteolytic enzymes, oral zinc, or oral pentoxifylline.

Clearly, more studies are needed in the area of prevention of radiation dermatitis; Zhang et al. (2013) point out that radiation dermatitis is the result of epidermal cell death and that future research regarding prevention should focus on agents that stimulate keratinocyte activity and epidermal regeneration.

Treatment

Wong et al. (2013) conclude, in their published guideline for prevention and treatment of radiation skin reactions, that there is insufficient evidence to support use of any specific products for treatment of radiation dermatitis. The authors reported on studies involving dressings, sucralfate cream, hydrocortisone 1%, honey, and trolamine; in the studies to date, none of these products reduced the time for resolution of radiation dermatitis.

Dry Desquamation

For patients with dry desquamation, the wound care nurse should continue to recommend preventive care including washing with pH-balanced soap, application of bland skin moisturizers twice daily, and the use of topical steroids such as mometasone for symptom management of burning, itching, and discomfort as outlined above.

Moist Desquamation

At present, little evidence is available to support the use of one dressing over another to promote healing of moist desquamation. The principles of moist wound healing should be used to guide dressing selection based on wound location, volume of exudate, presence or absence of bleeding, and the radiation oncologist's requirements regarding dressing removal for additional treatments. Guidelines for the treatment and management of radiation skin reactions do not recommend for or against hydrocolloids, hydrogels, or honey-impregnated dressings (Feight et al., 2011; Wong et al., 2013).

CLINICAL PEARL

There is insufficient evidence to recommend any specific products for treatment of radiodermatitis; dry desquamation should be managed with preventive measures (moisturizers and topical corticosteroids), and moist desquamation should be managed according to the principles of moist wound healing.

Late Radiation Toxicity

Wong et al. (2013) provide the only published guideline for late radiation toxicities. The available evidence focuses only on telangiectasia and cutaneous fibrosis. The guideline provides a weak recommendation for the use of pulse dye laser to improve visual appearance of telangiectasias and states that, at present, there is insufficient evidence to support use of pentoxifylline (800 mg/day) and vitamin E (1,000 IU/day) for treatment of fibrosis (Wong et al., 2013). Haubner et al. (2012) reviewed available literature related to wound healing in irradiated skin and concluded that at present the "...clinical challenge to optimize wound healing in irradiated patients remains" (p. 7). Strategies with limited evidence include the use of advanced wound dressings, negative pressure wound therapy, and hyperbaric oxygen therapy; in the future, therapy is predicted to include use of special dressings, injection of (multipotent) cells, topical administration of active substances, and the use of growth factors.

 Extravasation

Extravasation has been defined as the accidental leakage of fluid from a vein into the surrounding tissue (Pérez Fidalgo et al., 2012). In terms of chemotherapy, extravasation has been labeled a "dreaded" complication and a "preventable catastrophe" (Schulmeister, 2010). Fortunately, chemotherapy extravasation is now an uncommon event, occurring in only 0.1% to 6% of all patients who receive peripheral IV chemotherapy. The incidence is thought to be even lower among patients who receive chemotherapy via a central venous access device (0.3% to 4.7%) (Dest, 2010).

Risk Factors

Risk factors for extravasation can be classified as patient specific and procedure related. Patient-specific risk factors include the following: small, fragile veins; limited vein selection; history of multiple venipunctures; prior therapy with irritating or sclerosing drugs; sensory, cognitive, or communication deficits interfering with ability to report signs and symptoms of extravasation; difficult venous access (e.g., obese patient, prominent but mobile veins); predisposition to bleeding; and impaired perfusion (e.g., Raynaud's, superior vena cava syndrome, atherosclerosis related to advanced diabetes). Procedure-related risk factors include probing during IV catheter insertion, failure to adequately secure the IV catheter, placement of IV in site with minimal underlying tissue (e.g., dorsum of hand), use of rigid IV needle as opposed to pliable catheter, prolonged infusion, bolus infusion, high-pressure flow, and poorly placed central venous access device (Pérez Fidalgo et al., 2012; Polovich et al., 2009).

Pathology

Chemotherapeutic agents are classified as vesicants, irritants, or nonirritants, and the severity of tissue damage is related primarily to the irritant or vesicant properties of the specific agent involved (**Table 29-2**). Vesicant drugs exert damage to tissues in two different ways. The first category of vesicants cause tissue damage by binding to nucleic acids in the DNA of the healthy cells in the involved tissue, causing initial cell death; the damaged and dying cells release complexes that cause further damage and necrosis of the surrounding cells, causing cell death over an extended period of time. Drugs that fall into this category of vesicant include the anthracyclines (i.e., daunorubicin, doxorubicin, epirubicin, idarubicin), dactinomycin, mechlorethamine, and mitomycin. The second category of vesicants includes drugs that do not bind to the cellular DNA. These drugs undergo metabolism and are excreted more quickly compared to the other class of vesicants; thus, the injury does not persist over an extended period of time. Drugs in this category are also more easily neutralized compared to drugs that bind to DNA. Drugs included in this category of vesicants include paclitaxel and the plant alkaloids (vinblastine, vincristine, vindesine, vinorelbine).

TABLE 29-2 Classification of Chemotherapy Drugs According to Their Ability to Cause Local Damage after Extravasation

Vesicants	Irritants	Nonvesicants
DNA-binding compounds	Alkylating agents	Arsenic trioxide
Alkylating agents	Carmustine	Asparaginase
Mechlorethamine	Ifosfamide	Bleomycin
Bendamustine[a]	Streptozocin	Bortezomib
Anthracyclines	Dacarbazine	Cladribine
Doxorubicin	Melphalan	Cytarabine
Daunorubicin	Anthracyclines (other)	Etoposide phosphate
Epirubicin	Liposomal doxorubicin	Gemcitabine
Idarubicin	Liposomal daunorubicin	Fludarabine
Others (antibiotics)	Mitoxantrone	Interferons
Dactinomycin	Topoisomerase II inhibitors	Interleukin-2
Mitomycin C	Etoposide	Methotrexate
Mitoxantrone[a]	Teniposide	Monoclonal antibodies
Non–DNA-binding compounds	Antimetabolites	Pemetrexed
Vinca alkaloids	Fluorouracil	Raltitrexed
Vincristine	Platin salts	Temsirolimus
Vinblastine	Carboplatin	Thiotepa
Vindesine	Cisplatin	Cyclophosphamide
Vinorelbine	Oxaliplatin	
Taxanes	Topoisomerase I inhibitors	
Docetaxel[a]	Irinotecan	
Paclitaxel	Topotecan	
Others	Others	
Trabectedin	Ixabepilone	

[a]Single case reports describe both irritant and vesicant properties.

Used with permission from Pérez Fidalgo, J. A., García Fabregat, L., Cerbantes, J., et al. (2012). Management of chemotherapy extravasation: ESMO-EOPNS clinical practice guidelines. *Annals of Oncology*, *23*(supplement 7), vii 167–vii 173.

Drugs classified as irritants may cause inflammation and irritation to the vein when they are infused peripherally

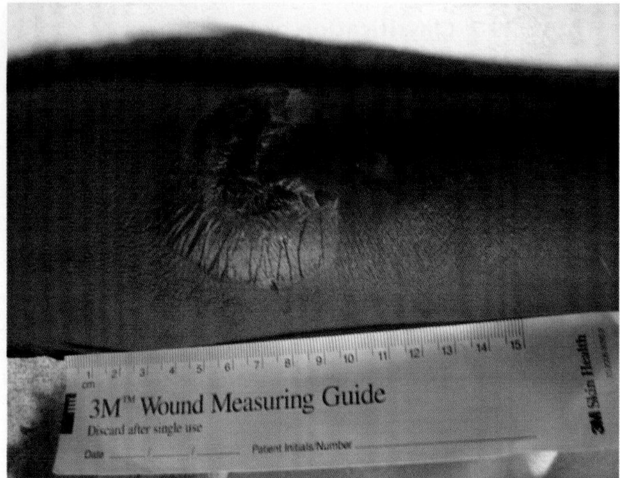

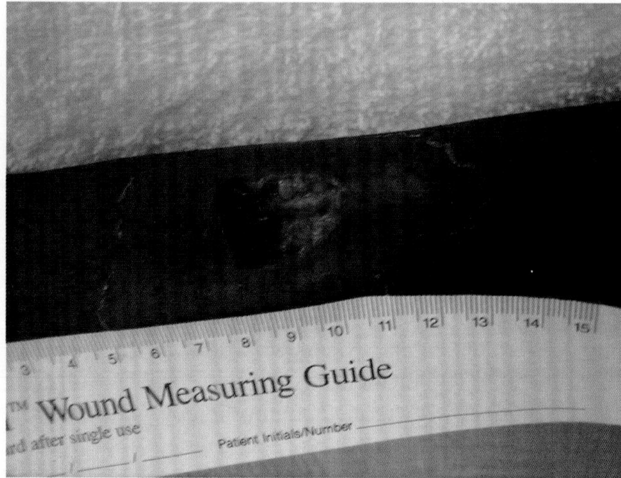

FIGURE 29-3. Extravasation injuries.

but do not cause significant cell death and tissue damage. At times, drugs that are classified as irritants may have vesicant properties. Drugs in this category include oxaliplatin, vinorelbine, and melphalan (Polovich et al., 2009).

Clinical Presentation

Initial symptoms of extravasation include complaints of burning, tingling, and pain at the infusion site; visual inspection at this point may reveal discernible swelling at the site. (Some extravasated drugs may not result in symptoms until hours or days later.) Later signs include blistering, necrosis, and ulceration (Fig. 29-3). The degree of tissue damage depends upon the specific drug administered, the concentration of the drug, and the amount of drug extravasated. In severe cases, the patient can experience nerve, tendon, and joint damage, loss of limb function, sensory impairment, disfigurement, and even loss of limb (Dest, 2010; Polovich et al., 2009; Schulmeister, 2010).

Diagnostics

Diagnosis initially is based on history of drug administration and patient complaint during the infusion.

Management

No randomized controlled studies have been conducted on management of extravasation injuries, due to ethical considerations; thus all recommendations are based on expert opinion and case reports. Whenever extravasation is suspected, the infusion should be stopped immediately and the prescribing health care professional should be notified. An attempt to aspirate any residual vesicant from the IV device using a 1- to 3-mL syringe should be attempted, and the IV should then be discontinued. At that point, either ice or heat should be applied, with the specific modality determined by the chemotherapeutic agent involved. Antidotes and treatments per institutional policy should then be administered (Polovich et al., 2009; Schulmeister, 2010). (See **Table 29-3** for management recommendations for specific agents.) To manage late side effects, particularly those related to DNA-binding agents, surgical debridement may be indicated. Signs that surgical debridement is indicated include pain or unresolved tissue necrosis persisting more than ten days after the extravasation (Polovich et al., 2009; Schulmeister, 2010).

The WOC nurse's role in management of extravasation injuries is to recommend topical therapy once initial treatment has been provided. Principles of moist wound healing should be followed, with specific recommendations based on the characteristics of the wound. No one dressing has been proven to be superior over another. It is common for plastic surgery to be involved and for skin grafting to be indicated in significant extravasation injuries; the wound care nurse should consult plastic surgery whenever the extravasation injury produces a full-thickness wound located over or adjacent to a tendon, bone, or joint.

TABLE 29-3 Extravasation Management

Drug Classification	Immediate Topical Therapy	Antidote
Alkylating agents	Ice	Sodium thiosulfate
Anthracyclines	Ice	Totect[a]
Antitumor antibiotics	Ice	No known antidote
Plant alkaloid or microtubular-inhibiting agents	Warm pack	Hyaluronidase
Taxanes	Ice	No known antidote

[a]Zinecard and generic dexrazoxane are neither indicated nor FDA approved for anthracycline treatment. There are no therapeutic equivalents to Totect. Currently, Totect is unavailable.

CLINICAL PEARL

The wound nurse's role in management of extravasation injuries is to recommend topical therapy based on moist wound-healing principles (once initial treatment protocols have been completed) and to initiate a plastic surgery consult if there is full-thickness damage over or adjacent to a tendon, bone, or joint.

Targeted Chemotherapy Skin Reactions

Targeted chemotherapy is the use of drugs or other chemicals that block cellular pathways and processes essential to cell growth and survival; drugs in this class include angiogenesis inhibitors, hormone therapies, signal transduction inhibitors, gene expression modulators, apoptosis inducers, immunotherapies, and toxin delivery molecules (National Cancer Institute, 2014). Specific medications currently available include epidermal growth factor receptor inhibitors (EGFR inhibitors) such as monoclonal antibodies and tyrosine kinase inhibitors, mammalian target inhibitors (mTOR), antiangiogenic agents, cytokines, and KIT and BCR-ABL inhibitors. This is an evolving area of cancer therapy and new drugs are continually being developed and brought to market; it is therefore beyond the scope of this chapter to list all of the medications in these classes.

CLINICAL PEARL

Targeted chemotherapies involve agents that block cellular pathways and processes essential to cell growth; skin reactions are common with these drugs and these reactions have been linked to tumor response and overall survival.

Although the mechanism of action is poorly understood, these agents can cause adverse skin and nail effects; the most commonly encountered skin reaction is a papulopustular rash. Hair changes, increased severity of radiation dermatitis, pruritus, fissures, and paronychia are all potential side effects of targeted therapies.

A positive correlation between the development of skin toxicity, including rash, has been linked to tumor response and overall survival. Several theories about this relationship have been advanced, but to date, no data have confirmed a causal relationship (Robert et al., 2012).

Prevalence/Incidence

The incidence of skin rash caused by targeted therapies varies based on the specific drug. In a recent meta-analysis, Qi et al. (2013) determined that the incidence of all stages of rash is 71.9% for anti-EGFR monoclonal antibodies; the incidence of high-grade rash resulting in treatment interruption was much lower (13.3%, range 6.3% to 25.3%). In another meta-analysis of 11 randomized controlled trials, Shameem et al. (2014) found the incidence of all grades of rash to be 27.3% for mTOR inhibitors, with a 1% incidence of high-grade rash necessitating treatment interruption.

Risk Factors

Risk factors for skin reactions related to targeted therapies differ depending upon the drug administered. For example, risk factors for the drug erlotinib include nonsmoking status, fair skin, and age >70 years. For cetuximab, male gender and age <70 appear to increase the risk for rash development. Rash is reported less commonly with low molecular weight tyrosine kinase inhibitors (5% to 9%) and more commonly with monoclonal antibodies (10% to 17%) (Lacouture et al., 2011).

Pathology

Targeted therapies are novel agents that block specific pathways affecting cellular function; the different drugs affect different areas of cellular pathways. For example, cetuximab binds to the extracellular portion of EGFR while erlotinib and gefitinib bind to the intracellular tyrosine kinase domain of EGFR. It is beyond the scope of this chapter to review the mechanism of action for each of the targeted therapies.

The exact pathologic mechanisms resulting in rash and other skin changes are dependent upon the specific medication; however, it should be noted that rash is an expected outcome with most of the targeted therapies. The antitumor mechanism of these drugs lies in their ability to target erroneously active or overexpression of growth factors by tumors. EGFR inhibitors, for example, target overexpression or aberrantly active EGFR in some tumors such as colorectal cancers. EGFR is essential to normal keratinocyte function, including the vital functions of the skin cell, such as the ability to proliferate, differentiate, migrate, and survive (Balagula et al., 2010). Thus, the pathogenesis of the rash and skin changes associated with targeted agents that inhibit EGFR is " ... marked alterations in growth and differentiation of the epidermis leading to altered corneocyte terminal differentiation....Other major changes are damage of the sebaceous glands and follicular infundibulum which generate cytokine release as well as inflammatory cell infiltration in periappendageal areas" (Chanprapaph et al., 2014, p. 2).

Shameem et al. (2014) predict increased incidence of skin reactions as newer agents are developed. Agents that are currently on the horizon include mTOR inhibitors, which work in a similar fashion to EGFR inhibitors. The exact etiology of mTOR rash is currently unknown, but it is thought to arise from inhibition of pathways that regulate cell growth and repair (Shameem et al., 2014).

Clinical Presentation

Skin changes associated with targeted therapies include rash, hand-foot skin reaction, xerosis, pruritis, and paronychia.

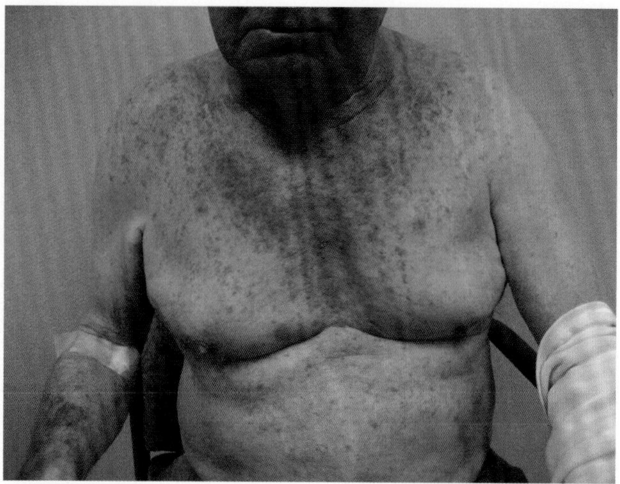

FIGURE 29-4. Papulopustular rash due to targeted chemotherapy.

Rash

The rash associated with targeted therapies has a classic presentation. The rash, which most commonly occurs within the first 2 weeks of therapy, presents as erythematous papules and pustules primarily along the seborrheic-rich areas on the face (nose, cheeks, nasolabial folds, chin, forehead, perioral region), scalp, and upper trunk. It less commonly will extend to the lower trunk, extremities, and buttocks. Initial presentation begins with edema, erythema, and sensory disturbances (pain, burning, and irritation). The next phase is eruption of the papulopustular rash (Fig. 29-4). During weeks 3 to 5, the rash is covered with crusts. In the second month, the papulopustular rash resolves, but there is persistent erythema, xerosis, and formation of telangiectasias in the areas previously affected by the rash.

Rash severity varies from patient to patient and typically waxes and wanes during the course of therapy. The rash is expected to resolve completely within four weeks following discontinuation of therapy. Rash severity is typically graded according to the National Cancer Institute's Common Terminology Criteria for Adverse Events (CTCAE) (**Table 29-4**) (Chen et al., 2012).

CLINICAL PEARL

Specific skin reactions associated with targeted chemotherapies include papulopustular rash, hand-foot skin reaction, xerosis, pruritis, and paronychia.

Hand-Foot Skin Reaction

Another type of skin reaction that may occur with targeted therapies is known as hand-foot skin reaction. These patients typically experience dysesthesia and paresthesia of the hands and/or feet that begin within the first 6 weeks of therapy, followed by development of tender lesions with or without blisters. The blisters are surrounded by an erythematous rim. The lesions are frequently located on areas subjected to pressure and friction, such as the distal tips of the fingers, the heels, and the skin over the metacarpophalangeal and interphalangeal joints. The lateral aspects of the soles, finger webs, and periungual regions can also be involved. Resolution of the blisters is followed by development of painful hyperkeratotic lesions. Hand-foot skin reaction is a distinct entity despite similar presentations of hand-foot syndrome associated with cytotoxic agents such as doxorubicin, 5-fluorouracil, and capecitabine (Fig. 29-5) (Balagula et al., 2010).

Xerosis

Xerosis is a late event that typically follows the rash associated with EGFR inhibitors. It presents as scaly, pruritic skin changes. If not treated effectively, the xerosis can progress to chronic xerotic dermatitis, which can lead to increased risk for superinfections. If the xerosis involves the hands and feet, the patient is at risk for development of painful fissures on the tips of the fingers, toes, and dorsal aspects of the interphalangeal joints (Balagula et al., 2010; Robert et al., 2012).

Pruritus

Pruritus often accompanies the rash associated with targeted therapies although the specific cause is not clearly

TABLE 29-4 Common Terminology Criteria for Adverse Events v4.0: Rash, Acneiform

Adverse Event	1	2	3	4	5
Rash, acneiform	Papules and/or pustules covering <10% BSA, which may or may not be associated with symptoms of pruritus or tenderness	Papules and/or pustules covering 10% to 30% BSA, which may or may not be associated with symptoms of pruritus or tenderness; associated with psychosocial impact; limiting instrumental ADL	Papules and/or pustules covering >30% BSA, which may or may not be associated with symptoms of pruritus or tenderness that limit self-care ADL; associated with local superinfection with oral antibiotics indicated	Papules and/or pustules covering any % BSA, which may or may not be associated with symptoms of pruritus or tenderness and are associated with extensive superinfection with IV antibiotics indicated; life-threatening consequences	Death

Definition: A disorder characterized by an eruption of papules and pustules, typically appearing on the face, scalp, upper chest, and back.
Reprinted from Chen, A. P., Setser, A., Anadkat, M. J., et al. (2012). Grading dermatologic adverse events of cancer treatments: The common terminology criteria for adverse events version 4.0. *Journal of the American Academy of Dermatology*, *67*(5), 1025–1039, Used with permission of Elsevier.

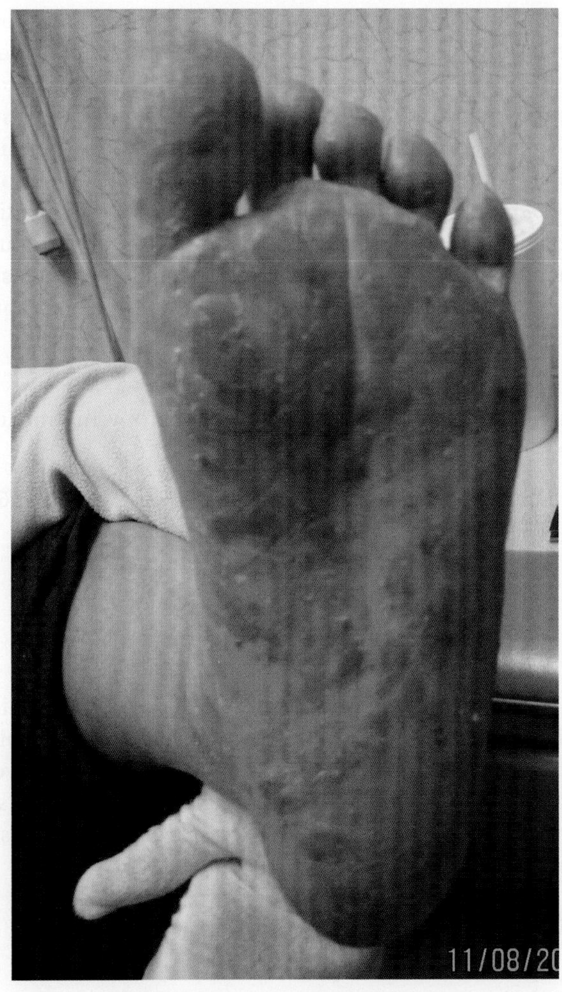

FIGURE 29-5. Hand-foot skin reaction.

defined. It is possible that the itching is a result of histamine released by mast cells. Careful assessment and treatment of dry skin are important for patients receiving EGFR inhibitors as pruritus can also be associated with dry skin. At this point, no studies have been undertaken to address the cause or treatment of pruritus associated with targeted therapies. Treatment at present is empiric and includes gentle skin care, antihistamines, topical menthol 0.5%–pramoxine 1%–doxepin 5%, and medium- to high-potency steroids (e.g., triamcinolone acetonide, 0.025% desonide 0.05%); second-line interventions include the use of gabapentin or pregabalin and may be used if first-line treatment strategies are ineffective (Lacouture et al., 2011).

Paronychia

Paronychia is a delayed reaction that occurs in 10% to 25% of patients following at least 4 weeks of targeted therapy. It is characterized by tender, edematous inflammation of the periungual folds. Initially, the lesions are aseptic but superinfections with purulence can occur. The inflammation can progress to a pyogenic granuloma-like lesion that gives the appearance of an infected ingrown nail.

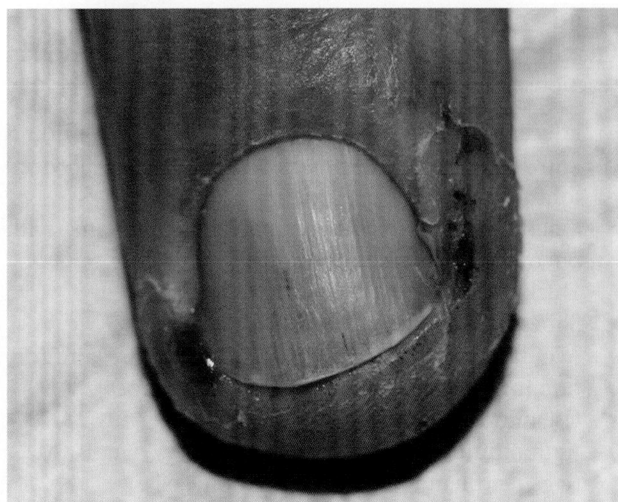

FIGURE 29-6. Paronychia.

This most often affects the toes but can also affect the fingers (Fig. 29-6) (Lacouture et al., 2011; Robert et al., 2012).

Management

There are two clinical practice guidelines that address evidence-based interventions for prevention and management of skin reactions to targeted therapies: the Multinational Association of Supportive Care in Cancer (MASCC) Skin Toxicity Study Group (2011) and a French interdisciplinary therapeutic algorithm (2012). Both guidelines stress the importance of routine preventive care unless there are patient-specific contraindications.

Rash

For prevention of the rash, patients should be prescribed hydrocortisone 1% with a moisturizer and sunscreen applied bid in addition to *either* doxycycline 100 mg bid for 6 weeks *or* minocycline 100 mg daily for 8 weeks. If a rash develops, a medium- to high-potency topical corticosteroid such as alclometasone 0.05% or fluocinonide 0.05% bid should be applied topically as well as clindamycin 1% topical. Systemic therapy for the patient with a rash should include doxycycline 100 mg bid OR minocycline 100 mg daily OR isotretinoin low dose (20 to 30 mg/day). Drugs not recommended by the guidelines include pimecrolimus 1% cream, tazarotene 0.05% cream, sunscreen as a single agent, tetracycline 500 mg bid, vitamin K1 cream, and acitretin. Other interventions supported by the guidelines include use of emollient moisturizing cream, perfume-free pH-balanced cleanser, cutting the nails straight but not too short, and nonaggressive shaving (Lacouture et al., 2011; Reguiai et al., 2012).

CLINICAL PEARL

Prevention and management of the rash associated with targeted chemotherapy agents include gentle skin care, moisturizers, sunscreen, topical corticosteroids, and doxycycline or minocycline.

Hand-Foot Skin Reaction

Preventive care for the individual at risk for hand-foot skin reactions includes the following:

- Education regarding symptoms; the patient should know to notify the health care team promptly if symptoms develop.
- Ongoing monitoring via full-body skin exam, with referral to podiatrist or orthotist if indicated.
- Thick cotton socks to help keep soles of feet dry.
- Shoes with padded insoles.
- Avoidance of excessive temperature, pressure, and friction (avoid long walks and constrictive shoes).
- Use of mild soap for bathing.
- Ammonium lactate 12% or heavy moisturizer (e.g., petroleum jelly) bid for prophylaxis.

Treatment of hand-foot skin reaction depends on the severity (grade) of the reaction. For Grade 1 reactions, current recommendations include urea cream 20% applied bid *and* clobetasol 0.05% applied daily, in addition to use of thick socks at night. For Grade 2 or 3 reactions, recommendations include (1) topical antibiotics for blisters and erosions; (2) topical corticosteroids (clobetasol 0.05% or fluocinonide 0.05%) applied bid to areas that are erythematous, inflamed, and painful; (3) topical keratolytic preparations (salicylic acid 6% or urea 20% to 40%) applied bid to hyperkeratotic areas *only*; and (4) pain management with systemic medications. (These measures should be used in addition to those already addressed for prevention and management of Grade 1 reactions.) For Grade 3 reactions, treatment should be interrupted until the severity is reduced to Grade 0 to 1 (Balagula et al., 2010; Gomez & Lacouture, 2011).

Xerosis

Guidelines for prevention of xerosis are straightforward and include use of tepid water for bathing (with bath oils or mild moisturizing soaps), regular use of moisturizing creams, and avoidance of direct sunlight and extremes in temperature.

Treatment guidelines are less clear but include the following as options:

- Occlusive emollient creams that are fragrance free and alcohol free; these include products that are petrolatum based and those that contain urea or colloidal oatmeal.
- Exfoliant products on scaly areas (e.g., ammonium lactate 12% or lactic acid cream 12%).
- Urea creams (10% to 40%) or salicylic acid (6%).
- Zinc oxide (13% to 40%).
- Severe xerosis: medium- to high-potency steroid creams (triamcinolone acetonide 0.025%, desonide 0.05%, fluticasone propionate 0.05%, alclometasone 0.05%).
- Avoid alcohol-containing lotions, retinoids, and benzoyl peroxide (Lacoutoure et al., 2011).

Pruritus

Prevention of pruritis includes the measures already listed for prevention of xerosis, which is a common contributing factor; in addition, patients should be counseled regarding the importance of gentle skin care. Treatment includes both topical agents (menthol-based products *or* pramoxine 0.5% *or* doxepin 1% *or* medium- to high-potency steroids, such as triamcinolone acetonide 0.025%, desonide 0.05%, fluticasone propionate 0.05%, or alclometasone 0.05%) and systemic agents (antihistamines, gabapentin/pregabalin if antihistamines are ineffective, or doxepin). Therapies that are *not recommended* include systemic steroids, topical antihistamines, topical lidocaine, and aprepitant (Lacouture et al., 2011).

Paronychia

Recommendations for prevention of paronychia include the following:

- Dilute bleach soaks (0.005%, i.e., 1/8 to 1/4 cup of 6% bleach to 3 to 5 gallons of water)
- Cutting nails straight but not too short
- Use of perfume-free pH-balanced cleansers
- Wearing comfortable shoes
- Wearing gloves for cleaning

Treatment recommendations include culturing the lesion to rule out superinfection, topical corticosteroids and anti-inflammatory dose of tetracycline (e.g., doxycycline 200 mg bid until resolution), and electrocautery, silver nitrate, or nail avulsion for excessive granulation tissue (Lacouture et al., 2011; Reguiai et al., 2012).

Palmar–Plantar Erythrodysesthesia (Hand-Foot Syndrome)

Palmar–plantar erythrodysesthesia (PPE) is a painful erythematous rash that occurs on the palms of the hands and the soles of the feet. The rash may progress to desquamation and bullae formation with resultant impairment in function. It is known by several other names including hand-foot syndrome, palmar–plantar erythema, acral erythema, and Burgdorf's reaction. It is associated with doxorubicin, capecitabine, docetaxel, cytarabine, and 5-fluorouracil (Kang et al., 2010; Latchford, 2010; von Moos et al., 2008).

CLINICAL PEARL

PPE (palmar–plantar erythrodysesthesia) is a painful erythematous rash on the palms of the hands and soles of the feet that may progress to desquamation and bullae formation with resultant impairment in function. Management of any open lesions is based on the principles of moist wound healing.

Prevalence/Incidence

The incidence of PPE has been reported to be between 6% and 42% of all patients treated with doxorubicin, capecitabine, docetaxel, cytarabine, 5-fluorouracil, cyclophosphamide, and vinorelbine. Capecitabine is the agent most commonly associated with PPE, with an incidence of 45% to 68% (Kang et al., 2010).

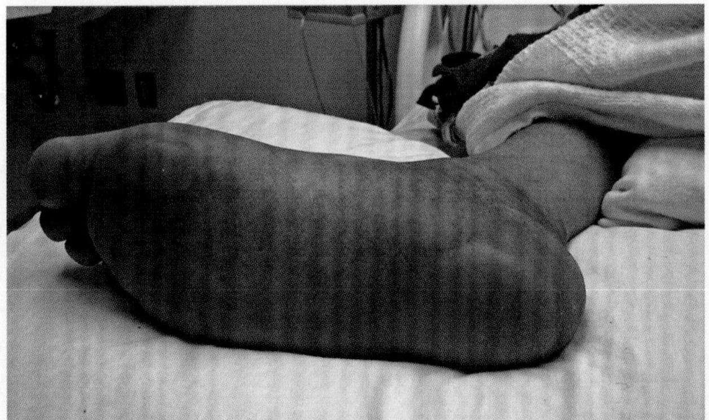

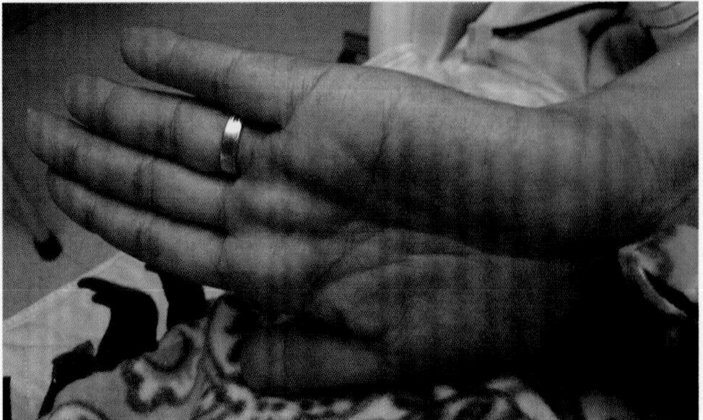

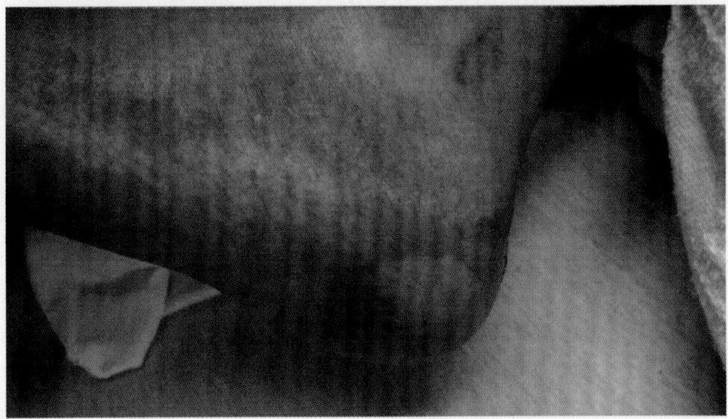

FIGURE 29-7. Palmar–plantar erythrodysesthesia.

Risk Factors

There are no specific risk factors for PPE; the potential for PPE is related primarily to the specific chemotherapeutic agent, the dose, and the schedule of administration (von Moos et al., 2008).

Pathology

The pathology of PPE is difficult to determine as it occurs with multiple chemotherapeutic agents with different mechanisms of action. However, the reaction has common features regardless of the associated chemotherapeutic agent. The areas involved are characterized by temperature gradients, a high concentration of eccrine glands, and exposure to significant friction and trauma. In one study of patients treated with pegylated liposomal doxorubicin (PLD), PLD fluorescence was detected by a dermatologic laser scanning microscope in deep sweat glands in the palms. The authors of this study concluded that the data suggest that the drug is transported to the skin surface via the sweat. Once the drug is deposited into the stratum corneum by the sweat, it generates free radicals that react with the epidermal cells to cause PPE (von Moos et al., 2008).

Clinical Presentation

The first symptom of PPE is a tingling sensation, followed by bilateral erythematous changes that are sharply demarcated. The erythema may progress to formation of bullae and desquamation. Patients with a dark complexion may present with hyperpigmentation and thickening of the skin that may result in stiffness. The hands and feet are most often affected, but other areas of the body may also be involved, including the axillae, groin, waist, inner surface of knees, posterior elbows, anterior folding lines of the wrists, sacral area, bra line, and other areas exposed to occlusion or friction (Fig. 29-7) (Latchford, 2010; von Moos et al., 2008).

Prevention and Management

There are no known preventive therapies. Pyridoxine was once thought to be effective in prevention of PPE but there are no randomized controlled trials that support its use. A recent double-blind placebo-controlled study showed no difference between the placebo group and the treatment group for any measures of efficacy (Kang et al., 2010). These investigators concluded that pyridoxine is not effective in the prevention of PPE and also expressed concern that pyridoxine may adversely affect the duration of response to hexamethylmelamine (Latchford, 2012; von Moos et al., 2008). General prevention measures are directed toward maintenance of healthy skin and prevention of skin trauma and are outlined in **Table 29-5**.

Treatment of PPE primarily involves dose reduction of the offending agent. The patient should be counseled to continue lifestyle prevention strategies, and analgesics should be prescribed as needed to control the pain (Latchford, 2012; von Moos et al., 2008). The wound care nurse may be consulted to assist with dressing recommendations for patients who have significant PPE. Dressing selection should be based on the principles of moist wound healing and is affected by the location of the lesions and volume

TABLE 29-5 Lifestyle Strategies for Prevention of Plantar–Palmar Erythrodysesthesia

- Keep areas well lubricated with emollient creams.
- Avoid skin irritants such as perfumes or alcohol.
- Protect the hands and feet with thick cotton socks and gloves.
- Avoid tight or constricting shoes or clothing.
- Avoid adhesives.
- Avoid activities that add pressure to areas at risk.
- Minimize perspiration.
- Wear protective gloves when performing household tasks.
- Pat skin dry; do not rub.
- Avoid direct sun exposure.
- Keep affected limbs elevated.

of drainage. Use of a nonadherent dressing (e.g., petrolatum gauze dressing) secured by wrap gauze is a reasonable choice in most situations; the dressing should be changed at least twice daily to allow for inspection of the skin.

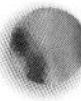

Cutaneous T-Cell Lymphoma (Mycosis Fungoides and Sézary Syndrome)

Mycosis fungoides (MF) and Sézary syndrome (SS) are common subtypes of cutaneous T-cell lymphoma. MF is the most commonly occurring of the two and is considered indolent. In contrast, SS is the aggressive leukemic variant; it can present as a progression of MF or can occur as new-onset lesions that progress rapidly (AlHothali, 2013; Jawed et al., 2014a).

CLINICAL PEARL

MF and SS are two subtypes of cutaneous T-cell lymphoma; MF is more common and is usually indolent, while SS is an aggressive leukemic variant.

Prevalence/Incidence

Cutaneous lymphomas represent 3.9% of all non-Hodgkin's lymphomas, and MF and SS account for 53% of these cutaneous lymphomas. The annual age-adjusted incidence is 6.4 to 9.6 cases per million in the United States. Older individuals are at greater risk (median age at diagnosis is 55 to 60), and the male:female ratio is 2:1 (Jawed et al., 2014a).

Risk Factors

Risk factors include exposure to agents that cause chronic antigenic stimulation, such as military herbicide exposure (Agent Orange) and occupational exposure to agents associated with the glass, pottery, and ceramics industries. Viral exposure is also theorized to play a causative role (AlHothali, 2013; Jawed et al., 2014a).

Pathology

The cause of MF/SS is unknown, although several theories have been proposed. As noted, environmental exposure is thought to play a contributing role through chronic antigen stimulation. This abnormal stimulation can lead to uncontrolled cell growth and accumulation of T cells in the skin. A second theory proposes that infection, specifically *Staphylococcus aureus*, may play a role in the development of MF. One study found that patients with MF and SS had a high rate of *S. aureus* colonization and that empiric antibiotic therapy was associated with clinical improvement. A third hypothesis is that immunosuppression and/or immunosuppressive therapy, such as occurs in HIV patients or after organ transplant, may on rare occasions precipitate the development of cutaneous T-cell lymphoma (AlHothali, 2013; Jawed et al., 2014a).

Clinical Presentation

MF has a classic presentation of patches or plaques on areas of the body that are not sun exposed. These areas may be well defined and pruritic and over time may progress to tumors. The disease is defined into four clinical stages. In stage 1, there are skin patches and plaques that cover either <10% body surface area (stage 1A) or more than 10% body surface area (stage 1B). Stage IIA disease is characterized by lymphadenopathy without nodal infiltration; Stage IIB is characterized by cutaneous tumors. The presence of generalized erythroderma is characteristic of Stage III disease. Pathologically positive lymph nodes are indicative of Stage IVA disease, while visceral disease characterizes Stage IVB.

SS, on the other hand, is characterized by the combination of circulating neoplastic T cells and erythroderma, with or without lymphadenopathy. Patients may also suffer from disabling pruritus. SS should be suspected in any patient who has atypical lymphocytes in the blood and an unexplained pruritic erythroderma (Fig. 29-8) (AlHothali, 2013).

Diagnostics

At the time of suspected initial diagnosis, the following studies should be performed: CBC with differential, chemistry panel, lactate dehydrogenase, and skin biopsy specimen for histology, immunophenotyping, and T-cell receptor gene rearrangement studies. In addition, Sézary cell count, circulating T-cell subsets and clonality, PET/CT scans, and/or lymph node biopsy should be performed. The results of these tests are essential for staging and treatment planning (Jawed et al., 2014a).

Management

Management is based on disease stage. The National Comprehensive Cancer Network (NCCN) has developed guidelines for the workup and management of MF/SS (*www.cutaneouslymphoma.stanford.edu/docs/nhl_3.2012_MFSS.pdf*). The reader is directed to this guideline for additional information.

In general, treatment for early disease is based on observational studies and case reports and includes the following topical agents: corticosteroids, nitrogen mus-

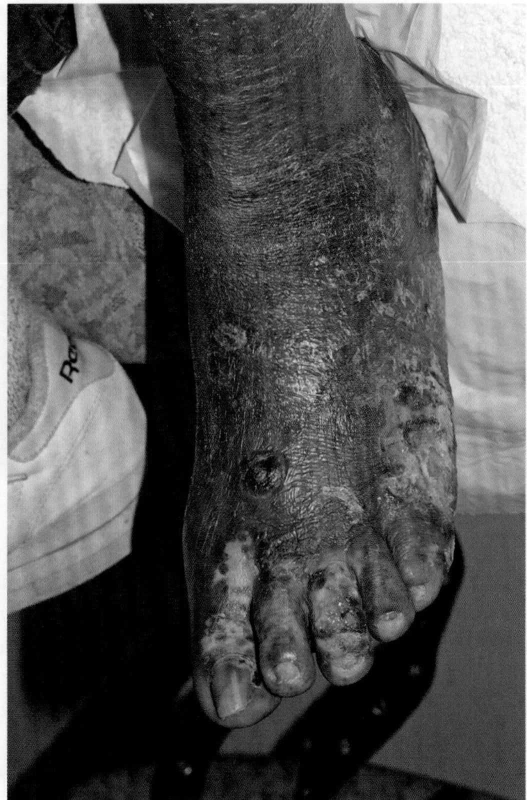

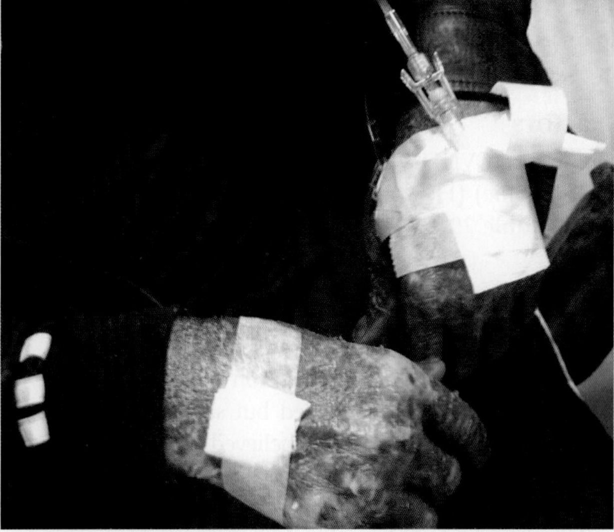

FIGURE 29-8. Sézary syndrome (pruritic erythroderma).

tard, local radiation, phototherapy, topical retinoids, and total skin electron beam therapy. More advanced disease or disease that fails to respond to topical therapy is treated with systemic therapy. Various forms of chemotherapy, immune therapy, targeted therapies, extracorporeal photopheresis, and, for advanced disease, stem cell transplant are mainstays of therapy (Jawed et al., 2014b; Weberschock et al., 2012).

The wound care nurse may be consulted for topical care recommendations as the patient experiences disease progression. In these cases, since the skin changes are due to tumor, the goal of care is palliation of symptoms. The role of the wound care nurse will center on addressing potential complicating factors such as prevention of pressure injury, infection prevention and control, debridement, exudate management, odor control, and appropriate topical care. Little has been written about the topical wound care of MF or SS, and no one dressing or treatment has been established as superior over another.

Graft versus Host Disease

Blood and marrow transplant (BMT) has been performed since the 1960s with the goal of providing cure for a variety of hematologic and solid tumors. There are several different types of transplants. Allogeneic transplants involve cells from a related donor or an unrelated volunteer. Autologous transplantation involves harvesting the patient's cells prior to the administration of high-dose chemotherapy and then reinfusing the patient's own cells following the high-dose chemotherapy. Syngeneic transplant is the use of cells from an identical twin.

Graft versus host disease (GVHD) is more often associated with allogeneic transplants. GVHD can be divided into two categories, acute and chronic. Acute GVHD usually affects three body systems (skin, liver, and gastrointestinal tract) and has been commonly defined as occurring within the first 100 days posttransplant. However, in 2005, the National Institutes of Health Consensus Project changed the classifications of GVHD. Classic acute GVHD is now defined as reactions occurring before day 100 while persistent, recurrent, or late-onset acute GVHD may occur after day 100. Chronic GVHD, on the other hand, occurs after the first 100 days and may involve any tissue, though most commonly the skin, eyes, oral cavity, GI tract, and liver are involved. Overlapping GVHD has symptoms of both acute and chronic GVHD (Chavan & El-Azhary, 2011; Hymes et al., 2012; Latchford, 2012).

CLINICAL PEARL

Graft versus host disease is usually associated with allogeneic transplants, may be either acute or chronic, and frequently results in skin pathology. A minority of patients experience severe cutaneous GVHD, which results in extensive moist desquamation.

Prevalence/Incidence

Acute GVHD is thought to occur in 90% of all allogeneic bone marrow transplant recipients; however, only about 50% of those will develop clinically significant disease. Of those patients with acute GVHD, survival approaches 60% or greater. For those who have severe acute GVHD, prognosis is grave (Latchford, 2010).

Chronic GVHD occurs in approximately 30% to 70% of all patients who undergo an allogeneic transplant. Median time to onset is 4 to 6 months with most occurring within the first 3 years posttransplant (Wu & Cowen, 2012).

Risk Factors

Risk factors for GVHD vary according to time of onset (acute vs. chronic) (Flowers et al., 2011). The risk factors are listed in Table 29-6.

Pathology

There continues to be controversy regarding the pathologic processes involved in acute and chronic GVHD. While some believe that chronic GVHD is an extension of acute GVHD, current evidence suggests two related but separate disease entities. Simply stated, acute GVHD is believed to represent an inflammatory response caused by a cytokine storm. Chronic GVHD, on the other hand, is not as well understood. Chronic GVHD pathology is thought to be similar to autoimmune diseases and possibly related to autoreactive T cells that have escaped negative selection by the thymus. A detailed discussion of the pathology of GVHD is beyond the scope of this chapter (Chavan & El-Azhary, 2011; Häusermann et al., 2008; Hymes et al., 2012; Latchford, 2012; Sung & Chao, 2013).

Clinical Presentation

Acute GVHD

Skin manifestations of GVHD typically present in the first 10 to 14 days posttransplant with a rash that begins acrally but eventually becomes generalized in distribution. The rash may be morbilliform or maculopapular and is generally symmetrical. The back and neck are commonly involved (Fig. 29-9). In severe cases, there is diffuse erythroderma and bullae formation with a positive Nikolsky sign, followed by extensive moist desquamation that resembles toxic epidermal necrolysis (TENS) (Fig. 29-10).

TABLE 29-6 Risk Factors for Acute and Chronic GVHD

Acute GVHD	Chronic GVHD
Age of recipient	Acute GVHD
GVHD prophylaxis	Older age
HLA matching between the donor and recipient (mismatched donor)	HLA matching between the donor and recipient (mismatched donor)
Intensity of the conditioning regimen	Donor gender (female donor with male recipient)
Graft composition	Use of peripheral blood as stem cell source
Donor gender (female donor with male recipient)	Use of donor lymphocyte infusion
Use of donor lymphocyte infusion	
Use of total body irradiation (TBI) in the conditioning regimen	

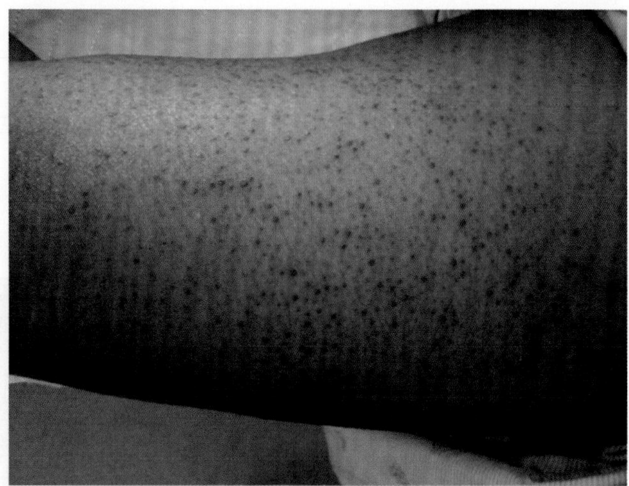

FIGURE 29-9. Rash secondary to acute GVHD.

Chronic GVHD

Chronic GVHD has a more subtle onset and variable presentation; possible signs and symptoms include the following (Fig. 29-11):

- Xerosis
- Keratosis pilaris–like lesions
- Ichthyosis
- Papulosquamous lesions
- Psoriasiform and pityriasis rosea–like skin changes
- Annular lesions
- Superficial erythema
- Lichenoid lesions
- Sclerotic changes with plaques
- Poikilodermatous changes

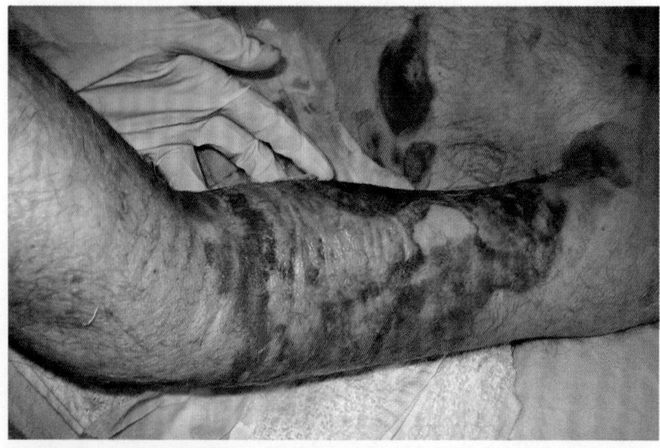

FIGURE 29-10. Extensive moist desquamation secondary to acute GVHD.

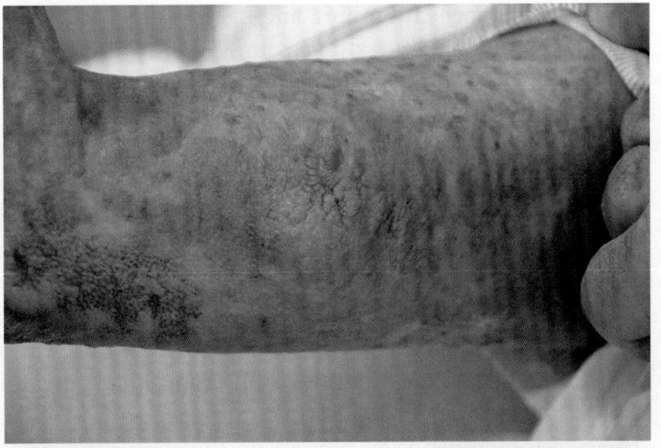

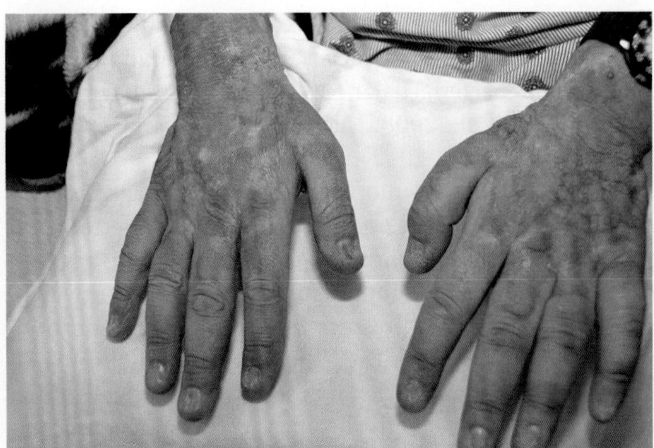

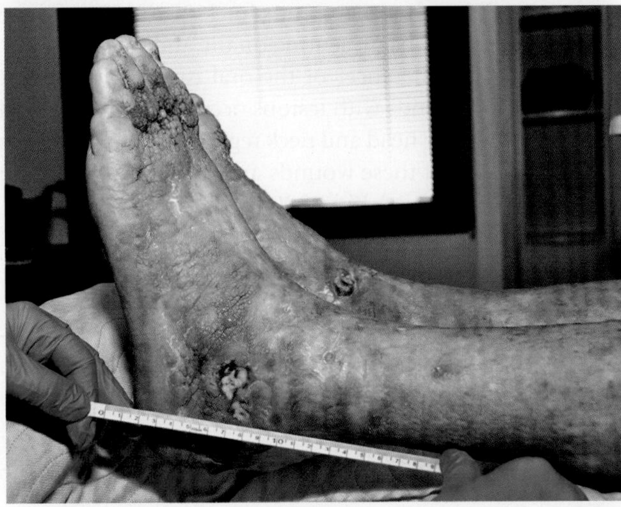

FIGURE 29-11. Skin and soft tissue changes due to chronic GVHD.

- Hair and nail changes (dystrophy, thickening or thinning, vertical ridging of nails, onycholysis, and scarring and nonscarring alopecia) (Häusermann et al., 2008; Hymes et al., 2012; Latchford, 2010; Wu & Cowen, 2012)

Diagnosis of both acute and chronic GVHD is based on clinical assessment and verified by skin biopsy.

Management of Acute GVHD

Management of acute GVHD is based on systemic therapy. Systemic management principles are listed in Table 29-7. The role of the wound care nurse will center on supportive care. Supportive care includes gentle cleansing; use of nonadherent dressings that absorb exudate, inhibit bacterial growth, and maintain a moist wound surface; and support surfaces that provide pressure redistribution, reduce shear and friction, and provide microclimate control.

CLINICAL PEARL

Management of acute GVHD includes systemic therapy to control the underlying process, topical therapy based on moist wound healing, and support surfaces that provide pressure redistribution, reduction in shear and friction, and microclimate control.

Management of Chronic GVHD

As is true of acute GVHD, systemic therapy is an essential element of management for chronic GVHD; supportive care is also critical to positive outcomes, and that is the role of the wound care nurse.

Supportive care includes *daily* bathing, use of appropriate antimicrobial agents when indicated, liberal use of emollient agents to keep the skin soft, and use of compression garments to manage venous insufficiency caused by

TABLE 29-7 Prevention and Treatment of Acute GVHD

Prevention	Treatment
Immunosuppression	Glucocorticoids for grades II–IV
Reduced-intensity conditioning regimens	Immune modulators
T-cell suppression or depletion in the donor marrow	Skin-targeted therapies: topical corticosteroids, topical tacrolimus 0.1% bid
	Phototherapy
	IVIG

soft tissue fibrosis. The importance of daily bathing cannot be stressed enough as a means for maintaining normal skin flora and bacterial balance (Chavan & El-Azhary, 2011; Häusermann et al., 2008; Latchford, 2010; Sung & Chao, 2013; Wu & Cowen, 2012).

The role of the wound care nurse in management of the patient with GVHD also involves dressing selection for patients with open wounds and recommendations regarding support surfaces. Support surfaces should be selected to provide maximum pressure redistribution in addition to microclimate control. The patient's level of mobility is a critical decision-making factor in support surface selection. Many times, patients with chronic GVHD have significant skin issues but continue to be ambulatory. Thus, surfaces must be chosen that provide pressure redistribution while maintaining the patient's mobility. Compression therapy or compression garments should be considered for all patients with fibrotic changes in the soft tissue as this will lead to venous insufficiency. At this time, there are no evidence-based guidelines or standards of care for the management of GVHD, and this remains an area where research is needed.

 Malignant Fungating Wounds

The term malignant fungating wound refers to those wounds that develop because of a malignant process. The National Cancer Institute defines a fungating lesion as

A type of skin lesion that is marked by ulcerations (breaks on the skin or surface of an organ) and necrosis (death of living tissue) and that usually has a "bad smell" (National Cancer Institute, n.d. a).

Skin metastases are indicative of advanced disease; median survival time following diagnosis of skin metastases has been reported as 7.98 months (Hu et al., 2008). These wounds are very difficult for clinicians, patients, and caregivers to manage; in addition, their presence is a constant reminder of the disease for the patient and family. Paramount when caring for patients with malignant fungating wounds is determination of the goal of care; generally, the goal is to manage symptoms rather than to resolve the wounds.

Prevalence/Incidence

There is no specific data regarding the incidence and prevalence of malignant fungating wounds, but it is estimated that between 5% and 10% of cancer patients will develop these lesions (Alexander, 2009a; Fromantin et al., 2014; Hu et al., 2008). Some cancers are more likely to cause a malignant fungating wound than others. In women, the tumor most likely to result in a malignant fungating wound is breast cancer; it is estimated that approximately 70% of all malignant fungating wounds are of breast origin. The most common sites for malignant fungating wounds resulting from breast cancer are the chest and abdomen, though these lesions may also present on the scalp, neck, upper extremities, and back. Women may also develop malignant fungating wounds from other malignancies, including melanoma (5% to 12%), colon cancer (9%), lung cancer (4%), and ovarian cancer (4%). The location of the malignant tumor wound may be indicative of the primary tumor. Melanoma wounds tend to occur on the lower extremities; colon wounds on the abdomen and pelvis; lung wounds on the chest wall, back, and scalp; and ovarian wounds on the abdomen and back.

In men, 32% of all fungating tumor wounds are caused by melanoma, with lesions presenting most commonly on the chest, back, and extremities. Lung cancer accounts for 24% to 29% of all malignant fungating wounds in men. These lesions most often present on the chest wall, back, and scalp. Colon cancer accounts for 11% to 19% of these wounds, with lesions presenting on the abdomen and pelvis. Squamous cell cancer of the oral cavity accounts for 11.5% of the wounds with lesions occurring in a localized distribution in the head and neck region. Renal cell tumors account for 4% of these wounds and generally present on the scalp (Rolz-Cruz & Kim, 2008).

Risk Factors

The only known risk factor for the development of a metastatic skin lesion is a cancer diagnosis, though some cancers are more likely than others to metastasize to the skin. In addition, some cancers present with direct extension to the skin (e.g., Paget's disease).

Pathology

Metastasis is a complex process that is dependent not only on the characteristics of the tumor but also on host response. Metastatic disease follows a specific distribution pattern dependent upon the tumor type.

Initially, a transforming event occurs that stimulates tumor cells to grow and expand. Nutrients are provided to the tumor by simple diffusion. As the tumor cells multiply, proangiogenic factors are secreted by the tumor, which stimulate development of a network of capillaries; this provides the support needed for further tumor growth. Penetration of the lymphatic and blood vessels is then enabled, which allows the tumor cells to enter into circulation. As the tumor cell enters into circulation, it can be deactivated by mechanical trauma or by the immune system. If the tumor cell survives, it will settle into the capillary bed of a selected organ; the site can be random or site specific depending on the tumor of origin. When the tumor cell reaches the capillary bed of the organ, extravasation of tumor cells occurs. The final step in the process occurs when the tumor cells proliferate at the new site and produce a new tumor.

Metastatic distribution can be completed by three processes. It can occur by mechanical tumor stasis, that is, metastatic extension into the surrounding tissue or the lymphatic drainage bed. Mechanical tumor stasis is the most common pattern of metastasis, accounting for 50%

to 60% of all distribution patterns. Metastatic distribution can also occur by site-specific attachment where the tumor cells target a specific organ and other regional areas are bypassed. The presence of a site-specific adhesion molecule dictates this type of metastatic pattern. The third way in which metastasis occurs is through a nonspecific pattern. This is commonly encountered with highly aggressive tumors. These tumors have the ability to adhere to vessel walls and establish themselves in many different sites (Rolz-Cruz & Kim, 2008).

Clinical Presentation

Malignant skin lesions may present either as ulcerative lesions or as raised nodules. The initial presentation may be painless skin nodules that vary in color from pale pink to purple. The lesion may involve only one nodule or multiple nodules, and the texture of the nodules can be either firm or rubbery. As the tumor proliferates, the lesion progresses to ulceration and cavity formation or to a raised lesion with a cauliflower-like (fungating) appearance (Fig. 29-12).

Diagnosis

Definitive diagnosis requires tissue biopsy to prove the presence of tumor cells.

Management

Management of these wounds centers on control of symptoms including exudate management, odor control, pain management, and control of bleeding. Since these wounds are caused by cancerous cells, *no topical therapy alone will result in wound closure.* For these wounds to resolve, systemic therapy in the form of chemotherapy, targeted therapy, biologic therapy, hormone therapy, or radiation therapy must be administered.

Cleansing

Wound cleansing is an important aspect of care for any wound, including a malignant tumor wound. Wound cleansing should be gentle so as not to cause increased pain or bleeding. Showering with copious amounts of water is a common and simple approach to cleansing of these challenging wounds. If the patient is unable to shower, irrigation with normal saline or warm tap water is also an acceptable method of cleansing. Topical antiseptic solutions have been considered contraindicated due to their toxicity to healthy tissues (Cochran & Jakubek, 2010; Draper, 2005).

Odor Control

While it is well documented that odor is problematic for patients with malignant wounds, there is no documented definitive cause of the odor. The odor is hypothesized to be due to some combination of the following: anaerobic bacteria supported by the breakdown of proteins in the necrotic tissue, aerobic bacteria, clinical infection, necrotic tissue, and/or the stagnant exudate contained within the dressings (Cochran & Jakubek, 2010).

Control of odor associated with malignant wounds has been accomplished in one of three ways: oral metronidazole, topical metronidazole, and use of advanced dressings or topical antiseptics. At present, there is insufficient evidence to prove that any one approach is superior. The current studies that have been published either are poorly powered or have flaws in methodology. In 2013, the Cochrane review published a paper, *Topical agents and dressings for fungating wounds*. This paper's final conclusion is that "There is insufficient evidence in this review to give a clear direction for practice with regard to improving quality of life or managing wound symptoms associated with fungating wounds. More research is needed" (Adderly & Holt, 2014, p. 2).

CLINICAL PEARL

Common issues with fungating malignant wounds include odor, exudate control, and control of bleeding; strategies shown in limited studies to be beneficial in odor control include topical metronidazole, medical grade honey, and silver dressings. Anecdotal reports suggest that Dakin's solution may also be of benefit.

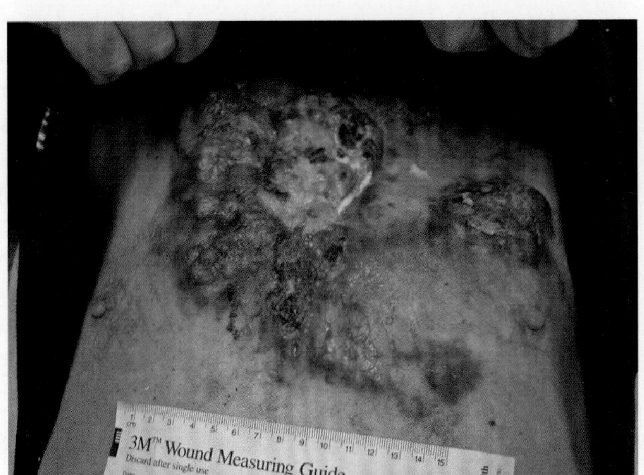

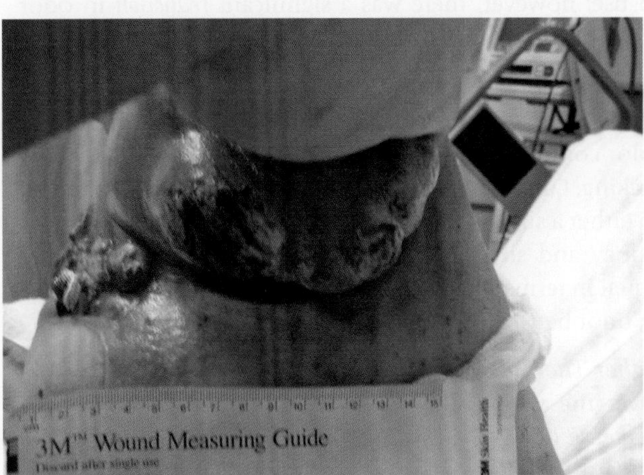

FIGURE 29-12. Malignant fungating wounds.

Metronidazole

Two studies compared the use of metronidazole to placebo. The first study was conducted in 1984 and compared oral metronidazole to placebo; six patients were treated in a crossover design and a significant reduction in odor was noted with metronidazole as compared to placebo. The investigators decided not to do a more in-depth study, because the beneficial effects of metronidazole were so great that they felt it would be unethical to withhold the drug (Ashford et al., 1984). Bower et al. (1992) compared metronidazole gel to placebo. In this study, eleven patients were enrolled and in every case, there was a statistically significant reduction in the assessment of odor. Case reports have reported similar findings in regard to the beneficial effects of both topical and oral metronidazole (Santos et al., 2010). At this time, topical metronidazole is the preferred route of administration due to the side effect profile of this medication (Alexander, 2009b). Metronidazole is available as a wound gel, which donates moisture to the wound bed and may be the preferred agent for wounds with minimal exudate. Metronidazole tablets have also been crushed and applied directly to the wound bed with improvement in odor being noted (Bauer et al., 2000).

Dakin's Solution

Topical dressings have also been used as a way to decrease odor from malignant fungating tumor wounds. The use of Dakin's solution either as a cleanser or applied to gauze and placed onto the wound bed twice daily can be effective as a deodorizer. The effect most likely is due to its negative effect on microorganisms. There is no published data on the strength, frequency of application, systemic absorption or comparison of Dakin's solution to other products. More research is needed on the use of Dakin's for odor control with fungating tumor wounds (Cochran & Jakubek, 2010).

Silver-Impregnated Dressings

One small study (n = 26) has demonstrated a significant reduction in odor with use of silver foam dressings as compared to foam dressings without silver. In this study, there was no increase in odor while standard foam dressings were in use; however, there was a significant *reduction* in odor with the silver foam dressing (Kalemikerakis et al., 2012).

Medical Grade Honey

Medical grade honey dressings have also been used for odor control though definitive data regarding benefits are lacking. Lund-Nielsen et al. (2011) randomized 69 patients to either a silver dressing or a honey dressing. In this study, honey and silver dressings were found to be essentially equal in terms of odor control, and no statistical difference in odor between the two groups was noted.

Other Therapies

Over the years, other therapies have been proposed to decrease odor of fungating tumor wounds. These include the use of charcoal dressings, yogurt, buttermilk, various antibiotic combinations, chlorophyllin copper complex, aromatherapy, sugar paste, baking soda, vanilla extract, vinegar, coffee granules, cat litter, larval therapy, vacuum-assisted closure, Chloromycetin, debridement, and cadexomer iodine. However, none of these products have demonstrated success in decreasing wound odor. In all cases, the cost of the dressing as well as the effectiveness must also be considered. Interventions should be directed at those that prevent malodor at the source rather than those that will mask the odor (Alexander, 2009b).

Exudate Management

Malignant wounds typically produce high volumes of exudate due to the increased capillary permeability caused by the disorganized tumor vasculature that is characteristic of these wounds. Autolysis of necrotic tissue within the wound bed is also responsible for a larger volume of exudate. Inflammation and edema are common with these wounds, which further increases the management challenge. As with all wounds, exudate management is a primary goal of topical therapy. Control of exudate is aimed not only at providing the optimum environment for the wound but also as a means to improve quality of life for the patient. At the same time, the clinician is challenged with the cost of advanced dressings with absorptive properties due to restrictions placed on the use of dressings for these types of wounds by third-party reimbursement.

There is no *ideal* dressing that has been defined for malignant wounds, but certain characteristics of wound dressings should be considered when choosing a wound dressing. These characteristics include nonadherence to the wound bed, conformability, ability to transfer excessive moisture away from the wound bed itself, high absorbency, and aesthetic acceptability (Alexander, 2009b; Cochran & Jakubek, 2011; Dowsett, 2008; Draper, 2005). For wounds that are slightly exudative, the application of a hydrogel dressing may be advisable. Alternatives would include simple and inexpensive nonadherent dressings such as those impregnated with petrolatum. Since healing is dependent on response to systemic therapy, the focus in topical therapy should be simply to provide coverage of the tumor and management of any exudate. At times, it may be appropriate to leave the minimally exudative wound open to air if there are confounding circumstances such as lack of third-party reimbursement or lack of caregiver support. Wounds that are more exudative may require the use of an alginate or foam dressing to contain the drainage. Other advanced dressings are also available and effective, but the clinician must consider cost and simplicity as well as absorptive capacity when making recommendations. Some authors have recommended the use of pouching systems to manage highly exudative wounds (Cochran & Jakubek, 2010); however, the complexity of placing a wound pouch in addition to the cost of these systems may make this option cost-prohibitive.

Control of Bleeding

Control of bleeding continues to be an important management goal. Malignant fungating wounds tend to bleed easily due to the fragility of the wound bed and erosion of capillaries by the tumor. There may also be impairment of the coagulation cascade due to the disease process and/or the treatments for the cancer (Alexander, 2009c; Cochran & Jakubek, 2011). The primary focus is on patient education to prevent bleeding. Patients and caregivers should be instructed on gentle cleansing. Additionally, atraumatic dressing removal is of paramount importance. If the dressing is adherent to the wound bed, it should be moistened prior to removal.

Measures to manage bleeding include the following:

- Direct pressure for 10 to 15 minutes
- Ice packs to the wound
- Use of topical coagulants or hemostatic agents (e.g., WoundSeal Powder, Gelfoam)
- Silver nitrate sticks
- Topical sucralfate suspension (Cochran & Jakubek, 2010)

If bleeding is heavy, patients should be instructed to seek professional assistance. In a controlled setting, antifibrinolytics, vasoconstrictors, ligation, and cauterization may be options to control heavy bleeding (Alexander, 2009c).

Pain Management

The first step in management of wound-related pain is a thorough assessment of the pain including the site, nature, duration, onset, frequency, and severity as well as the impact on the patient's life. Aggravating and alleviating factors should also be determined. Systemic pain medication continues to be the gold standard and should be prescribed by the primary health care team. Measures to ensure comfort with dressing changes should be undertaken including medication with short-acting pain medications prior to dressing changes, the use of nonadherent dressings, and decreased frequency of dressing changes. Topical anesthetics have been proposed as a means to improve patient comfort as well as the use of morphine in hydrogel. While there are several case reports on these products with malignant wounds, little evidence exists to support the use of these products in malignant lesions, and thus, their use remains off-label (Bergstrom, 2011; Cochran & Jakubek, 2010).

Conclusion

Wound and skin care for the cancer patient is an evolving area of practice as new therapies are implemented to eradicate cancer that affects basic cellular pathways. Many new drugs and therapies are on the horizon that will affect the skin and the way the patient responds to injury. The wound care nurse should assess each patient individually, consult the primary team for the effects of the therapeutic agents, and then address the skin change with evidence-based interventions if available. These wounds and skin changes are a unique challenge for the wound care nurse. By adhering to the basic principles of wound care, the wound nurse can choose appropriate therapies for this unique population.

CASE STUDIES

CASE STUDY

Mrs. R is a 76-year-old female with a diagnosis of Stage IV breast cancer, with a fungating tumor wound, who has been admitted to the hospital inpatient unit with neutropenic fever. The patient has never been seen by a wound care nurse in the past. She is newly diagnosed with her breast cancer and has not undergone a mastectomy or radiation due to her advanced disease. She has received her first course of chemotherapy (Taxol, Pertuzumab, and trastuzumab) 12 days ago.

The wound care nurse is consulted by the oncology team for wound care recommendations. The patient reports her usual care of her wound involves dabbing it with hydrogen peroxide once per day and then covering the area with paper towels. She states she has had the wound on her breast for about 6 months. She states she was afraid to go to the doctor, so she did not tell anyone about her wound. She states that since her chemotherapy, she has had an increase in odor from the wound.

On exam, the patient presents with a large fungating tumor wound on her left breast. The wound is 6 cm (l) × 5 cm (w) and located in the lateral aspect of the breast. The wound bed is 50% dry yellow slough tissue that is tightly adherent. The remainder of the wound is 50% pink tissue. The periwound skin is firm but not erythematous. There is a foul odor noted from the wound bed.

The patient's social history includes a history of smoking 1 ppd × 50 years. She also reports recent weight loss of 20# over the past 6 months.

Pertinent lab values include HBG of 6.8, WBC of 2.1, and PLT of 38. No nutritional lab values have been drawn. Cefepime 1 g q8h IV has been ordered to address her neutropenic fever.

Wound Care Nurse Interventions

The goal of care for this patient is control of symptoms including wound odor:

1. Wound culture.
2. Wound care order: Irrigate wound with 250 mL of normal saline under pressure. Apply metronidazole crushed tablets 250 mg, and cover with petrolatum gauze dressing. Top with bulky dressing and secure in nonadherent fashion q8h.

Outcome

On reevaluation 2 days later, no odor is noted in the patient's room. The patient reports she feels more comfortable. She states she thinks she can do the procedure at home independently. On hospital discharge, the patient was instructed to clean the wound in the shower if able rather than doing irrigations to the wound bed.

REFERENCES

Adderly, U. J. & Holt, I. G. S. (2014). Topical agents and dressings for fungating wounds. *Cochrane Database of Systematic Reviews*, doi:10.1002/14651858.CD003948.

Ashford, R., Plant, G., Maher, J., & Teares, L. (1984). Double-blind trial of metronidazole in malodorous ulcerating tumours. *The Lancet, 323*(8388), 1232–1233.

Alexander, S. (2009a). Malignant fungating wounds: Epidemiology, aetiology, presentation and assessment. *Journal of Wound Care, 18*(7), 273–280.

Alexander, S. (2009b). Malignant fungating wounds: Managing malodour and exudate. *Journal of Wound Care, 18*(9), 374–382.

Alexander, S. (2009c). Malignant fungating wounds: Key symptoms and psychosocial. *Journal of Wound Care, 18*(8), 325–329.

AlHothali, G. I. (2013). Review of the treatment of mycosis fungoides and Sézary syndrome: A stage-based approach. *International Journal of Health Sciences, 7*(2), 220–239.

American Cancer Society. (2014). *Cancer facts & figures 2014*. Retrieved April 8, 2014, from http://www.cancer.org/research/cancerfactsstatistics/cancerfactsfigures2014/index

Archambeau, J. O., Pezner, R., & Wasserman, T. (1995). Pathophysiology of irradiated skin and breast. *International Journal of Radiation Oncology Biology, 31*(5), 1171–1185.

Balagula, Y., Lacouture, M. E., & Cotliar, J. A. (2010). Dermatologic toxicities of targeted anticancer therapies. *Supportive Oncology, 8*(4), 149–161.

Bauer, C. Gerlach, M. A., & Doughty, D. (2000). Care of metastatic skin lesions. *Journal of Wound, Ostomy, and Continence Nursing, 27*(4), 247–251.

Bauer, C., Laszewski, P., & Magnan, M. (2015). Promoting adherence to skin care practices among radiation oncology patients. *Clinical Journal of Oncology Nursing, 19*(2), 196–203.

Bauer, S. M., & Bauer, C. (2009). The use of sodium hyaluronate for the treatment of radiation recall dermatitis. *Journal of Oncology Pharmacy Practice, 15*, 123–126.

Bergstrom, K. J. (2011). Assessment and management of fungating wounds. *Journal of Wound, Ostomy, and Continence Nursing, 38*(1), 31–37.

Berthelet, E., Truong, P. T., Musso, K., et al. (2004). Preliminary reliability and validity testing of a new skin toxicity assessment tool (STAT) in breast cancer patients undergoing radiotherapy. *American Journal of Clinical Oncology, 27*(6), 626–631.

Bower, M., Stein, R., Evans, T. R. J., et al. (1992). A double-blind study of the efficacy of metronidazole gel in the treatment of malodorous fungating tumours. *European Journal of Cancer, 28A*(4/5), 888–889.

Chanprapaph, K., Vachiramon, V., & Rattanakaemakorn, P. (2014). *Epidermal growth factor receptor inhibitors: A review of cutaneous adverse events and management. Dermatology Research and Practice*, Retrieved July 22, 2014 from http://www.hindawi.com/journals/drp/2014/734249/abs/

Chavan, R., & El-Azhary, R. (2011). Cutaneous graft-versus-host disease: Rationales and treatment options. *Dermatologic Therapy, 24*, 219–228.

Chen, A. P., Setser, ., Anadkat, M. J., et al. (2012). Grading dermatologic adverse events of cancer treatments: The common terminology criteria for adverse events version 4.0. *Journal of the American Academy of Dermatology, 67*(5), 1025–1039.

Cochran, S. & Jakubek, P. R. (2010). Malignant cutaneous disease. In M. L. Haas & G. J. Moore-Higgs (Eds.), *Principles of skin care and the oncology patient* (pp. 77–100). Pittsburg, PA: Oncology Nursing Society.

Dest, V. M. (2010). Systemic therapy-induced skin reactions. In M. L. Haas & G. J. Moore-Higgs (Eds.), *Principles of skin care and the oncology patient* (pp. 115–139). Pittsburg, PA: Oncology Nursing Society.

Dowsett, C. (2008). Exudate management: A patient-centered approach. *Journal of Wound Care, 17*(6), 249–252.

Draper, C. (2005). The management of malodour and exudate in fungating wounds. *British Journal of Nursing, 14*(11), S4–S12.

Feight, D., Baney, T., Bruce, S. et al. (2011). Putting evidence into practice: Evidence-based interventions for radiation dermatitis. *Clinical Journal of Oncology Nursing, 15*(5), 481–492.

Flowers, M. E., Inamoto, Y., Carpenter, P. A., et al. (2011). Comparative analysis of risk factors for acute graft-versus-host disease and for chronic graft-versus-host disease according to National Institutes of Health consensus criteria. *Blood, 117*(11), 3214–3219.

Fromantin, I., Watson, S., Baffie, A., et al. (2014). A prospective, descriptive cohort study of malignant wound characteristics and wound care strategies in patients with breast cancer. *Ostomy Wound Management, 60*(6), 38–48.

Gomez, P., & Lacouture, M. E. (2011). Clinical presentation and management of hand-foot syndrome skin reaction associated with sorafenib in combination with cytotoxic chemotherapy: Experience in breast cancer. *The Oncologist, 16*, 1508–1519.

Haubner, F., Ohmann, E., Pohl, F., et al. (2012). Wound healing after radiation therapy: Review of the literature. *Radiation Oncology, 7*(162). Retrieved October 6, 2014 from http://www.ro-journal.com/content/7/1/162

Häusermann, P., Walter, R. B., Halter, J., et al. (2008). Cutaneous graft-versus-host disease: A guide for the dermatologist. *Dermatology, 216*, 287–304.

Hopewell, J. W. (1990). The skin: Its structure and response to ionizing radiation. *International Journal of Radiation Biology, 57*(4), 751–773.

Hu, S. S., Chen, G. S., Lu, Y. W., et al. (2008). Cutaneous metastases from different internal malignancies: A clinical and prognostic appraisal. *Journal of the European Academy of Dermatology and Venereology, 22*, 735–740.

Hymes, S. R., Strom, E. A., & Fife, C. (2006). Radiation dermatitis: Clinical presentation, pathophysiology, and treatment 2006. *Journal of the American Academy of Dermatology, 54*(1), 28–46.

Hymes, S. R., Alousi, A. M., & Cowen, E. W. (2012). Graft-versus-host disease part I. Pathogenesis and clinical manifestations of graft-versus-host disease. *Journal of the American Academy of Dermatology, 66*(4), 515e1–515e18.

Jawed, S. I., Myskowski, P. L., Horwitz, S., et al. (2014a). Primary cutaneous T-cell lymphoma (mycosis fungoides and Sézary syndrome) Part I. Diagnosis: Clinical and histopathologic features and new molecular biologic markers. *Journal of the American Academy of Dermatology, 70*(2), 205e1–205e16.

Jawed, S. I., Myskowski, P. L., Horwitz, S., et al. (2014b). Primary cutaneous T-cell lymphoma (mycosis fungoides and Sézary syndrome) Part II. Prognosis, management, and future directions. *Journal of the American Academy of Dermatology, 70*(2), 223e1–223e17.

Kang, Y., Lee, S. S., Yoon, D. H., et al. (2010). Pyridoxine is not effective to prevent hand-foot syndrome associated with capecitabine therapy: Results of a randomized, double-blind, placebo-controlled study. *Journal of Clinical Oncology, 28*(24), 3824–3829.

Kalemikerakis, J., Vardaki, Z., Fouka, G., et al. (2012). Comparison of foam dressings with silver versus foam dressings without silver in the care of malodorous malignant fungating wounds. *Journal of BUON: Official Journal of the Balkan Union of Oncology, 17*(3), 560–564.

Lacouture, M. E., Anadkate, M. J., Bensadoun, R., et al. (2011). Clinical practice guidelines for the prevention and treatment of EGFR inhibitor-associated dermatologic toxicities. *Supportive Care Cancer, 19*, 1079–1095.

Latchford, T. M. (2010). Cutaneous effects of blood and marrow transplantation. In M. L. Haas & G. J. Moore-Higgs (Eds.), *Principles of skin care and the oncology patient* (pp. 167–194). Pittsburg, PA: Oncology Nursing Society.

Lewis, L., Carson, S., Bydder, S., et al. (2014). Evaluating the effects of aluminum-containing and non-aluminum containing deodorants on axillary skin toxicity during radiation therapy for breast cancer: A 3-armed randomized controlled trial. *International Journal of Radiation Oncology Biology Physics, 90*(4), 765–771.

Lund-Nielsen, B., Adamsen, ., Kolmos, H. J., et al. (2011). The effect of honey-coated bandages compared with silver-coated bandages on treatment of malignant wounds—A randomized study. *Wound Repair and Regeneration, 19*, 664–670.

McQuestion, M. (2010). Radiation-induced skin reactions. In M. L. Haas & G. J. Moore-Higgs (Eds.), *Principles of skin care and the oncology patient* (pp. 115–139). Pittsburg, PA: Oncology Nursing Society.

McQuestion, M. (2011). Evidence-based skin care management in radiation therapy: Clinical update. *Seminars in Oncology Nursing, 27*(2), e1–e17.

National Cancer Institute. (2014, April 25). Targeted cancer therapies. Retrieved July 22, 2014 from http://www.cancer.gov/cancertopics/factsheet/Therapy/targeted

National Cancer Institute. (n.d. a). NCI dictionary of cancer terms: fungating lesion. Retrieved June 28, 2014 from http://www.cancer.gov/dictionary?CdrID=367427

National Cancer Institute. (n.d. b). Radiation therapy for cancer. Retrieved July 16, 2014 from http://www.cancer.gov/cancertopics/factsheet/Therapy/radiation

Noble-Adams, R. (1999). Radiation-induced skin reactions 3: Evaluating the RISRAS. *British Journal of Nursing, 8*(19), 1305–1312.

Pérez Fidalgo, J. A., García Fabregat, L., Cerbantes, A., et al. (2012). Management of chemotherapy extravasation: ESMO-EOPNS clinical practice guidelines. *Annals of Oncology, 23*(Suppl 7), vii 167–vii 173.

Polovich, M., Whitford, J. M., & Olsen, M. (2009). *Chemotherapy and biotherapy Guidelines and recommendations for practice*. Pittsburg, PA: Oncology Nursing Society.

Qi, W., Sun, Y., Shen, Z., et al. (2013). Risk of anti-EGFR monoclonal antibody-related skin rash: An up-to-date meta-analysis of 25 randomized controlled trials. *Journal of Chemotherapy*, doi: 10.1179/1973947813Y.0000000155.

Reguiai, A., Bachet, J. B., Bachmeyer, C., et al. (2012). Management of cutaneous adverse events induced by anti-EGFR (epidermal growth factor receptor): A French interdisciplinary therapeutic algorithm. *Supportive Care Cancer, 20*, 1395–1404.

Robert, C., Sibaud, V., Mateus, C., et al. (2012). Advances in the management of cutaneous toxicities of targeted therapies. *Seminars in Oncology, 39*(2), 227–240.

Rolz-Cruz, G., & Kim, C. C. (2008). Tumor invasion of the skin. *Dermatologic Clinics, 26*, 89–102.

Schulmeister, L. (2010). Preventing and managing vesicant chemotherapy extravasations. *Supportive Oncology, 8*, 212–215.

Roy, I., Fortin, A., & Larochelle, M. (2001). The impact of skin washing with water and soap during breast irradiation: A randomized study. *Radiotherapy and Oncology, 58*, 333–339.

Santos, C. M. C., Pimenta, C. A. M., & Nobre, M. R. C. (2010). A systematic review of topical treatments to control the odor of malignant fungating wounds. *Journal of Pain and Symptom Management, 39*(6), 1065–1076.

Shameem, R., Lacouture, M., & Wu, S. (2014). Incidence and risk of rash to mTOR inhibitors in cancer patients—A meta-analysis of randomized controlled trials. *Acta Oncologica*, doi: 10.3109/0284186X.2014.923583.

Sung, A. D., & Chao, N. J. (2013). Concise review: Acute graft-versus-host disease: Immunobiology, prevention, and treatment. *Stem Cells Translational Medicine, 2*, 25–32.

von Moos, R., Thuerlimann, B. J., Aapro, M., et al. (2008). Pegylated liposomal doxorubicin-associated hand-foot syndrome: Recommendations of an international panel of experts. *European Journal of Cancer, 44*, 781–790.

Weberschock, T., Strametz, R., Röllig, L. M., et al. (2012). Interventions for mycosis fungoides. *Cochrane Database of Systemic Reviews*, doi: 10.1002/14651858.CD008946.

Wong, R. K.S., Bensadoun, R. J., Boers-Doets, C., B., et al. (2013). Clinical practice guidelines for the prevention and treatment of acute and late radiation reactions for the MASCC Skin Toxicity Study Group. *Supportive Care in Cancer, 21*, 2933–2948.

Wu, P. A., & Cowen, E. W. (2012). Cutaneous graft-versus-host disease—Clinical considerations and management. *Current Problems in Dermatology, 43*, 101–115.

Zhang, Y., Zhang, S., & Shao, X. (2013). Topical agent therapy for prevention and treatment of radiodermatitis: A meta-analysis. *Supportive Care in Cancer, 21*, 1025–1031.

QUESTIONS

1. Which radiation treatment used to eradicate cancer cells carries the least risk for radiation dermatitis?
- A. Using electron beams to treat lymph nodes
- B. Using cobalt 60 to target tissues only 1.5 cm below skin surface
- C. Using a tangential field or a bolus
- D. Daily radiation dose of 2 Gy per day

2. A wound care nurse is caring for cancer patients receiving radiation treatment. Which patient factor does NOT place the patient at greater risk for radiation dermatitis?
- A. Diabetes mellitus as a comorbid condition
- B. Age <50 years
- C. Diagnosis of renal failure
- D. History of smoking

3. A wound care nurse is describing the clinical presentation of radiation dermatitis to a patient receiving radiation for breast cancer. Which statement accurately describes the development of this condition?
- A. "There is frequently erythema developing following the first treatment that disappears within a few hours but returns with subsequent treatments."
- B. "Persistent erythema typically becomes manifest at about treatment day 4 to 5, assuming 1.8 to 2 Gy per treatment (single-dose fraction)."
- C. "Hyperpigmentation may develop at weeks 1 to 2 due to overactivity of the melanocytes."
- D. "Moist desquamation may develop once the total dose reaches 30 to 40 Gy, resulting in partial-thickness skin loss with exposure of the dermis."

4. The wound care nurse is teaching skin care to patients receiving radiation therapy. Which teaching point follows recommended guidelines?
   A. Clean the skin three times a day with mild soap and water.
   B. Expose the treatment area to sunlight as often as possible.
   C. Do not apply topical moisturizers, gels, or emulsions before treatment.
   D. Do not use corticosteroid creams to treat itching or irritation that develops.

5. The wound care nurse is treating a patient with dry desquamation. What present strategy is being used to treat this condition?
   A. Use of hyperbaric oxygen therapy
   B. Use of topical corticosteroids
   C. Use of solid gel dressings
   D. Use of negative pressure

6. What is the role of the WOC nurse in the management of extravasation injuries related to chemotherapy?
   A. Stop the infusion immediately and notify the prescribing health professional.
   B. Aspirate any residual vesicant from the IV device using a 1- to 3-mL syringe.
   C. Assist with surgical debridement
   D. Recommend topical therapy once initial "rescue" treatment has been provided.

7. A patient receiving targeted chemotherapy with an EGRF inhibitor presents with scaly, pruritic skin; she reports that she initially had a rash but that has now resolved. The patient's current skin condition should be documented as which of the following?
   A. Xerosis
   B. Hand-foot skin reaction
   C. Paronychia
   D. Papulopustular rash

8. A wound care nurse is caring for a patient diagnosed with grade 1 hand-foot skin reaction. What is a recommended treatment for this condition?
   A. Chemotherapy treatment interruption until severity is Grade 0
   B. Pain management with systemic medications
   C. Clobetasol 0.05% daily
   D. Topical keratolytic agents for hyperkeratotic lesions bid

9. A patient is diagnosed with Stage III cutaneous T-cell lymphoma (mycosis fungoides and Sézary syndrome). What finding is characteristic of this stage of the syndrome?
   A. Skin patches and plaques that cover <10% body surface area
   B. Lymphadenopathy without nodal infiltration
   C. Pathologically positive lymph nodes
   D. The presence of generalized erythroderma

10. What treatment is a recommended intervention used to manage a patient with malignant skin lesions?
   A. Providing vigorous wound cleansing
   B. Irrigating the wound with normal saline or warm tap water
   C. Managing bleeding with warm compresses to the wound
   D. Increasing the frequency of dressing changes

ANSWERS: 1.**D**, 2.**B**, 3.**A**, 4.**C**, 5.**B**, 6.**D**, 7.**A**, 8.**C**, 9.**D**, 10.**B**

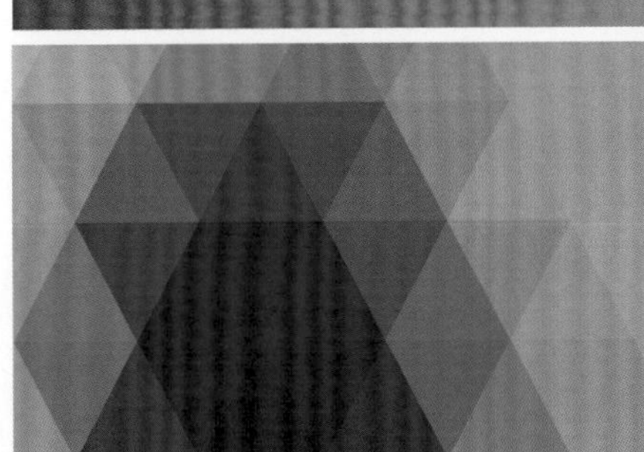

CHAPTER 30

Thermal Wounds

Burn and Frostbite Injuries

Yvette Mier

OBJECTIVES

1. Describe the pathology of burn injuries.
2. Define the following terms and discuss implications for management: zone of coagulation, zone of stasis, and zone of hyperemia.
3. Identify the criteria for referral to a burn center.
4. Describe the principles of topical therapy for thermal injuries.
5. Explain the pathology of frostbite injury and recommended management.

Topic Outline

 Introduction

Thermal wounds are unique in terms of pathology, evolution, and management, and all wound care nurses need to be knowledgeable regarding the basics of management and the indications for referral. The assessment and management of thermal injuries (burns and frostbite) are the focus of this chapter.

 Burn Wounds

Major burn injuries are one of the most severe and complex injuries the body can sustain. They create intense emotional responses in most people, including health care professionals. Associations with severe pain, sepsis, and death versus survival accompanied by gross disfigurement have been the images presented by the media for many years. Due to advances in burn care, this perception is now grossly inaccurate. Survival as the primary goal in burn care has essentially been achieved. At present, the major goal of burn care is to address and maximize quality of life (Herndon, 2012). This goal is best achieved with specialized care provided by a multidisciplinary team that includes doctors/surgeons, nurses (including the wound care nurse), physical, occupational and respiratory therapists, dieticians, social workers, case managers, pharmacists, and psychologists. Effective teams assure an equal voice for each team member, and all members understand each other's overlapping role in treating the patient as he or she moves from acute injury through recovery into long-term rehabilitation. This type of specialized, cohesive team is typically found in regional burn centers (Connor-Ballard, 2009; Simko & Culleton, 2013).

CLINICAL PEARL

Survival as a goal of burn care has essentially been achieved; at present, the major goals relate to maximizing quality of life.

Epidemiology

There are approximately 450,000 burn injuries treated in hospital emergency departments in the United States each year. Forty thousand of those individuals require hospital admission, and 30,000 require treatment at specialized burn centers. 30% to 40% of these patients are younger than 15 years; the average age of the pediatric burn patient is 32 months. Men are at greater risk for burn injuries than women (69% vs. 31%). Ethnic differences also exist: 59% of burn patients are Caucasian, 20% are African American, 14% are Hispanic, and 7% are of other ethnic backgrounds. Flame and scald injuries are most common (43% and 34%, respectively); other sources include contact burns (9%), electrical burns (4%), and chemical burns (3%), with the remaining classified as "other." The vast majority of burn injuries (72%) occur within the home; 9% occur as the result of occupational exposure, 5% occur in the street/highway, and 5% are recreational/sports-related injuries.

CLINICAL PEARL

Seventy-two percent of burn injuries occur in the home; flame and scald burns are the most common types of burns.

The annual health care cost associated with burn injuries is $7.5 billion. Current survival rate is 96.6% for adults and 99% for children. Death is more likely when the burn is associated with anoxic brain injury due to concomitant inhalation injury (Burn Incidence, 2013; Kliegman et al., 2011; Fire Deaths, n.d.).

Risk Factors

Groups at increased risk of burn injury include children <4 years of age, adults older than 65 years of age, individuals living in poverty and individuals living in rural areas. Smoking is the leading causative agent in residential fires, and 37% of fire-related deaths occur in homes without working smoke detectors. Alcohol consumption is associated with 40% of all residential fire deaths (Fire Deaths, n.d.).

Mechanisms of Burn Injury

Sources of burn injury include thermal burns, chemical burns, electrical burns, and radiation burns. The pathophysiology involved in each of these injuries is similar; however, each also has special considerations that guide treatment and recovery.

Thermal Burns

Thermal burns occur as the result of heat transfer, specifically through conduction, radiation, or convection. Conduction injuries occur when an object has direct contact with a heat source, such as touching a hot stove or being submerged in boiling water. Radiation involves the conversion of kinetic energy to electromagnetic energy, which then travels in space until it reaches an object and is converted back to kinetic energy. Examples of radiation-induced burn injuries would include those from a tanning bed or a heat lamp. Convection injuries involve heat carried by air currents. A burn caused by a flash explosion would be an example of this type of thermal burn (Carrougher, 1998).

Two factors determine the severity of a thermal burn injury: the temperature to which the tissue is heated and length of exposure to the elevated temperature (Carrougher, 1998). For example, water heated to 140 °F will produce a full-thickness burn in 3 seconds. Water heated to 156 °F will produce the same full-thickness burn in 1 second. In contrast to water, substances of a thicker consistency, such as grease or hot oil, will naturally have a longer contact time with the skin and will produce a deeper injury. Moving further along the same progressive viscosity spectrum, substances such as tar or candle wax would have the longest contact time with the skin and would produce the deepest burn. Of interest in this example, tar itself is not harmful and poses no health risks after it has cooled. Often by the time the burn injured patient reaches a medical facility for treatment, the tar has cooled and is no longer contributing to the severity of the burn. Tar is very difficult to remove, and its painful debridement is not immediately necessary; it can be left in place and removed over several days. (The best approach to tar removal is with the use of petrolatum jelly dressings changed every few hours.) Of course, if the tar burn covers a large surface area, the burn surgeon may elect to surgically remove the tar and associated devitalized tissue more quickly. While the depth of the burn cannot be ascertained until all of the tar is removed, these burns are almost always full thickness (Herndon, 2012).

CLINICAL PEARL

The severity of a thermal burn is determined by the temperature to which the tissue is heated and the length of exposure; thus, burns caused by viscous liquids are typically worse than those caused by water due to the greater time of exposure.

Chemical Burns

Chemical burns are caused by tissue exposure to noxious substances. The severity of the burn is directly proportional to the concentration and quantity of the agent, the length of time exposed, and the cutaneous toxicity of the agent itself. Chemical burns tend to progress until the agent is inactivated, either through tissue dissipation or dilution with sufficient amounts of water (Carrougher, 1998). Health care workers treating chemical burns should wear full personal protective equipment to prevent accidental self-exposure. Substances that cause chemical burns are classified based on pH, that is, as either alkalis or acids.

CLINICAL PEARL

Chemical burns tend to progress until the agent is inactivated (e.g., via copious irrigation with water); health care workers should wear full personal protective equipment when treating patients with chemical burns.

Alkali Burns

Alkalis are commonly found in industrial cleaning agents, oven cleaners, fertilizers, and cement. They generally produce more severe burns because they bind with cutaneous lipids to cause a reaction characterized by destruction of proteins and progressive necrosis and liquefaction of tissues, which permits the chemical to penetrate more deeply into the tissue (Evans, 2007). Copious irrigation with water is the initial treatment for this type of burn injury. Of note, within this category of burn injury, wet cement burns can be particularly challenging. Spills into workers' boots or gloves unfortunately do not become symptomatic for several hours; by that time, the injury is extensive and treatment often requires surgical debridement and grafting (Herndon, 2012).

Acid Burns

Acids are commonly found in household bathroom cleansers, swimming pool chemicals, and industrial drain cleaners. These burn injuries are characterized by coagulation necrosis and protein precipitation; these tissue reactions create a barrier within the exposed tissue that self-limits further penetration of the acid. Hydrofluoric acid (HF) burns constitute a major exception to this "rule of thumb" in management of acid burns. HF is the strongest known inorganic acid; it rapidly penetrates deeply into the tissue and acts as a metabolic poison that binds calcium and magnesium, which can produce cardiac dysrhythmias. As is true of cement burns, there is frequently a delay between exposure to HF and the onset of symptoms. When the patient does present for treatment, it is imperative to identify the concentration of the acid. The concentration can usually be found on the label of the container or on a Material Safety Data Sheet. Treatment of low-concentration HF burns involves copious irrigation with water and topical application of calcium gluconate gel. In burns involving higher concentrations, treatment can be as extreme as amputation or urgent surgical excision of the burned site (Evans, 2007; Herndon, 2012). Burns as small as 2% total body surface area (TBSA), with an HF concentration of 10%, can be potentially life threatening due to systemic hypocalcemia.

Vesicant Burns

Vesicant burns are typically associated with military injuries or terrorist attacks, and are considered a possible threat in the United States following the attacks on the World Trade Center on September 11, 2001. Vesicant agents include sulfur mustard, nerve gas, lewisite, and phosgene oxime. The exact mechanism of action for these agents is not completely understood; it is believed that they damage cellular DNA, causing progressive cellular necrosis. Clinical presentation usually involves pain, severe pruritus, and blister formation; when the blisters rupture, amber fluid is released and shallow ulcerations remain. Treatment is lavage with copious amounts of water. Injuries associated with vesicant-induced burns would be triaged in community hospitals prior to transfer to burn units (Atiyeh and Hayek, 2010; Carrougher, 1998; Herndon, 2012).

Electrical Burns

Electrical burn injuries are divided into four separate groups: high voltage (more than 1,000 V), low voltage (<1,000 V), lightning strikes, and electric arc injuries. The severity of an electrical burn is dependent on the type of current, the pathway of the flow, the resistance of the tissue involved, and the duration of contact. If the current flows through the heart, brain, or visceral organs, the damage can be devastating. It is important to note that complications associated with electrical burns can be immediate or delayed (Carrougher, 1998; Evans, 2007).

Voltage Injuries

Voltage injuries are the most common type of electrical burn and are usually associated with alternating current (AC). With AC, the electricity flows back and forth between the power source and the entry point on the patient's body.

This can cause cardiac dysrhythmias and/or skeletal muscle and diaphragmatic tetany. Direct current (DC) injuries are most commonly associated with lightning strikes; however, the use of direct current can also be found in industrial settings. Direct current injuries flow in one direction (Carrougher, 1998; Evans, 2007).

CLINICAL PEARL

The severity of an electrical burn is determined by the type of current, direction of flow, tissue resistance, and duration of contact; if the current flows through the heart, brain, or visceral organs, the damage can be devastating.

Electrical current always follows the path of least resistance through the body. It flows from the point of contact (entry wound) to the ground (exit wound). Tissue resistance is the most important factor in determining direction of flow and amount of heat generated. Different tissues offer different levels of resistance; the greater the resistance, the greater the amount of heat generated. Skin resistance varies based on the condition of the skin; thicker, callused, and even dirty skin has higher resistance than clean, wet skin. The path followed by the electrical current is usually along the nerves and blood vessels; however, the path can also be along the bones. As the electricity travels under the intact skin, heat is dissipated, which causes necrosis of the underlying tissue. If the heat is dissipated along the very dense bone, it causes necrosis of the adjacent muscle (Carrougher, 1998; Evans, 2007; Herndon, 2012).

Arc Burns

Arc burns occur when electricity flows alongside but external to the body; as the electricity jumps from the point of contact to the ground, it causes the air between the two points to become superheated. Arc burns are most commonly associated with high-tension wires. Since the body is never in contact with the actual current, there are no systemic electrical consequences (heart dysrhythmia); it is the joints in close proximity to the superheated air that are at highest risk for injury. Arc burns most frequently occur when the elbow is in a flexed position and present as visible burn wounds on the volar aspect of the wrist and the antecubital fossa (Carrougher, 1998; Evans, 2007; Herndon, 2012).

Compartment Syndrome

Electrical burns frequently require early surgical intervention, due to the development of compartment syndrome secondary to edema in the fascial compartments. Peripheral pulses must frequently be assessed; the patient must also be monitored for symptomatic progressive neuropathy and pain, which typically precedes pulse loss. Deep tissue necrosis following electrical injury must quickly be identified and treated to avoid life-threatening metabolic acidosis and myoglobinuria resulting in acute renal failure. Wide tissue debridement, fasciotomies, and even limb amputation may be necessary for survival (Carrougher, 1998; Evans, 2007; Herndon, 2012).

CLINICAL PEARL

When treating a burned extremity, vascular assessment is imperative. Be creative in the application of a dressing to this area so that the bedside nurse can check pulses and sensory function regularly without doing a complete dressing change.

Neurologic Symptoms

Neurologic symptoms occur in more than 50% of all cases involving electrical burns. Immediate symptoms can include para or quadriplegia and an altered level of consciousness. These symptoms usually resolve within a few days. Delayed symptoms can begin a few days after injury or several years later. Delayed symptoms include seizures, headaches, and memory loss. If the electrical burn involves the head, there is a high risk of ocular disorders, most commonly cataracts (Evans, 2007).

CLINICAL PEARL

Electrical burns are commonly associated with compartment syndrome, neurologic symptoms, and delayed complications.

Radiation Burns

Radiation burns are the rarest kind of burn. They occur with exposure to ionizing radiation. Tissue damage occurs when radiant energy is transferred to the body, stimulating the formation of highly reactive chemicals. When these chemicals interact with normal body chemicals, they form cellular toxins that target rapidly growing cells. The areas of the body with the most rapidly growing cells involve the skin, GI tract, and bone marrow. The severity of radiation damage is commensurate to the amount of exposed body surface and length of time exposed. Treatment involves decontamination and wound care (Carrougher, 1998; Herndon, 2012).

Inhalation Injury

Inhalation injury is the most common and lethal concomitant injury associated with burn injuries. The three types of inhalation injuries include carbon monoxide poisoning, upper airway inhalation injury, and lower airway inhalation injury. Carbon monoxide poisoning causes asphyxiation and is responsible for the majority of deaths associated with fires. Asphyxiation occurs prior to the burn injury, if a burn injury occurs at all (Evans, 2007).

Inhalation injuries involving the upper airway are heat related. Edema above the glottis develops rapidly and causes airway obstruction. Patients admitted with facial burns, singed nasal hairs, dyspnea, carbonaceous sputum, disorientation, anxiety, and/or hoarseness, should be monitored closely for airway edema. Intubation with mechanical ventilation is required until the edema is resolved (Carrougher, 1998; Evans, 2007).

CLINICAL PEARL

Inhalation injury is the most common and lethal concomitant injury associated with burn injury; thus, the nurse should closely monitor any patient with facial burns, singed nasal hairs, dyspnea, disorientation, anxiety, or hoarseness for airway edema.

Inhalation injuries involving the lower airway are usually the result of noxious chemicals produced from combustion reactions that occur during the normal course of a fire. This commonly occurs when the fire is located in a small, enclosed space. The noxious chemicals cause damage to the mucosa in the distal airways, which results in sloughing of the damaged mucosa 1 to 3 days post-injury. Clinically, the patient presents with distal airway obstruction, atelectasis, pneumonia and/or respiratory failure requiring mechanical ventilation with aggressive pulmonary toileting (Evans, 2007).

Pathophysiology and Management of Burn Injury

There are numerous medical conditions that, as a result of their pathophysiology, result in significant tissue loss. These include necrotizing fasciitis, Stevens-Johnson syndrome, epidermolysis bullosa, toxic epidermal necrolysis, and staphylococcal scalded skin syndrome. In all of these conditions, there is a period of acute physiologic stress, inflammation, edema, hypermetabolism, hemodynamic instability, core body temperature variations, glycolysis, proteolysis, and lipolysis. It can also be correctly argued that these responses are present in all critically ill trauma and surgical patients. However, burn injuries differentiate themselves from all of these cases based on the severity, length, and overall amplitude of the physiologic response (Townsend et al., 2012).

The pathophysiology and management of a thermal injury can be conceptualized as an ongoing process involving three stages: emergent, acute /wound management and rehabilitative. The first 72 hours is considered the "emergent phase." The focus of this phase is hemodynamic stabilization through fluid resuscitation and early wound management. This is followed by the acute wound management phase. As the name implies, the focus of this phase is wound management, which includes debridement and skin grafting along with general support for wound healing. When the wounds are healed, the final phase begins. The rehabilitative phase can last for months or years depending on the severity of the burn. The focus in this phase is on maximizing functional capacity and psychosocial adaptation and returning the patient to the highest quality of life possible (Evans, 2007).

CLINICAL PEARL

The major phases of burn injury and care are the emergent phase (fluid resuscitation and initial wound care), acute wound management (debridement and skin grafting along with nutritional support and glycemic control), and rehabilitation (physical and psychosocial support for resumption of lifestyle to greatest extent possible).

Generally, burns smaller than 30% TBSA produce a local response only. However, burns larger than 30% TBSA produce both a local and systemic pathologic response.

Local Response

The local response to injury is unique to burns and includes three zones of injury: zone of coagulation, zone of stasis, and zone of hyperemia (Fig. 30-1). The zone of coagulation is the point of the most severe damage. Tissue destruction in this area is irreversible due to the coagulation of cells and the denaturing of proteins. If damage extends through the dermis, it is a full-thickness burn injury. If the damage is confined to the tissue above the dermal appendages, the burn is a partial-thickness injury (Evans, 2007; Hettiaratchy & Dziewulski, 2004).

CLINICAL PEARL

Small burns (<30% TBSA) usually trigger only a local response; larger burns trigger both local and systemic responses.

Surrounding the zone of coagulation is the zone of stasis. This area is characterized by decreased tissue perfusion

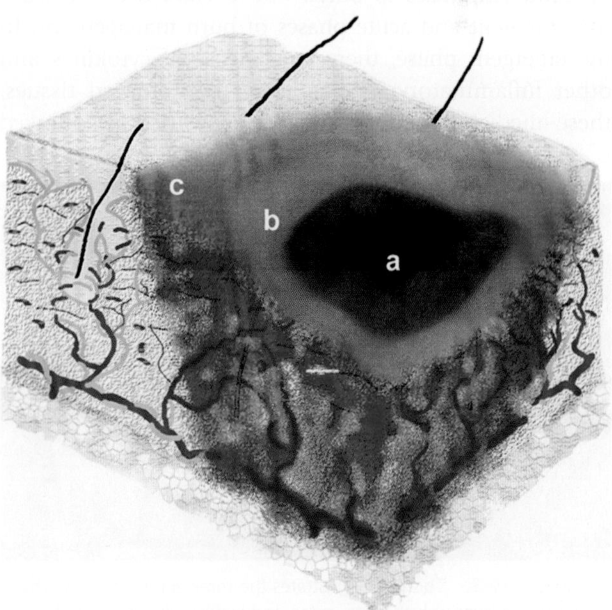

FIGURE 30-1. Zones of injury correlate to the depth of injury. "A" is the zone of necrosis. "B" is the zone of stasis. "C" is the zone of hyperemia. (Reprinted with permission from Mulholland, M. W., Maier, R. V., et al. (2006). *Greenfield's surgery scientific principles and practice* (4th ed.). Philadelphia, PA: Lippincott Williams & Wilkins.)

due to vessel constriction and thrombus formation producing transient ischemia. Tissue damage in this area is potentially reversible with appropriate fluid resuscitation, which promotes tissue perfusion. It is for this reason that the initial management of a burn injury focuses on this zone to preserve as much tissue as possible. However, pre-existing medical conditions can have a significant impact on the clinical course of the burn injury. Comorbidities such as diabetes, COPD, CHF, morbid obesity, and hypertension, and potential burn complications, such as infection, prolonged hypotension and edema, can all further compromise tissue perfusion and lead to irreversible tissue necrosis (Evans, 2007; Hettiaratchy & Dziewulski, 2004; Herndon, 2012; Orgill & Ogawa, 2013).

CLINICAL PEARL

There are three "zones" of burn injury: the central zone of coagulation (irreversible damage); a surrounding "zone of stasis," which may progress to tissue loss or may recover, depending on management; and an outer "zone of hyperemia," which heals in <21 days if managed appropriately.

The zone of hyperemia is the outermost area of burn injury. This area is characterized by vasodilation and inflammation, which manifests clinically as an outer zone of erythema. This zone is usually a partial-thickness injury and will thus heal in <21 days unless complicated by infection or prolonged hypoperfusion (Fig. 30-2) (Evans, 2007; Hettiaratchy & Dziewulski, 2004).

Systemic Response

Systemic responses to burns >30% TBSA occur in both the emergent and acute phases of burn management. In the emergent phase, there is a release of cytokines and other inflammatory mediators by the damaged tissues; these mediators cause initial vasoconstriction followed

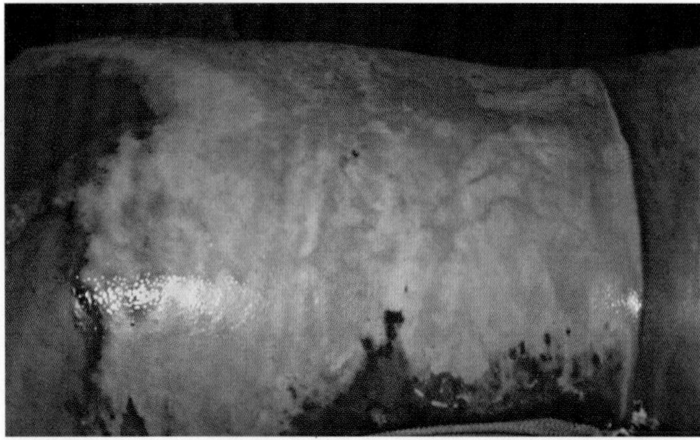

FIGURE 30-2. This photo illustrates the three zones of injury. The center of the burn, which appears tan and leathery, is the zone of necrosis. Surrounding that zone, notice the moist, pale, pink tissue. This is the zone of stasis. The outermost rim, which appears bright red, is the zone of hyperemia. (Reprinted with permission from Mulholland, M. W., Maier, R. V., et al. (2006). *Greenfield's surgery scientific principles and practice* (4th ed.). Philadelphia, PA: Lippincott Williams & Wilkins.)

by vasodilation and increased capillary permeability. The increased permeability permits plasma proteins to leak into the surrounding tissue, leading to changes in osmotic pressure that cause a significant loss of plasma into the tissues. The ultimate result is third spacing and the gross edema associated with burn injury, as well as the potential for severe hypovolemia and multisystem organ failure. Edema not only occurs at the site of injury but also is generalized throughout the body. Pulmonary edema can be a serious complication; even in the absence of an inhalation injury, the lungs are expressly susceptible to edema following a major burn (Evans, 2007; Herndon, 2012; Kliegman et al., 2011).

Fluid Resuscitation

Adequate fluid resuscitation during the emergent phase of burn management is imperative to prevention of multisystem organ failure. Loss of plasma volume (hypovolemia) translates into generalized hypoperfusion of all tissues including the heart, which results in decreased cardiac output. Decreased cardiac output in turn causes decreased blood flow to the kidneys and GI tract. Decreased blood flow to the kidney reduces glomerular filtration and, if left untreated, leads to tubular necrosis and acute renal failure. Decreased blood flow to the GI system causes mucosal atrophy, which limits the ability to absorb nutrients, and reduces peristalsis. Decreased peristalsis predisposes the patient to ileus and a type of stress ulcer known as a Cushing's ulcer. Diminished blood flow to the bowel mucosa also causes increased intestinal permeability, which adversely affects the function of the immune system; this is important because a healthy immune system is vital to surviving a major burn injury (Evans, 2007; Herndon, 2012). Fluid resuscitation is calculated based on the TBSA involved, age of the patient, presence or absence of inhalation injury, and preburn comorbidities.

CLINICAL PEARL

Prompt and adequate fluid resuscitation is essential to prevention of multisystem failure; aggressive nutritional support and glycemic control are also critical elements of systemic support because burn injuries result in a hypermetabolic state and impaired glucose metabolism.

Nutritional Support

As hemodynamic stability returns, and the patient moves from the emergent phase to the acute phase of burn management, there is a consistent release of catecholamines, glucocorticoids, glucagon, and dopamine. This slowly propels the patient into a hypermetabolic state, which ultimately leads to a catabolic state. It is for this reason that aggressive nutrition protocols are paramount to survival (Herndon, 2012).

Burn-injured patients sustain extreme metabolic stress, which persists for up to 3 years post injury. This means that nutritional needs must be continually monitored and met to avoid malnutrition. Patients who are unable to consume enough protein, fat, carbohydrate, vitamins (vitamin C and zinc), trace minerals and amino acids (glutamine and arginine) will require supplemental nutrition. This is essential because nutritional deficiencies impede fibroblast proliferation, collagen synthesis, and ultimately epithelial migration. When supplemental nutrition is required, as is the case in most large burns, enteral nutrition is preferred to parenteral nutrition. This is because enteral nutrition helps maintain the structural and functional integrity of the gastrointestinal tract. Enteral nutrition is started early to prevent atrophy of the villi within the GI tract. If enteral nutrition is delayed, the intervening atrophy of the villi results in reduced absorption and poor tolerance, which is manifest by diarrhea. There are numerous formulas that exist to calculate the specific needs of each patient; formulas take into account age, preburn or "dry" weight, depth of the burn, and percentage of the TBSA affected (Carrougher, 1998; Evans, 2007; Kavalukas & Barbul, 2010).

CLINICAL PEARL

The nurse managing a burn wound in an outpatient setting must not forget to monitor the individual for weight loss and to intervene as needed to manage the hypermetabolic state and to assure sufficient support for healing.

Management Hyperglycemia

Other postburn metabolic phenomena include impaired glucose metabolism and insulin sensitivity, which can last up to 12 months post injury. This is a difficult problem to manage in any patient; it is an immense problem in patients with a comorbid diagnosis of diabetes or prediabetes. Also of note, there is a 10- to 50-fold elevation in corticosteroid levels that persist up to 3 years after burn injury, which increases the risk of hyperglycemia and also renders the individual more susceptible to disease (Townsend et al., 2012; Somerset et al., 2014).

Persistent hypermetabolism and associated hyperglycemia are areas of active research in burn management. The beta adrenergic blocker, propranolol, is currently providing the most effective management of burn-induced catabolism. The optimal target for glucose control in burn-injured patients is elusive and a source of controversy. Maintaining blood glucose levels below 110 mg/dL through the administration of insulin reduces mortality, infection, and sepsis. It has also been proven to assist in the resolution of acute kidney injuries and in the weaning of patients from mechanical ventilation. Research also suggests that tight glucose control parlays into better outcomes in long-term rehabilitation. However, attempts to maintain glucose levels below 110 mg/dL are also associated with 4 times the number of serious hypoglycemic episodes and associated adverse events. Thus, maintaining blood glucose levels below 150 mg/dL is the more accepted target at present (Townsend et al., 2012).

Burn Wound Evaluation

The classification of burn injury severity is largely based on the size and depth of the injury. The location, however, is also an important factor to consider when determining severity.

Size (TBSA)

The size or extent of a burn injury is expressed in terms of the percentage of TBSA affected. Accurate assessment is essential as it guides initial management. TBSA is used both to calculate adequate fluid resuscitation and to predict the physiologic response. There are several methods of calculating TBSA. The most common method is known as "the rule of nines" (Fig. 30-3). The rule of nines divides the body into sections, with each section corresponding to a percentage of TBSA for an average adult. Because a child's body sections are proportioned differently than an adult's, a modified TBSA chart must be used. There is a child-specific chart based on the "rule of nines"; however, the pediatric Lund-Browder chart is more accurate and is more commonly used in assessing TBSA for a child (Fig. 30-4). If the burn pattern involves scattered, small areas, calculating TBSA can be more challenging. As a general rule, the area from the crease of the wrist to the crease of the base of the fingers (palm) on the patient's hand is considered 1% and total TBSA can be crudely calculated with this method. Accuracy of TBSA assessment varies, depending on the method chosen and

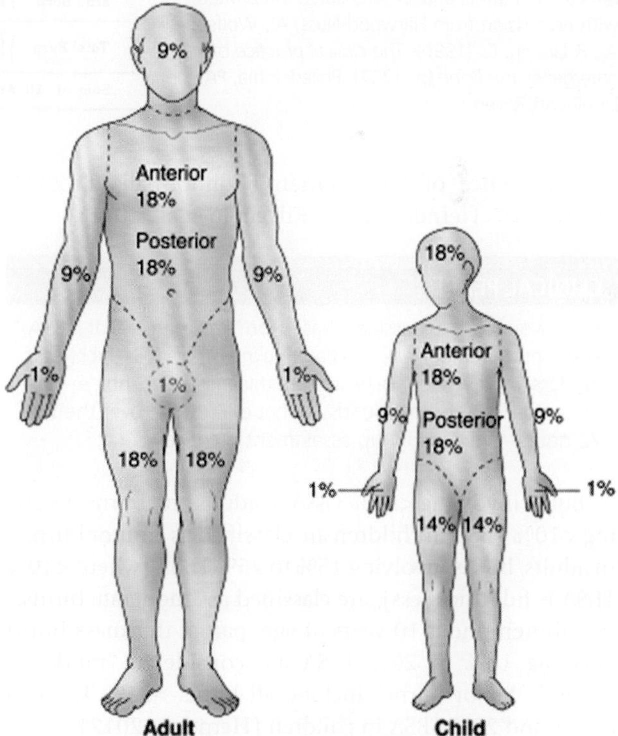

FIGURE 30-3. "The rule of nines" chart is used to determine percentage of TBSA affected in adults. The modified pediatric chart can be used to assess children; however, the pediatric Lund-Browder chart is preferred. (Reprinted with permission from Mulholland, M. W., Lillemoe, K. D., Doherty, G. M., et al. (2011) (Eds.), *Greenfield's surgery: Scientific principles & practice* (5th ed.). Philadelphia, PA: Lippincott Williams & Wilkins.)

BURN SHEET

Name________ Age______ Number______

Burn Record. Ages—Birth-7½ Date of Observation______

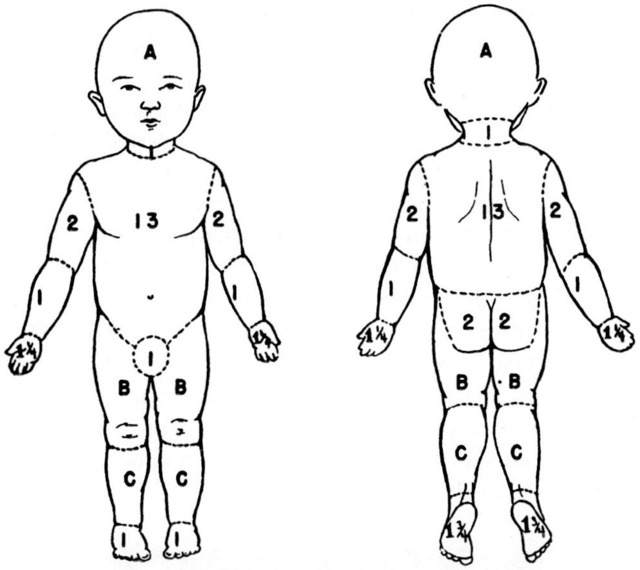

RELATIVE PERCENTAGES OF AREAS AFFECTED BY GROWTH

Area	Age 0	1	5
A = ½ of Head	9½	8½	6½
B = ½ of One Thigh	2¾	3¼	4
C = ½ of One Leg	2½	2½	2¾

% BURN BY AREAS

Probable 3rd° Burn { Head___ Neck___ Body___ Up. Arm___ Forearm___ Hands___
Genitals___ Buttocks___ Thighs___ Legs___ Feet___

Total Burn { Head___ Neck___ Body___ Up. Arm___ Forearm___ Hands___
Genitals___ Buttocks___ Thighs___ Legs___ Feet___

Sum of All Areas___ Probably 3rd°___ Total Burn___

FIGURE 30-4. The pediatric Lund-Browder chart is used to determine percentage of TBSA affected in infants and small children. (Reprinted with permission from Harwood-Nuss, A., Wolfson, A., & Linden, C. (1996). *The clinical practice of emergency medicine* (p. 1207). Philadelphia, PA: Lippincott-Raven.)

the experience of the clinician (Connor-Ballard, 2009; Evans, 2007; Herndon, 2012; Kliegman et al., 2011).

CLINICAL PEARL

Burn wounds are classified based on size (percent of TBSA) and depth (epidermal, partial thickness, or full thickness). In classifying a wound based on thickness, the nurse must remember that burn wounds continue to evolve over the first 72 hours—thus follow-up assessment is critical.

Burns involving <15% TBSA in adults and burns involving <10% TBSA in children are classified as "minor burns." In adults, burns involving 15% to 25% TBSA (where <10% TBSA is full thickness), are classified as "moderate burns." In children under 10 years of age, partial-thickness burns affecting 10% to 20% TBSA are considered "moderate burns." "Major burns" include all burns >25% TBSA in adults and 20% TBSA in children (Herndon, 2012).

CLINICAL PEARL

Burns involving <15% TBSA in adults and <10% TBSA in children are classified as "minor burns"; burns involving >25% TBSA in adults or >20% TBSA in children are considered "major burns."

Depth

Burn depth is based on clinical examination. It may involve the epidermis only, part or all of the dermis, or may extend through the subcutaneous tissue into the muscle and bone. Nomenclature remains a general source of confusion in the medical literature when describing burn injuries. This is important to rectify so that a common vocabulary can be applied to all burn injuries. This would not only facilitate accurate communication among providers but would also be important in training and education programs (Kearns et al., 2013).

Historically, description of a burn was based on degree of injury (first, second, third, or fourth); however, this is no longer the standard of care. Burns are now classified based on the level of tissue involvement: epidermal, partial thickness, or full thickness (Herndon, 2012).

Burns involving the epidermis only are not counted when calculating TBSA. They are red, hot, and painful, but do not blister and do not involve skin loss. They typically heal in 3 to 4 days. Sunburn is an example that falls into this category. Treatment is focused primarily on comfort measures: gentle cleansing, mild analgesics for pain management, loose clothing, and use of moisturizers (Evans, 2007; Helvig, 2002; Herndon, 2012).

CLINICAL PEARL

Burns involving only the epidermis (e.g., a nonblistering sunburn) are not counted when calculating TBSA.

Partial-Thickness Burns

Partial-thickness burns extend into but not through the dermis. They are divided into two categories: superficial and deep partial-thickness burns. In the first 72 hours post burn, it can be difficult to distinguish between superficial and deep injuries due to the dynamic evolution of the burn injury; thus, ongoing assessment is essential (Herndon, 2012).

Superficial partial-thickness burns are erythematous, very painful, and blanchable to touch. They are characterized by edema, blister formation, and weeping. Superficial partial-thickness burns heal spontaneously with moist wound care within 2 weeks. A scald or flash burn would be likely examples of this type of injury. Blisters <2 cm should be left intact; large blisters should be unroofed. It is only when a large blister is unroofed that depth can be determined as larger blisters are often deep partial-thickness injuries (Fig. 30-5) (Evans, 2007; Helvig, 2002; Herndon, 2012; Townsend et al., 2012).

CLINICAL PEARL

Blisters <2 cm diameter should be left intact; large blisters should be unroofed in order to accurately assess the depth of the burn.

Deep partial-thickness burns appear paler and drier and do not blanch to the touch. Some blistering may or may not be present as these wounds are frequently intermixed with superficial partial-thickness burns (Fig. 30-6). These injuries are treated with moist wound care and typically heal in

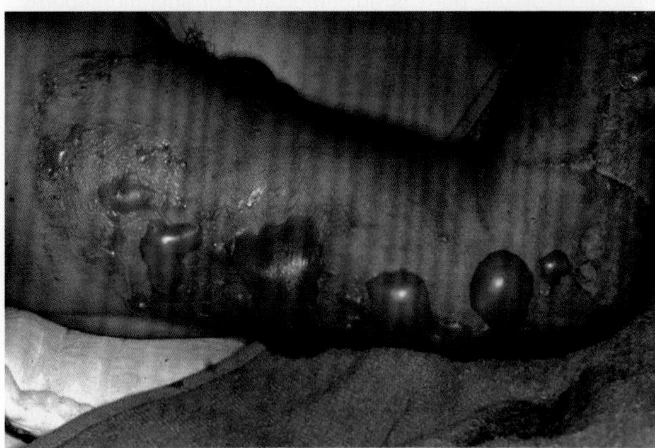

FIGURE 30-5. The partial-thickness burns on this patient's upper arm display the characteristic blisters common in this injury. In the area just below the elbow, loss of the epidermis is evident revealing a pink, moist wound bed. This is also consistent with a superficial partial-thickness burn. (Reprinted with permission from Britt, L. D., Peitzman, A., Barie, P., et al. (2012). *Acute care surgery*. Philadelphia, PA: Wolters Kluwer Health.)

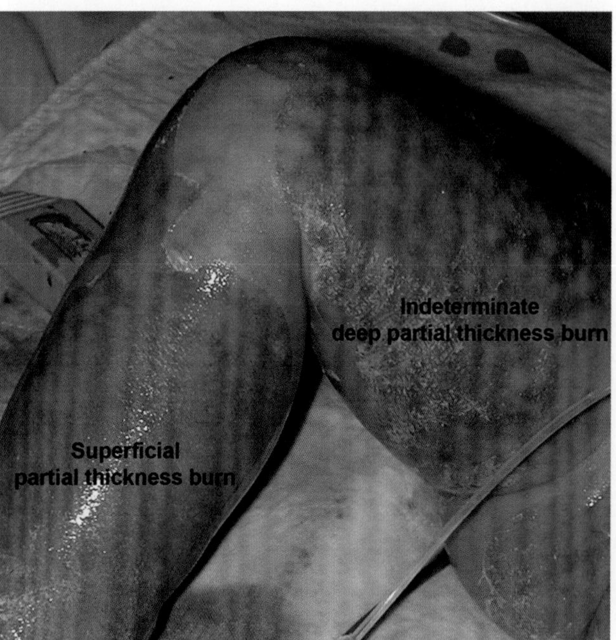

FIGURE 30-6. This photo illustrates both superficial and deep partial-thickness burns. Note the white, dry, patchy appearance on the deep partial-thickness burn compared to the consistent, moist pink appearance on the superficial partial-thickness burn. (Reprinted with permission from Mulholland, M. W., Maier, R. V., et al. (2006). *Greenfield's surgery scientific principles and practice* (4th ed.). Philadelphia, PA: Lippincott Williams & Wilkins.)

<21 days. Of note, burns that heal within 14 to 21 days exhibit reduced cohesion between the epidermis and dermis for up to 3 months. Therefore, intermittent formation of blisters in response to shearing from minor trauma is common during this time. If the injury takes longer than 21 days to heal, excision and grafting should be considered to prevent issues with hypertrophic scarring. This is particularly true if the injury is in proximity to a joint (Evans, 2007; Helvig, 2002; Herndon, 2012; Townsend et al., 2012).

CLINICAL PEARL

Most partial-thickness burns heal within 21 days with appropriate management; however, there is reduced cohesion between the epidermis and dermis for up to 3 months that results in blister formation in response to minor trauma.

Full-Thickness Burns

Full-thickness burns involve necrosis of the entire dermis and extend, at a minimum, into the subcutaneous tissue. The associated devitalized tissue is called eschar. Eschar can have different appearances depending on the depth and mechanism of the injury. Eschar appears dry, waxy, and white in thermal injuries producing coagulation of vessels in the subcutaneous tissue. If the burn extends into the deeper tissues (e.g., muscle), the appearance of the eschar may be brown, dry, leathery, and charred; this presentation is often associated with prolonged flame contact. Noncharred full-thickness burn eschar can have a mottled

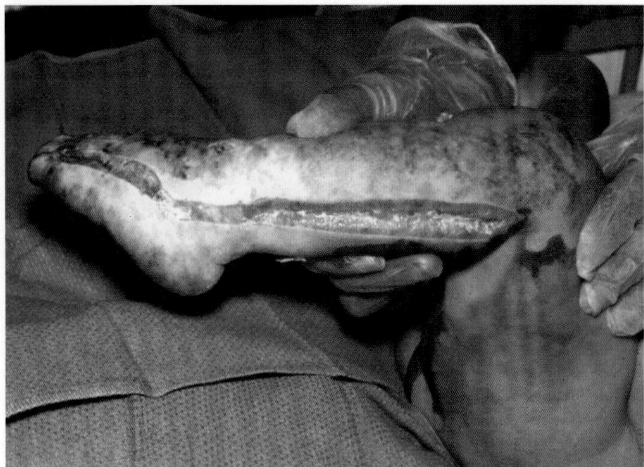

FIGURE 30-7. The full-thickness burns on the left leg and foot of this child display the leathery, dry eschar characteristic of full-thickness burns. Edema beneath the circumferential eschar necessitated the escharotomy incision evident in the midlateral line of the burned leg and the lateral aspect of the foot. (Reprinted with permission from Britt, L. D., Peitzman, A., Barie, P., et al. (2012). *Acute care surgery*. Philadelphia, PA: Wolters Kluwer Health.)

appearance (chemical burns) or a dry, cherry-red appearance (severe scald injuries). As burn-induced edema worsens, the eschar typically becomes very firm. If the eschar involves an extremity and is circumferential or close to circumferential, an emergent escharotomy is required to prevent acute arterial occlusion (Fig. 30-7). Full-thickness burns involve complete destruction of the nerves, and this fact has led to the commonly held belief that full-thickness burns are not painful. However, burns are rarely of uniform depth so what appears to be a full-thickness injury may actually include areas of painful, partial-thickness injury. Thus, the clinician must always assess the patient for pain as opposed to assuming that the wound is not painful. Full-thickness burns are treated with early excision and skin grafting to avoid secondary complications, such as infection and hypertrophic scarring (Evans, 2007; Helvig, 2002; Herndon, 2012; Townsend et al., 2012).

CLINICAL PEARL

Full-thickness burns involve eschar development; if the eschar involves an extremity and is circumferential (or close to circumferential), escharotomy is required to prevent ischemic damage. Ongoing assessment of perfusion is critical in management of patients with extremity burns; the wound nurse should assure access to pulse sites when dressing the burn.

Location

The location of a burn injury is also of critical importance. Burns involving the face require special care to prevent scarring and loss of function (Fig. 30-8). If the hands or feet are involved in the burn, care must be taken to preserve function and blood supply. Perineal burns require fastidious care; they are high risk for infection due to the presence of GI flora, which could cause the burn to evolve in depth. In addition, grafting is extremely difficult in this area, and graft failure rates are high. Burn injuries involving any joint require complex management. Grafting is almost always the best treatment because any scarring across the joint could lead to contractures. These patients need appropriate splinting, positioning, and range of motion exercises to ensure that function of the joint is preserved (Helvig, 2002).

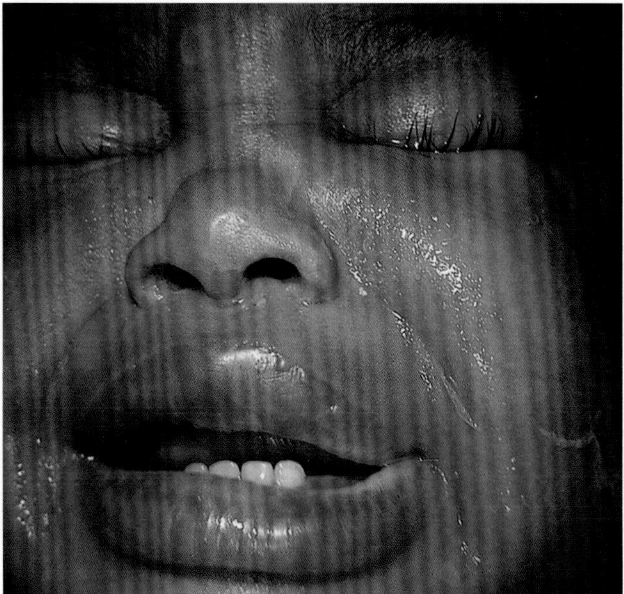

FIGURE 30-8. This facial burn is superficial partial thickness as evidenced by weeping, blistering, and edema. This child would need close monitoring of the airway; progressive edema could cause obstruction requiring mechanical ventilation. (Reprinted with permission from Fleisher, G. R., Ludwig, S., & Baskin, M. N. (2004). *Atlas of pediatric emergency medicine*. Philadelphia, PA: Lippincott Williams & Wilkins.)

CLINICAL PEARL

Location of the burn is an important consideration; burns involving the face, hands, feet, or joints require special care and consideration to minimize scarring and maintain normal function, and those involving the perineum require special care to prevent infection.

Nonaccidental Injury

The abuse of children, the elderly and dependent adults is a universal problem. It is not limited to any socioeconomic class, race, or religion. Abusers can include caregivers, family members, or institutional staff. It is estimated that up to 10% of all pediatric burns are the result of abuse (Hettiaratchy & Dziewulski, 2004). Thus, when evaluating a burn injury, the health care provider must consider whether the story told about how the injury occurred and the actual pattern of the burn correlate with one another.

Nonaccidental burn injuries can be the result of neglect or violent assault. Scald, flame and thermal contact burns are the types of burns most commonly associated with abuse. Scald burns that appear symmetrical, lack the

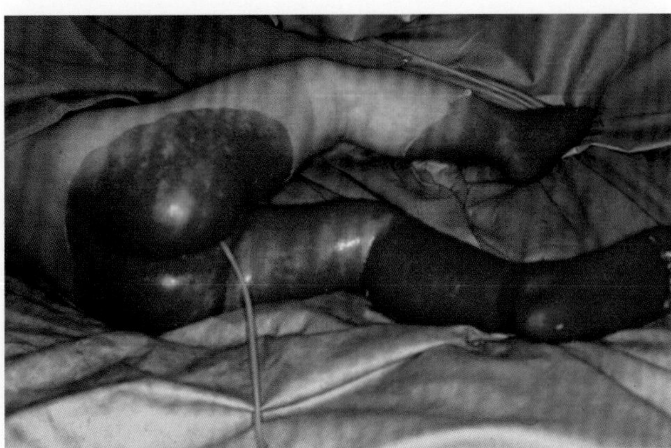

FIGURE 30-9. The distribution of the burns on this child (feet, legs, posterior thighs, buttocks, and perineum) is characteristic of abuse caused by intentional immersion scalding. Note the absence of splash burns. (Reprinted with permission from Britt, L. D., Peitzman, A., Barie, P., et al. (2012). *Acute care surgery*. Philadelphia, PA: Wolters Kluwer Health.)

presence of splash marks, and/or are on the buttocks and perineum should be of concern (Fig. 30-9). When an individual is intentionally submerged into hot liquid, there is a clear line of demarcation between the injured and healthy skin. Thermal burns caused as a result of intentional contact with a hot object, such as an iron, will "match" the exact shape of the object. An intentional burn from a cigarette appears deep and round; an accidental cigarette burn does not appear round because the natural reflex is to pull away. Any suspicion of nonaccidental injury should immediately trigger hospital admission and notification of social services (Hettiaratchy & Dziewulski, 2004; Mok, 2008).

CLINICAL PEARL

When evaluating a burn injury, the nurse must remember that abuse of children, elders, and dependent individuals is common, and must determine whether the clinical presentation matches the story being told.

Referral Criteria

The American Burn Association has established criteria to guide providers in making appropriate decisions regarding transfer of a patient to a specialized burn center. In spite of these guidelines, a recent retrospective study suggests that nearly 50% of all burn patients who meet the established criteria, are never transferred to a burn center (Fish and Bezuhly, 2012). Criteria for referral to a burn center are listed in Box 30-1. In the case of burn injury complicated by concomitant trauma, if the trauma poses greater immediate risk than the burn, the patient may be initially stabilized in a trauma center and then transferred to a burn unit. The decision in such situations is based on physician judgment, which should be consistent with the regional medical director plan and triage protocols (Burn Center Referral Criteria, 2006). The clinician should never hesitate to consult the staff of the closest burn center regarding patient

BOX 30-1. Criteria for Referral to Burn Center

1. Partial-thickness burns >10% TBSA
2. Burns that involve the face, hands, feet, genitalia, perineum, or major joints
3. Full-thickness burns in any age group
4. Electrical burns, including lightning injury
5. Chemical burns
6. Inhalation injury
7. Burn injury in patients with preexisting medical disorders that could complicate management, prolong recovery, or affect mortality
8. Any patient with burns and concomitant trauma (such as fractures) in which the burn injury poses the greatest risk of morbidity or mortality
9. Burn injured children in hospital without qualified personnel or equipment for the care of the children
10. Burn injury in patients who will require special social, emotional, or rehabilitative intervention

CLINICAL PEARL

The wound nurse must be knowledgeable regarding the criteria for referral to a burn center and must assure that all individuals who meet the criteria are appropriately referred and transferred. Wound nurses can safely treat burns that do not meet the criteria for referral.

management; they are happy to share their expertise and their input can help to assure optimal outcomes and prevent problems.

Wound care nurses can safely treat burn injuries that fall outside the ABA referral guidelines in local hospitals, and partial-thickness burns <10% TBSA can be treated in an outpatient setting (Townsend et al., 2012).

Burn Wound Care

The key elements of local burn wound care include pain management, wound cleansing, and dressing selection.

Pain Management

Before the start of any wound care procedure, preemptive pain management is essential. Pain associated with wound care is the shared experience of all burn injured patients. In addition to the effect on the patient's quality of life, the physiologic stress response to pain can actually compromise wound healing and prolong the recovery process. Because pain is a subjective sensation that is experienced differently by each individual, and because response to pain relief measures and medications is also variable, it is not possible to establish a universal protocol for managing pain in all burn patients. Unfortunately, this has led to a great deal of inconsistency in treatment of pain, and to the potential for under treatment. Thus, the wound care nurse needs to make pain assessment and management a very high priority when caring for burn patients.

CLINICAL PEARL

Preemptive pain management is a very high priority in burn care; pain management specialists should be consulted when needed for complex patients, such as those with a history of drug abuse.

Opioids are the drug of choice in treating pain during the acute phase, specifically intravenous (IV) morphine. Supplemental benzodiazepines given prior to dressing change procedures can promote relaxation and potentiate the effects of the morphine. Aspirin and nonsteroidal anti-inflammatory agents are avoided due to potential adverse effects on coagulation and the high risk of gastric ulcers (Connor-Ballard, 2009; Evans, 2007; Helvig, 2002).

As the wound heals, IV narcotics are slowly replaced with oral pain medications. Adequate pain management with oral medications alone must be achieved prior to discharge from the acute care setting. Once in the outpatient setting, hydromorphone and hydrocodone are commonly prescribed medications. Patients are given instructions to take the medication 30 minutes to 1 hour prior to the dressing change procedure to reduce pain. Short acting oral benzodiazepines, also to be taken prior to dressing change, are prescribed as necessary (Connor-Ballard, 2009; Evans, 2007; Helvig, 2002).

Physicians and nurses who are inexperienced in treating burn wounds can confuse opioid tolerance with addiction and can therefore be reluctant to prescribe or administer higher doses of narcotics. This reluctance is frequently even greater when the patient has a history of drug or alcohol abuse; many clinicians fail to realize that these patients have accelerated systemic clearance of narcotics and therefore require significantly higher doses of medications to achieve pain control (not a recreational high). The burn care team members must recognize that ineffective pain management leads to increased anxiety surrounding the dressing change procedure, which leads to a negative spiral in which anxiety further limits the effectiveness of any prescribed medication. Uncontrolled pain can also have long-term psychological consequences (Connor-Ballard, 2009; Helvig, 2002). Pain management specialists can be of tremendous benefit in assuring appropriate pain management for these complex patients, and should be consulted when available.

Cleansing

The goal of wound care is to maintain a clean, moist environment and prevent infection. Wound cleansing should be kept as simple as possible. Burn wounds are not sterile; however, meticulous attention to maintaining a clean environment while doing dressing changes is important in preventing infection. Therapy rooms where dressing changes are done should be kept warm as the burn injured patient has difficulty regulating core body temperature secondary to skin loss. Burn wounds can be cleaned with saline or a dermal cleanser. Larger burns can be gently washed in a clean shower with running water and mild soap. In the hospital setting, immersion hydrotherapy has largely been eliminated due to the risk of cross contamination and infection. Nonimmersion hydrotherapy using a table and shower head remains in use in many facilities; however, this technique is also associated with risks related to infection control, and protocols to eliminate risk must be instituted and followed. Loose, necrotic tissue can be trimmed away during the cleansing procedure (Helvig, 2002; Langschmidt et al., 2014).

Silver Dressings

Silver-based dressings have a long history in topical burn treatment. Silver is a broad-spectrum bactericidal agent that works by disrupting DNA replication. It is effective against both aerobic and anaerobic organisms, Gram-positive and Gram-negative bacteria, fungi and some viruses. Older formulations include silver nitrate and silver sulfadiazine (SSD); these dressings were considered the gold standard for decades and were effective in preventing infection. The major drawback in use of these agents is that they are rapidly inactivated by substances in the wound environment; thus, frequent dressing changes are necessary to maintain therapeutic levels of bactericidal activity. SSD remains the most widely recognized and commonly used topical burn-specific antimicrobial agent (Fish & Bezuhly, 2012; Gravante et al., 2009).

CLINICAL PEARL

Silver sulfadiazine is the most commonly used topical burn-specific antimicrobial agent; however, frequent dressing changes are needed to maintain therapeutic levels of bactericidal activity. In contrast, nanocrystalline silver dressings can maintain therapeutic antimicrobial levels for 3 to 7 days.

Nanocrystalline silver is the new gold standard in topical burn treatment, and the level of evidence supporting its use continues to grow. Silver in this form is more effective than SSD as it allows for the rapid yet sustained release of the silver ions into the wound bed. Dressings can provide therapeutic antimicrobial levels for 3 to 7 days, depending on the specific formulation and the volume of exudate. These dressings have been associated with reduced numbers of infections, reduced levels of pain related to dressing changes, and reduced length of hospital stay, all of which translate into improved clinical outcomes. Additionally, studies comparing SSD and nanocrystalline silver reveal a cost savings when costs are calculated based on overall wound care (including the cost of primary and secondary dressings, labor, and medications involved in the dressing change procedure). Nanocrystalline silver dressings are manufactured in various forms and can be found in high-density polyurethane mesh, hydrofibers, high performance fabric, or soft silicone foam. The effectiveness of one form versus another may depend on the property of the dressing in relation to the characteristics of the wound. For example, some research studies suggest that hydrofiber nanocrystalline dressings are more effective in highly exudative burn wounds as compared to high-density polyurethane mesh nanocrystalline dressings. Other research studies comparing various forms of silver dressings report no difference in days to healing, or infection; however, they do report differences in cost, ease of use and patient comfort related to specific dressings. In conclusion, more study is required before any conclusions or recommendations can be made as to the "best silver dressing" for burn care (Bauer et al., 2006; Besner et al., 2007; Fish & Bezuhly, 2012; Gravante et al., 2009; Rick et al., 2004; Townsend et al., 2012; Verbelen et al., 2014).

Honey-Based Dressings

Honey is one of the oldest documented wound care dressings; its beneficial effects appear to be due in part to its high osmolality, which inhibits bacterial growth. It is supported in the literature as effective against a broad spectrum of bacterial species, including *Pseudomonas aeruginosa.* This virulent and opportunistic species is often a worrisome problem in burn wounds; there is a high correlation between Pseudomonas burn colonization and skin graft failure. Therefore, current evidence suggests that honey can be a useful agent in the treatment of burn wounds infected with or at risk of infection with Pseudomonas (Fish & Bezuhly, 2012; Molan et al., 2002).

Sulfamylon Dressings

Mafenide acetate salve (Sulfamylon) is used, in limited capacity, on burn wounds; its use is based on the fact that it is a broad-spectrum antimicrobial agent that has the ability to penetrate eschar. However, application to any area of a burn wound with intact nerve endings may cause the patient additional pain. In addition, it cannot be used on large wounds because systemic absorption can lead to metabolic acidosis. It is most commonly used to treat deep partial or full-thickness burns to the ears or nose. These cartilaginous areas, which are not very vascular, benefit from the penetrating antimicrobial effects this agent provides (Townsend et al., 2012).

Biologic and Biosynthetic Dressings

Biologic and biosynthetic dressings are used to provide temporary coverage for wounds in which autografting is planned for definitive closure. They decrease the risk of infection, assist in regulation of core body temperature, decrease loss of fluid and proteins, and decrease overall metabolic stress. Commonly used biologic burn dressings include xenografts (pig skin) and allografts (fresh or cryopreserved cadaver skin). Xenografts are more readily available; however, allografts are considered superior as they more closely reproduce normal human skin function. Xenografts must be removed or allowed to slough prior to grafting. Allografts can act as a dermal substrate if the epithelium is removed or allowed to slough prior to grafting. Wound care involving these dressings includes daily gentle cleansing, coverage with a nonadherent gauze, and monitoring for rejection and/or signs of infection (Evans, 2007; Fish & Bezuhly, 2012; Townsend et al., 2012).

CLINICAL PEARL

Biologic and biosynthetic dressings are used to provide temporary coverage for burns in which grafting is planned for definitive closure.

Biosynthetic dressings are part biologic (usually animal) and part synthetic. The biosynthetic dressing most commonly used in burn management is Biobrane (Smith and Nephew). It is composed of porcine dermal collagen chemically bound to a nylon/silicone membrane. It is a flexible, temporary dressing used to treat partial-thickness burns and donor sites or excised full-thickness burns. It mimics the function of the skin with good fluid exchange and barrier protection. It is very flexible, which means it can be used in joint areas to allow for range of motion and normal function. Wound care is minimal. Following placement of the Biobrane, fluffed dressing and gauze wraps are applied and secured with elastic bandages to provide moderate level compression. The dressing should be left in place and undisturbed for 48 hours; at that point, the Biobrane is adherent to the wound bed and dressings are no longer needed. The area is monitored for infection until the Biobrane is removed approximately 14 days later, at which point the autograft is applied (Evans, 2007; Falanga and Lazic, 2011; Fish and Bezuhly, 2012).

Burn Wound Closure

Early excision and closure of burn wounds leads to improved outcomes, including reduced length of hospital stay, reduced numbers of infections, reduced incidence of hypertrophic scars, and reduced time for rehabilitation.

Autografts

The optimal closure of a burn wound is achieved with the patient's own skin (autologous grafting), which ideally occurs 3 to 4 days after injury. Split-thickness skin grafts (STSG) are harvested from healthy skin, with an average thickness of 0.008 to 0.0012 inches. STSG include the epidermis and a thin layer of the dermis. They can be applied as intact sheets or can be meshed to cover larger areas. Sheet grafts are used in locations that require better functional and cosmetic outcomes, such as the hands, feet, joints, face, and neck. Sheet grafts are frequently managed without a dressing in the initial postoperative period, since it is essential to closely monitor the newly placed graft for collection of fluid between the graft and the underlying wound bed. If fluid collects, it causes separation of the graft and the wound bed and failure of the graft. Any fluid accumulation must be promptly removed to promote graft adherence; this can be done through aspiration or by carefully rolling a cotton-tipped applicator over the top of the graft to express the fluid (Evans, 2007; Kliegman et al., 2011; Townsend et al., 2012).

CLINICAL PEARL

The optimal closure of a burn wound is achieved with the patient's own skin (autologous grafting), which ideally occurs 3 to 4 days after injury. The graft must be carefully monitored for any fluid accumulation between the graft and wound bed, which must be removed.

Meshed autologous skin grafts are used on larger burns; meshing facilitates coverage of a greater surface area. If the grafted area is an extremity or a joint, splints are applied to maintain a functional position. Post-operatively the meshed graft is dressed with a nonadherent layer to prevent shearing and a "bolster" dressing comprised of fluffed gauze soaked in 5% sulfamylon solution; the solution is reapplied every 2 to 3 hours to maintain efficacy. The bolster component of the dressing is designed to maintain approximation of the wound bed and the graft and is essential to normal healing and "take" of the graft. (The graft will survive only if it gets adequate blood supply from the wound bed through the ingress of capillary loops, and this process requires close adherence of the graft to the wound bed.) The initial dressing is typically left undisturbed for 5 to 7 days, at which time the dressings are removed to allow examination of the graft. Dressing changes at this time usually involve nonadherent products that support moist wound healing. Graft donor sites are treated as superficial partial-thickness burns. Dressing choice for donor sites varies greatly and ranges from Vaseline gauze to alginates to biosynthetic dressings (Evans, 2007; Orgill & Ogawa, 2013).

Full-thickness skin grafts (FTSG) are used only on small full-thickness burns, usually for reconstructive purposes. They are obtained from a full-thickness donor site where the donor skin is excised down to the subcutaneous tissue layer. Because they are thicker grafts, they are less prone to contractures and hypertrophic scarring. Donor sites are sutured closed and allowed to heal through primary intention or with placement of an STSG (Evans, 2007).

Cultured Epithelial Autografts

Cultured epithelial autografts (CEAs) have been used for many years in burns with >50% TBSA due to the limited availability of healthy donor sites. In this procedure, autologous keratinocytes are harvested and sent to a tissue lab to replicate over 3 to 4 weeks before transplantation. The epithelial cells are placed on a petrolatum-based dressing and applied to a viable wound bed. Reported success rates with CEAs alone are variable; however, recent literature reports high success rates when CEAs are used in conjunction with acellular dermal matrices. Wound care for CEAs is simple. The surgeon secures the CEA-impregnated dressing with staples and covers it with gauze. The dressing is left undisturbed for 7 to 10 days; care must be taken to avoid friction and mechanical stress at the fragile graft site. After that time, wound care is essentially the same as previously described for STSG (Evans, 2007; Fish & Bezuhly, 2012; Fang et al., 2014).

Staged Closure

In burns involving more than 30% TBSA, autologous skin grafting is not always an immediate option due to limited availability of uninjured skin. In these cases, wound closure is completed in staged procedures. The full-thickness burns are excised and, if autologous skin is not available for grafting, the open wound is covered with an acellular matrix dressing that replaces the lost dermis. This acellular dressing supports ingrowth of new blood vessels and formation of healthy granulation tissue. When autologous skin becomes available, the skin grafting procedure is completed. There are several products that are used in this capacity. The two most commonly used are Integra (Integra LifeSciences) and AlloDerm (LifeCell Corp.) (Evans, 2007; Fish & Bezuhly, 2012; Paul et al., 2001; Townsend et al., 2012).

Integra is a meshed bilayer matrix dressing that promotes neogenesis and collagen synthesis. The inner layer is composed of bovine collagen and chondroitin-6-sulfate. The outer layer is silicone sheeting, which is removed approximately 2 weeks following initial application. If there is skin appropriate for an autograft or a CEA is available at that time, grafting is done and is usually successful. Integra is advantageous because it can replace the entire dermis and can be applied directly over muscle or bone. Integra is particularly effective when used in combination with negative pressure wound therapy (NPWT). If the periwound skin integrity is insufficient to maintain NPWT, the Integra dressing is managed in the same manner as a fresh STSG (Evans, 2007; Fish & Bezuhly, 2012; Fang et al., 2014).

AlloDerm is an acellular matrix dressing derived from cryopreserved cadaver allograft. Because all of the epidermal and dermal cells are removed during processing, the final product is acellular and thus nonimmunogenic. Like Integra, it works as a scaffold to promote neoangiogenesis and collagen synthesis. However, it does have one major limitation; the STSG must be placed immediately following AlloDerm placement. Therefore, wound care associated with AlloDerm is exactly the same as wound care associated with a newly placed STSG. If a patient has limited donor skin availability and CEA is not available, this product may not be appropriate (Evans, 2007; Fish and Bezuhly, 2012).

Pressure Ulcers and Burn Patients

All patients with limited mobility are at risk for pressure ulcers. While no burn-specific literature exists, it is suspected that pressure ulcers are more problematic in the burn population due to initial hypovolemic shock followed by edema, hypermetabolism, nutritional deficits, wet dressings, and splinting with immobilization postgrafting procedures. Therefore, an aggressive pressure ulcer prevention program must be implemented. Education and involvement of the entire multidisciplinary team is vital. When the patient is too hemodynamically unstable to tolerate turning, it should be documented, and repositioning should be resumed as soon as tolerated. Precautions to avoid friction and shearing should be implemented, including low shear surfaces and use of appropriate lifting and repositioning devices. Physical and occupational therapists must be cognizant of pressure ulcer risk when constructing splints. The use of low or high air loss surfaces can be used to reduce pressure and promote evaporation of excessive moisture. When the patient is able to get out of bed, pressure relieving chair cushions should be used (Richard et al., 2004).

CLINICAL PEARL

Burn patients are thought to be at high risk for pressure ulcers; therefore, a comprehensive program of risk assessment and preventive interventions must be implemented.

Scar Formation

Full-thickness burn injuries heal through scar formation. Immediately after reepithelialization, healed skin appears pink, soft, and flat; with normal remodeling, the scar tissue remains flat. However, burn wounds are high risk for excessive scarring, either hypertrophic scar (HTS) or keloid; the likelihood of this increases as the depth of the burn increases. Hypertrophic or keloid scars become visible after a period of time that ranges from weeks to months (Carrougher, 1998).

CLINICAL PEARL

Burn wounds are high risk for excessive scarring, either hypertrophic scar (HTS) or keloid; the likelihood of this increases as the depth of the burn increases.

Hypertrophic Scar Formation

As noted, hypertrophic scar (HTS) formation is more common postburn injury as compared to other types of wounds. Risk factors that predict the formations of HTSs include age (children are at greater risk than adults), race (dark-skinned and very fair-skinned individuals are at greater risk), increased depth of burn injury, increased incidence of infection, and a prolonged number of days to healing. HTSs present as raised, thickened, firm scars that are reddish in color and that do not extend beyond the borders of the original injury (Fig. 30-10). Related complaints of pain and excessive pruritus are common (Herndon, 2012; Holland et al., 2012).

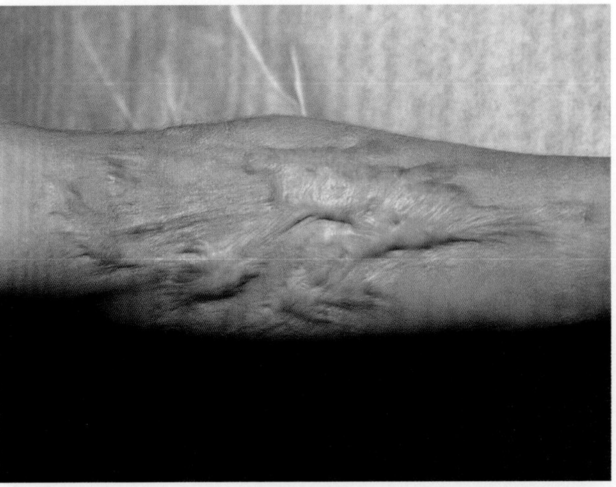

FIGURE 30-10. Hypertrophic irregular burn scar. (Reprinted with permission from Lugo-Somolinos, A., et al. (2011). *VisualDx: Essential dermatology in pigmented skin*. Philadelphia, PA: Wolters Kluwer Health.)

Treatment of hypertrophic scars is most effective if initiated early. The use of custom pressure garments has been the standard of care for many years (Fig. 30-11). Although there is little published evidence as to the exact mechanism of action for pressure garments, they have been shown to reduce scar thickness and redness as well as pruritus; in addition, pressure garment therapy is associated with reduced time to scar maturation. Garments should be worn 23 hours/day, which makes compliance with therapy sometimes challenging, especially with children. Patients and/or parents of patients must be educated and encouraged to be compliant with therapy and must understand the potential long-term ramifications of noncompliance (Evans, 2007; Herndon, 2012; Jones et al., 2008; Kliegman et al., 2011). Additional options for management of hypertrophic scars include topical silicone gel and silicone gel sheets, and intralesional injections of corticosteroid, all of which have been shown to be of benefit. In extreme cases,

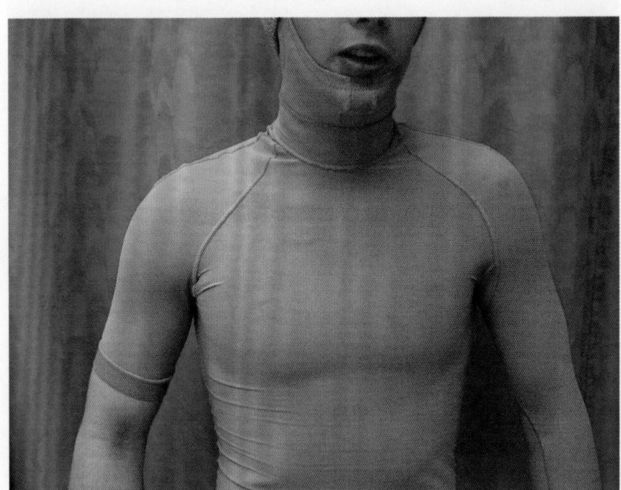

FIGURE 30-11. Custom, elastic pressure garments. Application of pressure garments helps prevent hypertrophic burn scarring. (Used with permission of Jobst Institute, Inc., Toledo, OH.)

surgical excision may be necessary for either cosmetic or functional improvement (Jones et al., 2008).

Keloid Formation

Keloid formation can occur spontaneously or in response to trauma. It is more common in dark-skinned individuals of African ancestry compared to lighter-skinned European descendants. Keloid scars appear as raised, firm, hyperpigmented nodules. They extend, sometimes dramatically, beyond the borders of the original injury. Treatment of keloids is difficult at best. There are reports of limited success with corticosteroid injection, chemotherapy agents, radiation, lasers, and surgical removal where a rim of keloid scar is left in place. Surgical removal, however, is usually not done unless the keloid becomes pendulous (Jones et al., 2008).

Pruritus

Itching is an irritating and often relentless phenomenon associated with healing and healed burn wounds. The exact etiology of the pruritus is not known though there are several theories as to cause. Increased histamine production is believed to be the primary source of itching and is thought to be related to inflammatory mediators produced during healing. Itching sensations are most intense immediately after the burn wound has healed and peaks 2 to 6 months later. Complaints of pruritus can last up to 18 months; itching that persists beyond that point is thought to have a psychogenic component. Treatment includes oral antihistamines, use of moisturizers to minimize dry skin, a cool air-conditioned environment, application of cool cloths, and compression garments (which are thought to decrease inflammation). Another less common measure is the administration of penicillin. This is based on evidence that most hypertrophic scars are colonized with *Staphylococcus aureus* and beta-hemolytic streptococcus when compared to nonhypertrophic scars (Herndon, 2012).

CLINICAL PEARL

Itching is an often relentless phenomenon associated with burn wounds; management includes moisturizers, antihistamines, pressure garments, cool cloths, and sometimes penicillin.

Traumatic Blisters in Reepithelialized Burn Wounds

Newly healed epithelium is thin and very fragile with markedly reduced cohesion between the epidermal and dermal layers; thus, minor trauma can cause small blisters to form. This can be very stressful to the patient as they are often emotionally vulnerable and fear setbacks. Patients need to be educated about blisters and reassured that the tensile strength of the epithelium will increase over time. Ruptured blisters should be treated with moist wound care (Herndon, 2012).

Psychosocial Adaptation Following Burn Injury

The traumatic nature of burn injuries has lasting physical and psychological consequences. Unfortunately, the burn patient's emotional and mental health needs are often obscured by the physical needs associated with survival. Long term, most of these patients need help in coming to terms with their changed body and psychological distress is common. Acute stress disorder, post-traumatic stress disorder and depression are observed in 45% of adult survivors. Risk factors for psychological disorders include the percentage of TBSA affected, length of hospital stay, preburn anxiety or depression disorders, and being female. There does not seem to be a correlation between the visibility of burn scars and psychological distress, but the literature does suggest that the degree of distress is related to the individual's subjective perception of how others see them. Those with a higher self-esteem preburn injury are much more likely to do well emotionally in the rehabilitative phase (Fish & Bezuhly, 2012; Logsetty et al., 2013).

CLINICAL PEARL

Acute stress disorder, post-traumatic stress disorder and depression are observed in 45% of adult survivors.

Psychosocial adaptation in the rehabilitation phase must be multifaceted and must openly address patient concerns. These concerns usually center on the ability to return to work, issues related to sexual function and sexual relationships, and the ability to return to preburn roles within the family. Adaptation is best supported through formal counseling, burn-specific support groups, and vocational retraining. In pediatric populations, a school re-entry program is necessary. These programs should be specific to the child's developmental level and educational needs. School staff and children should have the opportunity, before the patient returns, to obtain accurate information and to ask questions to reduce anxiety (Fish & Bezuhly, 2012; Kliegman et al., 2011).

CLINICAL PEARL

The Phoenix Society and World Burn Congress can offer invaluable support and resources for burn survivors; the wound nurse should encourage the individual to utilize available resources to optimize his/her mental health and adaptation.

Marjolin's Ulcers

Marjolin's ulcers are malignant ulcers, usually squamous cell, that develop in traumatized and chronically inflamed skin. Pathogenesis is not well understood; however, the biologic behavior of these malignancies is frequently more virulent than other types of skin cancers. Malignant transformation is most frequently associated with burn scars, but can also occur in scars associated with other chronic wounds. There is always a dormant period between the offending injury and the development of the ulcer. The average time to malignant transformation is 35 years post injury; although rare, acute onset can occur in weeks post injury. Treatment must be aggressive and usually includes radical excision in conjunction with radiation therapy (Copcu, 2009).

CLINICAL PEARL

Healed burns and donor sites are more susceptible to melanoma, and burn scars can also undergo malignant transformation (Marjolin's ulcer). Thus, instruction in sun protection should be a standard component of discharge teaching, and any nonhealing or deteriorating wound should be biopsied, as should recurrent wounds in previously healed burn sites.

Research and New Directions in Burn Care

The Multicenter Trial Group is a group established by the American Burn Association, with the objective of providing "best practice" data to guide burn management. Most of the studies published involve retrospective reviews of burn care in North America. It is believed this group will be the single biggest influence on the delivery of burn care over the next 10 years (Fish & Bezuhly, 2012).

The ability to accurately and expeditiously diagnose burn depth has a significant impact on clinical management and resultant outcomes. Current literature suggests that assessment based on clinical observation is only 70% accurate even among experienced burn surgeons. Noncontact laser Doppler imaging may be an answer to this problem. This technology provides a color perfusion map of the burn wound, which, in conjunction with physical exam, can improve accuracy in depth assessment. The imaging can be done daily during the emergent phase of burn management to evaluate dynamic changes in wound bed perfusion. The major barrier to implementing this technology is the associated high cost (Fish & Bezuhly, 2012; Herndon, 2012).

Expeditious closure of burn wounds is a major contributor to burn survival. Not only is closure vital, but the speed at which closure occurs affects the risk for life-threatening complications during the acute phase. Speed of closure also has long-term effects, specifically on the degree of scarring and on psychosocial adaptation in the rehabilitative phase. Thus, an ongoing area of research is identification of best and earliest approaches to burn closure. Currently, there are reports of success with cultured skin substitutes, platelet-rich plasma, and amniotic membranes (Boyce et al., 2006; Mohammadi et al., 2013).

Giving the patient the best cosmetic and functional outcome is a major focus when treating burn injuries. In reconstructive surgery, fat has been used as filler for many years. New research suggests that fat grafting could have additional benefits. Stem cells derived from fat cells are regenerative, and in vitro studies reveal a significant improvement in the texture, thickness and contours of the skin when treated with fat grafts. Current research involves ways to harvest, process and inject fat into injured sites (Ranganathan et al., 2013).

CLINICAL PEARL

Patients "see" themselves in the eyes of their caregivers and family members before they ever see a mirror; the wound nurse must monitor her/his facial expressions and must counsel the family regarding burn wound appearance when they begin to assist with dressing changes.

CASE STUDIES

CASE STUDY: 1

A 24-year-old male presents 72 hours post flash explosion involving gasoline. He was treated immediately after the incident in an urgent care center. He was instructed to change the dressing daily with silver sulfadiazine (SSD) and told to follow up in the wound center.

Wound Assessment: The patient is out of the emergent phase and is in the acute/wound care phase of management. His only comorbidity is tobacco abuse. Arm burns are not circumferential. Chest burn is epidermal only and thus not counted in TBSA assessment. TBSA is estimated at 9% with depth assessment categorized as superficial partial thickness. Patient has palpable radial pulses. He is afebrile with stable vital signs. PO intake is reported as "fair." It is safe to treat this patient on an outpatient basis. He will follow up in 3 days.

Wound Care Recommendations: Shower with mild soap and water. The possibility of any gasoline on the skin must be addressed. SSD is not the best choice, but it is not a wrong choice. The patient (who has no insurance) has already purchased several jars. Continue daily SSD dressing changes. Education regarding nutrition and smoking cessation provided. Patient given instructions to start high-protein diet and add a multivitamin and vitamin C 1,000 mg daily.

Day 6 (see figure):

Wound Assessment: Burn is not larger but more visible. Note intact hair follicles apparent in the arms. Patient is doing well. PO intake improved.

Wound Care Recommendations: Continue with current plan of care.

Day 9 (see figure):

Wound Assessment: Burns are largely healed.

Wound Care Recommendations: Moist wound care and protection from trauma. Patient will change dressing daily with wound gel and nonstick gauze.

Day 14 (see figure):

Wound Assessment: Burn is healed. Skin needs continued protection from trauma and routine application of moisturizing agents. No long-term compression therapy needed.

Wound Care Recommendations: Patient discharged with instructions: gentle skin care with moisturizer applied at least twice daily and protection from sun with use of protective clothes. Daily use of sunscreen starting in 2 weeks (skin too sensitive at present) for a minimum of 3 months.

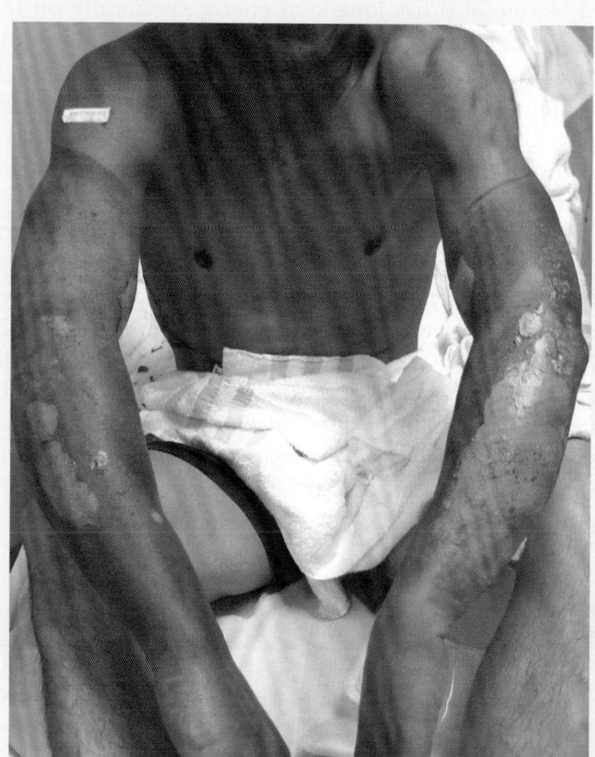

Day 6 post injury

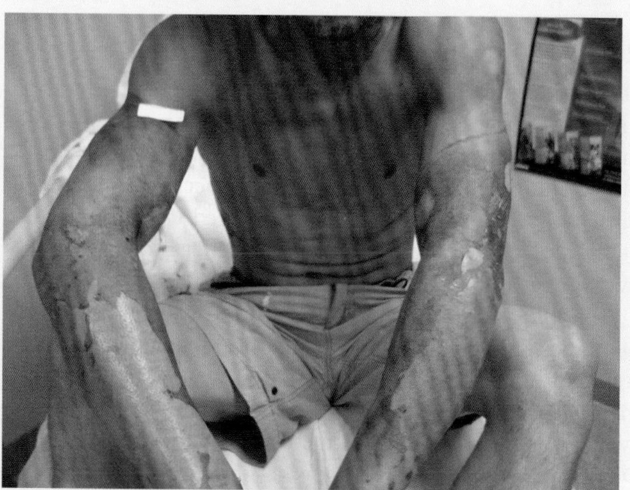

Day 9 post injury

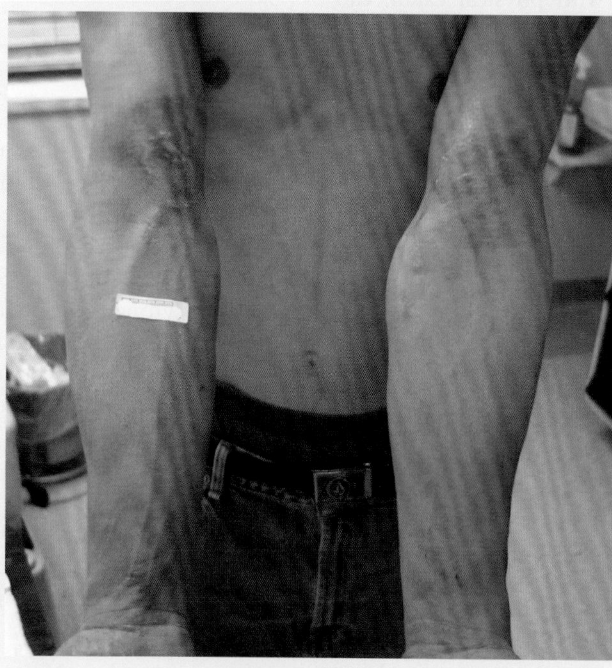

Day 14 post injury

CASE STUDY: 2

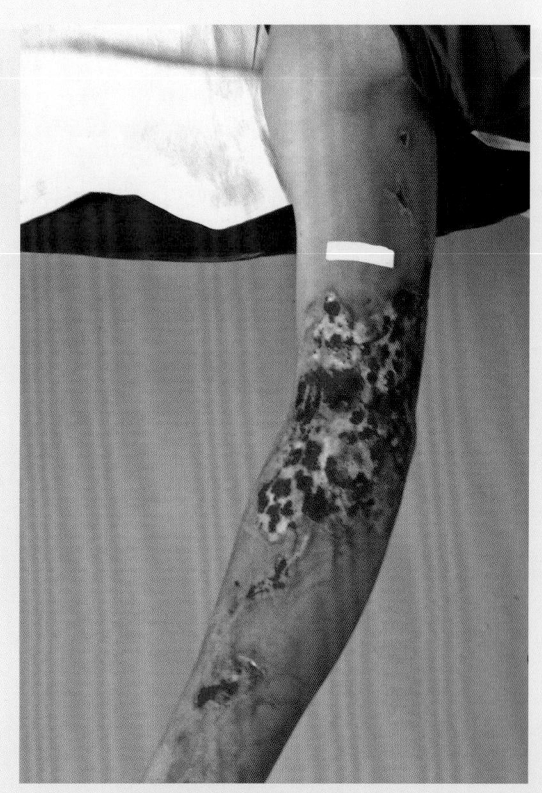

A 17-year-old male involved in motor vehicle accident. Left arm with thermal burn. Patient was admitted to a local hospital and stabilized. Wound care nurse consulted 3 days after injury.

Wound Assessment: Patient is out of the emergent phase and is in the acute/wound care phase. He has no comorbidities. The wound appears dry with white, leathery patches surrounded by red tissue indicating full thickness intermixed with deep partial thickness. TBSA is approximately 4%. The injury occurs over a major joint in an extremity. Patient has a palpable radial pulse. Patient meets criteria for transfer to a burn center.

Wound Care Recommendations: Wound cleansed with NS and a nanocrystalline silver dressing applied. Formal recommendation to transfer patient to a burn center made to attending physician. She was in agreement and patient was transferred within 24 hours. Follow-up report provided by the burn unit indicated that the patient was treated with surgical excision of the burn-injured tissue and placement of STSG.

CASE STUDY: 3

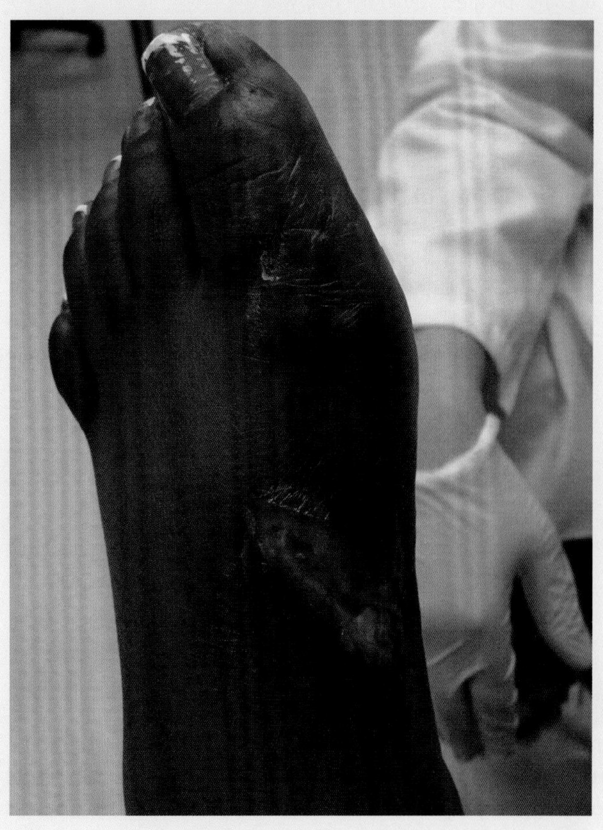

A 47-year-old female is referred from her primary care provider to an outpatient wound center for podiatry evaluation of burns to her feet. The burns occurred 5 days prior when she fell asleep in front of a space heater. Medical history includes non–insulin-dependent diabetes (A1c 6.2) and hypertension. She denies any history of tobacco use or alcohol use.

Wound Assessment: This patient is out of the emergent phase and in the acute/wound care phase. TBSA is 1% per foot. Burns in dark-skinned individuals are more difficult to evaluate than burns in lighter-skinned persons. Note the discoloration of the great toe—appears blistered—unable to determine accurate depth at this time. There is a similar burn to the right foot (not pictured). The burn to the left dorsal midfoot is characterized by eschar surrounded by pink tissue. This burn is full thickness. Bilateral lower extremities with +1 edema. Bilateral dorsalis pedal and posterior tibial pulses are Doppler identifiable only. Weinstein monofilament test reveals loss of protective sensation.

Wound Care Recommendations: Vascular status is unclear, and immediate referral to a vascular surgeon for an arterial duplex study was made. In the interim, toe blisters painted with betadine. Midfoot burn wounds treated with nanocrystalline silver dressing. Patient placed in offloading shoe. Education provided regarding role of nutrition and glucose control in wound healing.

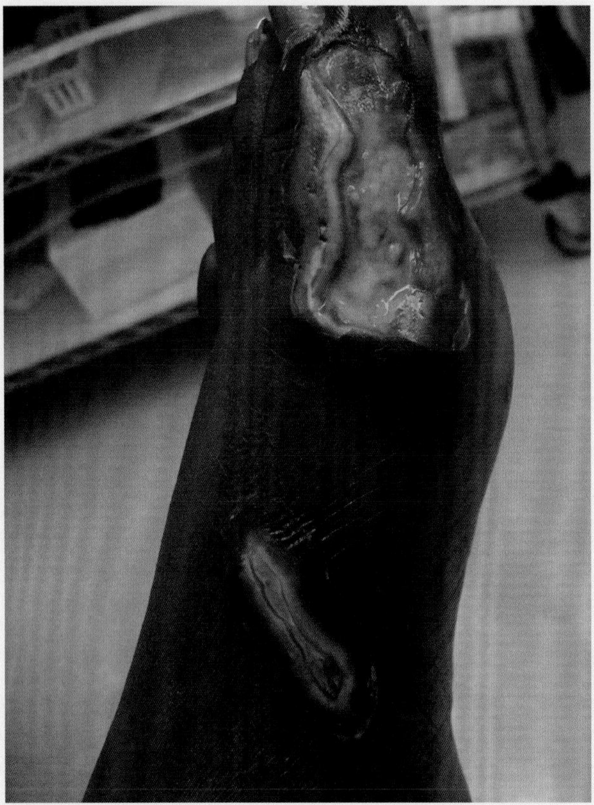

Postburn injury day 12. Arterial study revealed bilateral lower extremities with an ABI of 0.6. Vascular surgeon believes healing potential is marginal and would like to be reconsulted if wound does not progress within the next week.

Day 12 (see figure):

Wound Assessment: Right foot burns appear unchanged (not pictured). Left great toe foot blister now appears as dry pink tissue surrounding adherent slough. Depth of this burn is deep partial thickness.

Wound Care Recommendations: Wounds cleansed with NS and treated with nanocrystalline silver dressings. Due to ABI, recommended evaluation for adjunctive hyperbaric oxygen (HBO) therapy. Continued to educate patient regarding role of nutrition and glucose control in wound healing.

Postburn day 14:

Patient went for HBO evaluation and testing revealed good response to HBO therapy. HBO facility recommended 5 treatments per week for the next 6 to 7 weeks. However, patient reports she cannot afford her $100 per dive copay and declined therapy. No change in appearance of wounds.

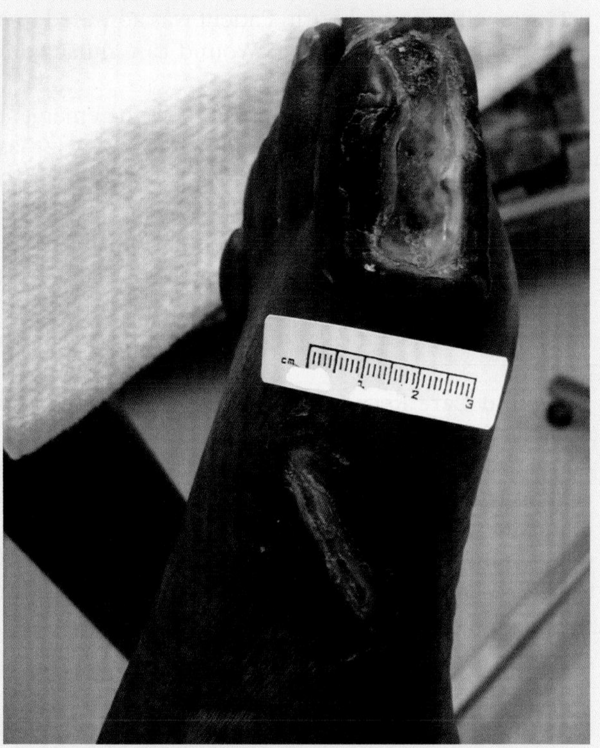

Postburn day 19

Day 19 (see figure):

Wound Evaluation: Deterioration of left great toe burn wound. Appearance is dry and leathery. No change in right foot burn wounds (not pictured).

Wound Care Recommendations: Reconsult vascular surgery. Wounds cleansed with NS and treated with nanocrystalline silver dressings.

Ultimate Outcome: Patient was admitted into the hospital for an arteriogram, and a stent was placed to left leg to improve blood flow. Unfortunately, the small vessels feeding the left great toe were calcified secondary to pathology associated with diabetes. Two days after discharge from the hospital, the patient's blood sugar spiked to 350. She was again admitted into the hospital for treatment. While there, the left foot became gangrenous and a life-saving below-the-knee amputation was done. The patient has since adapted well and has returned to her normal life with the aid of a prosthetic limb. The right foot healed completely.

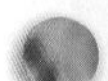 Frostbite

Frostbite is a traumatic injury that occurs when tissue temperature falls below freezing. It is a relatively common injury in the United States in the homeless population and among individuals living in lower socioeconomic urban areas. Additionally, frostbite is seen in association with outdoor winter recreational activities. It is a local injury that usually is seen on the extremities or the face. Predisposing factors include alcohol and drug use, mental illness, and motor vehicle accident or failure of a motor vehicle (Herndon, 2012; Koljonen et al., 2004; Woo et al., 2013).

CLINICAL PEARL

Frostbite is a relatively common injury in the homeless population and those living in lower socioeconomic urban areas; it is most likely to involve the face or extremities.

Pathophysiology

The pathophysiology of frostbite has two distinct mechanisms. The initial injury occurs at the time of exposure and involves cellular damage and death due to the formation of ice crystals. Depending on the speed at which the tissue temperature drops, ice crystal formation can be intracellular or extracellular; intracellular ice crystals are associated with rapid cooling and are more damaging. The second mechanism of injury in frostbite occurs following tissue thawing and involves thrombosis and progressive damage to the microcirculation, resulting in progressive tissue ischemia and dermal necrosis (Herndon, 2012; Koljonen et al., 2004).

CLINICAL PEARL

There are two pathologic mechanisms involved in frostbite: cell damage due to ice crystal formation and microcirculatory changes occurring following thawing.

Classification of Injury

Frostbite classification is based on depth and resembles burn classifications. It is classified as frostnip, superficial frostbite, and deep frostbite.

Frostnip

When a frostnip injury occurs, the skin becomes very pale and sensation is slowly lost. When rewarming occurs, the skin becomes hyperemic. Paresthesia can persist for several weeks, but there is no significant tissue damage with frostnip (Herndon, 2012; Koljonen et al., 2004).

Superficial Frostbite

Superficial frostbite is subdivided into first- and second-degree frostbite. With first-degree frostbite, there is partial freezing limited to the superficial layers of the epidermis; initial characteristics of first-degree frostbite include erythema, edema, and hyperemia. Superficial skin desquamation may occur 5 to 10 days post injury (Fig. 30-12), but there is no long-term tissue damage. With second-degree frostbite, there is freezing of the entire epidermis; these wounds are characterized by significant edema, erythema, and the formation of vesicles filled with clear fluid (Fig. 30-13). As these wounds evolve, there is skin loss (desquamation) and eschar formation.

CLINICAL PEARL

First-degree frostbite is manifest by erythema, edema, and superficial skin desquamation 5 to 10 days post injury, but no long-term damage. Second-degree frost bite is manifest by edema, erythema, and blister formation; these wounds evolve to skin loss and possible eschar formation.

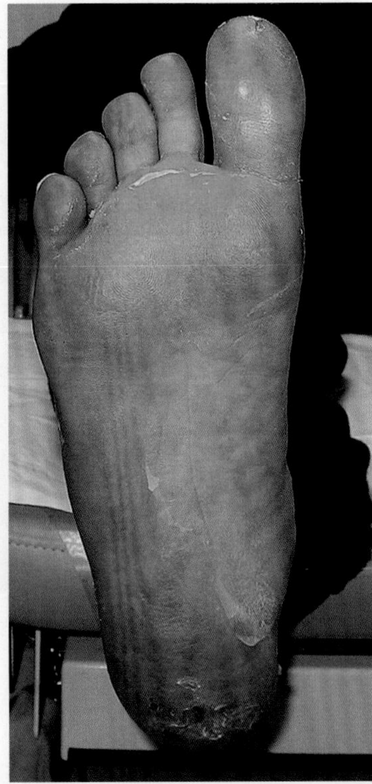

FIGURE 30-12. Superficial frostbite injury. (Reprinted with permission from The Podiatry Institute. (2012). *McGlamry's comprehensive textbook of foot and ankle surgery*, 2-Volume Set (4th ed.), Philadelphia, PA: Wolters Kluwer.

Deep Frostbite

Deep frostbite is subdivided into third- and fourth-degree classifications. Third-degree frostbite involves freezing injury of the entire skin, with extension into the subcutaneous tissue; it is manifested initially by the presence of violet-hued, hemorrhagic blisters. Skin necrosis ensues and appears blue-gray. Fourth-degree frostbite involves freezing of the skin, subcutaneous tissue, muscle, tendon and bone. There is rarely any edema. It initially appears mottled, cyanotic or deep red. As the injury progresses, the involved area appears dry, black and mummified (Fig. 30-14) (Koljonen et al., 2004).

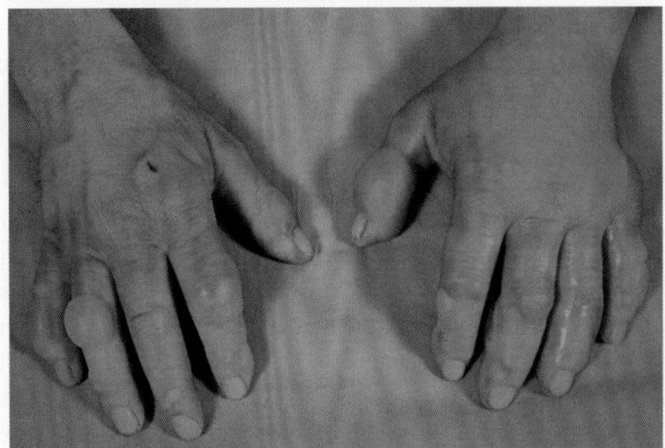

FIGURE 30-13. Frostbite with bullae formation. (Reproduced with permission from Berg, D., & Worzala, K. (2006). *Atlas of adult physical diagnosis*. Philadelphia, PA: Lippincott Williams & Wilkins.)

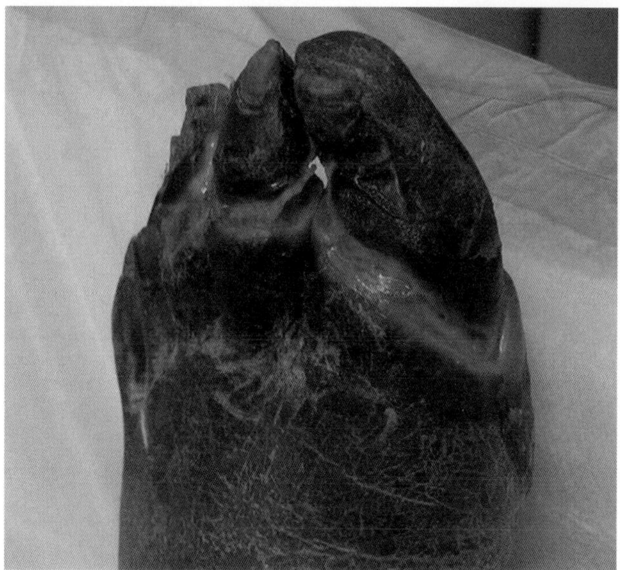

FIGURE 30-14. Demarcated fourth-degree frostbite with necrosis of the toes. (Photo courtesy of Scott Sherman, MD.)

Treatment

Initial treatment of a frostbite injury is to prevent further injury. For many years, field "first aid" recommended rubbing the injured area with snow; this is now known to cause further damage.

On-Site Interventions

Current recommendations for on-site interventions include removal of any jewelry (which conducts cold) and covering the patient in blankets until transport to a medical facility can be completed (Herndon, 2012; Koljonen et al., 2004).

Rewarming

The next phase of treatment involves rewarming. This is a painful procedure and the patient should be medicated accordingly. Rewarming should be carried out in a circulating water bath at a recommended temperature of 37 to 39°C. The patient is kept in the bath for approximately 30 minutes or until sensation returns and flushing is seen on the most distal aspect of the involved tissue. Prevention of intravascular thrombosis should be attempted with the use of antithromboxane agents, ibuprofen being the most common, and topical aloe vera gel (Herndon, 2012; Koljonen et al., 2004).

Postthaw Management

Postthaw management involves standard wound care for the injured tissue. There is evidence in the literature that hyperbaric oxygen therapy can be useful, even if there is a significant time lapse between the injury and initiation of HBO treatment. Surgery may ultimately be required but is delayed until there is a clear line of demarcation between the viable and devitalized tissue; this may take 1 to 3 months (Kemper et al., 2014; Herndon, 2012; Koljonen et al., 2004).

CLINICAL PEARL

Postthaw management of third- and fourth-degree frostbite involves standard wound care; HBOT may also be helpful. Debridement is delayed until there is a clear line of demarcation between viable and devitalized tissue, which may take 1 to 3 months.

Conclusion

All wound care nurses will, at some point in their career, be asked to consult on a burn wound or frostbite injury. Regardless of the severity of the injury, the wound care nurse will be expected to write wound care protocols and direct basic wound management. It is essential for the wound nurse to be knowledgeable regarding the criteria for transfer to a burn treatment center and to base recommendations on an understanding of the pathology underlying the wound, assessment of the tissue layers involved, and understanding of the three phases of burn management. Effective management of thermal injuries requires a multidisciplinary and holistic approach if optimal long-term outcomes are to be achieved.

CLINICAL PEARL

Do not be hesitant to call your regional burn unit for advice. Nurses and physicians in these specialized areas treat every day what is foreign to you. They would rather assist you on the front end than try and fix something done wrong on the back end.

REFERENCES

Atiyeh, B. S., & Hayek, S. N. (2010). Management of war-related burn injuries: Lessons learned from recent ongoing conflicts providing exceptional care in unusual places. *Journal of Craniofacial Surgery, 21*, 1529–1537.

Bauer, G. J., Caruso, D. M., Foster, K. N., et al. (2006). Randomized clinical study of hydrofiber dressing with silver or silver sulfadiazine in the management of partial-thickness burns. *Journal of Burn Care and Research, 27*, 298–309.

Besner, G. E., Paddock, H., Fabia, R., et al. (2007). Silver impregnated antimicrobial dressing reduces hospital length of stay for pediatric patients with burns. *Journal of Burn Care and Research, 28*, 409–411.

Boyce, S. T., Kagan, R. J., Greenhalgh, D. G., et al. (2006). Cultured skin substitutes reduce requirements for harvesting of skin autograft for closure of excised, full-thickness burns. *Journal of Trauma: Injury, Infection, and Critical Care, 60*, 821–824.

Burn Center Referral Criteria. (2006). *American Burn Association*. Retrieved April 14, 2014, from http://ameriburn.org

Burn Incidence and Treatment in the United States: 2013 Fact Sheet. (n.d.). Retrieved June 3, 2014, from http://ameriburn.org/resources_factsheet.php

Carrougher, G. J. (1998). *Burn care and therapy*. St Louis, MO: Mosby.

Connor-Ballard, P. (2009). Understanding and managing burn pain: Part 1. *American Journal of Nursing, 109*, 48–56.

Copcu, E. (2009). Marjolin's ulcer: A preventable complication of burns? *Plastic and Reconstructive Surgery, 124*, 156e–161e.

Evans, J. (2007). Massive tissue loss: Burns. In R Bryant. (Ed.), *Acute & chronic wounds: Current management concepts* (3rd ed., pp. 361–390). St Louis, MO: Elsevier/Mosby.

Falanga, V., & Lazic, T. (2011). Bioengineered skin constructs and their use in wound healing. *Plastic and Reconstructive Surgery, 127*, 75S–90S.

Fang, T., Lineaweaver, W., Sailes, F., et al. (2014). Clinical application of cultured epithelial autografts on acellular dermal matrices in the treatment of extended burn injuries. *Annals of Plastic Surgery, 73*(5), 509–515.

Fire Deaths and Injuries: Fact Sheet. (n.d.). Retrieved April 21, 2014, from https://www.cdc.gov/HomeandRecreationsSafety/Fire-Prevention/fires-factsheet.html

Fish, J. S., & Bezuhly, M. (2012). Acute burn care. *Plastic and Reconstructive Surgery, 130*, 349e–358e.

Gravante, G., Caruso, R., Sorge, R., et al. (2009). Nanocrystalline silver: A systematic review of randomized trials conducted on burned patients and an evidenced-based assessment of potential advantages over older silver formulations. *Annals of Plastic Surgery, 63*, 201–205.

Helvig, E. I. (2002). Managing thermal injuries within WOCN practice. *Journal of Wound, Ostomy, and Continence Nursing, 29*, 76–82.

Herndon, D. N. (2012). *Total burn care* (4th ed., p. 2, 6, 10, 17, 40, 42, 46). Retrieved from https://www.clinicalkey.com/

Hettiaratchy, S., Dziewulski, P., (2004). Pathophysiology and types of burns. *British Medical Journal, 328*, 1427–1429.

Holland, A. J., Chan, Q. E., Harvey, J. G., et al. (2012). The correlation between time to skin grafting and hypertrophic scarring following an acute contact burn in a porcine model. *Journal of Burn Care and Research, 33*, e43–e48.

Jones, I. S., Berman, B., Viera, M. H., et al. (2008). Prevention and management of hypertrophic scars and keloids after burns in children. *Journal of Craniofacial Surgery, 19*, 989–1006.

Kavalukas, S., Barbul, A. (2011). Nutrition and wound healing: An update. *Plastic and Reconstructive Surgery, 127*, 38S–43S.

Kearns, R., Holmes, J., & Cairns, B. (2013). Burn injury: What's in a name? Labels used for burn injury classification: A review of the data from 2000–2012. *Annals of Burns and Fire Disasters, 26*, 115–120.

Kemper, T. C., de Jong. V. M., Anema, H. A., et al. (2014). Frostbite of both first digits of the foot treated with delayed hyperbaric oxygen: a case report and review of literature. *Undersea and Hyperbaric Medicine, 41*(1), 65–70.

Kliegman, R. M., Stanton, B. F., St. Geme, J. W., et al. (2011). Burn injuries. In *Nelson textbook of pediatrics* (19th ed., p. 68). Retrieved from https://www.clinicalkey.com/

Koljonen, V., Anderson, K., Mikkonen, K., et al. (2004). Frostbite injuries treated in the Helsinki area from 1995 to 2002. *Journal of Trauma: Injury, Infection, and Critical Care, 57*, 1315–1320.

Langschmidt, J., Caine, P., Wearn, C., et al. (2014). Hydrotherapy in burn care: A survey of hydrotherapy practices in the UK and Ireland and literature review. *Burns, 40*(5), 860–864,

Logsetty, S., Hunter, T. A., Medved, M. I., et al. (2013). "Put on your face to face the world": Women's narratives of burn injury. *Burns, 39*, 1588–1598.

Mohammadi, A., Johari, H., Eskandari, S., (2013). Effects of amniotic membrane on graft take in extremity burns. *Burns, 39*, 1137–41.

Mok, J. Y. (2008). Non-accidental injury in children—An update. *Injury, 39*, 978–985.

Molan, P. C., Cooper, R., & Halas, E. (2002). The efficacy of honey in inhibiting strains of *Pseudomonas aeruginosa* from infected burns. *Journal of Burn Care and Rehabilitation, 23*, 366–370.

Monstrey, S., Verbelen, J., Hoeksema, H., et al. (2014). Aquacel Ag dressing versus Acticoat™ dressing in partial thickness burns: A prospective, randomized, controlled study in 100 patients. Part 1: Burn wound healing. *Burns, 40*(3), 416–427.

Orgill, D. P., & Ogawa, R. (2013). Current methods of burn reconstruction. *Plastic and Reconstructive Surgery, 131*(5), 827e–836e.

Paul, C. N., Hansen, S. L., Voight, D. W., et al. (2001). Using skin replacement products to treat burns and wounds. *Advances in Skin and Wound Care, 14*, 37–46.

Ranganathan, K., Wong, V. C., Krebsbach, P. H., et al. (2013). Fat grafting for thermal injury: Current state and future directions. *Journal of Burn Care and Research, 34*, 219–226.

Richard, R. L., Gordon, M. D., Gottschlich, M. M., et al. (2004). Review of evidenced-based practice for the prevention of pressure sores in burn patients. *Journal of Burn Care and Rehabilitation, 25*, 388–410.

Rick, C., Caruso, D. M., Foster, K. N., et al. (2004). Aquacel Ag in the management of partial-thickness burns: Results of a clinical trial. *Journal of Burn Care and Rehabilitation, 25*, 89–97.

Simko, L. M., & Culleton, A. (2013). Caring for patients with burn injuries. *Nursing, 43*, 26–34.

Somerset, A., Coffey, R., Jones, L., et al. (2014). The impact of prediabetes on glycemic control and clinical outcomes postburn injury. *Journal of Burn Care and Research, 35*, 5–10.

Townsend, C. M., Beauchamp, R. D., Evers, B. M., et al. (2012). Burns. In *Sabiston textbook of surgery* (19th ed., p. 21). Retrieved from https://www.clinicalkey.com/

Woo, E., Lee, J., Hur, G., et al. (2013). Proposed treatment protocol for frostbite: A retrospective analysis of 17 cases based on a 3-year single institution experience. *Archives of Plastic Surgery, 40*, 510–516.

QUESTIONS

1. The wound nurse is caring for a patient who was exposed to a product containing 10% hydrofluoric acid and has burns on 3% of his body. For what life-threatening condition would the nurse monitor this patient?

A. Hypocalcemia
B. Hyperkalemia
C. Hypophosphatemia
D. Hyponatremia

2. A patient is admitted to an acute care facility with electrical burns on 40% of his body caused by alternating current. This patient would be at risk for which of the following serious complications?

A. Cellular necrosis
B. Atelectasis
C. Compartment syndrome
D. Hypometabolism

3. A patient admitted to a burn unit with thermal injuries is in the "emergent phase" of the injury. What would be the primary focus of care during this phase of recovery?
   A. Debridement
   B. Hemodynamic stabilization
   C. Skin grafting
   D. Maximizing functional capacity

4. The burn team initially focuses on the zone of stasis when planning wound care. What is the rationale for this strategy?
   A. Tissue damage in this area is potentially reversible.
   B. Prevention of denaturing of proteins may prevent tissue damage.
   C. Full-thickness burns in this area must be treated first.
   D. The outermost area of burn injury requires the most aggressive therapy.

5. An adult sustained major burns in a home fire. What are the criteria for this classification of burns?
   A. Burns involve <10% TBSA.
   B. Burns involve <15% TBSA.
   C. Burns involve <15% to 25% TBSA with <10% full-thickness burns.
   D. Burns >25% TBSA.

6. A wound nurse caring for a patient with burns documents the following: Burns are erythematous, painful, and blanchable to touch, with edema, blister formation, and weeping present. What stage of burns is the nurse describing?
   A. Superficial burns
   B. Superficial partial-thickness burns
   C. Deep partial-thickness burns
   D. Full-thickness burns

7. Which burn injury can safely be treated in an outpatient setting based on the ABA referral guidelines?
   A. Burns that involve the hands
   B. Full-thickness burns
   C. Partial-thickness burns less than 10%
   D. Patients with partial-thickness burns and concomitant trauma

8. What drug of choice would the wound nurse recommend to treat pain during the acute phase of burn treatment?
   A. Intravenous morphine
   B. Aspirin
   C. Nonsteroidal anti-inflammatory agents
   D. Oral pain medications

9. A burn patient is scheduled to receive autografting for definitive closure of a partial-thickness burn. Which dressing would the wound nurse recommend to manage the burn as a temporary dressing prior to the autograft?
   A. Biobrane
   B. Sulfamylon dressing
   C. Honey-based dressing
   D. Silver dressing

10. Which type of graft, used for reconstructive purposes, would the wound nurse recommend for a small, full-thickness burn?
   A. Meshed autologous skin graft
   B. Full-thickness skin graft
   C. Cultured epithelial autograft
   D. Split-thickness skin graft

11. The WOC nurse recommends a meshed autologous skin graft for a large burn on a patient's knee area. Which action is performed correctly in this procedure?
   A. Preoperatively, the wound is dressed with a nonadherent layer to prevent shearing.
   B. Postoperatively, a "bolster" dressing is applied to the meshed graft comprised of gauze soaked in 10% saline solution.
   C. Since the grafted area is a joint, a splint is applied to maintain a functional position.
   D. The initial dressing is usually left undisturbed for 10 to 14 days, at which time dressings are removed to examine the graft.

12. The wound nurse documents third-degree frostbite in a hiker who got lost in the mountains. What clinical manifestation prompted this diagnosis?
   A. Superficial skin desquamation; no long-term tissue damage
   B. Formation of vesicles with clear fluid; skin loss and eschar formation
   C. Mottled, cyanotic or deep red skin turning dry, black, and mummified
   D. Initial presence of violet-hued, hemorrhagic blisters; skin necrosis occurs

13. Which intervention is a recommended treatment for frostbite victims?
   A. Rub the area vigorously with a towel or blanket.
   B. Pack the area in snow or use cool compresses on the area.
   C. Cover the patient in blankets until transport to medical facility.
   D. Place the patient in a cool bath for 30 minutes.

ANSWERS: 1.**A**, 2.**C**, 3.**B**, 4.**A**, 5.**D**, 6.**B**, 7.**C**, 8.**A**, 9.**A**, 10.**B**, 11.**C**, 12.**D**, 13.**C**

CHAPTER 31

Traumatic Wounds

Assessment and Management

David R. Crumbley and Lizabeth E. Andrew

OBJECTIVES

1. Describe the mechanisms of injury associated with common traumatic injuries.
2. Outline key considerations in management of traumatic wounds.
3. Describe the role of NPWT in management of traumatic wounds.
4. Explain the significance of compartment syndrome and management options.

Topic Outline

 Introduction

Traumatic injuries occur when an external or foreign object strikes the body. These injuries are commonly caused by motor vehicle crashes, bullets, natural disasters, explosive blasts, falls, and industrial accidents (Graybill et al., 2012). Traumatic wounds may damage bone and/or internal organs, are not created surgically, and always are viewed as contaminated and at risk for infection. This chapter presents an overview of the major causes of traumatic wounds, the management of these wounds, and complications that may arise.

 Causes of Traumatic Wounds

Motor Vehicle Accidents

Crashes and pedestrian accidents involving automobiles, trucks, and motorcycles cause multiple blunt force and deceleration injuries that may result in open and closed fractures, and injuries to the head, internal organs and vessels, spinal cord, and soft tissues. Blunt force trauma occurs when the body is propelled against objects within or outside the vehicle. Penetrating injuries cause skin or muscle damage and may involve bones, vessels, and internal organs.

Vehicular crash victims who suffer blunt force injuries may also have open wounds caused by surgical intervention.

In the event of a crush injury or fracture, the patient may undergo a fasciotomy to prevent or mitigate compartment syndrome of an extremity. Abdominal surgery may be required to control hemorrhage, repair damaged organs, prevent or treat abdominal compartment syndrome, and allow tissue swelling to resolve. Compartment syndrome and fasciotomy management are discussed later in this chapter, under the sections Compartment Syndrome and Management of Fasciotomy Wounds.

Bullet/Gunshot Wounds

When a bullet (also known as a missile or projectile) strikes tissue, the tissue is lacerated and crushed along the trajectory of the projectile (Cubano et al., 2013). As the projectile interacts with the tissue, it produces both a smaller permanent cavity and a larger temporary cavity. The permanent cavity involves an area of tissue necrosis proportionate to the size of the projectile, and can extend the length of the projectile's travel through the tissue. The temporary cavity is created by the lateral transfer of tissue as the projectile passes through it (Cubano et al., 2013) (Fig. 31-1). Elastic tissue, such as muscle, blood vessels, skin, and fat are pushed aside but usually rebound after the passage of the projectile; however, contusions and hemorrhaging of the muscle tissue may occur. In contrast, nonelastic tissues like bone and liver may fracture (Cubano et al., 2013; Lichte et al., 2010). Bone involvement can result in severe injury as the pieces of fractured bone create secondary missiles that cause additional trauma to surrounding tissues.

CLINICAL PEARL

Bullets and similar projectiles create both a smaller permanent cavity and a larger temporary cavity; the tissues involved in the temporary cavity may rebound and recover (soft tissue) or may fracture (bone and liver).

Injuries caused by firearms are often classified by the velocity of the projectile; however, the rule of thumb for care providers is to "treat the wound, not the weapon" (Cubano et al., 2013). Handguns cause low-velocity wounds; hunting rifles or military weapons cause high-velocity wounds (Lichte et al., 2010). However, velocity alone cannot predict tissue trauma. The potential for tissue trauma depends on the tissue involved, low-energy transfer versus high-energy transfer, and the nature of the projectile. In gunshot wounds, especially high-energy transfer wounds, tissue damage can be extensive, and the extent of damage may not be fully determined until 4 days after the initial injury (Edlich et al., 2010). The difficulty in determining the full extent of tissue damage is due to the fact that energy is transferred from the high-energy projectile to tissue adjacent to the area of initial impact. This tissue may appear to be healthy on initial examination but may become necrotic over subsequent hours and days. This delayed necrosis can be caused by vascular damage or by massive edema that compromises blood flow and tissue oxygenation; it can also be a result of bacterial contamination. This phenomenon is often termed "wound evolution" by military physicians, that is, the wound evolves over the first few days following injury.

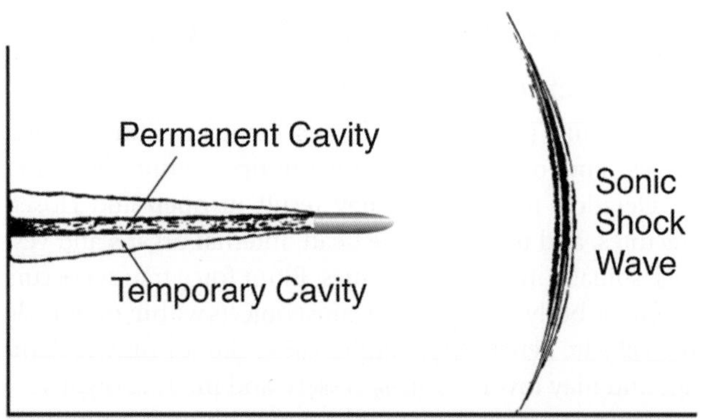

FIGURE 31-1. Projectile–tissue interaction, showing components of tissue injury. (Courtesy of Borden Institute Fort Sam Houston, TX.)

CLINICAL PEARL

In high-energy gunshot wounds, tissue damage can be extensive, and the extent of the damage may not be evident for several days postinjury.

Conversely, tissue that initially appears ischemic may improve over the first few days following injury, a phenomenon known in trauma and burn care as "tissue resuscitation." Tissue resuscitation involves recovery of tissue adjacent to the primary site; this tissue sustains trauma but may recover without progression to necrosis, depending on the care provided following the injury. For example, prompt and effective management of soft tissue edema can prevent the vascular compression that would cause tissue necrosis.

In summary, there is both direct injury that is irreversible, and indirect injury of the adjacent tissue and vasculature related to tissue transfer and to soft tissue swelling; this indirect injury may cause progressive tissue necrosis or, in some cases, may be reversed by prompt management of edema.

Blast Injuries

Blast injuries can be caused by military explosive munitions, improvised explosive devices (IEDs), or industrial accidents. Blast injuries can be categorized into four types: (1) primary, (2) secondary, (3) tertiary, and (4) quaternary injuries (Cubano et al., 2013). Proximity to the blast epicenter is a major determinant of the type of injury and the severity of injury (Fig. 31-2). Victims may experience all four types of injury depending upon the device and the proximity of the victim to the explosion. Musculoskeletal injuries are the most frequently occurring blast injuries (Hayda et al., 2004).

Primary blast injuries are caused by the sonic shockwave of the blast striking the body. These injuries take place

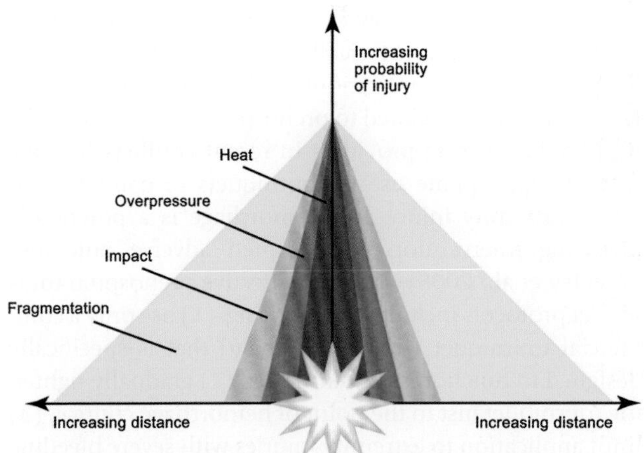

FIGURE 31-2. The probability of sustaining a given trauma is related to the distance from the epicenter of the detonation. (Courtesy of Borden Institute Fort Sam Houston, TX.)

relatively close to the source of explosion. This shockwave/overpressure force causes damage to hollow organs such as the lung, the gastrointestinal tract, and the ear. Secondary blast injuries occur when device fragments or debris are propelled through the air by the blast causing penetrating trauma, fragmentation injuries, and blunt trauma. Fragments from a terrorist's IED may contain objects such as marbles, nails, and glass. Figure 31-3 shows the mechanism of injury from a landmine and the propulsion of debris into the deep tissue. In blasts that occur in or near a building, penetrating wounds may be caused by fragments from the glass blown out of windows, or other debris from the building structure (Hayda et al., 2004). Tertiary blast injuries occur when the victim is thrown by the blast and strikes surrounding objects. Victims may suffer blunt and penetrating injuries, fractures, and traumatic amputations. Quaternary blast injuries are all other injuries including thermal injuries, injuries from toxic exposure, and any postincident events or exacerbations of chronic conditions (Centers for Disease Control and Prevention, 2012; Ramasamy et al., 2009).

Wounds Caused by Natural Disasters

Earthquakes, tornadoes, and hurricanes are natural disasters that collapse buildings and create falling debris. The debris and falling structures can cause serious injuries with extensive orthopedic trauma (fractured extremities) as well as internal damage. The most common injuries associated with earthquakes include open and closed fractures, crush injuries, and wound infections (Sonshine et al., 2012; *MMWR. Morbidity and Mortality Weekly Report, 2011*). Tornadoes and hurricanes can generate flying debris that causes penetrating wounds, especially near the storms' strong epicenters. Wounds caused by natural disasters may be contaminated with debris, soil, or contaminated water, and crush injuries and fractures may result in compartment syndrome. When large-scale natural disasters occur, especially in underdeveloped nations, the potential for wound complications is even greater, because the time from injury to treatment may extend from hours to days.

Management of Traumatic Wounds

Management of Bacterial Contamination

Bacterial contamination is a serious concern in the management of traumatic wounds. All traumatic wounds, regardless of mechanism of injury, should be considered contaminated due to the nonsterile nature of their occurrence and the environment where the injury occurs.

Bacterial contamination can occur in any environment where damaged soft tissue comes in contact with soil or debris. Wounds may be contaminated by bacteria from soil, especially when a blast projects soil deeply into soft tissue. Gunshot wounds and blast wounds may be contaminated with clothing, fragments from projectiles, or soil, and fecal contamination can occur when the bowel is perforated.

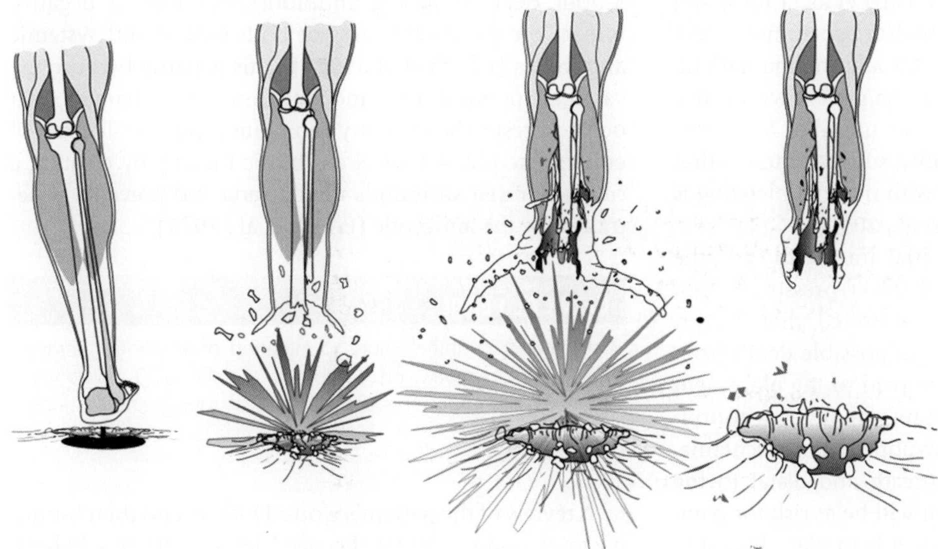

FIGURE 31-3. Mechanisms of injuries caused by antipersonnel landmines. (Courtesy of Borden Institute Fort Sam Houston, TX.)

A number of United States Service Members in Afghanistan who sustained significant blast injuries caused by IEDs were subsequently diagnosed with cutaneous mucormycosis, an aggressive fungal infection caused by soil contaminants projected deeply into the soft tissue by IEDs buried in the soil (Lewandowski et al., 2013). Mucormycosis is a life-threatening angioinvasive fungal infection that is difficult to eradicate. Following the Joplin, Missouri tornado in 2011, thirteen victims developed mucormycosis; five of the thirteen died. Since all victims were located in the area that sustained storm damage, their infections were associated with penetrating soft tissue trauma and multiple wounds caused by deadly tornadic winds (Fanfair et al., 2012).

A wound caused by glass or sharp metal exhibits less tissue damage and is more resistant to infection than a wound caused by blunt trauma (Edlich et al., 2010; Thacker et al., 1977). Sharp objects create less tissue damage, and less energy is necessary to create the wound; in contrast, blunt trauma wounds exhibit more damage to the wound edges because more force is needed to cause the tissue failure. The blunt trauma wound is created through compression and tension of the tissue rather than through shearing, which is the mechanism of injury with a sharp object. Because the object is blunt and not sharp, more tissue comes in contact with the wounding object and more damage is caused to the surrounding tissue (Edlich et al., 2010).

Initial Acute Management and Hemorrhage Control

The initial acute management of traumatic injuries focuses on life-threatening conditions that involve the patient's airway, breathing, and circulation; care is dictated by Advanced Trauma Life Support (ATLS) guidelines, with the goals of ensuring correct management and preventing complications (Lichte et al., 2010). Controlling hemorrhage is critical because it is a leading cause of death, second only to central nervous system injury. Hemorrhage from extremities is the leading preventable cause of mortality in combat casualties (Beekley et al., 2008; Bellamy et al., 1986), and internal bleeding caused by blunt and/or penetrating injury is a life-threatening complication for any trauma patient. Surgical intervention is necessary if the patient with active internal bleeding is hemodynamically unstable. Since surgery can increase the risk of mortality, surgical intervention may be postponed if the patient with internal bleeding is hemodynamically stable (Lichte et al., 2010).

Direct pressure is the best initial intervention if the source of bleeding is external. If direct pressure is not effective and bleeding cannot be controlled, then a tourniquet should be applied to prevent possible death from exsanguination. Attention must be paid to the placement and timing of the tourniquet because applying a tourniquet puts the patient at risk for hypoperfusion, ischemia, and necrosis of the tissue underneath and distal to the tourniquet placement. The patient will be at risk for compartment syndrome if the tourniquet is in place for more than 90 minutes (Beekley et al., 2008; Kam et al., 2001). Tourniquet use has historically been controversial due to the potential for complications such as those listed above. However, findings related to prehospital tourniquet use by military health care providers in recent conflicts indicate that the appropriate use of tourniquets in patients with severe extremity injury and hemorrhage is a potentially lifesaving intervention with limited adverse outcomes (Beekley et al., 2008). Safe and effective prehospital tourniquet protocols include the following: (1) use only a commercial tourniquet with a wide band that is specifically designed to function as a tourniquet, (2) gradually tighten the tourniquet just to the point of hemorrhage control, (3) limit application to extremity injuries with severe bleeding and apply the tourniquet proximal to the site of injury, (4) leave the tourniquet in place if transport time to a higher level of care is less than 30 minutes, (5) reassess tourniquet use after 30 minutes for possible removal and placement of a pressure dressing to prevent pain and tissue ischemia (when transport time greater than 30 minutes), (6) leave the tourniquet in place if the patient is unstable and in circulatory shock, (7) if tourniquet removal is advised, loosen carefully, apply pressure dressing, and leave the tourniquet in place in case of recurrent hemorrhage, (8) do not remove the tourniquet from an amputated or near amputated extremity, and (9) in mass casualty settings when tourniquet use is required, mark "TK" and application time clearly on patient's forehead or other prominent location (Doyle & Taillac, 2008).

Obtaining Wound History

Recording a thorough wound history is essential once life-threatening conditions have been mitigated and the patient is stable. A wound history should include the mechanism of injury as well as the time of injury; this information provides insight into the extent of injury and the potential for infection. The time from injury to initial treatment can impact the susceptibility of the wound to infection. Even a 3-hour delay initiating antibiotics can have a negative impact on the effectiveness of both topical and systemic antibiotics (Edlich et al., 1971). This is partly because the vascular permeability and inflammatory changes that occur in response to injury can reduce the effectiveness of either systemic or topical antibiotic therapy by creating a coagulum that surrounds the bacteria and prevents penetration by the antibiotic (Edlich et al., 1971).

CLINICAL PEARL

The time from initial injury to initiation of antibiotic therapy has a major impact on outcomes; a delay of 3 hours can significantly reduce the effectiveness of topical and systemic antibiotics.

A review of the patient's wound history and their immunization status informs the need for tetanus prophylaxis.

In traumatic wounds, the anaerobic bacterium *Clostridium tetani* (*C. tetani*) enters the body through the broken skin. *Clostridium tetani* infection can occur through puncture wounds or penetrating injuries, bites, burns, frostbite, or crush injuries or through necrotic tissue contaminated with soil, feces, or saliva (Afshar et al., 2011; Wood, 2004). Tetanus is a rare disease in the United States and Western Europe because of rigorous immunization programs. Individuals who have had a tetanus booster within the 5 years preceding injury may not require prophylaxis. Tetanus immunization is recommended if immunization status cannot be determined or if the wound is heavily contaminated. Tetanus prophylaxis is recommended for (1) wound management if the patient's most recent tetanus vaccination is greater than 5 years or if the patient's immunization status cannot be determined; (2) wounds contaminated with soil, feces, or saliva; (3) puncture wounds or avulsions; and (4) wounds caused by missiles, crush injuries, burns, and frostbite (Kretsinger et al., 2006a, 2006b). When working with populations outside the United States or Western Europe, tetanus prophylaxis is extremely important. Limited active immunization programs in underdeveloped countries are one cause for the high incidence of tetanus worldwide.

Wound Debridement and Irrigation

After initial trauma management and mitigation of life-threatening injuries and the completion of a thorough wound history, the wound should be debrided and irrigated. Debridement is paramount in establishing a healthy wound healing environment (Haury et al., 1978). Surgical debridement is necessary to remove nonviable tissue (skin, fat, fascia, bone, muscle, or tendon), which can harbor bacteria or may be heavily contaminated with soil or foreign bodies (Fig. 31-4). This nonviable tissue serves as a medium for anaerobic organisms, compromising the body's ability to fight infection, and potentially contaminating healthy tissue (Joint Theatre Trauma System Clinical Practice Guideline, 2012).

For larger and/or heavily contaminated wounds, debridement and irrigation are performed in the operating room under anesthesia to prevent additional pain for the patient and to permit wound exploration. Understanding the mechanism of injury and environment of the injury will help the surgeon to determine the degree of debridement and irrigation necessary. The extent of debridement required is determined by the surgeon's assessment of the wound and surrounding tissue; copious irrigation of the wound removes the foreign material and increases the accuracy of the assessment.

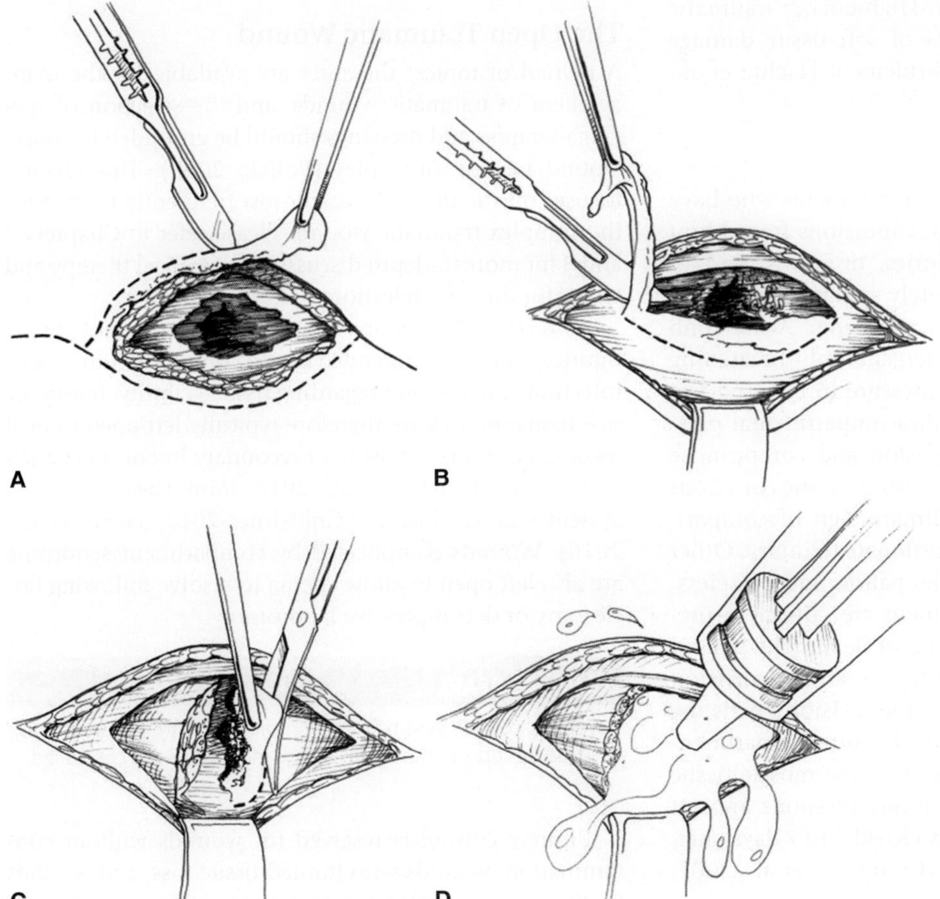

FIGURE 31-4. **(A)** Skin excision, **(B)** removal of fascia, **(C)** removal of avascular tissue, and **(D)** irrigation. (Courtesy of Borden Institute Fort Sam Houston, TX.)

There are a variety of acceptable approaches to irrigation, including bulb irrigation, pulsatile lavage, gravity irrigation, and high-pressure syringe irrigation using a 35-mL syringe and 19-gauge catheter (Graybill et al., 2012; Gross et al., 1972; Joint Theatre Trauma System Clinical Practice Guideline, 2012; Stevenson et al., 1976). Sterile normal saline, sterile water, sterile antibiotic solution, or potable water may be used for wound irrigation (Fernandez et al., 2004; Hall, 2007; Storer et al., 2012). Potable water may be used for irrigation outside of the operating room but would never be used within the operating room. A sterile isotonic solution is the preferred solution for irrigating large traumatic wounds (Joint Theatre Trauma System Clinical Practice Guideline, 2012).

Military medicine uses the term "wound evolution" to describe the changes in tissue viability that occur in traumatic large soft tissue injuries over the first 4 to 7 days following injury (Edlich et al., 2010; Joint Theatre Trauma System Clinical Practice Guideline, 2012). This change in tissue viability calls for a more frequent schedule of debridement and irrigation in the acute phase (<72 hours) and a less frequent debridement and irrigation schedule during the subacute phase (3 to 7 days) (Joint Theatre Trauma System Clinical Practice Guideline, 2012). This frequent debridement and irrigation schedule of every 24 to 48 hours allows for a more accurate assessment of tissue evolution. High-energy traumatic wounds have a greater amount of soft tissue damage and require more extensive debridement (Lichte et al., 2010).

Compartment Syndrome

Compartment syndrome can occur in patients who have suffered fractures, crush injuries, contusions from blunt trauma, arterial or venous injuries, or burns, and in patients whose wounds were acutely managed with tourniquets or pneumatic antishock garments. Acute limb compartment syndrome is an emergent limb-threatening syndrome caused by increased pressure in a closed fascial space that results in high intracompartmental pressures that reduce capillary perfusion and compromise tissue viability (Gourgiotis et al., 2007). In the conscious and unsedated patient, the hallmark sign of compartment syndrome is pain disproportionate to injury. Other clinical signs include paresthesia, pallor, and pulselessness. Early detection and treatment are critical to prevent muscle necrosis, amputation, or death. The patient may require a fasciotomy, which is a surgical incision into the affected muscular fascia; the incision opens the fascial compartment, which reduces intracompartmental pressures and restores perfusion to the muscle tissue (Gourgiotis et al., 2007). Fasciotomy incisions are not closed primarily; they are usually closed 3 to 7 days later, once the swelling has resolved (Gourgiotis et al., 2007; Pollak, 2008).

CLINICAL PEARL

Compartment syndrome is a common complication of traumatic injury and requires emergent intervention (such as fasciotomy) to prevent tissue necrosis caused by severe edema and vessel compression.

The critically injured trauma patient who suffers blunt or penetrating intra-abdominal injuries and/or requires massive resuscitation efforts is at risk for developing abdominal compartment syndrome, a life-threatening condition with a high mortality rate (Harrell & Melander, 2012). Treatment involves surgical decompressive laparotomy, which is the abdominal equivalent of fasciotomy (Anand & Ivatury, 2011). The fascia of the abdomen is not reapproximated immediately; a temporary closure is performed instead. This temporary closure may consist of (1) a skin-only closure (fascia is not closed), (2) use of a commercially available abdominal closure system, or (3) a system fashioned from sterile irrigation bags placed over the bowel with the use of negative pressure. Military medicine uses the term "temporizing" to describe this process of temporarily closing the abdominal compartment until bowel edema resolves and the fascia can be reapproximated (Anand & Ivatury, 2011; Navsaria et al., 2013; Vertrees et al., 2008).

The Open Traumatic Wound

A myriad of topical therapies are available for the management of traumatic wounds, and the selection of specific therapies and dressings should be grounded in sound wound healing principles (Pollak, 2008). This chapter focuses on the therapies used most frequently to manage the complex traumatic wound. Please refer to Chapters 7 and 8 for more in-depth discussions of topical therapy and tenets for dressing selection.

As discussed, primary closure of traumatic soft tissue injuries is not recommended due to contamination, risk of infection, and concern regarding tissue viability; traumatic soft tissue injuries are therefore typically left open to heal by delayed primary closure or secondary intention (Edlich et al., 2010; Graybill et al., 2012; Joint Theatre Trauma System Clinical Practice Guideline, 2012; Lichte et al., 2010). Wounds complicated by compartment syndrome are also left open to allow edema to resolve following fasciotomy or decompressive laporotomy.

CLINICAL PEARL

Wounds complicated by infection or compartment syndrome should be left open until infection and edema are controlled.

Primary closure is reserved for wounds without contamination, wounds with limited tissue loss, and wounds to the face. Complex traumatic wounds with extensive

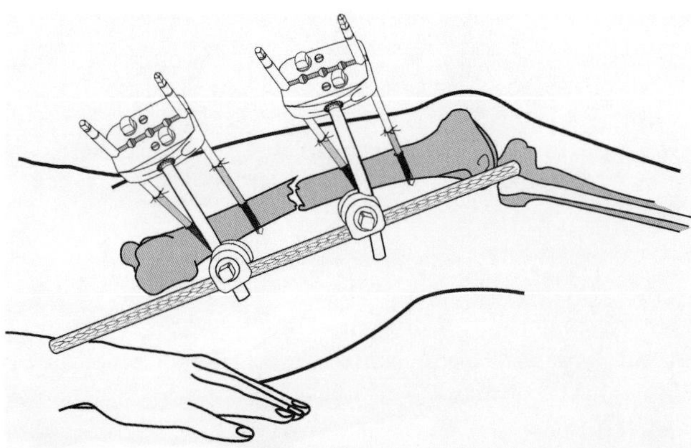

FIGURE 31-5. Frame applied and fracture grossly reduced. Lateral placement of stabilizing rod is preferred. (Courtesy of Borden Institute Fort Sam Houston, TX.)

tissue loss are frequently managed with delayed primary closure, a skin graft, or tissue flap (Edlich et al., 2010; Graybill et al., 2012; Joint Theatre Trauma System Clinical Practice Guideline, 2012; Lichte et al., 2010). Wounds left to heal by secondary intention are generally smaller, well approximated, and located in an area where cosmesis is less important (e.g., the trunk). Wounds healing by secondary intention take longer to heal as they must first fill with granulation tissue and then must undergo epithelial migration from the wound edges; secondary intention wound healing also produces more scar tissue than primary closure.

In delayed primary closure, wound closure is delayed to allow time for elimination of infection and management of edema (Edlich et al., 2010). The exact time for closure varies but may be as soon as 3 to 5 days after initial surgery (Edlich et al., 2010; Joint Theatre Trauma System Clinical Practice Guideline, 2012). Wounds with extensive soft tissue loss will require a skin graft or tissue flap to cover the defect (Graybill et al., 2012). If open traumatic wounds are complicated by concomitant fractures, the fractures must be stabilized with either internal or external fixation prior to or at the time of wound closure (Fig. 31-5).

To ensure the wound bed is free of contaminants and nonviable tissue, serial debridements and wound irrigations are continued until the wound bed is clean and the wound can be closed surgically. If the wound cannot be closed primarily, temporary coverage must be implemented to (1) protect and prepare the wound bed, (2) prevent contamination and desiccation of the wound, and (3) manage exudate. The technique of temporarily covering the wound awaiting delayed primary closure, skin graft, or tissue flap is often referred to as "temporizing" the wound.

Temporization of the Open Soft Tissue Injury/Negative Pressure Wound Therapy

Following thorough debridement of the traumatic wound, the surgeon may choose to cover the wound with fluffed moistened sterile gauze (antimicrobial or plain gauze) or may use a negative pressure wound therapy (NPWT) system with reticulated open cell foam dressings (NPWT/ROCF). A moistened sterile gauze dressing may be used in wounds where there is questionable tissue viability or extreme contamination necessitating frequent returns to the operating room every 24 hours for debridement and irrigation. Cavitary wounds should never be packed in a manner that would obstruct fluid egress from the wound; rather, they should be lightly filled, so that the gauze serves to wick the fluid out of the wound (Cubano et al., 2013). This approach is especially important when managing traumatic wounds with small openings.

NPWT/ROCF is the preferred coverage for the patient who will undergo less frequent debridement and irrigation (48 to 72 hours). Over the past 15 years, NPWT /ROCF has become the treatment of choice for military surgeons and trauma surgeons managing complex soft tissue wounds, penetrating trauma, open fractures, and fasciotomy incisions (Blum et al., 2012; Krug et al., 2011; Pollak, 2008). This approach is based on case studies, anecdotal evidence, and the demonstrated mechanisms of action and clinical benefits of NPWT: (1) reduction of wound fluid and edema, which enhances blood flow to the wound, (2) promotion of granulation tissue formation, (3) removal of inflammatory cytokines, (4) reduction of cross-contamination in the hospital, (5) reduction in time to definitive closure, and (6) reduction in frequency of painful dressing changes (Crumbley & Perciballi, 2007; Morykwas et al., 1997; Pollak, 2008; Venturi et al., 2005). These qualities make NPWT an important adjunct in the management of complex soft tissue injuries with significant tissue loss resulting in wounds that are contaminated, edematous, painful, and heavily exudative, and that often have irregularly shaped edges. NPWT bridges the wound until definitive closure is performed, simplifies the process of soft tissue coverage, and may reduce the need for major soft tissue reconstructive procedures (Bernabe et al., 2014; Dedmond et al., 2007; Stannard et al., 2010). Chapters 11 and 32 provide additional details regarding indications, contraindications, and guidelines for use of NPWT.

CLINICAL PEARL

NPWT has become the treatment of choice for military surgeons and trauma surgeons managing complex soft tissue wounds, penetrating trauma, open fractures, and fasciotomy incisions

NPWT dressings are changed every 48 to 72 hours in the complex soft tissue wound until the wound is clean and stable and ready for closure. Dressing changes usually are scheduled to coincide with routine debridements/irrigations in the operating room; this approach provides for effective pain control during dressing changes (Tarkin, 2008). Settings for NPWT range from 75 to 125 mm Hg of negative pressure. Continuous suction may be better tolerated than intermittent in the complex open wound as the switching off and on of negative pressure may be painful and may cause loss of an effective seal in wounds with a large surface area or high-volume exudate. In complex traumatic wounds with exposed bone, tendons, nerves, or vessels, it is important to prevent injury and desiccation of these structures; this can be done by applying a nonadherent layer over the structure that provides protection from the ROCF dressing (Baharestani et al., 2009; Graybill et al., 2012). In addition, a nonadherent layer should be used whenever there is concern for tissue adherence to the ROCF dressing during removal.

Military surgeons and trauma surgeons have found silver-impregnated foam NPWT dressing to be useful in wounds with high bacterial loads (Graybill et al., 2012; Tarkin, 2008). An alternative method for reducing bacterial or fungal burden in the traumatic wound is the application of wound chemotherapy in conjunction with NPWT/ROCF (Giovinco et al., 2010; Lewandowski et al., 2013). The technique of wound chemotherapy with NPWT/ROCF involves the infusion of substances into the wound during NPWT. A frequently used chemotherapy substance is a dilute Dakin's solution. United States Military surgeons have used a Dakin's solution of 0.025% sodium hypochlorite solution successfully in the management of an invasive fungal infection in the combat wounded (Lewandowski et al., 2013). The use of wound chemotherapy is not advised until staff has been trained and policies are in place to prevent the inadvertent delivery of wound chemotherapy solutions via alternative routes (IV, IM, or PO).

Antibiotic Beads

Antibiotic-impregnated polymethyl methacrylate (PMMA) beads are commonly placed in high-risk traumatic wounds with concomitant orthopedic injury; the beads are placed into the wound bed near the site of the orthopedic injury to prevent or mitigate osteomyelitis or other infectious processes (Large et al., 2012). NPWT with ROCF is also frequently used in these wounds, and there have been concerns that the concomitant use of NPWT might reduce the effectiveness of the beads. Large and colleagues (2012) conducted a study and found that antibiotic concentration in the wound was reduced by NPWT if there was no fascia or tissue between the NPWT dressing and the antibiotic beads. It is therefore recommended that a nonadherent dressing or tissue coverage be placed between the beads and the NPWT foam to prevent a reduction in antibiotic concentration (Joint Theatre Trauma System Clinical Practice Guideline, 2012).

Split-Thickness Skin Grafts

Large soft tissue wounds healing by second intention require a split-thickness skin graft for final closure of the wound. Skin grafting is delayed until the wound bed is healthy and free of nonviable tissue and infection and has granulated to near skin level. NPWT has replaced traditional bolster dressings as the preferred method for maintaining close adherence between the split-thickness graft and the underlying wound bed for complex wounds (Baharestani et al., 2009; Moisidis et al., 2004; Scherer et al., 2002). NPWT/ROCF is beneficial because it (1) provides downward pressure onto the graft promoting apposition to the wound bed, (2) prevents wound fluid from accumulating under the graft, (3) promotes a moist environment, and (4) seals the wound from outside contamination (Tarkin, 2008). Use of NPWT also protects the graft from shearing forces and works well in irregular areas. Once the skin graft has been harvested, it is passed through a meshing device; the graft is then placed onto the wound bed and secured in place, typically with circumferential staples (Fig. 31-6). A nonadherent dressing is placed over the split-thickness skin graft as an interface between the NPWT/ROCF dressing and the skin graft (Fig. 31-7). This is done to prevent adherence of the foam to the graft and subsequent lifting

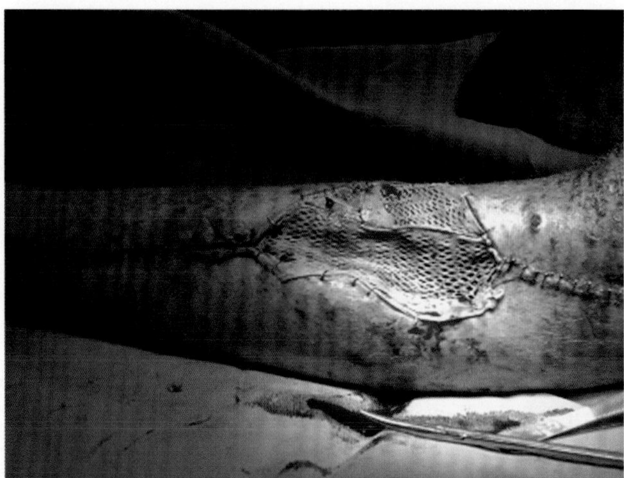

FIGURE 31-6. Split-thickness skin graft placed on open wound and secured with staples.

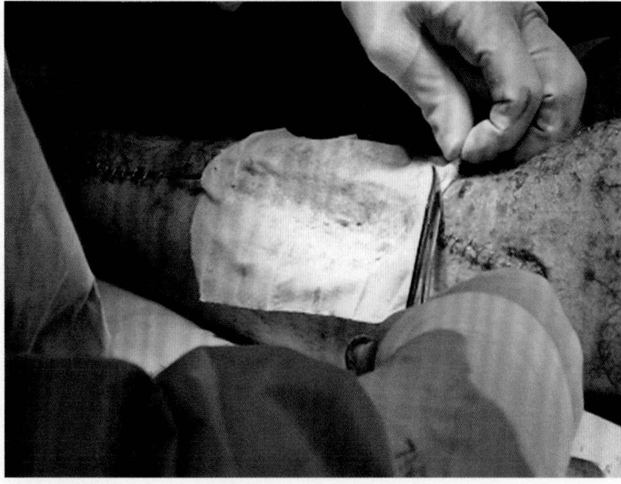

FIGURE 31-7. Nonadherent dressing applied over split-thickness skin graft.

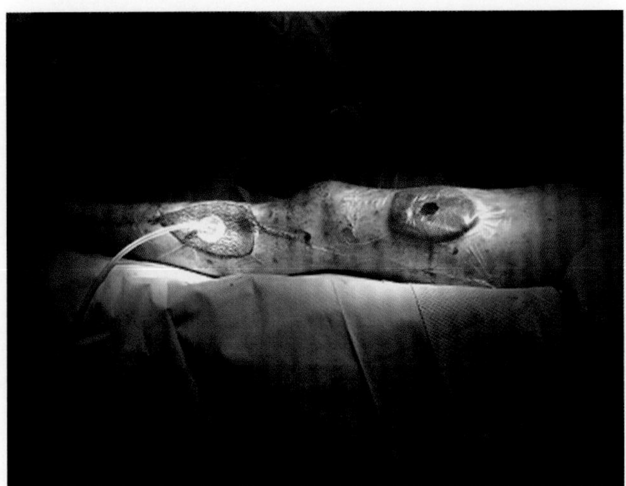

FIGURE 31-8. NPWT/ROCF dressing applied over skin graft.

of the graft during dressing removal (Fig. 31-8). Removal of the dressing most frequently occurs about 3 to 5 days postoperatively or when there is adequate graft take (Baharestani et al., 2009; Tarkin, 2008). Leaving the NPWT/ROCF dressing in place longer than 5 days is not recommended, since this may result in formation of hypergranulation tissue between the interstices of the meshed graft.

CLINICAL PEARL

Split-thickness skin grafts may be needed for coverage of large soft tissue defects, and NPWT is commonly used to maintain close adherence between the graft and the wound bed; a contact layer should be placed between the graft and the foam to prevent adherence of the graft to the foam.

Fasciotomy Wounds

Following a fasciotomy to an extremity, the incision/wound is left open to allow for the muscle edema to resolve (Fig. 31-9). If the wound edges are well approximated, the fasciotomy wound can be closed through delayed primary closure within 3 to 7 days postoperatively (Gourgiotis et al., 2007; Pollak, 2008). If the wound edges are not well approximated and delayed primary closure is not possible, the wound is closed by placing a skin graft over the defect.

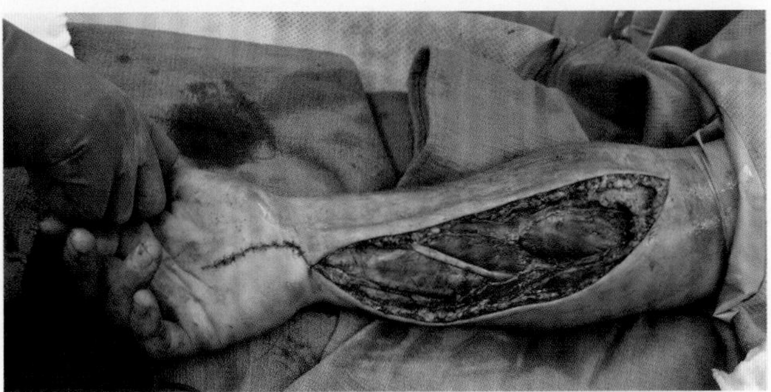

FIGURE 31-9. Fasciotomy performed due to compartment syndrome of forearm.

In all circumstances, the fasciotomy wound is initially left open and requires temporary coverage or bridging until the wound can be closed, through either delayed primary closure or a split-thickness skin graft. Temporary management of the open fasciotomy wound is frequently provided by NPWT/ROCF. NPWT/ROCF provides temporary coverage, a moist healing environment, less frequent dressing changes, and removal of excess fluid while the edema resolves (Morykwas et al., 2002; Tarkin, 2008; Yang et al., 2006). The surgeon may use a "crossed rubber band" technique with the NPWT system to keep the wound edges more closely approximated (Fig. 31-10). This process may improve the potential for delayed primary closure and reduce the need for skin grafting (Tarkin, 2008). This technique involves use of crossed rubber bands stapled to the wound edges to hold the wound edges in closer approximation. In this case, a nonadherent NPWT foam dressing is placed over the fasciotomy wound prior to application of the crossed rubber bands. If the nonadherent type NPWT foam dressing is not available, a nonadherent contact layer may be used as an interface between the fascia and the standard NPWT foam dressing. When the wound is ready for closure, the rubber bands and the NPWT nonadherent foam dressing are removed and the wound is closed primarily (Baharestani et al., 2009; Tarkin, 2008). If the fasciotomy wound is to be closed using a skin graft, then the NPWT/ROCF dressing may be used without a contact layer or nonadherent NPWT dressing; this approach may enhance granulation tissue formation over the muscle, which facilitates skin graft "take" (Stone et al., 2004).

Fasciotomy wounds of the abdomen, like fasciotomy wounds of the extremity, are left open to allow intrafascial edema to resolve. Management of the open abdominal fasciotomy wound most commonly involves use of an NPWT system (Navsaria et al., 2013). NPWT systems allow for temporary management of the open abdomen by (1) providing a closed environment that prevents desiccation of the abdominal contents, (2) removing excess wound fluid, and (3) reducing the amount of fascial retraction (Graybill et al., 2012; Navsaria et al., 2013; Vertrees et al., 2008). NPWT systems designed specifically for management of the complex open abdomen are commercially available. These commercially available systems consist of a fenestrated nonadherent film that is placed directly over

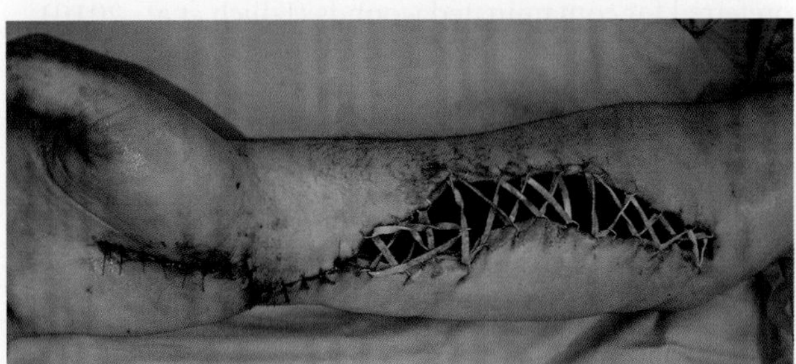

FIGURE 31-10. Vessel loop and staples used to approximate the tissues and minimize the area requiring a skin graft.

the abdominal viscera, a foam layer that is placed on top of the nonadherent film, an occlusive dressing covering the wound, and a negative pressure pump. The purpose of the fenestrated nonadherent film is to serve as a base layer that prevents adherence of the abdominal organ tissue to the ROCF dressing; this reduces the risk of fistula development. In addition, the fenestrations permit free egress of excess fluid out of the abdomen. When a commercial system is not available, IV bags or surgical towels can be used as the nonadherent base layer, followed by moistened gauze and an occlusive cover dressing. Negative pressure is then delivered by attaching wall suction to the dressing (Vertrees et al., 2008). These dressings should remain in place until abdominal edema resolves and delayed primary closure can be performed.

 Complications of Traumatic Wounds

Infection

Due to the nature of the high-risk traumatic wound, wound infection or osteomyelitis are always potential complications. High-risk wounds include grossly contaminated wounds; wounds with retained foreign material; wounds contaminated with organic material; wounds with devitalized tissue; wounds with delayed presentation; wounds to the foot or mouth; wounds with open fractures; wounds involving joint, tendon, or cartilage; and wounds involving an immunocompromised host (Moran et al., 2008). Adequate cleansing and meticulous technique are the most beneficial interventions to prevent wound infections (Moran et al., 2008). It is important to assess for signs and symptoms that could indicate infection in these high-risk wounds. Purulent drainage, fever, erythema, edema, pain, nonhealing wounds or fractures, and/or unexplained elevated blood glucose levels in the patient with diabetes are all indicators of infection and warrant further assessment. Treatment requires PO or IV antibiotics that are guided by wound or tissue culture findings; the adjunctive use of antimicrobial dressings or wound chemotherapy may also be necessary. Early administration of antibiotics is important as a delay in treatment lasting longer than 6 hours may allow bacteria to proliferate to levels sufficient to cause infection, and even a 3-hour delay may inhibit the effectiveness of systemic or topical antibiotics (Edlich, 1989; Edlich et al., 1971). Antibiotics administered via the IV route are preferred for contaminated wounds (Edlich et al., 2010).

CLINICAL PEARL

Complications of traumatic wounds include infection, heterotopic ossification (HO), PTSD, and major depression.

Heterotopic Ossification

HO is the formation of mature bone in nonosseous tissue, or simply put, deposition of bone in soft tissues (Melcer et al., 2011; Potter et al., 2006). Signs and symptoms of HO may include fever, chills, inflammation, impaired joint mobility, a palpable mass or bony spurs in soft tissue, and pain along pressure-sensitive areas of the injured/residual limb (Adams, 2014). HO is readily visible on radiograph and is most commonly found in the extremities of patients who have suffered traumatic injuries including blunt trauma, fractures, burns, traumatic brain injury, and spinal cord injury (Kaplan et al., 2004; Polfer et al., 2013). The exact etiopathogenesis of HO is unclear. HO has become more common with the increase in combat-related injuries and amputations occurring from the recent wars on terrorism. A few explanations for this recent increase in HO include: (1) the intensification of primary and secondary blast forces related to advancements in weaponry and explosives, (2) medical advances allowing patients to survive injuries that have previously been fatal, and (3) amputation close to or within the zone of injury, with the goal of preserving as much of the injured extremity as possible (Potter et al., 2006). Complications of HO formation include pain at the injury/amputation site, neurovascular entrapment, and skin breakdown caused by the use of prosthetics (Melcer et al., 2011; Polfer et al., 2013). HO can be limiting to the amputee by preventing prosthesis wear due to pain and/or skin breakdown. Resolution of symptoms may be managed conservatively through prosthetic adjustments, or in severe cases may require surgical excision of the offending bony formation (Melcer et al., 2011). Prophylactic nonsteroidal anti-inflammatory drug therapy may be beneficial in preventing HO formation (Potter et al., 2006).

Posttraumatic Stress Disorder/Major Depression

Posttraumatic stress disorder (PTSD) and major depression are prevalent among individuals suffering from major traumatic injury. In a large trauma center study, more than 40% of patients hospitalized following a traumatic injury suffered from PTSD or major depression, or both (Shih et al., 2010; Warren et al., 2014). PTSD and/or major depression place the trauma patient at risk for poor long-term outcomes that include physical disability, an increased risk for alcohol misuse, and a lower perceived quality of life (Heltemes et al., 2014; Shih et al., 2010). Early intervention is imperative to prevent and/or mitigate the effects of PTSD and depression in the trauma patient and provide the opportunity for a full recovery. Patients suffering from significant trauma and their family members should be screened for PTSD and/or depression, and referred to the appropriate provider. One easy-to-use screening device for PTSD that has been used effectively in both military and civilian trauma patients is the Primary Care PTSD screening tool (PC-PTSD). The PC-PTSD tool consists of four questions concerning recent nightmares, avoidance of situations, watchfulness/hypervigilance, and feelings of numbness or detachment from others or activities (Reese et al., 2012).

Conclusion

The major mechanisms for traumatic injury include motor vehicle crashes, gunshots, blasts, and natural disasters. Initial management of traumatic injury must focus on stabilizing the patient using measures dictated by ATLS guidelines. After the trauma patient is stabilized, it is important to obtain a through history regarding the nature of the wounding: time of injury, environment in which the injury occurred, and tetanus immunization status. The wound history will guide the treatment team in developing their initial management of the wound. In the acute traumatic wound, debridement of all nonviable tissue and thorough irrigation are critically important interventions for prevention of wound infection. Multiple debridements may be necessary in the first 4 to 7 days following a traumatic wound to ensure that all nonviable tissue is removed from the wound. These multiple debridements are necessary because the wound "evolves" over time and nonviable tissue will continue to declare itself during this time period. Patients who suffer crush injuries, fractures, arterial injuries, or burns and/or require application of tourniquets to control bleeding may also require fasciotomies to prevent compartment syndrome. Initially, most traumatic wounds must be left open because of the contaminated nature of these wounds. A temporary coverage for open traumatic wounds may be provided via NPWT/ROCF. NPWT/ROCF has become the industry standard for the management of open wounds until these wounds can safely be closed by delayed primary closure, skin graft, or tissue flap.

REFERENCES

Adams, L. (2014). Heterotopic ossification. *Radiation Therapist, 23*(1), 27–48.

Afshar, M., Raju, M., Ansell, D., et al. (2011). Narrative review: Tetanus—a health threat after natural disasters in developing countries. *Annals of Internal Medicine, 154*(5), 329–335.

Anand, R., & Ivatury, R. (2011). Surgical management of intra-abdominal hypertension and abdominal compartment syndrome. *The American Surgeon, 77*(Suppl 1), S42–S45.

Baharestani, M., Amjad, I., Bookout, K., et al. (2009). V.A.C. Therapy in the management of paediatric wounds: Clinical review and experience. *International Wound Journal, 6*(Suppl 1), 1–26.

Beekley, A., Sebesta, J., Blackbourne, L., et al. (2008). Prehospital tourniquet use in Operation Iraqi Freedom: Effect on hemorrhage control and outcomes. *Journal of Trauma, 64*(2), S28–S37.

Bellamy, R., Maningas, P., & Vayer, J. (1986). Epidemiology of trauma: Military experience. *Annals of Emergency Medicine, 15*(12), 1384–1388.

Bernabe, K., Desmarais, T., & Keller, M. (2014). Management of traumatic wounds and a novel approach to delivering wound care in children. *Advances in Wound Care, 3*(4), 335–343.

Blum, M., Esser, M., Richardson, M., et al. (2012). Negative pressure wound therapy reduces deep infection rate in open tibial fractures. *Journal of Orthopaedic Trauma, 26*(9), 499–505.

Centers for Disease Control and Prevention. (2012). Blast injuries: Fact sheets for professionals. National Center for Injury Prevention and Control Division of Injury Response. http://www.amtrauma.org/data/files/gallery/BlastInjuryResourcesFileGallery/Blast_InjuryRadiologic_Diagnosis.pdf

Crumbley, D., & Perciballi, J. (2007). Negative pressure wound therapy in a contaminated soft-tissue wound. *Journal of Wound, Ostomy, and Continence Nursing, 34*(5), 507–512.

Cubano, M., et al. (2013). *Emergency war surgery* (4th ed.). Fort Sam Houston, TX: Borden Institute. Digital edition may be found at http://www.cs.amedd.army.mil/borden/Portlet.aspx?ID=cb88853d-5b33-4b3f-968c-2cd95f7b7809

Dedmond, B., Kortesis, B., Punger, K., et al. (2007). The use of negative-pressure wound therapy (NPWT) in the temporary treatment of soft-tissue injuries associated with high-energy open tibial shaft fractures. *Journal of Orthopaedic Trauma, 21*(1), 11–17.

Doyle, G., & Taillac, P. (2008). Tourniquets: A review of current use with proposals for expanded prehospital use. *Prehospital Emergency Care, 12*(2), 241–256.

Edlich, R. (1989). General requirements for controlled clinical trials of antibiotic treatment of soft tissue lacerations. *Annals of Emergency Medicine, 18*(8), 900.

Edlich, R., Madden, J., Prusak, M., et al. (1971). Studies in the management of the contaminated wound. VI. The therapeutic value of gentle scrubbing in prolonging the limited period of effectiveness of antibiotics in contaminated wounds. *American Journal of Surgery, 121*(6), 668–672.

Edlich, R., Rodeheaver, G., Thacker, J., et al. (2010). Revolutionary advances in the management of traumatic wounds in the emergency department during the last 40 years: Part I. *Journal of Emergency Medicine, 38*(1), 40–50.

Fanfair, R., Benedict, K., Bos, J., et al. (2012). Necrotizing cutaneous mucormycosis after a tornado in Joplin, Missouri, in 2011. *New England Journal of Medicine, 367*(23), 2214–2225.

Fernandez, R., Griffiths, R., & Ussia, C. (2004). Effectiveness of solutions, techniques and pressure in wound cleansing. *JBI Reports, 2*(7), 231–270.

Giovinco, N., Bui, T., Fisher, T., et al. (2010). Wound chemotherapy by the use of negative pressure wound therapy and infusion. *Eplasty, 10*, e9.

Gourgiotis, S., Villias, C., Germanos, S., et al. (2007). Acute limb compartment syndrome: A review. *Journal of Surgical Education, 64*(3), 178–186.

Graybill, J., Stojadinovic, A., Crumbley, D., et al. (2012). Traumatic wounds: Bullets, blasts, and vehicle crashes. In R. Bryant & D. Nix (Eds.), *Acute and chronic wounds current management concepts* (4th ed.). St Louis, MO: Elsevier Mosby.

Gross, A., Cutright, D., & Bhaskar, S. (1972). Effectiveness of pulsating water jet lavage in treatment of contaminated crushed wounds. *American Journal of Surgery, 124*(3), 373–377.

Hall, S. (2007). A review of the effect of tap water versus normal saline on infection rates in acute traumatic wounds. *Journal of Wound Care, 16*(1), 38–41.

Harrell, B. R., & Melander, S. (2012). Identifying the association among risk factors and mortality in trauma patients with intra-abdominal hypertension and abdominal compartment syndrome. *Journal of Trauma Nursing, 19*(3), 182–189.

Haury, B., Rodeheaver, G., Vensko, J., et al. (1978). Debridement: An essential component of traumatic wound care. *American Journal of Surgery, 135*(2), 238–242.

Hayda, R., Harris, R., & Bass, C. (2004). Blast injury research: Modeling injury effects of landmines, bullets, and bombs. *Clinical Orthopaedics and Related Research, (422)*, 97–108.

Heltemes, K., Clouser, M., MacGregor, A., et al. (2014). Co-occurring mental health and alcohol misuse: Dual disorder symptoms in combat injured veterans. *Addictive Behaviors, 39*(2), 392–398.

Joint Theatre Trauma System Clinical Practice Guideline. (2012). Initial management of war wounds: Wound debridement and irrigation. http://www.usaisr.amedd.army.mil/clinical_practice_guidelines.html

Kam, P., Kavanagh, R., Yoong, F., et al. (2001). The arterial tourniquet: Pathophysiological consequences and anaesthetic implications. *Anaesthesia, 56*(6), 534–545.

Kaplan, F., Glaser, D., Hebela, N., et al. (2004). Heterotopic ossification. *Journal of the American Academy of Orthopaedic Surgeons, 12*(2), 116–125.

Kretsinger, K., Broder, K., Cortese, M., et al. (2006a). Preventing tetanus, diphtheria, and pertussis among adults: Use of tetanus toxoid, reduced diphtheria toxoid and acellular pertussis vaccine—recommendations of the Advisory Committee on Immunization Practices (ACIP) and recommendation of ACIP, supported by the Healthcare.

Kretsinger, K., Broder, K. R., Cortese, M. M., et al. (2006b). Infection Control Practices Advisory Committee (HICPAC), for use of Tdap among health-care personnel. *MMWR Morbidity and Mortality Weekly Report, 55*(RR-17), 1–36.

Krug, E., Berg, L., Lee, C., et al. (2011). Evidence-based recommendations for the use of Negative Pressure Wound Therapy in traumatic wounds and reconstructive surgery: Steps towards an international consensus. *Injury, 42*(Suppl 1), S1–S12.

Large, T., Douglas, G., Erickson, G., et al. (2012). Effect of negative pressure wound therapy on the elution of antibiotics from polymethylmethacrylate beads in a porcine simulated open femur fracture model. *Journal of Orthopaedic Trauma, 26*(9), 506–511.

Lewandowski, L., Purcell, R., Fleming, M., et al. (2013). The use of dilute Dakin's solution for the treatment of angioinvasive fungal infection in the combat wounded: A case series. *Military Medicine, 178*(4), e503–e507.

Lichte, P., Oberbeck, R., Binnebösel, M., et al. (2010). A civilian perspective on ballistic trauma and gunshot injuries. *Scandinavian Journal of Trauma, Resuscitation and Emergency Medicine, 18*, 35. doi:10.1186/1757-7241-18-35

Melcer, T., Belnap, B., Walker, G., et al. (2011). Heterotopic ossification in combat amputees from Afghanistan and Iraq wars: Five case histories and results from a small series of patients. *Journal of Rehabilitation Research and Development, 48*(1), 1–12.

Moisidis, E., Heath, T., Boorer, C., et al. (2004). A prospective, blinded, randomized, controlled clinical trial of topical negative pressure use in skin grafting. *Plastic and Reconstructive Surgery, 114*(4), 917–922.

Moran, G., Talan, D., & Abrahamian, F. (2008). Antimicrobial prophylaxis for wounds and procedures in the emergency department. *Infectious Disease Clinics, 22*(1), 117.

Morykwas, M., Argenta, L., Shelton-Brown, E., et al. (1997). Vacuum-assisted closure: A new method for wound control and treatment: Animal studies and basic foundation. *Annals of Plastic Surgery, 38*(6), 553–562.

Morykwas, M., Howell, H., Bleyer, A., et al. (2002). The effect of externally applied subatmospheric pressure on serum myoglobin levels after a prolonged crush/ischemia injury. *Journal of Trauma, 53*(3), 537–540.

Navsaria, P., Nicol, A., Hudson, D., et al. (2013). Negative pressure wound therapy management of the "open abdomen" following trauma: A prospective study and systematic review. *World Journal of Emergency Surgery, 8*(1), 4.

Polfer, E., Forsberg, J., Fleming, M., et al. (2013). Neurovascular entrapment due to combat-related heterotopic ossification in the lower extremity. *Journal of Bone and Joint Surgery (American Volume), 95*(24), e195(1–6).

Pollak, A. (2008). Use of negative pressure wound therapy for reticulated open cell foam for lower extremity trauma. *Journal of Orthopaedic Trauma, 22*(10), S142–S145.

Potter, B., Burns, T., Lacap, A., et al. (2006). Heterotopic ossification in the residual limbs of traumatic and combat-related amputees. *Journal of the American Academy of Orthopaedic Surgeons, 14*(10 Spec. No.), S191–S197.

Ramasamy, A., Hill, A., Hepper, A., et al. (2009). Blast mines: Physics, injury mechanisms and vehicle protection. *Journal of the Royal Army Medical Corps, 155*(4), 258–264.

Reese, C., Pederson, T., Avila, S., et al. (2012). Screening for traumatic stress among survivors of urban trauma. *Journal of Trauma and Acute Care Surgery, 73*(2), 462–468.

Scherer, L., Shiver, S., Chang, M., et al. (2002). The vacuum assisted closure device: A method of securing skin grafts and improving graft survival. *Archives of Surgery (Chicago, Ill.: 1960), 137*(8), 930–933.

Shih, R., Schell, T., Hambarsoomian, K., et al. (2010). Prevalence of posttraumatic stress disorder and major depression after trauma center hospitalization. *Journal of Trauma, 69*(6), 1560–1566

Sonshine, D., Caldwell, A., Gosselin, R., et al. (2012). Critically assessing the Haiti earthquake response and the barriers to quality orthopaedic care. *Clinical Orthopaedics and Related Research, 470*(10), 2895–2904.

Stannard, J., Singanamala, N., & Volgas, D. (2010). Fix and flap in the era of vacuum suction devices: What do we know in terms of evidence based medicine? *Injury, 41*(8), 780–786.

Stevenson, T., Thacker, J., Rodeheaver, G., et al. (1976). Cleansing the traumatic wound by high pressure syringe irrigation. *JACEP, 5*(1), 17–21.

Stone, P., Prigozen, J., Hofeldt, M., et al. (2004). Bolster versus negative pressure wound therapy for securing split-thickness skin grafts in trauma patients. *Wounds: A Compendium of Clinical Research and Practice, 16*(7), 219–223.

Storer, A., Lindauer, C., Proehl, J., et al. (2012). Emergency nursing resource: Wound preparation. *Journal of Emergency Nursing, 38*(5), 443–446.

Tarkin, I. (2008). The versatility of negative pressure wound therapy with reticulated open cell foam for soft tissue management after severe musculoskeletal trauma. *Journal of Orthopaedic Trauma, 22*(10), S146–S151.

Thacker, J., Stalnecker, M., Allaire, P., et al. (1977). Practical applications of skin biomechanics. *Clinics in Plastic Surgery, 4*(2), 167–171.

Venturi, M., Attinger, C., Mesbahi, A., et al. (2005). Mechanisms and clinical applications of the vacuum-assisted closure (VAC) device: A review. *American Journal of Clinical Dermatology, 6*(3), 185–194.

Vertrees, A., Greer, L., Pickett, C., et al. (2008). Modern management of complex open abdominal wounds of war: A 5-year experience. *Journal of the American College of Surgeons, 207*(6), 801–809.

Warren, A., Foreman, M., Bennett, M., et al. (2014). Posttraumatic stress disorder following traumatic injury at 6 months: Associations with alcohol use and depression. *Journal of Trauma and Acute Care Surgery, 76*(2), 517–522.

Wood, M. J. (2004). Toxin-mediated disorders: Tetanus, botulism, and diphtheria. In J. Cohen, et al. (Eds.), *Infectious diseases*. Philadelphia, PA: Mosby.

Yang, C., Chang, D., & Webb, L. (2006). Vacuum-assisted closure for fasciotomy wounds following compartment syndrome of the leg. *Journal of Surgical Orthopaedic Advances, 15*(1), 19–23.

QUESTIONS

1. Wound care nurses implement care for patients with various types of traumatic wounds. Which statement accurately describes the effect of these wounds on the human body?
   A. Blunt trauma injuries cause skin or muscle damage but do not usually affect bones, vessels, and internal organs.
   B. As a bullet interacts with the tissue, it produces both a smaller permanent cavity and a larger temporary cavity.
   C. Elastic tissue, such as muscle, blood vessels, skin, and fat may fracture and result in secondary injury.
   D. Handguns cause high-velocity wounds; hunting rifles or military weapons cause low-velocity wounds.

2. The wound care nurse documents that tissue adjacent to a gunshot wound that appeared healthy on examination has become necrotic eight hours later. What is the term for this phenomenon?
   A. "Tissue resuscitation"
   B. "Hidden necrosis"
   C. "Wound evolution"
   D. "Boomerang effect"

3. A wound care nurse working in a VA hospital cares for patients with various types of blast injuries. Which statement accurately describes the effect of a tertiary blast injury?
   A. The victim is thrown by the blast and strikes surrounding objects.
   B. The sonic shockwave of the blast strikes the body.
   C. Device fragments are propelled through the air and cause trauma.
   D. Thermal injuries and injuries from toxic exposure occur.

4. What type of injury is the most frequently occurring blast injury?
   A. Musculoskeletal injury
   B. Burn injury
   C. Wound infections
   D. Neurological injury

5. The wound care nurse is caring for patients who sustained significant blast injuries caused by a tornado. For what life-threatening secondary condition would the nurse monitor these patients?
   A. Delayed wound healing
   B. Viral infections
   C. Fungal infections
   D. Dehydration

6. A patient presents with hemorrhaging from a wound located on a lower extremity. What is the best initial intervention for this type of external bleeding?
   A. Tourniquet
   B. Bandages
   C. Surgical closure of the wound
   D. Direct pressure

7. A wound care nurse is applying a tourniquet to a patient injured in an automobile crash. What intervention is performed according to prehospital tourniquet protocols?
   A. If a commercial tourniquet is not available, use a soft cloth.
   B. Leave the tourniquet in place if transport time is under 30 minutes.
   C. Quickly tighten the tourniquet until hemorrhage stops.
   D. Remove the tourniquet immediately if the patient is unstable and in shock.

8. In which case would wound management with tetanus prophylaxis be recommended?
   A. The patient's most recent tetanus vaccination is greater than 2 years.
   B. The wound is contaminated with soil, feces, or saliva.
   C. The wound is a closed wound caused by blunt trauma.
   D. The wound is a pressure ulcer that becomes infected.

9. The wound care nurse monitors patients with traumatic wounds for signs of compartment syndrome. Which of the following is a sign of this condition?
   A. Rapid pulse
   B. Cyanosis
   C. Pain that is disproportionate to injury
   D. Neurological changes

10. For which type of wounds is primary closure the treatment of choice?
   A. Wounds to the face
   B. Soft tissue injuries
   C. Infected wounds
   D. Wounds complicated by compartment syndrome

11. What is one benefit of negative pressure wound therapy (NPWT)?
   A. Reduction of granulation tissue formation
   B. Increase in inflammatory cytokines
   C. Prevention of infection
   D. Reduction in time to definitive closure

12. The wound care nurse assesses a patient with a large soft tissue wound that is healing by secondary intention. Final closure of this wound is generally accomplished by:
    A. Antibiotic beads
    B. Split-thickness skin grafts
    C. NPWT with ROCF
    D. Fasciotomy

13. The wound care nurse documents heterotopic ossification (HO) in a patient's wound bed. What is a potential complication of HO?
    A. Neurovascular entrapment
    B. Occurrence of skin flaps
    C. Skin cancer
    D. Bone cancer

ANSWERS: 1.**B**, 2.**C**, 3.**A**, 4.**A**, 5.**C**, 6.**D**, 7.**B**, 8.**B**, 9.**C**, 10.**A**, 11.**D**, 12.**B**, 13.**A**

CHAPTER 32

Management of Surgical Wounds

C. Tod Brindle and Suzanne Creehan

OBJECTIVES

1. Describe the phases of healing for a closed surgical wound and implications for assessment of these wounds.
2. Discuss guidelines for prevention, prompt detection, and management of surgical wound complications, to include infection, dehiscence, and compartment syndrome.
3. Explain situations in which a surgical wound cannot be closed primarily and options for management of these open surgical wounds.
4. Explain indications for use of mesh in closure of abdominal wounds, the differences in unmodified and modified mesh, and implications for assessment and management of wounds with exposed mesh.
5. Describe assessment and management of open abdominal or chest wounds, to include modifications in standard wound care and in use of NPWT.

Topic Outline

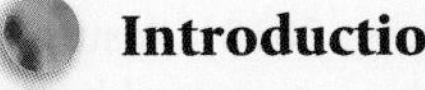
Introduction

Healing Process for Surgical Wounds
- Hemostasis and Inflammation
- Proliferative Phase
- Remodeling Phase

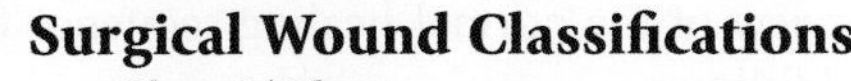
Surgical Wound Classifications
- Class I/Clean
- Class II/Clean–Contaminated
- Class III/Contaminated
- Class IV/Dirty Infected

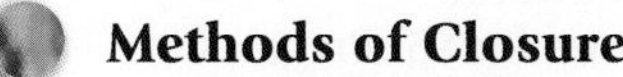
Methods of Closure
- Primary Closure
- Delayed Primary Closure (Tertiary Intention Wound Management)
- Secondary Intention
- Flap or Graft

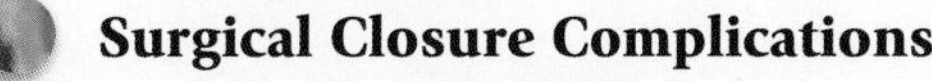
Surgical Closure Complications

Surgical Wound Assessment
- Day 1 to Day 4: Inflammation and Epithelial Resurfacing
- Day 5 to Day 9: Proliferative Phase
- Days 10 to 14: Continued Proliferation and Early Remodeling
- Day 15 and Beyond

Guidelines for Incisional Care

Indications and Guidelines for Management of Complex Wounds
- Incisional Negative Pressure Wound Therapy
  - Benefits of Incisional NPWT
  - Options for iNPWT
  - Indications for iNPWT
  - Complications and Contraindications for iNPWT
- Management of Complex Abdominal Wounds
  - Impact of Muscle Disruption
  - Management of the Open Abdomen
- Incisional Failure following Primary Closure
  - Mechanical Risk Factors
  - Biologic Risk Factors
- Management Decisions
  - Care Options
  - Critical Assessment Factors

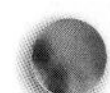

Introduction

According to the Centers for Disease Control and Prevention (CDC), approximately 51.4 million inpatient surgical procedures are performed annually in the United States; in addition, the most recent outpatient statistics indicate that an additional 19.9 million procedures are performed in hospital-based ambulatory surgical clinics and 14.9 million procedures are performed in free standing ambulatory surgery centers (CDC, 2009, 2014). The number of acute surgical wounds far exceeds that of chronic wounds; yet, chronic wound healing carries the burden of higher cost and greater impact on quality of life. Acute surgical wounds typically proceed "normally" through the phases of healing; however, surgical wounds are sometimes complicated by impaired healing and dehiscence due to intrinsic and extrinsic risk factors. Thus, the major goal in management of surgical wounds is to prevent complications and eliminate deterrents to healing (Franz et al., 2008).

> **CLINICAL PEARL**
>
> Surgical wounds usually heal normally; however, these wounds are sometimes complicated by impaired healing and dehiscence due to intrinsic and extrinsic risk factors.

Individuals undergo surgical procedures for a variety of purposes; electively, for management of complications related to acute disease or for repair of an injury. The reason for and timing of surgery can impact the outcome in terms of wound healing. In an elective situation, the date of surgery can be selected when the patient's health is in optimal condition; in this case, positive outcomes are very likely. In contrast, the patient who undergoes emergent surgery related to acute illness or injury is at risk for impaired healing due to the multiple physiologic stressors affecting the body. In addition, tissue that is already diseased, inflamed, or traumatized does not heal as well as healthy tissue.

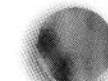

Healing Process for Surgical Wounds

As explained in Chapter 2, acute full-thickness injuries heal in a predictable manner through the overlapping stages of hemostasis, inflammation, proliferation, and remodeling. This also is the classic pathway for surgical wound healing (Cooper, 1990; Phillips, 2000). Surgical wounds proceed through the phases of repair in an orderly and timely manner when obstacles to healing are minimized and the host response is maximized. Healed surgical wounds are characterized by restoration of skin integrity through reepithelialization of the incision and full-thickness restoration in the tissue layers beneath. If an acute surgical wound has not adhered to the normal healing sequence in terms of symptoms, signs, or time to heal within a 4- to 6-week time frame, most authors agree that it is then labeled chronic (Lee & Hansen, 2009; Widgerow, 2013). The time point at which a surgical wound becomes chronic has been a long-standing topic of expert discussion. According to Widgerow (2013), surgical wounds should be labeled as "chronic" when they deviate from the normal healing trajectory as evidenced by symptoms, signs, or time to healing.

Ideally, acute surgical wounds undergo uncomplicated healing and rapid closure. The trajectory to healing is affected by intrinsic and extrinsic host factors as well as surgical skill and technique. Additionally, not all surgical wounds are located in healthy tissue, and the poor integrity of the tissue can cause delays in healing. Surgical wounds located in areas of significant trauma, such as crush injuries, or grossly contaminated wounds may require a longer than anticipated time to heal (Widgerow, 2013). A surgical wound that has not progressed to the anticipated healing end point of closure and displays characteristics such as bleeding, exudate production, and pain after a 4-week time period may be considered to be a chronic surgical wound (Widgerow, 2013).

A brief overview of the normal healing sequence for a surgical wound follows.

Hemostasis and Inflammation

Acute wound healing begins with establishment of hemostasis. The coagulation cascade is activated by vessel disruption and involves platelet aggregation to form a clot and vasoconstriction to control hemorrhaging and reduce blood loss. Surgeons augment these physiologic reflexes through use of the bovie and other electrocauterization tools. Vasoconstriction of the vessels in the surgical field is the immediate response to a surgical injury. Platelet activation produces two key results that are critical to both hemostasis and the inflammatory phase of repair: (1) fibrin clot formation, which seals the vessels to prevent bacterial invasion and serves as a temporary scaffolding for cell migration, and (2) the release of growth factors and cytokines that recruit the leukocytes needed for bacterial control and elimination of any damaged tissue. Once hemostasis is accomplished, the wound moves into the inflammatory phase of repair. This phase is supported by vasodilatation, which occurs within minutes following the initial vasoconstrictive response. The increased blood flow that accompanies the inflammatory phase is the basis for the edema, erythema, warmth, and pain that is characteristic of this phase of healing. The key cells during the initial phase of repair (hemostasis and inflammation) include platelets, neutrophils, and macrophages.

CLINICAL PEARL

The repair process for a surgical wound begins with platelet activation and clot formation, which seals the vessels to prevent bacterial invasion, provides a temporary scaffolding for cell migration, and releases the growth factors and cytokines that recruit the cells needed for repair.

Neutrophils are phagocytic leukocytes that are summoned to the wound site within hours of the injury and remain active up to several days. The phagocytic action primarily targets invading microorganisms; the neutrophils also produce superoxide, which enhances the effectiveness of systemic antibiotics (Sussman & Bates-Jensen, 2012). Macrophages arrive in the wound 2 to 3 days postinjury and play an important role in the inflammatory phase as well as the transition to the proliferative phase. Macrophages carry out a number of key functions: they secrete elastase and collagenase to break down damaged tissue, they destroy microorganisms through phagocytosis and release of nitric oxide, and they attract fibroblasts to the wound bed via chemotactic signaling (Goldman, 2004; Sussman & Bates-Jensen, 2012).

Proliferative Phase

In a surgical wound in which the wound edges are approximated with staples, sutures, or fibrin glue, the proliferative phase begins within 24 hours of injury and overlaps the inflammatory phase. The first component of the proliferative phase is epithelial resurfacing. Keratinocytes respond to cytokines released by the neutrophils, specifically by advancing from the wound edges to resurface the minor disruption in skin integrity (Chin et al., 2007). Because the epithelial defect is very limited in an approximated wound, initial epithelialization is typically complete within 2 days. Once epithelial resurfacing is complete, the bacterial barrier has been restored and wound dressings become optional.

CLINICAL PEARL

In a surgical wound closed primarily, the proliferative phase of repair begins within 24 hours and overlaps the inflammatory phase; the first component of the proliferative phase is epithelial resurfacing, followed by formation of sufficient granulation tissue to knit the underlying tissue layers together.

The second component of the proliferative phase is granulation tissue formation, which begins on day 3 to 5 postinjury, following and overlapping the inflammatory phase. The goal of the proliferative phase is to synthesize new tissue to fill the defect in the soft tissues (suture line). Granulation tissue formation involves the simultaneous production of new blood vessels and the synthesis of new connective tissue proteins (creation of an extracellular matrix). Angiogenesis begins with sprouting of new capillary buds from existing vessels located in the adjacent wound tissue; this neovascular network is ultimately responsible for delivery of oxygen-rich blood and nutrients to the wound. Simultaneously, a collagen matrix is being formed that provides the supportive architecture for the new vessels (Chin et al., 2007). The fibroblasts are responsible for synthesis of collagen and other connective tissue proteins that form the extracellular matrix (Chin et al., 2007). Deposition of collagen early in the healing process is crucial for successful wound closure; any failure of this process increases the risk for wound dehiscence, which most commonly occurs during post-op days 5 to 8 (Whitney, 2012). The newly formed collagen is type III, which lacks tensile strength; during the remodeling phase, the type III collagen is converted to type I collagen, which provides tensile strength.

In open wounds, contraction of the wound occurs at the same time that granulation tissue is being formed; contraction of the wound edges is accomplished through the work of myofibroblasts and acts to reduce the size of the defect (Chin et al., 2007). Contraction is generally beneficial in open wounds; however, if the open wound is located over a joint, contraction could result in limitation of mobility and function and is therefore undesirable (Greer et al., 2007). Contraction does not occur in surgical wounds where the edges are approximated.

Remodeling Phase

The various phases of wound healing overlap and occur somewhat simultaneously. The remodeling phase begins during the final days of the proliferative phase and involves breakdown of the type III collagen and replacement with type I collagen, which is characterized by an orderly and parallel pattern (Chin et al., 2007). The remodeling phase lasts from 3 weeks to 2 years postinjury.

CLINICAL PEARL

The maturation phase lasts from 3 weeks to 2 years post-surgery and involves breakdown of the type III collagen and replacement with type I collagen, which provides tensile strength.

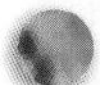 Surgical Wound Classifications

Surgical wounds are classified as classes I to IV based on the degree of sterility or contamination (Mangram, 1999; Menez, 2009). The classification may guide the surgeon's decision for primary, delayed primary, or secondary intention closure. The definitions are as follows:

Class I/Clean

Uninfected operative wound with no inflammation observed and no entry into respiratory, alimentary, genital, or urinary tract. Incision is closed primarily and if necessary drained with a closed drainage apparatus.

Class II/Clean–Contaminated

Respiratory, alimentary, genital, or urinary tract was entered under controlled conditions and without unusual contamination. No evidence of infection or major break in technique was encountered. The incision is closed primarily and if necessary drained with a closed drainage apparatus.

Class III/Contaminated

Open, fresh, accidental wounds; surgeries with major breaks in techniques or gross spillage from the GI tract; and incisions in which acute, nonpurulent inflammation occurs. These wounds are left open initially and later closed through delayed primary closure or left open to heal by secondary intention.

Class IV/Dirty Infected

Old traumatic wounds with retained devitalized tissue and those that involve existing clinical infection or perforated viscera. Microorganism(s) causing the infection were present in operative field before surgery. These wounds are left open to heal by secondary intention.

CLINICAL PEARL

Surgical wounds are classified based on the degree of contamination (from class I to class IV); clean wounds can usually be closed primarily, while dirty wounds and those with heavy bacterial loads are usually managed with delayed closure or left open to heal by secondary intention.

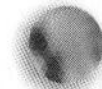 Methods of Closure

Primary Closure

Primary closure of a wound occurs when the edges of the wound are approximated by a surgeon and held in place by staples, sutures, or skin adhesives (Fig. 32-1). Primary closure implies each tissue layer is approximated and closed, including the dermis, subcutaneous layer, fascia, and muscle. Primary closure typically occurs at the conclusion of a surgical procedure, although it is a wound closure technique used for clean traumatic injuries as well. Placement of sutures or staples for tissue approximation is an additional form of injury; sutures and staples are intentionally placed foreign bodies. If the foreign body becomes infected or causes irritation, the wound rarely heals until the material is extruded or removed.

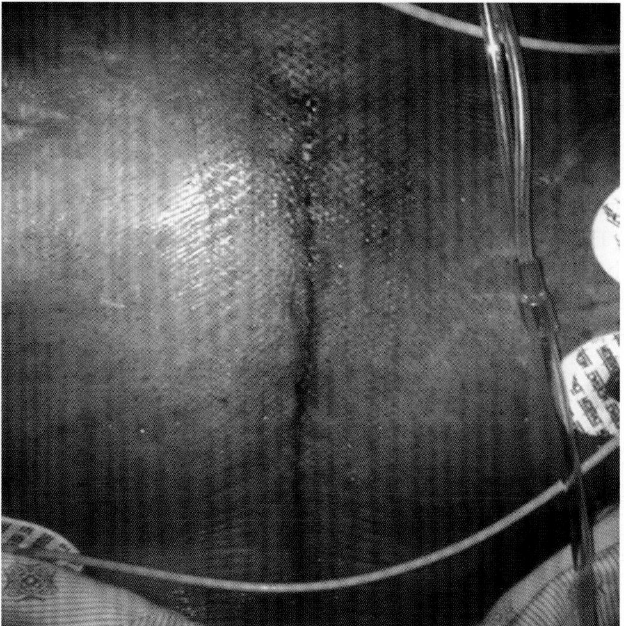

FIGURE 32-1. Wound closed by primary intention.

Primary repair should approximate the wound edges without causing strangulation of vessels within the wound (Franz et al., 2008). Lee and Hansen (2009) stress the importance of atraumatic tissue handling, selective cauterization of blood vessels, and avoidance of excessive tension at the suture/staple line in prevention of skin and soft tissue necrosis. Skin necrosis from vascular disruption or excessive closure tension leads to impaired healing and eventually a chronic open wound (Lee & Hansen, 2009). Primary closure is the preferred method of closure for clean wounds and wounds involving repair of injured structures such as nerves, tendons, and blood vessels when the zone of injury is small and the wound is clean; primary closure is contraindicated in the presence of tension, potential infection, and/or when the extent of injury is unclear (Lee & Hansen, 2009). Wounds with known or suspected colonization or infection $>10^5$ bacteria per gram of tissue should not be primarily closed (Franz et al., 2008).

Delayed Primary Closure (Tertiary Intention Wound Management)

Delayed primary closure was developed during World War II in an effort to reduce infection rates in traumatic war injuries (Wechter et al., 2005). Wounds were debrided

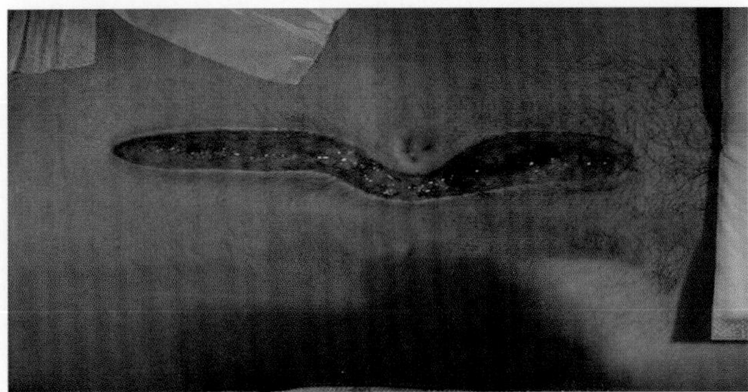

FIGURE 32-2. Wound for delayed primary closure.

and left open with packing for several days, then sutured closed. This practice change reduced the incidence of wound infections from 23% to 2% (Wechter et al., 2005). Today, delayed primary closure is used when there is a high level of contamination. The wound is left open until topical therapy has reduced the bacterial load and the likelihood of soft tissue infection (typically 2 to 5 days); at that point, the wound edges are approximated and closed with sutures, staples, or skin adhesives. Delayed closure may also be used prior to graft application; in this case, the delay is used to create a healthy bed of granulation tissue that will support the graft (Fig. 32-2).

CLINICAL PEARL

Delayed primary closure is used for heavily contaminated wounds; the wound is left open until bacterial loads have been controlled, at which point the wound edges are approximated and closed with sutures, staples, or skin adhesives.

Secondary Intention

Surgical wounds not closed primarily or with delayed primary closure are left open to heal by secondary intention (Fig. 32-3A and B). These wounds are treated with topical wound care to optimize the body's ability to fill the cavity or deficit with scar. This approach is indicated for heavily contaminated wounds, poorly perfused wounds, malignant wounds, wounds with necrosis or known infection, and wounds with extensive tissue loss in which attempted approximation would create excessive tension and increased risk for dehiscence (Greer et al., 2007). Surgical wounds most commonly left open to heal by secondary intention involve GI perforations, penetrating trauma wounds, perforated appendix, and compartment syndrome. Aggressive or serial debridement of necrotic tissue, elimination of malignant tissue, and eradication of infection may permit eventual surgical closure of wounds initially left open.

CLINICAL PEARL

Wounds left open to heal by secondary intention include those involving bowel perforation, penetrating trauma, and compartment syndrome; the focus in management of these wounds is on wound care to promote granulation tissue formation and epithelial resurfacing.

Flap or Graft

Another method of surgical closure involves placement of a graft or flap. Grafting can involve donor tissue from another species (biologics, heterograft, or xenograft), from another human being (allograft), or from the patient himself or herself (autograft). Autografts can be split thickness (the epidermis and part of the dermis), full thickness (the epidermis and dermis), or composite (skin and underlying tissue). Flaps involve closure of the defect with skin and soft tissue from another area of the body and include random flaps, axial/arterial flaps, musculocutaneous flaps, fasciocutaneous flaps, and free flaps. Grafts and flaps are typically reserved for situations involving large tissue defects and/or the inability to close the tissue primarily. In this case, the flap or graft serves to provide coverage of the wound base and in some cases also provides protection and coverage for exposed muscles, tendons, and bones or organs. Further discussion on this topic exceeds the intent of this chapter. Even though the decision to apply a graft or flap resides with the provider, the wound care clinician may be consulted as a member of the interdisciplinary team to assist in developing the plan of care for a grafted patient. In this case, it is important to assure stabilization of the graft, use of atraumatic dressings, and exudate management and to monitor for graft adherence and flap viability.

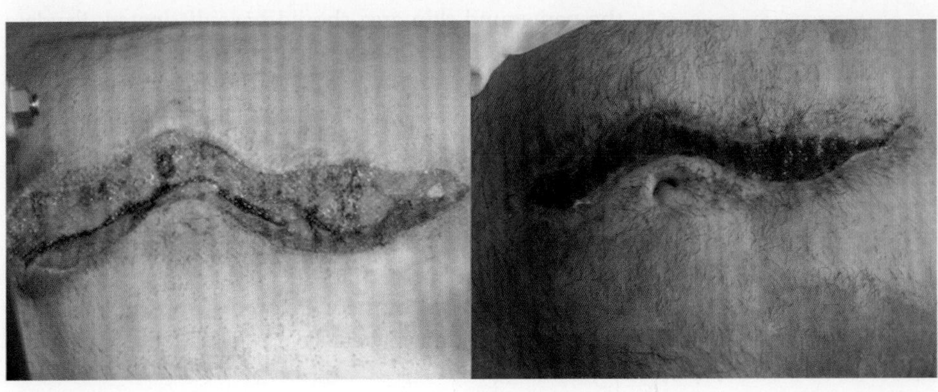

FIGURE 32-3. Wound healing by secondary intention.

 Surgical Closure Complications

Common complications involving surgically closed wounds include hematomas and seromas, incisional separation, and dehiscence; evisceration is a much less common event.

Post-op hematomas or seromas involve collections of clotted blood or serum between the tissue layers of the surgical wound and can exert sufficient pressure to interfere with perfusion of the adjacent tissue. Hematomas are of particular concern, because blood is an excellent medium for bacterial growth; thus, hematomas that are not quickly reabsorbed should be evacuated to avoid a free fluid collection of microorganisms (Franz et al., 2008). This can be accomplished by needle aspiration or placement of a drain. Franz et al. (2008) noted that wound hematomas are increasingly common due to the increased use of prophylactic and therapeutic anticoagulation and antiplatelet therapy in surgical patients (Nutescu et al., 2011).

CLINICAL PEARL

Hematomas provide an excellent medium for bacterial growth; hematomas that are not quickly reabsorbed should be evacuated by aspiration or placement of a drain.

Incisional separation is superficial; the skin edges are separated, but the deeper tissues remain approximated. The term dehiscence refers to separation of the skin and soft tissue layers and can be further classified as complete or incomplete. Complete dehiscence involves disruption of the fascia and often the peritoneum, whereas incomplete dehiscence is a separation of the epidermis, dermis, and subcutaneous tissue but not the fascia. Evisceration is protrusion of the intestine into the wound and requires an emergent response to maintain bowel viability (Doughty & Sparks-DeFriese, 2007).

CLINICAL PEARL

Dehiscence refers to separation of the skin and soft tissue layers and can be further classified as complete or incomplete. Evisceration involves protrusion of the bowel into the wound and requires emergent response to maintain bowel viability.

 Surgical Wound Assessment

Ongoing assessment of the surgical wound is a critical element of postoperative nursing management. Visual assessment of the incision and surrounding tissue and gentle palpation are key to determining progress in healing. Acute surgical wounds should proceed in an orderly and timely fashion through the phases of healing briefly described earlier, as well as more extensively in Chapter 2. Aligning surgical site assessment with the physical manifestations of the wound-healing process (inflammation, proliferation, and remodeling) will help determine if the wound is progressing as expected or not.

Day 1 to Day 4: Inflammation and Epithelial Resurfacing

The incision should be well approximated, with skin edges touching; the open edges are red in color. Periwound skin may appear mildly inflamed, may feel warm to the touch, and may be tender on palpation. Edema and erythema in the surrounding soft tissue are normal but should be resolving by days 3 to 4 postoperatively. If staples or sutures are present, mild inflammation of the staple and/or suture insertion sites is normal since they are intentionally placed foreign bodies (Bates-Jensen & Williams, 2012). Often, an equal and continuous halo of erythema may be seen around the wound margins; the erythema should not extend >2 cm beyond the wound edges and should steadily decrease in intensity.

A close look at the incision will reveal a new epithelial layer covering the incision at 48 to 72 hours postoperatively. This reflects epithelial resurfacing and indicates the wound is "closed," and the protective skin barrier function has been restored (Bates-Jensen & Williams, 2012).

CLINICAL PEARL

In assessing a closed surgical wound, the clinician should correlate clinical findings with physiologic events; for example, at 48 to 72 hours postoperatively, the incision is normally "closed" at the surface, and by days 5 to 8 postoperatively, a "healing ridge" should be palpable.

Initially, any exudate will be sanguineous, progressing to serosanguineous as vessel leakage subsides and extracellular serous fluid mixes with residual bloody serum. The volume of exudate should be limited.

Day 5 to Day 9: Proliferative Phase

The redness of the incision fades to a pink as capillary beds regress beneath the newly epithelialized surface; at the same time, the new epidermis is reestablishing normal thickness and the distinct epidermal layers. In a wound healing normally, the new epithelium is intact with no breaks in integrity. Any preexisting inflammation, edema, or erythema in the periwound skin area should have dissipated. Exudate should not be present (Bates-Jensen & Williams, 2012).

Beneath the surface, a collagen matrix is being established. Palpation along the entire length of the incision should reveal a stiffness or firmness to the tissue up to 1 cm on either side of the incision (Phillips, 2000); this is known as a healing ridge and is a normal expected outcome. In fact, lack of a healing ridge is an indicator of high risk for dehiscence or infection (Lee & Hansen, 2009); wound dehiscence most often occurs post-op days 5 to 8 and is likely linked to delayed or inadequate collagen deposition (Whitney, 2012).

Days 10 to 14: Continued Proliferation and Early Remodeling

As the proliferative phase continues, the sutures and staples can safely be removed and Steri-Strips may or may not be applied. The epithelial resurfacing is visible, the healing ridge is palpable, and surrounding tissue remains normal. There is no exudate at this point of surgical wound healing (Bates-Jensen & Williams, 2012).

Day 15 and Beyond

As capillary regression continues, the color of the incision continues to pale and ultimately the incision takes on a pearly gray appearance. As the collagen converts to type I and reorganizes in a patterned fashion, the healing ridge softens (Bates-Jensen & Williams, 2012). The final tensile strength of the healed incision is approximately 80% compared to its preinjured state.

Guidelines for Incisional Care

The primary purpose of a post-op incisional dressing is for protection against bacterial invasion, exudate absorption, and thermal insulation. Most authors and clinical experts agree that primary incisional wounds should be protected by a sterile occlusive dressing that provides protection against bacterial invasion. Sterile technique should be maintained when health care providers are changing the post-op dressing for the first 48 hours (Bates-Jensen & Williams, 2012; Whitney, 2012). Often the original dressing applied in the OR is left in place for the first 48 hours. However, if there is a need to change this original dressing due to soiling, dislodgement, or drainage, sterile supplies and technique are recommended. This first post-op sterile dressing change should be completed by whomever the hospital policy or physician's order denotes. After 48 to 72 hours, the individual may have the dressing removed and may be allowed to shower so long as epithelial resurfacing is complete. Conversely, if epithelial resurfacing has not occurred, reapplication of a sterile dressing with characteristics to promote reepithelialization is appropriate and may aid in reducing the risk of surgical site infection (SSI). This is consistent with the CDC guidelines for prevention of SSIs and guidelines from the United Kingdom (Leaper, 2008; Mangram, 1999).

CLINICAL PEARL

Clinical experts agree that primary incisional wounds should be protected by a sterile occlusive dressing that provides protection against bacterial invasion for the first 48 hours and until reepithelialization has occurred.

While there is general agreement that a fresh post-op incision should be covered by a sterile dressing and managed with sterile technique for the first 48 hours post-op, there is a lack of evidence supporting the use of one dressing over another. Common choices include sterile gauze and occlusive dressings. Although there are a substantial number of publications on this topic, clinical evidence supporting the choice for either gauze or occlusive dressings has been largely based on clinician preferences, case series, small cohort studies, and poorly powered randomized trials. In evaluating dressings that provide an occlusive or semiocclusive moist environment, versus dry dressings, there are no significant differences in the rate of SSI, patient comfort, or cost (Shinohara et al., 2008; Ubbink et al. 2008; Vogt et al., 2007). With the recent focus on SSI reduction as a quality improvement strategy mandated by Centers for Medicare and Medicaid Services (CMS), The Joint Commission (TJC), and payers, industry has brought to market a multitude of impermeable dressings, both with and without antimicrobial agents. The benefit of occlusion for preventing the ingress of bacteria is supported by Dealey (2005), along with the use of sterile occlusive dressings and sterile technique until resurfacing is complete. Pittman et al. (2005) published results of a small study comparing occlusive antimicrobial post-op dressings versus standard of care showing a 44% reduction in SSIs.

In addition, most wound care clinicians have come to prefer nonadherent dressings over the incision and to avoid the use of gauze, in an effort to minimize pain during dressing changes and to reduce the disruption of cells involved in healing. The National Institute for Health Care Excellence (NICE) (2008) guideline recommends the following: "cover the incision with an appropriate interactive dressing at the end of the operation," use sterile technique and sterile saline for wound cleansing up to 48 hours post-op, and refer to a "tissue viability nurse" for advice on appropriate dressings for the management of wounds healing by secondary intention (Orsted et al., 2010).

Sterile technique and dressings should be used when caring for fresh post-op wounds healing by delayed primary closure. The principles of moist wound healing (as covered in Chapter 7) should be followed. Since the goal of delayed primary closure is to reduce the bioburden of the wound, thorough irrigation with normal saline or a noncytotoxic wound cleanser should occur with each dressing change. Dressings that will provide an optimum environment for granulation tissue formation should be selected. Once the surgeon primarily closes the wound, the guidance for primary closure wounds should be followed.

Class III and IV surgical wounds are typically left open to heal by secondary intention, that is, by formation of granulation tissue, wound contraction, and epithelial resurfacing. Topical therapy for these wounds is based on the principles of wound bed preparation with the optimal dressing determined by the wound's characteristics, wound bed tissue type, absence or presence of dead space (undermining or tunneling), and the type and volume of exudate.

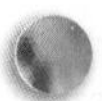

Indications and Guidelines for Management of Complex Wounds

Acute surgical wound care has developed and improved significantly over the course of the last decade; as a result, wound clinicians are frequently asked to recommend management and are expected to provide the evidence and research to support use of advanced therapies. Staying informed and up to date is not only a professional obligation but it also instills a level of confidence in the clinical recommendations the wound care clinician has to offer. The following sections provide an evidence-based perspective and clinical guidelines for the use of incisional negative pressure wound therapy (iNPWT), management of open abdomen and open chest, management of compartment syndrome, and appropriate use of biologic and synthetic mesh.

Incisional Negative Pressure Wound Therapy

First described by Kostiuchenok et al. (1986) and Khirurgii (1986–1991) and later popularized for clinical practice in 1997, negative pressure wound therapy has proven to be a major tool in management of complex wounds (Argenta & Morykwas, 1997; Morykwas et al., 1997). The application of negative pressure to open wounds has been shown to promote healing through its effects on the microcirculation, endothelial cell activation (Borquist et al., 2011; Chen et al., 2005; Wackenfors et al., 2004), removal of wound exudate and debris, stimulation of angiogenesis and collagen synthesis, and reduction in levels of proinflammatory cytokines and bacterial colony counts (Anesäter et al., 2011; Weigand & White, 2013). These beneficial effects are the basis for the use of NPWT in wounds healing by delayed primary closure or secondary intention and for wounds involving grafts and flaps. While the use of NPWT on open wounds is well established, its use on closed surgical incisions is more recent and less clear. It is also unknown whether there is a difference between use of traditional negative pressure wound therapy and newer disposable incisional management systems for closed incisions.

Benefits of Incisional NPWT

While surgical wound complications will be discussed in more detail later in this chapter, it is important for the sake of this discussion to recall that primary impediments to surgical wound healing involve dehiscence, infection, seroma, or hematoma. Additionally, risk factors that are direct correlates to these complications include edema, prolonged incisional drainage, and underlying comorbid conditions that compromise wound healing and development of tensile strength (Karlakki et al., 2013). The use of iNPWT is suggested to directly address these concerns.

First, it is important to discuss the anticipated benefits of negative pressure on a closed incision. This modality should be judged on its impact on the incidence of surgical site complications as opposed to its impact on incisional wound healing (Webster et al., 2012). A recent systematic review examined the impact of iNPWT on surgical site complication rates, that is, infection, dehiscence, seroma and hematoma formation, and reoperation rates, and on the reduction of incisional drainage (Ingargiola et al., 2013). The results varied based on the type of surgery, type of surgical closure, and patient characteristics; thus, the investigators were unable to make any definitive conclusions or recommendations.

Factors affecting the risk for dehiscence include the host's ability to synthesize collagen, the strength of the suture material, the closure technique, and factors that increase stress on the incision (e.g., obesity, coughing). One benefit of iNPWT is a reduction in lateral tension. An in vitro study by Wilkes et al. (2012) demonstrated a 50% reduction in lateral stress and 50% improvement in the tensile strength of the incision; this translates into reduced risk of dehiscence. In addition, Wilkes and colleagues found that iNPWT altered the distribution of forces to the tissue in a way consistent with normal intact skin. Specifically, the authors noted that, *without* the iNPWT, there was a tendency for the lines of stress to be directed toward the sutures, which resulted in a bowing effect, increased stress on the incision, and a possible increase in risk of hematoma as well as dehiscence.

Another potential benefit of iNPWT is a reduction in the duration of postoperative drainage, which is a known risk factor for SSIs. Stannard et al. (2006) conducted a randomized controlled trial evaluating duration of postoperative drainage in patients undergoing surgery for orthopedic trauma ($N = 44$) who were managed with NPWT as compared to those managed with pressure dressings. They found a significant reduction ($p = 0.03$) in drainage time in the patients randomized to iNPWT (1.6 days) versus pressure dressings (3.1 days). They subsequently studied patients with high-risk pelvic and lower extremity fractures, comparing a traditional postoperative dry incision dressing to iNPWT. Again, there was a significant reduction in duration of drainage among patients managed with iNPWT (iNPWT, 1.8 days; post-op dressing, 4.8 days; $p = 0.02$). Reddix et al. (2010) studied the impact of iNPWT on wound complications following acetabular surgery in obese individuals; they followed 19 patients with a body mass index (BMI) >40 kg/m^2, none of whom developed complications. These authors then conducted a comparative cohort study of 301 obese patients who required operative repair of an acetabular fracture. Outcomes were compared for 235 patients managed with iNPWT and 66 consecutive patients who underwent the same procedure prior to the introduction of iNPWT. The results suggested a reduction in the incidence of wound infections (1.27%) and dehiscence (0.426%) in the iNPWT group compared with the historical cohort's infection rate (6.06%) and wound dehiscence rate (3.03%). The authors concluded that more study was needed to validate these findings.

Stannard et al. (2012b) conducted a prospective multicenter randomized clinical trial involving patients with high-risk traumatic injuries of the lower extremity requiring surgical intervention. The patients were randomized to a standard care control group or the iNPWT intervention group. There was a statistically significant reduction in the number of infections in the iNPWT group ($p = 0.049$), and the relative risk for infection was 1.9 times higher for the control group (95% confidence, 1.03 to 3.55). The authors concluded that iNPWT should be used for patients with high-risk lower extremity traumatic injuries. This recommendation is supported by findings of other investigators (Stannard et al., 2012b).

While all studies to date support the use of iNPWT in management of patients undergoing complex orthopedic procedures (Brem et al., 2014), the benefit of iNPWT following other surgical procedures is less clear. Two retrospective, single-center chart reviews of patients undergoing potentially contaminated open colorectal surgery (Bonds et al., 2013) and abdominal wall reconstruction (AWR) (Condé-Green et al., 2013) report reductions in SSIs, dehiscence, and other wound complications in patients managed with iNPWT as compared to those managed with conventional therapy. However, a study by Pauli et al. (2013) failed to demonstrate a beneficial effect among patients undergoing repair of potentially infected ventral hernias. In their nonrandomized study of 119 patients, 70 of whom received standard wound dressings, and 49 of whom received iNPWT, there was no difference in 30-day SSI rates or in the severity of the SSIs reported. Interestingly, initial reports are more favorable for use of iNPWT in management of noncontaminated abdominal surgeries. In a pilot study evaluating iNPWT following cesarean section in obese females, there were no complications in the patients treated with iNPWT, as compared to 10.4% complication rates in the historical control group (Mark et al., 2013). There is additional evidence that iNPWT may be beneficial in the postoperative management of obese individuals. Grauhan et al. (2012) conducted a prospective randomized controlled trial involving 159 cardiac surgery patients with a BMI of 30 kg/m^2 or more. Seventy-five patients received iNPWT with the dressing removed on post-op day 6 to 7, and the 75 control patients received a standard postoperative gauze-based dressing that was removed on the second postoperative day. There was a statistically significant reduction in SSIs with iNPWT (4% iNPWT, 16% standard of care group); swab culture results revealed gram-positive flora for only 1 wound in the iNPWT group, as compared to 10 in the standard of care group.

CLINICAL PEARL

Potential benefits of iNPWT include reduced duration of drainage, reduced incidence of wound infections, and reduced tension on the suture line, which translates into reduced risk of dehiscence.

Options for iNPWT

Many of the early studies utilizing NPWT on closed incisions utilized traditional NPWT foam- or gauze-based systems with a contact layer to protect the skin. However, new developments in iNPWT technology give the clinician more options. Now, single-use (disposable) negative pressure therapy units are available from multiple manufacturers in both powered and nonpowered versions. In the above study by Grauhan et al. (2013), as well as a previous study by Colli (2011), *disposable* iNPWT systems were associated with a significant reduction in incidence of postoperative infection and wound seroma (Pachowsky et al., 2011). An in vitro comparative analysis was performed by Malmsjö et al. (2014) in which a disposable, battery-operated iNPWT device was compared to a traditional NPWT system utilizing a variety of foam and gauze combinations. The authors reported no significant differences in wound contraction, wound microvascular blood flow, or the delivery of measured levels of pressure to the tissues. Therefore, based on current evidence, the selection of a specific NPWT system should be based on clinical practice considerations, as outlined below.

Indications for iNPWT

Indications are based on the available evidence as well as assessment of individual patients' comorbidities and risk for wound complications. Based upon the aforementioned studies, surgical patients with high-risk lower extremity fractures and those undergoing cardiothoracic surgery have shown the greatest reduction in infection, seroma, and dehiscence rates. Additionally, patients at risk for delayed healing (such as obese patients or patients at risk for prolonged incisional drainage) should be considered for iNPWT. As of now, more evidence is needed to determine whether routine use of iNPWT is beneficial following contaminated procedures or abdominal closure.

CLINICAL PEARL

In selecting patients for iNPWT, the clinician should be aware that patients with high-risk lower extremity fractures and those undergoing cardiothoracic surgery have shown the greatest reduction in infection, seroma, and dehiscence rates; more study is needed to determine whether routine use of this therapy is beneficial following contaminated procedures or abdominal closure.

Selection Considerations for iNPWT

Exudate levels are a key consideration in selection of traditional versus disposable systems. Disposable iNPWT systems manage exudate through evaporative loss, an absorptive dressing, or a relatively small external canister; they are intended for management of wounds with minimal-to-moderate exudate. Large or copiously draining wounds would likely overwhelm the capacity of these dressings or their associated canisters. Therefore, the clinician should consider the anticipated volume of drainage and the probable duration of drainage when determining the best system to use. In addition, the clinician should consider that large amounts of continued drainage may be indicative of developing complications. The clinician must review manufacturers' guidelines for each system used in her or his system to include the volume of drainage accommodated by the dressing or canister and whether the canister can be changed independent of the dressing.

Cost is another consideration and is typically reduced considerably with use of disposable systems. In a wound with limited exudate, the one-time fee and up to 7-day wear time is of major benefit, especially in the ambulatory surgery setting and the outpatient setting. The ability to discharge a patient following ambulatory surgery and to schedule the first postoperative dressing change for the outpatient setting eliminates the need for home health and frequent dressing changes. Cost is also a key consideration in selection of NPWT for an indigent patient who requires, but does not qualify for, traditional NPWT at home.

CLINICAL PEARL

In selecting a specific system for iNPWT, the clinician must consider volume of exudate, cost, and the patient's need for mobility and for discretion.

Enhanced mobility and the ability to wear the system discreetly are popular features of the disposable systems and additional reasons for selection when there is limited exudate. The new disposable systems are considerably smaller and may either fit into a pocket or be secured to the body via an arm or leg strap. These systems have significantly shorter drainage tubing lengths and can often be applied in a manner that minimizes or eliminates visibility to others, unlike traditional NPWT systems that are more bulky and often require a shoulder carry sling. This may facilitate greater compliance, especially among teens and young adults, who may be sensitive to therapy that is visible in social situations.

Selection between a powered versus nonpowered iNPWT systems is a matter of personal choice, as there is no evidence to suggest any difference in clinical performance between the two systems. It may be ease of use or comfort level that is the deciding factor. Some of the new nonpowered versions offer a variety of negative pressure setting options to allow for customization of the NPWT, where powered disposables often have only one default pressure setting. Additionally, since these systems vary in their design, clinicians should determine and consider the expected battery life versus the projected length of pressure delivery in spring-loaded nonpowered versions.

Complications and Contraindications for iNPWT

Since 2007, the FDA reported 12 deaths and 174 injury reports related to traditional negative pressure wound therapy (US Food and Drug Administration, 2007) (http://www.fda.gov/MedicalDevices/Safety/AlertsandNotices/ucm244211.htm), primarily due to bleeding and infection. Although there are inherently different levels of risk related to use of NPWT for closed incisions, the clinician should be aware of potential risk factors and contraindications for iNPWT.

Relative contraindications to the use of iNPWT include signs and symptoms of active infection or hematoma. In a retrospective study by Hansen et al. (2013), factors associated with treatment failure included INR > 2, history of previous hip surgeries, and therapy lasting >48 hours. The elevated INR is likely related to the potential for hematoma formation; however, there are limited data supporting use of iNPWT for seroma prevention. The authors concluded that previous hip surgeries may cause soft tissue deficits that affect the risk of failure. The use of iNPWT for more than 48 hours is not believed to increase the incidence of failure; rather, prolonged use may be a clinical indication of poor wound healing and a higher risk of failure. In summary, clinicians must always carefully assess the wound and patient to determine appropriateness of iNPWT.

Management of Complex Abdominal Wounds

The abdominal wall is a dynamic and intricate system of muscle and connective tissue; any alteration in the physical structure of the abdominal wall results in a change in muscle physiology and function. The centrally located rectus abdominis muscle is divided vertically by a thick band of connective tissue known as the linea alba, which serves as the primary insertion site for the muscles of the abdominal wall: the external oblique, internal oblique, and transversus abdominis muscles. Additionally, multiple layers of fascia encase the abdominal wall, primarily the anterior and posterior rectus fascia (Fig. 32-4).

CLINICAL PEARL

The abdominal wall is a dynamic system of muscle and connective tissue; any alteration (such as occurs during laparotomy) results in altered muscle physiology and function. For example, primary closure delayed more than 7 to 10 days may result in lateralization requiring AWR.

Impact of Muscle Disruption

The abdominal wall has multiple functions: maintenance of upright posture, spine stabilization, complex movements, protection of the abdominal viscera, respiration, and Valsalva maneuver. The function of the abdominal muscles is greatly affected by disruption during laparotomy. When an incision is made through the linea alba, the release of the weight causes lateralization of the rectus muscle and corresponding fascia. Lateralization of the abdominal wall is defined as movement of the rectus muscle and its associated fascia away from the midline over time (Björck and Wanhainen, 2014). Lateralization

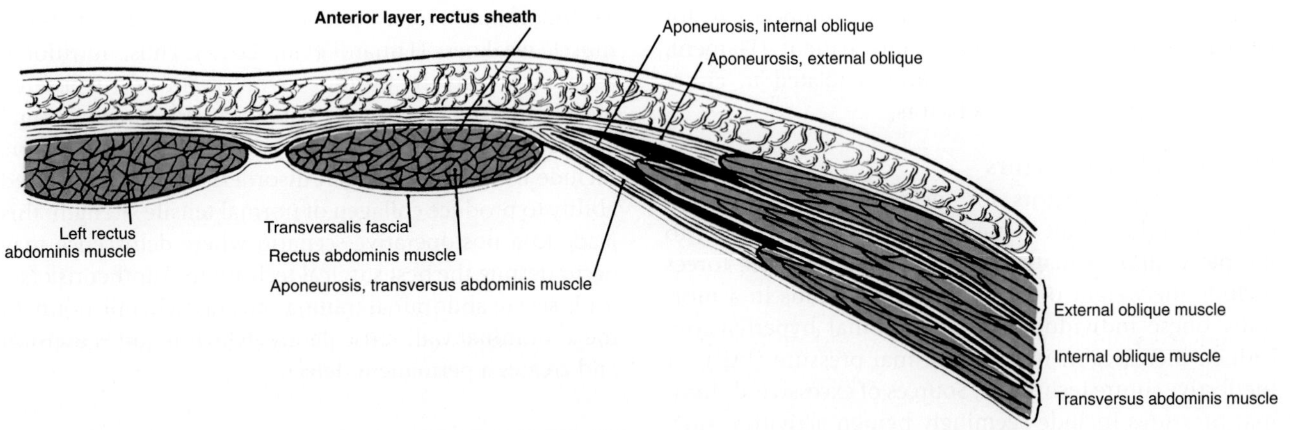

FIGURE 32-4. Cross section of the abdominal wall.

causes a marked reduction in load applied to the oblique muscles, which eventually results in atrophy (Criss et al., 2014). The main goal following open abdominal procedures is to approximate the rectus and fascia in order to reestablish abdominal wall structure and function. In patients with abdominal wall defects (congenital, traumatic, or postoperative), simple approximation is not possible, and it is necessary to reconstruct the abdominal wall. This requires use of structures capable of replicating the function of skin, fascia, and muscle whenever possible (Ger, 2009). Criss et al. (2014) used dynamometry to demonstrate a physiologic return of abdominal wall function 6 months following AWR with a corresponding statistically significant increase in patient quality of life. Positive outcomes of AWR are largely dependent upon surgeon technique, proper selection of reinforcing mesh, and the patient's comorbidities and inherent ability to heal.

Management of the Open Abdomen

In situations in which approximation of the abdominal wall is not possible at the time of surgery, purposeful and effective management of the open abdomen is essential. Situations in which the abdomen must be left open include prevention or treatment of abdominal compartment syndrome (ACS), damage control for life-threatening intra-abdominal bleeding, and management of severe intra-abdominal sepsis (Demetriades and Salim, 2014). Specific approaches to management of the open abdomen are typically driven by the surgeon and are beyond the scope of this chapter. It should be noted, however, that the longer the abdomen remains open, the greater the risk of complications. Kaplan et al. (2005) found that leaving the abdomen open for 7 to 10 days usually resulted in sufficient lateralization and adhesion formation to prevent primary closure. This is consistent with the findings of Rausei and colleagues, who reported that reducing the time that the abdomen remained open was associated with a greater likelihood of closure and a decrease in complications (Rausei et al., 2014). Conditions resulting in prolonged bowel edema, such as peritonitis and sepsis, are associated with increased risk of ACS if the rectus is closed prematurely; these patients may require a significant delay in wound closure, which results in a chronic open abdomen. Fortunately, negative pressure wound therapy has been used effectively in many of these situations to reduce edema and inflammation, thus permitting primary closure at a much earlier point (Plaudis et al., 2012). However, in some cases, the rectus cannot be approximated, and the resulting muscle atrophy will necessitate future AWR to reestablish normal function. Many techniques are used to reconstruct the abdominal wall, including advanced techniques such as separation of components, use of biologic materials, mesh traction, zipper closures, and dynamic sutures (Burlew et al., 2011; Demetriades & Salim, 2014). However, a detailed discussion of the various surgical techniques is beyond the scope of this chapter.

CLINICAL PEARL

NPWT has been used effectively to reduce edema and inflammation associated with open abdominal wounds, thus permitting primary closure at a much earlier point.

Incisional Failure following Primary Closure

As noted previously, incisional failure is a common and significant postoperative complication, and risk of incisional failure is influenced both by surgical technique (e.g., material used to approximate the tissues) and by the patient's comorbidities and ability to heal normally. In a wound left open to the fascia, incisional failure may result in evisceration; in an abdominal wound that is closed to the skin, failure ranges from superficial skin dehiscence (partial dehiscence), to dehiscence down to the fascia (full dehiscence), to dehiscence of the fascia, to frank evisceration. Failure may also be manifest as postoperative hernia formation; the linea alba is the most common site for hernia formation in the laparotomy patient (Flament, 2006). Generally, incisional failure is related to either mechanical or biological risk factors.

Mechanical Risk Factors

Mechanical risk factors for incisional failure include conditions that result in application of excessive force to the newly approximated rectus and fascia. These forces include the weight of the abdominal pannus in a morbidly obese individual, intra-abdominal hypertension, sudden increases in intra-abdominal pressure (IAP), or ineffective suture technique. Sources of excessive abdominal pressures include seemingly benign activities, such as endotracheal suctioning, coughing/deep breathing, or changes in position from lying to sitting. Excessive pressures may also result from abnormal bowel wall edema, intra-abdominal hypertension, and ACS. To manage these risks, surgeons may elect to use either synthetic or biologic mesh to support and reinforce the abdominal wall, with the goal of preventing incisional failure and hernia formation or recurrence. Primary suture closure alone has been shown to be inferior to mesh repair in prevention of incisional failure, and hernia recurrence is higher when mesh is not utilized (Luijendijk, 2000; Sauderland et al., 2009). Of particular interest to WOC nurses, the creation of an ostomy has been shown to create a midline shift toward the contralateral side, which alters rectus muscle thickness and innervation and increases mechanical stress on the suture line. Ostomy creation is also thought to increase the risk of incisional hernia (Timmermans et al., 2014).

Biologic Risk Factors

Biologic risk factors for incisional failure include comorbidities that alter fibroblast function and collagen synthesis, for example, ischemia, smoking, corticosteroid use, chronic obstructive pulmonary disease, morbid obesity, and infection (Timmermans et al., 2014). Obesity can be viewed as both a mechanical and biologic risk factor for incisional failure, which is alarming given the marked increase in the percentage of children and adults who are obese or morbidly obese. From 2011 to 2012, 8.1% of infants and toddlers, 16.9% of 2- to 19-year-olds, and 34.9% of adults over the age of 20 were reported to be obese (Ogden et al., 2014). Obesity is found to be highest in non-Hispanic blacks, followed by Hispanics and non-Hispanic whites, and may vary according to socioeconomic status (http://www.cdc.gov/obesity/data/adult.html). Obesity increases the mechanical stress on the incision; in addition, many obese individuals are found to have protein malnutrition, which compromises their ability to synthesize new connective tissue proteins. Malnutrition not only impedes wound healing and increases the risk of wound infection but also has been shown to increase the risk of pulmonary complications in abdominal surgery patients secondary to expiratory muscle weakness (Lunardi et al., 2012). Thus, nutritional assessment and the prompt involvement of a registered dietitian in the care of any patient at risk for nutritional compromise are essential. Less common risk factors include congenital collagen disorders leading to reduced ability to produce collagen of normal tensile strength; this leads to a postoperative scenario where dehiscence may occur despite the best surgical technique. Another risk factor is severe abdominal trauma causing ischemic injury to the abdominal wall musculature, which requires excision and creates a permanent defect.

CLINICAL PEARL

Risk factors for incisional failure include mechanical factors that increase stress on the suture line (such as morbid obesity, coughing, suctioning, or position changes) and biologic risk factors that impair healing (such as smoking, malnutrition, and steroid use).

Management Decisions

When consulted regarding the management of an open abdominal wound, the clinician must first conduct a focused history and physical, with specific attention paid to the operative note. In reviewing the operative note, the nurse should note the type of surgery performed, any impact to the abdominal organs, reports of any complications, and the type of closure (closure to fascia level, approximation of all tissue and skin layers, or skin-only closure). It is essential to correlate the structures visualized in the wound base with an understanding of the type of closure. In abdominal wounds that have been closed to fascia level, the clinician should see intact, well-approximated fascial sutures in the wound base, as well as healthy subcutaneous tissue and dermis along the sidewalls of the wound (Fig. 32-5). In the presence of an intact fascial closure with no evidence of dehiscence or suture line tension, the underlying abdominal organs are effectively protected. In contrast, a fascial closure that is only partially intact due to areas of dehiscence can result in exposure of the bowel (Fig. 32-6). In progressive incisional failure and dehiscence, frank evisceration may occur

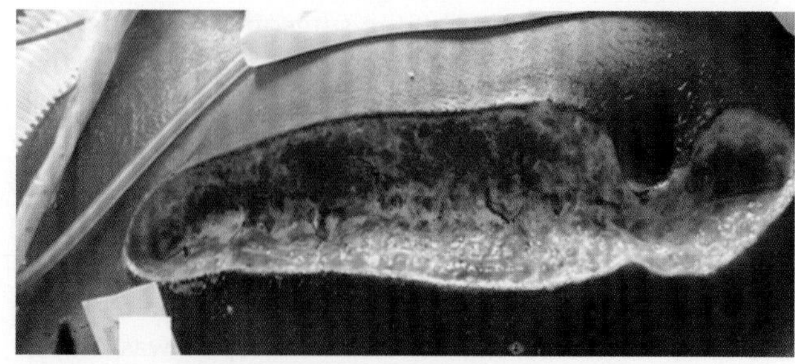

FIGURE 32-5. Wound closed to fascia level.

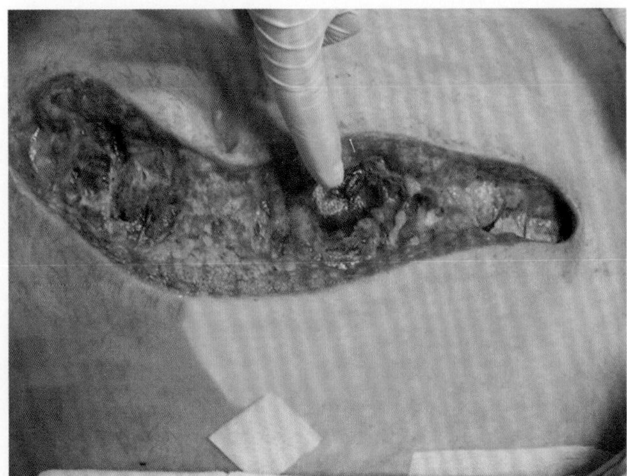

FIGURE 32-6. Wound closed to fascia level with partial dehiscence.

(Fig. 32-7), or there may be abdominal wall dehiscence with exposure of underlying abdominal organs (Fig. 32-8). Each of these situations requires a different approach to wound management. Finally, skin-only closure can look identical to primary closure, but they are very different and require different management (Fig. 32-9). A skin-only closure is used when primary fascial closure is not possible; skin flaps are raised to provide superficial coverage of the large wound defect in order to decrease the risk of postoperative complications such as enteroatmospheric fistula formation. In these two scenarios, therapy options and expectations are inherently different based upon the anatomy underlying the

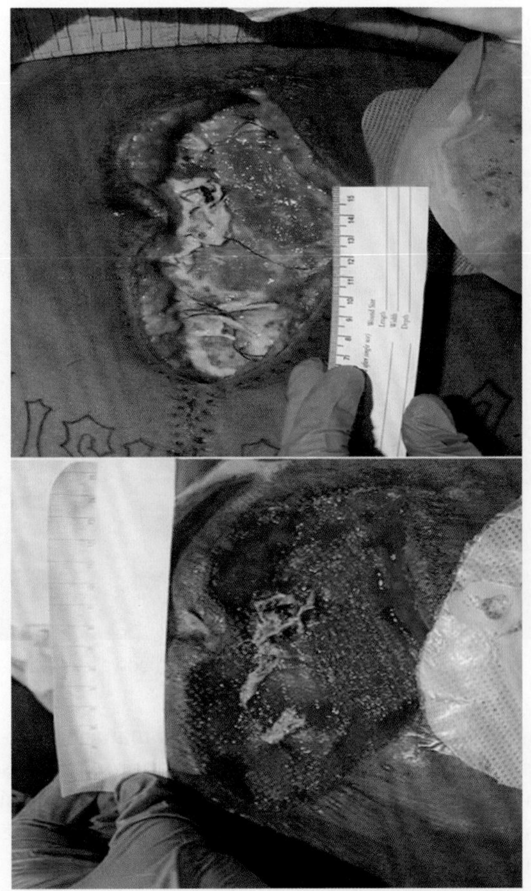

FIGURE 32-8. Abdominal wound dehiscence with partial organ exposure.

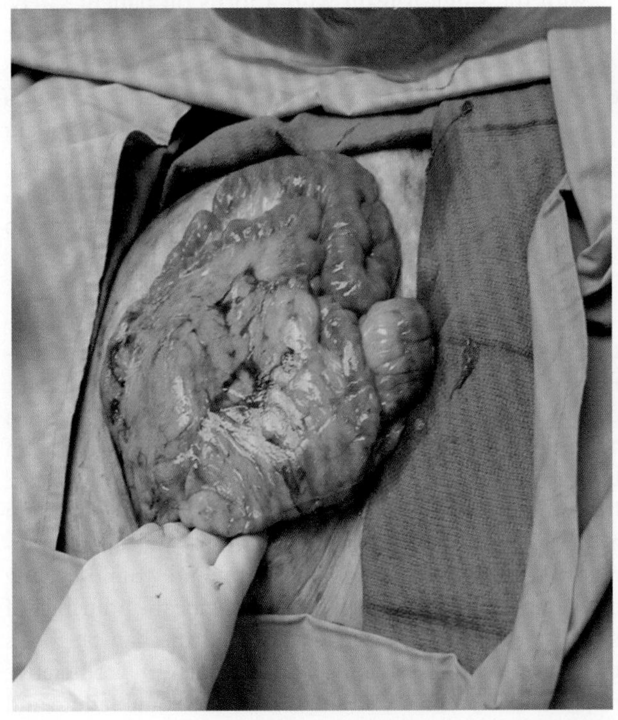

FIGURE 32-7. Evisceration.

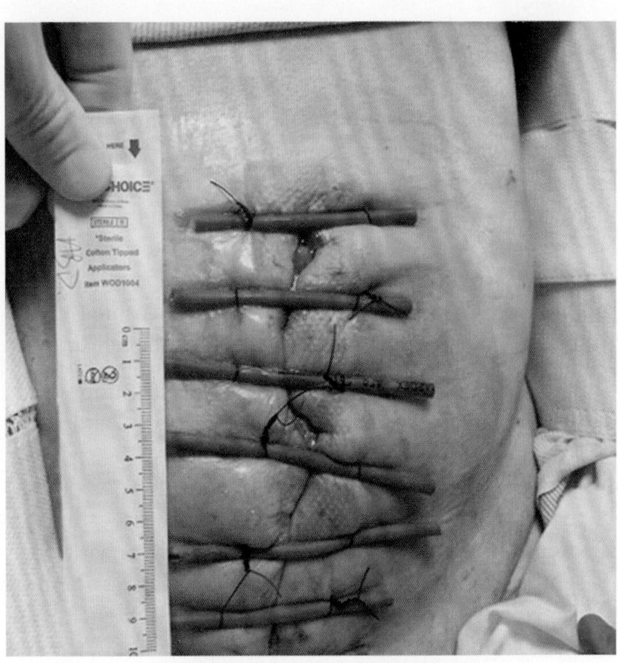

FIGURE 32-9. Skin-only closure.

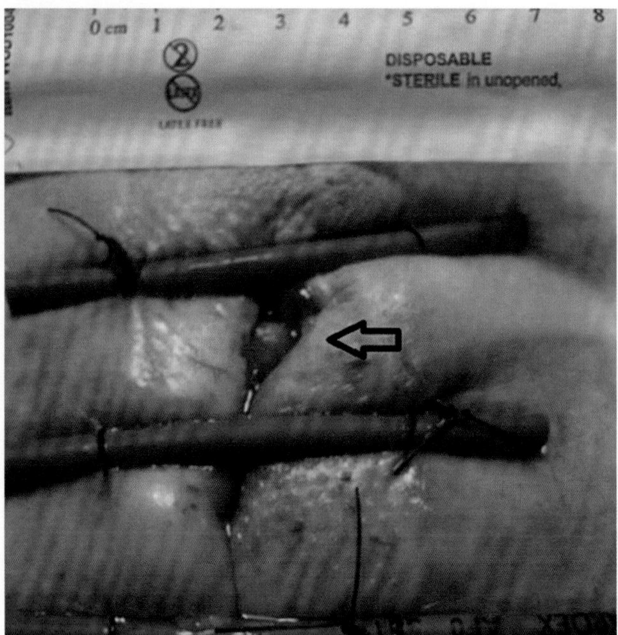

FIGURE 32-10. Skin-only closure with bowel exposure.

skin incision. For example, a request to manage an at-risk incision with iNPWT would require appropriate assessment of the incision in a skin-only closure for any signs of bowel exposure (Fig. 32-10) in order to determine the safety of such therapy and to provide protection of any sensitive structures during wound care.

CLINICAL PEARL

In assessing an open abdominal wound and making recommendations for care, it is essential to correlate the structures visualized in the wound base with the type of closure.

Care Options

Before providing wound care recommendations on the postoperative abdominal wound, the wound care clinician should ensure that there is clear communication with the surgeon regarding any structures exposed in the wound bed and the ultimate plan of care for the patient. When complex wounds are presented, a bedside meeting for direct discussion and visualization of the structures is warranted. Depending on the specific wound and type of abdominal wall closure (AWC), the plan of care may include one or more of the following:

1. Primary closure of all tissue/skin layers: support for healing and prevention of complications, either via advanced incisional dressings or via iNPWT.
2. Primary fascial and skin closure with the use of synthetic or biologic mesh. The wound care clinician should be aware of common complications with both synthetic and biologic mesh to enhance assessment of the closed incision. The location of placement of the mesh should be known so that in the case of incisional failure and mesh exposure, the anatomy can be more readily identified. Supportive wound care may involve either iNPWT or advanced incisional dressings.
3. Delayed primary fascial closure: Use of a temporary open abdomen technique such as intra-abdominal NPWT may be utilized to achieve a rapid reduction in edema and enhanced neoangiogenesis in preparation for delayed primary closure.
4. Closure of the abdominal wall to fascia level using reinforced biologic mesh or bridged biologic mesh; the patient returns from surgery with an open abdominal wound to the layer of the reinforced mesh closure. The goal is to promote ingrowth of granulation tissue and incorporation of the mesh into the granulation tissue, which will allow for secondary or delayed primary closure of the skin and subcutaneous tissues. The mesh placement location should be known so that the wound clinician can accurately identify any separation or disintegration of the mesh and can distinguish the mesh from other underlying structures. Management frequently involves traditional NPWT with careful attention to protection of any exposed mesh.
5. Open abdominal wound with exposed abdominal organs (viscera) and possibly omentum, due to inability to close the abdominal wall. Inflammatory adhesions and/or granulation may result in the exposed organs (small and large intestine, liver) becoming one large visceral mass without distinguishable anatomy (otherwise known as a "frozen abdomen"). Goal is either a skin-only closure or granulation over the exposed structures with or without absorbable mesh in preparation for eventual skin graft closure. Topical therapy for wounds with exposed organs requires coordination with the surgical team with a focus on patient safety, maintenance of acceptable levels of moisture and core body temperature, and complication prevention.
6. In cases in which the abdominal wound is open for a prolonged period of time, the clinician and the patient should be aware that without correction of the abdominal wall defect and achievement of complete fascial closure, the patient will likely need additional surgery 3 to 6 months in the future for definitive AWR.

Principles of wound assessment and wound bed preparation were thoroughly discussed in Chapters 3 and 7 and therefore will not be described in detail here. However, specific considerations for the provision of topical therapy for open abdominal wounds include identification and protection of the anatomical structures involved and of any exposed mesh. Interestingly, there is a correlation between the load strain achieved by the closure of the abdominal wall/reestablishment of normal anatomical alignment and wound-healing outcomes. Culbertson et al. (2011) describe the principles of mechanotransduction, whereby normal mechanical forces impact on cellular signaling and thus on the proliferative response of fibroblasts. In the case of incisional failure and hernia development, this alteration in normal mechanical

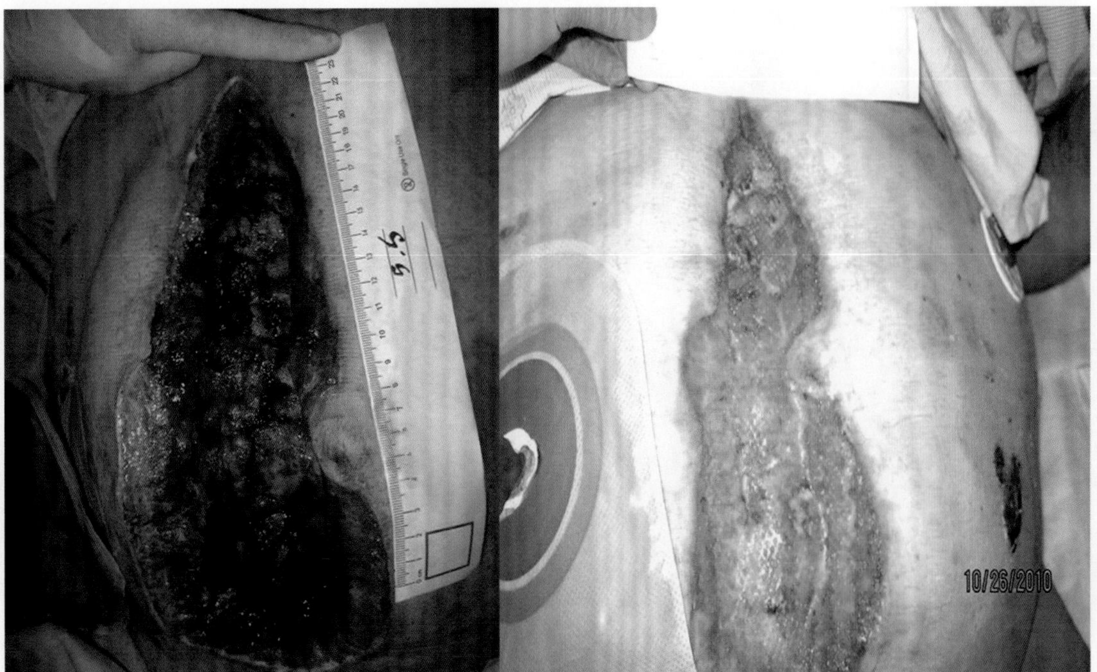

FIGURE 32-11. Tension-free fascial closure with subsequent granulation.

load may interfere with normal cell signaling and thus may impair normal wound healing (Culbertson et al., 2011).

CLINICAL PEARL

Specific considerations in providing care for open abdominal wounds include identification and protection of the anatomical structures involved and of any exposed mesh.

For abdominal wounds that are open to the fascial sutures, assessment is focused on the continued approximation of the fascial closure, the viability of the tissue, any signs of abdominal distention, and the presence of developing necrosis or signs and symptoms of infection. Patients with intact fascial closures may be managed with the principles of traditional wound bed preparation and attention to systemic factors affecting healing capacity (Fig. 32-11). However, certain principles of wound bed preparation should be modified dependent upon wound presentation. For example, instrumental debridement should *never* be performed when it involves the fascial suture line as this may cause dehiscence or evisceration. In these cases, unless warranted by the surgeon's evaluation, noninstrumental approaches to debridement (such as autolysis) and dressings to reduce bacterial loads are usually more appropriate. Additionally, signs of active dehiscence should be reported to the surgeon immediately in order to determine the plan of care, and the wound care clinician should reassess the appropriateness of current topical therapy recommendations based upon the possible exposure of underlying structures such as bowel (Fig. 32-12). Mesh exposure and management are discussed later in the chapter.

CLINICAL PEARL

Patients with intact fascial structures can be managed with traditional principles of wound bed preparation; however, instrumental debridement of the fascial suture line should *never* be performed due to risk for dehiscence or evisceration.

Since the underlying viscera is protected in wounds closed at the fascial level, wound care follows the accepted principles of wound bed preparation and support of granulation tissue. Additionally, while there are no level one studies to support its use in all cases, an abdominal binder is often recommended for at-risk patients to provide support during activities associated with increased IAP. The wound care clinician should assess tension exerted on the wound edges as well as viability of the tissue present in the wound and the quantity of granulation tissue.

Following so-called contaminated surgeries, such as colorectal surgery or laparotomy following a perforation, ostomy creation, or bowel resection, the wound is often left open to heal by secondary intention in order to monitor for signs or symptoms of infection and viability of the subcutaneous tissues. However, clinicians often make the mistake of assuming the only way to heal these wounds is via the formation of large amounts of scar tissue. In actuality, techniques that promote approximation of the edges of the granulating wound while preventing the creation of dead space can improve both clinical and aesthetic outcomes. Once it is determined that the wound is proliferating well with ample granulation tissue and there is no evidence of infection, either delayed primary closure or a variety of surgical "wick" techniques should be considered. Figure 32-13

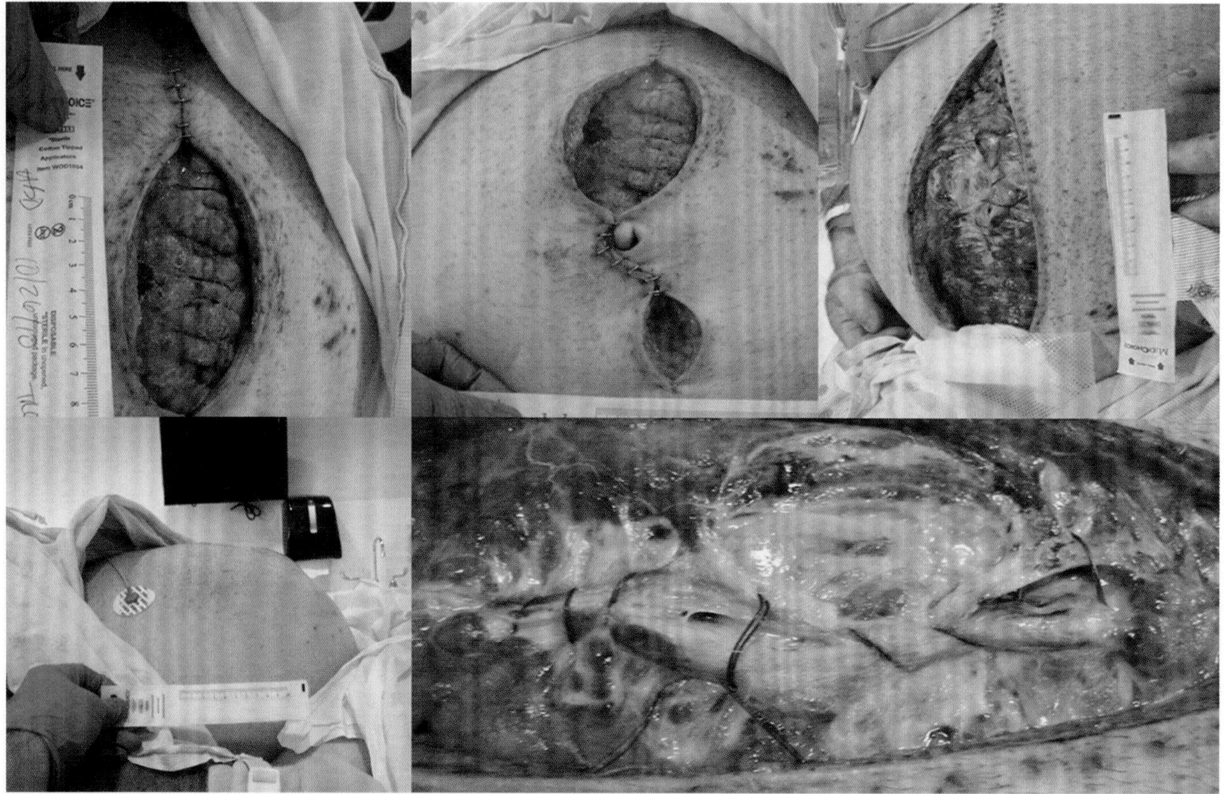

FIGURE 32-12. Progressive abdominal distention and dehiscence.

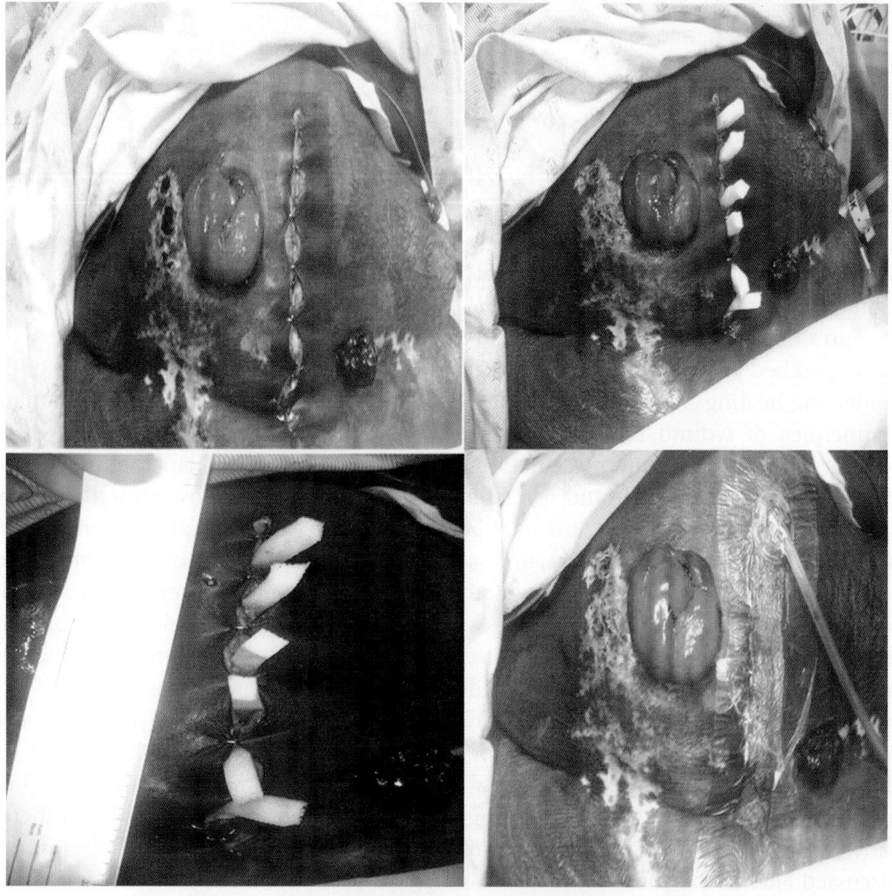

FIGURE 32-13. Interrupted surgical technique with "wicks."

shows an example of interrupted incisional closure in the OR combined with use of NPWT sponges as "wicks"; the sponges were dipped into antimicrobial solution and packed into the full-thickness openings down to the fascial closure, in an attempt to minimize wound size while allowing for continued wound monitoring. Figure 32-14 shows a wick technique used for a morbidly obese patient following heart transplantation. This patient underwent 1 week of standard NPWT to produce adequate granulation tissue followed by interrupted incisional closure and use of NPWT sponges as wicks. The wicks were changed routinely with reduction in depth as the wound filled with granulation tissue. (While this was not an abdominal wound, the management technique was the same.) This promotes granulation as well as closure of the wound edges, while managing exudate and providing ongoing monitoring for infection. A myriad of options for wound bed management are available that are based on the principles of moist wound healing; the specific option should be selected based on wound characteristics and individualized patient assessment.

CLINICAL PEARL

In managing large open wounds, techniques that promote wound edge approximation while preventing the creation of dead space can improve both clinical and aesthetic outcomes.

Critical Assessment Factors

When assessing and making recommendations for chronic open abdominal wound management, one of the most important questions is whether any new anastomoses or enterotomies were created during surgery. This question is most important in preventing development of an enteroatmospheric (enterocutaneous) fistula, which is a devastating complication for the patient and a major challenge for the care team. While there are many causes of fistula listed in the literature, 85% of the time fistulas occur as the result of an anastomotic leak. The wound care clinician should discuss the location of any new anastomoses or the existence of any incidental enterotomies created and closed during surgery. It is particularly important to determine whether any anastomoses or repaired enterotomies

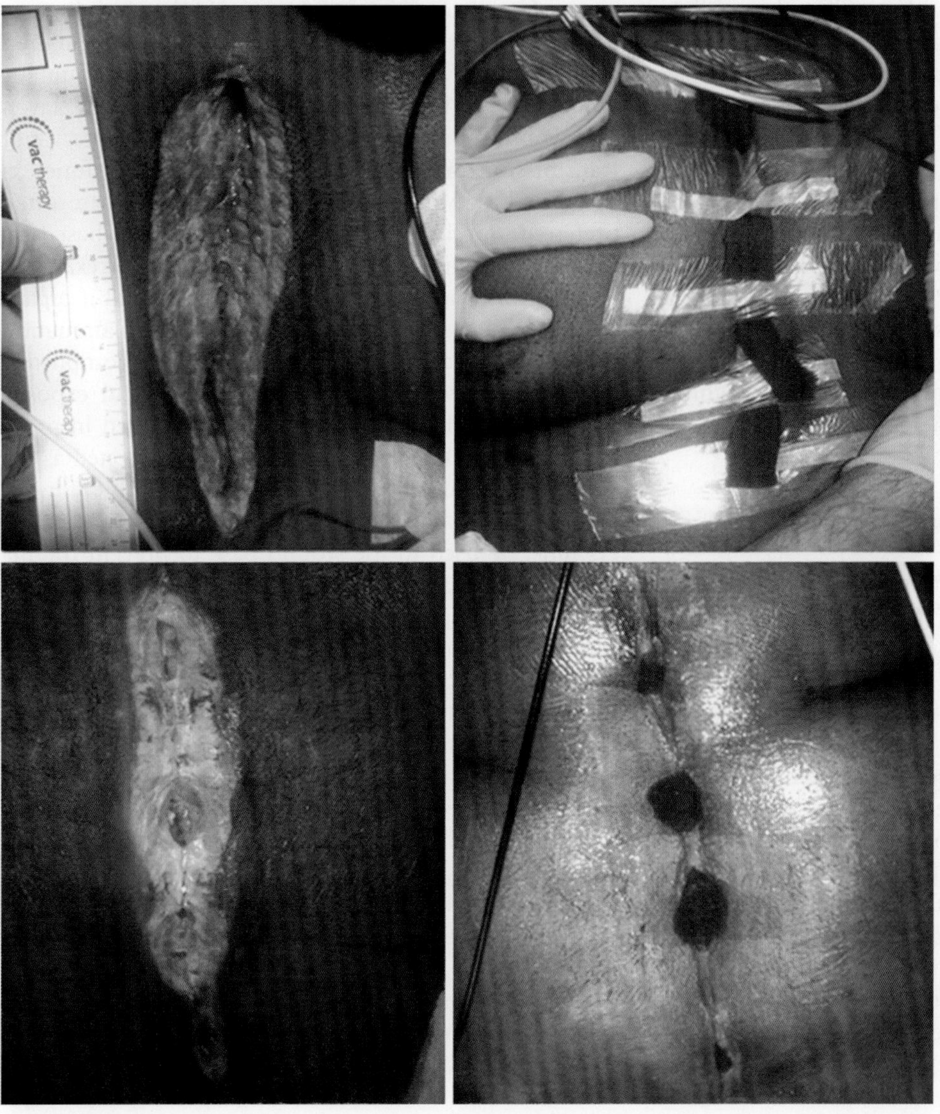

FIGURE 32-14. "Wick" technique in patient S/P heart transplant.

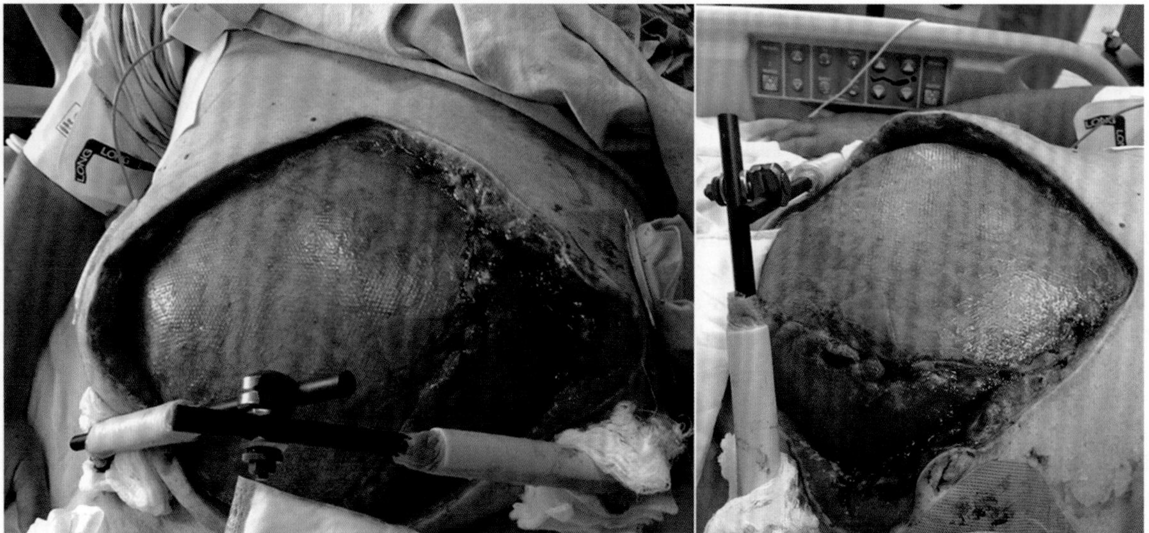

FIGURE 32-15. Open abdomen with residual omentum under Vicryl mesh.

are "buried" or superficial. Often, the surgeon will attempt to protect these sites by placing them deep in the abdominal cavity (assuming that the bowel is sufficiently mobile). In situations where any new anastomoses or repairs are covered by omentum or placed deep in the abdominal cavity and away from the wound surface, more advanced therapies such as negative pressure wound therapy can be safely utilized (Fig. 32-15A and B). Multiple studies indicate that, with proper understanding and application of NPWT, there is relatively low risk for an NPWT-induced ECF in this situation. However, when there is a superficial anastomosis or enterotomy, NPWT is usually considered *contraindicated* due to risk of fistula formation. If NPWT *is* used in this type of situation, it is critical to use low-pressure settings and to protect the wound surface with a contact layer (or several nonadherent contact layers) or a nonadherent layer of foam.

CLINICAL PEARL

When managing an open abdominal wound, the clinician must determine whether there are any new anastomoses or repaired enterotomies that lie close to the wound surface; if so, NPWT should be either avoided or used with contact layers and low-pressure settings.

When working with exposed bowel or organ structures, there are no evidence-based, dressing-specific topical therapy recommendations. Instead, the clinician should keep the following principles in mind: atraumatic, autolytic, and normothermic wound care or atraumatic, autolytic, antimicrobial, and normothermic wound care, with attention to minimizing the frequency of dressing changes. The wound care clinician should *never* perform sharp debridement over organ structures secondary to the risk of inadvertent trauma, enterotomy, or bleeding. Due to the excellent perfusion of the abdominal viscera, autolysis usually provides sufficient debridement of any necrotic tissue. In cases of the chronic open abdomen, there are a number of options for topical therapy: advanced wound dressings, NPWT with atraumatic application technique and nonadherent contact layer, and wound pouching. Due to the high moisture vapor transmission rate and poor insulation/barrier function of gauze-based products, advanced dressings are often preferred. Specific therapy decisions must be based on thorough patient and wound assessment. For example, a moist warm wound environment is essential if organs are exposed, in order to prevent serosal inflammation and wound bed desiccation. This can be accomplished with many products; volume of exudate and exposed structures are the key factors to be considered in product selection. Often transparent films are selected as the cover dressing due to their ability to trap ambient moisture and maintain wound bed temperature. Contact layers must be used in the wound base to prevent trauma to exposed organs; silicone contact layers are preferred as they will not change their structure or function over time. Unfortunately, some petrolatum-based products may actually adhere to the wound bed over time, with dehydration or dilution of the petrolatum. Between the contact layer and the secondary dressing, appropriate packing materials include rolled gauze or large sheets of alginate or hydrofiber. In wounds with very little exudate, hydrogels may be the most appropriate option. The clinician must always consider safety issues in selecting products for wound care; for example, when selecting filler and wicking agents for wounds with extensive undermining, the goal is to reduce the number of dressing pieces used and to clearly communicate with subsequent care providers how many dressing pieces have been placed into the wound.

CLINICAL PEARL

When working with wounds with exposed bowel or organ structures, the clinician must adhere to the principles of atraumatic, normothermic, autolytic, and (if indicated) antimicrobial wound care.

Often, the chronic open or frozen abdomen is managed with NPWT due to the ability to create robust granulation tissue in a relatively short amount of time. Again, this therapy should only be chosen if there are no known superficial anastomoses or enterotomy closure sites present and following discussion with the surgeon. As noted before, if NPWT is used in this situation, it is critical to use nonadherent dressings in the wound bed and to assure atraumatic dressing/sponge removal. In determining the level of protection needed, the clinician must consider the presence of omental coverage and the volume of granulation tissue covering the wound bed and the underlying organs. In addition to assuring appropriate use of nonadherent contact layers or foam, whenever there are exposed organs or anastomoses close to the surface of the wound, the clinician should initiate negative suction at settings much lower than the standard settings recommended by the manufacturer. Initial settings of −25 mm Hg to −50 mm Hg should be utilized, with slow titration to higher levels based upon wound presentation and amount of granulation.

In situations where NPWT is not recommended due to the presence of anastomoses or enterotomies, and use of advanced dressings is not feasible due to the large wound surface area, wound pouches or fistula pouches should be considered. Benefits include the terrarium-like environment created by the pouch, along with the ability to manage high levels of exudate and to access the wound frequently for assessment (if necessary). These pouches have multiple port sites, which can be placed to bedside drainage systems, thus managing very large volumes of exudate. Another option is to connect the pouching system to wall suction on a low setting; if this is contraindicated for any reason, it must be clearly communicated to the staff. An additional advantage provided by pouching systems is protection of the periwound skin and prevention of periwound moisture–associated skin damage and the associated increase in risk of infection (Colwell et al., 2011). One potential negative consideration in use of pouching systems for chronic open abdomen management is that sterile packaging may or may not be available; the use of a clean pouch should be first discussed with the surgeon to determine appropriateness of use. In most cases, this is not a problem since an open abdomen is already colonized with bacteria. In extreme cases involving massive bowel wall edema secondary to peritonitis and ACS, a large pouching system may be used to accommodate the eviscerated organs (Fig. 32-16). Such a complex patient requires definitive collaboration between the wound clinician and the surgeon.

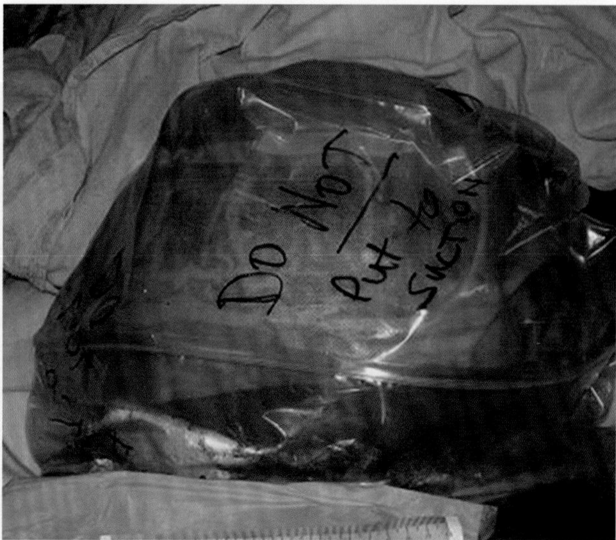

FIGURE 32-16. Open abdominal wound managed with large wound pouch.

Abdominal Nightmare: Fistula Development

Enterocutaneous fistulas (ECF) are characterized by the connection of the bowel to the skin, whereas enteroenteric fistulas involve two or more segments of the bowel (such as an ileocolonic fistula), and enteroatmospheric fistulas (EAF) are a connection between the bowel and the air, such as with a complex open abdomen (Brindle, 2012). Fistula management is discussed in detail in Chapter 34; the discussion in this chapter is limited to description of a technique for isolating the fistula and the enteric output from the wound bed, thus permitting use of NPWT to the wound if indicated.

CLINICAL PEARL

Enterocutaneous fistulas are characterized by connection of the bowel to the skin, while enteroatmospheric fistulas involve connection of the bowel to an open wound.

Multiple techniques for fistula isolation have been described in the literature (Brindle & Blankenship, 2007; Brindle, 2012). However, a more novel technique is gaining acceptance based on its ability to provide complete fecal stream diversion and to allow for skin grafting in the presence of a high-output small bowel EAF. Figures 32-17 and 32-18 illustrate two cases in which the Brindle and Whelan glove isolation technique was used successfully (Brindle, 2012; Brindle & Whelan, 2011). While not a new concept, previous attempts to attach a collection bag or plastic bag conduit to the open fistula were wrought with limitations in wear time and leakage. Brindle and Whelan's technique, on the other hand, has been shown to provide up to 1 week of fecal diversion at a time, while allowing for repetitive dressing changes of the surrounding wound. The isolation is best created in

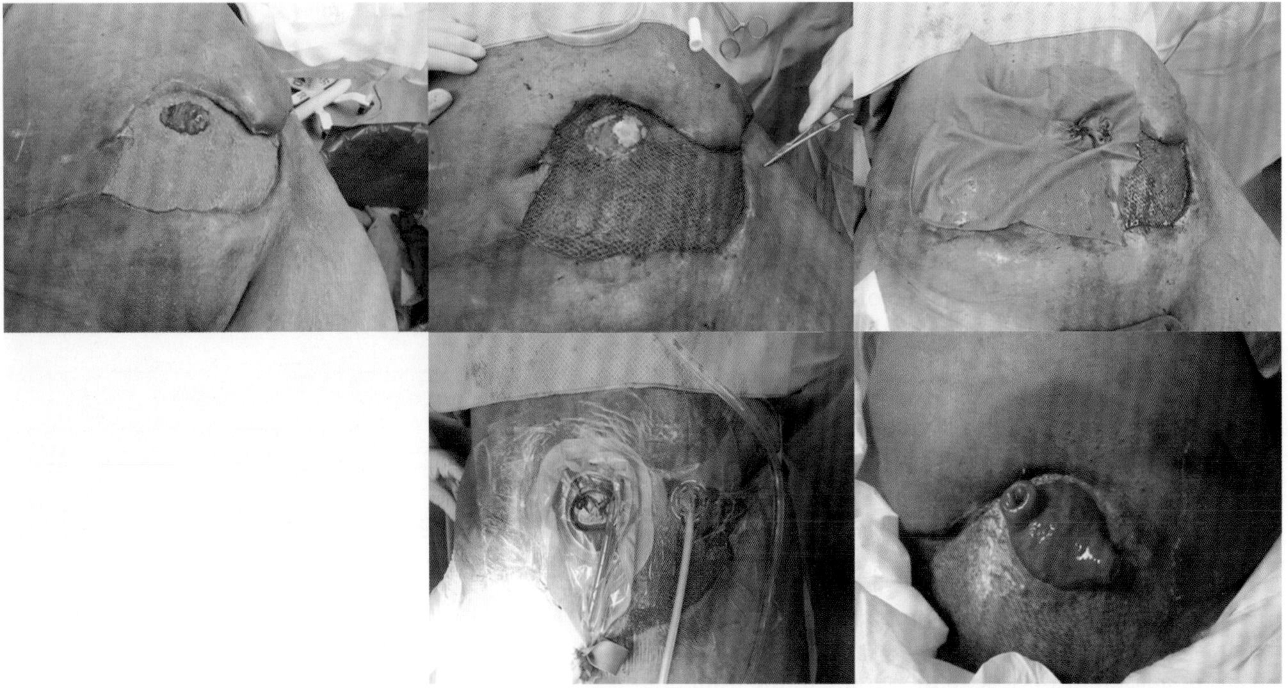

FIGURE 32-17. Glove technique for isolating enteric fistula from open wound.

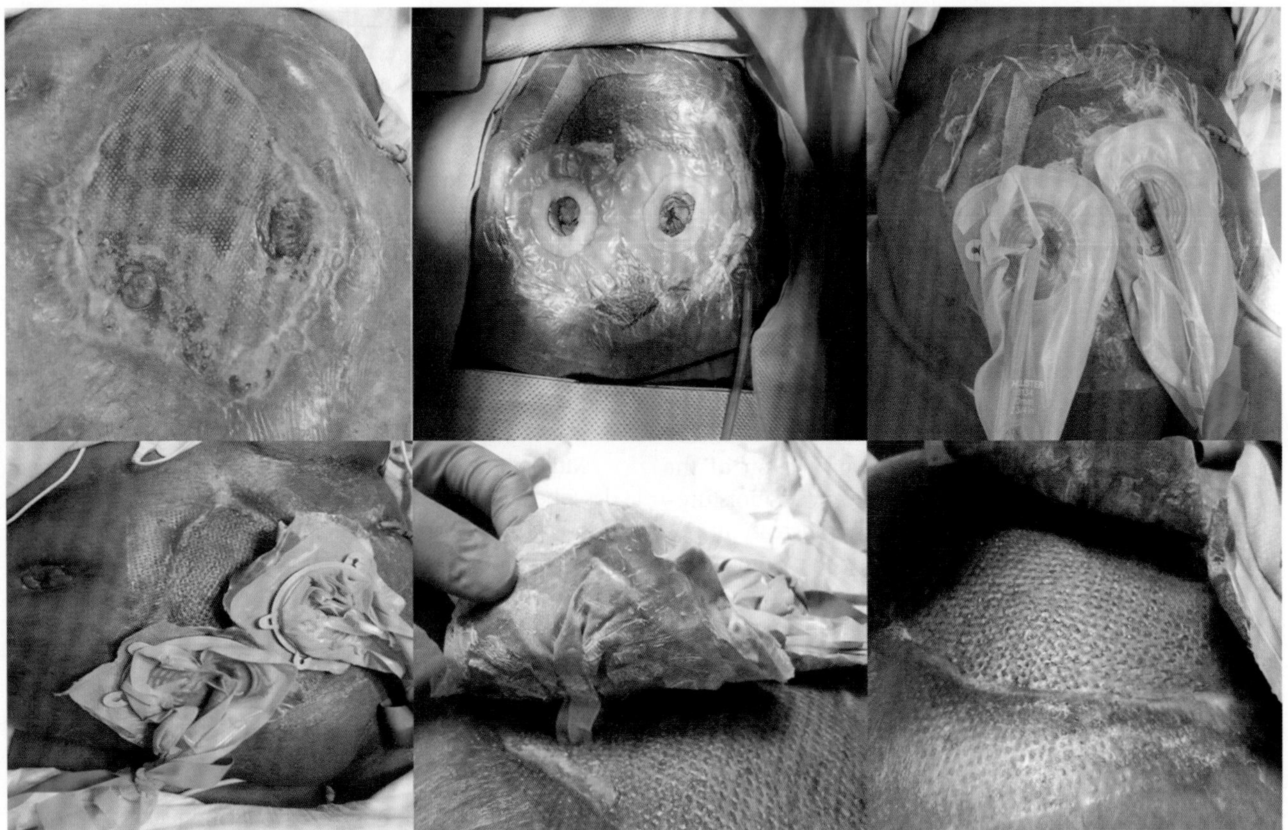

FIGURE 32-18. Glove technique for isolating enteric fistula in open wound.

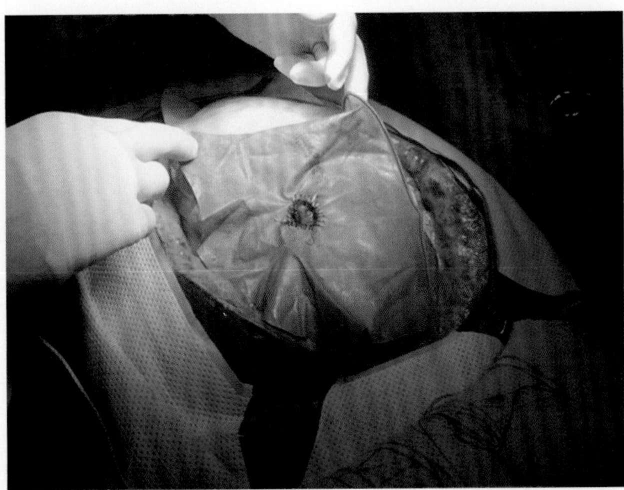

FIGURE 32-19. Surgical attachment of open glove square to os of fistula.

the operating room. A latex orthopedic glove is opened and trimmed to create a square platform; a 3-0 polydioxanone suture (PDS; Ethicon) is then used to attach the glove platform to the fistula os by a tight running suture (Fig. 32-19). Care should be taken to ensure a tight seal as this is the primary protection against leakage. Once the glove is applied, it should be held straight up in the air, to allow for negative pressure therapy to be applied circumferentially to the surrounding wound. The transparent film is applied similarly around the glove so that the glove projects upward through the negative pressure dressing. In order to create an intact vacuum seal, the glove is then glued down to the surrounding transparent film using Liquid Bonding Cement (Torbot, Cranston, RI). Once this is done, the negative pressure system can be initiated to create an intact seal, while the fistula remains open to the air. An ostomy appliance can then be applied to the glove. Since ostomy products were not meant to stick to latex gloves, the liquid bonding cement is again used to glue one side of an extended wear 4-inch barrier ring to the glove (Adapt Ring #7806, Hollister, Libertyville, IL) allowing the pouch to be applied on top. Subsequently, stool is diverted into the ostomy appliance, and carefully cutting around the glove allows for negative pressure dressing changes. Otherwise, the glove isolation may be surrounded with absorptive dressings, for frequent wound evaluation if needed. This isolation is not dependent on the outside dressing used, allowing for fecal stream diversion and frequent monitoring of the wound bed when NPWT is not utilized (Fig. 32-20). This technique is still being studied but appears to be promising as it provides absolute diversion of the fecal stream and may benefit the surgeon in very difficult circumstances.

CLINICAL PEARL

Effective management of an enteric fistula emptying into an open wound bed frequently requires isolation of the fistula; one technique gaining increasing acceptance involves use of a surgical glove to provide complete diversion of the fecal stream.

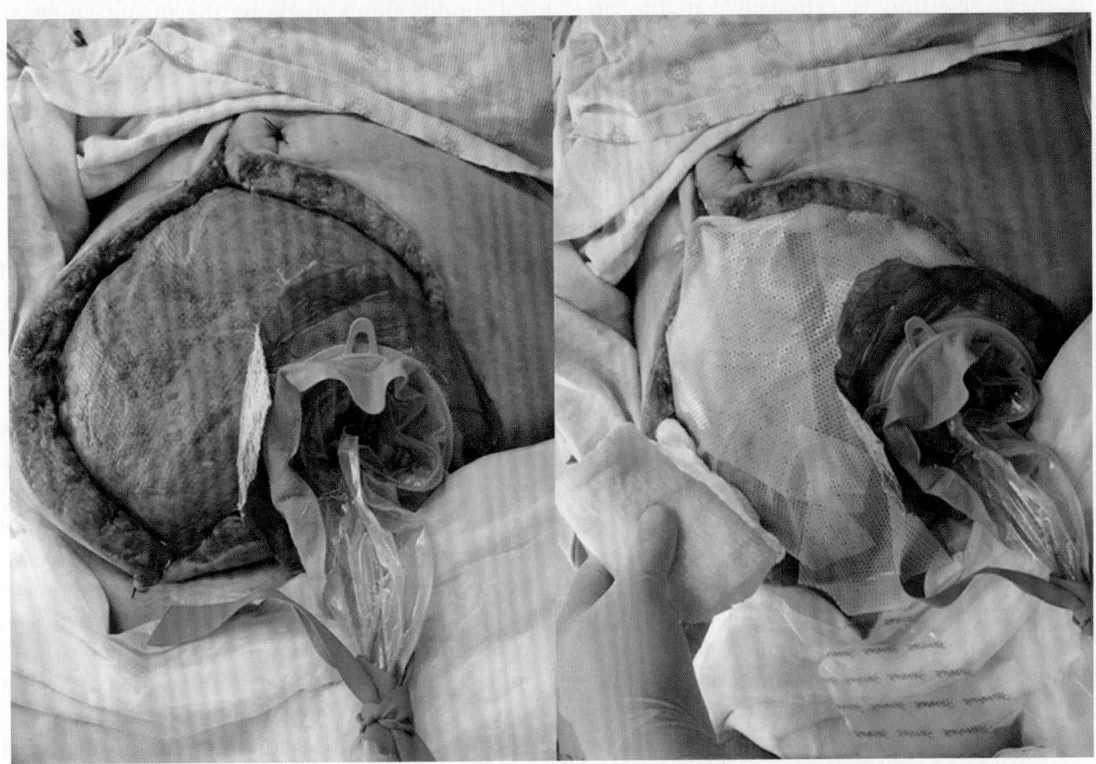

FIGURE 32-20. Glove isolation technique with advanced wound dressings.

Management of Wound Closed with Mesh

Synthetic and biologic mesh products are frequently used to reduce the risk of incisional failure and hernia development or recurrence. Luijendijk (2000) described the superiority of mesh repair over primary suture closure in reducing hernia recurrence, and this is supported by the Cochrane Collaboration (2009), which reported hernia recurrence rates of 33% with primary suture repair, as compared to 16.4% with mesh closure. Additional factors influencing recurrence were reported by Satterwhite (2012) and include the following: history of more than two prior hernia repairs, postoperative complications such as infection, overlay mesh placement, use of human-derived allograft, and surgeon technique ($p < 0.05$). While potentially reducing the risk of incisional failure and hernia recurrence, mesh is not without its own inherent risks. Specifically, wound infections were found to be more frequent in patients undergoing mesh repair than in patients closed with primary suture repair (Weber et al., 2010; Burger, 2004; Korenkov, 2002; Saunderland et al., 2009).

Both synthetic and biologic mesh products are utilized to strengthen/support the abdominal wall, to close a defect in the rectus abdominis that cannot be primarily approximated, or to serve as a bridge between large rectus defects in order to protect the underlying viscera. Selection of the specific mesh to be used is largely surgeon specific, based both on available evidence and personal experience. Unfortunately, the strength of evidence supporting mesh selection is extremely variable and some of the data available are limited to animal studies; thus, evidence-based guidelines await further research. At present, biologics are frequently selected rather than synthetics in the following situations: when there is contamination, when there are concerns regarding injury to the bowel, when the patient has comorbidities that increase the risk of infection or impaired healing, or when large surface areas are involved (Diaz, 2009; Franz, 2011; Rosen, 2010).

CLINICAL PEARL

Mesh products (both synthetic and biologic) are used to strengthen the abdominal wall, close a muscle defect that cannot be approximated, or to serve as a bridge over large muscle defects to protect the underlying viscera.

Unfortunately, for wound healing clinicians, there are no data regarding the best options for topical therapy in wounds with mesh products. Exposure of synthetic mesh is usually indicative of impaired healing and infection, and surgical excision is usually warranted (Fig. 32-21). Therefore, the surgeon should be notified immediately if there is suspected mesh exposure within a dehisced abdominal wound.

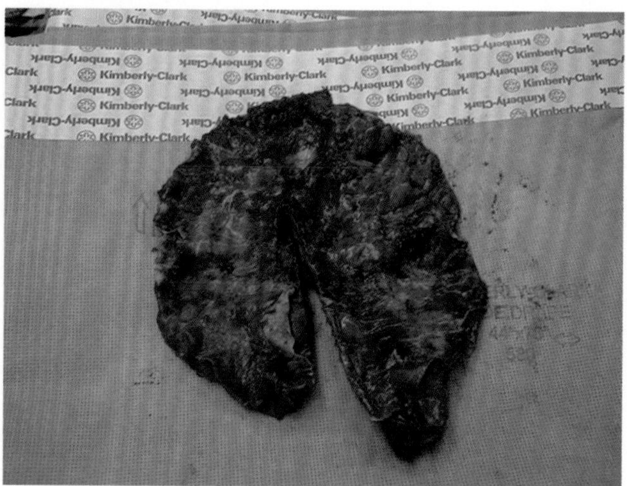

FIGURE 32-21. Mesh removed from open wound.

Types of Mesh

In order to discuss wound assessment, topical therapy selection, and management of abdominal wounds with exposed biologics, the clinician must first understand what a biologic mesh is and the expected response of the host to an implanted biologic.

Biologic meshes are acellular extracellular matrix (ECM) products. The matrix comprises collagen, elastin, glycoproteins, and retained vascular channels from cadaveric, bovine, or porcine sources. The source of the ECM, the method in which the tissue was harvested, and any chemical modifications made by the manufacturer all impact the response of the host. Ideally, an implanted biologic is compatible with the host tissue and provides support for regeneration and remodeling of the host tissue. This means that the product must not cause a significant inflammatory response, because this would result in resorption of the biologic secondary to protease degradation. In addition, it is crucial to avoid a generalized immune or foreign body response, as this would lead to encapsulation and impaired performance. Thus, an important determinant of how the body will respond to these products is the level of antigenicity that remains following product preparation and preservation.

As reported by Franz (2011), immunogenic response is largely tied to the presence of alpha-gal epitopes or expression proteins that remain following attempts by the manufacturer to "wash away" the tissues' genetic information. Since there are multiple biologic mesh options on the market, it can be daunting for the wound care practitioner to try and remember the details of each individual product, especially when the average wound clinician does not have much experience with the products used in AWR. There are actually three critical assessment factors: surgical location of the mesh, whether the name brand mesh being used is modified or unmodified, and whether the name brand mesh being used is cross-linked or non–cross-linked.

Answering these assessment questions will provide guidance in terms of anticipated time until granulation, and what to expect from both a visual and olfactory presentation of the mesh.

A mesh that is *unmodified* indicates that the manufacturer decellularized the biologic tissue, but otherwise did not alter its structural make up, or the orientation of its collagen structures. These unmodified meshes are less likely to cause immunogenic responses and are more readily vascularized by the surrounding tissue. The con for the unmodified non–cross-linked meshes is decreased strength and resistance to bacterial degradation, with increased reports of laxity and hernia recurrence over time. *Modified* meshes indicate that the manufacturer, after standard removal of cellular materials, chemically changed the structural integrity of the product, for example, by chemically cross-linking the collagen. Increasing the cross-links provides greater resistance to bacterial protease degradation and also provides increased strength and reduced risk of laxity. However, this cross-linking and chemical modification ultimately leaves behind greater numbers of immunogenic substances, increasing the body's inflammatory response to the mesh and resulting in possible encapsulation or resorption of the material. At this time, there are no studies to determine which product is better suited for AWR, and in most institutions, surgeons have a variety of options and select these products based on the needs of the individual patient.

CLINICAL PEARL

Biologic mesh products can be unmodified and non–cross-linked; these products create less of an immunologic response but may lead to laxity over time. In contrast, products that are modified and cross-linked provide greater structural support but also cause more potential for an immunogenic reaction.

Assessment Guidelines

For the wound care clinician, it is a little bit more simplified. When a mesh is exposed in the wound bed, the clinician should ascertain the product name and should then determine its source and preparation, which will provide immediate guidance in terms of expectations and assessment parameters. A nonmodified, non–cross-linked mesh will typically show evidence of granulation within 7 to 14 days, while a modified, heavily cross-linked mesh may take greater than 4 weeks to show signs of granulation. This is important because, as a mesh begins to granulate, it often appears to be disintegrating or breaking down within the wound bed. Therefore, if a nonmodified, non–cross-linked mesh presents with small areas of granulation and many areas of apparent disintegration at 8 days, this would be indicative of normal progression (Figs. 32-22 and 32-23). However, if a heavily cross-linked and modified mesh appears to be falling apart at 8 days, it may be a sign that the mesh is not incorporating or is being actively degraded by bacterial collagenases. All biologic meshes produce an odor, which is sometimes profound and often mistaken for fistula formation. However, the more heavily cross-linked meshes and porcine-derived meshes tend to have a stronger odor in our experience. Thorough assessment is necessary to determine if there are any other signs or symptoms of bacterial proliferation associated with an increasingly odiferous wound and whether antimicrobial therapy is required. The mesh should appear flat and taut in the wound bed, with no evidence of buckling. When the mesh buckles or folds in on itself, it is no longer adherent to the underlying wound bed and therefore cannot be appropriately vascularized. This separation of the mesh from the wound bed can lead to seroma formation or abscess formation under the mesh, which can ultimately result in mesh destruction and removal (Fig. 32-24). If buckling is seen, this should be reported to the surgeon immediately.

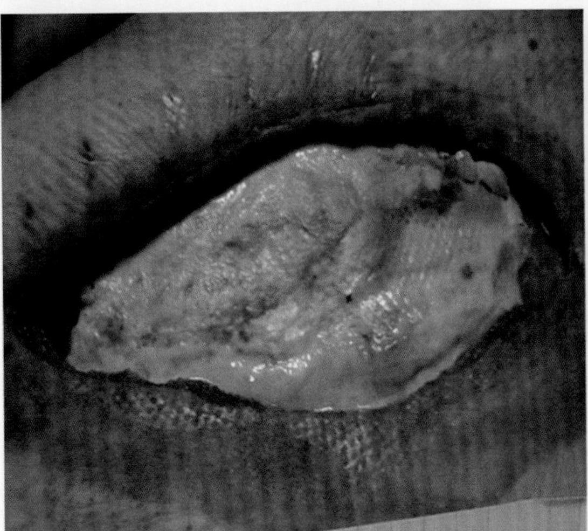
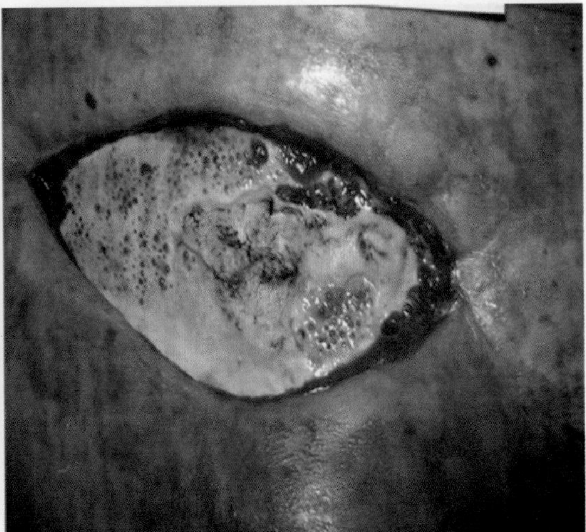

FIGURE 32-22. Progressive vascularization of non–cross-linked mesh.

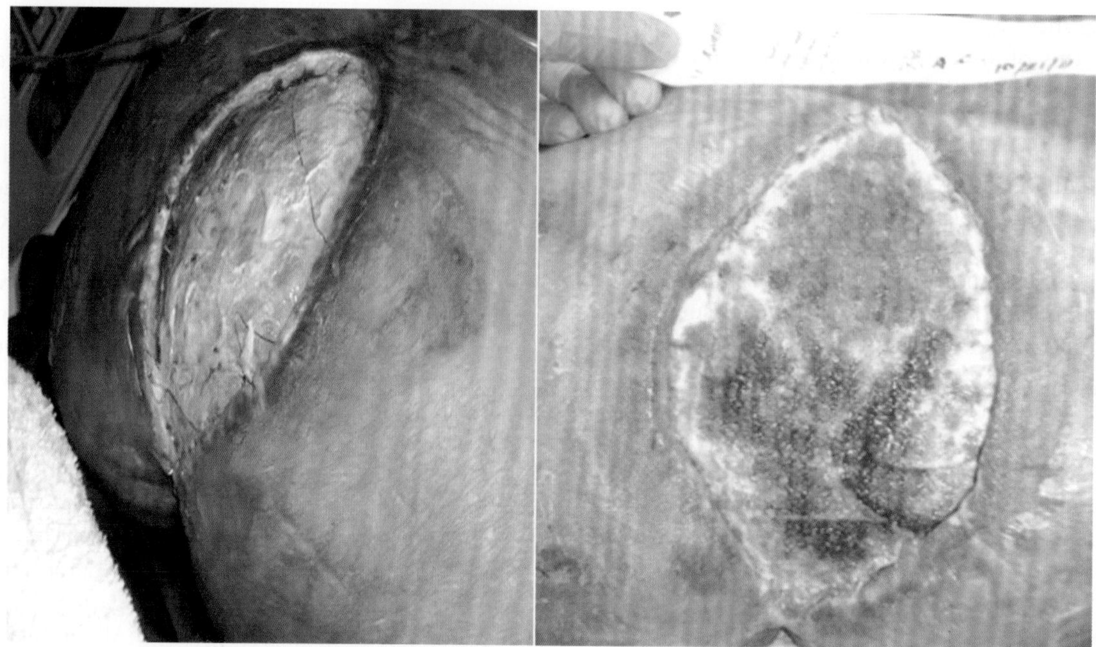

FIGURE 32-23. Progressive vascularization of non–cross-linked mesh.

> **CLINICAL PEARL**
>
> A nonmodified, non–cross-linked mesh typically granulates within 7 to 14 days, while a modified and cross-linked mesh may require >4 weeks to granulate. Thus, the wound care clinician must know what type of mesh has been used in order to provide knowledgeable assessment.

Topical Therapy Guidelines

In providing topical therapy, it is important to understand that biologic meshes were never intended to be exposed in a wound bed. Mesh was designed to either provide secondary structural support to a wound managed with primary closure or provide primary coverage of an abdominal wall defect. In either case, the therapeutic goal is to cover the mesh

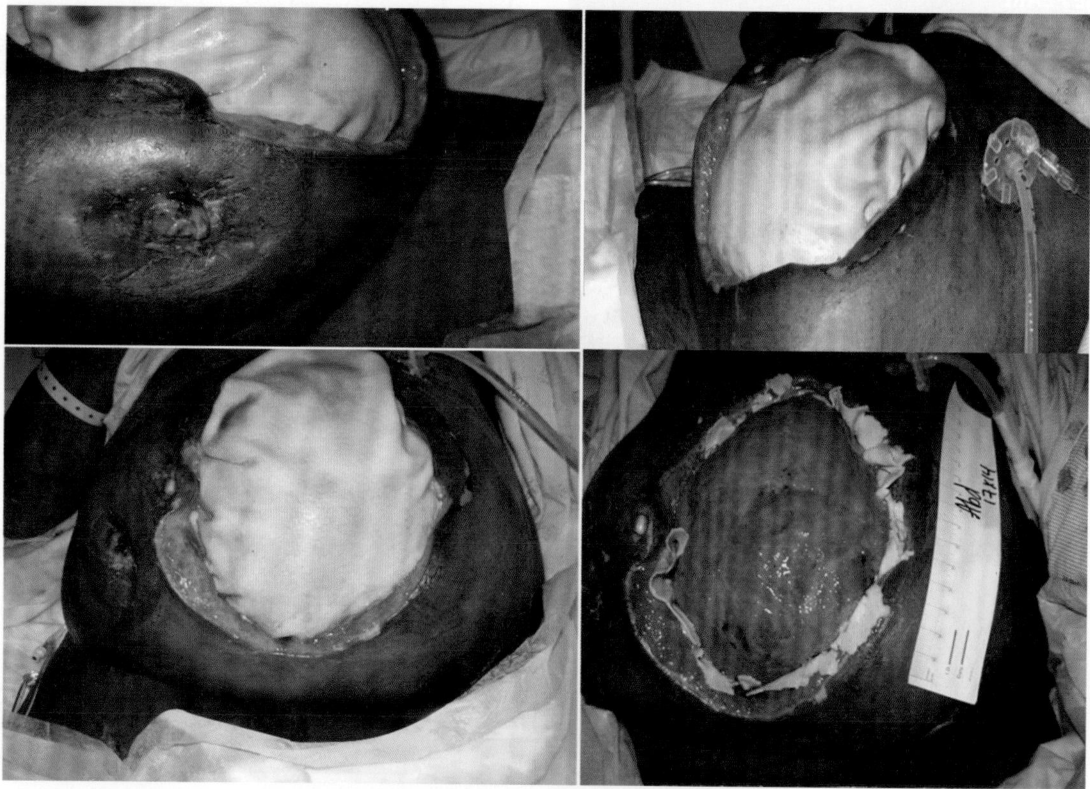

FIGURE 32-24. Mesh that is buckling and has to be removed.

with the patient's own tissues, which promotes granulation, moisture management, and protection against bacterial invasion. Topical therapy for a wound with exposed mesh requires creation of an environment that prevents mesh desiccation, controls bioburden, and protects against trauma. The clinician needs to assess the mesh for the amount of surface area exposed and volume of drainage, as larger areas of exposure will require more attention to maintaining adequate levels of moisture. Additionally, wound care providers should be aware that, depending on the manufacturer's harvesting techniques, the edge of the biologic has inherent structural weakness and may not support sutures. Surgeons typically need to take a larger "bite" of the mesh when securing it to the abdominal wall. When sutures are visible in the wound, the clinician needs to assess for suture security with each dressing change.

Bioburden assessment is a constant requirement. Although biologic mesh is considered preferable to synthetic mesh in contaminated wounds because of its greater resistance to infection, biologic mesh may still get infected. Attention to patient symptomatology is critical for prompt identification of increasing bacterial loads. One important reminder for the wound care clinician that is different from traditional wound bed preparation is the following: as the biologic mesh begins to granulate, there may be residual areas that never become viable, and these areas will ultimately slough out of the wound. During this process, the nonviable mesh looks very similar to necrotic slough; however, the wound care clinician should never provide sharp debridement since the underlying mesh may be adherent to bowel, and debridement may result in accidental enterotomy (Fig. 32-25). Debridement of any nonviable or nongranulating mesh should be accomplished conservatively via autolytic techniques over time.

The wound clinician also needs to understand that there are *no* evidence-based recommendations for appropriate topical therapy to be utilized with biologic mesh, either from the manufacturer or in the literature. The following recommendations are therefore based upon principles of wound care, biology of the mesh, and anecdotal reports.

First, since biologic mesh is a conglomeration of connective tissue proteins and since ingrowth of granulation tissue is dependent on fibroblast activity, cytotoxic and debriding products should be avoided. Examples of products to avoid would be the application of topical endogenous collagenases, cytotoxic concentrations of antimicrobials such as ¼, ½, or full-strength Dakin's solution, hydrogen peroxide, and acetic acid. Instead, the focus of wound bed preparation for wounds with exposed biologic mesh is on thorough irrigation, maintenance of a moist wound surface, minimizing the frequency of dressing changes, reducing the risk of trauma, and reducing bioburden (when indicated). NPWT is frequently used in the management of open wounds with biologic mesh; however, the practitioner may need to modify "standard procedures" to assure maintenance of sufficient moisture at the wound surface and to prevent trauma with dressing removal. For example, hydrophilic sponges or moisture-retentive contact layers containing petrolatum may be needed to maintain adequate hydration and to prevent trauma to large areas of exposed biologic mesh. Wounds with large volumes of exudate or wounds involving small areas of exposed mesh may benefit from NPWT using hydrophobic foam or gauze. Suction settings are typically set between −75 and −125 mm Hg to manage exudate, provide constant moisture and a temperature-controlled environment, and to reduce the risk of bacterial exposure from frequent dressing changes and multiple provider interactions.

CLINICAL PEARL

In managing a wound with exposed mesh, the nurse should avoid use of any products that could cause breakdown of connective tissue proteins; this includes enzymes (collagenase) and antiseptics (e.g., Dakin's solution or acetic acid).

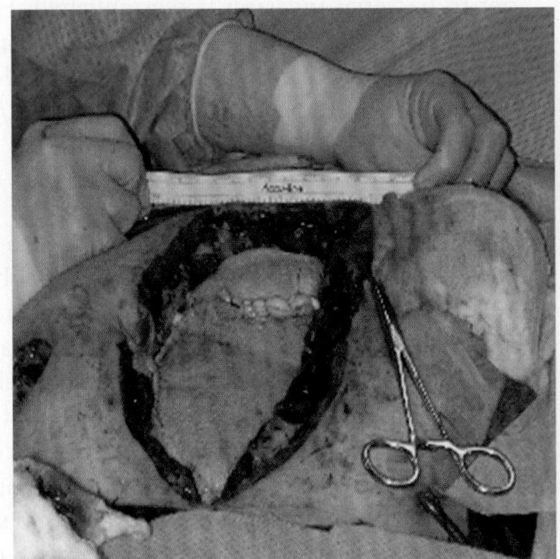

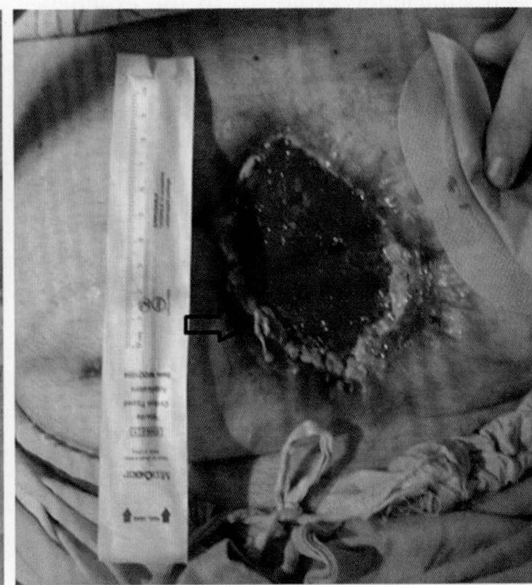

FIGURE 32-25. Nonviable residual mesh.

In all wounds, high-volume irrigation is mandatory, for example, 500 to 1,000 mL of warm normal saline removed by bedside suction (Yankauer). In cases where there is suspicion of high bioburden, it is critical to reduce bacterial counts in order to decrease the risk of mesh degradation by bacterial collagenases and endotoxins. If high levels of bioburden are suspected, high-volume irrigation should be continued, with either saline or a noncytotoxic solution such as diluted and stabilized hydrochlorous acid or polyhexamethylene biguanide. However, the use of these products should be short term as their use with biologic mesh has not been sufficiently studied. Dry wounds with mesh exposure and high levels of bacteria may benefit from use of a wound pouching system to maintain moisture and normothermia, along with use of ionic silver hydrogel. Due to the rapid inactivation of silver in the presence of wound plasma, topical products should be applied multiple times daily for sufficient antimicrobial effect. For wounds with moderate-to-high volumes of exudate, either silver alginates or hydrofibers may be selected. It should be noted that Silvadene cream (silver sulfadiazine) should be avoided in open abdominal wounds, especially those with large surface areas, as the risk of heavy metal toxicity and systemic absorption is considerable due to the product's high silver concentration (parts per million). High release silvers also have the potential of staining the mesh, which may interfere with visual assessment. Possible silver alternatives include noncytotoxic broad-spectrum topical antimicrobials such as cadexomer iodine, pathogen-binding (hydrophobic bonding) mesh, Manuka honey, or products known to be bacteriostatic such as LevaFiber technology or methylene blue–gentian violet polyvinyl alcohol foams. As noted, there are presently no evidence-based guidelines to determine the most appropriate product. Additional options that may be considered by the wound care provider include negative pressure wound therapy with instillation; theoretical benefits include reports of antibiofilm activity and enhanced promotion of granulation tissue as compared to standard negative pressure. Its use with exposed biologic mesh, however, has not been sufficiently explored. In the experience of the authors, standard moist wound healing provides adequate support for both autolysis and granulation tissue formation. Because heavily cross-linked modified meshes do not granulate for over a month, there may be a greater need for antimicrobial agents to reduce the risk of infection. One important caveat in management of all biologic meshes is the strict avoidance of wet-to-dry dressings; their high moisture vapor transmission rates, lack of bacterial barrier protection, and propensity to cause mechanical debridement increase the risk for desiccation or traumatic destruction of the mesh, with a resultant increase in risk of infection.

CLINICAL PEARL

In management of any open abdominal wound with exposed mesh, topical therapy should include high-volume irrigation with warmed saline to reduce bacterial loads.

 Management of Poststernotomy Wound and Open Chest

Care of the patient poststernotomy from cardiothoracic surgery involves similar considerations as described above in management of the open abdomen. In the case of the poststernotomy wound, the surgeon must close and stabilize the sternum, followed either by primary closure of the muscle, soft tissues, and skin or by delayed secondary closure (initial closure to fascial level followed by later closure of the full-thickness wound) (Chang et al., 2013). In selected cases involving surgical complications, the surgeon may opt to leave the chest open and delay sternal closure until the patient has been stabilized. Each clinical situation will be addressed from the standpoint of important assessment and management principles.

Primary Closure

Wounds closed primarily reflect successful closure of the sternum, fascia, muscle, subcutaneous tissue, and skin. Typical protocols for incisional management include sterile dressing application in the operating room with removal 48 to 72 hours following the operative procedure and subsequent daily cleansing either with plain tap water or, in some facilities, with antimicrobials such as chlorhexidine gluconate (CHG). As mentioned earlier in the chapter, high-risk patients may benefit from the application of iNPWT to the closed incision after surgery. Assessment criteria for the closed sternal incision involves evaluation of epithelialization, signs of underlying complications such as seroma or hematoma, signs of infection (increasing erythema, induration, warmth, pain, and drainage; elevated white blood cell count; elevated C-reactive protein), or evidence of tissue necrosis (e.g., necrosis of adipose tissue, especially in obese individuals, or necrosis of the sternum itself following harvesting of the left internal mammary artery). Following complete epithelialization of the incision, the natural biologic barrier to bacterial invasion is reestablished. However, epithelialization does not signify complete healing, as there may be failure to form sufficient granulation tissue for healing of the underlying soft tissues and/or failure of bony union of the sternum.

Sternal Healing

The sternum itself may take upward of 3 to 6 months to heal despite adequate soft tissue closure (Cohen & Griffin, 2002), making sternal approximation and reinforcement the most important aspect of wound management long term; if the sternum does not heal appropriately, the patient experiences long-term instability of the chest wall. Sternal dehiscence is most often due to infectious complications but can also be caused by noninfectious impediments to wound healing; in a study involving 12,380 sternotomies, the incidence of infectious dehiscence was 2.4% compared to 0.39% for noninfectious dehiscence. Risk factors for noninfectious sternal dehiscence include obesity, National Heart Association Severity Score class IV, diabetes mellitus, chronic obstructive pulmonary disease, chronic cough, smoking, internal mammary artery harvesting, prolonged duration of cardiopulmonary bypass, and excessive blood transfusions during the postoperative period (Olbrecht et al., 2006; Tekumit et al., 2009). Another major factor leading to noninfectious dehiscence is sternal motion and instability occurring during the days and weeks following surgery. Sternal closure technique has also been identified as a contributing factor, though controversy exists as to the best technique for ensuring stability of the sternum and preventing late nonunion, reoperation, or mediastinitis. For example, Tekumit et al. (2009) found no statistically significant difference in complication rates between patients closed with single loop closure and those closed with figure-of-eight wired closure techniques. Patients presenting with nonunion of the sternum had higher rates of mediastinitis, osteomyelitis, and chronic instability and also a higher mortality rate.

CLINICAL PEARL

Assessment of a closed sternal wound must include inspection and palpation to detect indicators of sternal closure breakdown, for example, sternal movement during respiration and coughing, sternal click, sudden onset of increasing pain, bubbling along the closure line, and/or exudate. The clinician should *avoid* any aggressive probing of undermined or tunneled areas.

Assessment Sternal Healing

Due to the significance of sternal separation and failure to heal, manual palpation of the sternum is recommended in addition to the standard assessment for evidence of skin or soft tissue infection. The clinician should place one finger on each side of the sternal incision and should feel for sternal movement during inspiration/expiration and coughing. The clinician should also listen and feel for an audible sternal click, which indicates that the sternal edges are moving against each other. Sudden onset of increasing pain is another potential indicator of sternal separation. Any indicators of sternal movement should be reported to the surgeon. The ability to express seropurulent exudate, clear amber exudate, or old bloody drainage should be reported to the surgeon since these findings are indicators of infection, seroma, or necrotic fat. If there is partial skin dehiscence, the clinician should assess for signs of underlying air movement, bubbling, or disappearance of any irrigated saline. The clinician should strictly *avoid* aggressive probing of any undermined or tunneled areas, as forceful exploration could result in subsequent dehiscence or entrance into a deeper cavity. In addition, the clinician should *use caution* in placing wicking material into blind tunnels, as the difference between barometric pressure and intrathoracic pressure in wounds with sternal separation may result in a sucking chest wound, which could cause the packing strip to be sucked into the deep recesses of the wound or chest cavity and out of the visual field of the clinician.

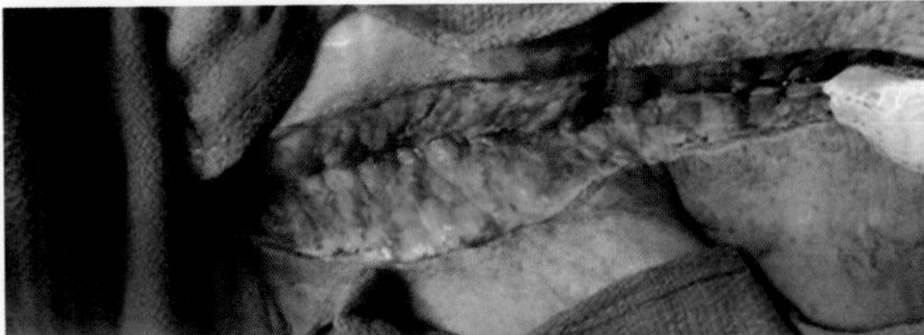

FIGURE 32-26. Wound closed to subcutaneous tissue level.

Sternal dehiscence may heal on its own or may require surgical intervention. In a retrospective study by Nazerali et al. (2014), investigators found complete sternal healing with no evidence of mediastinitis in 57 high-risk patients who underwent rigid sternal fixation using a variety of sternal fixation plate devices. Their results suggest that prophylactic use of rigid fixation may safely be considered in high-risk cases, especially those prone to mediastinitis. In the case of chronic dehiscence and nonunion, debridement with rewiring or debridement with muscle flaps is often required (Olbrecht et al., 2006).

Sternal Closure with Open Chest Wound

Sternal closure with an open full-thickness wound may be the best surgical approach for patients at high risk for impaired healing or infection or the patient who has undergone multiple sternotomies (Figs. 32-26 to 32-29). This approach allows the surgical team to monitor the patient for any signs or symptoms of infection, necrosis, or wound deterioration and provides for immediate intervention. The goal in management of this wound is establishment of sufficient granulation tissue to allow for secondary closure or, in some cases, delayed primary

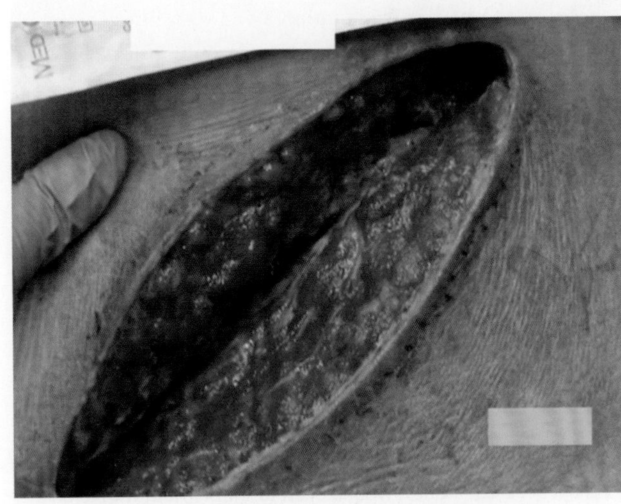

FIGURE 32-27. Chest wound closed to fascia level.

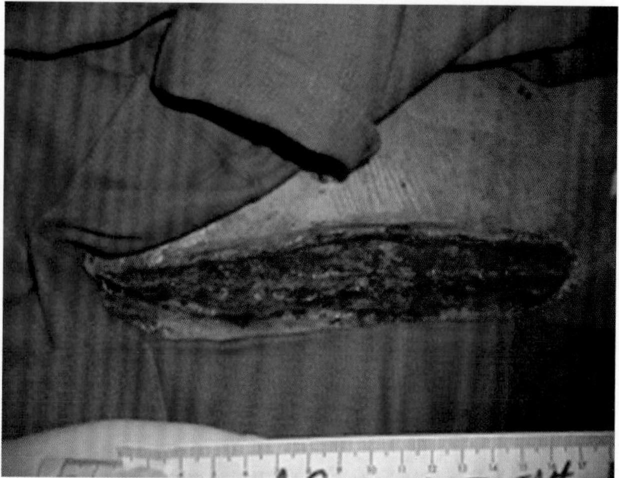

FIGURE 32-28. Chest wound closed to the sternum.

closure. When managing these wounds, the wound care clinician must provide appropriate wound bed preparation and moist wound healing and must also monitor for closure of the sternum. In many cases, the sternum and sternal wires are exposed, necessitating sterile technique for dressing changes in addition to assessment for proper sternal approximation and any signs of sternal nonunion or dehiscence. The clinician should provide several minutes of direct visualization of the sternum during normal breathing or any episodes of coughing and should be alert to any signs of fluctuation. Other than visual confirmation of sternal movement, dehiscence may be evidenced as an audible sucking sound during breathing. Minor separation may be manifest by signs of bubbling along the sternal closure. Finally, disappearance of the saline into the chest cavity during wound irrigation is another ominous sign. If any evidence of sternal fluctuation is found, the surgeon should be notified so that the plan of care can be reviewed or altered.

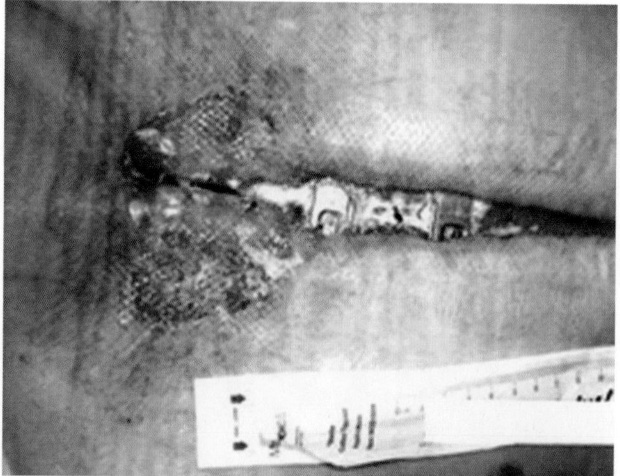

FIGURE 32-29. Chest wound open to the sternum with talon exposure.

Often, NPWT is selected in these situations to provide sternal stability, prevent frequent changes in intrathoracic pressure changes, and decrease the risk of retained wound exudate in the thoracic cavity. There are some modifications in standard wound care that should be incorporated when there is sternal separation: gentle cleansing with normal saline and avoidance of high-volume irrigations to prevent retention of fluid in the chest cavity and clear documentation of the number, type, and location of packing materials to prevent inadvertent retention of dressings. When NPWT is not the recommended treatment choice (e.g., in wounds complicated by infection or necrosis), the clinician should recommend a packing material that provides sufficient absorptive capacity to meet the wound's needs, while allowing for ease of removal and prevention of retained dressings.

CLINICAL PEARL

Modified NPWT may be indicated for wounds with sternal separation, to provide increased stability and to reduce the risk of retained exudate in the thoracic cavity.

When no sternal fluctuation is seen, and the primary sternal closure is deemed to be stable, the clinician can be more aggressive in implementation of traditional wound-healing principles. One exception to foundational recommendations for wound bed preparation would be to avoid sharp debridement along the sternal closure. This is because there is frequently a layer of fascia over the wires that may be mistaken for necrosis. Additionally, inappropriate debridement of the sternal closure may result in sternal wire rupture, debridement of the fascia, and increased risk of sternal dehiscence.

An anecdotal finding for patients with full-thickness wounds following hardware insertion is the patient's experience of pain. Frequently, patients undergoing implantation of a ventricular access device (VAD, LVAD, RVAD, BiVAD) or total artificial heart (TAH) report little to no pain with sternal wound dressing changes but exhibit hypersensitivity of the periwound skin, especially in response to adhesive removal. Thus, measures should be implemented to reduce the risk of pain and medical adhesive–related skin injury (MARSI) (McNichol et al., 2013) in these patients, such as the use of contact layers, periwound skin protectants, use of silicone-based or gel-based adhesive removers, and limiting the skin surface covered by adhesive products.

Cardiac surgery patients are also at higher risk for bleeding because they are typically anticoagulated on a variety of agents; therefore, their coagulation levels can change suddenly, and they may require repeated laboratory studies prior to wound care. In some cases, wound care may need to be delayed or postponed past manufacturer or organizational guidelines for dressing change frequency due to concerns regarding bleeding. The wound care clinician should always have a plan for establishing hemostasis in the event of acute bleeding, such as the use of kaolin-impregnated gauze agents (QuickClot, Z-Medica, Connecticut), cellulose-based products (Surgicel/Surgifoam, Ethicon, Somerville, NJ), or cautery agents such as silver nitrate. Additionally, primary dressings should be selected based on their nonadherent quality. Good options include nonadherent contact layers with and without NPWT, alginates, hydrofibers, and hydrogels; strict *avoidance* of wet-to-dry dressings is essential. Finally, patients who are status post–heart transplantation require systemic immunosuppressive agents and are therefore at greater risk for infection; many are also malnourished, and this also delays wound healing and increases the risk of infection. For these patients, advanced biomodulating dressings may be indicated at an earlier point in the management process to minimize the effects of the proinflammatory and antiangiogenic wound environment. Complex therapies such as noncontact low-frequency ultrasound have also been shown to be beneficial in these cases by reducing inflammation and promoting angiogenesis.

Open Chest with Delayed Sternal Closure

While the closed sternal incision, the open superficial sternal wound, and the deep full-thickness chest wound are all within the scope of practice for the wound care clinician, open-chest management (OCM) is decidedly the surgeon's domain. However, wound care clinicians are often asked for recommendations regarding management of these complex wounds; therefore, the wound care nurse needs to be knowledgeable regarding the principles underlying appropriate management. In cases where the sternum cannot be closed with usual surgical techniques, plastic surgery consultation is required. The wound care clinician should be knowledgeable regarding the following: reasons for delayed sternal closure; principles of sternal stabilization, sternal padding, and ventricular protection; and the principles underlying successful use of NPWT for OCM.

Indications

Delayed sternal closure has been used successfully for high-risk cardiac surgery patients and was first described by Riahi et al. (1975). One major reason for leaving the chest open immediately following cardiac surgery is to allow sufficient space for the edematous heart to beat; this is particularly important when the patient is hemodynamically unstable and at risk for further compromise if the sternum is approximated (Takayama et al., 2006). Specifically, patients with uncontrollable hemorrhage, intractable arrhythmias, reperfusion myocardial edema, implantable ventricular assist devices, or intra-aortic balloon pumps often benefit from OCM (Boeken et al., 2011a, 2011b). A retrospective study found no difference in infectious complications between a control group managed with primary sternal closure and an OCM group, despite the fact that the OCM group were higher acuity and required frequent reentries for management of bleeding (Dyke et al., 2014). Considering the low incidence of infection and associated complications, the researchers suggest that delayed closure is likely to be utilized more frequently in the future (Boeken et al., 2011a, 2011b). Similarly, a study of trauma patients undergoing emergent thoracotomy found no statistically significant difference in the rate of infections or survival between temporary OCM versus definitive closure. However, the open-chest patients had significantly lower peak inspiratory pressures compared to their closed counterparts (Lang et al., 2011).

Neonatal and pediatric studies support similar indications for the use of an open-chest technique following cardiac surgery (Erek et al., 2012; Woodward et al., 2011). Because of the small size of their chests, newborns are at risk for decompensation related to tamponade-like effects. Vojtovic and colleagues (2009) evaluated 23 neonates following biventricular correction surgery and found that chest closure decreased stroke volume, arterial blood pressure, cardiac output, and oxygenation secondary to decreased lung compliance. These risks are compounded by the relative difficulty of assessing for subtle changes that may develop days after closure. However, delayed sternal closure is not without its risks in this population. In an 8-year retrospective study of neonates undergoing primary sternal closure versus delayed closure using either skin-only or membrane-assisted closure, mortality was higher in the delayed sternal closure groups than the primary skin closure. While there were no reported differences in sternal wound complications among the three groups, the overall postoperative course was found to be far more complex in the delayed sternal closure group (Erek et al., 2012). Mortality in the study was associated with age, preoperative condition, bypass time >180 minutes, and cross-clamp time >99 minutes; these data suggest that the increased mortality in the delayed closure group may be more indicative of the critical patient condition that necessitated the delayed sternal closure than the technique itself.

In all cases of delayed sternal closure, the surgical team must monitor the patient daily for indications that the patient is ready for closure. Most often, the patient is assessed for hemodynamic stability, blood gas studies reflecting appropriate oxygenation without the need for aggressive respiratory support, decreasing lactate levels, no evidence of bleeding or sepsis, sufficient mean arterial pressure and systolic arterial pressures, and a total negative fluid balance. If the patient does not meet these indicators or if sudden decompensation occurs following attempted closure, the sternum may be again left open. Whenever the sternum must be left open, safely temporizing this wound becomes a priority.

Management Guidelines

Principles for safe management of the open chest involve stabilization of the open sternal edges, sternal padding, and myocardial protection. Specific recommendations for management have not been established, and surgeon preference often guides the plan of care. A mesh membrane is frequently placed temporarily to provide myocardial protection and to reduce the development of adhesions to the pericardium. It is particularly important to keep the often jagged edges of the cut sternum stabilized and separated; inadvertent downward movement or contact with the myocardium may result in ventricular laceration. If ventricular laceration is not treated immediately, death may result secondary to profuse bleeding or massive air embolism (Spain, 2004). Methods for stabilizing the sternum vary; one approach is use of rigid plastic stents, which are sometimes created from large gauge syringes (Hashemzadeh & Hashemzadeh, 2009; Ozker et al., 2012). In pediatric patients, multiple techniques have been described including the use of rib spreaders, stents, or struts (Pye and McDonnell, 2010). When sternal supports are chosen, the pericardial cavity is typically not packed with other materials; this permits ongoing visualization during any emergent events.

CLINICAL PEARL

Principles for safe management of the open chest involve stabilization of the open sternal edges, sternal padding, and myocardial protection.

If the sternal bone is too poor quality to accommodate a rigid support, or the surgeon believes closure is not feasible, chest packing may be utilized instead. In this case, multiple contact layers are utilized (with or without an underlying membrane) to provide protection of the myocardium, and the chest is then packed with sterile gauze. This provides multiple layers of protection between the sternal edges and the underlying organs to prevent trauma. The patient does need to be monitored for signs of tamponade, which can occur should the pericardial space be packed too tightly or when packing is required because of active bleeding. In the event of bleeding, radiopaque hemostatic gauze rolls are typically utilized (Combat Gauze, Z-Medica, Connecticut). Newer devices have been developed to provide progressive approximation of the sternum; they capitalize on the ability to stabilize the sternum, while eliminating the need for the aforementioned devices currently being utilized in an off-label fashion. Santini et al. (2012) described their experience with an implantable, temporary sternal spreader, which allowed for progressive closure using a rotating wire mechanism outside of the chest. They reported safe and effective closure in all patients, although the small sample size limits the impact of these findings.

With all of the above techniques, a sterile, transparent material is typically chosen to cover the skin bridge and provide an occlusive seal. Products utilized for coverage include standard transparent films, iodine-impregnated transparent films, and silastic patches or polytetrafluoroethylene (PTFE) mesh sutured to the patient's skin (Boeken et al., 2011). Dressing change frequency ranges from 24 to 72 hours depending on the patient's age and clinical status (Ozker et al., 2012). These changes are done using strict sterile technique, either in the OR at the bedside. Typically, high-volume irrigations of the chest cavity are indicated using warm normal saline, Betadine, or antibiotic solutions (Estrera et al., 2008; Hashemzadeh & Hashemzadeh, 2009; Yasa et al., 2010). Direct involvement and/or supervision by the attending surgeon should be provided during any dressing change.

Negative pressure wound therapy has been utilized in management of the open chest, and the wound care clinician may be called upon to provide advice regarding safe application and suction settings for adult and pediatric patients. A critical first step in these situations is to ascertain the safety of NPWT use when there is exposed myocardium and to provide protection against ventricular laceration or heart rupture.

Multiple porcine studies have been conducted to test the impact of NPWT on open chest wounds. In a study evaluating the effects of NPWT on normal, reperfused, and ischemic myocardium following various degrees of lower anterior descending (LAD) coronary artery occlusion, NPWT was found to significantly increase microvascular blood flow in all three conditions (Lindstedt et al., 2007a, 2007b). In this porcine model, a sternal spreader was used to maintain open chest status, while NPWT foam was directly applied to the myocardium at a setting of −50 mm Hg. Investigators found a statistically significant increase in myocardial blood flow with the use of NPWT in all situations, including the ischemic myocardium ($p > 0.05$). When applying NPWT to an open chest, the clinician should be cognizant of findings regarding the impact of NPWT on the thoracic cavity and the heart. Torbrand et al. (2008) described two major findings: (1) only the anterior aspect of the myocardium in direct contact with the NPWT system is impacted, and pressure readings on the posterior aspect of the heart and the pleural space are unaffected, and (2) this difference in anterior and posterior pressure causes the right ventricle to be pulled upward toward the sternum where it might be exposed to the sharp sternal edges and at risk for potential rupture (Torbrand et al., 2008). The researchers go on to state that this does not preclude NPWT use but does indicate a need for cautious application of this therapy to the open chest. Specifically, multiple contact layers are suggested to separate the sternal edges from any underlying structures. In clinical studies in humans, NPWT has demonstrated benefit in management of the open chest associated with delayed sternal closure and in clearance of mediastinitis. Gustafsson et al. (2003) reported on 4,124 sternotomy procedures over a 3-year period. During this time, 9 patients had sternal rewiring after early dehiscence, 4 patients had sternal instability with immediate application of NPWT and subsequent primary closure after the first NPWT change (due to negative cultures), and 40 patients presented with deep sternal wound infections and received NPWT after intraoperative assessment. The authors describe attention to revision of sternal edges, debridement of frank necrosis or infected tissues, and clearance of any adherences or sharp edges along the right ventricle or left hemisternum. Negative pressure was applied after first covering the ventricle, lung tissue, grafts, and all sternal edges with multiple layers of paraffin gauze; one piece of polyurethane foam was placed between the sternal margin, and a second piece was placed within the subcutaneous wound space. The foam was cut larger than the space between the sternal edges and sized to overlap the skin edges to ensure security and immobilization of the wound edges. The authors describe subsequent clearance of all mediastinitis with effective closure in all 40 patients and state that NPWT is considered the treatment of choice for this condition.

Bleeding is a potential complication of NPWT in patients with open chest wounds since most of these patients are anticoagulated with elevated international normalized ratio (INR) levels. Clinical staff caring for the patient with NPWT need to be educated on the signs and symptoms of active bleeding and appropriate response (immediate cessation of therapy along with measures to accomplish hemostasis). Bleeding in the open chest wound may be due to venous bleeding from the wound margins, periosteal bleeding from the sternum, or arterial bleeding from graft failure or ventricular injury. Additionally, "hidden" bleeding is a concern. In a case series comparing the effectiveness of gauze-based versus foam-based NPWT fillers, a blood clot that developed between the contact layers and the gauze resulted in cardiac tamponade necessitating emergent dressing change. The authors concluded that gauze-based NPWT seemed to be as clinically effective as foam-based NPWT, but noted a greater risk for overpacking the chest cavity with gauze as compared to foam (Rajakaruna & Marchbank, 2011).

CLINICAL PEARL

There are multiple case series that demonstrate the benefit and safety of NPWT for adults or neonates undergoing delayed primary closure of chest wounds due to congenital anomalies or mediastinitis. Modifications in standard techniques may be required to prevent complications such as bleeding.

Early indications of success with NPWT to the open chest and mediastinitis led to further comparative studies on its use and impact on mortality. A study of 46 patients with mediastinitis treated with NPWT who were subsequently closed without any additional tissue flaps were compared to 4,781 patients undergoing coronary artery bypass grafting (CABG) during the same time period without mediastinitis. The authors found similar survival rates at 1, 3 and 5 years for the patients undergoing NPWT with eventual rewiring and those who had primary closure following CABG (Sjogren et al., 2005). There are multiple case series that demonstrate the benefit and safety of NPWT for neonates undergoing delayed primary closure due to congenital anomalies or mediastinitis. Lower suction settings are usually recommended for these patients (Kodohama et al., 2008), and one case report describes deterioration of cardiac parameters when pressure was increased to −75 mm Hg, which was alleviated when the pressure was reduced to −25 mm Hg (Lindstedt et al., 2008a, 2008b, 2008c, 2008d; Oeltjen et al., 2009). This underscores the importance of individualizing suction settings for both adults and children based on the patient's hemodynamic response. With children as well as adults, complete protection of the myocardium with multiple contact layers is essential; the periwound skin must also be thoroughly protected since current recommendations include sizing the foam larger than the wound so that it overlaps onto the skin to provide greater stability for the wound. Finally, the NPWT suction setting may need to be titrated to avoid interference with the function of percutaneous chest tubes. In cardiac surgery, there are often at least three chest tubes inserted: mediastinal, pleural, and myocardial. Chest tubes are placed to low wall suction (typically −20 mm Hg) via the use of pleurevacs to evacuate blood and serous fluid from the chest cavity. However, in the presence of an open chest wound or open communication in a primarily closed sternal wound, NPWT may interfere with delivery of suction to the chest tubes; in this case, the NPWT suction setting should be reduced until acceptable chest tube function is achieved (in coordination with the cardiothoracic surgeon or intensivist). When the connection between the wound and the thoracic space has closed, or when the chest tubes are no longer necessary, the NPWT suction may be increased to appropriate levels.

Surgical Wound Complications

Surgical Site Infections

SSIs are the second most commonly reported hospital-acquired infection (HAI) in the United States, representing 17% of all infections and an approximate 300,000 SSI per year (CDC, 2013; US Department of Health and Human Services, 2013). The incidence of SSI is between 2% and 5% of all inpatient surgeries with an associated 3% mortality and 2 to 11 times higher risk of death and long-term disability (Anderson et al., 2008). SSI increases the length of stay (LOS) by 7 to 10 days, increases readmission rates, and costs the U.S. Healthcare System upward of $10 billion annually.

CLINICAL PEARL

SSIs are the second most commonly reported hospital-acquired infection in the United States and are associated with marked increase in risk of death or long-term disability.

SSI as Quality Indicator

SSI has become a national quality indicator due to the immense costs, morbidity, and mortality associated with an infection. SSI surveillance and prevention initiatives have evolved since the 1980s with a focus worldwide on decreasing the rates of SSI via adherence to best practices for prevention. One issue related to use of SSI as a quality indicator is the complexity surrounding risk for and development of infection and the difficulty in accurately measuring adherence to prevention guidelines. Biscione (2009) stated that, in order for SSI rates to accurately reflect the quality of care provided by different facilities and surgeons, reporting measures must be able to adjust for risk based on case mix and acuity of patient populations. Moreover, there is disagreement as to the percentage of HAIs that could be achieved with the implementation of all available prevention initiatives. Despite these issues, it is clear that our responsibility as clinicians is to implement all possible best practices in order to achieve the lowest SSI rate possible.

Current Guidelines for SSI Prevention

Today, there are many resources available to aid facilities and clinicians in the fight against SSI. Professional societies such as the Society for Healthcare Epidemiology of America (SHEA), the Infectious Diseases Society of America (IDSA), the Association for Professionals in Infection Control and Epidemiology, The Joint Commission, and the Institute of Healthcare Improvement (IHI) provide excellent resources and guidelines for decreasing HAIs (Bates et al., 2014; Berrios-Torres, 2009; Yokoe et al., 2008). One of the most widely utilized tools is the Surgical Care Improvement Project (SCIP) guidelines. In 2006, the Medicare and Medicaid Services and Centers for Disease Control and Prevention collaborated to develop the SCIP (Bratzler & Hunt, 2006). SCIP guidelines focus on the prevention of four major surgical complications: SSI, venous thromboembolism, cardiac events, and respiratory complications (Rosenberger et al., 2011). For SSI, SCIP recommendations include the following:

- Prophylactic antibiotic administration within 1 hour of surgical procedure or, for vancomycin, within 2 hours of procedure.
- Selection of proper antibiotic
- Discontinuation of antibiotics within 24 hours after surgery (48 hours in the case of cardiac surgery)
- Controlling postoperative 6 AM glucose levels in cardiac surgery patients
- No hair removal; or hair removal conducted with use of clippers or depilatories (no razors)
- Urinary catheter removal 1 to 2 days after surgery
- Appropriate perioperative temperature management

These measures focus on process measures for the prevention of SSI and specifically on preoperative, intraoperative, and postoperative interventions. However, studies to date fail to show a consistent relationship between adherence to SCIP measures and SSI rates, which is troublesome as SCIP measure compliance is publicly reported and tied to hospital reimbursement (Cataife et al., 2014; Haynes et al., 2009; Rasouli et al., 2013; Stulberg et al., 2010; Tillman et al., 2013). Awad (2012) concluded that the SCIP guidelines are not all inclusive, may produce invalid rates or comparisons, and subsequently do not accurately guide the public in choosing where to receive their care. Despite the debate on these measures, there is continued focus on pay-for performance and pay-for value initiatives including SCIP. A program that has been validated and shown to improve care delivery through outcomes assessment and clinician feedback is the National Surgical Quality Improvement Program (NSQIP). NSQIP offers program support (including data collection and analysis) for all facility types from academic to rural facilities; the benefit of this data is that it is risk and case adjusted, based on direct medical chart information, and includes 30-day outcomes (http://site.acsnsqip.org). Multiple studies have shown that adherence to the NSQIP program has resulted in improved outcomes, decreased lengths of stay, reduced mortality (by 27%), reduced complication rates (by 45%), and cost savings (Guillamondegui et al., 2012; Hall et al., 2009; Ingraham et al., 2010; McNelis & Castaldi, 2014).

Additional guidelines and recommendations for the prevention of SSI can be found on the CDC website (http://www.cdc.gov/HAI/ssi/ssi.html), which includes resources such as the National Healthcare Safety Network (www.cdc.gov/nhsn/), the nation's most widely used health care–associated infection tracking system. Impending changes associated with the Affordable Care Act indicate that SSI and infection prevention will be a quality and safety mandate that is tied to readmission rates and that requires an interprofessional approach and a culture of infection prevention (Pyrek, 2014).

SSI prevention is as important in ambulatory surgery as in acute care settings. Owens et al. (2014) provided a retrospective analysis of outpatient surgical procedures complicated by SSI that required a postsurgical acute care visit within 14- and 30-day follow-up periods. The researchers found that the overall rate of significant infections was low in the databases queried (3.09/1,000 at 14 days, and 4.84/1,000 at 30 days); however, when one considers the number of outpatient surgeries performed each year, the numbers may be more significant than initially appreciated.

Infection Classification

Prevention and identification of SSIs is predicated on the understanding that infections occur in three distinct areas: organ space, deep tissue, and superficial tissues, and that the causative factors, preventive measures, clinical presentation, and treatment vary based on location. The criteria for specific classification of each infection as determined by the CDC may be found at the following website: http://www.cdc.gov/nhsn/pdfs/pscmanual/9pscssicurrent.pdf.

Endogenous Versus Exogenous Pathogens

The pathogens responsible for infection arise from one of two sources, endogenous or exogenous. Endogenous organisms are the patient's own flora and originate from the skin, mucous membranes, or gastrointestinal system; they typically cause infection in the area(s) where they normally reside. Occasionally, infection from a distant source can result in a secondary infection at the surgical site. When the source of the infection is not from the host itself, the source is considered exogenous. Exogenous sources include medical personnel, breaks in surgical technique, the physical environment (including ventilation), and the equipment utilized during the surgical procedure (CDC).

Risk Factors for SSI

Patient risk factors are another important consideration in the prevention and management of SSI. Patient factors that increase the risk for infection include increased age, obesity, poor nutrition, diabetes mellitus, previous surgical infection, duration of surgery, excessive blood loss, chronic obstructive pulmonary disease, connective tissue disease, steroid use, smoking, peripheral vascular disease, renal insufficiency, and noncompliance with appropriate antibiotic prophylaxis. There is increasing evidence that risk factors for infection may differ somewhat based upon the type of surgery. For example, Fowler et al. (2005) reviewed the records of >300,000 patients undergoing CABG and identified the following risk factors for infection: BMI 30 to 40 kg/m^2, diabetes mellitus, previous myocardial infarction, urgent operative status, hypertension, cardiogenic shock, dialysis dependence, perfusion time in the OR of 200 to 300 minutes, and immunosuppressive therapy. In a study involving orthopedic patients, Jain et al. (2014) found diabetes and smoking to be most predictive of SSIs. Smoking deserves special mention as a risk factor; smokers are reported to have a higher incidence of both infectious and noninfectious wound-healing complications across all surgical specialties when compared to nonsmokers. On the positive side, laparoscopic procedures are associated with a decreased SSI rate when compared with open procedures in colon and gastric surgery (Imai et al., 2008) and in gynecological surgeries for cancer. Using the NSQIP database, 6,854 laparoscopic patients were studied with 5.4% incidence of SSI; open laparotomy presented a 3.5 times higher risk of infection, and the major risk factors were identified as obesity, ascites, preoperative anemia, American Society of Anesthesiologists score of Class 3 or greater, hypoalbuminemia, preoperative weight loss, and respiratory comorbidities (Mahdi et al., 2014). Even the technique for wound closure and the materials used to approximate the tissues have been identified as having a significant impact on infection development.

Interventions

One of the most critical strategies for infection prevention is consistent and appropriate hand hygiene on the part of all health team members; despite advancing technology, no single intervention has more impact than routine hand hygiene both before and after any patient encounter.

CLINICAL PEARL

One of the most critical strategies for infection prevention is consistent and appropriate hand hygiene on the part of all health team members.

Appropriate use of topical antimicrobial agents for presurgical bathing, site preparation, and postoperative site care are also critically important in reducing SSI rate. One particular biguanide antiseptic, CHG, is widely used due to its documented ability to reduce the levels of potentially dangerous pathogens on the skin surface and thereby to reduce the incidence of HAIs. CHG's molecular design allows this cationic molecule to readily bind to organic structures, thus providing a prolonged antimicrobial benefit (Wilson et al., 2004). CHG has replaced traditional antiseptics such as povidone–iodine (PVI) and ethanol–alcohol due to studies showing superior benefit across a variety of surgical procedures (Edmiston et al., 2010; Guzel et al., 2008). In a systematic review by Lee et al. (2010a), CHG outperformed PVI in prevention of SSIs in over nine randomized controlled trials and was also more cost-effective. Darouchie and colleagues (2010) found SSI rates in PVI cases to be consistently higher than their CHG comparator, and Borer et al. (2007) found that a body wash with 4% CHG could effectively reduce the levels of the most virulent organisms such as *Acinetobacter baumannii*. The reduction in HAI associated with use of CHG was not limited to SSI but included a reduction in central line–associated bloodstream infections (CLABSI), catheter-associated urinary tract infections (CAUTI), multidrug-resistant organism (MDRO) infections, and ventilator-associated pneumonia (VAP) (Evans et al., 2010; Montecalvo et al., 2012; Timsit et al., 2009). Climo et al. (2013) conducted a large, multicentered, cluster-randomized trial comparing bathing with a 2% no-rinse CHG daily bathing cloth to bathing with the same manufacturer's non-CHG bathing cloth; they found a 23% lower rate of MDRO acquisition (p=0.003), 28% reduction in CLABSI (p=0.007), and a 53% reduction in central catheter–associated bloodstream infections.

Because of the overwhelming evidence supporting use of CHG in adults and in children over the age of 2 months, CHG has become the "product of choice" for preoperative bathing and decolonization, surgical site preparation, and daily skin cleansing (Milstone et al., 2013). While the majority of studies show minimal adverse events associated with daily use of an antiseptic such as CHG, the long-term effects of daily bathing with CHG are unknown. This is typically not a problem for the short stay acute care patient; however, long-term care and long-term acute care patients could have longer exposure times. It should be noted that while CHG is universally recommended for the reduction of SSI, it should not be used on the face or in areas where contact with mucous membranes could occur; it is not currently recommended for use in the perineal area and is not indicated for CAUTI prevention. Presently, both the Association for Practitioners in Infection Control (APIC) and CDC guidelines recommend early catheter removal, gentle meatal cleansing, stabilization of the catheter, meticulous management of the drainage system and spout, and maintenance of a closed system as critical elements in a CAUTI prevention program.

CLINICAL PEARL

CHG has become the "product of choice" for preoperative bathing and decolonization, surgical site preparation, and daily skin cleansing for adults and children over the age of 2 months.

Patients and clinicians frequently ask about the time frame for safely showering or bathing after surgery and specifically about any data regarding postoperative showering and subsequent SSI development. A Cochrane Review investigated the impact of early postoperative bathing (within the first 48 hours) and delayed bathing or showering (after 48 hours); studies involving dirty, contaminated, or open wounds were excluded. They found only one randomized controlled trial involving patients who had undergone minor skin excision procedures ($N = 857$); there was no statistically significant difference in infection rates between those patients who showered or bathed in the initial 48 hours and those who delayed showering or bathing until >48 hours post-op (Toon et al., 2013). Due to the lack of evidence, surgical patients are commonly instructed to avoid submerging their wounds in any body of water until closure is complete. Additionally, many clinicians prefer the use of occlusive surgical dressings until epithelialization is complete, due to the potential for bacterial invasion up until the point when the skin's bacterial barrier has been reestablished. However, these preferences and recommendations have not yet been validated by research.

The recommended guidelines for SSI prevention include the application of a sterile dressing over the closed incision in the operating room and maintaining this dressing until 48 hours postoperatively at which time it can be discontinued. The specific postoperative dressing is not specified, and there is currently no evidence to support use of dressings beyond 48 hours. However, as our patients become increasingly vulnerable, the focus on SSI prevention becomes more intense, and the array of dynamic and specialized antimicrobial dressings continues to expand, we need to determine whether a topically applied dressing can provide protection against SSI.

First, the wound clinician must realize that, at best, an antimicrobial dressing plays an adjunctive role in prevention and that any impact will be limited to the skin and underlying tissues, not the deep tissues or organ space. In 2008, the National Institute of Health and Clinical Excellence (NICE) released guidelines that addressed the use of dressings for SSI prevention. Over eight randomized controlled trials were presented, representing a variety of topical dressings; none of them found any statistically significant difference in the incidence of SSI related to specific dressings. However, none of the RCTs evaluated antimicrobial dressings; they compared moist wound-healing products such as films, alginates, petrolatum gauze, and transparent films to either sterile gauze dressings or leaving the wound open to air. It is reasonable to consider the use of an antimicrobial barrier dressing to prevent postoperative bacterial penetration, as similar strategies have been found to provide great success in the prevention of other HAIs; specifically, CLABSI rates have been reduced by the use of CHG-impregnated topical dressings (Timsit et al., 2009). As organ space and deep SSIs are typically related to factors such as pre-op skin preparation or intraoperative technique, dressing use may be most beneficial in supporting epithelial resurfacing and preventing postoperative contamination.

Typically, epithelialization is complete within 48 to 72 hours, which significantly reduces the risk of bacterial invasion; thus, dressings are typically discontinued at the 2nd to 3rd postoperative day. Multiple comorbidities affecting healing, incomplete epithelialization determined by visual inspection, and/or persistent drainage are indicators of increased risk for infection; from a clinical perspective, antimicrobial dressings may be warranted in these patients. Incisions located within a skin fold, such as the abdomen or groin, may also present increased risk for infection and incisional breakdown and may also benefit from use of an antimicrobial dressing. Siah and Yatim (2011) evaluated 166 patients managed either with an occlusive antimicrobial dressing or with their incisions left open to air. There were statistically significant differences found between the two groups ($p < 0.001$) in bacterial colonization at days 5 to 7 postoperatively; incisions in the control group (those left open to air) were 4.1 times more likely to be contaminated with bacteria (95% CI is 1.884, 8.964) than those managed with antimicrobial dressings. With normal healing, the benefits of antimicrobial dressings may be negligible. However, in "at-risk" patients and those with persistent drainage or delayed epithelialization, antimicrobial dressings may reduce the bioburden at the incision and may help to reduce superficial SSIs. Unfortunately, we cannot accurately predict at the time of surgery which patients will experience delayed wound healing and may benefit from an antimicrobial dressing, and routine use of these dressings is associated with some increase in the cost of care. However, given the tremendous expense and morbidity associated with SSIs, and the comparatively low cost of an antimicrobial dressing, use of these dressings would be cost-effective even if there is only a limited reduction in SSI rates. At present, given the lack of evidence, antimicrobial dressing use is likely best reserved for high-risk patients and those with evidence of delayed healing. This approach is supported by various authors and groups, who advocate the use of prophylactic antimicrobial dressings with severely immunocompromised patients, wounds located near the genitals, poorly perfused wounds, or when the patient has a virulent MDRO isolated in culture. In these cases, international consensus recommendations support the use of antimicrobials on wounds for up to 2 weeks even in the absence of any signs of infection (Cutting et al., 2009; International Consensus, 2012).

CLINICAL PEARL

We currently lack evidence regarding the effects of antimicrobial dressings; most experts recommend their use for high-risk patients and those with evidence of delayed healing.

At present, there is insufficient evidence to suggest a particular dressing for the prevention of SSI, due primarily to the need for adequately powered studies with large sample sizes (Schwartz et al., 2014). Options for antimicrobial dressings and the advantages and disadvantages of each are discussed in detail in other publications (Weir & Brindle, 2015) and in Chapter 10. As already discussed, iNPWT is one treatment modality that has been associated with a reduction in wound-healing complications, including infection (Adogwa et al., 2014; Grauhan et al., 2014).

Compartment Syndrome

The bilateral upper extremities, shoulders, and bilateral lower extremities have multiple compartments of connective tissue and muscle that encase neurovascular structures. The fascial sheaths of the upper and lower extremity compartments are tightly wrapped around these muscle systems, creating individual tissue compartments surrounded by inelastic covers. These compartments are very susceptible to changes in pressure, due either to exterior forces (such as overly tight circumferential dressings) or to interior forces (such as bleeding or edema). When pressure within the compartment rises, the vessels are compressed; the end result is ischemia leading to tissue necrosis, neurologic deficits, muscle necrosis, ischemic contractures, infection, delayed healing, and possibly amputation (Egro et al., 2014). Risk factors for compartment syndrome include fracture, vascular lesions, crush injuries, blunt trauma causing contusions, peritonitis, burns, and prolonged muscular effort. Interestingly, compartment syndrome of the gluteus muscles due to pressure injury has also been reported, typically following long surgical procedures (Osteen & Haque, 2012). While the development of compartment syndrome generally involves the lower extremities and the forearms, compartment syndrome may occasionally develop in the hands following intravenous medication administration or in the abdomen.

CLINICAL PEARL

While compartment syndrome usually involves the lower extremities and forearms, this complication occasionally develops in the abdomen.

Presentation and Diagnosis

Symptoms of compartment syndrome include disproportionate pain in relation to the trauma, pain that increases and is generally not relieved by the administration of pain medication, tight, painful presentation of the muscle compartment, and the development of sensory deficits distal to the site of injury (Uzel et al., 2013). Rarely, compartment syndrome has been reported to be atraumatic; therefore, the clinician should be alert to the development of new-onset, localized, and severe edema coupled with any other indicators for compartment syndrome (Blanchard et al., 2013). In the presence of third-degree burns or intra-abdominal hypertension, the presentation may also involve profound hemodynamic instability. In addition to physical assessment, direct measurement of compartment pressures and serologic laboratory evaluations may be indicated. Compartment pressures are frequently used in diagnosis, especially when the clinical picture is unclear; however, studies have shown that one-time compartment pressure recordings have a high false-positive rate and cannot be used as the sole diagnostic criterion (Whitney, 2012). In the case of ACS, continuous pressure measurements may be utilized in the intensive care unit and can provide trending data that help determine the need for surgical intervention. Specifically, an increase in IAP > 20 mm Hg is associated with the development of organ failure, and readings >30 mm Hg are associated with a fourfold increase in the risk of sepsis and death in burn patients (Strang et al., 2014). Laboratory analysis includes measurement of lactate, myoglobin, and uric acid levels since these correlate with the metabolically induced changes associated with increasing compartment pressures (Mitas et al., 2014). Lactate levels > 3.0 mm/L are indicative of increasing tissue hypoxia and may indicate the need for fasciotomy, and elevated uric acid levels are associated with advanced ischemic damage. Myoglobin and bilirubin levels may also be elevated but these levels are dependent upon the scope of the injury and therefore do not function as independent variables. Additionally, evaluation of blood chemistries reflecting end-organ dysfunction, such as renal failure, is used to guide management.

CLINICAL PEARL

Patients experiencing compartment syndrome often require fasciotomy, which results in large, copiously draining wounds with exposed musculature.

Treatment

Treatment for compartment syndrome varies depending on severity and may involve conservative monitoring or noninvasive testing, intravenous hypertonic mannitol, or surgical intervention; in severe cases, immediate intervention is required to reduce pressures in the affected compartment (Ross, 2001). A fasciotomy (surgical incision to divide the fascia encasing the muscle compartment) is typically performed. This procedure allows for distention of the edematous musculature and for removal of blood or accumulating fluids. The surgery typically results in a large open wound, with copious drainage; depending on location, there may also be muscle and organ exposure. Initial management typically involves the use of highly absorptive dressings and frequent assessment of the musculature; the muscle should be beefy red and should contract if tapped or flicked. If there is minimal muscular contraction, or a dusky, blue, or gray appearance, the surgeon should be notified immediately; vascular evaluation is required and an extension of the fasciotomy may be needed. Once muscle viability has been established, dressing selection should be based on the need for edema reduction and exudate control. Negative pressure wound therapy is commonly used for management of compartment syndrome. Following reduction of tissue edema and resolution of the acute event, the wounds may either be primarily closed or be allowed to granulate with subsequent application of a skin graft.

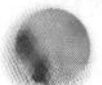

Conclusion

The management of surgical wounds requires collaboration and coordination between all members of the health care team to improve patient outcomes. Care recommended or provided by the wound care clinician ranges from simple to complex but always includes systemic measures for support of wound healing and topical therapy based on the principles of moist wound healing. Common complications of surgical wounds include infection and incisional breakdown; in addition, some complicated surgical procedures result in open abdominal or open chest wounds that present multiple challenges in management. Management of these wounds requires an interdisciplinary team and clear understanding of the surgical procedure and the structures exposed in the wound bed; frequently advanced therapies such as NPWT and biologic dressings are indicated, and standard care must be modified in order to protect exposed structures and minimize the risk of fistula formation while promoting wound healing.

REFERENCES

Adogwa, O., Fatemi, P., Perez, E., et al. (2014). Negative pressure wound therapy reduces incidence of post-operative wound infection and dehiscence after long-segment thoracolumbar spinal fusion: A single institutional experience. *Spine Journal.* doi: 10.1016/j.spinee.2014.04.011.

Anderson, D. J., et al. (2008). Strategies to prevent surgical site infections in acute care hospitals. *Infection Control and Hospital Epidemiology, 29*, s51–s61.

Anesäter, E., Borgquist, O., Hedstrom, E., et al. (2011). The influence of different sizes and types of wound fillers on wound contraction and tissue pressure during negative pressure wound therapy. *International Wound Journal, 8*(4), 336–342.

Argenta, L. C., Morykwas, M. J. (1997). Vacuum-assisted closure: A new method for wound control and treatment: Clinical experiences. *Annals of Plastic Surgery, 38*, 563–577.

Awad, S. S. (2012). Adherence to surgical care improvement project measures and post-operative surgical site infections. *Surgical Infections, 13*(4), 234–237.

Bates-Jensen, B., & Williams, J. (2012). Management of acute surgical wounds. In C Sussman. & B Bates-Jensen. (Eds.), *Wound care: A collaborative practice manual for health professionals* (4th ed., pp. 215–229). Baltimore, MD: Lippincott Williams & Wilkins.

Bates, O. L., O'Connor N., Dunn, D., et al. (2014). Applying STAAR interventions in incremental bundles: Improving post-CABG surgical patient care. *Worldviews on Evidence-Based Nursing, 11*(2), 89–97.

Berríos-Torres, S. I. (2009). Surgical site infection (SSI) toolkit: Activity C: ELC prevention collaboratives. Retrieved from http://www.cdc.gov/HAI/pdfs/toolkits/SSI_toolkit021710SIBT_revised.pdf

Biscione, F. M. (2009). Rates of surgical site infection as a performance measure: Are we ready? *World Journal of Gastrointestinal Surgery, 1*(1), 11–15.

Björck, M., & Wanhainen, A. (2014). Management of abdominal compartment syndrome and the open abdomen. *European Journal of Vascular and Endovascular Surgery*,47(3), 279–287.

Blanchard, S., Griffin, G. D., Simon, E. L. (2013). Atraumatic painless compartment syndrome. *American Journal of Emergency Medicine, 31*, 1723.e3-4. Available from http://dx.doi.org/10.1016/j.ajem/2013.08.008.

Boeken, U., Assmann, A., Mehdiani, A., et al. (2011a). Open chest management after cardiac operations: Outcome and timing of delayed sternal closure. *European Journal of Cardio-thoracic Surgery, 40*, 1146–1150.

Boeken, U., Feindt, P., Schurr, P., et al. (2011b). Delayed sternal closure (DSC) after cardiac surgery: Outcome and prognostic markers. *Journal of Cardiac Surgery, 26*, 22–27.

Bonds, A. M., Novick, T. K., Dietert, J. B., et al. (2013). Incisional negative pressure wound therapy significantly reduces surgical site infection in open colorectal surgery. *Diseases of the Colon and Rectum, 56*(12), 1403–1408.

Borer, A., Gilad, J., Porat, N., et al. (2007). Impact of 4% chlorhexidine whole-body washing on multidrug-resistant *Acinetobacter baumannii* skin oclonisation among patients in a medical intensive care unit. *Journal of Hospital Infection, 67*, 149–155.

Borquist, O., Anesäter, E., Hedström, E., et al. (2011). Measurements of wound edge microvascular blood flow during negative pressure wound therapy using thermodiffusion and transcutaneous and invasive laser Doppler velocimetry. *Wound Repair and Regeneration, 19*, 727–733.

Bratzler, D. W., & Hunt D. R. (2006). The surgical infection prevention and surgical care improvement projects: National initiatives to improve outcomes for patients having surgery. *Clinical Infectious Diseases, 43*(3), 322.

Brem, M. H., Bail, H. J., Biber, R. (2014). Value of incisional negative pressure wound therapy in orthopedic surgery. *International Wound Journal, 11*(Suppl 1), 3–5.

Brindle, C. T. (2012). Enterocutaneous fistulas: Current concepts in management. In A. Losken & J. E. Janis (Eds.), *Advances in abdominal wall reconstruction*. St. Louis, MO: Quality Medical Publishing.

Brindle, C. T., & Blankenship, J. (2009). Management of complex abdominal wounds with small bowel fistulae: Isolation techniques and exudate control to improve outcomes. *Journal of Wound Ostomy and Continence Nursing, 36*(4), 396–403.

Brindle, C. T., & Whelan, J. (2011, June). Novel solutions for the management of enterocutaneous and enteroatmospheric fistulas to allow for skin grafting. Podium Presentation at Annual Abdominal Wall Reconstruction Conference, Washington DC.

Burger, J., Luijendijk, R., Hop, W., et al. (2004). Long-term follow-up of a randomized controlled trial of suture versus mesh repair of incisional hernia. *Annals of Surgery, 240*(4), 578–583.

Burlew, C., Moore, E., Cuschier, J., et al. (2011). Sew it up: A Western Trauma Association multi-institutional study of enteric injury management in the post-injury open abdomen. *Journal of Trauma—Injury Infection and Critical Care, 70*(2), 273–277.

Cataife, G., Weinberg, D. A., Wong, H. H., et al. (2014). The effect of Surgical Care Improvement Project (SCIP) compliance on surgical site infections (SSI). *Medical Care, 52*(2 Suppl), 266–273.

Centers for Disease Control and Prevention (CDC). (2014). FastStats, Inpatient surgery. Retrieved from http://www.cdc.gov/nchs/fastats/inpatient-surgery.htm

Centers for Disease Control and Prevention. (2009). U.S. outpatient surgeries on the rise. Retrieved from http://www.cdc.gov/nchs/pressroom/09newsreleases/outpatientsurgeries.htm

Chang, E., Festekjian, J. H., Ardehali, A., et al. (2013). Chest wall reconstruction for sternal dehiscence after open heart surgery. *Annals of Plastic Surgery, 71*(1), 84–87.

Chen, S. Z., Li, J., Li, X. Y., et al. (2005). Effects of vacuum assisted closure on wound microcirculation: An experimental study. *Asian Journal of Surgery, 28*(3), 211–217.

Chin, G., Schultz, G. Diegelmann, R., et al. (2007). Biochemistry of wound healing in wound care practice. In P Sheffield. & C Fife. (Eds.), *Wound care practice* (2nd ed. (pp. 53–78). Flagstaff, AZ: Best Publishing Company.

Climo, M. W., Yokoe, D. S., Warren, D. K., et al. (2013). Effect of daily chlorhexadine bathing on hospital-acquired infection. *New England Journal of Medicine, 368*, 533–542.

Cohen, D. J., Griffin, L. V. (2002). A biomechanical comparison of three sternotomy closure techniques. *Annals of Thoracic Surgery, 73*, 563–568.

Colli, A. (2011). First experience with a new negative pressure incision management system on surgical incisions after cardiac surgery in high risk patients. *Journal of Cardiothoracic Surgery, 6*, 160. Retrieved from http://www.cardiothroacicsurgery.org/content/6/1/160

Colwell, J., Ratliff, C., Goldberg, M., et al. (2011). Moisture associated skin damage. Part 3: Peristomal MASD and periwound MASD: A consensus. *Journal of Wound Ostomy and Continence Nursing, 38*(5), 541–555.

Condé-Green, A., Chung, T. L., Holton, L. H., et al. (2013). Incisional negative-pressure wound therapy versus conventional dressings following abdominal wall reconstruction: a comparative study. *Annals of Plastic Surgery, 71*(4), 394–397.

Cooper, D. (1990). The physiology of wound healing. In D Krasner. (Ed.), *Chronic wound care: A clinical source book for healthcare professionals* (pp. 1–10). King of Prussia, PA: Health Management Publications.

Criss, C. N., Petro, C. C., Krpata, D. M., et al. (2014). Functional abdominal wall reconstruction improves core physiology and quality of life. *Surgery, 156*(1), 176–182.

Culbertson, E., Xing, L., Wren, Y., et al. (2011). Loss of mechanical strain impairs abdominal wall fibroblast proliferation, orientation, and collagen contraction and function. *Surgery, 150*(3), 410–417.

Cutting, K., White, R., Hoekstra, H. (2009). Topical silver-impregnated dressings and the importance of the dressing technology. *International Wound Journal, 6*, 396–402.

Darouiche, R. O., Wall, M. J., Itani, K. M. F., et al. (2010). Chlorhexidine-alcohol versus povidone-iodine for surgical-site antisepsis. *New England Journal of Medicine, 362*, 18–26.

Dealey, C. (2005). General principles of wound management. In *The care of wounds* (3rd ed). Oxford, UK: Blackwell Science.

Demetriades, D., & Salim, A. (2014). Management of the open abdomen. *Surgical Clinics of North America, 94*(1), 131–153.

Diaz, J., Conquest, A., Ferzoco, S., et al. (2009). Multi-institutional experience using human acellular dermal matrix for ventral hernia repair in a compromised surgical field. *Archives of Surgery, 144*(3), 209–215.

Doughty, D., & Sparks-DeFriese, B. (2007). Wound Healing Physiology. In R. Bryant & D. Nix. (Eds.), *Acute and chronic wounds current management concepts* (3rd ed., pp. 434–445). St. Louis, MI: Elsevier Mosby.

Dyke, C., Aronson, S., Dietrich, W., et al. (2014). Universal definition of perioperative bleeding in adult cardiac surgery. *Journal of Thoracic and Cardiovascular Surgery, 147*(5), 1458–1463.

Edmiston, C. E., Okoli, O., Graham, M. B., et al. (2010). Evidence for using chlorhexidine gluconate preoperative cleansing to reduce the risk of surgical site infection. *AORN Journal, 92*(5), 509–518.

Erek, E., Yalcinbas, Y. K., Turkekul, Y., et al. (2012). Indications and risks of delayed sternal closure after open heart surgery in neonates and early infants. *World Journal of Pediatric and Congenital Heart Surgery, 3*(2), 229–235.

Egro, F. M., Jaring, M. R., Khan, A. F. (2014). Compartment syndrome of the hand: Beware of innocuous radius fractures. *Eplasty, 14*, 46–51.

Estrera, A. L., Porat, E. E., Miller, C. C., III, et al. (2008). Outcomes of delayed sternal closure after complex aortic surgery. *European Journal of Cardio-Thoracic Surgery, 33*, 1039–1042.

Evans, H. L., Dellit, T. H., Chan, J., et al. (2010). Effect of chlorhexidine whole-body bathing on hospital-acquired infections among trauma patients. *Archives of Surgery, 145*(3), 240–246.

Flament, J. B. (2006). Functional anatomy of the abdominal wall. *Surgery, 77*, 401–407. doi: 10.1007/S00104-006-1184-5.

Fowler, V. G., O'Brien, S. M., Muhlbaier, L. H., Corey G. R., et al. (2005). Clinical predictors of major infections after cardiac surgery. *Circulation, 112*(Suppl 1), I-358-I-365.

Franz, M., Berndt, A., Grun, K., et al. (2011). Expression of extra domain A-containing fibronectin in chronic cardiac allograft rejection. *Journal of Heart and Lung Transplant, 30*(1), 86–94.

Franz, M., Robson, M., Steed, D., et al. (2008). Guidelines to aid healing of acute wounds by decreasing impediments of healing. *Wound Repair and Regeneration, 16*, 723–748.

Ger, R. (2009). The clinical anatomy of the anterolateral abdominal wall musculature. *Clinical Anatomy, 22*(3), 392–397.

Goldman, R. (2004). Growth factors and chronic wound healing: past, present and future. *Advances in Skin and Wound Care, 17*(1), 24–35.

Grauhan, O., Arashes, N., Tutku, B., et al. (2014). Effect of surgical incision management on wound infection in a post sternotomy patient population. *International Wound Journal* (Suppl 1), 6–9.

Grauhan, O., Navasardyan, A., Hofmann, M., et al. (2012). Prevention of poststernotomy wound infections in obese patients by negative pressure wound therapy. *Journal of Thoracic and Cardiovascular Surgery, 145*(5), 1387–1392.

Greer, D., Smith, J., & McCorvey, D. (2007). Principles of surgical wound management. In P Sheffield. & C Fife (Eds.), *Wound Care Practice* (2nd ed. pp. 251–275). Flagstaff, AZ: Best Publishing Company.

Guillamondegui, O. D., Gunter O. L., Hines, L., et al. (2012). Using the national surgical quality improvement program and the Tennessee surgical quality collaborative to improve surgical outcomes. *Journal of the American College of Surgery, 214*(4), 709–714.

Gustafsson, R. I., Sjögren, J., Ingemansson, R. (2003). Deep sternal wound infection: A sternal-sparing technique with vacuum-assisted closure therapy. *Annals of Thoracic Surgery, 76*, 2048–2053.

Guzel, A., Ozekinci, T., Ozkan, U., et al. (2008). Evaluation of the skin flora after chlorhexidine and povidone-iodine preparation in neurosurgical practice. *Surgical Neurology*. Retrieved from www.sciencedirect.com. doi: 10.1016/j.surneu.2007.10.026.

Hall, B. L., Hamilton B. H., Richards, K., et al. (2009). Does surgical quality improve in the American College of Surgeons National Surgical Quality Improvement Program: An evaluation of all participating hospitals. *Annals of Surgery, 250*(3), 363–376.

Hansen, E., Durinka, J. B., Cosanzo, J. A., et al. (2013). Negative pressure wound therapy is associated with resolution of incisional drainage in most wounds after hip arthroplasty. *Clinical Orthopaedics and Related Research, 47*(1), 3230–3236.

Hashemzadeh, K., Hashemzadeh, S. (2009). In hospital outcomes of delayed sternal closure after open cardiac surgery. *Journal of Cardiac Surgery, 24*, 30–33.

Haynes, A. B., et al. (2009). A surgical safety checklist to reduce morbidity and mortality in a global population. *New England Journal of Medicine, 360*, 491–499.

Imai, E., Ueda, M., Kanao, K., et al. (2008). Surgical site infection risk factors identified by multivariate analysis for patient undergoing laparoscopic, open colon, and gastric surgery. *American Journal of Infection Control, 36*, 727–731.

Ingargiola, M. J., Daniali, L. N., Lee, E. S. (2013). Does the application of incisional negative pressure therapy to high-risk wounds prevent surgical site complications? A systematic review. *Eplasty, 20*(13), e49.

Ingraham, A. M., Richards, K. E., Hall, B. L., et al. (2010). Quality improvement in surgery: The American College of Surgeons national Surgical Quality Improvement Program approach. *Advances in Surgery, 244*, 251–267.

International Consensus. 2012. *Appropriate use of silver dressings in wounds. An expert working group consensus*. London, UK: Wounds International. Available from www.woundsinternational.com.

Jain, R. K, Shukla, R., Singh, P., et al. (2014). Epidemiology and risk factors for surgical site infections in patients requiring orthopedic surgery. *European Journal of Orthopaedic Surgery and Traumatology*. doi: 10.1007/s00590-014-1475-3.

Kadohama, J., Akasaka, N., Nagamine, A., et al. (2008). Vacuum-assisted closure for pediatric post-sternotomy mediastinitis: Are low negative pressures sufficient? *American Journal of Thoracic Surgery, 85*(3), 1094–1096.

Kaplan, M., Barnwell, P., Orgill, D., et al. (2005). Guidelines for the management of the open abdomen: Recommendations from a multidisciplinary expert advisory panel. *Wounds, 17*(Suppl), S1–S24.

Karlakki, S., Brem, M., Giannini, S., et al. (2013). Negative pressure wound therapy for management of the surgical incision in orthopaedic surgery: A review of evidence and mechanisms for an emerging indication. *Bone and Joint Research, 2*, 276–284.

Khirurgii, V. (1986–1991). The Kremlin papers: A collection of published studies complementing the research and innovation of wound care.

Korenkov, M., Sauerland, S., Arndt, M., et al. (2002). Randomized clinical trial of suture repair, polypropylene mesh or autodermal hernioplasty for incisional hernia. *British Journal of Surgery, 89*(1), 50–56.

Kostiuchenok, II, Kolker V. A., Karlov, V. A. 1986. The vacuum effect in the surgical treatment of purulent wounds. *Vestnik Khirurgii, 9*, 18–21.

Lang, J. L., Gonzalez, R. P., Aldy, K. N., et al. (2011). Does temporary chest wall closure improve survival for trauma patients in shock after emergent thoracotomy? *Journal of Trauma, 70*(3), 705–709.

Leaper, D. (2008). NICE guideline prevention of surgical site infection. Retrieved from http://guidance.nice.org.uk/CGT74/Guidance/pdf/English

Lee, C., & Hansen, S. (2009). Management of acute wounds. *Surgical Clinics of North America, 89*, 659–676. doi: 10.1016/j.suc.2009.03.005.

Lee, I., Agarwal, R. K., Lee, B. Y., et al. (2010a). Systemic review and cost analysis comparing use of chlorhexidine with use of iodine for preoperative skin antisepsis to prevent surgical site infection. *Infection Control and Hospital Epidemiology, 31*(12), 1219–1229.

Lee, K. N., Seo, D. M., Hong, J. P. (2010b). The effect and safety after extended use of continuous negative pressure of 75 mm Hg over mesh and allodermis graft on open sternal wound from oversized heart transplant in a 3-month-old infant. *International Wound Journal, 7*, 379–384.

Lindstedt, S., Paulsson, P., Mokhtari, A., et al. (2008a). A compare between myocardial topical negative pressure levels of −25 mm Hg and −50 mm Hg in a porcine model. *BMC Cardiovascular Disorders, 8*, 14.

Lindstedt, S., Malmsjo, M., Ingemansson, R. (2007a). Blood flow changes in normal and ischemic myocardium during topically applied negative pressure. *Annals of Thoracic Surgery, 84*, 568–573.

Lindstedt, S., Malmsjo, M., Ingemansson, R. (2007b). No hypoperfusion is produced in the epicardium during application of myocardial topical negative pressure in a porcine model. *Journal of Cardiothoracic Surgery, 2*, 53. Available from http://www.cardiothoracicsurgery.org/content /2/1/53

Lindstedt, S., Malmsjo, M., Ingemansson, R. (2008b). Evaluation of continuous and intermittent myocardial topical negative pressure. *Journal of Cardiovascular Medicine, 9*(8), 813–819.

Lindstedt, S., Malmsjo, M., Sjogren, J., et al. (2008c). Impact of different topical negative pressure levels on myocardial microvascular blood flow. *Cardiovascular Revascularization Medicine, 9*, 29–35.

Lindstedt, S., Malmsjo, M., Gesslein, B., et al. (2008d). Topical negative pressure effects on coronary blood flow in a sternal wound model. *International Wound Journal, 5*(4), 503–509.

Luijendijk, R., Hop, W., van den Tol, M., et al. (2000). A comparison of suture repair with mesh repair for incisional hernia. *New England Journal of Medicine, 343*(6), 392–398.

Lunardi, A., Miranda, C., Silva, K., et al. (2012). Weakness of expiratory muscles and pulmonary complications in malnourished patients undergoing upper abdominal surgery. *Respirology, 17*(1), 108–113.

Mahdi, H., Gojayev, A., Buechel, M., et al. (2014). Surgical site infection in women undergoing surgery for gynecologic cancer. *International Journal of Gynecological Cancer, 24*(4), 779–786.

Malmsjö, M., Huddleston, E., Martin, R. (2014). Biological effects of a disposable, canisterless negative pressure wound therapy system. *Eplasty, 2*(14), e15.

Mangram, A. (1999). Guideline for prevention of surgical site infection. *Infection Control and Hospital Epidemiology, 20*, 97–134. doi: 10.1016/S0196-6553(99)70088-X.

Mark, K. S., Alger, L., Terplan, M. (2013). Incisional negative pressure therapy to prevent wound complications following caesarian section in morbidly obese women. A pilot study. *Surgical Innovation, 21*, 345–349. doi: 10.1177/1553350613503736.

McNelis, J., Castaldi, M. (2014). The National Surgery Quality Improvement Project (NSQIP): A new tool to increase patient safety and cost efficiency in a surgical intensive care unit. *Patient Safety in Surgery, 8*(19). doi: 10.1186/1754-9493-8-19.

McNichol, L., Lund, C., Rosen, T., et al. (2013). Medical adhesives and patient safety: State of the science, consensus statements for the assessment, prevention, and treatment of adhesive related skin injuries. *Journal of Wound Ostomy and Continence Nursing, 40*(4), 365–380.

Menez, J. (2009). Perioperative nursing care. In H Craven. (Ed), *Core curriculum for medical-surgical nursing* (4th ed. pp. 157–171). Pittman, NJ: Anthony Jannetti, Inc.

Milstone, M., Elward, A., Song, X., et al. (2013). Daily chlorhexidine bathing to reduce bacteraemia in critically ill children: A multicenter, cluster-randomised crossover trial. *Lancet, 381*(9872), 1099–1106.

Mitas, P., Verjrazka, M., Hruby, J., et al. (2014). Prediction of compartment syndrome based on analysis of biochemical parameters. *Annals of Vascular Surgery, 28*, 170–177.

Montecalvo, M. A., McKenna, D., Yarrish, R., et al. (2012). Chlorhexidine bathing to reduce central venous catheter-associated bloodstream infection: Impact and sustainability. *American Journal of Medicine, 125*(5), 505–511.

Morykwas, M. J., Argenta, L. C., Shelton-Brown, E. I., et al. (1997). Vacuum-assisted closure: A new method for wound control and treatment animal studies and basic foundation. *Annals of Plastic Surgery, 38*, 553–562.

National Institute for Health and Care Excellence (2008). Surgical site infection: Prevention and treatment of surgical site infection. Retrieved from http://www.nice.org.uk/guidance/cg74/chapter/1-Guidance

Nazerali, R. S., Hinchcliff, K., Wong, M. S. (2014). Rigid fixation for the prevention and treatment of sternal complications. *Annals of Plastic Surgery, 72*, Suppl 1, 227–230.

Nutescu, E. A., Bathija, S., Sharp, L. K., et al. 2011. Anticoagulation patient self-monitoring in the United States. *Pharmacotherapy, 31*(12), 1161–1174.

Oeltjen, J. C., Panos, A. L., Salerno, T. A., et al. (2009). Complete vacuum-assisted sternal closure following neonatal cardiac surgery. *Journal of Cardiac Surgery, 24*, 748–750.

Ogden, C., Carroll, M., Flegal, K. (2014). Prevalence of childhood and adult obesity in the US. *Journal of American Medical Association, 311*(8), 806–814.

Olbrecht, V. A., Barreiro, C. J., Bonde, P. N., et al. (2006). Clinical outcomes of noninfectious sternal dehiscence after median sternotomy. *Annals of Thoracic Surgery, 82*, 902–908.

Orsted, H., Keast, D., Kuhnke, J. et al. (2010). Best practice recommendations for the prevention and management of open surgical wounds. *Wound Care Canada, 8*(1), 6–34.

Osteen, K. D., Haque, S. H. (2012). Bilateral gluteal compartment syndrome following right total knee revision: A case report. *Ochsner Journal, 12*, 141–144.

Owens, P. L., Barrett, M. L., Raetzman, S., et al. (2014). Surgical site infections following ambulatory surgery procedures. *JAMA, 311*(7), 709–716.

Ozker, E., Saritas, B., Vuran, C., et al. (2012). Delayed sternal closure after pediatirc cardiac operations; single center experience: A retrospective study. *Journal of Cardiothoracic Surgery, 7*, 102.

Pachowsky, M., Gusinde, J., Klein, A., et al. (2011). Negative pressure wound therapy to prevent and treat surgical incisions after total hip arthroplasty. *International Orthopaedics, 36*, 719–722.

Pauli, E. M., Krpata, D. M., Novitsky, Y. W., et al. (2013). Negative pressure therapy for high-risk abdominal wall reconstruction incisions. *Surgical Infections, 14*(3), 270–274.

Phillips, S. (2000). Physiology of wound healing and surgical wound care. *ASAIO Journal, 46*, S2–S5.

Pittman, J., Tape, J., Pelliccia, J., et al. (2005). Comparative study of the use of antimicrobial barrier film dressing in post-operative incision care. *Journal of Wound, Ostomy, and Continence Nursing, 32*(25), S25.

Plaudis, H., Rudzats, A., Melberga, L., et al. (2012). Abdominal negative pressure therapy: A new method in countering abdominal compartment syndrome and peritonitis—Prospective study and critical review of the literature. *Annals of Intensive Care, 2*(Suppl 1), S23. Retrieved from http://www.annalsofintensivecare.com/content/2/S1/S23

Pye, S., McDonnell, M. (2010). Nursing considerations for children undergoing delayed sternal closure after surgery for congenital heart disease. *Critical Care Nurse, 30*, 50–61.

Pyrek, K. (2014). *Policy update: Infection prevention is part of the mandate for quality and safety*. Infection Control Today. Retrieved from http://www.infectioncontroltoday.com/articles/2014/01/2014-policy-update-infection-prevention-is-part-of-the-mandate-for-quality-and-safety.aspx

Rajakaruna, C., & Marchbank, A. (2011). Gauze-based negative pressure wound therapy to infected deep sternotomy wound complicated by cardiac tamponade: A case report. *International Wound Journal, 8*, 96–98.

Rasouli, M. R., Jaberi, M. M., Hozack, W. J., et al. (2013). Surgical Care Improvement Project (SCIP): Has its mission succeeded? *Journal of Arthroplasty, 28*, 1072–1075.

Rausei, S., Dionigi, G., Boni, L., et al. (2014). Open abdomen management of intra-abdominal infections: Analysis of a twenty-year experience. *Surgical Infections, 15*(3), 200–206.

Reddix, R. N., Jr, Leng, X. I., Woodall, J., et al. (2010).The effect of incisional negative pressure therapy on wound complications after acetabular fracture surgery. *Journal of Surgical Orthopaedic Advances, 19*(2), 91–97.

Riahi, M., Tomatis, L. A., Schlosser, R. J., et al. (1975). Cardiac compression due to closure of the median sternotomy in open heart surgery. *Chest, 67*, 113–114.

Rosen, M., Fatima, J., Sair, M. (2010). Repair of abdominal wall hernias with restoration of abdominal wall function. *Journal of Gastrointestinal Surgery, 14*(1), 175–185.

Rosenberger, L. H. H, Politano, A. D., Sawyer, R. G. (2011). The surgical care improvement project and prevention of poster-operative infection, including surgical site infection. *Surgical Infections, 12*(3), 163.

Ross, D. (2001). Compartment syndrome. In P. L. Swearingen & J. H. Keen. *Manual of critical care nursing* (4th ed). St. Louis, MO: Mosby.

Santini, F., Onorati, F., Telesca, M., et al. (2012). Preliminary experience with a new device for delayed sternal closure strategy in cardiac surgery. *International Journal of Artificial Organs, 35*(6), 471–476.

Satterwhite, T., Miri, S., Chung, C., et al. (2012). Outcomes of complex abdominal herniorrhaphy: Experience with 106 cases. *Annals of Plastic Surgery, 68*(4), 35–38.

Sauderland, S., Walgenbach, M., Habermalz, B., et al. (2011). Laparoscopic vs open surgical techniques for ventral hernia repair. *Cochrane Database Systematic Reviews*, (3), CD00778.

Schwartz, J., Goss, S., Facchin, F., et al. (2014). A prospective two-armed trial assessing the efficacy and performance of silver dressing used postoperatively on high-risk, clean surgical wounds. *Ostomy/Wound Management, 60*(4), 30–40.

Shinohara, T., et al. (2008). Prospective evaluation of occlusive hydrocolloid dressing versus conventional gauze dressing regarding the healing effect after abdominal operations: randomized controlled trial. *Asian Journal of Surgery, 31*(1), 1–5.

Siah, C. J., Yatim, J. (2011). Efficacy of total occlusive ionic silver-containing dressing combination in decreasing risk of surgical site infections: an RCT. *Journal of Wound Care, 20*(12), 561–568.

Spain, K. (2004). Use of deep hypothermic circulatory arrest following ventricular laceration: A case report. *AANA Journal, 72*(3), 193–195.

Stannard, J., Gabriel, A., Lehner, B. (2012a). Use of negative pressure wound therapy over clean closed surgical incisions. *International Wound Journal, 9*(Suppl 1), 32–39.

Stannard, J. P., Robinson, J. T., Anderson, E. R., et al. (2006). Negative pressure wound therapy to treat hematomas and surgical incisions following high-energy trauma. *Journal of Trauma, 60*, 1301–1306.

Stannard, J. P., Volgas, D. A., McGwin, G, 3rd., et al. (2012b). Incisional negative pressure wound therapy after high-risk lower extremity fractures. *Journal of Orthopaedic Trauma, 26*(1), 37–42.

Strang, S. G., Van Lieshout, E. M., Breederveld, R. S., et al. (2014). A systematic review on intra-abdominal pressure in severely burned patients. *Burns, 40*, 9–16.

Sussman, C., & Bates-Jensen, B. (2012). Skin and soft tissue anatomy and wound healing physiology. In C Sussman. & B Bates-Jensen. (Eds.), *Wound care: A collaborative practice manual for health professionals* (pp. 17–52). Baltimore, MD: Lippincott Williams & Wilkins.

Takayama, H., Leone, R. J., Aldea, G. S., et al. (2006). Open chest management after heart transplantation. *Texas Heart Institute Journal, 33*, 306–309.

Tekumit, H., Cenal, A. R., Tataroglu, C., et al. (2009). Comparison of figure-of-eight and simple wire sternal closure techniques in patients with non-microbial sternal dehiscence. *Anadolu Kardiyoloji Dergisi, 9*, 411–416.

Tillman, M., Wehbe-Janek, H., Hodges, B., et al. (2013). Surgical care improvement project and surgical site infections: Can integration in the surgical safety checklist improve quality performance and clinical outcomes? *Journal of Surgical Research, 184*, 150–156.

Timmermans, L., Deerenberg, E., Lamme, B., et al. (2014). Parastomal hernia is an independent risk factor for incisional hernia in patients with an end colostomy. *Surgery, 155*(1), 178–183.

Timsit, J. F., Schwebel, C., Bouadma, L., et al. (2009). Chlorhexidine-impregnated sponges and less frequent dressing changes for prevention of catheter-related infection in critically ill adults: A randomised controlled trial. *JAMA, 301*(12), 1231–1241.

Toon, C. D., Sinha, S., Davidson, B. R., et al. (2013). Early versus delayed post-operative bathing or showering to prevent wound complications. *Cochrane Database of Systematic Reviews*. doi: 10.1002/1465/1858.CD010075.pub2.

Torbrand, C., Ingemansson, R., Gustafsson, L., et al. (2008). Pressure transduction to the thoracic cavity during topical negative pressure therapy of a sternotomy wound. *International Wound Journal, 5*, 579–584.

Ubbink, D., Vermeulen, H., Goossens, A., et al. (2008). Occlusive versus gauze dressings for local wound car in surgical patients: A randomized clinical trial, *Archives of Surgery, 143*(10), 950–955.

United States Department of Health and Human Services. (2013). National action plan to prevent health care-associated infections: Road map to elimination. Available from http://www.health.gov/hai/pdfs/hai-action-plan-acute-care-hospitals.PDF

United States Food and Drug Administration. (2007). Safety communication: Negative pressure wound therapy. Available from: http://www.fda.gov/MedicalDevices/Safety/AlertsandNotices/ucm244211.htm

Uzel, A. P., Bulla, A., Henri, S. (2013). Compartment syndrome of the thigh after blunt trauma: A complication not to be ignored. *Musculoskeletal Surgery, 97*, 81–83.

Vogt, D. et al. (2007). Moist wound healing compared with standard care of treatment of primary closed vascular surgical wound: A prospective randomized controlled study. *Wound Repair and Regeneration, 15*, 624.

Vojtovic, P., Reich, O., Selko, M., et al. (2009). Haemodynamic changes due to delayed sternal closure in newborns after surgery for congenital cardiac malformations. *Cardiology in the Young, 19*, 573–579.

Wackenfors, A., Sjögren, J., Gustafsson, R., et al. (2004). Effects of vacuum-assisted closure therapy on inguinal wound edge microvascular blood flow. *Wound Repair and Regeneration, 12*, 600–606.

Weber, G., Baracs, J., Horvath, O. (2010). "Onlay" mesh provides significantly better results than "sublay" reconstruction: Prospective randomized multicenter study of abdominal wall reconstruction with sutures only, or with surgical mesh: Results of 5-year followup. *Magyar Sebeszet, 63*(5), 302–311.

Webster, J., Scuffham, P., Sherriff K. L., et al. (2012). Negative pressure wound therapy for skin grafts and surgical wounds healing by primary intention. *Cochrane Database of Systematic Reviews, 4*, CD009261.

Wechter, M., Pearlman, M, & Hartmann, K. (2005). Reclosure of the disrupted laparotomy wound: A systematic review. *Obstetrics & Gynecology, 106*(2), 376–383. doi: 10.1097/01.AOG.000017114.75338.06.

Weigand, C., White, R. (2013). Microdeformation in wound healing. *Wound Repair Regeneration, 21*, 793–799.

Weir, D., & Brindle, C. T. (2015). Wound dressings. In R. Hamm (Ed.), *Text and atlas of wound diagnosis and treatment*. New York, NY: McGraw-Hill.

Whitney, J. (2012). Surgical wounds and incision care. In R Bryant. & D Nix. (Eds.), *Acute and chronic wounds current management concepts* (4th ed pp. 469–471). St. Louis, MI: Elsevier Mosby.

Widgerow, A. (2013). Surgical wounds. In M Flanagan. (Ed), *Wound healing and skin integrity: Principles and practice* (pp. 224–241). West Sussex, UK: Wiley-Blackwell.

Wilkes, R. P., Kilpadi, D. V., Zhao, Y., et al. (2012). Closed Incision Management with Negative Pressure Therapy (CIM): Biomechanics. *Surgical Innovation, 19*(1), 67–75.

Wilson, C. M., Gray, G., Read, J. S., et al. (2004). Tolerance and safety of different concentrations of chlorhexidine for peripartum vaginal and Infant washes: HIVNET025. *Journal of Acquired Immune Deficiency Syndromes, 35*(2), 138–143.

Woodward, C. S., Son, M., Calhoon, J., et al. (2011). Sternal wound infection sin pediatric congenital cardiac surgery: A survey of incidence and preventative practice. *Annals of Thoracic Surgery, 91*, 799–804.

Yasa, H., Lafci, B. B., Yilik, L., Bademci, M., et al. (2010). Delayed sternal closure: An effective procedure for life-saving in open-heart surgery. *Anadolu Kardiyoloji Dergisi, 10*, 163–167.

Yokoe, D. S., Mermel, L. A., Anderson, D. J., et al. (2008). A compendium of strategies to prevent healthcare-associated infections in acute care hospitals. *Infection Control and Hospital Epidemiology, 29*, S12–S21.

QUESTIONS

1. A surgical wound that is beginning to develop granulation is in what phase of wound healing?
   A. Hemostasis
   B. Inflammatory
   C. Proliferative
   D. Remodeling

2. The wound care nurse is assessing an open surgical abdominal wound; the surgical record indicates that there was nonpurulent inflammation related to gross spillage from the GI tract. This wound would fall into which of the following classifications?
   A. Class I
   B. Class II
   C. Class III
   D. Class IV

3. Which type of wound would be most likely to heal by primary intention?
   A. A perforated appendix
   B. A clean stab wound
   C. A GI perforation
   D. Compartment syndrome

4. Upon assessment of a patient's surgical wound on day 2 post-op, the wound care nurse documents the following: "Incision is well approximated, partial epithelialization; no drainage. Periwound skin slightly warm and edematous; tender to touch. No induration and no significant erythema." Which of the following represents the most accurate assessment?
   A. All findings normal for this phase of healing (inflammation, which lasts 1 to 4 days postoperatively).
   B. There is evidence of delayed healing and developing wound infection.
   C. There is a failure of granulation tissue formation, which normally begins immediately postinjury and can be palpated as a healing ridge.
   D. The wound lacks tensile strength and is at high risk for dehiscence.

5. Which of the following is a known benefit of incisional negative pressure wound therapy (iNPWT)?
   A. Endothelial cell deactivation
   B. Increase in levels of proinflammatory cytokines
   C. Increase in lateral tension
   D. Stimulation of angiogenesis and collagen synthesis

6. Which factor is a key consideration in the selection of traditional versus disposable iNPWT systems?
   A. Cost
   B. Exudate
   C. Patient preference
   D. Granulation tissue

7. The wound care nurse would advise a patient with which type of abdominal wall closure (AWC) that surgery 3 to 6 months in the future may be needed for definitive abdominal wall reconstruction?
   A. A patient with primary closure of all tissue/skin layers
   B. A patient with primary fascial and skin closure with the use of mesh
   C. A patient with delayed primary fascial closure
   D. A patient with open abdominal wound with exposed abdominal organs

8. What is the most common cause of fistula formation in wounds?
   A. Anastomotic leak
   B. Debridement of the wound
   C. Infection
   D. Trauma

9. Which management strategy would the wound care nurse recommend for a patient with a chronic open abdominal wound?
   A. NPWT used on a high-pressure setting
   B. Autolytic atraumatic wound care methods
   C. Sharp debridement of necrotic tissue
   D. Strict avoidance of wound or fistula pouches

10. The wound care nurse is caring for a patient whose surgeon used a biologic mesh when closing the surgical incision. Mesh lowers the risk of:
    A. Infection
    B. Granulation tissue overgrowth
    C. Hernia development
    D. Incisional pain

11. Which statement accurately describes a reaction to the use of mesh in a surgical wound bed?
    A. A nonmodified, non–cross-linked mesh will typically show evidence of granulation within 7 to 14 days.
    B. A modified, heavily cross-linked mesh may take 1 to 2 weeks to show signs of granulation.
    C. If a heavily cross-linked and modified mesh appears to be falling apart day 28, it may be a sign that the mesh is not incorporating or is being degraded.
    D. The more heavily cross-linked meshes and porcine-derived meshes tend to have less of an odor during healing.

12. Which topical therapy would the wound care nurse recommend when biologic mesh is used in a wound bed?
    A. Use of debriding products
    B. Application of topical endogenous collagenases
    C. Use of hydrogen peroxide or acetic acid
    D. Thorough irrigation of the wound

13. In cases of delayed sternal closure, the surgical team must monitor the patient daily for indication that the patient is ready for closure, such as:
    A. Increasing lactate levels
    B. Hemodynamic stability
    C. Total positive fluid balance
    D. Decompensation upon attempted closing

14. Which of the following is a Surgical Care Improvement Project (SCIP) recommendation for the prevention of surgical site infection (SSI)?
    A. Prophylactic antibiotic administration within 1 hour of surgical procedure
    B. Discontinuation of antibiotics within 36 hours after surgery
    C. Hair removal at the site of surgery with a razor
    D. Urinary catheter use for 1 week after surgery

15. Patients experiencing compartment syndrome often require fasciotomy. What type of wound results from this corrective procedure?
    A. Small wound healing by primary intention
    B. Large wounds with minimal exudate
    C. Wounds with exposed musculature
    D. Wounds with heavy bleeding and fistula formation

ANSWERS: 1.**C**, 2.**C**, 3.**B**, 4.**A**, 5.**D**, 6.**B**, 7.**D**, 8.**A**, 9.**B**, 10.**C**, 11.**A**, 12.**D**, 13.**B**, 14.**A**, 15.**C**

CHAPTER 33

Palliative Wound Care

Kevin R. Emmons and Barbara A. Dale

OBJECTIVES

1. Explain the similarities and differences in hospice care and palliative care.
2. Describe the philosophy of palliative care and the implications for care.
3. Discuss modifications in standard pressure ulcer prevention protocols that may be indicated for the palliative care patient.
4. Explain skin changes that are common at end of life and that increase the risk for skin breakdown.
5. Describe guidelines for management of wounds commonly found in the palliative care population, to include pressure ulcers, leg ulcers, skin tears, and fungating wounds.

Topic Outline

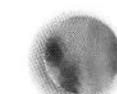 Introduction

As noted throughout this text, in most situations, the goal of wound management is complete wound healing, and each aspect of assessment and treatment is geared toward that outcome. This "healing" goal and expectation is reflected in the common caveat that a wound that fails to show measureable improvement in the first 2 to 4 weeks of therapy must be reevaluated and management must be changed. From this perspective, a nonhealing wound represents a failure of wound management. This focus on healing is appropriate in most cases; however, for some patients and situations, it is inappropriate and can actually compromise appropriate care. In particular, there are many patients whose wound care is much better approached from a palliative care perspective. This requires the wound care team to shift their approach from a singular goal of "wound healing" to a more comprehensive focus on patient-focused goals such as improved quality of life, stabilization of the wound, or a decrease in odor, pain, and exudate. It is important to clarify that palliative wound care is not a singular protocol or care pathway devoid of wound healing outcomes.

Rather, palliative wound care is a concept and approach that can be integrated and applied across the continuum of care.

> **CLINICAL PEARL**
>
> Palliative care requires the wound team to shift their approach from a singular goal of "wound healing" to a more comprehensive focus on patient-focused goals such as improved quality of life.

Palliative Care Overview

The World Health Organization (2011) defines palliative care as "an approach that improves the quality of life of patients and their families facing the problems associated with life-threatening illness, through the prevention and relief of suffering by means of early identification and impeccable assessment and treatment of pain and other problems, physical, psychosocial and spiritual". The Worldwide Palliative Care alliance adds further clarification, stating that palliative care is: (1) applicable early within a course of illness, (2) needed in chronic care as well as life-threatening/limiting conditions, (3) not limited by time or prognosis, (4) needed at all levels of care, and (5) not limited to any one setting (WPCA & WHO, 2014). In a comprehensive analysis on palliative care, it was concluded that palliative care should be thought of early within a chronic disease trajectory (Hui et al., 2013).

Palliative versus Hospice Care

Palliative care is often confused with hospice care, and there are commonalities; however, hospice care is limited to patients at the end of life, while palliative care has a much broader application (Meghani, 2004). Unfortunately, the confusion between palliative care and hospice care has resulted in negative perceptions and stigma; many people interpret palliative care as meaning loss of hope or withdrawal of active treatment. These inaccurate and negative perceptions have limited acceptance and implementation of the palliative care framework and philosophy. Therefore, Hui et al. (2012, 2013) recommend use of the alternative term, supportive care, for palliative care provided during early stages of chronic diseases. This change in nomenclature may be an important nuance that promotes patient, family, and provider acceptance. However, at this time, the accepted term is palliative care, and this chapter addresses concepts and strategies for palliative wound care.

> **CLINICAL PEARL**
>
> Hospice care is limited to end-of-life care, while palliative care has much broader application and is *not* limited to end of life.

Principles of Palliative Care

The concept of palliative care is dynamic and will continue to evolve over time (Meghani, 2004), and it is anticipated that the concept of palliative wound care will also evolve as science progresses. Several articles describing palliative wound care emphasize the importance of symptom management, wound stabilization, measures to reduce suffering, and strategies to improve quality of life as important aspects of palliative wound care (Ennis & Meneses, 2005; Langemo et al., 2007; Hughes et al., 2005). Ferris et al. (2007) concluded that palliative wound care includes therapies aimed at (1) effective communication, decision making, and care delivery, (2) stabilization of the wound, (3) minimizing risk of infection and wound progression, (4) managing issues that cause patient and family suffering, and (5) optimizing function and quality of life as long as possible. A comprehensive concept analysis on the evolution of palliative wound care defined it as a holistic and integrated approach to care that provides symptom management, improves psychosocial well-being, is multidisciplinary, is driven by patient/family goals, and is integrated into everyday care practice (Emmons & Lachman, 2010).

> **CLINICAL PEARL**
>
> Palliative wound care is a holistic approach to care that provides symptom management, improves psychosocial well-being, is multidisciplinary, is driven by patient/family goals, and is integrated into everyday practice.

Indications for Palliative Care

A common challenge is determining when to implement a palliative wound care approach in the nonterminally ill patient. Emmons and Lachman suggest that a palliative approach is appropriate whenever outcomes shift from a primary focus on wound healing to a focus on symptom control and relief of suffering, with the ultimate goal of improving quality of life and psychosocial well-being; they note that it is not necessary to completely abandon the goal of healing (Emmons & Lachman, 2010). In fact, excellence in palliative wound care promotes healing to the extent that repair is possible (Maida et al., 2012). Scenarios in which palliative wound care may be beneficial include the following: situations in which symptom management is challenging and a major focus; chronic debilitating disease or advanced illness; severe malnutrition and dehydration; chronic long-standing wounds; unclear or unknown etiology when the diagnostic workup required to determine etiology is inconsistent with overall care priorities; extremely large wounds in which healing is unlikely; uncorrectable pathology; and, of course, terminal illness (Emmons & Lachman, 2010; Letizia et al., 2010; Maida, 2013).

> **CLINICAL PEARL**
>
> A palliative approach is appropriate when the goal shifts from wound healing to a focus on symptom control—it is not necessary to completely abandon the goal of wound healing.

Palliative Wound Care

Palliative care is obviously the best approach for wounds with very limited potential for healing; however, at present, clinicians do not have any objective measures for identifying these wounds. A Wound Healing Probability Tool was developed some years ago to aid clinicians in determining a wound's likelihood of healing (Table 33-1) (FRAIL, 2002), based on factors known to impact on repair. The higher the score on the tool (i.e., the greater the number of impediments to healing affecting the individual), the less likely the wound is to heal. While the tool has not been validated by rigorous studies, clinicians may elect to use this tool to guide decision making as to whether palliation might be a better focus and priority for the individual than a single-minded emphasis on wound healing.

Wounds have been shown to negatively impact the individual's quality of life, with degree of impact determined by symptom presence and severity as well as psychosocial responses (Emmons, 2012). Common wound-related symptoms that impact quality of life include chronic wound pain, episodic wound pain, odor, drainage, itching, and bleeding (Alvarez et al., 2007; Emmons, 2012; Langemo et al., 2007; McDonald & Lesage, 2006). Poorly controlled wound-related symptoms may in turn result in psychosocial responses that further impair quality of life, such as fear, anxiety, depression, anger, and concerns regarding burden on others (Alvarez et al. 2007; Eisenberger & Zeleznik, 2003). Therefore, a critical aspect of palliative wound care is effective symptom control, which in turn improves quality of life and psychosocial well-being.

TABLE 33-1 Healing Probability Assessment Tool (FRAIL, 2002)

- Wound(s) is over 3 months old or is a reoccurrence of a preexisting breakdown
- The patient spends 20 or more hours of a day in a dependent position (chair or bed)
- The patient is incontinent of urine
- The patient is incontinent of feces
- The patient has lost >5% of baseline weight, or 10 pounds, in the past 90 days
- The patient does not eat independently
- The patient does not walk independently
- The patient has a history of falls within last 90 days
- The patient is unable/unwilling to avoid placing weight over wound(s) site(s)
- Wound is associated with complications of diabetes mellitus
- Wound is associated with peripheral vascular disease (PVD)
- Severe chronic obstructive pulmonary disease (COPD)
- End-stage renal, liver, or heart disease
- Wound is associated with arterial disease
- The patient has diminished range of motion (ROM) status nonresponsive to rehabilitative services
- The patient has diminished level of mental alertness demonstrated by muted communication skills and inability to perform activities of daily living (ADLs) independently
- Wound is full thickness with presence of tunneling
- Blood values indicate a low oxygen-carrying capacity
- Blood values indicate an exhausted or decreasing immune capacity (i.e., low lymphocyte count)
- Blood values indicate below normal visceral protein levels that have not responded to nutritional support efforts (i.e., low prealbumin, transferrin, retinol-binding protein, and albumin)

From FRAIL. (2002). Palliative wound care: Palliative wound care and healing probability assessment tool. http://www.frailcare.org/images/Palliative%20Wound%20Care.pdf

CLINICAL PEARL

Common wound-related symptoms that impact quality of life include pain, odor, drainage, itching, and bleeding.

Palliative Wound Care Patient Exemplar

An example of a nonterminally ill patient who is an excellent candidate for palliative wound care is a patient on a ventilator with a nonhealing wound who is not a candidate for surgery, has severe malnutrition, and has a highly exudative wound. In this case, the wound care nurse should clearly document that the likelihood of complete wound healing is unlikely at the present time, due to the presence of multiple concomitant factors that impair wound healing. She or he should establish a wound care plan focused on stabilizing the wound, preventing infection, controlling symptoms, and optimizing the patient physiologically. When and if the patient improves physiologically, wound improvement is likely to be seen, and goals may be modified to include a focus on repair. This scenario highlights the need for realistic and clearly articulated care goals and a plan of care that emphasizes symptom management but does not abandon the goal of healing.

Developing a Palliative Plan of Care

An essential aspect of palliative wound care is the focus on the whole patient rather than a focus solely on the wound. When developing a plan of care, the clinician must gather and organize all pertinent information to create an accurate and comprehensive clinical picture. This provides the foundation for discussions that involve the patient, family, and other members of the health care team and that result in informed rational decisions regarding the plan of care. In addition to the current and past medical history, laboratory data, physical exam and wound assessment, the clinician must gather scenario specific information that addresses the patient's quality of life, wound-related symptomatology and concerns, and patient and family preferences, goals, and values.

An open conversation exploring the impact of the illness and the wound and the patient's and family's perceptions and concerns helps to elicit important information for goal setting and care planning. Specific questions should be asked regarding wound-related symptoms, such as "What is bothering you the most (pain, odor, drainage, bleeding, frequent dressings, etc.)?" The family should be queried as well, since their concerns may be somewhat different; for example, the patient may be most concerned about pain, while the family may be very distressed by odor and drainage. In addition to physical symptomatology, the nurse should ask about factors such as cosmesis, social isolation, functional impairment or limitations related to the wound, and burden of care. Once the nurse has developed a clear picture of the issues and concerns of most importance to the patient and family, those concerns can be prioritized in order of importance to the patient and family and probable responsiveness to interventions. It is critically important to help the patient and family establish realistic goals with achievable outcomes. For example, if the patient and family identify wound healing as a high priority goal but the nurse knows that healing is not likely at the present time due to ongoing chemotherapy and nutritional compromise, the nurse should explain the conditions required for healing and should redirect the goals to wound stabilization and symptom management *until* blood counts and nutritional status return to normal, at which point the care focus can be shifted to wound healing. This underscores the point that goals and interventions will change in response to the disease trajectory and patient response to medical and surgical management. It is also important for the nurse to explain that the wound care provided will be evidence based and will support healing but will be modified based on the patient's overall condition and the patient's and family's priorities at any given point in time. Thus, wound healing may be *one* of the goals, but it is not the *primary* goal of palliative wound care.

CLINICAL PEARL

Goals and interventions in palliative care change in response to the disease trajectory and patient response to management; wound healing may be *one* of the goals, but it is not the *primary* goal.

Skin Changes at End of Life

As previously noted, palliative wound care is often associated with end-of-life care. With advanced illness and at end of life, significant changes in bodily systems occur, each of which has an impact on skin integrity. Although skin changes at the end of life were documented over 100 years ago (Charcot, 1877), it was not until recently that this issue received more focus among clinicians and in the literature. For example, the Kennedy Terminal Ulcer (KTU) was first described in 1989 as unavoidable skin breakdown that occurs at end of life. The characteristics of KTU include (1) location on the sacrococcygeal area, (2) sudden onset of deeply discolored skin in the shape of a butterfly or pear, (3) rapid progression despite appropriate management (from deep purple, red, black, or blue area to clearly necrotic wound), and (4) irregular borders (Kennedy, 1989). The KTU was the first wound hypothesized to be the result of hypoperfusion associated with multiorgan failure such as occurs during the dying process. Once these ulcers develop, there is rapid enlargement; within a short window of time, a moist necrotic area forms over the center of the well-demarcated area, regardless of pressure redistributing interventions (Langemo & Black, 2010; Yastrub, 2010) (Fig. 33-1).

CLINICAL PEARL

Kennedy Terminal Ulcer was first described in 1989 as unavoidable skin breakdown that occurs at end of life and is characterized by rapid onset and progression despite appropriate preventive care.

In more recent literature, skin changes at end of life have been described as skin failure for consistency with terminology related to other end-of-life changes such as cardiac and renal failure. Skin failure is defined as "an event in which the skin and underlying tissue die due to hypoperfusion that occurs concurrent with severe dysfunction or failure of other organ systems" (Langemo & Brown, 2006). In 2008, an interdisciplinary panel of 18 wound experts convened to develop a consensus statement on the changes that occur at the end of life (Skin Changes at Life's End [SCALE]) (Sibbald et al., 2009, 2010). SCALE can be attributed to reduced soft tissue perfusion, decreased tolerance to external insults, and impaired removal of metabolic wastes. Risk factors and signs and symptoms associated with SCALE include suboptimal nutrition, loss of appetite, weight loss, cachexia and wasting, low serum albumin/prealbumin, low hemoglobin, and dehydration. At end of life, the dying process may compromise the homeostatic mechanisms of the body, including perfusion; when cardiac output is reduced, the body attempts to protect vital organs by shunting blood away from the skin

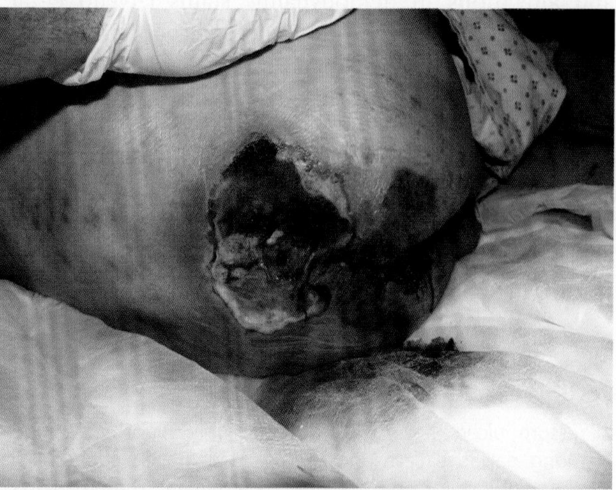

FIGURE 33-1. A rapidly evolving unstageable pressure ulcer with suspected deep tissue injury on sacrum.

resulting in peripheral tissue hypoperfusion (White-Chu & Langemo, 2012). Diminished tissue perfusion is the most significant risk factor for SCALE. Most of the skin has collateral vascular supply, but the most distal locations (fingers, toes, ears, and nose) lack collaterals; these areas are therefore more susceptible to hypoperfusion and to pressure damage, even if the pressure is of minimal intensity and limited duration. Thus, mechanical insults that would normally be well tolerated (limited pressure, shear, and friction) can lead to skin hemorrhage, gangrene, infection, skin tears, and pressure ulcers (Sibbald et al., 2009). A major conclusion from the SCALE consensus panel was that not all pressure ulcers are avoidable (Sibbald et al., 2009, 2010, 2011).

CLINICAL PEARL

Skin changes at end of life are also sometimes classified as "skin failure," for consistency with terminology relating to other organ systems at end of life (e.g., cardiac failure or renal failure).

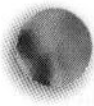

Common Wounds in the Palliative Care Population

Pressure Ulcers

Pressure ulcers are the most commonly reported wound in hospice and palliative care (Maida et al., 2012), with prevalence estimated as between 13% and 47% (Graves & Sun, 2013). These numbers are not surprising, given the fact that hospice and palliative care patients are high risk due to the disease trajectory and (for hospice patients) the impact of terminal illness on perfusion status. Factors contributing to pressure ulcer risk among all palliative care patients include the following: deteriorating physical condition/increasing frailty, immobility, decreased nutritional and fluid intake, fecal and/or urinary incontinence, changes in sensory perception and levels of consciousness, and alterations in hemodynamic status (Ayello et al., 2015). Neurological or noncancer diagnosis, previous pressure ulcers, older age, and caregiver frailty have also been shown to be increased risk factors in the development of new pressure ulcers in home health and hospice palliative care patients (Burt, 2013; Reifsnyder & Magee, 2005). In addition to being higher risk for pressure ulcer development, palliative care and hospice care patients are at risk for impaired healing, due to the same factors that contribute to ulcer development.

CLINICAL PEARL

Pressure ulcers are the most commonly reported wound among palliative care and hospice patients; in addition to being high risk for pressure ulcer development, these patients are high risk for impaired healing.

Risk Assessment

The Braden Scale for Predicting Pressure Sore Risk is a reliable validated tool and has been shown to positively reflect risk in the palliative care patient (Bolton, 2007). However, the Braden scale does not consider other physiologic conditions that may increase risk in palliative care patients such as severe organ dysfunction. In contrast, the Hunters Hill Marie Curie Center pressure sore risk assessment tool (Hunters Hill Tool) was designed specifically for use in the palliative care setting (Chrisman, 2010). The Hunters Hill Tool includes the primary risk factors addressed by the Braden Scale and Norton Scale but also considers existing skin condition. As of this date, this tool has not been tested for interrater reliability, and there is only limited research regarding its validity. Recent literature points to additional factors, particularly perfusion status, in the development of pressure ulcers at end of life (Coleman et al., 2013); further research is needed in regards to the impact of reduced tissue perfusion on pressure ulcer development in this population, and the implications for risk assessment and prevention.

Prevention

Pressure ulcer prevention is of vital importance in palliative care; however, the specific components of the program must be modified to meet the needs of the individual patient. Information gained from the overall patient assessment, the total risk assessment score, and the risk assessment subscores should be used to formulate a very specific prevention program that addresses the individual's needs and priorities (Bolton, 2007). For example, a typical prevention program for the patient with low mobility subscale scores would include a pressure redistribution surface and routine turning and repositioning (VandenBosch et al., 1996). In the general patient population, these measures are usually sufficient to protect the tissues against ischemic damage. However, in palliative care patients who have compromised tissue perfusion, pressure ulcers may develop despite these interventions, because "even lower (levels of) applied pressure may be sufficient to induce ulceration" (Lyder & Ayello, 2008, p. 3).

Thus, palliative care and hospice care patients must be recognized as a high-risk group for whom accepted preventive measures may be insufficient. In addition, specific aspects of preventive care may be inconsistent with the patient's care goals and priorities. These will be discussed individually.

Turning and Positioning

It is widely accepted that keeping the head of the bed at or lower than 30 degrees reduces pressure in the sacrococcygeal area and helps to protect the vulnerable tissues in this anatomic region and that q2–4h repositioning is a key pressure ulcer prevention measure (Wound, Ostomy, Continence Nurses Society, 2010). However, patients may require higher degrees of head of bed elevation due to pain or to compromised pulmonary or cardiovascular status and may refuse turning due to pain and the desire to be left undisturbed once they get comfortable. Appropriate interventions for these patients might include obtaining a higher-level pressure redistribution support surface, reducing turning frequency, and augmenting the turning program with small weight shifts or use of pillows and/or folded towels to reduce pressure over vulnerable areas (Krapfl & Gray, 2008). Premedicating patients 20 to 30 minutes prior to scheduled position changes may also be very helpful in meeting the dual goals of pressure ulcer prevention and maintenance of patient comfort (EPUAP & NPUAP, 2009). When pain precludes routine turning and repositioning, nursing documentation should include a notation regarding reasons for not turning the patient and compensatory interventions (e.g., Patient refused turning 10 PM till 6 AM due to pain and unwillingness to be disturbed—verbalizes awareness that failure to turn increases risk of skin breakdown. Will contact MD regarding adjustments in pain medication; minor weight shifts provided Q 2 hours in attempt to minimize ischemic damage. The patient remains on high-level air support surface.)

CLINICAL PEARL

Measures to prevent pressure ulcer development are of critical importance for the palliative care or hospice patient; however, specific interventions (such as turning frequency and nutritional management) may require modification if comfort goals have been determined higher priority than skin care goals.

Support Surfaces

Support surfaces should be selected based on the patient's mobility in bed and willingness to be turned, comfort factors, need for microclimate control, and environmental factors. All patients found to be at risk for developing pressure ulcers should be placed on a pressure redistribution surface, and those who cannot be turned and repositioned frequently should be placed on an alternating pressure overlay or mattress if tolerated. Some patients find the shifts in position produced by alternating pressure surfaces to be uncomfortable and may prefer a nonpowered surface. In general, the staff should "strive to reposition the patient at least every 4 hours if on a pressure redistributing support surface or viscoelastic foam and every 2 hours on a regular mattress" (EPUAP & NPUAP, 2009, p. 37). Regardless of the type of support surface being used, heels should always be floated using heel protectors or pillows under the calves (EPUAP & NPUAP, 2009).

Nutrition

In general, a low nutrition score on the pressure ulcer risk assessment tool prompts the clinician to implement supportive interventions that will increase intake of the fluids, calories, protein, and vitamins necessary for wound healing and/or pressure ulcer prevention. In the palliative care setting, aggressive nutritional interventions may not be appropriate. Nausea, anorexia, and weight loss are common manifestations in palliative care individuals and at end of life. Families and caregivers may see their family member deteriorating and not understand that loss of appetite and reduced food and fluid intake is common with chronic illness and at end of life. They may even request or demand supplemental nutrition such as tube feedings. Open communication with caregivers is essential and should include the fact that use of alternatives such as hand feeding and oral supplements is usually preferable to enteral feedings, even if the overall intake is poor. Enteral nutrition can provide for basic nutritional needs and would *seem* to be the ideal solution to situations in which oral intake is inadequate; however, there are a number of complications associated with enteral feedings, and studies on advanced dementia patients have shown little to no benefit in reducing risk or promoting healing of pressure ulcers (Hanson, 2013; Teno et al., 2012). Hand feeding or comfort feeding can help reduce symptoms such as dry mouth, hunger, and thirst as well as providing an opportunity for patient caregiver interaction. Oral care aids in reducing mouth pain and improving taste (Langemo & Black, 2010). Small frequent meals and lifting of any dietary restrictions (such as glucose or salt restriction) has also been shown to be beneficial in improving nutritional intake. However, it may not always be possible to assure adequate intake of fluids and nutrients, and the patient's goals must always determine the priorities in care, including nutritional management (Posthauser, 2007).

CLINICAL PEARL

Hand feeding or comfort feeding can help reduce symptoms such as dry mouth, hunger, and thirst and may provide better outcomes than enteral feedings, which are associated with a number of complications and have not been shown to significantly improve healing.

In summary, pressure ulcer prevention is of great importance in the palliative care setting, for a number of reasons. First, skin breakdown can add to the patient's discomfort, level of morbidity, and risk of mortality. Secondly, pressure ulcer development increases the level of skilled and formal care required, which can adversely affect the patient's quality of life (Brink et al., 2006). Finally, caregivers often see the development of a pressure ulcer as an indicator of poor care by themselves and/or staff. In most cases, use of appropriate support surfaces, routine use of heel elevation devices, and diligent attention to modified repositioning programs is effective in maintaining skin integrity. However, the basic concept of palliative care is holistic care directed by patient and caregiver goals; thus, in some situations, pressure ulcers may be unavoidable (e.g., situations in which the patient is cachectic, the tissues are poorly perfused, and the patient and family elect comfort as a higher priority than maintenance of skin integrity). It is critically important to document decisions regarding care priorities and reasons for modified positioning. In addition, there should be ongoing documentation of skin status; staff and caregivers should be taught to incorporate skin inspection into routine care and activities of daily living. Any observation of impending or actual breakdown should be promptly reported to the patient and family, with further discussion as to care priorities (aggressive skin care vs. comfort care). Consistent priorities in care are to (1) comply with patient wishes and overall goals, (2) help to maintain or improve quality of life, and (3) facilitate reduction of burdensome symptoms.

Malignant Wounds

In some patients with advanced cancer, the tumor extends to and invades the skin (Figs. 33-2 to 33-4). In 2012, 36% of hospice patients had a primary diagnosis of cancer (National Hospice and Palliative Care Organization, 2013), and it is estimated that 5% to 19% of all patients with a malignant neoplasm diagnosis will develop a skin lesion (Sibbald et al., 2011). Thirty percent of patients with metastatic breast cancer develop cutaneous lesions (Ladizinski et al., 2014), with 62% of fungating wounds found on the breast. Head and neck cancers account for another 24% (Bergstrom, 2011).

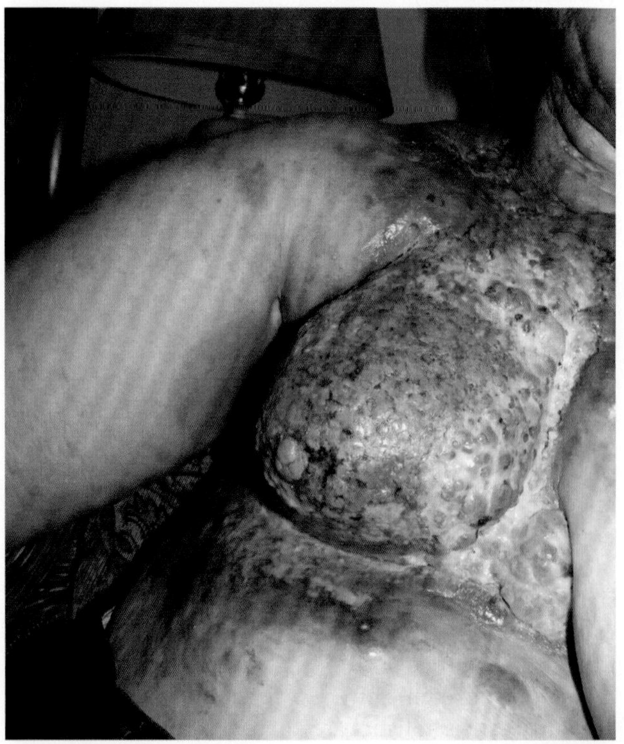

FIGURE 33-2. Malignant fungating wound of the left breast with associated lymphedema.

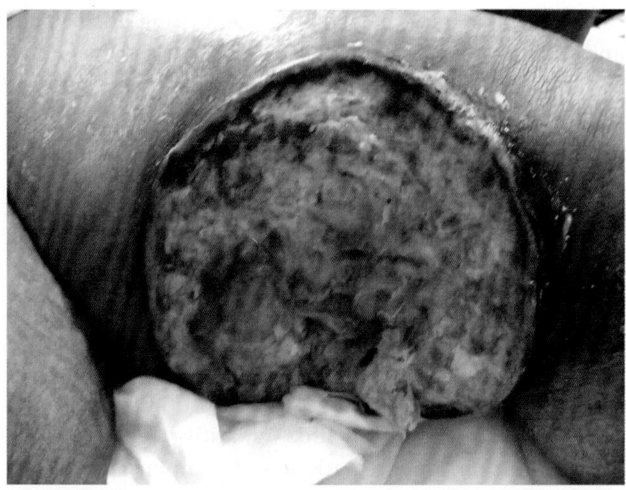

FIGURE 33-3. Ulcerative malignant wound on the left inner thigh.

CLINICAL PEARL

Five to nineteen percent of patients with a malignancy develop metastatic skin lesions, and 30% of patients with metastatic breast cancer develop these lesions.

A fungating wound is defined as "the infiltration and proliferation of malignant cells into the skin and its supporting blood and lymph vessels" (Bergstrom, 2011, p. 31). These cutaneous malignant wounds can be further classified as either ulcerative or fungating depending on the growth pattern. Ulcerative tumors form craters while proliferative tumors form a nodular fungus or cauliflower-type lesion referred to as fungating (Langemo, 2012). All malignant wounds produce both physical and emotional stress for patients and caregivers due to the symptoms and the appearance of the wound. The most commonly reported symptoms associated with malignant wounds are odor, drainage, bleeding, and pain (Bergstrom, 2011). Management of these

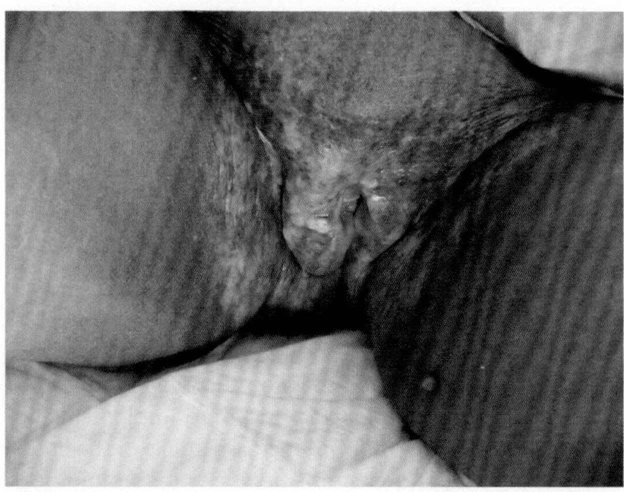

FIGURE 33-4. Malignant fungating wound of the vulva.

symptoms can be easily adapted and applied in the care of other wound etiologies such as pressure ulcers and leg ulcers.

Odor

A common and very distressing symptom reported by patients and caregivers is wound odor. Patients typically report feeling embarrassed and stigmatized because of wound odor, which leads to social isolation; this in turn can increase feelings of hopelessness and depression (Lo et al., 2012). Odor control can be attained by reducing the necrotic tissue and bacterial loads within the wound. Reducing the overall bacterial load is particularly helpful in reducing wound odor. Thorough irrigation of the wound with copious amounts of potable (drinkable) water can help reduce bacterial counts in the wound. If the patient is able to shower, allowing free indirect flow of water across the wound bed is another effective approach to reduction of bacterial loads (Bergstrom, 2011). Dressings such as cadexomer iodine, gentian violet, and silver products can help reduce odor by providing an antimicrobial effect; these dressings are also generally cost-effective since most can stay in place for a longer period of time. Antiseptic solutions such as sodium hypochlorite or acetic acid are inexpensive and effective, but they can cause burning or tingling at the site and periwound irritation and discomfort (due to pH levels); in addition, they add to caregiver burden because they must be changed daily (Merz et al., 2011). To reduce the risk of periwound irritation and pain at the site, a contact layer or base layer of moist saline gauze can be used with the sodium hypochlorite or acetic acid moistened gauze as a secondary layer. Of note, sodium hypochlorite is thrombolytic and may increase topical bleeding and should therefore be used cautiously with friable wounds (Ayello et al., 2015). Antiseptic solutions should be used for a short period of time to quickly reduce bacterial loads, thereby reducing symptom burden. Then the use of advanced antimicrobial dressings with longer wear time can be implemented for sustained bacterial suppression. Advanced antimicrobial and moisture retentive dressings may also contribute to reduced bacterial loads and reduced odor, by supporting autolytic debridement and through direct antimicrobial action (unless there is significant immune dysfunction).

CLINICAL PEARL

Topical metronidazole and antimicrobial dressings are first-line approaches to management of odor with fungating malignant wounds; antiseptics such as dilute Dakin's solution may also be used on a short-term basis.

Another very effective approach to odor control is use of topical metronidazole, which has been shown to effectively reduce and control wound odor within 14 days (Alexander, 2009). Metronidazole is commercially available with a prescription as a gel, powder, paste, cream, or tablet. The gel, paste, or creams can be applied directly to the malignant wound in a thick layer, which promotes a moist wound healing environment, decreases dry cracking lesions, reduces trauma with removal of the dressing, and promotes autolytic debridement of nonviable tissue. Tablets can be dissolved in potable water and used to irrigate the wound, or the solution can be used to soak gauze used to pack or cover the wound. Tablets can also be crushed and sprinkled on the wound surface and then covered with petrolatum gauze and a dry bulky dressing. If the nurse crushes a tablet, he or she must be sure to wear a mask or crush the tablets in a bag, as metronidazole particles are harmful to pleural tissue. Charcoal dressings are available but are infrequently used due to cost and the need to secure the dressing circumferentially with tape (so that the odor molecules are forced through the charcoal as opposed to being allowed to escape from the sides of the dressing). Room deodorizers and other types of aromatherapy can also be used to mask any odors, such as essential oils (peppermint, lavender, lemon, etc.), scented candles, or charcoal. Kitty litter or coffee grounds placed in containers around the home or under the patient's bed has also been cited as a useful adjunct to odor control (Merz et al., 2011).

Drainage

Drainage from malignant wounds is frequently copious, and, along with odor, is frequently embarrassing for the patient. In addition, the copious amount of drainage can cause periwound irritation and breakdown. The periwound skin should be routinely protected with moisture barrier creams or ointments or with liquid barrier films. Measures to reduce bacterial counts and to eliminate necrotic tissue also help to reduce drainage to a manageable level. Once bacterial counts are reduced and odor is controlled, exudate can be managed with a wide variety of dressings that are nonadherent, conformable, and absorptive. Unfortunately, malignant wounds are frequently located in difficult to dress areas such as the chest wall, axilla, or head and neck region. Soft gentle adhesive foam dressings are frequently a good choice for smaller wounds with low-to-moderate volumes of exudate. Larger wounds with higher-volume drainage may require alginate or hydrofiber dressings as the primary dressing in addition to secondary gauze dressings for additional absorption; stockinette-like tube bandages or binders can be useful for securing dressings when tape is not appropriate.

Bleeding

The realistic fear of bleeding and/or hemorrhage can be worrisome to the palliative care patient, their caregivers, and health care providers as bleeding is often difficult to manage. Bleeding occurs frequently in malignant wounds because cancer cells stimulate angiogenesis, thus increasing vascularity; in addition, associated pathologies (e.g., thrombocytopenia, disseminated intravascular coagulopathy [DIC], and malnutrition) (Recka et al., 2012) are common and can also increase the risk of bleeding. These wounds are very friable because the quality of the new vasculature is poor with haphazard connections and leaky dilated vessels (Recka et al., 2012). Slight trauma to the wound bed caused by dressing changes, cleansing, stretching or cracking of the skin and wound, and frequent movement can all contribute to bleeding. Major bleeding episodes are usually due to the wound's proximity to large vessels, such as in head and neck wounds. Tumor growth can cause pressure on vessels, leading to erosion and leaks or to major bleeding episodes.

CLINICAL PEARL

Bleeding is a common and frightening complication associated with fungating malignant wounds; calcium alginate dressings can be used to control minor oozing, but major bleeding usually requires hemostatic foams or gauze.

Prevention of bleeding should be a priority in management of malignant wounds. Maintaining a moist wound surface via use of nonadherent topical products reduces the risk of trauma and thereby reduces the incidence of episodic bleeding. Selection of methods to control bleeding is dependent on access to specific products and medications. Common topical agents to treat bleeding include natural hemostatic agents, coagulants, sclerosing agents, vasoconstrictors, fibrinolytic inhibitors, and astringents (Woo & Sibbald, 2010). Control of minor generalized oozing can be achieved with calcium alginate dressings. The calcium found within these dressings helps promote the clotting cascade and thereby eliminates bleeding. Most brands of calcium alginate can also be found in a rope structure that easily accommodates the often irregular contours of malignant and fungating wounds. Considerations when using alginates for hemostasis is that the coagulation of blood may cause the dressing to stick to the wound bed, which can lead to recurrent bleeding upon alginate removal. It is therefore best to leave the base layer of alginate in the wound during subsequent dressing changes and to allow the alginate to gradually separate from the wound and to be removed with gentle wound irrigations. For large areas of active bleeding, gelling hemostatic foams and hemostatic surgical gauze are better options, though more expensive and not as readily available. These hemostatic dressings can be applied in layers and left in place. Epinephrine-soaked gauze can also be applied topically; it causes vasoconstriction of vessels, thus helping to control bleeding. Antifibrinolytic medication (e.g., tranexamic acid and aminocaproic acid) can be taken orally or in some cases applied topically (Recka et al., 2012) for management of low pressure bleeding; however, these medications are more costly and require a prescription. For pinpoint minor bleeding, silver nitrate is a quick and easy intervention that cauterizes exposed vessels. In severe cases that may cause significant distress, surgical and radiologic procedures can be performed. However, in some scenarios when bleeding cannot be stopped, the implementation of nonpharmacologic and comfort measures to reduce distress are imperative. Collection devices such as wound or ostomy pouching systems can contain large amounts of blood and can be easily emptied. Finally, patients and their caregivers can be instructed to keep dark towels and dark sheets on hand to mask the color and to reduce anxiety associated with bleeding and/or hemorrhage.

Pain

Pain management, a central aspect of palliative care, can be difficult to manage, and wound-related pain is no exception. The principles of wound-related pain management have been discussed in detail in Chapter 7, and these principles and strategies are equally effective for management of pain in palliative care patients; for example, use of the World Health Organization (WHO) pain control ladder is beneficial in management of any patient with chronic pain. Persons who would benefit from palliative care often have concurrent conditions requiring effective pain management via control with long-acting and breakthrough pain medications. Uncontrolled general chronic pain can exacerbate and potentiate other pain such as wound-related pain. A thorough pain assessment to determine triggering and relieving factors is an essential first step in determining whether the pain is persistent or associated primarily with procedures or dressing changes. Persistent pain is managed with around the clock analgesics. Procedure-related pain can be significantly reduced with the following strategies: premedication, use of nonadherent dressings, gentle technique, less frequent dressing changes, and allowing the patient to call "time-outs" during dressing changes if needed. Patients and providers alike often look for topical solutions to reduce wound-related pain. Morphine in hydrogel can be an effective pain reliever, and it has little to no systemic absorption (Emmons et al., 2014). Other topical anesthetics (lidocaine and EMLA cream) may provide intermittent pain relief but can be accompanied by transient burning and systemic absorption with chronic use.

CLINICAL PEARL

A thorough pain assessment and aggressive pain management are critical components of care for the palliative care patient.

Skin Tears

Prevention of skin tears in palliative care involves the same principles and strategies as skin tear prevention for the general population. Most skin tears occur as a result of falls, adhesive removal, assistance with activities of daily living (bathing, dressing, turning, and repositioning), and trauma incurred during transfers (e.g., bumping the extremities against side rails or wheelchair parts). Interventions to prevent skin tears are essentially the same for palliative care and usual care patients; however, palliative care patients are usually higher risk and require greater awareness and more attentive preventive care. Meticulous skin care with pH balanced cleansers, routine use of emollients and lotions, gentle handling techniques to reduce friction and shear, and proper transfer/reposition techniques are some of the interventions that can easily be implemented. Instructing caregivers to keep the patient's and their own nails trimmed is an often overlooked measure. Protective sleeves and leggings are commercially available and very beneficial; simple alternatives include stockinette and athletic socks with the toes cut out. Tape should be avoided whenever possible; devices and dressings should be secured with wrap gauze, binders, stretch net, stockinette, mastectomy bras, or nonadhesive, self-stick tapes. In providing topical care, the nurse should avoid any dressings with aggressive adhesives; good options for management include use of contact layer dressings covered by dry gauze and secured with wrap gauze (extremity wounds), or gentle adhesive foam dressings (trunk wounds) (LeBlanc & Baranoski, 2011).

CLINICAL PEARL

In providing topical care, the nurse should avoid use of aggressive adhesives and should use wrap gauze to secure dressings on extremity wounds.

Lower Leg Ulcerations

A history of leg ulcers and/or active lower limb ulcers is not uncommon in the palliative care population; simple preventive measures should be continued for those with a history of lower-extremity ulcers (and those known to be at risk), and active wounds should be managed based on symptomatology. Differential assessment is paramount in the management of any lower leg ulcers to confirm etiologic factors, because the management of these wounds differs significantly based on the causative factors. For example, venous ulcers are typically best managed by elevation and compression, whereas arterial ulcers are best managed with limited activity and dependent positioning until (and unless) revascularization can be implemented. Neuropathic ulcers are most often seen on the plantar surface of the foot in an individual with diabetes; essential elements of management *when the goal is healing* include consistent offloading along with tight glucose control. For the palliative care patient, the primary goals in the management of a leg ulcer are pain control and prevention of infection. Pain is the most often reported symptom with venous and arterial ulcers (Pieper et al., 2009); however, as noted, measures to relieve the pain differ based on etiology. For example, arterial ulcer pain is relieved in part by dependency, while patients with venous ulcers find relief with elevation. Patients with neuropathic ulcers may have nighttime or rest pain (paresthesias) that may require pharmacologic management. Interventions to address pain in each of these individuals would vary greatly; thus, differentiation is vitally important.

Venous Leg Ulcers

Patients with venous leg ulcers can experience pain related to the underlying venous insufficiency, pain caused by the ulcer itself, or skin irritation and discomfort caused by the high-volume exudate associated with a venous leg ulcer. Standard pain management therapies for venous leg ulcers can be utilized in the palliative care patient unless contraindicated (compression, leg elevation, and oral analgesics if needed). The large amount of drainage can be managed with highly absorptive dressings and use of moisture barrier ointments or liquid barrier films for periwound skin protection. Patients with respiratory diagnoses and patients with heart failure often cannot tolerate compression therapy due to the risk of increased pulmonary distress caused by increased venous return (increased preload). To control drainage and edema, a trial of modified low-level compression bandaging may be implemented (Wound Ostomy Continence Nurses Society, 2014). Short-stretch bandages may be a good alternative to multilayer compression if the patient is unable to tolerate normal compression levels; however, short-stretch bandages are only effective in the ambulatory patient (Wound Ostomy Continence Nurses Society, 2011). It should be noted that long-stretch bandages, such as ACE-type bandages, do not require the patient to be ambulatory but do not provide consistent effective compression; tubular elasticated dressings provide 10 mm Hg compression with each layer and are generally more effective than Ace Bandages and also easier for the home caregiver to apply. If the patient's status improves over time to the point where she or he can tolerate higher compression, then more traditional methods and levels of compression therapy can be provided.

Arterial and Gangrenous Wounds

Pain associated with arterial or developing gangrenous leg ulcers is typically treated systemically. As ischemia progresses, the pain can become intense. When a vascular consult is implausible, topical care is based on the status of the wound. If the wound is open and most of the wound bed is viable, principles of moist wound healing should be utilized; maintenance of a moist wound bed prevents tissue desiccation, which causes increased pain. In contrast, the wound that is primarily covered with dry stable eschar or dry gangrene should be dressed with dry dressings or kept open to air to keep the area dry (Wound Ostomy Continence Nurses Society, 2014) to prevent infection and/or progression from dry gangrene to wet gangrene. When managing dry eschar or dry gangrene, some clinicians advocate daily application of povidone iodine solution or a liquid film barrier and allowing it to dry, with the goal of reducing topical bacteria while maintaining dry stable eschar (Wound Ostomy Continence Nurses Society, 2014). The nurse should be aware that the appearance of dry eschar or gangrene is often overwhelming to the patient or caregiver. Simply covering the area with loose dry dressings is appropriate and can reduce the emotional pain associated with visualizing a necrotic area (Fig. 33-5).

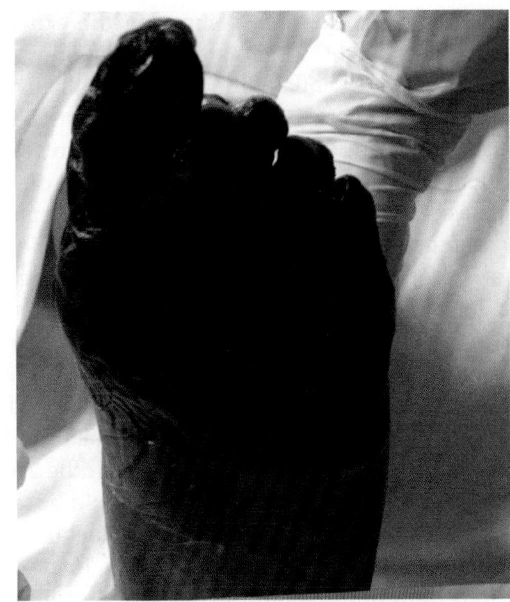

FIGURE 33-5. Dry gangrene of the left foot.

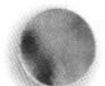 Conclusion

The emergence of palliative wound care is due in part to the fact that people are living longer with more severe and chronic diseases, and the plan of care frequently needs to shift to palliative goals rather than healing. However, healing goals are not abandoned; rather, they are reprioritized within the context of palliation first and healing second. Providers of wound care must have the knowledge to develop a plan of care that is appropriate within the context of the person's health status.

CASE STUDY

PALLIATIVE WOUND CARE CASE

A 43-year-old female with a primary diagnoses of HIV/AIDS was admitted to home health hospice. A wound care consult was requested for assessment and management of wound odor related to a neck wound. Upon physical examination, a large fungating wound was noted on the left side of the neck. Significant odor was noted upon exam. The malignant wound deeply invaded into the neck cavity and had significant white, yellow, and black necrosis. There was a 3-cm tunnel noted at about 7 o'clock. Exudate was mild and able to be contained with daily gauze dressings prior to assessment. The periwound assessment revealed old radiation burns and dry desquamation.

Wound odor was the primary reason for this consult. After speaking with patient and family, it became clear that the problems were more extensive. Our conversation started with questions asking about how this wound had affected the patient and her family. This revealed that the patient was embarrassed to be seen outside with gauze wrapped around her neck and with a terrible strong odor. As a result, this patient became socially isolated in her house. We then explored other things that bothered her such as the drainage and the burden of dressing changes and trying to keep them in place. The discussion then transitioned into the patient's and family's goals. We listed and prioritized them as follows: (1) control odor, (2) have cosmetically appealing dressing, (3) find easy to apply dressings that are painless upon removal, and lastly (4) regain ability to go to a restaurant and movie without feeling embarrassed about the wound. During this time,

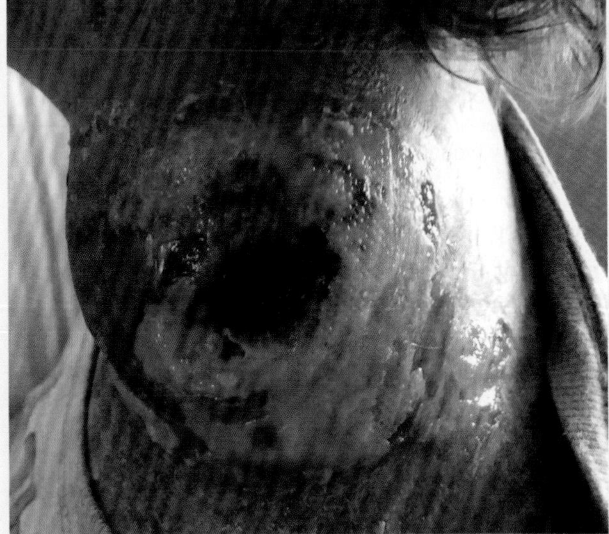

Malignant fungating wound on the neck.

we discussed the fact that tumor wounds would not shrink without treatment (which had been stopped). We explored the possibility of the wound continuing to grow and the potential for other issues such as itching and the possibility of bleeding.

A plan was then developed for each of the goals. Cleansing lightly in the shower was recommended. A topical metronidazole cream was chosen as the antimicrobial and deodorizing agent. This was chosen because the wound did not have significant drainage, and this product was available through the providing pharmacy. The metronidazole cream would provide a cooling sensation, a moist environment that would support autolytic debridement (to the extent physiologically possible), and atraumatic removal of the cover dressing. The cover dressing selected was a thin foam dressing with a soft silicone adhesive. This dressing reduced the topical layer to a single thin layer as opposed to a bulky gauze wrap; the soft silicone adhesive foam also reduced the flaky irritated skin that had developed following radiation. Finally, a "stretchy" loose fitting head band was used to keep the dressing in place during frequent movement and to provide a final appealing look for the patient. She could choose any color to match her outfit. Options were also discussed for the management of bleeding (both oozing and major bleeding) and for management of increasing odor and drainage (should this become a problem).

Follow-up

Within 4 days, the odor had almost completely subsided. The patient reported that she frequently left the house with family, and she no longer had fears related to uncontrolled wound symptoms.

As the patient's disease process progressed and she became homebound, the plan of care also changed until her death. Drainage had increased, and a silver alginate was chosen as the topical dressing with soft silicone adhesive foam cover dressings, which contained both odor and drainage.

This case exemplifies the need to explore what is important to the patient and family. Here, social isolation was the main issue and was caused by wound odor and the need for bulky conspicuous dressings. The plan of care was driven by the patient and family with the collaboration of the wound care nurse. Fears regarding healing and wound progress were discussed, and options were developed to alleviate concerns. Ultimately, this plan of care focused on improving quality of life by giving the patient back the freedom to leave the house without the burden of uncontrolled symptoms.

REFERENCES

Alexander, S. (2009). Malignant fungating wounds: managing pain, bleeding and psychosocial issues. *Journal of Wound Care, 18*(10), 418–425.

Alvarez, O. M., Kalinski, C., Nusbaum, J., et al. (2007). Incorporating wound healing strategies to improve palliation (symptom management) in patients with chronic wounds. *Journal of Palliative Medicine, 10*(5), 1161–1189.

Ayello, E. A., Sibbald, R. G., Woo, K. Y., et al. (2015). Skin alterations. In M. Matzo & D. W. Sherman (Eds.), *Palliative care nursing: Quality care to the end of life* (4th ed., pp. 627–647). New York: Springer.

Bergstrom, K. (2011). Assessment and management of fungating wounds. *Journal of Wound, Ostomy, & Continence Nursing, 38*(1), 31–37.

Bolton, L. (2007). Which pressure ulcer risk assessment scales are valid for use in the clinical setting? *Journal of Wound, Ostomy, & Continence Nursing, 34*(4), 368–381.

Brink, P., Smith, T. F., & Linkewich, B. (2006). Factors associated with pressure ulcers in palliative home care. *Journal of Palliative Medicine, 9*, 1369–1375.

Burt, T. (2013). Palliative care of pressure ulcers in long-term care. *Annals of Long-Term Care, 21*(3), 20–28.

Chrisman, C. A. (2010). Care of chronic wounds in palliative care and end of life patients. *International Wound Journal, 7*(4), 214–235.

Coleman, S., Gorecki, C., Nelson, E. A., et al. (2013). Patient risk factors for pressure ulcer development: Systematic review. *International Journal of Nursing Studies, 50*(7), 974–1003.

Charcot, J. M. (1877). *Lectures on the diseases of the nervous system* (Vol. 1). London, UK: New Sydenham Society.

Eisenberger, A., & Zeleznik, J. (2003). Pressure ulcer prevention and treatment in hospices: A qualitative analysis. *Journal of Palliative Care, 19*(1), 9–14.

Emmons, K. R. (2012). *Wounds at the end of life: Wound symptoms and severity, quality of life, and patient-reported symptoms and preferences for care* (Doctoral Dissertation). Drexel libraries e-repository and archives. http://hdl.handle.net/1860/3757

Emmons, K. R., Dale, B., & Crouch, C. (2014). Palliative wound care part 2: Application of principles. *Home Healthcare Nurse, 32*(4), 201–222.

Emmons, K. R., & Lachman, V. L. (2010). Palliative wound care: A concept analysis. *Journal of Wound, Ostomy, and Continence Nursing, 37*(6), 639–644.

Ennis, W. J., & Meneses, P. (2005). Palliative care and wound care: 2 emerging fields with similar needs for outcomes data. *Wound, 17*(4), 99–104.

European Pressure Ulcer Advisory Panel and National Pressure Ulcer Advisory Panel (EPUAP and NPUAP). (2009). *Prevention and treatment of pressure ulcers: Quick reference guide*. Washington DC: National Pressure Ulcer Advisory Panel.

Ferris, F. D., Al Khateib, A. A., Fromantin, I., et al. (2007). Palliative wound care: Managing chronic wounds across life's continuum: A consensus statement from the International Palliative Wound Care Initiative. *Journal of Palliative Medicine, 10*(1), 37–39.

FRAIL. (2002). *Palliative wound care: Palliative wound care and healing probability assessment tool*. Retrieved from http://www.frailcare.org/images/Palliative%20Wound%20Care.pdf

Graves, M. L., & Sun, V. (2013). Providing quality wound care at the end of life. *American Journal of Hospice & Palliative Nursing, 15*(2), 66–74.

Hanson, L. C. (2013). Tube feeding versus assisted oral feeding for persons with dementia: Using evidence to support decision-making. *Annals of Long-Term Care, 21*(1), 16–28.

Hui, D., De La Cruz, M., Mori, M. et al. (2013). Concepts and definitions for "supportive care," "best supportive care," "palliative care," and "hospice care" in the published literature, dictionaries, and textbooks. *Supportive Care in Cancer, 21*(3), 659–689.

Hui, D., Mori, M., Parsons, H., et al. (2012). The lack of standardized definitions in the supportive and palliative oncology literature. *Journal of Pain and Symptom Management, 43*(3), 582–592.

Hughes, R. G., Bakos, A. D., O'Mara, A., & Kovner, C. T. (2005). Palliative wound care at the end of life. *Home Health Care Management & Practice, 17*(3), 196–202.

Kennedy, K. L. (1989). The prevalence of pressure ulcers in an intermediate care facility. *Decubitus, 2*(2), 44–45.

Krapfl, L. A., & Gray, M. (2008). Does regular repositioning prevent pressure ulcers?. *Journal of Wound, Ostomy and Continence Nursing, 36*(6), 571–577.

Ladizinski, B., Alavi, A., Jambrosic, J., et al (2014, July). Cancers mimicking fungal infections. *Advances in Skin & Wound Care, 27*(7), 301–309.

Langemo, D. K. (2012). General principles and approaches to wound prevention and care at end of life: An overview. *Ostomy Wound Management, 58*(5), 24–34.

Langemo, D. K., Anderson, J., Hanson, D., et al. (2007). Understanding palliative wound care. *Nursing, 37*(1), 65–66.
Langemo, D. K., & Black, J. (2010). Pressure ulcers in individuals receiving palliative care: A National Pressure Ulcer Advisory Panel White Paper©. *Advances in Skin & Wound Care, 23*(2), 59–72.
Langemo, D. K., & Brown, G. (2006). Skin fails too: Acute, chronic, and end-stage skin failure. *Advances in Skin and Wound Care, 19*(4), 206–211.
LeBlanc, K., & Baranoski, S. (2011). Skin tears: State of the science: Consensus statements for the prevention, prediction, assessment, and treatment of skin tears. *Advances in Skin & Wound Care, 24*(S9), 2–15.
Letizia, M., Uebelhor, J., & Paddack, E. (2010). Providing palliative care to seriously ill patients with nonhealing wounds. *Journal of Wound, Ostomy, & Continence Nursing, 37*(3), 277–282.
Lo, S. F., Hayter, M., Hu, W. Y., et al. (2012). Symptom burden and quality of life in patients with malignant fungating wounds. *Journal of Advanced Nursing, 68*(6), 1312–1321.
Lyder, C. H., & Ayello, E. A. (2008). Pressure ulcers: A patient safety issue. In R. G. Hughes (Eds.), *Patient safety and quality: An evidence-based handbook for nurses* (pp. 1–33). Rockville, MD: Agency for Healthcare Research and Quality. Retrieved from http://www.ncbi.nlm.nih.gov/books/NBK2650/
McDonald, A., & Lesage, P. (2006). Palliative management of pressure ulcers and malignant wounds in patients with advanced illness. *Journal of Palliative Medicine, 9*(2), 285–295.
Maida, V. (2013). Wound management in patients with advanced illness. *Current Opinion in Supportive and Palliative Care, 7*(1), 73–79.
Maida, V., Ennis, M., & Corban, J. (2012). Wound outcomes in patients with advanced illness. *International Wound Journal, 9*(6), 683–692.
Meghani, S. H. (2004). A concept analysis of palliative care in the United States. *Journal of Advanced Nursing, 46*(2), 152–161.
Merz, T., Klein, C., Uebach, B., et al. (2011). Fungating wounds-multidimensional challenge in palliative care. *Breast Care, 6*, 21–24.
National Hospice and Palliative Care Organization. (2013). *NHPCO's facts and figures. Hospice care in America* 2013 ed. Alexandria, VA: National Hospice and Palliative Care Organization. Retrieved August 12, 2014, from http://www.nhpco.org/sites/default/files/public/Statistics_Research/2013_Facts_Figures.pdf
Pieper, B., Vallerand, A. H., Nordstrom, C. K., et al. (2009). Comparison of bodily pain. Persons with and without venous ulcers in an indigent care clinic. *Journal of Wound, Ostomy, Continence Nursing, 36*(5), 493–502.
Posthauser, M. E. (2007). The role of nutritional therapy in palliative care. *Advances in Skin & Wound Care, 20*(1), 32–33.
Recka, K., Montagnini, M., & Vitale, C. A. (2012). Management of bleeding associated with malignant wounds. *Journal of Palliative Medicine, 15*(8), 952–954.
Reifsnyder, J., & Magee, H. (2005). Development of pressure ulcers in patients receiving home hospice care. *Wounds, 17*(4), 74–79.
Sibbald, R. G., Goodman, L., Woo, K. Y., et al. (2011). Special considerations in wound bed preparation 2011: An update. *Advances in Skin and Wound Care, 24*(9), 415–438.
Sibbald, R. G., Krasner, D. L., & Lutz, J. (2010). SCALE: Skin changes at life's end: Final Consensus Statement: October 1, 2009©. *Advances in Skin & Wound Care, 23*(5), 225–236.
Sibbald, R. G., Krasner, D. L., Lutz, J., the SCALE Expert Panel. (2009). *Skin changes at end of life: Final consensus document*. New York, NY: Gaymar Industries.
Teno, J. M., Gozalo, P., Mitchell, S. L., et al. (2012). Feeding tubes and the prevention or healing of pressure ulcers. *Archives of Internal Medicine, 172*(9), 697–701.
VandenBosch, T., Montoye, C., Satwicz, M., et al. (1996). Predictive validity of the Braden Scale and nurse perception in identifying pressure ulcer risk. *Applied Nursing Research, 9*(2), 80–86.
White-Chu, E. F., & Langemo, D. (2012). Skin failure: Identifying and managing an underrecognized condition. *Annals of Long-Term Care, 20*(7), 28–32.
Woo, K. Y., & Sibbald, R. G. (2010). Local wound care for malignant palliative wounds. *Advances in Skin & Wound Care, 23*(9), 417–428.
World Wide Palliative Care Alliance (WPCA) and World Health Organization (WHO). (2014). Global atlas of palliative care at the end of life. London, UK: Worldwide Palliative Care Alliance.
World Health Organization. (2011). *WHO definition of palliative care*. Geneva, the Switzerland: World Health Organization.
Wound, Ostomy, Continence Nurses Society. (2010). *Guideline for prevention and management of pressure ulcers*. Mt Laurel, NJ: WOCN.
Wound Ostomy Continence Nurses Society. (2011). Guideline for management of wounds in patients with lower-extremity venous disease. *WOCN Clinical Practice Guideline Series No. 4*. Mount Laurel, NJ: WOCN.
Wound Ostomy Continence Nurses Society. (2014). *Guideline for management of wound in patients with lower-extremity arterial disease*. Mount Laurel, NJ: WOCN.
Yastrub, D. J. (2010). Pressure or pathology: Distinguishing pressure ulcers from the Kennedy Terminal Ulcer. *Journal of Wound, Ostomy, & Continence Nursing, 37*(3), 249–250.

QUESTIONS

1. A wound care nurse recommends palliative care for a patient with terminal cancer who has a nonhealing pressure ulcer. Which statement accurately describes a principle of palliative wound care?

A. Palliative care is applicable only to life-threatening conditions.
B. Palliative care is limited to the long-term care setting.
C. Palliative care is applicable early within a course of illness.
D. The focus of palliative care is wound healing.

2. What is the biggest difference between palliative care and hospice care?

A. Hospice care is limited to end-of-life care.
B. Palliative care focuses on wound healing.
C. Hospice care is more appropriate for patients with chronic conditions.
D. Palliative care denotes the withdrawal of active treatment.

3. Which of the following meets the Kennedy Terminal Ulcer criteria for unavoidable skin breakdown occurring at the end of life?
A. Location on the extremities
B. Slow progression from pink color to clearly necrotic tissue
C. Circular shape
D. Rapid progression despite appropriate care

4. Which end-of-life condition is the most significant risk factor for SCALE (Skin Changes at Life's End)?
A. Undernutrition
B. Hypoperfusion
C. Impaired removal of metabolic wastes
D. Cachexia

5. Which type of wound occurs most frequently in hospice and palliative care?
A. Pressure ulcers
B. Malignant wounds
C. Skin tears
D. Lower leg ulcerations

6. Which of the following measures to prevent pressure ulcer development is appropriate for the palliative or hospice patient?
A. Keeping the head of the bed higher than 30 degrees
B. Avoiding the use of pillows or folded towels to reduce pressure
C. Using higher-level pressure redistribution support systems
D. Increasing turning frequency

7. Pressure ulcer prevention is of great importance in the palliative care setting. Which measure helps to accomplish this goal?
A. Use enteral feedings instead of hand feeding to improve healing ability.
B. Reposition patients on pressure redistributing support surfaces every 4 hours.
C. Reposition patients on regular mattresses every hour.
D. Avoid floating heels with heel protectors or pillows.

8. Which of the following is a first-line approach to the management of odor with fungating wounds?
A. Charcoal dressings
B. Topical metronidazole and antimicrobial dressings
C. Long-term irrigation with antiseptic solutions
D. Soaking the wound in a basin of potable water

9. The wound care nurse is providing palliative care to a patient with a small very shallow pressure ulcer that has a low volume of exudate. What dressing would be the best choice?
A. Alginate or hydrofiber dressing + gauze and tape
B. Dry gauze dressings
C. Gentle adhesive foam dressing
D. Wet-to-dry gauze dressings

10. The wound care nurse is choosing a dressing for a leg ulcer with a large area of active bleeding. What would be the best choice?
A. Silver nitrate followed by wet-to-dry gauze
B. Hydrofiber dressing + wrap gauze
C. Adhesive foam dressing
D. Gelling hemostatic foam

11. The wound care nurse is managing a patient on palliative care who has arterial leg ulcers. What management technique is recommended?
A. Limited activity
B. Elevation
C. Compression
D. Tight glucose control

ANSWERS: 1.**C**, 2.**A**, 3.**D**, 4.**B**, 5.**A**, 6.**C**, 7.**B**, 8.**B**, 9.**C**, 10.**D**, 11.**A**

CHAPTER 34

Fistula Management

Denise Nix and Ruth A. Bryant

OBJECTIVES

1. Describe causative and contributing factors to fistula development.
2. Describe guidelines for medical management of the patient with an enterocutaneous fistula.
3. Outline criteria and guidelines for promotion of spontaneous fistula closure.
4. Explain the significance of pseudostoma formation in the patient with a fistula.
5. Discuss indications for surgical closure of a fistula.
6. Develop and implement individualized management plan for the fistula patient that provides for containment of drainage and odor and protection of perifistular skin.

Topic Outline

Introduction

A fistula (plural fistulas or fistulae) is an abnormal passage between two or more epithelialized surfaces that results in communication between one body cavity or hollow organ and another hollow organ or the skin (Bryant & Best, 2015). An enterocutaneous fistula (ECF) refers to an opening from the intestine to the skin. Although ECFs *can* be located *within* a wound, they should not be confused with a draining wound, surgically placed drain site, or wound dehiscence.

The mortality rates for patients with ECFs range from as low as 5.5% to as high as 30%; death is most often due to sepsis, malnutrition, or fluid and electrolyte imbalance (Kaur & Minocha, 2000; Li et al., 2003; McNaughton et al., 2010). Although the true incidence of ECF development is unknown, Teixeira et al. (2009) reported an incidence of 1.5% in a large study involving 2,373 trauma patients who required laparotomy. They also found that patients with ECFs required significant hospital resources with a statistically significant increase in intensive care unit length of stay (28.5 ± 30.5 vs. 7.6 ± 9.3 days, $p = 0.004$), hospital length of stay (82.1 ± 100.8 vs. 16.2 ± 17.3 days, $p < 0.001$), and mean hospital charges ($539,309 vs. $126,996, $p < 0.001$).

An interdisciplinary team is needed to meet the needs of the patient with a fistula (Canadian Association for Enterostomal Therapy [CAET], 2009). Most authors suggest that essential team members include wound/ostomy nurse, dietitian, pharmacist, nurse, social worker, surgeon, and physician (Haffejee, 2004; Hollington et al., 2004; Lal et al., 2006). Other team members include pain specialists, radiologists, physiotherapists, and occupational therapists (Lal et al., 2006; Oneschuk & Bruera, 1997). ECF management is one of the most difficult clinical challenges for the wound/ostomy nurse. It can also be the most rewarding experience once the patient's quality of life is restored through individualized, unique, and best practice interventions.

Clinical Presentation and Classification

Fever and abdominal pain are the initial indicators of a possible fistula (Nussbaum & Fischer, 2006); however, these are nonspecific indicators. The definitive indicator of a cutaneous fistula is the passage of gastrointestinal (GI) secretions or urine into an open wound bed or through an unintentional opening onto the skin. Manifestations of a fistula tract terminating in the vagina include passage of urine (vesicovaginal fistula) or passage of gas, feces, and/or purulent and extremely malodorous drainage (rectovaginal or enterovaginal fistula). Irradiation-induced rectovaginal fistulas often are preceded by diarrhea, passage of mucus and blood rectally, a sensation of rectal pressure, and a constant urge to defecate (Saclarides, 2002). Fistulas between the intestinal tract and the urinary bladder (e.g., colovesical fistula) present with passage of gas or stool-stained urine through the urethra.

CLINICAL PEARL

The definitive indicator of a cutaneous fistula is the passage of GI secretions or urine into an open wound bed or through an unintentional opening onto the skin.

The pH of the effluent may suggest the origin of the fistula tract. For example, extremely acidic fluid (pH 1.0 to 3.0) suggests a gastric fistula, whereas highly alkaline output (7.8 to 8) is consistent with a pancreatic fistula (Huether, 2002).

TABLE 34-1 Fistula Classification

	Designation	Characteristics
Location	Internal	Tract contained within body
	External	Tract exits through skin
Involved structures (not inclusive)	Colon to vagina	Colovaginal
	Intestine to skin	Enterocutaneous
	Bladder to vagina	Vesicovaginal
	Colon to skin	Colocutaneous
	Rectum to vagina	Rectovaginal
	Colon to vagina	Colovaginal
Volume	High output	>500 mL/24 h
	Moderate output	200–500 mL/24 h
	Low output	<200 mL/24 h
Complexity	Simple	Short direct tract, no abscess, no other organ involvement
	Complex	Type 1—abscess, multiple organ involvement Type 2—opens into the base of a wound

Modified from Bryant, R., & Best, M. (2015). Management of draining wounds and fistulas. In R. Bryant & D. Nix (Eds.), *Acute and chronic wounds: Current management concepts* (5th ed.). St. Louis, MO: Mosby. (In Print.)

Most clinicians describe and classify fistulas according to location, involved structures, and volume of effluent. Although less frequently used, fistulas may also be classified by complexity (see Table 34-1). Mucous fistulas are surgically created openings into the defunctionalized section of bowel; they secrete mucus only, which is relatively easy to contain with dressings or pouches, and they do not increase morbidity or mortality. They are therefore not further discussed in this chapter.

CLINICAL PEARL

Fistulas are typically "named" for the organ of origin and the organ of termination; for example, an ECF is one from the bowel to the skin, and a colovesical fistula is one from the colon to the vagina.

Etiologic Factors

ECFs commonly develop postoperatively, due to anastomotic breakdown, but can also occur spontaneously, as a result of inflammatory bowel disease, cancer, or diverticulitis. The risk of fistula formation is further increased when one of these conditions is complicated by malnutrition, sepsis, hypotension, vasopressors, or corticosteroids (Nussbaum & Fischer, 2006).

Approximately 25% of fistulas develop spontaneously and are associated with an intrinsic intestinal disease (cancer, radiation, diverticulitis, inflammatory bowel disease, appendicitis) or external trauma. Spontaneous fistulas are generally resistant to spontaneous closure. Patients treated for a pelvic cancer are particularly vulnerable to ECFs due to radiation damage; the fistula may develop immediately following radiation or years later (Tran & Thorson, 2008). An analysis of 41 publications reported that 17% of patients receiving pelvic radiation developed ECFs, and the average time frame for fistula development was 3.4 years following completion of radiation therapy (Meissner, 1999). Irradiation-induced ECFs are more likely to occur in patients who receive higher radiation doses (>5,000 cGy), smoke cigarettes, or have atherosclerosis, hypertension, diabetes mellitus, advanced age, pelvic inflammatory disease, or previous pelvic surgery (Hollington et al., 2004; Saclarides, 2002; Tran & Thorson, 2008).

CLINICAL PEARL

Most ECFs occur postoperatively, as a result of anastomotic breakdown; however, fistulas may also develop spontaneously as a result of inflammatory bowel conditions (e.g., diverticulitis, Crohn's disease, radiation enteritis) or trauma.

The majority of ECFs (75% to 85%) are iatrogenic (inadvertently induced from a medical procedure); these fistulas develop postoperatively due to anastomotic breakdown (Nussbaum & Fischer, 2006). A key risk factor for anastomotic breakdown is malnutrition (Mäkelä et al., 2003; Telem et al., 2010). Additional risk factors for postoperative ECF development include existing conditions such as inflammatory bowel disease, cancer, or previous radiation therapy. Surgery-related risk factors include inadequate blood supply, poor suture technique, inadequate bowel prep (e.g., emergency surgery), extensive lysis of adhesions, and trauma surgery (Kassis & Makary, 2008; Nussbaum & Fischer, 2006; Wong et al., 2004). The method of anastomosis (stapled or hand-sewn) has not proven to be a predictor of ECF after surgery for trauma (Demetriades et al., 2002; Kirkpatrick et al., 2003). Patients scheduled for elective surgical procedures should receive adequate nutrition preoperatively in order to minimize the risk of anastomotic breakdown. When emergency surgery is necessary, prevention strategies include adequate intravenous fluids, circulatory support, keeping the patient warm, and broad-spectrum antibiotics (Kassis & Makary, 2008; Maykel & Fischer, 2003). If there are concerns regarding delayed healing of the intestinal anastomosis due to poorly controlled morbidities and extensive intra-abdominal infection, a temporary stoma may be created proximal to the anastomosis to protect the anastomosis during healing; the stoma is closed once healing is complete. In the past, temporary stomas were commonly performed following bowel resection and anastomosis due to traumatic injury; this is no longer standard, as most of these anastomoses have been shown to heal in a timely manner. Interestingly, recent studies indicate that diversion following colonic anastomosis for penetrating colonic injury did not reduce the incidence of septic complications, including abscess and fistula (Demetriades et al., 2001).

Medical Management

Management for this patient population requires a clear understanding of the underlying pathophysiology, astute assessment skills, knowledge about management alternatives and options, competent technical skills, diligent follow-up, and persistence. A comprehensive and effective interdisciplinary approach is required to reduce complications and achieve closure (Bryant & Best, 2015). Spontaneous closure of an ECF is defined as closing with medical management within 6 to 8 weeks (Teixeira et al., 2009). Wong et al. (2004) report 90% of simple type 1 fistulas close spontaneously, whereas <10% of complex type 2 fistulas close spontaneously. Additional factors that correlate with spontaneous closure include postoperative occurrence, low output, absence of sepsis, and adequate nutrition (Campos et al., 1999; Nussbaum & Fischer, 2006). When sepsis is controlled and appropriate nutritional support is provided, approximately 19% to 40% of all fistulas close spontaneously with medical management. The majority of ECFs that close spontaneously do so within 5 weeks (Kassis & Makary, 2008).

CLINICAL PEARL

Only a limited percentage (19% to 40%) of fistulas close spontaneously, even with optimal management; those that do close spontaneously usually do so within 5 to 6 weeks.

Objectives of ECF management are described below and include: (1) maintenance of fluid and electrolyte balance; (2) measures to minimize fistula output; (3) control of infection; (4) nutritional support; (5) definition of the fistula tract; and (6) skin protection and containment of effluent.

Maintenance of Fluid and Electrolyte Balance

Each day 8 to 10 L of fluid flows through the jejunum, depending on oral intake. In the intact functioning intestine, 98% of this fluid is (re)absorbed, leaving only 100 to 200 mL of fluid to be excreted in the stool. Development of a fistula permits abnormal fluid losses, with volume of loss determined in part by size of the fistulous opening and in part by anatomic location within the bowel. For example, fistulas located in the proximal small bowel are generally high output, while fistulas occurring in the colon are typically low output. When providing fluid replacement, the prescribing provider must consider both the volume and the composition of the fistulous drainage, both of which are impacted by fistula location within the GI tract. Severe metabolic disturbances have been noted with ECF output >200 mL/day due to loss of hydrogen, chloride, sodium, and potassium ions (Arebi & Forbes, 2004; Makhdoom et al., 2000). Careful monitoring of tissue perfusion, weight, urine, and fistula output is necessary to evaluate fluid balance. Adequate fluid and electrolyte replacement is critical to prevent hypovolemia and circulatory failure in the patient with a high-output ECF (Makhdoom et al., 2000).

Measures to Minimize Fistula Output

A key intervention for promotion of spontaneous closure is to minimize the amount of fluid flowing through the fistula tract, that is, to reduce oral and enteral intake. This may be done by making the patient NPO (nothing by mouth), or by limiting oral and/or enteral intake to the amount needed to keep the intestinal mucosa healthy. Significantly reduced oral/enteral intake minimizes fistula output by decreasing luminal contents, GI stimulation, and pancreaticobiliary secretion. Administration of H_2 antagonists (e.g., cimetidine), frequently used to prevent stress ulcerations, also decreases gastric, biliary, and pancreatic secretions. Despite this reduction in secretions, H_2 receptors have not been shown to affect either the number of ECFs that close spontaneously or the time to ECF closure (Arebi & Forbes, 2004; Evenson & Fischer, 2006).

Somatostatin and its analog, octreotide, are known to decrease intestinal output in some situations, and have been used as adjunctive therapy in the treatment of ECF. Somatostatin is administered through continuous intravenous infusion due to its short half-life of 1 to 2 minutes. Octreotide's half-life is almost 2 hours, and it is administered three times daily subcutaneously (Makhdoom et al., 2000). In the past, there was lack of consensus as to whether these medications increased closure rates or decreased time to closure (Arebi & Forbes, 2004; Fagniez & Yahchouchy, 1999; Hesse et al., 2001; Sancho et al., 1995; Torres et al., 1992). More recently, a systematic review and meta-analysis conducted by Coughlin et al. (2012) concluded that somatostatin analogs appear to decrease the duration of ECFs (time to closure) and hospital stays, though there was no reduction in number of fistulas that closed and no reduction in fistula-related mortality. Octreotide is not recommended for routine use due to reports of precipitated villous atrophy, interruption of intestinal adaptation, and acute cholecystitis. Some authors recommend a 5- to 8-day trial, with discontinuation of the octreotide if there is no significant reduction in fistula output within that time frame (Draus et al., 2006).

CLINICAL PEARL

Measures to promote spontaneous closure of ECFs include nutritional support, limited oral/enteral intake to reduce the volume of fistula output, and possibly negative pressure wound therapy (NPWT) (to promote wound healing).

Control of Infection

Uncontrolled sepsis and sepsis-associated malnutrition have been shown to be important determinants of mortality in the patient with an ECF (Dubose & Lundy, 2010; Lynch et al., 2004). Symptoms may include localized and then diffuse abdominal pain, ileus, and fever. Presence of abscess can be detected with computed tomographic scanning or ultrasound. CT-guided drainage is the initial management of choice in patients presenting with spontaneous or postoperative intra-abdominal abscess. This can obviate the need for early operative intervention. As seen in Figure 34-1, if a fistula develops, a definitive procedure can be deferred with the drain left in place to control further abscess formation (Davis et al., 2000; Lynch et al., 2004). Abscess contents should be cultured after percutaneous or surgical drainage, to assure appropriate antibiotic therapy (Wong et al., 2004).

CLINICAL PEARL

Somatostatin analogs have been shown to reduce the time to fistula closure and the length of hospital stay, but do not increase the number of fistulas that close spontaneously.

Definition of the Fistula Tract

Once the patient is stabilized, definition of the fistula tract should be undertaken. The fistula should be assessed for point of origin, condition of adjacent bowel, presence of

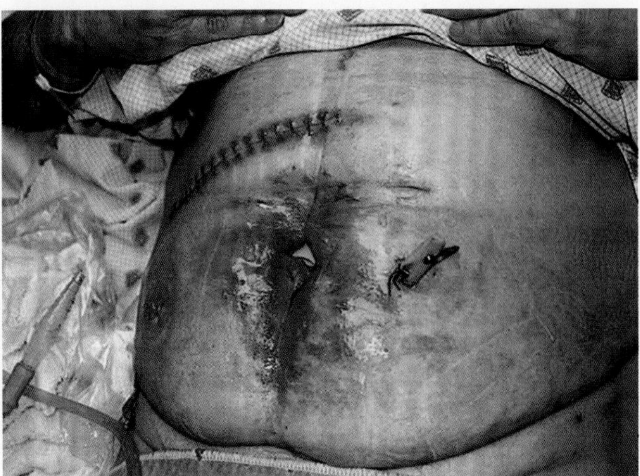

FIGURE 34-1. ECF (small bowel to skin); extensive skin damage due to enzymatic drainage; drain in place for abscess management. (Reproduced with permission from Davis, M., et al. (2000). Options for managing an open wound with draining enterocutaneous fistula, *Journal of Wound Ostomy and Continence Nursing, 27*(2), 118–123.)

abscess, and any distal obstruction or bowel discontinuity. This can be accomplished with a range of radiological examinations: fistulagram, ultrasonography, magnetic resonance imaging (MRI), positive emission tomography (PET) scan, or computerized tomography (Arebi & Forbes, 2004; Schecter et al., 2009).

Nutritional Support

As previously discussed, adequate nutritional support is an essential component of effective management; it is critical to keep the patient in positive nitrogen balance to promote healing of the fistula tract. The route of nutritional support depends on the patient's ability to ingest sufficient quantities, the location of the fistula tract, the absorptive capacity of the bowel mucosa, and the patient's tolerance.

The use of total parenteral nutrition (TPN), accompanied by simultaneous "bowel rest," has revolutionized the care of the fistula patient by allowing for the delivery of nutrition while simultaneously minimizing fistula effluent; this enhances patient management and the potential for spontaneous closure (Dubose & Lundy, 2010). On the negative side, the delivery of TPN through central venous catheters is associated with an appreciable rate of bacteremia and line sepsis. In one study conducted by Wong and colleagues (2004), positive blood cultures were obtained from 24.6% of 88 catheters utilized to deliver TPN to patients undergoing nonoperative management of enteric fistulas.

There is currently increased interest in the use of *enteral* nutrition for prevention and management of patients with ECFs, based on the role of enteral intake on the health and integrity of the intestinal mucosa; low-volume enteral intake can prevent translocation of bacteria; maintain the normal structural, immunologic, and hormonal integrity of the GI tract; and reduce cost relative to TPN (Dubose & Lundy, 2010). During a small retrospective study, Collier et al. (2007) noted that early postoperative initiation of enteral nutrition (≤4 days) resulted in a lower fistula formation rate than did nutritional approaches involving later initiation of enteral feedings (9% vs. 26%, respectively). Researchers also noted that the use of early enteral nutrition resulted in earlier primary abdominal closure and lower hospital charges.

CLINICAL PEARL

Nutritional support is a critical element of effective fistula management; the goals of nutritional management are to maintain positive nitrogen balance (usually through TPN), maintain the integrity of the intestinal mucosa (usually through low-volume enteral intake), and minimize fistula output (usually through reduced oral/enteral intake).

In selected patients, enteral nutrition may be used to maintain nutritional status while promoting fistula closure. It is now known that approximately 4 feet of healthy small intestine (in the adult) are needed to meet nutritional needs via the enteral route (Knechtges & Zimmermann, 2009). Therefore enteral nutrition may be feasible for the patient whose fistula is located in the most proximal or distal portion of a functional GI tract; if the fistula is located in the most proximal segment of the bowel, the enteral feeding must be administered distal to the fistula. Many types of enteral solutions are available, and a dietician should be consulted to recommend the most appropriate solution and administration procedure so that GI intolerance (e.g., diarrhea, abdominal distention) can be avoided.

Skin Protection and Containment

Establishing and maintaining skin protection and containment of the fistula effluent can be a challenging and yet rewarding experience. It is beneficial for WOC nurses managing the patient with an ECF to frequently remind themselves of the four general principles presented by Rolstad and Wong (2004).

1. Assess the pouching system and seal frequently; expect to make changes in the management system.
2. Build flexibility into the care plan.
3. Innovate, using the easiest, most practical approach first.
4. Recognize that care of the patient is frequently provided by inexperienced caregivers.

Skin protection and effluent containment should be initiated as soon as the fistula develops and is not contingent upon medical diagnosis. Goals for topical management of the ECF are listed in Box 34-1 (Bryant & Best, 2015). Methods and techniques for skin protection and containment will be described in the intervention section of the chapter and are presented in **Tables 34-2** and **34-3**.

CLINICAL PEARL

Skin protection and effluent containment should be initiated as soon as the fistula develops and is not contingent upon medical diagnosis nor the medical plan of care.

BOX 34-1. Goals for Topical Management of the ECF

- Perifistular skin protection
- Containment of effluent
- Odor control
- Patient comfort
- Accurate measurement of effluent
- Patient mobility
- Ease of care
- Cost containment

TABLE 34-2 Fistula Products and their Indications

Product/Accessory	Action	Indications
Skin barrier wipes, wands, or sprays	Provides a protective film to skin	**Low-output fistulae**—provides protective layer to skin. Used in combination with dressings **High-output fistulae**—used in combination with pouches, suction systems, and NPWT to protect against adhesive trauma
Moisture barrier creams, ointments, or pastes	Repels moisture and protects skin	**Low-output fistulae**—provides protection to skin around fistula. May be used in combination with dressings **High-output fistulae**—not indicated. Does not provide enough protection with high-output effluent. Contraindicated with the use of any adhesive products (i.e., pouches), as creams will not allow products to adhere to skin
Pectin barrier rings, strips, and pastes	Provides physical barrier to effluent/stool	**Low-output fistulae**—provides skin protection against effluent **High-output fistulae**—used to fill in uneven surfaces for pouching or as a part of the pouching system
Pouches	Contain effluent/stool and odor from fistula	**Low-output fistulae**—where odor is a problem or the patient prefers to change pouch as opposed to dressings **High-output fistulae**—used to contain stool and odor
Suction systems	Contain effluent in combination with low intermittent suction and dressings or pouches	**Low-output fistulae**—not indicated **High-output fistulae**—where pouching systems to gravity drainage are not effective due to large amounts of liquid effluent. Not a long-term solution
NPWT	Direct pressure closure	**Low-output fistulae**—not indicated **High-output fistulae**—where closure is a possibility. No abscess can be present. The patient must receive bowel rest and nutritional support, e.g., TPN. There should be no evidence of epithelial cells on opening of fistula (no evidence of pseudostoma formation)
Dressings	Absorb drainage	**Low-output fistulae**—used in combination with other skin protectants such as skin barrier wipes, barrier creams and pastes, and pectin wafers **High-output fistulae**—not indicated

NPO, nothing by mouth; NPWT, negative pressure wound therapy; TPN, total parenteral nutrition.

TABLE 34-3 Fistula Containment Options Based on Output and Need for Access

Output volume	<100 mL	<100 mL	>100 mL or dressing change > every 4 h	>100 mL or dressing change > every 4 h
Need for odor control	No	Yes	Yes or no	Yes or no
Need for frequent access	Yes/no	Yes/no	Yes	No
Containment options	Absorptive dressings and perifistular skin protectant (e.g., ointment, paste barrier)	Charcoal cover dressing (placed over absorptive dressings) with environmental deodorants and frequent dressing changes OR Ostomy pouch	Wound management system with window emptied frequently or attached to bedside bag OR Two-piece ostomy pouch emptied frequently Two-piece urostomy pouch emptied frequently or attached to bedside bag (urinary or fecal spout)	Pouching systems OR Closed systems with suction or attached to straight drainage NPWT

 Fistula Management for the WOC Nurse

Methods and strategies for fistula management are guided by a thorough assessment; the parameters first described by Boarini and Bryant (1986) remain the standard for fistula assessment today (Bryant & Best, 2015; CAET, 2009).

Assessment

In addition to determining the type of fistula, assessment must include abdominal contours, fistula opening, effluent characteristics, and the condition of the perifistular skin. Each dressing or pouch change represents an opportunity to reevaluate the fistula and to modify the care plan accordingly. All assessments, reassessments, interventions, responses to interventions, and management and follow-up plans should be documented (see Box 34-2).

BOX 34-2. Documentation for the WOC Nurse

Focused Assessment
- Fistula source (see Table 34-1)
- Pain
- Fistula opening
  - Location
  - Length and width
  - Height (retracted, skin level, protruding)
- Perifistular skin integrity
  - Intact
  - Impaired (erythema, maceration, candidiasis, denudement)
- Abdominal contours and proximity of fistula to: scars, skin folds, bony prominences, drains, or ostomies
- Output/effluent
  - Volume
  - Consistency
  - Color
  - Odor
- Containment system and frequency of changes

Interventions
- Emotional support
- Changes in containment method/procedure with rationale (if any change required)
- Education of patient/family
  - Normal versus impaired skin
  - Signs of infection
  - Containment procedure

Evaluation
- Indicators of progress in closure (or impediments, such as pseudostoma formation)
- Effectiveness of containment system
  - Wear time without leakage
  - Perifistular skin intact or improved
  - Odor control
  - Effects on patient mobility
  - Ease of care
- Patient/family response to interventions
  - Patient satisfaction
  - Comfort
  - Level of activity
  - Learning

Follow-up Plan
- Approximate day of next visit
- Instruction for staff between visits (including what to do if questions/concerns arise)

Progress toward/Impediments to Spontaneous Closure

A critical aspect of assessment is evaluation of progress toward and impediments to spontaneous closure (see Box 34-3). Progress in closure is evidenced by reduced output through the fistula tract along with increased fecal output through the distal bowel (rectum or stoma); thus, fistula output should be monitored, as should the output from any stoma, and the patient with an intact distal bowel should be routinely queried regarding bowel movements. Any indicators of abscess formation (e.g., increasing abdominal tenderness, fever, or purulent drainage mixed with the fecal output) must be promptly reported so that intervention can be initiated. The nurse must also be alert to development of a stomatized fistula, also known as a pseudostoma or an epithelialized stoma; this occurs when the anterior wall of the bowel becomes adherent to the abdominal wall and the fistula tract undergoes mucosal eversion. The end result is a permanent opening into the bowel that must be closed surgically; thus, observation of a "stoma" in the wound bed requires prompt MD notification (see Fig. 34-2).

CLINICAL PEARL

Assessment of the individual with a fistula must include the volume and characteristics of the output, the contours of the abdominal wall and fistula opening, and indicators of progress toward or impediments to spontaneous closure.

Abdominal Contours and Fistula Opening

The fistula opening and abdominal contours should be assessed while the patient is standing, sitting, and lying down if possible. If the pannus is large, more positions may be necessary to observe the changes in perifistular contours that occur with shifts in position of the pannus. Skin contours should be noted, and the abdomen should be inspected for irregular skin surfaces that are created by scars, creases, bony prominences, or other obstacles such as sutures/staples, incisions (dehisced or intact), or stomas. The location of the ECF should be identified, and visible openings should be measured (length and width in cm) and documented. The level at which the fistula empties in relation to the skin (or wound) surface is of critical importance. The fistula opening may be retracted (lower than skin level), level with the skin, above the level of the skin, or in a deep wound (see Fig. 34-2). If the fistula empties directly onto the skin and is level with the skin, a convex pouching system is usually required; in contrast, a

BOX 34-3. Factors that Prevent Spontaneous Closure

- Compromised distal suture line/anastomosis (i.e., tension on suture line, improper suturing technique, inadequate blood supply to anastomosis)
- Distal obstruction
- Foreign body in fistula tract or suture line
- Epithelium-lined tract contiguous with skin (pseudostoma)
- Presence of tumor or disease in site
- Previous irradiation to site
- Crohn's disease
- Abscess
- Hematoma

Adapted from Bryant, R., & Best, M. (2015). Management of draining wounds and fistulas. In R. Bryant & D. Nix (Eds.), *Acute and chronic wounds: Current management concepts* (5th ed.). St. Louis, MO: Mosby. (In Print.)

fistula that has undergone mucosal maturation (pseudostoma formation) and that protrudes above the level of the skin may enable a better pouch seal. The opening might also contain a drain, as seen in Figure 34-1, for drainage of an abscess.

CLINICAL PEARL

A "pseudostoma" occurs when the anterior wall of the bowel becomes adherent to the abdominal wall, and the fistula tract undergoes mucosal eversion to create an epithelium-lined tract. Pseudostoma development requires MD notification because it means the fistula will have to be closed surgically.

Assessment of all these parameters will help determine the level of skin protection required, as well as the flexibility, size, and shape of adhesive barrier needed for effective protection of the perifistular skin and avoidance of any areas that could compromise the adhesion of the pouching system or cause discomfort to the patient.

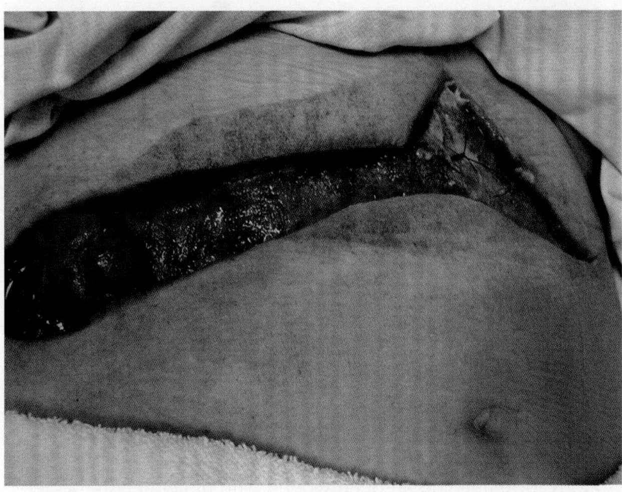

FIGURE 34-2. Pseudostoma in deep wound.

Effluent Characteristics

Assessment of fistula effluent (source, volume, odor, consistency, composition) influences topical management selection by providing insight into the degree of risk for perifistular skin breakdown and odor as well as the type of pouch closure needed. For example, an odorous fistula producing effluent with semi-formed consistency is most likely originating from the left transverse or descending colon. Effluent from the transverse or descending colon will be less damaging to the skin than is output from the small intestine or stomach. (See Fig. 34-1 for illustration of skin damage related to small bowel drainage.) Thus, the primary goals of topical management for that patient would be containment of effluent and odor control.

ECF output *volumes* >100 mL over 24 hours usually require a pouch or suction or both. In contrast, the ECF with minimal output can often be managed with the application of a perifistular moisture barrier and an absorptive dressing. However, in the presence of odor, even the patient with a low-output fistula may prefer a containment pouch for odor control. It should be noted that odor may originate from numerous sources, including fecal drainage, exudate, necrotic or infected tissue, soiled dressings, and/or chemicals used during treatment.

CLINICAL PEARL

There are multiple options for containment of fistula effluent and perifistular skin protection; the best option for an individual patient is determined by the volume and characteristics of the output and the abdominal contours.

Consistency of effluent is particularly important to selection of a pouching system because it influences the type and number of skin barriers needed as well as the type of drainage outlet required to efficiently empty the pouch. For example, liquid effluent is much more corrosive than is thick effluent and is much more likely to result in premature erosion of the skin barrier; thus, liquid effluent requires the most durable skin barrier/protectant. Liquid effluent is easier to empty from a spout rather than clamp type closure.

Constant exposure of the epidermis to moisture, enzymes, extremes in pH, and mechanical trauma frequently leads to perifistular skin damage. Denudation of perifistular skin is a common complication in fistula patients and often is present when the patient is first seen with the fistula. Perifistular skin is also at risk for fungal infection as a consequence of moisture entrapment against the skin and antibiotic precipitated changes in the normal skin flora. Candidiasis is a common secondary complication and requires treatment with a topical antifungal agent. See Chapter 17 of the wound core curriculum for additional information regarding differential assessment and management of periwound MASD.

In addition to visual inspection, valuable information can be obtained from the patient and nursing staff. For example, patient reports of burning or stinging sensations around the fistula commonly indicate denudation or erosion of the epidermis, and the patient who requires frequent dressing or pouch changes is at risk for skin damage from mechanical injury in addition to damage from exposure to the effluent.

Interventions and Containment Strategies

Fistulas can be managed with skin protection and either dressings or containment devices (pouches, suction, negative pressure). There are a wide number of products available, and the appropriate selection is based on patient assessment. Principles of management warrant repetition: begin with the easiest approach based on assessment and sound rationale, reassess frequently and be flexible, and expect that needs will change. Interventions should be based on established principles and rationale, should include measures for skin protection and containment as well as patient and family support and education, and should be appropriately documented (see Box 34-2). **Tables 34-2** and **34-3** present factors to consider when selecting containment methods.

CLINICAL PEARL

The recommended approach to determining the best system for effluent containment and skin protection is to begin with the simplest approach and modify as needed.

Skin Protectants and Barriers

Skin protectant products are available in many types and forms (**Table 34-2**). Major types include moisture barrier creams, ointments or pastes; solid pectin-based adhesive wafers, rings, or strips; hydrocolloid or karaya-formulated rings; barrier (ostomy) paste formulated with or without alcohol; barrier powder; and liquid barrier film products (skin sealant wipes, wands, and sprays with or without alcohol). As previously stated, product selection must always be based on assessment and a clear understanding of the patient's needs and the properties and indications for use of the various products. For example, moisture barrier products are appropriate only for low-output fistulas managed with dressings. Pectin-based barrier wafers, rings, strips, and paste are widely used to protect the skin and improve adhesion of pouching systems and NPWT systems. Barrier powder is used to treat denuded skin. Liquid barrier film products (also known as skin sealants) are primarily used to protect the skin against adhesive trauma. **Table 34-2** provides indications and contraindications for use of each type of barrier product.

CLINICAL PEARL

Moisture barrier ointments are used to protect the skin against moisture and drainage but are appropriate only for low-output fistulas managed with absorptive products; liquid barrier films are used primarily to protect against adhesive trauma; and pectin-based pouches, rings, and pastes are used to promote an effective pouching system and to protect the skin against enzymatic drainage.

Pectin-Based Barrier Products

Most containment pouches have an integrated solid skin barrier attached to the pouch by the manufacturer. Barrier pastes, strips, or rings are frequently needed adjunct products that are used to fill skin defects and create a flatter pouching surface, add convexity, or provide caulking to ensure a effective pouch seal. If the skin is weepy, barrier powder may be lightly applied (as shown in Fig. 34-3) to absorb moisture and improve adhesion of the barrier and pouch to the damaged skin. It is important to realize that application of excessive amounts of powder will impair adhesion. When the skin is extremely denuded, application of the powder can be followed by application of an alcohol-free liquid barrier film; these steps can be repeated up to three times to create a dry surface or crust. When applied and removed appropriately, most of these pectin barrier products are safe to use on damaged as well as intact skin. It should be noted that liquid barrier films (skin sealants) must be allowed to dry so solvents can escape before other products are applied. Some barrier films and barrier pastes contain alcohol and can cause great discomfort when used on damaged skin; the wound/ostomy nurse must provide clear protocols and ongoing staff education to assure that alcohol-free products are the "standard of care" for damaged skin. Great care must be taken to prevent medical adhesive–related skin damage (MARSI) as described in Chapter 17 of the wound core curriculum.

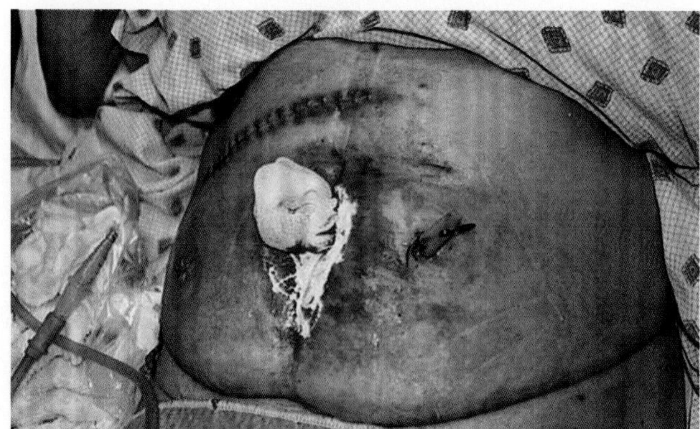

FIGURE 34-3. Pectin powder dusted onto weeping damaged skin; excess powder removed to avoid compromised adhesion of pouch. (Reproduced with permission from Davis, M., et al. (2000). Options for managing an open wound with draining enterocutaneous fistula, *Journal of Wound Ostomy and Continence Nursing, 27*(2), 118–123.)

CLINICAL PEARL

Pectin powder can be dusted onto areas of denuded skin to create a gummy protective layer; it is important to avoid excessive powder application as this would interfere with adhesion of the pouch.

Absorptive Dressings and Moisture Barriers

Fistulas that are nonodorous with low-volume output (<100 mL/day) and fistulas located in deep creases or anatomical locations that make pouching impossible may require management with dressings and moisture barriers. In these situations, the perifistular skin is protected with a liquid barrier film or a moisture barrier ointment (petrolatum, dimethicone, or zinc oxide–based ointment or paste), and absorptive dressings are then applied. The frequency of changes and reapplication of dressings and barriers is determined by the volume of drainage and the specific products being used. Absorptive dressings include gauze (sponges or strip packing), alginates, hydrofibers, foams, and combinations. When packing is required (e.g., wounds with depth, tunnels, or undermined areas), the wound or ostomy nurse must select a dressing that can be completely retrieved from the wound. If the volume of drainage is such that the dressing must be changed more frequently than every 4 to 8 hours, pouching or closed suction should be considered.

Closed Suction

Closed suction systems can provide skin protection, drainage containment, and odor control, and have been used for years as a reliable and cost-effective method for managing high-output fistulas, or fistulas that are too difficult to pouch (Jeter et al., 1990; Jones & Harbit, 2003; Kordasiewicz, 2004). The wound and surrounding skin are gently cleansed; the periwound skin is then protected with a liquid barrier film and/or hydrocolloid barrier strips. Any major skin defects adjacent to the wound can be filled with barrier strips or paste to improve adhesion of the dressing. The wound base is covered by several layers of moistened gauze to prevent damage to the wound surface by the suction catheter; suction catheters are then placed near the fistula orifice and stabilized with additional layers of moistened gauze. The entire wound is then covered with a transparent adhesive dressing, and paste is applied around the suction catheters, if needed to obtain a secure seal. The suction catheters are then connected to wall suction at a low level of continuous suction (see Fig. 34-4A–C). A Hemovac can provide the suction for short periods to increase the patient's mobility. Effluent must be liquid if suction is to be effective; thick or

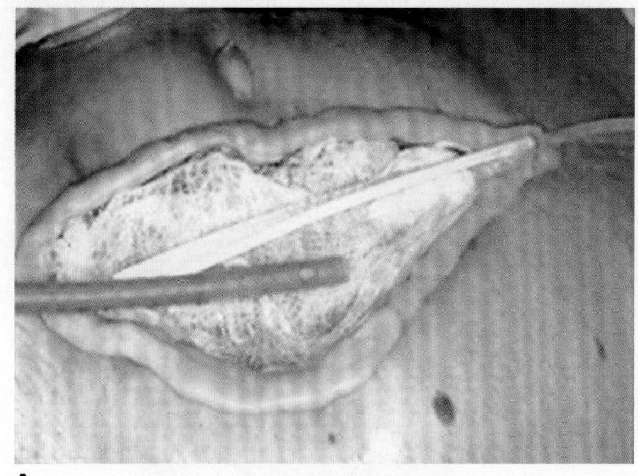

A

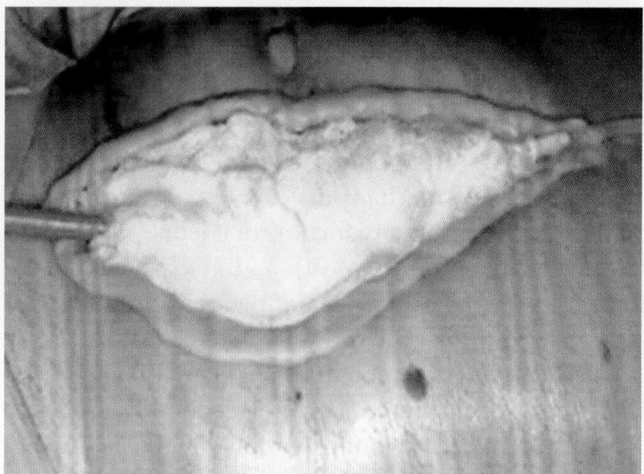

B

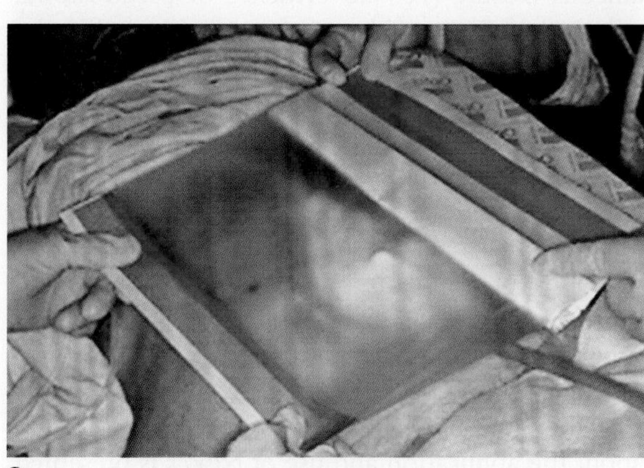

C

FIGURE 34-4. **A–C.** Closed suction procedure.

particulate effluent will occlude the catheter. Typically, these systems are changed every 2 to 3 days to prevent leakage and to permit wound assessment.

CLINICAL PEARL

Closed suction is sometimes a good option for the patient who is not a good candidate for pouching; it provides effective drainage containment and skin protection, but is used only short-term because it severely limits patient mobility.

It must be emphasized that a catheter that is inserted into the fistula tract will act as a foreign body and may interfere with healing and even increase fistula output. On the other hand, a catheter coiled in a defect above the orifice or in the open wound surrounding the fistula opening will not inhibit closure. Because firm tubes can injure fragile tissue, only soft, flexible suction catheters should be used with fistulas. Suction systems should be considered a short-term intervention because of the limitations placed on patient mobility and the time-intensive nature of the care (Dearlove, 1996; Nishide, 1997; Pontieri-Lewis, 2005).

CLINICAL PEARL

A catheter inserted into the fistula tract acts as a foreign body and prevents wound closure.

Negative Pressure Wound Therapy

NPWT incorporates a sponge or gauze and subatmospheric pressure (suction) to promote closure of fistula tracts, the removal and containment of effluent, and/or wound healing. The mechanisms involved in promotion of wound healing include reduction in edema (with associated improvement in perfusion), and mechanical deformation of cells, which has been shown to stimulate the wound repair process. NPWT systems have built-in sensors to alert caregivers to potential and actual breaches in the integrity of the system. NPWT is frequently used for fistulas located in open wounds so long as the following conditions are met: the fistula exhibits the potential for spontaneous closure (i.e., no evidence of pseudostoma formation); there is no evidence of exposed bowel in the wound base; and there is no evidence of abscess or distal obstruction. Caution should be used to prevent any additional fistula formation, that is, a contact layer or the nonporous "white" foam should be used in contact with the wound bed. If the effluent is too thick for suction, or if the fistula has "stomatized" but the wound still needs NPWT for promotion of granulation tissue formation, there are techniques that segregate the fistula for management with pouching while permitting continued use of NPWT for promotion of wound healing (Bruhin et al., 2014; CAET, 2009; Reed et al., 2006) (see Box 34-4). Further information about the application and use of NPWT is presented in Chapter 11 of the wound core curriculum.

BOX 34-4. Procedure for Isolating a Fistula for NPWT

1. Assemble equipment: Ostomy pouch and supplies, NPWT supplies, skin barrier ring, skin barrier paste, transparent dressing.
2. Prepare ostomy/fistula pouch as described in Box 34-5. Apply bead of paste to back of pouch around opening.

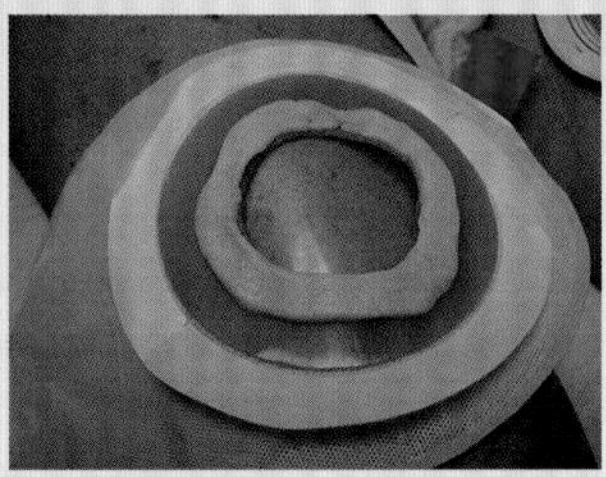

3. Cut a ring out of NPWT sponge dressing material slightly larger than the stomatized fistula; place into wound bed around fistula opening.

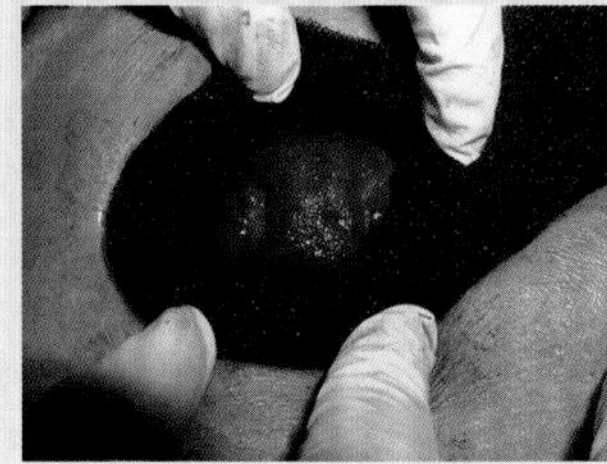

4. Optional: Place skin barrier ring right around fistula and over the NPWT sponge ring; apply bead of paste directly around fistula to caulk area between fistula and barrier ring.
5. Proceed to dress the wound utilizing NPWT procedure/protocol. Initiate suction and assure secure seal.

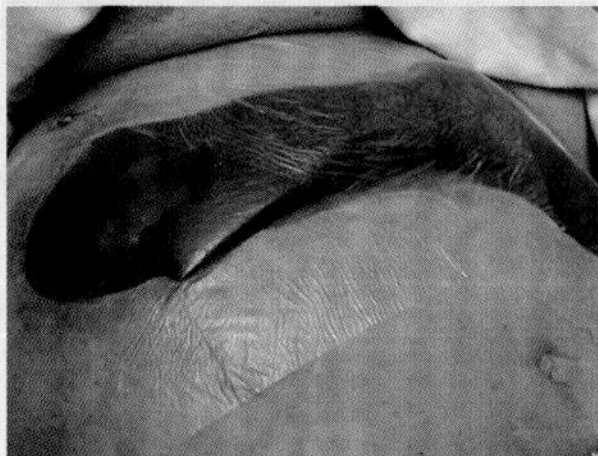

6. Cut an opening in the transparent dressing over fistula.

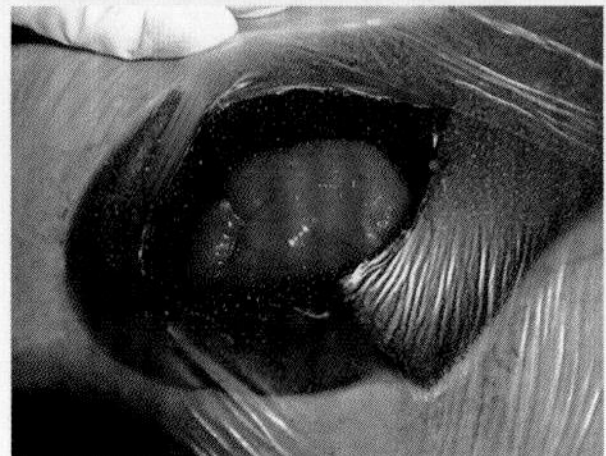

7. Apply the pouch over the fistula on top of the NPWT dressing; close the end of the pouch.

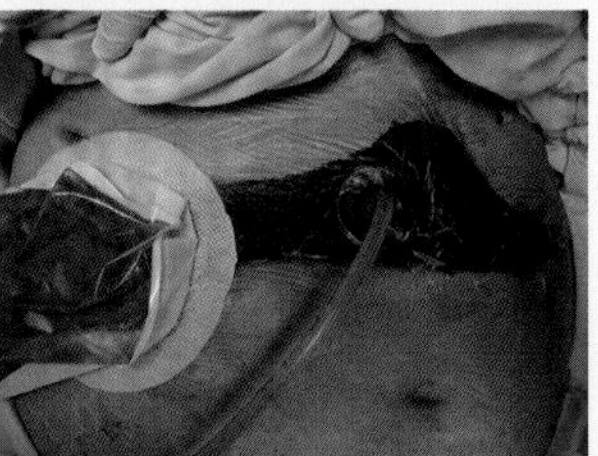

Photos courtesy of: Terri Reed and Diana Economon

CLINICAL PEARL

NPWT can be used to promote wound healing and fistula closure so long as there are no impediments to spontaneous closure; a contact layer or nonporous foam should be used in contact with the wound bed to prevent any additional trauma.

Pouching Systems

Fistula pouches, ostomy pouches (pediatric or adult), retracted penis pouches, and fecal incontinence collectors have all been used for fistula management. Most are preattached to solid-wafer skin barriers. Additional pectin skin barrier products may be required to caulk edges, fill creases, and/or add convexity (see Table 34-2).

When the fistula is located adjacent to an incision, the attached barrier of the pouch sometimes needs to be placed over the incision to prevent leakage onto the incision. When applied and removed appropriately, these products will protect rather than harm an incision. A simple strategy for protection of the incision is to place steristrips or tape strips over the suture line or staple line prior to application of the pouching system.

Strategies to promote adhesion of the pouch to the perifistular skin include assurance of a dry surface; a moist surface will impair pouch adhesion. Pectin barrier powders (NOT talc or corn starch) may be used to absorb moisture from denuded skin and to create a dry surface that supports pouch adherence. The amount of skin barrier powder used should be just enough to absorb the moisture and create a gummy or dry surface; too much powder will impair the adhesion of the pouch. Severely denuded skin may benefit from the "crusting" procedure, as described previously.

CLINICAL PEARL

If a pouching system or NPWT dressing extends over the suture or staple line, steristrips or tape strips should be placed over the incision for protection prior to application of the dressing or pouching system.

Medical adhesive products approved for the skin should be used according to manufacturers' instructions and only when needed. Medical adhesives can be used to enhance the tack of an existing adhesive, extend the adhesive surface on a pouch, or to compensate for the reduced adhesion caused by the application of skin barrier powder onto denuded perifistular skin. Medical adhesives are formulated as liquids/cements, medical adhesive sprays, and adhesive strips, rings, and sheets. Some adhesive products contain potential irritants or allergens, such as latex and/or alcohol; therefore, it is critical for the wound or ostomy nurse to carefully evaluate any adhesive product being considered for use in terms of indications, contraindications, and guidelines for use. Adhesive liquids and sprays must be allowed to dry completely in order for solvents to evaporate and the adhesive product to become tacky (Bryant, 1994, Bryant & Best, 2015).

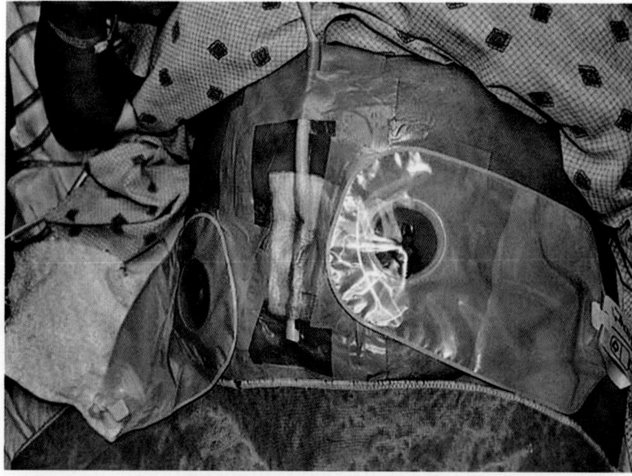

FIGURE 34-5. Two pouches used for separate fistulas. (Reproduced with permission from Davis, M., et al. (2000). Options for managing an open wound with draining enterocutaneous fistula, *Journal of Wound Ostomy and Continence Nursing, 27*(2), 118–123.)

If two drainage/fistula sites are too far apart to be included in one pouching system, two pouches may be necessary (see Fig. 34-5) (Davis et al., 2000). When the fistula is located in a deep wound (see Fig. 34-2), it may be helpful to select a pouching system with an integrated window/access cap that facilitates adjunct use of a wound filler dressing such as an alginate or an antimicrobial or saline-moistened gauze. A pattern and procedure for preparation, removal, and application of the pouching system should be created, dated, and kept in the patient's room with instructions and supplies. Figure 34-6 and Box 34-5 present examples of a pattern and pouch change procedure.

Pouching System Adaptations

There are situations in which adaptations of standard pouching techniques are required. Pouching system

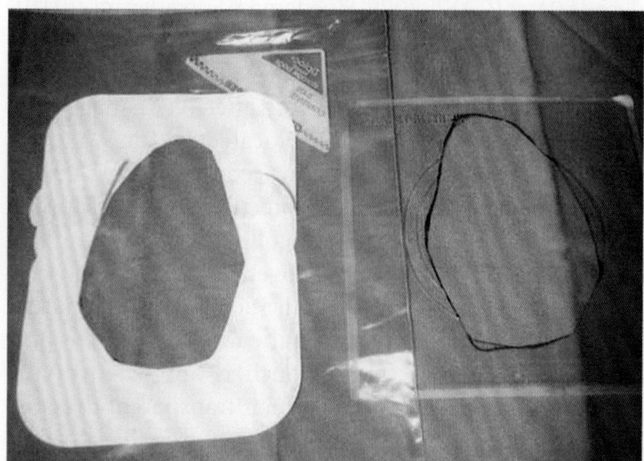

FIGURE 34-6. Pattern for fistula pouch. (Reproduced with permission from Davis, M., et al. (2000). Options for managing an open wound with draining enterocutaneous fistula, Journal of Wound Ostomy and Continence Nursing, 27(2), 118–123.)

BOX 34-5. Fistula Pouch Change Procedure

1. Assemble equipment
   Pouch with integrated skin barrier, pattern, skin barrier paste, scissors, closure device or attachment for bedside bag, water, soft gauze.
2. Prepare pouch.
   A. Trace pattern onto skin barrier surface of pouch. Note: the pattern should provide at least ¼ inch "clearance" of the wound edges (to prevent undermining of drainage under edge of pouch).
   B. Pull the anterior pouch surface away from posterior surface to avoid accidentally cutting hole in pouch surface.
   C. Cut out skin barrier surface according to tracing.
   D. Remove protective backing(s) from the pouch.
3. Remove and apply the pouch.
   A. Remove the pouch, using "push–pull" technique; gently press down on skin with one hand while pulling up on the pouch with the other.
   B. Discard the pouch and save closure clip or attachment device for bedside bag.
   C. Control any discharge with soft gauze.
   D. Clean the skin with water or gentle skin cleanser (without emollients that may impair adhesion of the pouch).
   E. Dry gently and thoroughly.
   F. Position the patient so abdomen has minimal wrinkles and folds (usually supine).
   G. Apply paste around the fistula. Fill in any uneven skin surfaces with paste, barrier rings, or skin barrier strips as needed.
   H. Apply a new pouch, centering fistula/wound site in opening.
   I. Close the bottom of the pouch with clip or attach to bedside bag.

adaptations (e.g., bridging, saddlebagging, and troughing) have been previously described and illustrated by Bryant (1994), and are recognized internationally over two decades later (CAET, 2009; Hoedema & Suryadevara, 2010). These techniques will be briefly described and illustrated (Figs. 34-7 to 34-9).

Troughing (Fig. 34-7) is a very effective management technique when the fistula is located within an open wound and routine pouching procedures are ineffective. The periwound skin is first protected with overlapping strips of pectin barrier or hydrocolloid wafer and/or barrier paste. The wound is then covered with a transparent adhesive dressing; prior to application of the transparent dressing, an opening is cut into the most dependent portion of the dressing and a pouch is applied over the opening. The opening in the pouch/transparent dressing unit must be placed at the junction between the skin and the inferior aspect of the wound, and must be wider than the diameter of the wound at that point. Since most wounds for which the trough procedure is required are very large, it is helpful to apply the transparent adhesive

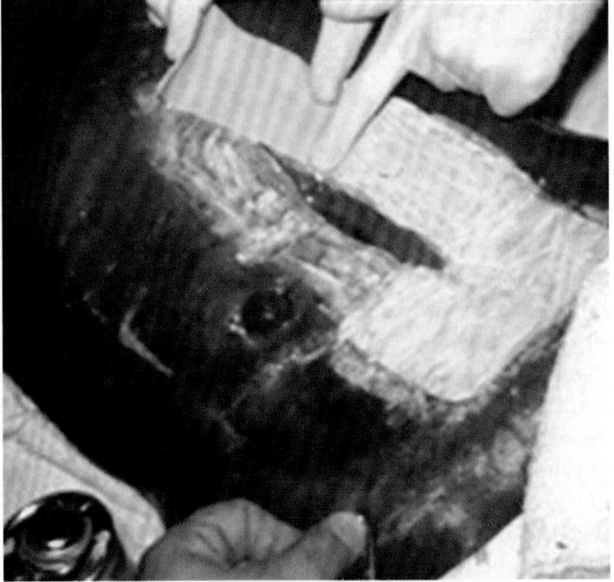

A

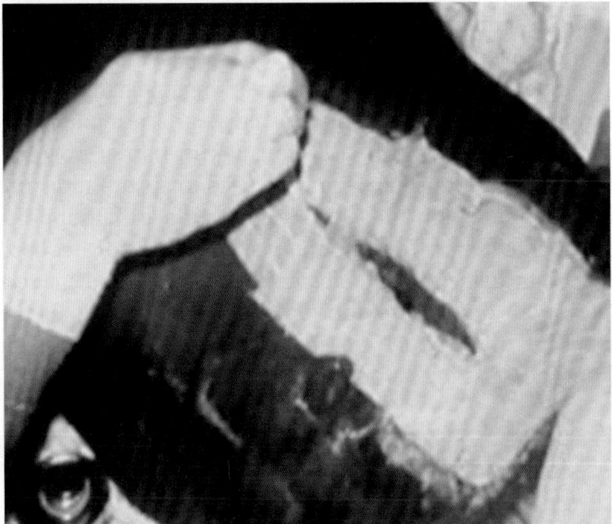

B

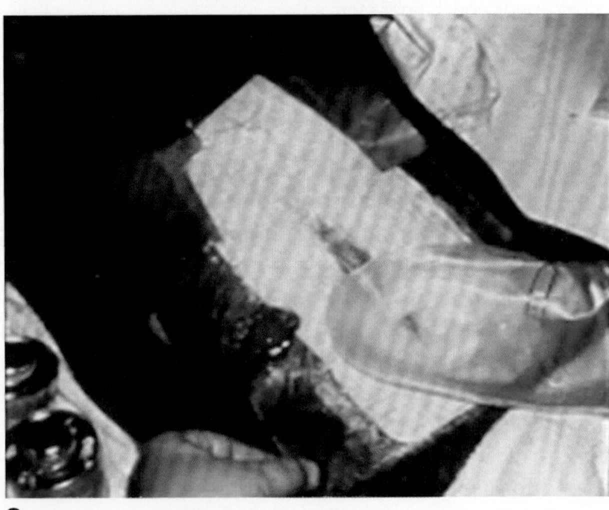

C

FIGURE 34-7. **A–C.** Troughing procedure.

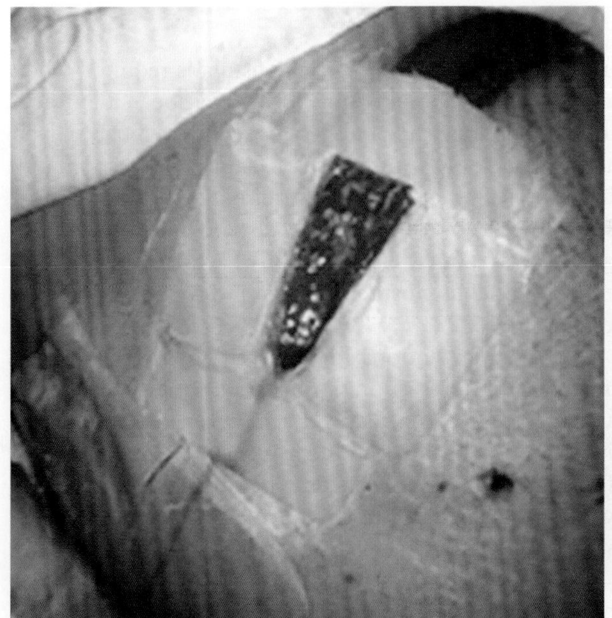
A

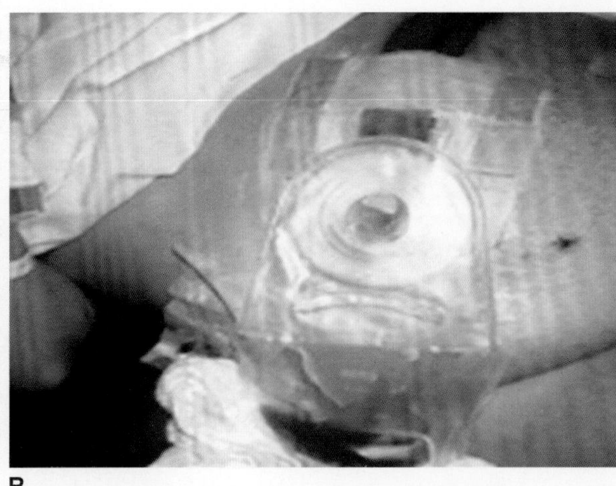
B

FIGURE 34-8. **A** and **B.** Bridging.

dressing in overlapping strips. (Typically the strips are applied from "bottom" to "top"; the bottom strip is the one with the opening and the pouch.) Since most of these fistulas are high output, it is helpful to select a pouch with a spout that can be connected to gravity drainage (or to wall suction if needed) (Bryant, 1994; Hoedema & Suryadevara, 2010).

CLINICAL PEARL

Troughing can frequently be used to provide effective skin protection and containment of effluent for patients in whom a secure pouch seal cannot be maintained.

A common concern in management of fistulas located within open wounds and managed either by pouching or troughing is the impact of small bowel drainage on the healing process. Fortunately, the enzymes in small bowel fluid do not attack the newly formed collagen and blood vessels that comprise granulation tissue, and the very low bacterial counts in small bowel fluid minimize the risk of infection. Clinicians consistently observe that wounds with fistulas continue to heal at the expected rate despite exposure to small bowel effluent.

Bridging (Fig. 34-8) may be used when the fistula is located at the inferior aspect of a long vertically oriented wound or at the most lateral aspect of an extensive horizontally oriented wound. The goal is to isolate the fistula from the remainder of the wound so that the fistula can be managed with pouching or troughing and the wound can be managed with moist wound healing or packing. Steps in the bridging procedure are as follows: (1) Identify a point slightly above (or medial to) the fistula at which the bridge will be "built." (2) Apply 1-inch strips of pectin barrier or hydrocolloid wafer in layers to create a structure that fills the wound at that point and extends slightly above skin level. (The white foam used for NPWT therapy can also be used to create a bridge that fills the wound and extends slightly above the skin surface.) (3) Cut a strip of pectin barrier or hydrocolloid wafer that is 1-inch wide (to match the width of the bridge) and long enough to cover the diameter of the wound and 2 inches of skin on either

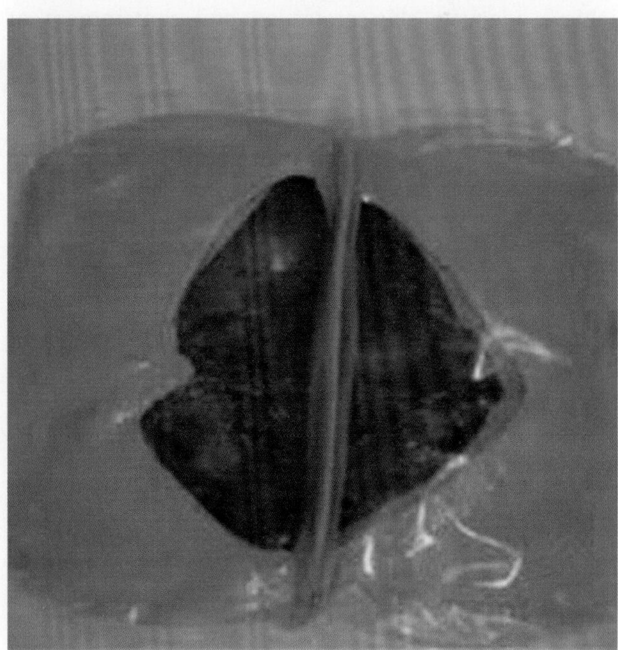

FIGURE 34-9. Saddlebagging: Example of two fistula pouches connected together along the adhesive surface to make one larger adhesive surface.

side of the wound. Place the covering strip over the bridge and onto the surrounding skin. (4) Proceed with pouching or troughing of the fistula and management of the remaining wound according to moist wound healing principles (Bryant, 1994; Hoedema & Suryadevara, 2010).

CLINICAL PEARL

Wounds continue to heal at the expected rate despite exposure to small bowel effluent.

Saddlebagging (Fig. 34-9) is a technique in which two pouches are attached at the skin barrier adhesive edges of each pouch to create one pouch with a larger adhesive surface than standard pouches (Bryant, 1994; CAET, 2009). This technique may be necessary for larger fistulas or fistulas within a large wound that need to be pouched.

Education and Emotional Support

Education and emotional support are critical aspects of the plan of care and its effectiveness. Patients report feelings of loss of control, frustration, embarrassment, hopelessness, isolation, and demoralization due to prolonged hospitalization, financial concerns, alterations in body image, and uncertain outcomes (Haffejee, 2004; Kaushal & Carlson, 2004; Kozell & Martins, 2003; Lloyd et al., 2006; Renton et al., 2006). Unfortunately, these feelings are exacerbated by the inability to eat normally, the possibility/probability of additional surgical procedures, the trial and error process so often required to achieve adequate skin protection and containment of effluent, and the prolonged care trajectory (Kozell & Martins, 2003).

CLINICAL PEARL

Education and emotional support are critical aspects of care for the patient with a fistula and his/her family.

Open communication with the patient and family will decrease anxiety, increase trust, and facilitate independence (Cobb & Knaggs, 2003; Kaushal & Carlson, 2004; Kozell & Martins, 2003). Education should be individualized based on goals of care, specific management approaches, and the patient's needs and learning style. Whenever possible, the patient should learn by participating in his/her care to gain back his/her independence and sense of control. It is important for the wound or ostomy nurse to help the patient and family to establish realistic goals and expectations, and to understand that fistula management and educational needs change over time (Burch & Buchan, 2004; Kozell & Martins, 2003).

Surgical Closure

Surgical intervention to close the fistula is required when impediments to spontaneous closure have been identified, and/or when the fistula fails to close spontaneously. Given the fact that only a minority of fistulas close spontaneously, surgical intervention is required for closure of most fistulas. Surgical procedures may also be indicated for palliation (Nussbaum & Fischer, 2006). Factors known to prevent spontaneous closure are listed in Box 34-3 (Bryant & Best, 2015).

Surgical interventions for ECFs either divert the fecal stream (without resection of the fistula) or provide definitive resection of the fistula tract. Diversion techniques divert the stool away from the fistula site without removal of the fistula by creating a stoma proximal to the fistula or by anastomosing (end-to-end or side-to-side) the two segments of bowel on each side of the fistula. This approach is required when resection of the fistula is not possible or appropriate, such as in the presence of extensive or recurrent malignancy or inadequate perfusion in the vicinity of the fistula due to previous surgery, scar formation, or prior irradiation. The process of resection involves removal of the diseased tissue and fistula tract followed by end-to-end anastomosis of the intestine. To protect the anastomosis, diversion of the fecal stream through a temporary stoma may be indicated. If the fistula involves the colon and the distal colon and rectum are not suitable for anastomosis or the anal sphincters are not competent, a permanent stoma with a Hartmann pouch may be the safest procedure. Enteric fistulas communicating with the urinary tract will always require diversion of the fecal stream proximal to the fistula site to prevent urinary tract infections and pyelonephritis. Timing of surgery depends on the patient's status. Surgery for a type 1 fistula is appropriate when the patient is nutritionally and metabolically stable, the fistula tract has been free of infection for 6 to 8 weeks, and the abdominal wall and peritoneal cavity have returned to a relatively soft, supple, pliable state; the goal is to maximize the potential for successful closure of the fistula, and to minimize the potential for additional complications, including recurrent fistula formation. Judicious timing is warranted for surgical closure of complex type 2 fistulas; surgery is usually delayed for 3 to 6 months, which is extremely frustrating for the patient and family. The wound/ostomy nurse must be able to explain to the patient and family that the extensive intra-abdominal infection associated with the original bowel perforation or anastomotic breakdown resulted in formation of extensive scar tissue within the abdominal cavity (obliterative peritonitis), and that it takes a number of months for the scar tissue to soften enough for the surgeon to separate the loops of bowel and remove the fistula tract without risking additional injury to the bowel and additional fistula formation. Nutritional, metabolic and immunologic status should be restored prior to surgery (Wong et al., 2004); for the patient with an ECF, this usually means that TPN will be required until the fistula is closed. However, the restrictions on oral intake are usually liberalized once it is clear that the fistula will not close spontaneously and that surgical intervention will be required; typically patients are allowed to eat and drink small amounts for pleasure and to keep the bowel mucosa healthy, as discussed earlier.

CLINICAL PEARL

Surgical closure is required for fistulas with known impediments to healing, and for those that "fail" medical management (i.e., fail to close within 5 to 6 weeks of comprehensive management); surgical intervention is usually delayed for several months to permit softening of intra-abdominal adhesions.

Vesicovaginal, Rectovaginal, or Enterovaginal Fistulas

While the vast majority of fistulas involve openings between two loops of bowel or between the bowel and the skin, fistulous openings can also develop between the bladder, rectum, or small bowel and the vagina. Fistulas between the bladder and vagina are typically managed initially by urinary diversion (indwelling urethral or suprapubic catheter or nephrostomy tubes), followed by surgery to close the fistula tract. The urine draining continually from the vagina is usually managed with absorptive pads; alternatively, a balloon-tipped catheter can be placed in the vagina and connected to a leg bag. (If the diameter of the vaginal vault exceeds the diameter of the inflated balloon, causing the catheter to constantly slip out of place, the catheter can be threaded through a baby nipple so that the tip of the catheter rests just above the base of the nipple; the baby nipple/catheter unit is then folded and gently inserted into the vagina so that the base of the nipple rests within the introitus to minimize leakage.) This technique can also be used for management of enterovaginal fistulas; because the drainage is thicker, it is necessary to use a large diameter catheter. Rectovaginal fistulas are typically managed by fecal diversion to permit healing of the fistula tract. For the patient who is not a candidate for surgical intervention, the focus of management should be measures to minimize vaginal contamination, specifically, titration of fiber and fluid intake to maintain soft formed stool that will not pass through the narrow fistulous tract. The patient can also be counseled to use mild antiseptics approved for intravaginal use to reduce or eliminate odor (e.g., TrimoSan).

Conclusions

Caring for a patient with a fistula is one of the most challenging, and rewarding, situations the WOC nurse will encounter (Hoedema & Suryadevara, 2010; McNaughton et al., 2010; Schaffner et al., 1994). Effective management requires a clear understanding of the anatomy of the fistula tract and plan of care, ongoing assessment regarding progress in closure or evidence of failure to close, creativity in developing an effective strategy for containment of effluent and odor, and consistent support and education for the patient and family. The key ingredients to positive outcomes when managing a patient with a fistula are patience; persistence; interdisciplinary collaboration; close surveillance; excellent communication with the patient, family, and colleagues; and a little ingenuity.

REFERENCES

Arebi, N., & Forbes, A. (2004). High output fistula. *Clinics in Colon and Rectal Surgery, 17*(2), 89–98.

Boarini, J., & Bryant, R. A. (1986). Fistula management. *Seminars in Oncology Nursing, 2*, 287.

Bryant, R. (1992). Management of drain sites and fistulas. In R. Bryant (Ed.), *Acute and chronic wounds: Nursing management*. St. Louis, MO: Mosby.

Bryant, R., & Best, M. (2015). Management of draining wounds and fistulas. In R. Bryant & D. Nix (Eds.), *Acute and chronic wounds: Current management concepts* (5th ed.). St. Louis, MO: Mosby. (In Print.)

Bruhin, A., Ferreira, F., Chariker, M., et al. (2014). Systematic review and evidence based recommendations for the use of negative pressure wound therapy in the open abdomen. *International Journal of Surgery, 12*(10), 1105–1114.

Burch, J., & Buchan, D. (2004). Support and guidance for failure and enterocutaneous fistula care. *Gastrointestinal Nursing, 2*(7), 25–32.

Campos, A. C., Andrade, D. F., Campos, G. M., et al. (1999). A multivariate model to determine prognostic factors in gastrointestinal fistulas. *Journal of the American College of Surgery, 188*(5), 483–490.

Canadian Association for Enterostomal Therapy (CAET). (2009). Best practice recommendations for management of enterocutaneous fistulae.

Cobb, A., & Knaggs, E. (2003). The nursing management of enterocutaneous fistulae: A challenge for all. *British Journal of Community Nursing, 8*(9), S32–S38.

Collier, B., Guillamondegui, O., Cotton, B., et al. (2007). Feeding the open abdomen. *Journal of Parenteral and Enteral Nutrition, 31*(5), 410–415.

Coughlin, S., Roth, L., Lurati, G., et al. (2012). Somatostatin analogues for the treatment of enterocutaneous fistulas: A systematic review and meta-analysis. *World Journal of Surgery, 36*(5), 1016–1029.

Davis, M., Dere, K., Hadley, G., et al. (2000). Options for managing an open wound with draining enterocutaneous fistula. *Journal of Wound, Ostomy, and Continence Nursing, 27*(2), 118–123.

Dearlove, J. L. (1996). Skin care management of gastrointestinal fistulas. *Surgical Clinics of North America, 76*(5), 1095–1109.

Demetriades, D., Murray, J. A., Chan, L., et al. (2001). Committee on Multicenter Clinical Trials. American Association for the Surgery of Trauma penetrating colon injuries requiring resection: Diversion or primary anastomosis? An AAST prospective multicenter study. *Journal of Trauma, 50*(5), 765–775.

Demetriades, D., Murray, J. A., Chan, L. S., et al. (2002). Hand sewn versus stapled anastomosis in penetrating colon injuries requiring resection: A multicenter study. *Journal of Trauma, 52*(1), 117–121.

Draus, J. M. Jr., Huss, S. A., Harty, N. J., et al. (2006). Enterocutaneous fistula: Are treatments improving? *Surgery, 140*(4), 570–576; discussion 576–578.

Dubose, J., & Lundy, J. (2010). Enterocutaneous fistulas in the setting of trauma and critical illness. *Clinics in Colon and Rectal Surgery, 23*(3), 182–189.

Evenson, A. R., & Fischer, J. E. (2006). Current management of enterocutaneous fistula. *Journal of Gastrointestinal Surgery, 10*(3), 455–464.

Fagniez, P. L., & Yahchouchy, E. (1999). Use of somatostatin in the treatment of digestive fistulas. *Digestion, 60*(Suppl. 3), 65.

Haffejee, A. A. (2004). Surgical management of high output enterocutaneous fistulae: A 24 year experience. *Current Opinion in Clinical Nutrition and Metabolic Care, 7*, 309–316.

Hesse, U., Ysebaert, B., & de Hemptinne, B. (2001). Role of somatostatin-14 and its analogues in the management of gastrointestinal fistulae: Clinical data. *Gut, 49*(Suppl. IV), iv11.

Hoedema, R., & Suryadevara, S. (2010). Enterostomal therapy and wound care of the enterocutaneous fistula patient. *Clinics in Colon and Rectal Surgery, 23*(3), 161–168.

Hollington, P., Maurdsley, J., Lim, W., et al. (2004). An 11 year experience of enterocutaneous fistulae. *British Journal of Surgery, 91*, 1046–1051.

Huether, S. (2002). The cellular environment: Fluids and electrolytes, acids and bases. In K. McCance & S. Huether (Eds.), *Pathophysiology: The biologic basis for disease in adults and children* (4th ed.). St. Louis, MO: Mosby.

Jeter, K. F., Tintle, T. E., & Chariker M. (1990). Managing draining wounds and fistulae: New and established methods. In D. Krasner (Ed.), *Chronic wound care: A clinical source book for healthcare professionals* (pp. 240–246). King of Prussia, PA: Health Management.

Jones, E. G., & Harbit, M. (2003). Management of an ileostomy and mucous fistula located in a dehisced wound in a patient with morbid obesity. *Journal of Wound, Ostomy, and Continence Nursing, 30*(6), 351.

Kassis, E. S., & Makary, M. A. (2008). Enterocutaneous fistula. In J. S. Cameron (Ed.), *Current surgical therapy* (9th ed.). St. Louis, MO: Mosby.

Kaushal, M., & Carlson, G. L. (2004). Management of enterocutaneous fistulae. *Clinics in Colon and Rectal Surgery, 17*(2), 79–87.

Kaur, N., & Minocha, V. (2000). Review of a hospital experience of enterocutaneous fistula. *Tropical Gastroenterology, 21*(4), 197.

Kirkpatrick, A. W., Baxter, K. A., Simons, R. K., et al. (2003). Intra-abdominal complications after surgical repair of small bowel injuries: An international review. *Journal of Trauma, 55*(3), 399–406.

Knechtges, P., & Zimmermann, E. M. (2009). Intra-abdominal abscesses and fistulae. In T. Yamada et al. (Eds.), *Textbook of Gastroenterology, Vol II* (6th ed.). Philadelphia, PA: Lippincott Williams & Wilkins.

Kordasiewicz, L. M. (2004). Abdominal wound with fistula and large amount of drainage status after incarcerated hernia repair. *Journal of Wound, Ostomy, and Continence Nursing, 31*(3), 150.

Kozell, K., & Martins, L. (2003). Managing the challenges of enterocutaneous fistulae. *Wound Care Canada, 1*(1), 10–14.

Lal, S., Teubner, A., & Shaffer, J. L. (2006). Review article: intestinal failure. *Alimentary Pharmacology and Therapeutics, 24*, 19–31.

Li, J., Ren, J., Zhu, W., et al. (2003). Management of enterocutaneous fistulae: 30-Year clinical experience. *Chinese Medical Journal, 116*(2), 171–175.

Lloyd, D. A. J., Gabe, S. M., & Windsor, A. C. J. (2006). Nutrition and management of enterocutaneous fistula. *British Journal of Surgery, 93*, 1045–1055.

Lynch, A. C., Delaney, C. P., Senagore, A. J., et al. (2004). Clinical outcome and factors predictive of recurrence after enterocutaneous fistula surgery. *Annals of Surgery, 240*(5), 825–831.

Mäkelä, J. T., Kiviniemi, H., & Laitinen, S. (2003). Risk factors for anastomotic leakage after left-sided colorectal resection with rectal anastomosis. *Diseases of the Colon and Rectum, 46*(5), 653–660.

Makhdoom, Z. A., Komar, M. J., & Still, C. D. (2000). Nutrition and enterocutaneous fistulas. *Journal of Clinical Gastroenterology, 31*(3), 195.

Maykel, J. A., & Fischer, J. E. (2003). Current management of intestinal fistulas. In J. L. Cameron (Ed.), *Advances in surgery*. St. Louis, MO: Mosby.

McNaughton, V., Canadian Association for Enterostomal Therapy ECF Best Practice Recommendations Panel, Brown, J., et al. (2010). Summary of best practice recommendations for management of enterocutaneous fistulae from the Canadian Association for Enterostomal Therapy ECF Best Practice Recommendations Panel. *Journal of Wound, Ostomy, and Continence Nursing, 37*(2), 173–184.

Meissner, K. (1999). Late radiogenic small bowel damage: Guidelines for the general surgeon. *Digestive Surgery, 16*, 169.

Nishide, K. (1997). Development of closed-suction pouch drainage for giant fistulae: A report on two cases. *WCET Journal, 17*(1), 16–19.

Nussbaum, M. S., & Fischer, D. R. (2006). Gastric, duodenal and small intestinal fistulas. In C. J. Yeo, et al. (Eds.), *Shackelford's surgery of the alimentary tract* (6th ed.). St. Louis, MO: Saunders.

Oneschuk, D., & Bruera, E. (1997). Successful management of multiple enterocutaneous fistulae in a patient with metastatic colon cancer. *Journal of Pain and Symptom Management, 14*(2), 121–124.

Pontieri-Lewis, V. (2005). Management of gastrointestinal fistulae: A case study. *Medical-Surgical Nursing, 14*(1), 68–72.

Reed, T., Economon, D., & Wiersema-Bryant, L. (2006). Colocutaneous fistula management in a dehisced wound: A case study. *Ostomy Wound Management, 52*(4), 60–64, 66.

Renton, S., Robertson, I., & Speirs, M. (2006). Alternative management of complex wounds and fistulae. *British Journal of Nursing, 15*(16), 851–853.

Rolstad, B., & Wong, W. D. (2004). Nursing considerations in intestinal fistulas. In P. A. Cataldo, & J. M. MacKeigan (Eds.), *Intestinal Stomas: Principles, Techniques, and Management* (2nd ed.). New York, NY: Marcel Dekker.

Saclarides, T. J. (2002). Rectovaginal fistula. *Surgical Clinics of North America, 82*, 1261.

Sancho, J. J., di Costanzo, J., Nubiola, P., et al. (1995). Randomized double-blind placebo-controlled trial of early octreotide in patients with postoperative enterocutaneous fistula. *British Journal of Surgery, 82*(5), 638–641.

Schaffner, A., Hocevar, B. J., & Erwin-Toth, P. (1994). Small-bowel fistulas complicating midline surgical wounds. *Journal of Wound, Ostomy, and Continence Nursing, 21*, 161–165.

Schecter, W. P., Hirshberg, A., Chang, D. S., et al. (2009). "Enteric fistula" principles of management. *Journal of the American College of Surgeons, 209*(4), 484–491.

Teixeira, P. G., Inaba, K., Dubose, J., et al. (2009). Enterocutaneous fistula complicating trauma laparotomy: A major resource burden. *American Surgeon, 75*(1), 30–32.

Telem, D. A., Chin, E. H., Nguyen, S. Q., et al. (2010). Risk factors for anastomotic leak following colorectal surgery: A case–control study. *Archives of Surgery, 145*(4), 371–376.

Torres, A. J., Landa, J. I., Moreno-Azcoita, M., et al. (1992). Somatostatin in the management of gastrointestinal fistulas. A multicenter trial. *Archives of Surgery*, 127(1), 97–99, discussion 100.

Tran, N. A., & Thorson, A. G. (2008). Rectovaginal fistula. In J.L. Cameron (Ed.), *Current surgical therapy* (9th ed.). St. Louis, MO: Mosby.

Wong, W. D., et al. (2004). Management of intestinal fistulas. In P. A. Cataldo & J. M. MacKeigan (Eds.), *Intestinal stomas: Principles, techniques, and management* (2nd ed.). New York, NY: Marcel Dekker.

QUESTIONS

1. The wound care nurse suspects that a patient's surgical wound is developing a fistula. Which of the following is the definitive indicator of a cutaneous fistula?
   A. Fever and infection in the wound bed
   B. Abdominal pain and wound dehiscence
   C. Blood migrating from a wound bed to the gastrointestinal tract
   D. Passage of gastrointestinal secretions or urine into an open wound bed

2. A patient is diagnosed with an enterocutaneous fistula with a high-output volume. Which statement correctly defines this diagnosis?
   A. A passage is created from the intestine to the skin, and the volume is >500 mL/24 h.
   B. A passage is created from the colon to the vagina, and the volume output is >500 mL/24 h.
   C. A passage is created from the bladder to the vagina, and the volume output is 200 to 500 mL/24 h.
   D. A passage is created from the colon to the skin, and the volume output is <200 mL/24 h.

3. The wound care nurse is assessing the wound of a patient diagnosed with a type 1 complex fistula. What data regarding the fistula would the nurse document in the patient record?
   A. Fistula with a short direct tract, no abscess, no other organ involvement
   B. Fistula with an abscess, with multiple organ involvement
   C. Fistula that opens into the base of the wound
   D. Fistula with a tract that is contained within the body

4. What is the etiology of the majority of enterocutaneous fistulas (ECFs)?
   A. Bowel disease
   B. Diverticulitis
   C. Surgical procedures
   D. External trauma

5. The wound care nurse is planning care for a patient with an enterocutaneous fistula (ECF). What is a key initial step in managing a patient with ECF?
   A. Administer H_2 antagonists to decrease ECF closure time.
   B. Use a 2-week trial of octreotide to reduce fistula output.
   C. Limit oral or enteral intake to amount keeping intestinal mucosa healthy.
   D. Force fluids to decrease gastric, biliary, and pancreatic secretions.

6. A patient is diagnosed with an intra-abdominal abscess following a CT scan. What is the initial management of choice for this patient?
   A. CT-guided drainage
   B. Surgical intervention
   C. Pharmacological management
   D. Keeping the patient NPO for 3 days

7. Which of the following assessment findings indicates that the patient will require surgical closure?
   A. Output exceeding 750 mL/24 h.
   B. Evidence of mucosal eversion/pseudostoma formation.
   C. History indicates fistula has been present >14 days.
   D. Hypertrophic granulation tissue in wound bed.

8. The wound care nurse is recommending products for patients with fistulas. Which product is used correctly?
   A. Moisture barrier cream for a high-output fistula
   B. Negative pressure wound therapy (NPWT) for a low-output fistula
   C. Suction system for a low-output fistula
   D. Pouch for a high- or low-output fistula

9. A patient presents with a fistula that has an output volume <50 mL with a need for odor control. What would be a good containment option for this patient?
   A. Wound management system with window emptied frequently
   B. Closed system with suction
   C. Charcoal dressings over dressings with environmental deodorants
   D. Absorptive dressings (e.g., calcium alginate dressings)

10. The wound care nurse is teaching a patient how to change a fistula pouch. Which of the following is a recommended step in this procedure?
    A. Trace the pattern onto the skin barrier surface of the pouch providing at least ¼ inch clearance of wound edges.
    B. Trace the pattern onto the skin barrier of the pouch being careful to size the opening to match the contours of the wound exactly.
    C. Remove the pouch by pulling off the skin quickly while applying gentle pressure on skin with one hand.
    D. Clean the skin with an alcohol wipe or skin cleanser with an emollient and dry gently and thoroughly.

11. The wound care nurse is isolating a fistula for negative pressure wound therapy (NPWT). What step would the nurse take after fitting the sponge around the fistula opening and covering the wound with a transparent drape?

A. Apply the negative pressure suction control device directly over the fistula.
B. Adhere the NPWT ring to the wound bed with the skin barrier ring and paste.
C. Cut an opening in the transparent dressing over the fistula and apply the pouch.
D. Place the suction catheter on the transparent dressing and initiate suction.

12. A patient's fistula is located in an open wound, and routine pouching procedures have been ineffective. What pouching system adaptation would the wound care nurse recommend?

A. Saddlebagging.
B. Bridging.
C. Troughing.
D. The pouching system should be discontinued.

ANSWERS: 1.**D**, 2.**A**, 3.**B**, 4.**C**, 5.**C**, 6.**A**, 7.**B**, 8.**D**, 9.**C**, 10.**A**, 11.**C**, 12.**C**

CHAPTER 35

Nursing Management of the Patient with Percutaneous Tubes

Jane Fellows and Michelle C. Rice

OBJECTIVE

Apply assessment and nursing management techniques to address the complex care needs of a patient with percutaneous tubes.

Topic Outline

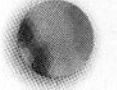

Gastrostomy and Jejunostomy Tubes
- Comparative Complication Rates
- Routine Tube Care
- Managing Skin Complications
- Hypertrophic Granulation
- Tube Replacement
- Pediatric Considerations

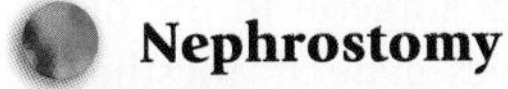

Nephrostomy Tubes

Biliary Tubes

Conclusions

Percutaneous tube placement into body organs or spaces is a means for drainage of fluids, maintaining an opening into an organ where obstruction exists, or providing for instillation of fluids, medication, or feeding through the tube. The tubes are usually placed by a physician in surgery, via endoscopy or interventional radiology. The WOC nurse is often consulted for management of these tubes and the complications that may occur with them. Knowledge of the location, purpose, and desired outcome of the tube placement is essential to effectively manage the care of patients with these tubes.

The use of percutaneous tubes is common in the adult and pediatric patient populations across acute care, long-term care, and home care settings. Increasingly they are being used for pain relief and symptom management in palliative care (Requarth, 2011). Common types of these tubes are gastrostomy, jejunostomy, biliary, and nephrostomy.

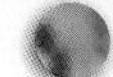

Gastrostomy and Jejunostomy Tubes

Nasogastric tubes (NGT) are the simplest to insert in the gastrointestinal (GI) tract and the least invasive, but they carry a higher risk for dislodgment and aspiration leading to pneumonia (Hsu et al., 2009). When feeding through the tube or decompression of the GI tract is needed for more than a few weeks, a percutaneous tube is inserted. NGT are indicated for short-term use. Common indications for gastrostomy tube (GT) insertion are obstructing head and neck cancer, benign and malignant esophageal disease, neurologic dysfunction, trauma, and respiratory failure.

GTs have been reported in the literature since the 1800s. Dr. Martin Stamm developed a surgical procedure for placement of a tube directly into the stomach, which is still used today. The standard Stamm gastrostomy involves circumferential purse-string sutures to stabilize the tube within the lumen of the stomach and affix the stomach to the anterior abdominal wall. A later technique developed by Witzel involves creating a serosal tunnel as well as an abdominal wall tunnel through which the tube passes. This is useful when the stomach has been altered so that it cannot be secured to the abdominal wall such as after a gastric bypass surgery or resection of esophageal cancer (Gaurav, 2014). Variations on these open surgical procedures remained the standard of care for feeding or gastric decompression until the 1980s when a procedure for percutaneous endoscopic gastrostomy (PEG) was developed.

PEG is a method of placing a tube into the stomach through the skin, aided by endoscopy (Fig. 35-1). A PEG with a jejunal extension tube can be placed through a preexisting PEG to facilitate more distal feeding while also providing an avenue for gastric decompression when necessary.

PEG tube placement is one of the most common endoscopic procedures performed today, and an estimated 100,000 to 125,000 are performed annually in the United States (Gaurav, 2014).

PEG is now considered the method of choice for enteral access due to the simplicity, effectiveness, and lower cost of the procedure (Miller et al., 2014). However, PEG is not always clinically appropriate, and some of the possible contraindications include the following:

- Uncorrected coagulopathy or thrombocytopenia
- Upper tract obstruction or malformation
- Severe ascites
- Hemodynamic instability
- Sepsis
- Intra-abdominal perforation
- Active peritonitis
- Abdominal wall infection at the selected site of placement
- Gastric outlet obstruction (if PEG tube is being placed for feeding)
- Severe gastroparesis (if PEG tube is being placed for feeding)
- History of total gastrectomy

When a PEG is not feasible for the patient, radiologic placement is a possible alternative. This was first described in the literature in the mid-1980s (Duszak, 2014) and avoids the use of an endoscope and is not contraindicated in the presence of upper tract obstruction. It uses fluoroscopy and ultrasound to identify the stomach, and a GT with a balloon is secured against the gastric mucosa with an external bumper on the skin (Fig. 35-2). If gastroesophageal reflux or delaying gastric emptying is a problem, another feeding tube option is a percutaneous gastrojejunal tube (Fig. 35-3). This tube has a balloon and an external skin bumper. There is an extension that is guided through the duodenum and into the jejunum for feeding. These tubes will have a gastric port that can be used for medication or fluid administration or decompression of the stomach and one for the jejunal feeding. A study of 124 patients requiring conversion from a GT to gastrojejunal tube showed a significantly higher success rate using the radiologic placement procedure rather than nonradiologic procedures (Kim et al., 2010). These radiologic procedures require providers with training in interventional radiology, which is not always an option in all facilities.

Both the PEG and radiologic procedures can be done with sedation rather than anesthesia making the procedure safer for the patient, and the time for initial feedings is not delayed. If feeding in the stomach is not possible due to surgical absence of the organ, severe gastroparesis, or gastric outlet obstruction, radiologic intervention is used to place a feeding tube directly into the jejunum. This tube is secured with a stabilizer sutured to the skin.

For those patients who are not candidates for PEG or radiologic procedures, surgical approaches offer the advantage of direct visualization of tube placement into the intended organ (stomach or jejunum). An open laparotomy or laparoscopy is done by a surgeon in the operating room, and the patient receives general anesthesia.

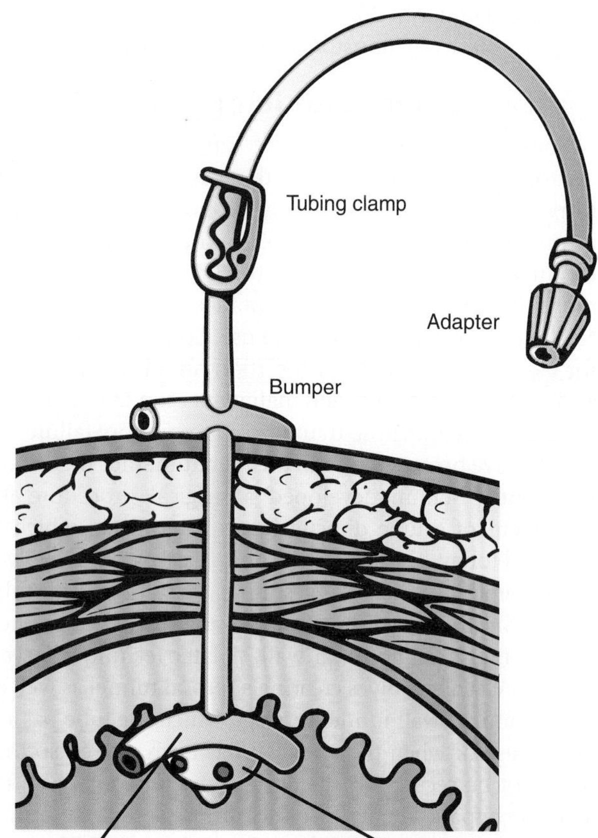

FIGURE 35-1. PEG tube with internal and external bumper. (*Essentials for nursing practice* (8th ed., pp. 926–926), copyright Elsevier, 2015.)

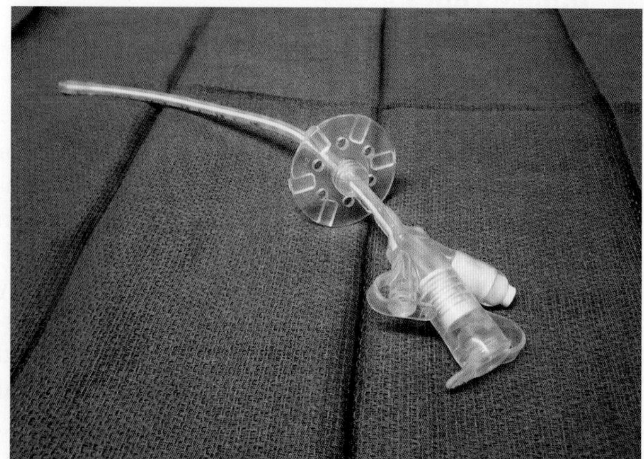

FIGURE 35-2. Balloon-tipped gastrostomy tube. (Courtesy of Jane Fellows, MSN, RN, CWOCN.)

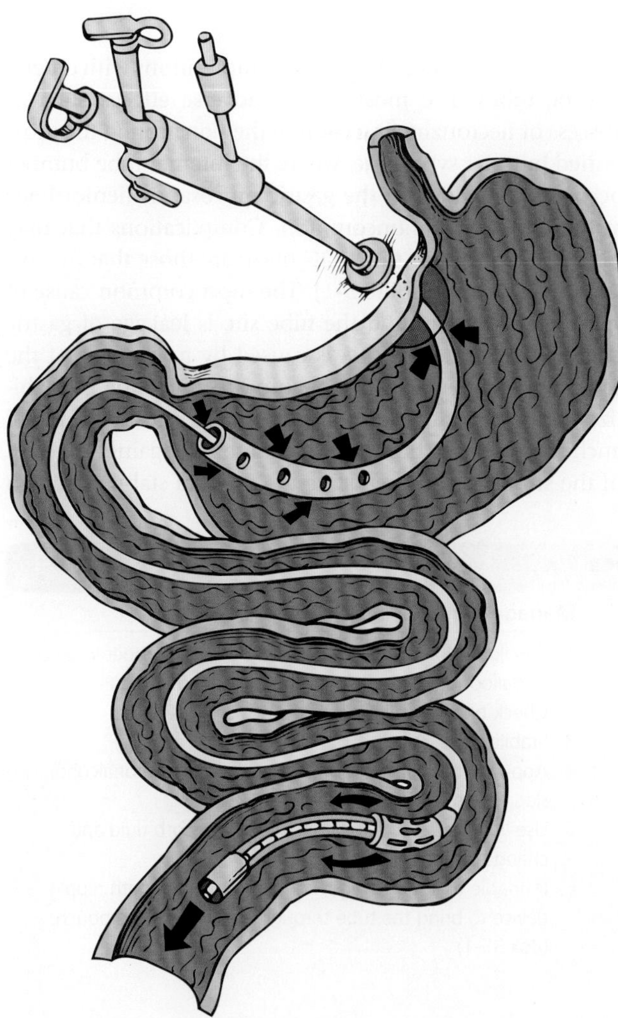

FIGURE 35-3. PEG with jejunal extension. (*Essentials for nursing practice* (8th ed., pp. 926–926), copyright Elsevier, 2015.)

During the surgical approach, the stomach or jejunum is identified following a laparotomy incision or insertion of the laparoscope. The laparoscopic approach offers smaller incision size, less pain, and decreased risk of incisional hernia (Mizrahi et al., 2014). The appropriate feeding tube is secured within the lumen of the targeted organ and brought out through a separate stab incision. If a patient is scheduled for an open or laparoscopic abdominal surgery and it is expected that a feeding tube may be needed, it should be placed at the time of the surgery.

Comparative Complication Rates

There are many potential complications with these procedures, and most of the patients are malnourished and have significant comorbidities. However, the complication rates are relatively low. The complication rates reported in the literature vary, but it seems generally accepted to be 1% to 3% for PEG placement, 8% to 10% with radiologic procedures, and 7% to 15% with surgical procedures (Miller, 2014). Complications associated with percutaneous endoscopic approaches include endoscopic trauma and perforation of the GI tract, bleeding, skin and soft tissue infection, injury to intra-abdominal viscera such as the liver or colon, tube dislodgment, and fistula creation. Radiologic placement has many of the same risks as do endoscopically placed tubes, but there is no risk of upper tract trauma from the endoscope. Surgically placed tubes are associated most commonly with skin and soft tissue infection, incisional hernia, bleeding, inadvertent removal of the tube, and complications associated with general anesthesia. Issues with inadvertent injury to surrounding intra-abdominal viscera are very rare due to the better visibility during the procedure. In a study comparing laparoscopic versus open laparotomy, the laparoscopic surgery took longer to perform, but the complication rate was higher in the open surgery group (Mizrahi et al., 2014).

Routine Tube Care

Following placement of percutaneous tubes, the external bolster should generally be left in place for at least 4 days. After 4 days, there should be 1/2 to 1 cm of laxity left between the entry point and the bumper of the tube to prevent ulceration of the gastric mucosa or pressure damage to the skin under the bumper. Due to the possibility of edema at the tube site, positioning of the tube should be observed frequently for the first 48 hours after insertion (Miller et al., 2014). Evidence for most effective site care is lacking, but patient education materials recommend that the site be washed with mild soap and water, rinsed well with water, and dried daily. One gauze drain sponge may be placed under the bumper unless it sutured in place to absorb any drainage from the site. The use of a dressing after the first week is optional if there is no drainage around the tube site. It is important to know how much fluid was put in the balloon at the time of placement (if the tube is a balloon tube) and what manufacturer made the tube. The manufacturer's Web sites have specific information about their tubes and recommendations about how often to check the fluid levels in the balloon. If leakage is a problem, check the balloon for fluid and refill the balloon to the level placed at the time of the tube insertion. Use sterile water to fill the balloon (Simons, 2013).

CLINICAL PEARL

If there is crusting around the opening, use a water-moistened cotton-tipped applicator to gently remove.

The time before the tube can be used for feeding varies with the procedure performed and the preference of the provider. When feeding is allowed, it is important to routinely flush the tube to prevent clogging from occurring. It should be flushed with 30 mL water before and after each feeding and every 4 to 6 hours when the patient has continuous feedings. Use 10 mL water to flush before and after giving each medication. If liquid medication is not available, the medication should be finely crushed and mixed with water (Simons & Remington, 2013). If the tube does become clogged, try the following:

- Be sure the tube is not kinked.
- Milk the tube to remove any mechanical obstruction.
- Aspirate any fluid from the tube and then instill 10 mL warm water with a 60-mL catheter tip syringe and pull back and forth on the plunger to try to dislodge the obstruction.
- If it is still clogged, repeat the above step with one pancreatic enzyme tablet and one sodium bicarbonate tablet crushed and mixed in 5 mL of water (WOCN, 2008).
- If the tube cannot be unclogged, contact the physician. Instrumentation or replacement may be necessary.

Managing Skin Complications

There are many types of possible complications with enteral feeding tubes. The most serious adverse effects, such as abscess or necrotizing infection in the skin around the tube; buried bumper syndrome, where the internal tube bumper becomes imbedded in the gastric mucosa; or hemorrhage at the tube site, are uncommon. Complications that may require a consult for the WOC nurse are those that involve skin breakdown (Table 35-1). The most common cause of skin breakdown around the tube site is leakage of gastric contents on the skin. This is caused by movement of the tube that may enlarge the opening in the skin. To stabilize the tube, gently pull up on the tube until the internal anchoring device (bumper) or balloon is against the wall of the stomach and then slide the external stabilizer down

TABLE 35-1 Complications Associated with Enteral Tubes

Type	Contributing Factors	Management
Irritant dermatitis	Leakage of gastric secretions Tube displacement Improper balloon inflation Inadequate tube stabilization Recent weight loss Increased abdominal pressure related to chronic cough, constipation, hypertonicity/spasticity Presence of granulation tissue/hyperplasia Inability to decompress gastric content (i.e., burp) Delayed gastric motility Body structure changes (spinal stenosis, scoliosis) Failure of tract closure related to inadequate wound healing	1. If balloon-tipped tube is in place, check for proper inflation of balloon and add fluid if amount inadequate 2. Check balloon volume weekly 3. Stabilize the tube 4. Apply barrier ointment, such as zinc oxide or nonalcohol skin sealant to irritated skin 5. Use light gauze, or foam dressings to absorb fluid and change whenever wet 6. If unable to stop leakage, consider pouching with nipple device to bring the tube through the front of the pouch (Box 35-1)
Device-related pressure ulcer	Excess tension of the bumper against the skin Failure to rotate bumper after initial insertion Location of tube in a skin fold Weight gain or increased girth Sutured bumpers	1. Ensure the stabilizer rests comfortably against the skin without excess tension 2. Rotate bumper daily if appropriate 3. Consider eliminating the need for the bumper by utilizing a tube anchoring device 4. Depending on characteristics of the ulcer, consider the following: Skin barrier powder, sheet hydrocolloid, or absorptive dressing 5. Ask primary care provider if suture removal is an option
Fungal infection	Chronic moisture in the area of the tube Deep skin fold around the tube On systemic antibiotics Receiving immunosuppression medications	1. Keep the skin dry 2. Use moisture barrier creams or no-sting liquid skin barrier 3. Apply topical antifungal medication twice daily and continue for 2 wk after rash is resolved 4. Recommend systemic treatment if topical is not effective
Cellulitis	Invasive procedure Immunosuppression Diabetes Inappropriate or excessive handling of tube Chronic steroid use	1. Observe the skin for erythema, induration, purulent drainage 2. Assess pain with palpation 3. Recommend a systemic antibiotic if indicated by assessment
Hypertrophic granulation tissue	Moist friable tissue at the site where the tube enters the abdomen. Tissue is composed of connective tissue and tiny blood vessels and bleeds easily	1. Stabilize the tube if the etiology is felt to be a tube that is not secured 2. Consider use of silver nitrate cautery, steroid crème (triamcinolone 0.5% tid) or antimicrobial foam

BOX 35-1. Procedure for Pouch Application around the Gastrostomy Tube

Equipment:
Ostomy pouch
Scissors
Skin barrier powder
Wet and dry cloths
No sting skin prep
Cotton-tipped applicators
Gloves
Catheter holder device
Water-resistant tape

Directions:

1. Clamp tube and turn off feeding.
2. Remove the pink tape from around the tube where it exits the pouching system and gently remove the pouch using adhesive remover or warm water. Be careful not to pull or dislodge the tube.
3. Clean the skin with water and pat dry. Cleanse the area under the tube bumper by inserting a cotton-tipped applicator between sutures. Sprinkle skin barrier powder under the bumper to protect the skin.

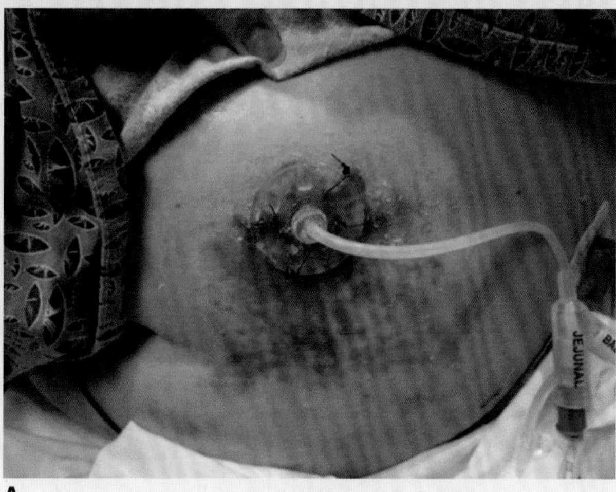

A

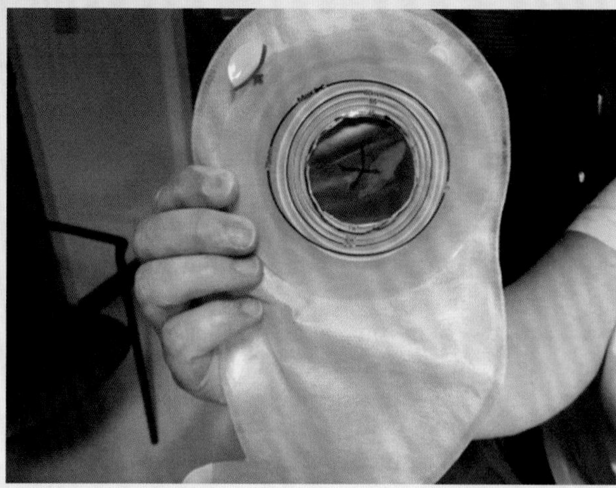
B

4. If there is any skin breakdown **(A)**, sprinkle skin barrier powder on the skin, rub in, and seal with no-sting liquid skin barrier.
5. Cut an opening in skin barrier of the one-piece pouching system to fit around the bumper. Cut an X-shaped opening on the front of the pouch so the gastrostomy tube can be pulled through **(B)**.
6. Place catheter holder device over X cut in front of the pouch to secure the tube and avoid leakage **(C)**. Instructions come with each device. Cut a hole in the nipple large enough to pull the tube through **(D)**.

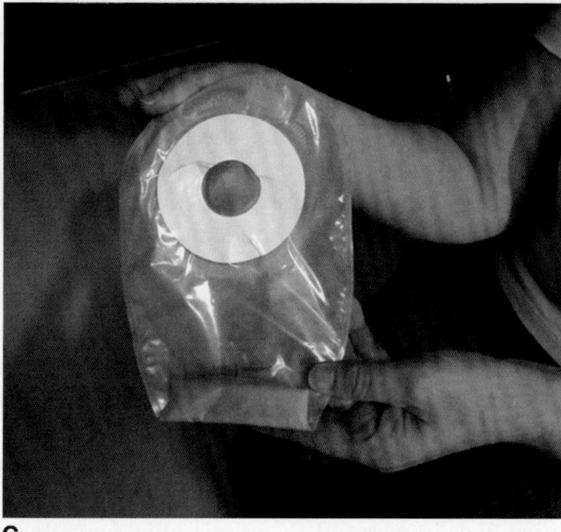
C

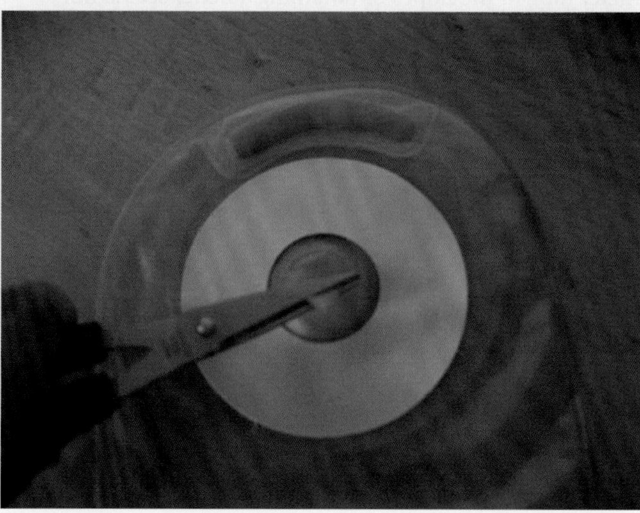
D

BOX 35-1. Procedure for Pouch Application around the Gastrostomy Tube (*Continued*)

7. Pull tube through the opening and place the pouch on the skin. Make sure the skin is dry before placing the pouch **(E)**. Use pink tape around the tube where it exits the pouch to seal the opening in the nipple **(F)**.

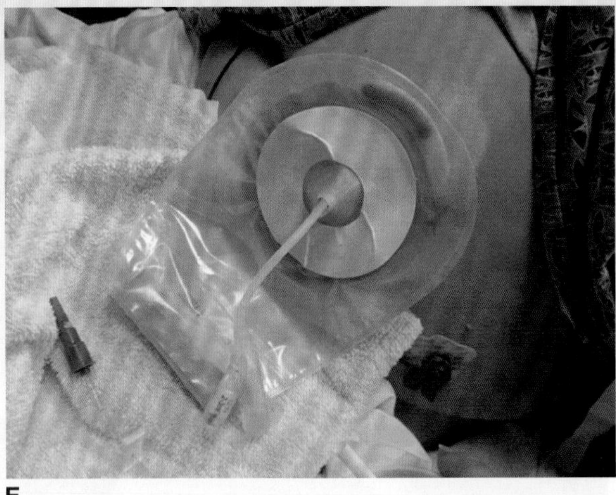

E

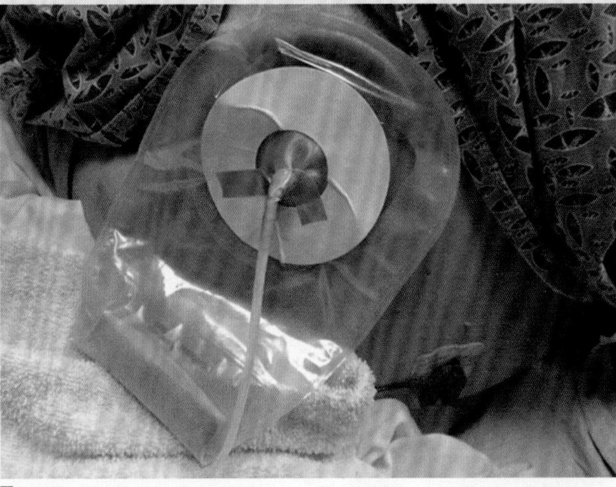

F

to rest comfortably on the skin without excess tension (WOCN, 2008). If there is an external stabilizer sutured to the skin with a jejunostomy and the sutures are no longer intact, it may be necessary to have these replaced. This tube is not secured with an internal bumper or a balloon, so it will migrate if sutures are not present. If there are sutures in the bumper of a PEG tube stabilizer, they may impede the ability to care for the skin and prevent skin complications such as irritant dermatitis and device-related pressure ulcers. It is appropriate to ask if these can be removed after healing has taken place. If there is no external bumper, the use of a commercial stabilizing device to secure the tube (Fig. 35-4) or taping the tube in place may prevent movement. With a balloon-tipped tube, loss of water in the balloon will cause migration of the tube. Replacing a leaking tube with a larger diameter tube in the hopes of obtaining a better seal is not effective and is contraindicated (Stayner et al., 2012). This will further enlarge and distort the leaking tube tract. In rare cases of persistent leakage, the tube must be removed and placed in a different site allowing the original site to close.

FIGURE 35-4. Drain tube attachment device. (Courtesy of Hollister Incorporated.)

CLINICAL PEARL

It is recommended that the amount of water in the balloon is checked weekly and replaced with the correct amount.

Hypertrophic Granulation

It is thought that a poorly secured tube or one that migrates easily in and out of the skin opening may be a causative factor in the development of hypergranulation tissue around an enteral tube. Leakage of fluid, use of hydrogen peroxide, and poor fitting low-profile GT may also contribute to this overgrowth of tissue. The tissue itself is moist and often is friable, which contributes to leakage of formula and enteral fluid round the tube creating a cycle of leakage being both cause and effect. In some cases, it is painful to touch and may bleed easily. The presence of this tissue is not considered a serious complication, but there are reports in the literature linking it to wound infection and cellulitis around the tube (Rahnemai-Azar et al., 2014). A wide variety of treatment options from the application of topical antimicrobial agents and steroid creams to cauterization with silver nitrate and surgical removal have been described in the literature, but the evidence is anecdotal. Nurses in one community health district in the United Kingdom described a care routine for those persons ($n = 25$) in homes or care facilities with GTs and an overgrowth of granulation tissue around them. They used an antimicrobial cleanser and an antimicrobial foam dressing around the tube for 6 weeks and checked on them at 2-week intervals. At the end of the first 2 weeks, one third ($n = 8$) of the patients no longer had hypergranular tissue present. At the end of 6 weeks, the problem was resolved in six additional patients. The remaining patients received a silver alginate under a foam dressing, and if that did not resolve the hypergranulation, a steroid cream was applied (Warriner & Spruce, 2014). When hypergranulation tissue is present, it is important to stabilize the tube to reduce movement of the tube in the tract. In addition, clinicians use silver nitrate cautery, steroid cream (triamcinolone 0.5% applied tid), or an antimicrobial such as silver in or with a thin foam dressing. Silver nitrate sticks should be used with care to avoid getting the silver nitrate on intact skin as this may cause a burning sensation. More than one application may be needed. In extreme cases, surgical excision of the tissue may be required (WOCN, 2008).

Tube Replacement

GTs may become accidentally dislodged for a variety of reasons. The stabilizer may have loosened, water may have leaked from the balloon, inadvertent traction is placed on the tube, or the patient may have pulled it out. The latter cause is usually secondary to an altered mental state. In these patients, a low-profile tube may be appropriate (Fig. 35-5). The low-profile tube may also be used as a replacement tube when the patient wishes to have one for convenience and ease of concealing the tube under clothing. It is required to measure the stoma tract; there are measuring devices that determine the size tract for low-profile tube needed. This is especially important as a child is growing and may need to order another size tube. GT replacement may be done by a nurse, but verification of workplace policies and regulations of the state board of nursing should guide the decision to do this. In a healthy person, the tract in which the GT is placed would be healed in 2 to 3 weeks. The patients requiring enteral access for feeding are usually malnourished and have chronic conditions that may interfere with healing, so it is advisable to wait 4 to 6 weeks before a nurse should attempt tube replacement (McGinnis, 2013). There is a risk of inserting the tube in the peritoneum if the tract is not healed. When a tube is dislodged unexpectedly after 6 weeks from original placement, it must be replaced as soon as possible before the tract and the opening in the skin begins to close (Box 35-2). For patients at home, a family member may be taught to do this to avoid loss of access. Placing a tube into the opening will solve the immediate problem of maintaining the tract, but the tube should not be used until proper placement has been ascertained by return of gastric fluid through the tube (Juern & Verhaalen, 2014). Replacement GTs are preferred, but a Foley catheter may be used if a GT is not available. The Foley catheter is more readily available and is a less expensive option, but the lumen of the catheter will be smaller and it is less durable, so replacement with a GT should be done when one is available (Ojo, 2013).

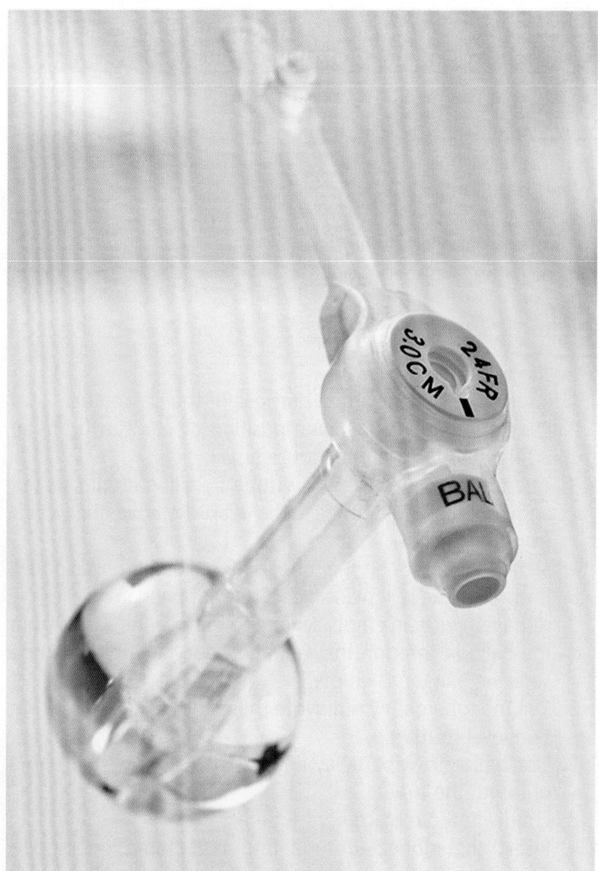

FIGURE 35-5. Low-profile gastrostomy tube. (MIC-KEY™ G Feeding Tube is a Registered Trademark or Trademark of Halyard Health, Inc. or its affiliates. Image copyright © 2014 HYH. All rights reserved.)

CLINICAL PEARL

The patient should understand that when the tube falls out they should replace the tube immediately or seek medical attention for replacement.

Pediatric Considerations

The use of enteral feeding tube is a widely used, effective, and standard means of meeting the nutritional needs of child with a dysfunctional GI tract or who is unable to take oral nutrition (Hannah, 2013). The procedure is considered minimally invasive, and patients are discharged a short time after the procedure (Rollins et al., 2013). However, the procedure is not without risks and complications. A review of the literature demonstrates that patients with GTs have significant number of complications and emergency department (ED) visits for nonurgent tube issues. According to Pemberton et al. (2013), anywhere from 11% to 26% of pediatric patients have complications after GT placement. Common complications include leakage, peristomal skin breakdown, dislodgment, and hypergranulation tissue. The management of these complications is the same as for adult patients with a feeding tube. Tube dislodgment may be

BOX 35-2. Procedure for Gastrostomy Tube Exchange with a Balloon-Tipped Tube

Equipment:
Replacement gastrostomy tube of the same size as the one being removed
Water-based lubricant
Empty 10-mL syringe
10-mL syringe filled with water
60-mL catheter-tipped syringe
Gauze pads
Gloves

Directions:
1. Inform the patient of the purpose of the procedure.
2. Place the patient in supine position or elevate the head 30 degrees, as the patient prefers.
3. Test the balloon on the new tube by filling it with water, and ascertain that there is no leak. Remove the water from the balloon.
4. Slide the bumper up the tube to make sure it moves easily.
5. If the old tube is in place (i.e., it has not been inadvertently removed), use an empty syringe to remove the water from the balloon through the aspiration port. Reaspirate to be sure the balloon is empty.
6. Pull the tube gently out. Note the length of the tube from skin level to the tip.
7. Use gauze to wipe away any gastric contents that come out with the tube.
8. Lubricate the replacement tube.
9. Insert the lubricated tube into the stoma opening a couple of centimeters past the length of the tube that was removed.
10. Fill the balloon with water.
11. Pull the tube up until you feel resistance against the stomach wall.
12. Slide the bumper down the tube so that there is only 2 to 3 mm of space between the bumper and the skin. The tube should be able to be turned around freely in the opening.
13. Use the 60-mL syringe to aspirate gastric contents to affirm correct placement.
14. If no gastric contents can be aspirated, connect the tube to a bedside drainage bag and wait 20 minutes to see if the contents drain.
15. If there is no drainage in 20 minutes, tube placement should be confirmed with an abdominal radiograph in the oblique position using contrast.
16. Do not start feeding or flush the tube until there is confirmation of intragastric placement.

decreased with a low-profile tube, and these are used frequently in pediatric patients. A retrospective study by Novotny et al. (2009) of 223 young children who received a standard PEG (n = 110) versus a low-profile PEG (n = 113) showed a significant decrease in tube dislodgment with the low-profile tube and no difference in infection rate. There was also a significantly decreased length of hospital stay in the low-profile tube group. There was not a difference in ED visits for minor complications with the tubes.

According to a 4-year prospective study by Goldberg et al. (2010), infection developed in 37% of patients with the majority taking place during the first 15 days after placement. Hypergranulation tissue was noted in 68% of children with a recurrence in 17% of patients after receiving treatment. A 2009 retrospective cross-sectional descriptive study by Saavedra et al. (2009) showed that over a 23-month period, 77 patients had 181 ED visits for complaints related to the GT. Dislodgment of the GT occurred in 62% of the patients, and 75% of the visits were for GT replacement. In a study of 247 patients treated at a tertiary children's hospital, Correa et al. (2014) found that 20% of patients accounted for 44 ED visits within the first 30 days of discharge for complaints of leaking, mild clogs, and hypergranulation (hyperplasia) tissue. During the time period of 31 to 365 days postdischarge, 40 additional patients returned to the ED a total of 71 times for potentially avoidable visits.

It is clear that care of these children creates substantial stress for family caregivers. Specific education and support needs to be directed to the patients and their families in order to decrease the number of potentially avoidable visits to the ED. This is an area in which a WOC nurse can have tremendous impact on patient and caregiver quality.

Nephrostomy Tubes

Percutaneous nephrostomy tubes are inserted through the skin and into the renal pelvis of the kidney to facilitate drainage of urine after a partial or complete obstruction has occurred. Indications for use include tumors, strictures, dilations, and kidney stone removal. The tube exits through the flank and is connected to extension tubing and drains into a leg or bedside drainage bag (Clinical Center NIH, N.D., p. 3). Important factors in the management of this tube include tube stabilization to prevent pulling, kinking, or dislodgment; possible tube flushing with MD order; prevention of skin irritation; and signs of infection (ACI Urology Network-Nursing, 2012).

Tube stabilization can be accomplished with the use of a commercial catheter holder. Tape may also be used if commercial devices are not available. When securing the tube, consider the tube angle to prevent kinking.

In some instances, flushing of the tube may be needed if there is an absence of urine; persistent flank pain; or presence of clots, debris, or sediment (ACI Urology Network-Nursing, 2012). Consult facility protocols and/or physician guidelines for this practice. Generally, 5 to 10 mL of sterile, normal saline is flushed into the tube. Do not force the saline into the tube. After saline is instilled, reconnect to straight drainage. If unable to instill saline, the physician must be notified.

During the first 2 weeks postprocedure, sterile gauze nephrostomy dressings should be kept dry and be changed daily and as needed for drainage. For sensitive skin, consider the use of adhesive remover to loosen the dressing. If a sterile transparent dressing is in use, it must be changed every 3 days. After the initial 2-week period, the dressing should be changed twice per week and if wet or lifting off (Clinical Center NIH, N.D.). If skin irritation occurs, consider the use of an alcohol-free liquid skin barrier to protect the area. If a fungal rash appears to be present, use an antifungal powder rather than an ointment or cream. If there appears to be sensitivity to the adhesive, consider a dressing with a silicone backing.

Patient and family education includes how to flush the tube if ordered by MD, signs of infection, skin care, how to use and care for a leg or bedside drainage bag, and how often the nephrostomy tube will be changed (usually every 2 to 3 months).

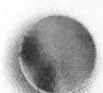 Biliary Tubes

Biliary tubes are necessary when an alternate method of draining bile from the hepatobiliary system is needed. Often, the bile ducts are blocked, resulting in a buildup of bile in the liver that can lead to jaundice, nausea, vomiting, itching, fever, dark urine, and infection (Cote Robson, 2009; Box 35-3). Blockages are caused by tumors, strictures, and gallstones. The thin tube is inserted through the skin into the bile ducts by an interventional radiologist and is connected to a small drainage bag. This procedure is also known as a percutaneous transhepatic cholangiogram (Goodwin & Burnes, 2010).

Management of the biliary tube includes adequate securement of the tube to prevent kinking or dislodgment, flushing of the tube with MD order, dressing changes, and keeping the drain bag below the waist to facilitate proper drainage (Cote Robson, 2009).

Dressing changes should be done weekly and whenever wet or soiled. For sensitive skin, consider the use of adhesive remover to loosen the dressing. If skin irritation develops, an alcohol-free liquid skin barrier may be used to protect the area. Flushing the tube is done twice daily with 10 mL of sterile saline. Never force the saline into the tube. If there is inability to instill, pain occurs, or leakage at the exit site occurs, the physician must be notified (Cote Robson, 2009).

Patient and caregiver education must include routine care of the catheter, assessment of catheter integrity, signs of infection, and signs and symptoms of a blockage.

BOX 35-3. Signs and Symptoms of Biliary Tube Blockage

Leakage at exit site
Decrease in bile drainage output
Inability to flush the tube
Fever, chills, nausea, and increased jaundice

Cote Robson, P. M. (2009). *Caring for your biliary drainage catheter.* Memorial Sloan-Kettering Cancer Center. Retrieved August 30, 2014, from http://www.mskcc.org/cancer-care/patient-education/resources/caring-your-biliary-drainage-catheter

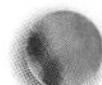 Conclusions

The provision of adequate nutrition support in the hospital setting is the standard of care. The use of the gut for feeding that is provided through enteral access is preferred to the use of parenteral nutrition whenever possible (Miller, 2014). It carries benefits physiologically for the patient as well as decreases the significant risks associated with parenteral nutrition. Patients with higher acuity are candidates for enteral access through endoscopic, radiologic, and surgical techniques available in various care settings. The WOC nurse must know what procedures may be done in his or her practice setting to be prepared for managing the care of these patients and those with other types of percutaneous tubes. Caregiver support and patient education are essential for those patients leaving the hospital with percutaneous tubes, and the WOC nurse can play an important role in preparing both patients and caregivers for discharge (see Care of Feeding Tubes, Appendix I).

REFERENCES

ACI Urology Network-Nursing. (2012). Nursing management of patients with nephrostomy tubes, guidelines and patient information templates. Retrieved from http://www.aci.health.nsw.gov.au/__data/assets/pdf_file/0011/165917/Nephrostomy-Tubes-Toolkit.pdf

Clinical Center NIH. (N.D.). Caring for your percutaneous nephrostomy tube. Retrieved August 30, 2014, from http://www.cc.nih.gov/ccc/patient_education/pepubs/percneph.pdf

Correa, J. A., Fallon, S. C., Murphy, K. M., et al. (2014). Resource utilization after gastrostomy tube placement: Defining areas of improvement for future quality improvement projects. *Journal of Pediatric Surgery*, DOI: http://dx.doi.org/10.1016/j.jpedsurg.2014.06.015

Cote Robson, P. M. (2009). *Caring for your biliary drainage catheter.* Memorial Sloan-Kettering Cancer Center. Retrieved August 30, 2014, from http://www.mskcc.org/cancer-care/patient-education/resources/caring-your-biliary-drainage-catheter

Duszak, R. (2014). Percutaneous gastrostomy and jejunostomy. http://emedicine.medscape.com/article/1821257-overview

Gaurav, A. (2014). Percutaneous endoscopic gastrostomy (PEG) tube placement. http://emedicine.medscape.com/article/149665-overview

Goldberg, E., Barton, S., Xanthopoulos, M. S., et al. (2010). A descriptive study of complications of gastrostomy tubes in children. *Journal of Pediatric Nursing,* 25(2), 72–80. DOI: 10.1016/j.pedn.2008.07.008

Goodwin, M., & Burnes, J. (2010). Biliary drainage. Retrieved August 30, 2014, from http://www.insideradiology.com.au/pages/view.php?T_id=90#.VATKc_ldWSo

Hannah, E. (2013). Everything the nurse practitioner should know about pediatric feeding tubes. *Journal of the America Association of Nurse Practitioners*, 25, 567–577.

Hsu, C. W., Sun, S. E., Lin, S. L., et al. (2009). Duodenal versus gastric feeding in medical intensive care unit patients: A prospective, randomized, clinical study. *Critical Care Medicine*, 37, 1866–1872.

Juern, J., & Verhaalen, A. (2014). Gastrostomy-tube exchange. *New England Journal of Medicine, 370*, e28. DOI: 10.1056/NEJMvcm1207131

Kim, C. Y., Patel, M. B., Miller, M. J., et al. (2010). Gastrostomy-to-gastrojejunostomy tube conversion: Impact of the method of original gastrostomy tube placement. *Journal of Vascular Interventional Radiology*, *21*(7), 1031–1037.

McGinnis, C. (2013). Replacing gastrostomy tubes. *Critical Care Nurse, 33*(5),75–76.

Miller, K. R., McClave, S. A., Kiraly, L. N., et al. (2014). A tutorial on enteral access in adult patients in the hospitalized setting. *Journal of Parental and Enteral Nutrition, 38*(3), 282–294.

Mizrahi, I., Garg, M., Divino, C. M., et al. (2014). Comparison of laparoscopic vs open approach to gastrostomy tubes. *Journal of the Society of Laparoendoscopic Surgeons, 18*(1), 28–33.

Novotny, N. M., Vegeler, R. C., Breckler, F. D., et al. (2009). Percutaneous endoscopic gastrostomy buttons in children: Superior to tubes. *Journal of Pediatric Surgery, 44*(6), 1193–1196.

Ojo, O. (2013). Balloon gastrostomy tubes for long-term feeding in the community. *British Journal of Nursing, 20*(1), 34–38.

Pemberton, J., Frankfurter, C., Bailey, K., et al. (2013). Gastrostomy matters—The impact of pediatric surgery on caregiver quality of life. *Journal of Pediatric Surgery, 48*(5), 963–970.

Rahnemai-Azar, A., Rahnemai-Azar, A., Naghshizadian, R., et al. (2014). Percutaneous endoscopic gastrostomy: Indications, technique, complications and management. *World Journal of Gastroenterology, 20*(24), 7739–7751.

Requarth, J. (2011). Image-guided palliative care procedures. *Surgical Clinics of North America, 91*(2), 367–402.

Rollins, H., Nathwani, N., & Morridson, D. (2013). Optimising wound care in a child with an infected gastrostomy exit site. *British Journal of Nursing, 22*, 1275–1279.

Saavedra, H., Loske, J. D., Shanley, L., et al. (2009). Gastrostomy tube related complaints in the pediatric emergency department identifying opportunities for improvement. *Pediatric Emergency Care, 25*(11), 728–732.

Simons, S., & Remington, R. (2013). The percutaneous endoscopic gastrostomy tube: A nurse's guide to PEG tubes. *Medsurg Nursing, 22*(2), 77–83.

Stayner, J. L., Bhatnagar, A., McGinn, A. N., et al. (2012). Feeding tube placement: Errors and complications. *Nutrition in Clinical Practice, 27*(6), 738–748.

Warriner, L., & Spruce, P. (2014). Managing overgranulation tissue around gastrostomy sites. *British Journal of Nursing, 21*(5), S20–S25.

WOCN. (2008). *Management of gastrostomy tube complications for adult and pediatric patients.* Mount Laurel, NJ.

QUESTIONS

1. The nurse is assessing a patient who has a nasogastric tube (NGT) in place following gastric surgery. What complication should the patient be monitored for?
- A. Fluid and electrolyte imbalance
- B. Aspiration pneumonia
- C. Constipation
- D. Gastroesophageal reflux

2. A percutaneous endoscopic gastrostomy (PEG) tube may be contraindicated in a patient with the following diagnosis?
- A. Severe ascites
- B. Ulcerative colitis
- C. Peptic ulcer
- D. Crohn's disease

3. The nurse is assessing a patient who has severe gastroesophageal reflux for placement of a feeding tube. What type of tube would be most appropriate for this patient?
- A. Percutaneous endoscopic gastrostomy (PEG) tube
- B. Nasogastric tube (NGT)
- C. Stamm gastrostomy tube
- D. Percutaneous gastrojejunal tube

4. A patient who is undergoing abdominal surgery will need a feeding tube. When would the surgeon place the tube?
- A. Prior to surgery
- B. During surgery
- C. The day after surgery
- D. Two to three weeks after surgery

5. Which complication is most commonly associated with surgically placed gastrostomy tubes as opposed to percutaneous endoscopic?
- A. Incisional hernia
- B. Perforation of the GI tact
- C. Injury to intra-abdominal viscera
- D. Fistula creation

6. A patient is scheduled for placement of a feeding tube in interventional radiology. What potential complication is avoided by using this method instead of the endoscopic method?
- A. Bleeding
- B. Soft tissue infection
- C. Upper tract trauma
- D. Liver trauma

7. The nurse is teaching a patient routine tube care for a newly placed percutaneous endoscopic gastrostomy (PEG) tube. What statement follows recommended guidelines for this care?
- A. Following placement of the tube, the external bolster will be left in place for 1 week.
- B. A water-resistant dressing should be placed over the tube and insertion site and left in place for 48 hours.
- C. The site of the tube should be washed with mild soap and water, rinsed well with water, and dried daily.
- D. One gauze drain sponge may be placed under the bumper of a tube that is sutured in place to absorb any drainage from the site.

8. The nurse is providing care for a patient with a gastrostomy tube. What is a recommended intervention when using the tube to administer feedings or medication?
   A. Flush the tube with 60 mL water before and after each feeding.
   B. Use 10 mL water to flush the tube before and after giving medications.
   C. Flush the tube with water every 8 hours with continuous feedings.
   D. Dilute all feedings with water to be sure the tube does not become clogged.

9. What would be the first intervention when a feeding tube becomes clogged?
   A. Milk the tube to remove any mechanical obstruction.
   B. Aspirate fluid from the tube and instill 20 mL warm water into the tube.
   C. If the tube remains clogged after instilling water, use pancreatic enzyme table and sodium bicarbonate table crushed and mixed in 10 mL water.
   D. Use a 60-mL catheter filled with air and pull back and forth on the plunger to dislodge the obstruction.

10. What is the priority intervention when hypergranulation tissue is present around a feeding tube placement site?
    A. Cleaning the area around the tube with hydrogen peroxide
    B. Stabilizing the tube to reduce movement of the tube in the tract
    C. Replacing the tube with another type of tube
    D. Removing the tissue by rubbing briskly with an alcohol-soaked gauze

11. Which of the following would the nurse recognize as indication of biliary tube blockage?
    A. Increase in bile drainage output
    B. A change in the color of the drainage
    C. Cyanosis
    D. Inability to flush the tube

12. What type of tube would be used for a patient who needs kidney stone removal?
    A. Nephrostomy tube
    B. Biliary tube
    C. Gastrostomy tube
    D. Jejunostomy tube

ANSWERS: 1.**B**, 2.**A**, 3.**D**, 4.**B**, 5.**A**, 6.**C**, 7.**C**, 8.**B**, 9.**A**, 10.**B**, 11.**D**, 12.**A**

GLOSSARY

Abscess a localized collection of pus surrounded by inflamed tissue, usually due to an infectious process.

Acanthosis diffuse epidermal hyperplasia (thickening of the skin).

Acanthosis nigricans asymmetric velvety thickening and hyperpigmentation of the skin chiefly on the neck, axilla, groins, and other body folds.

Achilles tendon long, strong tendon in the back of the leg, which attaches the calf muscle (gastrocnemius and soleus) to the heel.

Acral skin nonhairy skin located primarily on the hands, feet, and parts of the face.

Acute limb ischemia acute limb ischemia is any sudden decrease or worsening of limb perfusion that threatens tissue viability. Pulselessness, pallor, paresthesias, paralysis, and coolness are typical characteristics of an acutely ischemic limb.

Acute lipodermatosclerosis acute lipodermatosclerosis is characterized by pain and tenderness in the medial aspect of the leg. It is thought to be the result of venous insufficiency and to be the acute counterpart of chronic lipodermatosclerosis, a hallmark of venous disease.

AFO an ankle–foot orthosis. A splint used to control the position of the foot relative to the tibia.

Air plethysmography (APG) measures venous reflux, obstruction, and poor calf muscle pump function, which are associated with poor venous return. The air plethysmograph consists of a 35-cm-long polyurethane tubular air chamber that surrounds the entire leg. The air chamber is inflated with air at 6 mm Hg and connected to a pressure transducer/amplifier and a recorder or computer. Changes in the volume of the leg as a result of filling or emptying of veins produce corresponding changes in the pressure of the air chamber.

Albumin any protein with water solubility, which is moderately soluble in concentrated salt solutions and experiences heat coagulation (protein denaturation). Serum albumin is the most abundant blood plasma protein and is produced in the liver and forms a large proportion of all plasma protein.

Allodynia a painful response to a normally innocuous stimulus (as in an intolerance to bedsheets touching legs).

Ambulatory venous hypertension develops when abnormalities occur in any part of the system (i.e., calf muscle pump dysfunction and/or incompetent valves and perforating veins in the superficial, perforator, or deep vein systems). This leads to reflux of blood through this incompetent system.

Angiography diagnostic or therapeutic radiography of the heart and blood vessels using a radiopaque contrast medium.

Angioplasty use of a balloon to open or enlarge the lumen in a blood vessel. It is commonly done to treat stenosis of arteries due to atherosclerosis. Often, during the procedure, atherectomy and/or insertion of a stent may be performed.

Ankle brachial index (ABI) a noninvasive vascular assessment technique providing an objective indicator of arterial perfusion to a lower extremity. The ABI is a ratio obtained by dividing the higher of each ankle's systolic pressure by the higher of the brachial systolic pressures. If blood flow is normal, the pressure in the ankle should equal or be slightly higher than that in the arm.

Ankle flare see malleolar flare.

Antibacterial an agent that inhibits the growth of bacteria.

Antibiotic a substance that has the capacity to destroy or inhibit bacterial growth.

Anticoagulant a drug that delays clotting but does not dissolve existing clots: may prevent new clots from forming and existing clots from enlarging.

Antiembolism compression stockings (AECS) antiembolism stockings (AECS), also referred to as graduated compression stockings or thromboembolic deterrent stockings (TEDS), are often used as a noninvasive measure to prevent DVT in bedbound/immobile patients and surgical patients. AECS provide graduated pressures, which are generally 18 mm Hg at the ankle, 14 mm Hg at the calf, 8 mm Hg at the popliteal area, 10 mm Hg at the lower thigh, and 8 mm Hg at the upper thigh.

Antimicrobial an agent that inhibits the growth of microbes.

Antiplatelet an antiplatelet drug is a member of a class of pharmaceuticals that decreases platelet aggregation and inhibits thrombus formation.

Antiseptic an agent that prevents or inhibits growth of microorganisms.

APACHE II a severity of disease classification system that uses a point score based upon initial values of 12 routine physiologic measurements, age, and previous health status to provide a general measure of severity of disease.

Arterial pertaining to one or more arteries. Arteries are vessels carrying oxygenated blood to tissues.

Arterial insufficiency lack of sufficient blood flow via the arteries to the extremities, which can be caused by cholesterol deposits (atherosclerosis), clots (emboli), or damaged, diseased, or weak vessels.

Arteriogram an x-ray film of an artery injected with a dye.

Arteriosclerosis a common disorder of the arteries marked by thickening, hardening, and loss of elasticity of the walls of blood vessels.

Arthrodesis the surgical fixation of a joint by a procedure designed to accomplish fusion of the joint surfaces by promoting the proliferation of bone cells; called also artificial ankylosis.

Articular cartilage the smooth white, firm connective tissue covering ends of bones, thus creating joints.

Arthritis destructive process affecting a joint. This may result in pain, deformity, and restricted function. It may also be asymptomatic. There are many different causes ranging from injury to a joint, to infection, to autoimmune conditions.

Asymptomatic LEAD LEAD that presents without the typical or classic symptoms of intermittent claudication in the leg.

Atherectomy removal of plaque from the lumen of a vessel.

Atheroma abnormal fatty deposits in an artery; fatty degeneration of the inner lining of the artery.

Atherosclerosis plaques of cholesterol, fats, and other elements that are deposited in the walls of large- and medium-sized arteries. The walls of the vessels become thick and hardened, leading to narrowing, which reduces circulation to organs and other areas normally supplied by the artery.

Athlete's foot (*tinea pedis*) dermatophytic infection of feet characterized by erythema, chronic peeling of skin, fissuring of web spaces between toes, maceration, and blistering.

Atrophie blanche dermal sclerosis with dilated abnormal vasculature with ivory-white plaques on the ankle or foot and hemosiderin-pigmented borders.

Atypical leg pain lower-extremity exertional discomfort that does not consistently occur at a predictable, reproducible distance, and is not resolved with rest or limiting exercise.

Autonomic dysfunction (also known as dysautonomia) hallmarks due to sympathetic failure are impotence (in men) and a fall in blood pressure during standing (i.e., orthostatic hypotension). Excessive sympathetic activity can present as hypertension or a rapid pulse rate.

Autonomic neuropathy causes changes in digestion, bowel and bladder function, sexual response, and perspiration. It can also affect the nerves that serve the heart and control blood pressure. Autonomic neuropathy can also cause hypoglycemia unawareness, a condition in which people no longer experience the warning signs of hypoglycemia.

Avascular lacking in blood supply; synonyms are dead, devitalized, necrotic, and nonviable. Specific types include slough and eschar.

Bacteremia presence of bacteria in the blood.

Bates-Jensen Wound Assessment Tool (BWAT) tool formerly called the Pressure Sore Status Tool (PSST).

Bedsore see pressure ulcer.

Bioburden refers to the diversity, virulence, and interaction of organisms with each other and the body.

Biofilm a polysaccharide matrix in which organisms attach, live, and multiply on wound surfaces; can affect wound healing by creating chronic inflammation or infection.

Biological wound coverings human or animal tissue used as temporary wound coverings.

Biological dressings include:

Isografts. From genetically identical human (i.e., identical twin).

Allografts. From genetically dissimilar human.

Donor's skin. Skin banked from the patient.

Cadaver skin. Skin from a cadaver.

Xenografts. Skin from another species (e.g., pig skin).

Amniotic membrane. From the amniotic tissue from a fetus.

Artificial skin substitutes. Examples include Integra Artificial Skin, BioBrane, Apligraf, and Dermagraft.

Biomarker for biomonitoring purposes, a biomarker is the presence of any substance or a change in any biological structure or process measured as a result of exposure. Many biomonitoring studies focus on chemical substances or their metabolites as biomarkers.

Bisphosphonates structural analogs of pyrophosphates. They have a pharmacologic activity specific for bone, due to the strong chemical affinity of bisphosphonates for hydroxyapatite, a major inorganic component of bone.

Blanchable a vascular response showing a white or pale area created when blood is pressed away, and when pressure is released, a normal color returns.

Body mass index (BMI) a mathematical formula to assess relative body weight. BMI is calculated as weight in kilograms divided by the square of the height in meters (kg/m^2).

Bony prominences a bony elevation or projection on an anatomical structure.

Bottoming out a method of checking the adequacy of support surfaces. When a hand is placed (palm up) under the surface and below a bony prominence and less than an inch of material is felt, the support surface is fully compressed and not adequate for pressure redistribution. The National Pressure Ulcer Advisory Panel (NPUAP) has recently discounted this technique as a way to measure support surface efficacy. Nevertheless, it is still commonly used in conversation and in practice. The consulting editors suggest that this is but a single evaluative point in a complex assessment of support surface efficacy.

Bowel and bladder program an individualized plan for controlling bowel and bladder activity. Programs vary from person to person according to their underlying conditions, individual preferences, and needs.

Bowel management system a pouch or catheter system designed to collect fecal effluent.

Braden Scale a pressure ulcer risk assessment scale that addresses sensory perception, moisture, activity, mobility, nutrition, friction, and shear.

Braden Q Scale adaptation of the Braden Pressure Ulcer Risk Assessment Scale for use in the pediatric population.

Bunion/bunionette a localized swelling at either the medial or dorsal aspect of the first joint of the big toe, caused by an inflamed bursa due to pressure, shear, and friction. (Bunionette involves localized swelling at the lateral aspect of the 5th toe.)

C-reactive protein (CRP) CRP is a protein found in the blood. It is a marker for inflammation.

Calf muscle pump dysfunction varying degrees of dysfunction of the calf muscle pump as it sends venous blood back to the heart.

Callus a common, usually painless thickening of the skin at locations of pressure or friction.

Cavus foot high arches.

Cellulitis a diffuse, acute inflammation and infection of the skin and subcutaneous tissue that signifies a spreading infectious process.

Certified pedorthist (C-Ped.) pedorthists design, manufacturer, fit, and/or modify shoes and foot orthoses to alleviate foot problems caused by disease or injury. Board-certified pedorthists are trained in foot anatomy and construction of shoes and foot orthotic devices.

Charcot deformity, neuropathic fracture, neuropathic osteoarthropathy a Charcot joint is a progressive condition of the musculoskeletal system characterized by joint dislocations, pathologic fractures, and debilitating deformities. This disorder results in progressive destruction of bone and soft tissues at weight-bearing joints and may cause significant disruption of the bony architecture in its most severe form. Charcot arthropathy can occur at any joint; however, it occurs most commonly in the lower extremity at the foot and ankle.

Charcot joint (tabetic arthropathy) a neuropathic joint commonly associated with tabes dorsalis or diabetic neuropathy.

Charcot-Marie-Tooth disease usually characterized by weakness of the peroneal leg muscles and commonly resulting in a high-arched foot with marked claw toes.

Chelation an intravenous treatment designed to bind heavy metals in the body to treat heavy metal toxicity. Chelation therapy describes the use of chelating agents to detoxify poisonous metal agents such as mercury, arsenic, and lead by converting them to a chemically inert form that can be secreted without further interaction with the body.

Chilblain a mild form of cold injury marked by localized redness, burning, and swelling on exposed body parts, especially in cool, damp climates. The affected skin sometimes blisters or ulcerates. Insufficient blood flow into small vessels in the skin contributes to the formation of chilblains.

Chlamydia pneumonia an obligate, intracellular bacterium that is pathogenic in humans.

Cholesterol a white, crystalline substance that is found in animal tissues and some foods. It is normally synthesized by the liver, is an important constituent of cell membranes, and is a precursor to steroid hormones. Its level in the bloodstream can influence the pathogenesis of certain conditions such as atherosclerosis and coronary artery disease.

Chronic heart failure (CHF) occurs when the heart is unable to pump an adequate blood supply to meet the body's metabolic needs, leading to inadequate tissue perfusion; vascular, cardiac, and pulmonary congestion; and diminished functional capacity.

Chronic venous disorders morphological and functional abnormalities of the venous system.

Chronic venous insufficiency characterized by symptoms or signs produced by venous hypertension as a result of structural or functional abnormalities of veins.

Circulation movement of blood through the arteries and veins. It is maintained by the pumping of the heart and influenced by the elasticity and extensibility of the arterial walls, peripheral resistance in the small arteries, and the quantity of blood in the body.

Classic claudication consistent and reproducible, lower-extremity symptoms that are usually confined to the calf muscles (can affect the thigh or buttocks) and are brought on by exercise and only relieved by rest (see intermittent claudication).

Claw toes deformity caused by flexion contractures involving both proximal and distal interphalangeal joints.

Collagen an insoluble fibrous protein that is the chief constituent of the fibrils of connective tissue. It forms the white inelastic fibers of the tendons, ligaments, bones, and cartilage.

Colonized the presence and growth of bacteria on the surface of the skin without any evident tissue damage.

Complex decongestive physiotherapy use of a range of very gentle, rhythmic, pumping movements of the fingers to move the skin in the direction of lymph flow based on the underlying structure and physiology of the lymphatic system and used in conjunction with compression wraps.

Compression pump a device that enhances venous return by propelling blood out of the leg.

Compression therapy application of sustained, external pressure to the affected lower extremity to control edema and aid the return of venous blood to the heart. Compression may be achieved by wraps, stockings, or pneumatic compression pumps. Compression wraps are available as single or multilayer component systems. Some wraps are reusable. Multilayer systems combine elastic and inelastic layers. Compression may be classified as inelastic/short stretch or elastic:

> ***Inelastic/short stretch.*** Includes garments, boots, or wraps with limited to no elasticity that provide low resting pressures; ambulation is needed to achieve a therapeutic level of compression; and the product does not expand during ambulation. As the calf muscle expands during walking, pressure is created by the muscle pressing against the bandage/wrap; at rest, limited compression is provided.
>
> ***Elastic.*** Long-stretch wraps or stockings; pressure is sustained under the product without ambulation, adjusts to changes in limb volume, and provides compression while resting or walking.

Computed tomographic angiography (CTA) CTA is a medical imaging test that requires intravenous injection of a contrast agent and uses x-ray–based techniques to visualize the inside lumen of arteries to identify the anatomic location of stenosis or occlusions.

Contamination the entry of bacteria, other microorganisms, or foreign material into a previously clean or sterile wound or skin.

Contralateral affecting the opposite side of the body.

Corns (clavus) a small conical callosity caused by pressure over a bony prominence, usually on a toe. A hyperkeratosis, that is, a thickening of the normal keratin of the skin. Corns are either hard (helomata dura) and usually on the top of the toes or soft (helomata mollia) and between the toes.

Crepitus grinding most often produced by joint surfaces not being smooth.

Critically colonized level of bacterial proliferation that interferes with wound healing; intermediate between the category of colonization and infection into viable tissues.

Critical limb ischemia (CLI) CLI is defined as limb pain occurring at rest or impending limb loss due to severely compromised blood flow in the affected limb. The term should be used for all patients with chronic ischemic rest pain (inadequate resting perfusion), ulcers, or gangrene attributable to objectively proven arterial occlusive disease. The term CLI implies chronicity and is to be distinguished from acute limb ischemia, which is commonly due to an embolism.

Culture a laboratory test involving the growth of bacteria or other cells in a special growth broth. Cultures are grown to identify an organism and find out which antibiotics are effective in combating that organism.

Cuticle where the skin of the dorsal surface of the toe (eponychium) and the nail plate meet.

Cytotoxic a substance that kills or damages tissue cells.

Debridement removal of devitalized tissue. Types of debridement:

Autolytic debridement. Removal of devitalized tissue accomplished by use of moisture-retentive dressings.

Biodebridement. The use of maggots to remove necrotic tissue from a wound.

Enzymatic (chemical) debridement. Removal of devitalized tissue by the application of proteolytic enzymes.

Mechanical debridement. Removal of devitalized tissue from a wound by physical forces.

Sharp debridement. Removal of devitalized tissue by a sharp instrument such as a scalpel.

Decubitus ulcer see pressure ulcer.

Dependent pain occurs when the extremity is lower than the level of the heart.

Dermatitis inflammation of the epidermis and dermis.

Diabetic neuropathy most commonly occurring chronic complication of diabetes. There are three types—sensory, autonomic, and motor.

Sensory neuropathy. Causes a dulling of the sensations of pain, temperature, and pressure, especially in the lower legs and feet; places the individual at risk for unrecognized trauma. Can also cause neuropathic pain, which typically requires treatment with drugs.

Autonomic neuropathy. Altered function of the nerves controlling sweat gland function and constriction and dilation of the blood vessels; common sequelae include dry cracked feet and persistent high volume blood flow to the feet.

Motor neuropathy. Biomechanical and muscle alteration resulting in weakened intrinsic foot muscles and leading to anatomic deformity.

Diastasis dislocation or separation of two normally attached bones between which there is no true joint (as in a Charcot foot).

Doppler scanning Doppler velocity waveform analysis uses continuous-wave Doppler ultrasound to record arterial pulsations in various lower-extremity arteries.

Dorsalis pedis artery the continuation of the anterior tibial artery of the lower leg. It starts at the ankle joint, divides into five branches, and supplies various muscles of the foot and toes.

Dorsiflexion bending the foot upward or toward the shin.

Dressings materials applied to a wound for various reasons, including protection, absorption, and drainage.

Types of dressings:

Alginate dressing. Highly absorbent, biodegradable dressing derived from nonwoven absorptive dressing manufactured from seaweed.

Cadexomer iodine. Absorbs exudate and particulate matter from the surface of granulating wounds and releases iodine as exudate is absorbed.

Collagenase. Enzymes that break the peptide bonds in collagen, promoting debridement.

Honey. Manuka honey used for antimicrobial effects; can be effective on antibiotic-resistant strains of bacteria while promoting healing.

Silver. Antimicrobial dressing; may be incorporated into foam, alginate, and other dressings.

Collagen. Collagen products may accelerate wound repair, comes in various forms (e.g., gels, pastes, powders).

Film dressing. A clear, adherent, nonabsorptive, polymer-based dressing that is permeable to oxygen and water vapor but not to water.

Foam dressing. A sponge-like polymer dressing that may be impregnated or coated with other materials and has absorptive properties.

Gauze dressing. A weave, usually made of cotton or synthetics, that is absorptive and permeable to water, water vapor, and oxygen. The gauze may be impregnated with petrolatum, antiseptics, or other agents.

Hydrocolloid dressing. A type of dressing containing gel-forming agents, such as sodium carboxymethylcellulose (NaCMC) and gelatin. In many products, these are combined with elastomers and adhesives and applied to a carrier—usually polyurethane foam or film—to form an absorbent, self-adhesive, waterproof wafer.

Hydrogel dressing. A water-based, nonadherent gel. Some contain pectin and sodium carboxymethylcellulose in a clear, viscous vehicle containing propylene glycol. The dressing has the ability to absorb excess exudate from exuding wounds but donate moisture to dry necrotic tissue or slough.

Normothermic dressing. A moisture-retentive wound cover that insulates the open wound and helps maintain tissue temperature at a normal level, preserving blood supply and oxygen to the affected area.

Dressing Techniques:

Continuously moist saline gauze. A technique whereby gauze is moistened with normal saline to maintain a moist environment.

Wet-to-dry saline gauze. A technique whereby gauze is moistened with normal saline, applied wet to the wound and allowed to dry, then removed when adhered to the wound bed. As the dressing is removed, the wound is non-selectively debrided.

Duke Boot an inelastic compression wrap comprised of a primary dressing (when ulcer is present), Unna's boot paste, and self-adherent wrap applied at full stretch.

Duplex ultrasound test combining traditional ultrasound with Doppler ultrasonography. Traditional ultrasound uses sound waves that bounce off blood vessels to create images. Doppler examines how sound waves reflect off moving objects such as blood.

Dynamic support surface a powered support surface that is designed to cyclically change its support characteristics such as alternating pressure or lateral rotation.

Dysesthesia pain or uncomfortable sensations after being touched by an ordinary stimulus or even in the absence of stimulation, described as a "burning sensation," "sunburn-like," or "skin tingles."

Dysgeusia a distorted or altered sense of taste.

Dyslipidemia a disorder of lipoprotein metabolism. Dyslipidemias may be manifested by elevated blood levels of total cholesterol, low-density lipoprotein (LDL) cholesterol, and triglycerides and a decrease in the high-density lipoprotein (HDL) cholesterol level.

Edema a local or generalized condition that involves the abnormal pooling of fluid in body tissues.

Electrical stimulation the use of an electrical current to transfer energy to a wound. The type of electricity that is transferred is controlled by the electrical source.

Electromagnetic therapy application of electromagnetic radiation or pulsed electromagnetic fields (PEMF) to the body.

Embolus obstruction or occlusion of a vessel by a transported clot of foreign matter.

Endovascular surgery minimally invasive types of surgery that use small incisions to access blood vessels.

Epibole also clinically referred to as rolled-over edges, is often seen in chronic wounds with poor healing dynamics.

Epithelialization the process of becoming covered with or converted to epithelium.

Erysipelas type of skin infection (cellulitis).

Erythema a redness of the skin due to dilation of the superficial capillaries. Types of erythema are as follows:

Blanchable erythema. Reddened area that temporarily turns white or pale when pressure is applied with a fingertip. Blanchable erythema over a pressure site is usually due to a normal reactive hyperemic response.

Nonblanchable erythema. Redness that persists when fingertip pressure is applied. Nonblanchable erythema over a pressure site is a symptom of a Stage I pressure ulcer.

Eschar black or brown necrotic devitalized tissue; tissue can be loose or firmly adherent, hard, soft, or soggy.

Exercise ankle brachial index (ABI) an ABI is recorded after exercise and used to assess the functional severity of claudication. A drop in ankle pressure after exercise is diagnostic of LEAD. The degree of drop in the ankle pressure or ABI and the duration of recovery to preexercise levels provide valuable information about the overall state of lower-extremity arterial perfusion.

Extrinsic factor a factor outside the body that contributes to the development of a pressure ulcer.

Exudate any fluid that has been extruded from a tissue or its capillaries, such as fluid, cells, or cellular debris, which has escaped from blood vessels and has been deposited in tissue surfaces. It is characteristically high in protein and white blood cells.

Fibrinogen a protein involved in coagulation. Fibrinogen reacts with other molecules to produce blood clots.

Fissure any cleft or groove, normal or otherwise, especially a crack-like break in the skin.

Fistula an abnormal passage from an internal organ to the body surface or between two internal organs.

Foot anatomy *Forefoot.* composed of the five toes (called phalanges) and their connecting long bones (metatarsals).

Midfoot. Has five irregularly shaped tarsal bones and forms the foot's arch. The bones of the midfoot are connected to the forefoot and the hindfoot by muscles and the plantar fascia ligament.

Hindfoot. Is composed of three joints and links the midfoot to the ankle. The top of the talus is connected to the two long bones of the lower leg. The heel bone is the largest bone in the foot and it joins the talus to form the subtalar joint.

Friction the force of two surfaces moving across one another, such as the mechanical force exerted when skin is dragged across a coarse surface such as bed linens.

Full-thickness tissue loss ulceration extending through dermis to involve subcutaneous tissue and possibly muscle/bone.

Gait manner of walking. Can be normal or abnormal, such as antalgic (painful) gait where the stance phase is shortened.

Gangrene, dry gangrene, moist gangrene necrosis or death of tissue, usually the result of deficient or absent blood supply.

Goniometer an instrument for measuring angles.

Gout arthritic condition caused by excessive uric acid in the bloodstream. Gout can produce acutely painful joints when the uric acid crystallizes in the lining of a joint. It can also lead to long-term stiffness and, occasionally, soft mineral deposits beneath the skin.

Granulocyte colony–stimulating factor (G-CSF) is a blood growth factor that stimulates the bone marrow to produce more infection-fighting white blood cells (neutrophils).

Hallux the big toe, or great toe.

Hallux flexus hammer toe of the big toe.

Hallux rigidus a condition in which there is stiffness in the metatarsophalangeal joint of the big toe.

Hallux valgus deviation of the tip or main axis of the big toe toward the outer side of the foot.

Hallux varus deviation of the main axis of the big toe to the inner side of the foot.

Hammer toe a toe that is permanently flexed downward, due to a flexion contracture involving the proximal interphalangeal joint.

Hazard ratio (HR) HR is a measure of how often an event occurs in one group compared to another group over time that is expressed as a ratio. An HR of 1 means there is no difference between the groups. HRs greater or less than 1 means the event occurs more or less often in a group.

Healing a dynamic process involving synthesis of new tissue for repair of skin and soft tissue defects.

Hemosiderin staining pressure exerted on the lower leg veins results in loss of protein and red blood cells into the subcutaneous tissues. The blood is broken down into hemosiderin, a yellowish brown granular pigment, which can cause a brownish discoloration of the ankles and lower legs.

Heterotopic bone formation heterotopic ossification (HO) is the formation of lamellar bone (which may mature with time) where bone does not usually form, such as in soft tissues. May be a complication of pressure ulcers or traumatic injury.

High-density lipoprotein (HDL) HDL cholesterol is known as the good cholesterol because a high level of HDL cholesterol seems to have a protective effect.

High-pressure irrigation mechanical removal of wound debris by irrigation with fluid at 8 to 15 pounds per square inch (psi).

High-sensitivity C-reactive protein (hs-CRP) a test that can measure very low levels of CRP.

Homocysteine an amino acid in the blood. A high homocysteine level is related to a higher risk of coronary heart disease, stroke, and peripheral vascular disease. At high levels, homocysteine can damage the walls of arteries and contributes to blocking blood vessels.

HMG-Co-A reductase inhibitors (statin drugs) statins are a group of drugs commonly used to lower LDL cholesterol. These drugs block the liver's ability to produce cholesterol. In rare instances, they can cause damage to the liver and muscle.

HSMN (Hereditary sensory and motor neuropathy, known generically as Charcot-Marie-Tooth after one of its variants) an inherited progressive condition. It exists in various forms.

Hydrotherapy use of whirlpool, pulsatile lavage or submersion in water for wound cleansing.

Hyperalgesia an increased response to a painful stimulus.

Hyperbaric oxygenation the administration of oxygen under greater than normal atmospheric pressure (usually two to three times absolute atmospheric pressure).

Hypergranulation hyperplasia of granulation tissue is believed to occur as a result of an extended inflammatory response, recognized by its friable red appearance.

Hyperkeratosis thickening of the horny layer of the epidermis or mucous membrane.

Hyperlipidemia an excess of lipids in the blood.

Hypertension (high blood pressure) a common disorder, often without symptoms, in which blood pressure is higher than 140 mm Hg systolic or 90 mm Hg diastolic.

Hypoalbuminemia an abnormally low amount of albumin in the blood. A value less than 3.5 mg/dL is clinically significant. Low serum albumin may be due to inadequate protein intake, active inflammation, or serious hepatic and renal disease and is associated with pressure ulcer development.

Hyponychium junction between the distal end of the toenail and toenail bed; point at which "free nail border" begins.

Incidence the proportion of at-risk persons who develop a pressure ulcer over a specific period of time.

Incontinence-associated dermatitis (IAD) an inflammation of the skin caused by prolonged or recurrent contact between urine and/or stool and the perineal or perigenital skin.

Induration abnormal hardening of tissues.

Infection typical definitions of infection are based on acute infection, such as the presence of bacteria or other microorganisms in sufficient quantity to damage tissue or impair healing. For example, acute wounds can be classified as infected when the wound tissue contains 10^5 (100,000) or more microorganisms per gram of tissue. Typical signs and symptoms of infection include purulent exudate, odor, erythema, warmth, tenderness, edema, pain, fever, and elevated white cell count. However, in chronic wounds, these acute clinical signs of infection may not be present; rather, chronic wounds often display more subtle signs and symptoms such as increasing pain over time, change in exudate or presence of necrotic tissue, delayed healing, poor quality of granulation tissue, unusual odor, or new areas of breakdown.

Infrared dermal thermometry provides an inexpensive, convenient, and objective noninvasive measurement of inflammation, which can be effectively used in all stages of neuropathic foot and wound care.

Insensate foot loss of protective sensation due to peripheral neuropathy.

Interphalangeal joints joints between the bones of the toe.

Interface pressure force per unit area that acts perpendicularly between the body and the support surface. This parameter is affected by the stiffness of the support surface, the composition of the body tissue, and the geometry of the body being supported.

Intermittent claudication the classical symptom of LEAD, is reproducible muscle discomfort in the lower limb brought on by exercise and relieved only by approximately 10 minutes' rest. The symptoms most commonly are localized in the calf muscle but can also affect the thigh or buttocks.

Intermittent claudication distance. Distance walked until the onset of claudication or pain-free walking distance.

Absolute claudication distance. Distance walked at which the pain becomes so severe that the patient has to stop walking (i.e., maximal walking distance).

International normalized ratio (INR) INR is a standardized system of reporting prothrombin time based on a referenced calibration.

Intertriginous an area where opposing skin surfaces touch and may rub, such as skin folds of the groin, axilla, and breasts.

Intertrigo an inflammation of the top layers of skin caused by moisture, bacteria, or fungi in the folds of the skin.

Irrigation mechanical cleansing by a stream of fluid.

Ischemia poor blood supply to an organ or part, often marked by pain and organ dysfunction.

Ischemic rest pain ischemic pain is often described as a throbbing pain, dull ache, or numbness that typically worsens when the patient elevates the leg and in the evenings or nights while lying supine. The pain is relieved by lowering the leg to a dependent position due to mild improvement in the arteriolar blood flow caused by the effects of gravity. Ischemic rest pain might also be described as a burning pain in the arch or distal foot that occurs while the patient is recumbent and is relieved when the feet/legs are returned to a dependent position.

Isometric exercise contraction of a muscle without body movement (i.e., the muscle contracts but does not change in length).

Isotonic exercise contraction of a muscle by moving weight a distance, as in weight lifting.

Keratinization the process by which the epidermis forms its outer protective layer, the stratum corneum; conversion into keratin or keratinous tissue.

Keratolytic agents agents that soften, separate, and cause desquamation of the cornified epithelium or horny layer of skin.

L-arginine L-arginine is a precursor to nitric oxide, which is a compound in the body that promotes dilation of blood vessels.

Lancinating pain characterized by piercing or stabbing sensations.

Ligament a tough, stabilizing soft tissue structure that connects bones on either side of a joint.

Linton procedure an open surgical technique to interrupt the flow of incompetent perforator veins. This surgical approach has subsequently been modified due to significant complication rates, including poor healing of incisions in diseased skin and recurrent ulceration.

Lipoprotein a special blood protein designed to carry fat and cholesterol. Common lipoproteins are HDL (high-density lipoprotein), LDL (low-density lipoprotein), and chylomicrons.

Lipodermatosclerosis induration and hyperpigmentation of the lower third of the leg that often occurs in patients who have LEVD and is related to chronic inflammation. A frequent clinical presentation is an "apple-core" or "inverted champagne bottle" appearance to the lower leg.

Loss of protective sensation (LOPS) degree of neuropathy beyond which the patient has a measurably increased risk for diabetic foot ulceration.

Low-density lipoprotein (LDL) a lipoprotein particle in the blood responsible for depositing cholesterol into the lining of the artery.

Low-level laser therapy use of low-level lasers or light-emitting diodes to alter cellular function.

Lunula crescent-shaped opaque area at the base of the toenail and fingernail.

Lymphangitis inflammation of the lymphatic vessels, commonly seen as red streaks on skin near a focus of infection.

Lymphedema swelling of the subcutaneous tissues caused by obstruction of the lymphatic system. Is a result of fluid accumulation and may arise from surgery, radiation, or the presence of a tumor in the area of the lymph nodes. Over time, this results in firming or hardness of the tissue that is characterized by fibrosis and scarring.

Magnetic resonance angiography (MRA) a noninvasive test avoiding the use of iodinated contrast agents, which gives detailed anatomic information, including graft patency, and is often used to plan the best percutaneous or surgical strategy.

Mallet toe flexed deformity due to contracture of the distal interphalangeal joint, typically resulting in formation of a callus at the tip of that toe.

Malleolar flare (ankle flare) visible capillaries from distension of small veins around the medial malleolar area.

Manual lymphatic drainage (MLD) MLD or combined decongestive therapy (CDT) is a "retraining" of the lymph to make it flow faster and more efficiently. MLD facilitates the removal of metabolic wastes, excess water, large protein molecules, and foreign substances from the tissues through the lymph system. MLD is part of complex decongestive therapy that involves compression therapy, exercise, and skin care. MLD can be used for lymphedema and in some patients with mixed lymphedema/lipedema.

Matrix reproductive layer of nail.

Medical adhesive–related skin damage (MARSI) damage to the skin resulting from the use of medical adhesives. Includes contact dermatitis, allergic dermatitis, maceration, folliculitis, and mechanical damage such as skin tears, friction blisters, and epidermal stripping.

Medial malleolus the medial prominence of the ankle, which is usually a part of the distal tibia.

Metabolic syndrome (MetS) a consensus from the International Diabetes Foundation and American Heart Association/National Heart, Lung, and Blood Institute defined MetS as the presence of any three of the following criteria: elevated waist circumference according to population- and country-specific definitions, elevated triglycerides (≥150 mg/dL), HDL cholesterol <40 mg/dL for men and <50 mg/dL for women, BP ≥130/85, and fasting glucose 100 mg/dL or greater.

Metatarsalgia a cramplike burning pain that focuses in the region of the metatarsal bones of the foot.

Metatarsals long bones of the midfoot proximal to the toes (phalanges). They are numbered from one to five, five being behind the little toe.

Methylmalonic acid (MMA) an important component in diagnosing vitamin B_{12} deficiency anemia.

Moisture-associated skin damage (MASD) injury to the skin caused by repeated or sustained exposure to moisture in the form of water, urine or stool, perspiration, mucus, or saliva.

Moisture-retentive dressings dressings that allow wounds to remain moist.

Moisture vapor transmission rate (MVTR) a measure of the passage of water vapor through a substance.

Monofilament Semmes-Weinstein monofilaments are calibrated nylon monofilaments. These monofilaments produce a characteristic force perpendicular to the contacting surface and are identified by manufacturer-assigned numbers that range from 1.65 to 6.65. The higher the value of the monofilament, the stiffer and more difficult it is to bend.

Motor neuropathy biomechanical and muscle alteration leading to anatomic deformity.

Muscular pain described as "dull ache," "night cramps," "band-like sensation," "drawing sensation," spasms, and "toothache-like."

Necrotic tissue tissue that has died and has therefore lost its usual physical properties and biological activity. Also called "devitalized tissue."

Negative pressure wound therapy (NPWT) assists in wound closure by applying localized negative pressure to the surface and margins of the wound. This negative pressure therapy is applied to a special dressing positioned in the wound cavity or over a flap or graft. The negative pressure helps in removing fluids from the wound.

Neonatal Skin Condition Score (NSCD) score for overall skin condition of newborns, ranging from very low birth weight premature babies to full-term well babies.

Neonatal Skin Risk Assessment Scale (NSRAS) NSRAS is based on the Braden Q and may be helpful in predicting skin breakdown risk among neonates.

Neuroischemic presence of neuropathy plus ischemia. The neuroischemic foot (which may occur in patients with diabetes) is especially prone to traumatic ulceration, infection, and gangrene.

Neuroma a benign growth of nerve tissue; can cause nerve compression and significant pain.

Neuropathy see peripheral neuropathy.

Neuropathic osteoarthropathy deterioration of a joint or joints resulting from deprivation of sensory and autonomic feedback in the musculoskeletal and neurovascular systems.

Neurotraumatic theory this hypothesis states that Charcot joint is due to unperceived trauma or injury to an insensate foot. The sensory neuropathy renders the patient unaware of the osseous destruction that occurs with ambulation. This microtrauma leads to progressive destruction and damage to bone and joints.

Neurovascular theory this hypothesis of Charcot etiology suggests that the underlying condition causes development of an autonomic neuropathy. This neuropathy causes the extremity to receive an increase in blood flow. The increased blood flow leads to osteopenia due to a mismatch in bone destruction and synthesis.

Niacin a water-soluble form of vitamin B, which lowers LDL cholesterol and triglyceride levels, and is effective in raising HDL cholesterol levels.

Nitric oxide and anodyne therapy (monochromatic infrared photo energy [MIRE]) use of the anodyne therapy system (ATS) appears to elevate nitric oxide locally so that blood flow can be increased directly at the site of application. This increase in blood flow is the basis of the therapeutic benefits of the ATS on pain and neuropathy.

Nongranulating absence of granulation tissue; wound surface appears smooth as opposed to granular. For example, in a wound that is clean but nongranulating, the wound surface appears smooth and red as opposed to berry-like.

Nonhealing wound a wound that fails to progress to healing in a defined time frame.

Noninvasive refers to a test or treatment that does not require breaking the skin or entering a cavity or organ of the body.

Occlusion a blockage in a canal, artery, vein, or passage of the body.

Offloading the effective reduction of pressure and stress from repetitive walking at areas of highest foot pressure such as over the plantar surfaces and the bony areas of the forefoot.

Onychochauxis localized hypertrophy of the entire nail plate characterized by a hyperkeratotic, discolored, nontranslucent nail plate; subungual keratosis and debris are often present.

Onychoclavus sometimes painful, hyperkeratotic process that is most commonly located under the distal nail margin of the great toe.

Onychia inflammation in the fingernail or toenail.

Onychocryptosis nail plate pierces the lateral nail fold and causes inflammation with or without accompanying granulation tissue, tenderness at rest, and pain on ambulation or with pressure of the digit (ingrown toenail).

Onychodystrophy dystrophic changes in the fingernail or toenails, such as malformation or discoloration.

Onychogryphosis enlargement of the fingernails or toenails accompanied by increased thickening and curvature—ram's horn.

Onycholysis separation or loosening of a fingernail or toenail from its nail bed.

Onychomycosis fungal infection of the fingernails or toenails that results in thickening, roughness, and splitting of the nails, usually due to *T. rubrum*; also called tinea unguium.

- DSO—distal end; most common
- WSO—white superficial; surface of the nail plate
- PSO—proximal subungual;least common
- Candidal—entire nail plate involved; most common.

Onychophosis localized or diffuse hyperkeratotic tissue of varying degrees that develops on the lateral or proximal nail folds, in the space between the nail folds and the nail plate, or even subungually.

Orthotic an externally applied device (e.g., splint or insole) used to control the position and/or function of a body part.

Os calcis (calcaneus) heel bone.

Osteoarthritis the commonest form of arthritis. Also known as "wear and tear" arthritis. Often this remains localized to just one or two joints. It only affects musculoskeletal tissues.

Osteoarthropathy deterioration of a joint or joints resulting from deprivation of sensory feedback in the musculoskeletal system.

Osteomyelitis inflammation of bone and marrow, usually caused by pathogens entering the bone during an injury or surgery.

Pain measurement scales visual analog and faces rating scales used to measure pain.

Panniculitis acute inflammation of the subcutaneous layer of fat.

Paresthesia abnormal neurological sensations described as "pins and needles," "electric-like," "numb aching feet," or "as if my feet have been in ice water," "knife-like," or shooting pains.

Partial-thickness wound confined to the superficial skin layers; damage does not penetrate below the dermis and may be limited to the epidermal layers only.

Paronychia infection at the edge of the nail, usually the result of an ingrown toe nail.

Pedorthist specialist in prescription footwear.

Pes planus flat feet. It is commonly found in patients who develop symptomatic acquired adult flatfoot deformity.

Percutaneous transluminal angioplasty (PTA) a procedure used to enlarge the lumen of an occluded blood vessel by passing a balloon catheter through the skin, into the vessel, and through the vessel to the site of the lesion where the tip of the balloon is inflated to expand the lumen of the vessel. Stenting is commonly performed along with PTA to improve/maintain the vessel expansion.

Peripheral arterial disease a disease that results from narrowing of the arteries that supply the extremities. Risk factors include atherosclerosis and diabetes.

Peripheral arterial occlusive disease (PAOD) PAOD is one of the several terms that are used to refer to disease caused by narrowing and/or obstruction of large peripheral arteries. Other commonly used terms include peripheral vascular disease (PVD), peripheral arterial disease (PAD), and lower extremity arterial disease (LEAD).

Peripheral neuropathy

Sensory neuropathy. A common disorder characterized by tingling, aching, burning, and searing discomfort beginning in the toes and spreading to the soles of the feet and then to the tops of the feet, the ankles, and, on occasion, the knees. Numbness of the feet, which is usually also painful, frequently occurs. There may be loss of protective sensation and impaired temperature perception.

Motor neuropathy. Biomechanical and muscle alteration results in weakened intrinsic foot muscles leading to anatomic deformity.

Phlebotonic having a toning action on the veins.

Photoplethysmography (PPG) a noninvasive test that assesses blood flow by emitting an infrared light into the tissue that is reflected by the red blood cells in superficial vessels and is detected by the transducer. The amount of reflected light corresponds to pulsatile changes and tissue blood volume to provide a functional assessment of tissue perfusion.

Plantar fasciitis inflammation involving the fascia of the sole of the foot.

Plantar ulcer a full-thickness breakdown on the plantar surface of the foot.

Plastazote a foam made of a cross-linked polyethylene material, which is characterized by its ability to deform over time based on the ongoing force to which it is exposed. This means that this material will mold to the shape to which it is exposed. For this reason, Plastazote has many uses, such as arch supports (particularly for diabetics), lining braces, and inserts for amputee limbs.

Plantigrade foot walking on the entire sole of the foot.

Point prevalence the method used most commonly to measure prevalence. It measures the proportion of people who have a pressure ulcer at a specific point in time.

Posterior tibial artery one of the parts of the popliteal artery of the leg. It divides into eight branches, which supply blood to different muscles of the lower leg, foot, and toes and is situated midway between the medial malleolus and the medial process of the calcaneal tuberosity.

Pressure redistribution ability of a support surface to distribute load over the contact areas of the human body to reduce the overall pressure and avoid areas of focal pressure.

Pressure ulcer localized injury to the skin and/or underlying tissue usually over a bony prominence, as a result of pressure or pressure in combination with shear.

Avoidable pressure ulcer. An individual developed a pressure ulcer, but either risk factors were not assessed or interventions to decrease the risk were not implemented.

Unavoidable pressure ulcer. An individual developed a pressure ulcer despite the fact that risk factors were assessed and interventions were implemented to decrease the risk.

Proprioceptive sense the biofeedback from the extremities, which tells the brain where and in what position the body is in. Proprioception is critical in balance.

Prostaglandins one of a number of hormone-like substances participating in a wide range of body functions such as contraction and relaxation of smooth muscle, dilation and constriction of blood vessels, control of blood pressure, and modulation of inflammation.

PSI (pounds per square inch) a unit of pressure, in this case, the pressure exerted by a stream of fluid, against one square inch of skin or wound surface.

Pulsatile lavage a delivery of irrigation fluid in rapid, discrete pulses. Disposable, battery-powered units deliver variable irrigation pressures and concurrent suction. The pulsing of the irrigation fluid may increase the amount of debris removed. Concurrent suction immediately removes irrigation fluid, which has been contaminated by contact with the wound.

Pulse volume recordings (PVR) PVR is a noninvasive technique that uses plethysmography to measure changes in the lower limb volume with each cardiac cycle and provides a waveform representing the arterial pressure. Normal waveforms are triphasic; biphasic waveforms are typical of mild atherosclerosis. Monophasic waveforms indicate severe occlusive disease.

Purpura a disorder with bleeding beneath the skin or mucous membranes that causes black and blue spots (ecchymosis) or pinpoint bleeding.

Qualitative wound culture swabbing the wound surface with a moistened swab and processing the swab to determine the predominant organism that is present on the wound surface.

Quantitative tissue biopsy processing a specimen of wound tissue to determine the number of bacteria present. The quantitative level of bacteria is reported as organisms per gram of wound tissue.

Raynaud's vasoconstriction and reduced blood flow to the hands and feet in response to cold or stress.

RCTs (randomized control trials) quantitative, comparative, controlled experiments in which investigators study two or more interventions in a series of individuals who receive them in random order.

Receiver operating characteristic (ROC) ROC analysis is used to evaluate the performance of diagnostic tests to determine their accuracy in classifying individuals as diseased or nondiseased. An ROC curve is a plot of the sensitivity on the *y* axis against specificity on the *x* axis for varying values of the threshold/cutoff value of the test used to classify individuals. The area under the curve is a summary measure that averages diagnostic accuracy across the spectrum of test values.

Relative risk (RR) a statistical measure of the risk of disease or death occurring in a group exposed to a causative/risk factor or intervention compared to a similar group not exposed to the causative/risk factor or intervention.

Reliability the consistency of a set of measurements or measuring instrument.

Reticular veins reticular veins are deeper, darker-in-color veins that form bluish networks that crisscross over the thighs and lower legs.

Revascularization the process of restoring blood flow to an organ or tissue, such as in bypass surgery.

Rheumatoid arthritis a chronic and progressive systemic disease, especially common in women, characterized by stiffness and inflammation of the joints and sometimes leading to deformity and disability.

Ringworm any of a number of contagious fungal skin diseases characterized by ring-shaped scaly itching patches on the skin.

Risk assessment assessment to determine which, if any, risk factors are present that might contribute to the development of skin ulceration.

RSD reflex sympathetic dystrophy, also known as regional pain syndrome. A condition that results following surgery or an injury, characterized by significant pain (often burning in nature and widespread), which is present most of the time and may be worsened by extremes of temperature. The skin often becomes red, swollen, and hypersensitive. Light pressure over an affected area may result in very severe and immediate pain. Joints in the area will become stiffened and may develop contractures. If this complication occurs, it requires early and aggressive treatment with mobilization of the affected joint and often nerve blocks to reduce the action of the nerves that are driving the process.

Rutoside a flavonoid (plant-based substance) with antioxidant properties.

Sclerotherapy a strong solution (the sclerosant) is injected directly into the venules, causing inflammation of the walls of the vessel to make them disappear over a few weeks to months.

Segmental pressure measurements similar to the ABI test, with the addition of two or three additional blood pressure cuffs. A Doppler measures the blood pressure at each cuff location on the leg. A significant drop in pressure between two adjacent cuffs indicates a narrowing of the artery or blockage along the arteries in this portion of the leg.

Semiquantitative wound swab a standard procedure for determining the relative number of organisms colonizing wound tissue. The bacterial colonization results are reported as minimal, moderate, or extensive.

Sepsis a condition in which the body is fighting a severe infection that has spread via the bloodstream.

Sesamoids a bone that is enveloped within a tendon, as in the two bones under the metatarsal bone.

Shear the mechanical force that is parallel rather than perpendicular to an area. Shear may play a role in triangularly shaped or tunneled sacral pressure ulcers. Force per unit magnitude of the area acting parallel to the surface of the body. This parameter is affected by pressure, the coefficient of friction between the materials contacting each other, and how much the body interlocks with the support surface.

Sinus tract course or path of tissue destruction occurring in any direction from the surface or edge of the wound; results in dead space with potential for abscess formation. Also sometimes called "tunneling." (Can be distinguished from undermining by the fact that sinus tract involves a small portion of the wound edge, whereas undermining involves a significant portion of the wound edge.)

Skin barriers creams, ointments, pastes, and film-forming skin protectants.

Slough soft moist avascular (devitalized) tissue; may be white, yellow, tan, or green; may be loose or firmly adherent.

Squamous cell carcinoma (Marjolin's ulcer) a malignant new growth that arises from epithelial cells and has a cuboid appearance. When arising within a chronic ulcer, it is commonly referred to as Marjolin's ulcer.

Stanozolol an anabolic steroid.

Statistically significant a result is called statistically significant if it is unlikely to have occurred by chance.

Subfascial endoscopic perforator surgery (SEPS) a minimally invasive surgical technique for the ablation of incompetent perforator veins in the lower leg.

Subungual exostosis benign tender bony proliferation, most commonly on the great toe, which usually produces hypertrophy of the entire nail bed such that the appearance of the nail is an "inverted U" with incurvation of the medial and lateral aspects of the nail plate.

Subungual hematoma a collection of blood under the nail as a result of trauma.

Support surfaces surfaces that are used to widely distribute body weight pressure over the dependent surface.

Types of Support Surfaces

Replacement mattresses. Mattresses with pressure redistribution features that can be placed on an existing bed frame in lieu of the standard mattress. Mattress replacements may be static or dynamic.

Overlays. General term used to describe support surfaces placed on top of a standard hospital mattress. They may be constructed of foam, water, gel, air, or a combination of these materials. Mattress overlays may be static or dynamic.

Nonpowered (static). Devices designed to provide support characteristics that remain constant, that is, do not cycle in time. Examples include foam overlays, cushions, and water mattresses.

Foam. Thick foam slab with a textured surface designed to be placed on top of the standard hospital mattress to reduce pressure by enveloping the body. Its effectiveness is influenced by its thickness, density, and stiffness. Foam overlays should be at least 3 to 4 inches to be effective for reducing pressure. Two-inch foam is generally used for comfort only.

Water. A vinyl mattress or overlay composed of interconnected compartments that are filled with water to distribute pressure uniformly over the support surface to create a flotation effect.

Gel. Made of a viscous fluid that conforms to the contours of the body, allowing greater immersion into the surface. Microflow also "flows" with patient movement, reducing the effects of shear.

Air. A vinyl mattress or overlay that is inflated with a blower to provide pressure reduction.

Powered (dynamic). Devices that are powered with a pump that inflates mattress cells in an alternating cycle.

Alternating air-filled overlay. Mattress or overlay with interconnecting air cells that cyclically inflates and deflates to produce alternating high- and low-pressure intervals. Cells with larger depth and diameter produce greater pressure relief over the body.

Beds

Specialty beds. Beds with pressure redistribution features that are used in place of regular hospital.

Air-fluidized feature. Class of support surfaces that uses a high rate of air blown to fluidize fine particulate material (such as glass beads) to "float" the patient on the surface.

Low–air loss feature. A series of interconnected woven fabric pillows or sections that allow some air to escape through the support surface. The pillows or sections can be inflated or deflated to adjust the level of pressure relief.

Kinetic therapy feature. Beds that are designed to provide continuous passive motion or oscillation therapy, which is believed to enhance removal of respiratory secretions. They may be available with a low–air loss surface with a firm, slightly padded surface.

Surfactants a surface-active agent that reduces the surface tension of fluids to allow greater penetration.

Tarsal tunnel syndrome a condition characterized by irritation of the tibial nerve behind the medial malleolus (inside of the ankle).

Tendon the "business end" of a muscle. This tough unyielding tissue allows a muscle (of varying length) to exert pull across a joint.

Tendonitis inflammation of the outer layers of a tendon. The underlying tendon may be entirely healthy.

Tendinosis wear and tear/degenerative changes existing throughout the substance of a tendon. The tendon is unhealthy and may be more prone to rupture.

Telangiectasia (telangiectases) tortuous, spidery distended, blue to red capillary veins visible under skin.

Test accuracy number of overall correct true positive and true negative results.

Test sensitivity the probability of a diagnostic test correctly identifying the presence of true disease (i.e., correctly measures true positives). Highly sensitive tests provide few false-negative results.

Test specificity the probability of a diagnostic test correctly identifying the absence of disease (i.e., correctly measures true negatives). Highly specific tests provide few false-positive results.

Thrombolysis dissolution (lysis) of a thrombus (blood clot) usually involving an enzyme (plasmin); catalyzed cleavage of chemical bonds holding the thrombus together.

Thrombophilia hematologic disorders that increase the tendency to form venous clots.

Thrombus blood that has clotted in the heart or a blood vessel.

TIMPS tissue inhibitors of matrix metalloproteinases.

Tinea pedis (athlete's foot) dermatophytic infection of the feet with erythema, chronic peeling of skin, fissuring of web spaces between toes, maceration, and possibly blistering.

Tissue anoxia reduction of oxygen levels below normal. Can be a direct result of ischemia.

Toe brachial index (TBI) TBI is an index calculated by dividing the systolic blood pressure in the great toe by the higher of the brachial systolic blood pressures from the right or left arms.

Toe pressure a toe pressure is a systolic pressure that is measured on the great toe (or second toe if the great toe is absent or cannot be used due to pain or wounds). The toe pressure is typically measured by PPG using a small digital cuff. Toe pressures may be more accurate in patients with calcified ankle arteries.

Topical oxygen therapy (TOT) involves the application of oxygen to a cutaneous wound.

Total contact cast a casting technique that is used to heal diabetic foot ulcers and to protect the foot during the early phases of Charcot fracture dislocations. The cast is used to heal diabetic foot ulcers by distributing weight along the entire plantar aspect of the foot. It is applied in such a way to intimately contact the exact contour of the foot, hence the designation "total contact cast."

Transcutaneous oxygen pressure ($TcPO_2$) this pressure reflects the amount of oxygen coming out through the skin, which, in turn, reflects the amount of oxygen delivered to the skin by the blood.

Transcutaneous oxygen measurement/transcutaneous oximetry (TCOM) transcutaneous oximetry evaluates the delivery of oxygen to tissue by measuring oxygen pressure at the skin surface over a localized area of heat-induced hyperemia and provides a functional assessment of ischemia.

Triglycerides triglycerides are a major form of fat in the blood. Hormones, such as insulin, regulate the release of triglycerides from fatty tissue to meet the body's need for energy.

Triggers for VLU external events or exacerbating factors that lead to VLU.

Tunneling see sinus tract.

Undermining area of tissue destruction extending under intact skin along the periphery of a wound; commonly seen in shear injuries. Can be distinguished from sinus tract by fact that undermining involves a significant portion of wound edge.

Unna's boot static inelastic zinc-impregnated bandage with or without calamine.

Validity concerned with the study's success at measuring what the researchers set out to measure.

Variceal bleeding bleeding that occurs in dilated blood vessels, sometimes at the site of varicosities.

Varicose veins swollen and twisted veins that appear blue and appear close to the surface of the skin. They may bulge, throb, and cause the legs to feel heavy and to swell. Varicose veins may occur in almost any part of the body but are most often seen in the back of the calf or the inside of the leg between the groin and the ankle.

Vascularization the process where body tissues develop small blood vessels (capillaries). It can be a natural occurrence or the result of surgical intervention.

Vein ablation radiofrequency ablation and endovenous laser ablation. Laser ablation is performed by making a tiny puncture (percutaneous) through the skin through which a laser is passed into the saphenous vein. The laser is activated and applies very localized heat to the inner vein wall inducing thermal damage that permanently blocks the vein and it becomes closed. Saphenous reflux is eliminated.

Vein stripping a surgical procedure done under general or local anesthetic to remove varicose veins. The surgery involves making one or more incisions upon the desired area, usually the groin and ankle, followed by insertion of thin wire-like instrument at the incision into the vein. The instrument then removes or "strips" the vein by pulling it out through the incision.

Venography also called **phlebography**. A procedure in which an x-ray of the veins, a venogram, is taken after a special dye is injected into the bone marrow or veins.

Venous dermatitis a red itchy rash on the lower legs that occurs as a result of tissue inflammation caused by venous insufficiency.

Venous eczema the resulting increased permeability of capillary walls with LEVD allows proteins to infiltrate the interstitial spaces, which is irritating. This irritant reaction causes eczema, with or without the presence of an ulcer. Erythema is often a feature of venous eczema due to the dilation of capillaries in response to the irritant effect.

Venous insufficiency a condition in which the veins do not efficiently return blood from the lower limbs back to the heart. It usually involves one or more veins. The valves in the veins usually channel the flow of blood towards the heart. When these valves are damaged, the blood leaks and pools in the legs and feet. Symptoms include swelling of the legs and pain in the extremities (i.e., dull aching, heaviness, or cramping).

Venous leg ulcers ulcers caused by chronic venous insufficiency; full-thickness skin loss; sometimes called varicose or stasis ulcers.

Verrucous plantaris warts.

Index

Note: Page numbers followed by t indicate tables; those followed by f and b indicate figures and boxes, respectively.

D

CCS0317